Lung Cancer

Lung Cancer

EDITED BY

Jack A. Roth, MD, FACS

Professor and Bud Johnson Clinical Distinguished Chair
Department of Thoracic and Cardiovascular Surgery
Professor of Molecular and Cellular Oncology
Director, W.M. Keck Center of Innovative Cancer Therapies
Chief, Section of Thoracic Molecular Oncology
The University of Texas MD Anderson Cancer Center, Houston, TX, USA

Waun Ki Hong, MD, DMSc (Hon)

American Cancer Society Professor
Samsung Distinguished University Chair in Cancer Medicine
Professor and Head, Division of Cancer Medicine
Professor, Department of Thoracic/Head and Neck Medical Oncology
The University of Texas MD Anderson Cancer Center, Houston, TX, USA

Ritsuko U. Komaki, MD, FACR, FASTRO

Professor, Department of Radiation Oncology
Gloria Lupton Tennison Distinguished Endowed Professor in Lung Cancer Research
The University of Texas MD Anderson Cancer Center, Houston, TX, USA

ASSOCIATE EDITORS

Anne S. Tsao, MD

Associate Professor, Director, Mesothelioma Program
Director, Thoracic Chemo-Radiation Program
Department of Thoracic/Head and Neck Medical Oncology
The University of Texas MD Anderson Cancer Center, Houston, TX, USA

Joe Y. Chang, MD, MS, PhD

Professor, Clinical Section Chief, Department of Radiation Oncology
Director of Stereotactic Radiotherapy Program
The University of Texas MD Anderson Cancer Center, Houston, TX, USA

Shanda H. Blackmon, MD, MPH, FACS

Associate Professor, Weill Cornell Medical College
Chief, Division of Thoracic Surgery, Houston Methodist Hospital
Clinical Assistant Professor, The University of Texas MD Anderson Cancer Center
Houston, TX, USA

FOURTH EDITION

WILEY Blackwell

Published by John Wiley & Sons, Inc., Hoboken, New Jersey.
Published simultaneously in Canada.

Library of Congress Cataloging-in-Publication Data

Lung cancer (Roth)
Lung cancer / edited by Jack A. Roth, Waun Ki Hong, Ritsuko Komaki ; associate editors: Anne S. Tsao, Joe Y. Chang, Shanda H. Blackmon. – Fourth edition.
p. ; cm.
Includes bibliographical references and index.
ISBN 978-1-118-46874-6 (cloth)
I. Roth, Jack A., editor. II. Hong, Waun Ki., editor. III. Komaki, Ritsuko, editor. IV. Title.
[DNLM: 1. Lung Neoplasms–diagnosis. 2. Lung Neoplasms–therapy. WF 658]
RC280.L8
616.99′424–dc23

2014005807

Cover image: courtesy of Joe Y. Chang and James D. Cox
Cover design by Modern Alchemy

Set in 9.5/12pt Meridien by Aptara Inc., New Delhi, India
Printed and bound in Singapore by Markono Print Media Pte Ltd

10 9 8 7 6 5 4 3 2 1

Contents

Contributors

Christopher G. Azzoli, MD
Visiting Assistant Professor, Department of Medicine
Harvard Medical School
Massachusetts General Hospital
Boston, MA, USA

Sonia L. Betancourt Cuellar, MD
Department of Diagnostic Radiology
The University of Texas MD Anderson Cancer Center
Houston, TX, USA

Shanda H. Blackmon, MD, MPH, FACS
Associate Professor, Houston Methodist Hospital, Weill Cornell Medical College of Cornell University, Houston, TX, USA
Clinical Assistant Professor, The University of Texas MD Anderson Cancer Center
Houston, TX, USA

Lauren Averett Byers, MD, MS
Assistant Professor, Department of Thoracic/Head and Neck Medical Oncology
The University of Texas MD Anderson Cancer Center
Houston, TX, USA

David P. Carbone, MD, PhD
Thoracic Oncology Center
James Comprehensive Cancer Center
Ohio State University Medical Center
Columbus, OH, USA

Tina Cascone, MD, PhD
Resident Physician
Department of Medicine, Division of Medical Education
Barnes-Jewish Hospital/Washington University School of Medicine in St. Louis
St. Louis, MO, USA

Joe Y. Chang, MD, MS, PhD
Professor
Clinical Section Chief, Department of Radiation Oncology
Director of Stereotactic Radiotherapy Program
The University of Texas MD Anderson Cancer Center
Houston, TX, USA

Caleb T. Chu, MD, MPH
The University of Texas MD Anderson Cancer Center
Houston, TX, USA

James D. Cox, MD
Professor, Department of Radiation Oncology
The University of Texas MD Anderson Cancer Center
Houston, TX, USA

Millie Das, MD
Clinical Assistant Professor, Division of Oncology
Stanford University/Stanford Cancer Institute
Stanford, CA, USA
Staff Oncologist
VA Palo Alto Heath Care System
Palo Alto, CA, USA

Patricia M. de Groot, MD
Assistant Professor, Department of Diagnostic Radiology
The University of Texas MD Anderson Cancer Center
Houston, TX, USA

Steven M. Dubinett, MD
Chief of Pulmonary and Critical Care Medicine
Professor of Medicine and Pathology
Director of UCLA Lung Cancer Research Program
Division of Pulmonary and Critical Care Medicine
University of California at Los Angeles
Los Angeles, CA, USA

George A. Eapen, MD
Associate Professor, Department of Pulmonary Medicine
The University of Texas MD Anderson Cancer Center
Houston, TX, USA

Jeremy J. Erasmus, MD
Professor, Department of Diagnostic Radiology
The University of Texas MD Anderson Cancer Center
Houston, TX, USA

Renata Ferrarotto, MD
Department of Thoracic/Head and Neck Medical Oncology
The University of Texas MD Anderson Cancer Center
Houston, TX, USA

Justin Gainor, MD
Clinical Fellow, Hematology/Oncology
Dana Farber Cancer Institute/Massachusetts General Hospital
Boston, Massachusetts, USA

Amol J. Ghia, MD
Assistant Professor, Department of Radiation Oncology
The University of Texas MD Anderson Cancer Center
Houston, TX, USA

Kathryn A. Gold, MD
Assistant Professor, Department of Thoracic/Head and Neck Medical Oncology
The University of Texas MD Anderson Cancer Center
Houston, TX, USA

Daniel Gomez, MD
Assistant Professor, Department of Radiation Oncology
The University of Texas MD Anderson Cancer Center
Houston, TX, USA

Peter Hammerman, MD, PhD
Assistant Professor of Medicine, Harvard Medical School, Boston, MA, USA
Department of Medical Oncology, Dana-Farber Cancer Institute, Boston, MA, USA
Broad Institute of Harvard and MIT, Cambridge, MA, USA

Mohamed Hassanein, PhD
Research Assistant Professor of Medicine
Division of Allergy, Pulmonary and Critical Care Medicine
Vanderbilt University Medical Center
Nashville, TN, USA

John V. Heymach, MD, PhD
Chair, Department of Thoracic/Head and Neck Medical Oncology
The University of Texas MD Anderson Cancer Center
Houston, TX, USA

Waun Ki Hong, MD, DMSc (Hon)
American Cancer Society Professor
Samsung Distinguished University Chair in Cancer Medicine
Professor and Head, Division of Cancer Medicine
Professor, Department of Thoracic/Head and Neck Medical Oncology
The University of Texas MD Anderson Cancer Center
Houston, TX, USA

Karen Suchanek Hudmon, DrPH, MS, RPh
Associate Head for Operations, Department of Pharmacy Practice
Professor of Pharmacy
Purdue University
Indianapolis, IN, USA

Marcin Imielinski, MD, PhD
Broad Institute of Harvard and MIT, Cambridge, MA, USA
Department of Pathology, Massachusetts General Hospital
Boston, MA, USA

Puneeth Iyengar, MD, PhD
Assistant Professor, Department of Radiation Oncology
University of Texas Southwestern, Medical Center
Dallas, TX, USA

David Mark Jablons, MD
Professor and Chief Thoracic Surgery, UCSF Department of Surgery
Nan T. McEvoy Distinguished Professor of Thoracic Surgical Oncology
Ada Distinguished Professor of Thoracic Oncology
Program Leader Thoracic Oncology
UCSF Helen Diller Family Comprehensive Cancer Center
University of California
San Francisco, CA, USA

Rachel Jen, MD, FRCPC
Respiratory Division
Department of Medicine
University of British Columbia
Vancouver, British Columbia, Canada

Humam Kadara, PhD
Assistant Professor, Department of Translational Molecular Pathology
Division of Pathology and Laboratory Medicine
The University of Texas MD Anderson Cancer Center
Houston, TX, USA

Shaf Keshavjee, MD, MSc, FRCSC, FACS
Surgeon in Chief, UHN
James Wallace McCutcheon Chair in Surgery
Professor, Division of Thoracic Surgery & Institute of Biomaterials and Biomedical Engineering
University of Toronto
Toronto, ON, Canada

Edward S. Kim, MD
Chair, Solid Tumor Oncology and Investigational Therapeutics
Donald S. Kim Distinguished Chair for Cancer Research
Levine Cancer Institute
Carolinas HealthCare System
Charlotte, NC, USA

Lucia Kim, MD, PhD
Associate Professor, Department of Pathology
Inha University School of Medicine
Incheon, South Korea

Min P. Kim, MD
Assistant Professor
Weill Cornell Medical College
Department of Surgery
Division of Thoracic Surgery
Houston Methodist Hospital
Houston, TX, USA

Ritsuko U. Komaki, MD, FACR, FASTRO
Professor, Department of Radiation Oncology
Gloria Lupton Tennison Distinguished Endowed Professor in Lung Cancer Research
The University of Texas MD Anderson Cancer Center
Houston, TX, USA

Johannes R. Kratz, MD
Resident, Department of Surgery
Massachusetts General Hospital
Boston, MA, USA

Stephen Lam, MD, FRCPC
Professor of Medicine
University of British Columbia
Chair, Lung Tumour Group
BC Cancer Agency
Vancouver, BC, Canada

Donald R. Lazarus, MD
Interventional Pulmonology Fellow
Department of Pulmonary Medicine
The University of Texas MD Anderson Cancer Center
Houston, TX, USA

J. Jack Lee, PhD, MS
Professor, Department of Biostatistics
The University of Texas MD Anderson Cancer Center
Houston, TX, USA

Jay M. Lee, MD
Chief, Division of Thoracic Surgery
Associate Professor of Surgery
UCLA Lung Cancer Research Program
Jonsson Comprehensive Cancer Center
David Geffen School of Medicine at UCLA
Los Angeles, CA, USA

Zhongxing Liao, MD
Professor and Clinical Director, Department of Radiation Oncology
The University of Texas MD Anderson Cancer Center
Houston, TX, USA

Jie Lin, PhD
Department of Epidemiology
The University of Texas MD Anderson Cancer Center
Houston, TX, USA

Steven H. Lin, MD, PhD
Assistant Professor, Department of Radiation Oncology
The University of Texas MD Anderson Cancer Center
Houston, TX, USA

Geoffrey Liu, MD, FRCPC
Associate Professor
Princess Margaret Hospital/Ontario Cancer Institute;
Department of Medicine, Medical Biophysics, and Epidemiology
University of Toronto
Toronto, ON, Canada

Paolo Macchiarini, MD, PhD
Professor of Regenerative Surgery, Director of Advanced Center of Translational Regenerative Medicine, Director of European Airway Institute and Senior Consultant of Division Ear, Nose and Throat (CLINTEC)
Karolinska University Hospital
Stockholm, Sweden

Edith M. Marom, MD
Professor, Department of Diagnostic Radiology
The University of Texas MD Anderson Cancer Center
Houston, TX, USA

Erminia Massarelli, MD, PhD, MS
Assistant Professor
Department of Thoracic Head and Neck Medical Oncology
The University of Texas MD Anderson Cancer Center
Houston, TX, USA

Matthew Meyerson, MD, PhD
Department of Medical Oncology, Dana-Farber Cancer Institute, Boston, MA, USA
Broad Institute of Harvard and MIT, Cambridge, MA, USA
Department of Pathology, Brigham and Women's Hospital
Boston, MA, USA

Kathryn F. Mileham, MD
Solid Tumor Oncology
Levine Cancer Institute
Carolinas HealthCare System
Charlotte, NC, USA

Reginald F. Munden, MD, DMD, MBA
Professor and Chair, Department of Radiology
The Houston Methodist Hospital
Houston, TX, USA

Vassiliki A. Papadimitrakopoulou, MD
Professor, Department of Thoracic/Head and Neck Medical Oncology
The University of Texas MD Anderson Cancer Center
Houston, TX, USA

Mauricio Pipkin, MD
Thoracic Surgery Clinical Fellow
UHN
University of Toronto
Toronto, ON, Canada

Katherine M.W. Pisters, MD
Professor, Department of Thoracic/Head and Neck Medical Oncology
The University of Texas MD Anderson Cancer Center
Houston, TX, USA

Alexander V. Prokhorov, MD, PhD
Professor, Department of Behavioral Science
The University of Texas MD Anderson Cancer Center
Houston, TX, USA

Xia Pu, PhD
Department of Epidemiology
The University of Texas MD Anderson Cancer Center
Houston, TX, USA

David C. Rice, MB, BCh, BAO, FRCSI
Professor of Surgery
Department of Thoracic and Cardiovascular Surgery
The University of Texas MD Anderson Cancer Center
Houston, TX, USA

Kenneth E. Rosenzweig, MD
Chairman and Professor, Department of Radiation Oncology
Icahn School of Medicine at Mount Sinai
New York, NY, USA

Jack A. Roth MD, FACS
Professor and Bud Johnson Clinical Distinguished Chair
Department of Thoracic and Cardiovascular Surgery
Professor of Molecular and Cellular Oncology
Director, W.M. Keck Center of Innovative Cancer Therapies
Chief, Section of Thoracic Molecular Oncology
The University of Texas MD Anderson Cancer Center
Houston, TX, USA

Pierre Saintigny, MD, PhD
Assistant Professor, Department of Thoracic/Head and Neck Medical Oncology
The University of Texas MD Anderson Cancer Center
Houston, TX, USA

Francesco Sammartino, MD
General Surgeon, Department of General and Mininvasive Surgery
San Giovanni di Dio Hospital
Orbetello, Italy

Sherven Sharma, PhD
Professor, Division of Pulmonary and Critical Care Medicine
Department of Medicine
UCLA Lung Cancer Research Program
David Geffen School of Medicine at UCLA
West Los Angeles VA
Los Angeles, CA, USA

Alice Shaw, MD, PhD
Assistant Professor, Department of Medicine, Harvard Medical School
Massachusetts General Hospital
Boston, MA, USA

George R. Simon, MD, FACP, FCCP
Professor of Medicine and Oncology
Section Chief: Translational Research
Department of Thoracic/Head & Neck Medical Oncology
The University of Texas MD Anderson Cancer Center
Houston, TX, USA

Heath D. Skinner, MD, PhD
Assistant Professor, Department of Radiation Oncology
The University of Texas MD Anderson Cancer Center
Houston, TX, USA

Matthew A. Steliga, MD
Associate Professor of Surgery
Division of Thoracic Surgery
University of Arkansas
Little Rock, AR, USA

Sonal Sura, MD
Radiation Oncologist, Queen Hospital Center
Icahn School of Medicine at Mount Sinai
New York, NY, USA

Roman Thomas, MD
Department of Translational Genomics
Center of Integrated Oncology Köln – Bonn
University of Köln
Köln, Germany

Robert D. Timmerman, MD
Professor, Departments of Radiation Oncology and Neurosurgery
University of Texas Southwestern, Medical Center
Dallas, TX, USA

William Travis, MD
Attending Thoracic Pathologist, Department of Pathology
Memorial Sloan-Kettering Cancer Center
New York, NY, USA

Anne S. Tsao, MD
Associate Professor
Director, Mesothelioma Program
Director, Thoracic Chemo-Radiation Program
Department of Thoracic/Head and Neck Medical Oncology
The University of Texas MD Anderson Cancer Center
Houston, TX, USA

Ming-Sound Tsao, MD, FRCPC
Thoracic Pathologist and Professor
University Health Network, Princess Margaret Cancer Centre
Department of Laboratory Medicine and Pathobiology
University of Toronto
Toronto, ON, Canada

Heather Wakelee, MD
Assistant Professor of Medicine, Division of Oncology
Stanford University/Stanford Cancer Institute
Stanford, CA, USA

Howard West, MD
Medical Director, Thoracic Oncology Program
Swedish Cancer Institute
Seattle, WA, USA

William N. William Jr, MD
Assistant Professor
Chief, Head and Neck Section
Department of Thoracic/Head and Neck Medical Oncology
The University of Texas MD Anderson Cancer Center
Houston, TX, USA

Ignacio I. Wistuba, MD
Professor and Chair, Department of Translational Molecular Pathology
Anderson Clinical Faculty Chair for Cancer Treatment and Research
Division of Pathology and Laboratory Medicine
University of Texas MD Anderson Cancer Center
Houston, TX, USA

Xifeng Wu, MD, PhD, MS
Chair and Professor, Department of Epidemiology
Director, Center for Translational and Public Health Genomics
Betty B. Marcus Chair in Cancer Prevention
University of Texas MD Anderson Cancer Center
Houston, TX, USA

Preface

The publication of the fourth edition of *Lung Cancer* is occurring 20 years after the first edition. Looking back on those 20 years, the editors see major advances in our understanding of the molecular alterations in cells that cause lung cancer, the development of drugs targeted to specific gene mutations that drive lung cancer growth, identification of biomarkers that predict outcome and response to treatment, technological innovations in surgery and radiation therapy that improve outcomes, and developing more effective strategies in primary and secondary lung cancer prevention. Progress, particularly in targeted molecular and immunological therapeutics, has accelerated over the past five years since publication of the third edition.

One of the hallmarks of this book has been an attempt to concisely summarize recent major advances in lung cancer clinical research and treatment for the clinician. The editors and authors have attempted to describe state-of-the-art prevention, diagnosis, and treatment in the context of the newest developments in research and clinical care. The senior editors also felt it was appropriate to include a group of younger experts on the editorial board. We welcome the next generation of innovators and leaders in the field of lung cancer basic, translational, and clinical research.

The editors once again emphasize that advances are possible because of the work of those dedicated to translational research and rigorously conducted clinical trials. We are optimistic that progress will continue at a rapid pace and that deaths from lung cancer will continue to decline.

The Editors

Preface

CHAPTER 1

Smoking Prevention and Cessation

Alexander V. Prokhorov[1] *and Karen Suchanek Hudmon*[2]

[1]Department of Behavioral Science, The University of Texas MD Anderson Cancer Center, Houston, TX, USA
[2]Department of Pharmacy Practice, Purdue University, Indianapolis, IN, USA

Overview

It is well established that tobacco use is a leading cause of disease and death worldwide, and smoking is the primary risk factor for the development of lung cancer [1]. A considerable body of knowledge has been gained with respect to environmental, personal, and behavioral factors leading to smoking initiation and development of tobacco dependence. Two key elements of successful tobacco control are prevention and cessation. According to the 2012 Surgeon General's Report, prevention of tobacco use among adolescents and young adults is a matter of particular importance [2]. The dramatic downward trends in tobacco use rates among youth, observed since the mid-1990s, have stalled; furthermore, the use of smokeless tobacco is increasing among some age groups [2]. A variety of strategies, including policy change and education, have been shown to positively impact tobacco prevention [3]. Cessation of tobacco use provides extensive health benefits for everyone, regardless of age, sex, ethnicity, or health status [4]. Evidence-based treatment for smoking cessation includes behavioral counseling in conjunction with one or more FDA-approved pharmaceutical aids for cessation. The US Public Health Service *Clinical Practice Guideline for Treating Tobacco Use and Dependence* advocates a five-step approach to smoking cessation (Ask about tobacco use, Advise patients to quit, Assess readiness to quit, Assist with quitting, and Arrange follow-up) [5]. Systematic referral of patients who use tobacco to helpful resources, such as telephone quitlines, is recently emerging as a feasible and promising approach. Health care providers are encouraged to provide at least brief interventions at each encounter with a patient who uses tobacco [5].

Introduction

In 2011, an estimated 19% of adults in the United States were cigarette smokers [6], and in 2012, 17% of high-school seniors smoked at least 1 cigarette in the past 30 days [7]. This is despite the fact that five decades ago, the former US Surgeon General C. Everett Koop stated that cigarette smoking is the "chief, single, avoidable cause of death in our society and the most important public health issue of our time" [8]. Cigarette smoking is associated with nearly 443 000 deaths each year, including more than 49 000 deaths from exposure to secondhand smoke [9]. The economic implications are enormous: more than $75 billion in medical expenses and $81 billion in loss of productivity, as a result of premature death, are attributed to smoking each year [10]. While the public often associates tobacco use with elevated cancer risk, the

Lung Cancer, Fourth Edition. Edited by Jack A. Roth, Waun Ki Hong and Ritsuko U. Komaki.

negative health consequences are much broader. The 2004 Surgeon General's Report on the health consequences of smoking provides compelling evidence of the adverse impact of smoking and concluded that smoking harms nearly every organ in the body [11] (Table 1.1). In 2000, 8.6 million persons in the United States were living with an estimated 12.7 million smoking-attributable medical conditions [12]. There is convincing evidence that stopping smoking is associated with immediate as well as long-term health benefits, including reduced cumulative risk for cancer. This is true even among older individuals and among patients who have been diagnosed with cancer [13].

Of key importance, often undermined by health professionals, is the primary prevention of smoking initiation among youth. Indeed, 99% of first use of tobacco occurs by 26 years of age [2]. Thus, nearly all tobacco use starts in childhood or adolescence. Although a substantial decline in tobacco use rates among youth has been observed since the mid-1990s, this favorable trend appears to have stalled in the recent years, especially in smokeless tobacco use [7]. Tobacco use among adolescents is not just a social phenomenon. Rapidly developing physiological dependence on nicotine prevents many adolescents from quitting tobacco products; as such, about 80% of adolescent smokers will smoke into adulthood [2]. Each year, more than 1 million new tobacco users emerge in the United States. In his foreword to the 2012 Surgeon General's report, the Director of the Centers for Disease Control and Prevention, Dr Thomas R. Frieden, indicated that preventing smoking and smokeless tobacco use among young people is crucial to ending the epidemic of tobacco use [2].

Tobacco and lung cancer

In the United States, approximately 85% of all lung cancers occur among people who smoke or who have smoked [14]. Lung cancer is fatal for most patients, with the estimated number of deaths of lung cancer projected to exceed 1.3 million annually early in the third millennium [15]. Lung cancer is the leading cause of cancer-related deaths

Table 1.1 Health consequences of smoking (USDHHS SGR report, 2004)

Cancer	Acute myeloid leukemia Bladder Cervical Esophageal Gastric Kidney Laryngeal Lung Oral cavity and pharyngeal Pancreatic
Cardiovascular diseases	Abdominal aortic aneurysm Coronary heart disease (angina pectoris, ischemic heart disease, myocardial infarction, sudden death) Cerebrovascular disease (transient ischemic attacks, stroke) Peripheral arterial disease
Pulmonary diseases	Acute respiratory illnesses – Pneumonia Chronic respiratory illnesses – Chronic obstructive pulmonary disease – Respiratory symptoms (cough, phlegm, wheezing, dyspnea) – Poor asthma control – Reduced lung function in infants exposed (in utero) to maternal smoking
Reproductive effects	Reduced fertility in women Pregnancy and pregnancy outcomes – Premature rupture of membranes – Placenta previa – Placental abruption – Pre-term delivery – Low infant birth weight Infant mortality (sudden infant death syndrome)
Other effects	Cataract Osteoporosis (reduced bone density in postmenopausal women, increased risk of hip fracture) Periodontitis Peptic ulcer disease (in patients who are infected with *Helicobacter pylori*) Surgical outcomes – Poor wound healing – Respiratory complications

Source: [11].

among both men and women in the USA, with 174 470 estimated newly diagnosed cases and 162 460 deaths each year [16,17]. The number of deaths due to lung cancer exceeds the annual number of deaths from breast, colon, and prostate cancer combined [18]. Recent advances in technology have enabled earlier diagnoses, and advances in surgery, radiation therapy, imaging, and chemotherapy have produced improved responses rates. However, despite these efforts, overall survival has not been appreciably affected in 30 years, and only 12–15% of patients with lung cancer are being cured with current treatment approaches [19]. The prognosis of lung cancer depends largely on early detection and immediate, premetastatic stage treatment [20]. Prevention of lung cancer is the most desirable [21]. The causal role of cigarette smoking in lung cancer mortality has been irrefutably established in longitudinal studies, one of which lasted as long as 50 years [15]. Tobacco smoke, which is inhaled either directly or as secondhand smoke, contains an estimated 4000 chemical compounds, including 69 substances that are known to cause cancer [22]. Tobacco irritants and carcinogens damage the cells in the lungs, and over time the damaged cells may become cancerous. Cigarette smokers have lower levels of lung function than nonsmokers [23, 24], and quitting smoking greatly reduces cumulative risk for developing lung cancer [25, 26].

The association of smoking with the development of lung cancer is the most thoroughly documented causal relationship in biomedical history [27]. The link was first observed in the early 1950s through the research of Sir Richard Doll [28], whose pioneering research has, perhaps more so than any other epidemiologist of his time, altered the landscape of disease prevention and consequently saved millions of lives worldwide. In two landmark US Surgeon Generals' reports published within a 40-year interval (in 1964 and in 2004), literature syntheses further documented the strong link between smoking and cancer. Compared to never-smokers, smokers have a 15–30 times elevated risk of developing lung cancer, and more than 90% of lung cancers are attributable to smoking [29]. The risk for developing lung cancer increases with younger age at initiation of smoking, greater number of cigarettes smoked, and greater number of years smoked [30]. Findings are mixed in regards to the susceptibility of developing lung cancer in males or females for a given history of smoking [31].

Secondhand smoke and lung cancer

While active smoking has been shown to be the main preventable cause of lung cancer, secondhand smoke contains the same carcinogens that are inhaled by smokers [22, 32]. Consequently, there has been a concern since the release of the 1986 US Surgeon General's Report, which concluded that secondhand smoke causes cancer among nonsmokers and smokers. Although estimates vary by exposure location (e.g., workplace, home), the 2006 Surgeon General's Report estimates that 60% of children and 40% of nonsmoking adults were exposed to secondhand smoke [33]. Secondhand exposure to tobacco smoke kills more than 3000 adult nonsmokers from lung cancer [33]. According to Glantz and colleagues, for every eight smokers who die from a smoking-attributable illness, one additional nonsmoker dies because of secondhand smoke exposure [34].

Since 1986, numerous additional studies have been conducted and are summarized in the 2006 US Surgeon General's Report on *The Health Consequences of Involuntary Exposure of Tobacco Smoke.* The Report's conclusions based on this additional evidence are consistent with the previous reports: exposure to secondhand smoke increases risk of lung cancer. More than 50 epidemiologic studies of nonsmokers' cigarette smoke exposure at the household and/or in the workplace showed an increased risk of lung cancer associated with secondhand smoke exposure [33]. This means that 20 years after secondhand smoke was first established as a cause of lung cancer in lifetime nonsmokers, the evidence supporting smoking cessation and reduction of secondhand smoke exposure continues to mount. Eliminating secondhand smoke exposure at home, in the workplaces, and other public places appears to be essential for reducing the risk of lung cancer development among nonsmokers [33].

Smoking among lung cancer patients

Tobacco use among patients with cancer is a serious health problem with significant implications for morbidity and mortality [35]. Evidence indicates that continued smoking after a diagnosis of cancer has substantial adverse effects on treatment effectiveness [36, 37], overall survival [38], risk of second primary malignancy [39, 40], and increases the rate and severity of treatment-related complications such as pulmonary and circulatory problems, infections, impaired wound healing, mucositis, and xerostomia [41].

Despite the strong evidence for the role of smoking in the development of cancer, many cancer patients continue to smoke [42, 43]. Specifically, about one third of cancer patients who smoked prior to their diagnoses continue to smoke, and among patients who received surgical treatment of lung cancer 30% were abstinent at follow-up [44]. It is estimated that more than one half of former smokers resume regular smoking after surgical treatment for lung cancer [45]. Therefore, among patients with smoking-related malignancies, the likelihood of a positive smoking history at and after diagnosis is high [46].

Patients who are diagnosed with lung cancer may face tremendous challenges and motivation to quit after a cancer diagnosis can be influenced by a range of psychological variables [47]. Schnoll and colleagues reported that continued smoking among patients with head, neck, or lung cancer is associated with lesser readiness to quit, having relatives who smoke at home, greater time between diagnoses and assessment, greater nicotine dependence, lower self-efficacy, lower risk perception, fewer perceived pros and greater cons for quitting, more fatalistic beliefs, and higher emotional distress. Lung cancer patients should be advised to quit smoking, but once they are diagnosed, some might feel that there is nothing to be gained from quitting [48]. Smoking cessation should be a matter of special concern throughout cancer diagnosis, treatment, and the survival continuum, and the diagnosis of cancer should be used as a "teachable moment" to encourage smoking cessation among patients, family members, and significant others [43].

Forms of tobacco

Smoked tobacco

Cigarettes have been the most widely used form of tobacco in the United States for several decades, yet in recent years, cigarette smoking has been declining steadily among most population subgroups [6]. The number of former US smokers has exceeded the number of current smokers since 2002 [49]. Nineteen percent (43.8 million) of US adults were current cigarette smokers in 2011; of these, 77.8% (34.1 million) smoked every day, and 22.2% (9.7 million) smoked some days [6]. The prevalence of smoking varies considerably across populations (Table 1.2), with a greater proportion of men (21.5%) than women (16.5%) reporting current smoking. Persons of Asian or Hispanic origin exhibited the lowest prevalence of smoking (9.9 and 12.9%, respectively). American Indian/Alaska natives exhibited the highest prevalence (31.5%). Also, the prevalence of smoking among adults varies widely across the regions in the United States, ranging from 15.0% in the West to 21.8% in the Midwest [6]. According to the 2012 Monitoring the Future report, 17% of high school students reported smoking in the past 30 days [7]. Data from the 2011 National Youth Tobacco Survey indicated that among high-school males reported 12.9% used smokeless tobacco and 15.7% smoked cigars. These figures are of particular concern because nearly 90% of smokers begin smoking before the age of 18 years [50].

Other common forms of smoked tobacco in the United States include cigars, pipe tobacco, and bidis. Cigars represent a roll of tobacco wrapped in leaf tobacco or in any substance containing tobacco [51]. Popularity of cigars has somewhat increased over the past decade [50]. The latter phenomenon is likely to be explained by a certain proportion of smokers switching cigarettes for cigars and by adolescents' experimentation with cigars [50]. In 1998, approximately 5% of adults had smoked at least one

Table 1.2 Percentage of persons aged ≥ 18 years who were current cigarette smokers,[a] by selected characteristics – National Health Interview Survey, United States, 2011

Characteristic	Category	Men (n = 14,811)	Women (n = 18,203)	Total (n = 33,014)
Age group (yrs)	18–24	21.3	16.4	18.9
	25–44	24.5	19.7	22.1
	45–64	24.4	18.5	21.4
	≥ 65	8.9	7.1	7.9
Race/ethnicity[b]	White	22.5	18.8	20.6
	Black	24.2	15.5	19.4
	Hispanic	17.0	8.6	12.9
	American Indian/Alaska Native	34.4	29.1	31.5
	Asian[c]	29.7	5.5	9.9
Education[d]	0–12 years (no diploma)	30.5	25.1	25.5
	GED[e]	47.5	45.2	45.3
	High school graduate	27.9	23.8	23.8
	Associate degree	21.4	17.5	19.3
	Some college (no degree)	25.2	20.0	22.3
	Undergraduate degree	9.8	8.7	9.3
	Graduate degree	5.2	4.8	5.0
Poverty level[f]	At or above	20.2	15.6	20.6
	Below	33.6	25.7	29.9
	Unknown	19.4	11.4	18.4
Total		21.6	16.5	19

[a]Persons who reported having smoked at least 100 cigarettes during their lifetime and at the time of the interview reported smoking every day or some days; excludes 86 respondents whose smoking status was unknown.
[b]Excludes 61 respondents of unknown race. Unless indicated otherwise, all racial/ethnic groups are non-Hispanic; Hispanics can be of any race.
[c]Excludes Native Hawaiians or Other Pacific Islanders.
[d]Persons aged ≥25 years, excluding 173 persons whose educational level was unknown.
[e]General Educational Development Certificate.
[f]Calculated on the basis of US Census Bureau 2010 poverty thresholds.
Source: [52].

cigar in the past month [53]. The nicotine content of cigars sold in the United States ranges from 5.9 to 335.2 mg per cigar [54], while cigarettes have a narrow range of total nicotine content, between 7.2 and 13.4 mg per cigarette [55]. Therefore, one large cigar, which could contain as much tobacco as an entire pack of cigarettes, is able to deliver enough nicotine to establish and maintain physical dependence [56].

Pipe smoking has been declining steadily over the past 50 years [57]. It is a form of tobacco use seen among less than 1% of Americans [57]. Bidi smoking is a more recent phenomenon in the United States. Bidis are hand-rolled brown cigarettes, imported mostly from Southeast Asian countries, that are wrapped in a *tendu* or *temburni* leaf [58]. Visually, they somewhat resemble marijuana joints, which might make them attractive to certain population groups. Bidis are available in multiple flavors (e.g., chocolate, vanilla, cinnamon, strawberry, cherry, mango, etc.), which might make them particularly attractive to younger smokers. A survey of nearly 64 000 people in 15 states in the United States revealed that young people (18–24 years of age) reported higher rates of ever (16.5%) and current (1.4%) use of bidis than among older adults (ages 25 plus years). With respect to sociodemographic characteristics, the use of bidis is most common among males, African Americans, and concomitant cigarette smokers [59]. Although featuring less tobacco than standard cigarettes, bidis expose their smokers to considerable amounts of hazardous compounds. A smoking machine-based investigation found that bidis deliver three times the amount of carbon monoxide and nicotine and almost five times the amount of tar found in conventional cigarettes [60].

Smokeless tobacco

Smokeless tobacco products, also commonly called "spit tobacco," are placed in the mouth to allow absorption of nicotine through the buccal mucosa. Spit tobacco includes chewing tobacco and snuff. Chewing tobacco, which is typically available in loose leaf, plug, and twist formulations, is chewed or parked in the cheek or lower lip. Snus, commonly available as loose particles or sachets (resembling tea bags), has a much finer consistency and is generally held in the mouth and not chewed. Most snus products in the United States are classified as moist snuff. The users park a "pinch" (small amount) of snuff between the cheek and gum (also known as dipping) for 30 minutes or longer. In contrast dry snus, which is typically sniffed or inhaled through the nostrils, is used less commonly [61].

In 2004, an estimated 3.0% of Americans 12 years of age or older had used spit tobacco in the past month, with males using it at higher rates (5.8%) than women (0.3%) [62]. The prevalence of spit tobacco is the highest among 18- to 25-year-olds and is substantially higher among American Indians, Alaska natives, residents of the southern states, and rural residents [63]. The consumption of chewing tobacco has been declining since the mid-1980s; conversely, in 2005, snus consumption increased by approximately 5% over the previous year [63], possibly because tobacco users are consuming snus instead of cigarettes in locations and situations where smoking is banned.

While cigarette consumption in the United States continues to decline, promotion for and consumption of smokeless tobacco products is increasing [64]. A recent report indicated that between 2005 and 2011, sales of moist snus products increased by 65.6%. Sales of pouched and flavored forms of moist snus increased by 333.8% and 72.1%, respectively, and contributed to 28% and 59.4% of the total growth in the moist snus category respectively. Increased sales of flavored and discounted snuff raise concerns about use and appeal to youth [64] and warrant strong prevention programs addressing these tobacco products.

Recent developments on the tobacco market

Over the past decade, the tobacco industry has substantially increased its repertoire of potentially harmful products. The industry is broadly advertising new potentially reduced-exposure tobacco products (PREPs). These products are typically marketed as an "alternative to conventional cigarettes," implying that they are likely to cause less harm than traditional forms of tobacco (i.e., cigarettes) or decrease exposure to toxic compounds in the PREPs' smoke. These PREPs include modified-tobacco cigarettes (e.g., Omni, Advance), cigarette-like items (e.g., Accord, Eclipse), and smokeless tobacco products (e.g., Ariva, Exalt) [65].

The oral formulations of tobacco are available as small sachets of flavored tobacco (Camel Snus, Marlboro Snus), lozenges containing compressed low-nitrosamine tobacco powder (Ariva, Stonewall), or a dissolvable of finely grained tobacco with additives (Camel Orbs, Strips, and Sticks) that are often marketed as cigarette substitutes for situations where smoking is prohibited. Smokeless tobacco products reduce exposure to the harmful products associated with combustion, but do not substitute for a smoker's own brand of cigarette. Research has shown that noncombustible PREP use for typical smokers does not offer sufficient nicotine to suppress withdrawal symptoms, and therefore smokers are unlikely to switch from cigarettes [66]. Overall, no sufficient evidence has been obtained regarding these products' harmful effects [67]. It is clear, however, that all these nicotine-containing products possess addition potential. This, in turn, makes them dangerous with respect to engaging young people in tobacco use and possibly lifelong nicotine dependence.

There is public health concern about smoking tobacco through hookah (aka waterpipe, shisha, narghile, qalyan, etc.). In this smoking device, tobacco smoke passes through water in a special container before it is inhaled. Hookah smoking is becoming rapidly widespread in the United States, especially among young people [68–74]. For example, among college students, hookah smoking rates are second to the frequency of conventional cigarette use [75]. Importantly, many hookah users believe that this type of smoking is safer than cigarettes [76]. Research indicates though that hookah use is no less harmful than cigarette smoke, it may lead to the known tobacco-attributable diseases, and can interfere with successful quitting due to nicotine addiction [77].

Electronic cigarettes (or e-cigarettes) are another rapidly spreading form of unregulated nicotine delivery in the United States. An e-cigarette is a battery-operated device containing nicotine, various flavors, and other chemicals. The e-cigarette appearance resembles that of conventional cigarettes. Once switched on, the e-cigarette turns the chemical compounds into a vapor that is inhaled by the user in a way similar to smoking a regular cigarette. The laboratory analysis has detected toxic compounds such as diethylene glycol (used in antifreeze) and carcinogens (including nitrosamines) [78]. The particular public health concern regarding this type of product is in the appeal to modern youth who are highly interested in technology [79]. Young e-cigarette users are likely to develop nicotine addiction and may switch to conventional cigarettes later in life.

Factors explaining tobacco use

Smoking initiation

In the United States, smoking initiation typically occurs during adolescence. From mid-1990 to 2004, the past-month prevalence had decreased by 56% in 8th graders, 47% in 10th graders, and 32% in 12th graders [80]. In recent years, however, this downward trend has decelerated [80]. The downward trend is unlikely to be sustained without steady and systematic efforts by health care providers in preventing initiation of tobacco use and assisting young smokers in quitting.

A wide range of sociodemographic, behavioral, personal, and environmental factors have been examined as potential predictors of tobacco experimentation and initiation of regular tobacco use among adolescents. For example, it has been suggested that the prevalence of adolescent smoking is related inversely to parental socioeconomic status and adolescent academic performance [81]. Other identified predictors of adolescent smoking include social influence and normative beliefs, negative affect, outcome expectations associated with smoking, resistance skills (self-efficacy), engaging in other risk-taking behaviors, exposure to smoking in movies, and having friends who smoke [82–87].

Although numerous studies have been successful in identifying predictors of smoking initiation, few studies have identified successful methods for promoting cessation among youth, despite the finding that in 2005, more than half of high school cigarette smokers have tried to quit smoking in the past year and failed [88]. These results confirm the highly addictive nature of tobacco emphasizing the need for more effective methods for facilitating cessation among the young.

Smoking prevention

After decades of research, it became clear that only comprehensive, concerted efforts may lead to successful prevention of tobacco use among youth. Among the major conclusions of the 2012 Surgeon General's report, there is one that states the following: "Coordinated, multicomponent interventions that combine mass media campaigns, price increases including those that result from tax increases, school-based policies and programs, and statewide or community-wide changes in smoke-free policies and norms are effective in reducing the initiation, prevalence, and intensity of smoking among youth and young adults" [2]. Indeed, it "takes a village" to prevent tobacco use successfully, and healthcare providers represent a key group in this multicomponent system.

There are multiple ways for a healthcare provider to be engaged in smoking prevention among youth. First and foremost, efforts to prevent tobacco use should be applied routinely in the medical practice. Asking about tobacco use, advising to quit or not to start and assisting in adopting a non-smoking tobacco lifestyle through evidence-based materials and resources should become an indispensable component of patient care. It is essential to work with parents of young children to eliminate all secondhand smoke from the children's environment. A recent study, conducted among a predominantly low-socioeconomic status Mexican-American community, indicated very low knowledge about secondhand smoke exposure and associated health consequences [89]. A series of culturally sensitive, printed materials effectively increased this knowledge and practically eliminated secondhand smoke from the targeted Mexican-American households [89]. In addition to these direct health-enhancing effects, such elimination is likely to help in prevention of smoking initiation among children and adolescents.

Because young people do not seem to respond positively to telephone tobacco quitlines [90], it would be important to consider alternative resources designed specifically for the young audiences. Among them, Internet-based resources should be considered [91]. Healthcare providers need to be familiar with contemporary approaches to helping young patients make the right decisions to avoid initiation of tobacco use. Referral to these resources should be integrated into healthcare practice. Furthermore, as highly respected members of their communities, healthcare providers are positioned to make a difference in tobacco use prevention among youth beyond their medical practices. One possible highly rewarding direction of their activities could be advocating for smoking prevention programs in schools. Despite the criticism of school-based education programs aimed at prevention of tobacco use [92], these programs appear to represent an indispensable part of the systematic, comprehensive approach to reducing tobacco use among youth. It is imperative to realize that children, adolescents, and young adults are special population groups with unique needs and requirements that are often simply unmet or underappreciated.

In his systematic review of school-based programs, Dr Brian Flay, an internationally recognized expert in the area of smoking prevention among youth, outlined several key characteristics of effective school-based programs that were able to produce long-term effects [93]. He concluded that school-based programs can have long-term effects of practical importance if they: (a) include 15 or more educational sessions over multiple years, including sessions in high school; (b) use the social influence model and interactive delivery methods; (c) include components on norms, commitment not to use, intentions not to use, and training and practice in the use of refusal and other life skills; and (d) use peer leaders in some role. Such programs, Dr Flay concludes, are able to reduce smoking onset by 25–30%. A combination of school-based programs with community programs can dramatically reduce smoking onset (by 35–40%) by the time teens graduate from high school.

We would like to add to this analysis that the school-based programs should to be culturally sensitive, to better resonate of the needs with the culturally diverse adolescent populations in the United States. Program developers should be mindful of literacy levels in general, and health literacy in particular, among their target populations. The latter notion is of particular importance due to the fact that youth with the lowest literacy skills tend to be at the highest risk for smoking initiation and lifelong nicotine dependence. Finally, it is critically important to realize that we live in the era of technology. Therefore, using the interactive multimedia programs delivered via Internet, use of social networks (Facebook, Twitter, YouTube, etc.) highly popular among young populations, as well as programs and apps for smart phones, is becoming absolutely essential and standard for making smoking prevention programs attractive, effective, and sustainable. Our own evidence-based bilingual (English and Spanish) smoking prevention and cessation program for youth, called ASPIRE (A Smoking Prevention InteRactive Experience;

www.mdanderson.org/aspire), is based on many of the aforementioned principles [91, 94, 95]. It is currently being disseminated to 29 states in the United States with consistently positive feedback from the participating communities. For example, of the nearly 15 000 student participants, 92% said they learned new tobacco facts, 83% said the program influenced their decision not to use tobacco, 91% said they have a greater understanding of the effects of tobacco, and 77% said they would recommend ASPIRE to a friend/family member.

Nicotine addiction

Nicotine, the addictive component of tobacco, reaches the brain rapidly (within 10–20 seconds) [96] and produces a wide range of pharmacologic effects [97, 98]. Nicotine stimulates the release of neurotransmitters, inducing pharmacologic effects, such as pleasure and reward (dopamine), arousal (acetylcholine, norepinephrine), cognitive enhancement (acetylcholine), appetite suppression (norepinephrine), learning and memory enhancement (glutamate), mood modulation and appetite suppression (serotonin), and reduction of anxiety and tension (3-endorphin and GABA) [99]. Upon entering the brain, a bolus of nicotine activates the dopamine reward pathway, a network of nervous tissue in the brain that elicits feelings of pleasure and stimulates the release of dopamine.

In the absence of nicotine, the dependent patient experiences symptoms of withdrawal that can range from mild to severe. Although withdrawal symptoms are not the only consequence of abstinence, most quitters do experience withdrawal and cravings upon cessation [100], and relapse is common [101]. In general, most withdrawal symptoms manifest within 1–2 days after quitting, peak within the first week, and subside within 2–4 weeks [100]. The near-immediate calming effect of nicotine reported by many users is usually associated with alleviation of withdrawal effects rather than the direct effects of nicotine. This rapid dose-response, along with the short half-life of nicotine (approximately 2 hours), underlies tobacco users' frequent, repeated administration, thereby perpetuating tobacco use and establishment of dependence. Tobacco users become proficient in titrating their nicotine levels throughout the day to avoid withdrawal symptoms, to maintain pleasure and arousal, and to modulate mood. Withdrawal symptoms can include irritability/frustration/anger, anxiety, difficulty concentrating, restlessness/impatience, depressed mood/depression, insomnia, impaired performance, increased appetite/weight gain, and cravings [100].

Tobacco initiation, use, and dependence are hypothesized to result from an interplay of many factors (including pharmacologic, genetic, social and environmental, and learned/conditioned factors) [98]. Some of these factors are shared within families, either environmentally or genetically. Studies of families consistently demonstrate that compared to family members of nonsmokers, family members of smokers are more likely to be smokers also. However, in addition to shared genetic predispositions, it is important to consider environmental factors that promote tobacco use – siblings within the same family share many of the same environmental influences as well as the same genes. Because a myriad of factors contribute to tobacco use and dependence, tobacco control initiatives (e.g., community-based efforts) as well as tobacco cessation counseling services (provided at the individual level) should be multi-faceted [102].

Benefits of quitting

The reports of the US Surgeon General on the health consequences of smoking, released in 1990 and 2004, summarize abundant and significant health benefits associated with giving up tobacco [11, 103]. Benefits noticed shortly after quitting (e.g., within 2 weeks to 3 months), include improvements in pulmonary function and circulation. Within 1–9 months of quitting, the ciliary function of the lung epithelium is restored. Initially, patients might experience increased coughing while the lungs clear excess mucus and tobacco smoke particulates. With just a few months, smoking cessation leads to measurable improvements in lung function. Over time, patients experience decreased coughing, sinus congestion, fatigue, shortness of breath, and risk for pulmonary infection. One year post-cessation, the excess risk for coronary heart disease is reduced to half that of continuing smokers. After 5–15 years, the risk for stroke is reduced to a rate similar to that of people who are lifetime nonsmokers, and 10 years after quitting, an individual's chance of dying of lung cancer is approximately half that of continuing smokers. Additionally, the risk of developing mouth, larynx, pharynx, esophagus, bladder, kidney, or pancreatic cancer is decreased. Finally, 15 years after quitting, a risk for coronary heart disease is reduced to a rate similar of that of people who have never smoked. Smoking cessation can also lead to a significant reduction in the cumulative risk for death from lung cancer for males and females.

A growing body of evidence indicates that continued smoking after a cancer diagnosis has substantial adverse effects. Smoking reduces the overall effectiveness of treatment, causing complications with healing, exacerbating treatment side effects, increasing risk of developing second primary malignancy, and decreasing overall quality of life and survival rates. As such, smoking cessation should be considered an essential component of cancer treatment for all types of cancer – including, but not limited to, cancers of the lung [42].

Smoking cessation interventions

Effective and timely administration of smoking cessation interventions can significantly reduce the risk of smoking-related disease. Recognizing the complexity of tobacco use is a necessary first step in developing effective interventions and trials for cessation and prevention.

Health care providers are uniquely positioned to assist patients with quitting, having both access to quitting aids and commanding a level of respect that renders them particularly influential in advising patients on health-related issues. To date, physicians have received the greatest attention in the scientific community as providers of tobacco cessation treatment. Although less attention has been paid to other health care providers such as pharmacists, nurses, and respiratory therapists, they too are in a unique position to assist with quitting and are situated to initiate behavior change among patients or complement the efforts of other providers.

A meta-analysis of 29 studies determined that compared with smokers who do not receive an intervention from a clinician, patients who receive a tobacco cessation intervention from a physician clinician or a nonphysician clinician are 2.2 and 1.7 times as likely to quit smoking at 5 or more months post-cessation, respectively [101]. To assist clinicians with providing cessation treatment, the US Public Health Service has published a *Clinical Practice Guideline for the Treatment of Tobacco Use and Dependence* [101]. The *Guideline* is based on a systematic review and analysis of relevant scientific literature, yielding a series of recommendations and strategies to assist clinicians with delivering treatment for tobacco use and dependence. The update emphasizes the importance of identification of tobacco users by health care providers and offering at least brief treatment interventions to every patient who uses tobacco. Among the most effective approaches for quitting are behavioral counseling and pharmacotherapy, used alone or, preferably, in combination [101]. Effectiveness of the various behavioral and pharmaceutical strategies for cessation is shown in Table 1.3.

Behavioral counseling

Behavioral interventions play an integral role in smoking cessation treatment, either alone or in conjunction with pharmacotherapy [101]. These interventions, which include a variety of methods ranging from self-help materials to individual cognitive-behavioral therapy, enable individuals to more effectively recognize high-risk smoking situations, develop alternative coping strategies, manage stress, improve problem-solving skills, and increase social support. The *Clinical Practice Guideline* outlines a five-step framework that clinicians can apply when assisting patients with quitting. Health care providers should: (a) systematically identify all tobacco users, (b) strongly advise all tobacco users to quit, (c) assess readiness to

Table 1.3 Efficacy of treatment methods for tobacco use and dependence

Treatment method	Estimated odds ratio[a] (95% CI)	Estimated abstinence[b] rate (95% CI)
Behavioral interventions		
Advice to quit		
No advice to quit	1.0	7.9
Physician advice to quit	1.3 (1.1–1.6)	10.2 (8.5–12.0)
Clinician intervention		
No counseling by a clinician	1.0	10.2
Counseling by a nonphysician	1.7 (1.3–2.1)	15.8 (12.8–18.8)
Counseling by a physician	2.2 (1.5–3.2)	19.9 (13.7–26.2)
Format of smoking cessation counseling		
No format	1.0	10.8
Self-help	1.2 (1.0–1.3)	12.3 (10.9–13.6)
Proactive telephone counseling[c]	1.2 (1.1–1.4)	13.1 (11.4–14.8)
Group counseling	1.3 (1.1–1.6)	13.9 (11.6–16.1)
Individual counseling	1.7 (1.4–2.0)	16.8 (14.7–19.1)
Pharmacotherapy interventions		
Placebo	1.0	13.8
First-line agents		
Bupropion SR	2.0 (1.8–2.2)	24.2 (22.2–26.4)
Nicotine gum (6–14 weeks)	1.5 (1.2–1.7)	19.0 (16.5–21.9)
Nicotine inhaler	2.1 (1.5–2.9)	24.8 (19.1–31.6)
Nicotine lozenge (2 mg)	2.0 (1.4–2.8)	24.2[d]
Nicotine patch (6–14 weeks)	1.9 (1.7–2.2)	23.4 (21.3–25.8)
Nicotine nasal spray	2.3 (1.7–3.0)	26.7 (21.5–32.7)
Varenicline (2 mg/day)	3.1 (2.5–3.8)	33.2 (28.9–37.8)
Second-line agents[e]		
Clonidine	2.1 (1.2–3.7)	25.0 (15.7–37.3)
Nortriptyline	1.8 (1.3–2.6)	22.5 (16.8–29.4)
Combination therapy		
Patch (>14 weeks) + *ad lib* nicotine (gum or nasal spray)	3.6 (2.5–5.2)	36.5 (28.6–45.3)
Nicotine patch + bupropion SR	2.5 (1.9–3.4)	28.9 (23.5–35.1)
Nicotine patch + nortriptyline	2.3 (1.3–4.2)	27.3 (17.2–40.4)
Nicotine patch + nicotine inhaler	2.2 (1.2–3.6)	25.8 (17.4–36.5)

[a]Estimated relative to referent group.
[b]Abstinence percentages for specified treatment method.
[c]A quitline that responds to incoming calls and makes outbound follow-up calls. Following an initial request by the smoker or via a fax-to-quit program, the clinician initiates telephone contact to counsel the patient.
[d]One qualifying randomized trial; 95% CI not reported in 2008 *Clinical Practice Guideline*.
[e]Not approved by the US Food and Drug Administration as a smoking cessation aid; recommended by the USPHS *Guideline* as a second-line agent for treating tobacco use and dependence.
Reprinted from [108], with permission. Data from [101].

make a quit attempt, (d) assist patients in quitting, and (e) arrange follow-up contact. The steps have been described as the 5 A's: Ask, Advise, Assess, Assist, and Arrange. Due to the possibility of relapse, health care providers should also provide patients with brief relapse prevention treatment. Relapse prevention reinforces the patient's decision to quit, reviews the benefits of quitting, and assists the patient in resolving any problems arising from quitting. In the absence of time or expertise for providing more comprehensive counseling, clinicians are advised to (at a minimum), ask about tobacco use, advise tobacco users to quit, and refer these patients to other resources for quitting, such as a toll-free tobacco cessation quitline (1–800-QUIT NOW, in the United States).

Tobacco quitlines are telephone services that provide tobacco cessation counseling, generally at no cost, to the caller. Quitlines have proliferated in recent years, providing comprehensive interventions that can reach patients who might otherwise have limited access to medical treatment because of geographic location, financial resources or lack of insurance. In clinical trials, telephone counseling services for which at least some of the contacts are initiated by the quitline counselor have been shown to be effective in promoting abstinence [101, 104], and these results have been shown to translate into real-world effectiveness [105]. The addition of medication to quitline counseling significantly improves abstinence rates compared to medication alone [106]. In some states, clinicians can submit a fax-referral form, on behalf of a patient, to the quitline. This form initiates a process whereby a quitline counselor then contacts the patient directly. Up to 30% success rates have been shown for patients who complete all follow-up sessions. However, most physicians are unfamiliar with quitline services, and clinician referrals are low – yet even the busiest of clinicians can serve an important role by simply asking about tobacco use, advising patients who smoke to quit, and referring patients who are ready to quit to a quitline for more comprehensive counseling (Ask-Advise-Refer) [107].

Clinicians should also attempt to become familiar with local, community-based resources for tobacco cessation, such as group programs that might be offered through local hospitals or clinics. For some patients, an internet-based cessation program might be preferred, such as www.quitnet.com, an online quitting community where quitters can share experiences and support each other in achieving their cessation goals. Patients now have more options for obtaining assistance; clinicians should advise patients to utilize as many services as needed to achieve long-term success.

Our group has recently developed QuitMedKit©, a free iOS app, designed to assist healthcare providers in effective counseling and treatment of tobacco dependence among their patients. This program provides state-of-the-art knowledge on behavioral counseling, pharmacological treatments for nicotine dependence and is based on the *Clinical Practice Guideline*. QuitMedKit© is available in the Apple iTunes store and is compatible with iPhone, iPod touch, and iPad. It requires iOS 4.3 or later and is optimized for iPhone 5.

Pharmaceutical aids for smoking cessation

According to the *Clinical Practice Guideline for Treating Tobacco Use and Dependence* [101], all patients attempting to quit should be encouraged to use one or more effective pharmacotherapy agents for cessation except in the presence of special circumstances. These recommendations are supported by the results of more than 100 controlled trials demonstrating that patients receiving pharmacotherapy are approximately twice as likely to remain abstinent long-term (greater than 5 months) when compared to patients receiving placebo (Table 1.3) [101, 108]. Although one could argue that pharmacotherapy is costly and might not be a necessary component of a treatment plan for each patient, it is the most effective known method for maximizing the odds of success for any given quit attempt, particularly when combined with behavioral counseling [101].

Currently, seven marketed agents have an FDA-approved indication for smoking cessation in the United States: five nicotine replacement therapy (NRT) formulations (nicotine gum, nicotine lozenge, transdermal nicotine patches, nicotine nasal spray, and nicotine oral inhaler), sustained-release bupropion, and varenicline. These are described in brief below, and summaries of the prescribing information for each medication are provided in Table 1.4. For more details, readers are referred to the manufacturer's prescribing information.

Table 1.4 FDA-approved medications for smoking cessation

	Nicotine Replacement Therapy (NRT) Formulations						
	Gum	Lozenge	Transdermal Patch	Nasal Spray	Oral Inhaler	Bupropion SR	Varenicline
Product	**Nicorette[1], Generic** OTC 2 mg, 4 mg original, cinnamon, fruit, mint, orange	**Nicorette Lozenge,[1] Nicorette Mini Lozenge,[1] Generic** OTC 2 mg, 4 mg cherry, mint	**NicoDerm CQ[1], Generic** OTC (NicoDerm CQ, generic) Rx (generic) 7 mg, 14 mg, 21 mg (24-hour release)	**Nicotrol NS[2]** Rx Metered spray 0.5 mg nicotine in 50 mcL aqueous nicotine solution	**Nicotrol Inhaler[2]** Rx 10 mg cartridge delivers 4 mg inhaled nicotine vapor	**Zyban[1], Generic** Rx 150 mg sustained-release tablet	**Chantix[2]** Rx 0.5 mg, 1 mg tablet
Precautions	• Recent (≤2 weeks) myocardial infarction • Serious underlying arrhythmias • Serious or worsening angina pectoris • Temporomandibular joint disease • Pregnancy[3] and breastfeeding • Adolescents (<18 years)	• Recent (≤2 weeks) myocardial infarction • Serious underlying arrhythmias • Serious or worsening angina pectoris • Pregnancy[3] and breastfeeding • Adolescents (<18 years)	• Recent (≤2 weeks) myocardial infarction • Serious underlying arrhythmias • Serious or worsening angina pectoris • Pregnancy[3] (Rx formulations, category D) and breastfeeding • Adolescents (<18 years)	• Recent (≤2 weeks) myocardial infarction • Serious underlying arrhythmias • Serious or worsening angina pectoris • Underlying chronic nasal disorders (rhinitis, nasal polyps, sinusitis) • Severe reactive airway disease • Pregnancy[3] (category D) and breastfeeding • Adolescents (<18 years)	• Recent (≤ 2 weeks) myocardial infarction • Serious underlying arrhythmias • Serious or worsening angina pectoris • Bronchospastic disease • Pregnancy[3] (category D) and breastfeeding • Adolescents (<18 years)	• Concomitant therapy with medications or medical conditions known to lower the seizure threshold • Severe hepatic cirrhosis • Pregnancy[3] (category C) and breastfeeding • Adolescents (<18 years) **Warning:** • Black-boxed warning for neuropsychiatric symptoms[4] **Contraindications:** • Seizure disorder • Concomitant bupropion (e.g., Wellbutrin) therapy • Current or prior diagnosis of bulimia or anorexia nervosa • Simultaneous abrupt discontinuation of alcohol or sedatives/benzodiazepines • MAO inhibitor therapy in previous 14 days	• Severe renal impairment (dosage adjustment is necessary) • Pregnancy[3] (category C) and breastfeeding • Adolescents (<18 years) **Warnings:** • Black-boxed warning for neuropsychiatric symptoms[4] • Cardiovascular adverse events in patients with existing cardiovascular disease

(*continued*)

Table 1.4 (*Continued*)

	Nicotine Replacement Therapy (NRT) Formulations						
	Gum	Lozenge	Transdermal Patch	Nasal Spray	Oral Inhaler	Bupropion SR	Varenicline
Dosing	*1st cigarette ≤30 minutes after waking:* 4 mg *1st cigarette >30 minutes after waking:* 2 mg Weeks 1–6: 1 piece q 1–2 hours Weeks 7–9: 1 piece q 2–4 hours Weeks 10–12: 1 piece q 4–8 hours • Maximum, 24 pieces/day • Chew each piece slowly • Park between cheek and gum when peppery or tingling sensation appears (~15–30 chews) • Resume chewing when tingle fades • Repeat chew/park steps until most of the nicotine is gone (tingle does not return; generally 30 min)	*1st cigarette ≤30 minutes after waking:* 4 mg *1st cigarette >30 minutes after waking:* 2 mg Weeks 1–6: 1 lozenge q 1–2 hours Weeks 7–9: 1 lozenge q 2–4 hours Weeks 10–12: 1 lozenge q 4–8 hours • Maximum, 20 lozenges/day • Allow to dissolve slowly (20–30 minutes for standard; 10 minutes for mini) • Nicotine release may cause a warm, tingling sensation • Do not chew or swallow • Occasionally rotate to different areas of the mouth • No food or beverages 15 minutes before or during use • Duration: up to 12 weeks	<u>*10 cigarettes/day:*</u> 21 mg/day × 4 weeks (generic) 6 weeks (NicoDerm CQ) 14 mg/day × 2 weeks 7 mg/day × 2 weeks <u>*≤10 cigarettes/day:*</u> 14 mg/day × 6 weeks 7 mg/day × 2 weeks • May wear patch for 16 hours if patient experiences sleep disturbances (remove at bedtime) • Duration: 8–10 weeks	1–2 doses/hour (8–40 doses/day) One dose = 2 sprays (one in **each** nostril); each spray delivers 0.5 mg of nicotine to the nasal mucosa • Maximum – 5 doses/ hour or – 40 doses/ day • For best results, initially use at least 8 doses/day • Do not sniff, swallow, or inhale through the nose as the spray is being administered • Duration: 3–6 months	6–16 cartridges/day Individualize dosing; initially use 1 cartridge q 1–2 hours • Best effects with continuous puffing for 20 minutes • Initially use at least 6 cartridges/day • Nicotine in cartridge is depleted after 20 minutes of active puffing • Inhale into back of throat or puff in short breaths • Do NOT inhale into the lungs (like a cigarette) but "puff" as if lighting a pipe • Open cartridge retains potency for 24 hours • No food or beverages 15 minutes before or during use • Duration: 3–6 months	150 mg po q AM x 3 days, then 150 mg po bid • Do not exceed 300 mg/day • Begin therapy 1–2 weeks prior to quit date • Allow at least 8 hours between doses • Avoid bedtime dosing to minimize insomnia • Dose tapering is not necessary • Can be used safely with NRT • Duration: 7–12 weeks, with maintenance up to 6 months in selected patients	Days 1–3: 0.5 mg po q AM Days 4–7: 0.5 mg po bid Weeks 2–12: 1 mg po bid • Begin therapy 1 week prior to quit date; alternatively, the patient can begin therapy and then quit smoking between days 8–35 of treatment • Take dose after eating and with a full glass of water • Dose tapering is not necessary • Dosing adjustment is necessary for patients with severe renal impairment • Duration: 12 weeks; an additional 12-week course may be used in selected patients

	• Park in different areas of mouth • No food or beverages 15 minutes before or during use • Duration: up to 12 weeks						
Adverse Effects	• Mouth/jaw soreness • Hiccups • Dyspepsia • Hypersalivation • Effects associated with incorrect chewing technique: – Lightheadedness – Nausea/vomiting – Throat and mouth irritation	• Nausea • Hiccups • Cough • Heartburn • Headache • Flatulence • Insomnia	• Local skin reactions (erythema, pruritus, burning) • Headache • Sleep disturbances (insomnia, abnormal/vivid dreams); associated with nocturnal nicotine absorption	• Nasal and/or throat irritation (hot, peppery, or burning sensation) • Rhinitis • Tearing • Sneezing • Cough • Headache	• Mouth and/or throat irritation • Cough • Headache • Rhinitis • Dyspepsia • Hiccups	• Insomnia • Dry mouth • Nervousness/difficulty concentrating • Rash • Constipation • Seizures (risk is 0.1%) • Neuropsychiatric symptoms (rare; see Precautions)	• Nausea • Sleep disturbances (insomnia, abnormal/vivid dreams) • Constipation • Flatulence • Vomiting • Neuropsychiatric symptoms (rare; see Precautions)
Advantages	• Might satisfy oral cravings • Might delay weight gain • Patients can titrate therapy to manage withdrawal symptoms • Variety of flavors are available	• Might satisfy oral cravings • Might delay weight gain • Easy to use and conceal • Patients can titrate therapy to manage withdrawal symptoms • Variety of flavors are available	• Provides consistent nicotine levels over 24 hours • Easy to use and conceal • Once daily dosing associated with fewer compliance problems	• Patients can titrate therapy to rapidly manage withdrawal symptoms	• Patients can titrate therapy to manage withdrawal symptoms • Mimics hand-to-mouth ritual of smoking (could also be perceived as a disadvantage)	• Easy to use; oral formulation might be associated with fewer compliance problems • Might delay weight gain • Can be used with NRT • Might be beneficial in patients with depression	• Easy to use; oral formulation might be associated with fewer compliance problems • Offers a new mechanism of action for patients who have failed other agents

(*continued*)

Table 1.4 *(Continued)*

	Nicotine Replacement Therapy (NRT) Formulations						
	Gum	Lozenge	Transdermal Patch	Nasal Spray	Oral Inhaler	Bupropion SR	Varenicline
Disadvantages	• Need for frequent dosing can compromise compliance • Might be problematic for patients with significant dental work • Patients must use proper chewing technique to minimize adverse effects • Gum chewing may not be socially acceptable	• Need for frequent dosing can compromise compliance • Gastrointestinal side effects (nausea, hiccups, heartburn) might be bothersome	• Patients cannot titrate the dose to acutely manage withdrawal symptoms • Allergic reactions to adhesive might occur • Patients with dermatologic conditions should not use the patch	• Need for frequent dosing can compromise compliance • Nasal/throat irritation may be bothersome • Patients must wait 5 minutes before driving or operating heavy machinery • Patients with chronic nasal disorders or severe reactive airway disease should not use the spray	• Need for frequent dosing can compromise compliance • Initial throat or mouth irritation can be bothersome • Cartridges should not be stored in very warm conditions or used in very cold conditions • Patients with underlying bronchospastic disease must use with caution	• Seizure risk is increased • Several contraindications and precautions preclude use in some patients (see Precautions) • Patients should be monitored for potential neuropsychiatric symptoms[4] (see Precautions)	• May induce nausea in up to one third of patients • Patients should be monitored for potential neuropsychiatric symptoms[4] (see Precautions)
Cost/day[5]	2 mg or 4 mg: $1.89–$5.48 (9 pieces)	2 mg or 4 mg: $3.05–$4.38 (9 pieces)	$1.52–$3.40 (1 patch)	$4.12 (8 doses)	$7.35 (6 cartridges)	$2.38–$6.22 (2 tablets)	$5.96–$6.50 (2 tablets)

[1]Marketed by GlaxoSmithKline.

[2]Marketed by Pfizer.

[3]The US Clinical Practice Guideline states that pregnant smokers should be encouraged to quit without medication based on insufficient evidence of effectiveness and theoretical concerns with safety. Pregnant smokers should be offered behavioral counseling interventions that exceed minimal advice to quit.

[4]In July 2009, the FDA mandated that the prescribing information for all bupropion- and varenicline-containing products include a black-boxed warning highlighting the risk of serious neuropsychiatric symptoms, including changes in behavior, hostility, agitation, depressed mood, suicidal thoughts and behavior, and attempted suicide. Clinicians should advise patients to stop taking varenicline or bupropion SR and contact a healthcare provider immediately if they experience agitation, depressed mood, and any changes in behavior that are not typical of nicotine withdrawal, or if they experience suicidal thoughts or behavior. If treatment is stopped due to neuropsychiatric symptoms, patients should be monitored until the symptoms resolve.

[5]Wholesale acquisition cost from Red Book Online. Thomson Reuters, September 2012.

Abbreviations: MAO, monoamine oxidase; NRT, nicotine replacement therapy; OTC, over-the-counter (non-prescription product); Rx, prescription product.

For complete prescribing information, please refer to the manufacturers' package inserts.

Nicotine replacement therapy

In clinical trials, use of an NRT significantly increases quitting rates, compared to placebo [101]. The main mechanism of action of NRT products is thought to be a stimulation of nicotine receptors in the ventral tegmental area of the brain, which results in dopamine release in the nucleus accumbens. The rationale for use of NRT is to reduce the physical withdrawal symptoms and to alleviate the physiologic symptoms of withdrawal, so the smoker can focus on the behavioral and psychological aspects of quitting before fully abstaining from nicotine. Key advantages of NRT are that patients are not exposed to the carcinogens or other toxic compounds found in tobacco and tobacco smoke. NRT provides slower onset of action than nicotine delivered via cigarettes, thereby eliminating the near-immediate reinforcing effects of nicotine obtained through smoking (Figure 1.1).

Because the efficacy of the various NRT formulations (gum, lozenge, transdermal patch, inhaler, nasal spray) are similar [101], selection should be based on patient preference. With the exception of the nicotine patch, which is dosed once a day, all NRT formulations require frequent administration to ensure adequate concentrations of nicotine to alleviate withdrawal. To maximize chances for success, clinicians should advise patients to take the full recommended number of doses each day and continue to adhere to the recommended regimen for the entire course of therapy. There are no specific contraindications to NRT use, but because nicotine stimulates the sympathetic nervous system and leads to increases in heart rate, myocardial contractility, and blood pressure, NRT products should be used with caution in patients who have serious arrhythmias, underlying serious or worsening angina pectoris, or a recent (within 2 weeks) myocardial infarction [101]. Because the blood levels of nicotine associated with the recommended doses of NRT products are generally lower than those attained through smoking, most experts contend that the risks associated with NRT use in patients with cardiovascular disease are minimal relative to the significant risks associated with continued smoking [112].

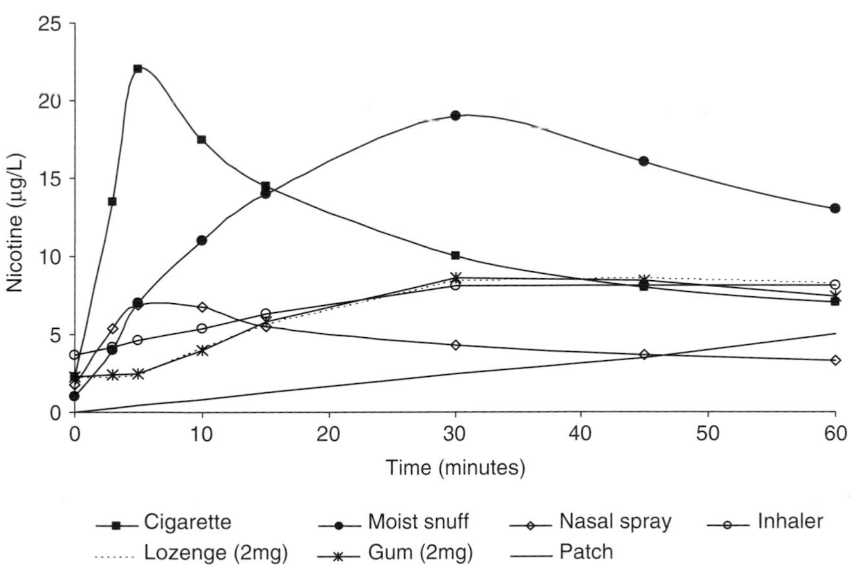

Figure 1.1 Plasma nicotine concentrations for various nicotine-containing products. *Source:* Reprinted from [108], with permission. Copyright © 1999–2014 The Regents of the University of California. All rights reserved. Plasma nicotine concentration curves derived from references [109–111].

Sustained-release bupropion

Initially marketed as an atypical antidepressant, sustained-release bupropion is hypothesized to facilitate smoking cessation by inhibiting the reuptake of dopamine and norepinephrine in the central nervous system [101] and acting as a nicotinic acetylcholine receptor antagonist [113]. These neurochemical effects are believed to modulate the dopamine reward pathway and reduce the cravings for nicotine and symptoms of withdrawal [101].

Because seizures are a dose-related toxicity associated with bupropion, this medication is contraindicated in patients with underlying seizure disorders and in patients receiving concurrent therapy with other forms of bupropion (Wellbutrin, Wellbutrin SR, and Wellbutrin XL). Bupropion also is contraindicated in patients with anorexia or bulimia nervosa and in patients who are undergoing abrupt discontinuation of alcohol or sedatives (including benzodiazepines) due to the increased risk for seizures. The concurrent administration of bupropion and a monoamine oxidase (MAO) inhibitor is contraindicated. At least 14 days should elapse between discontinuation of an MAO inhibitor and initiation of treatment with bupropion [114]. The incidence of seizures associated with the recommended 300 mg/day dose of the sustained-release formulation when used in the treatment of depression was 0.1% (1/1000) among patients without a previous history of seizures. For this reason, bupropion should be used with extreme caution in patients with a history of seizure, cranial trauma, patients receiving medications known to lower the seizure threshold, and patients with underlying severe hepatic cirrhosis.

In July 2009, the FDA mandated that the prescribing information for all bupropion-containing products include a black-boxed warning to highlight the risk of serious neuropsychiatric events, including but not limited to depression, suicidal ideation, suicide attempt, and completed suicide. All patients being treated with bupropion should be observed for neuropsychiatric symptoms including changes in behavior, hostility, agitation, depressed mood, and suicide-related events, including ideation, behavior, and attempted suicide. Patients should be advised to stop taking bupropion and contact a healthcare provider immediately if agitation, hostility, depressed mood, or changes in thinking or behavior that are not typical for the patient are observed, or if the patient develops suicidal ideation or suicidal behavior. Ongoing monitoring and supportive care should be provided until symptoms resolve [114].

Varenicline

The efficacy of varenicline, a partial agonist selective for the $\alpha4\beta2$ nicotinic acetylcholine receptor [115, 116], is believed to be the result of sustained, low-level agonist activity at the receptor site combined with competitive inhibition of nicotine binding. The partial agonist activity induces modest receptor stimulation, which leads to increased dopamine levels, thereby attenuating the symptoms of nicotine withdrawal. In addition, by competitively blocking the binding of nicotine to nicotinic acetylcholine receptors in the central nervous system, varenicline inhibits the surges of dopamine release that occur following the inhalation of tobacco smoke. The latter effect might be effective in preventing relapse by reducing the reinforcing and rewarding effects of smoking [116].

Similar to bupropion, in 2009 the FDA mandated that the prescribing information for varenicline include a black-boxed warning to highlight the risk of serious neuropsychiatric events, including but not limited to depression, suicidal ideation, suicide attempt and completed suicide. All patients being treated with varenicline should be observed for neuropsychiatric symptoms including changes in behavior, hostility, agitation, depressed mood, and suicide-related events, including ideation, behavior, and attempted suicide. Patients should be advised to stop taking varenicline and contact a healthcare provider immediately if agitation, hostility, depressed mood, or changes in thinking or behavior that are not typical for the patient are observed, or if the patient develops suicidal ideation or suicidal behavior [117].

More recently, a warning/precaution related to use among patients with known cardiovascular disease was added to the manufacturer's labeling for varenicline. Specifically, patients should be instructed to notify their health care provider if they notice any new or worsening cardiovascular symptoms and to seek immediate medical attention if they experience signs and symptoms of myocardial infarction or stroke. Although a meta-analysis of 15 clinical trials (including a trial in patients with stable cardiovascular disease) demonstrated that cardiovascular events were infrequent overall, some were reported more frequently in patients treated with varenicline, and these events occurred primarily among patients with known cardiovascular disease. In both the clinical trial and meta-analysis, however, all-cause and cardiovascular mortality was lower among patients treated with varenicline [117].

Combination therapy

While the use of a cessation medication approximately doubles the likelihood that a patient will successfully quit smoking, improvements in long-term quit rates are needed. Based on data from eight clinical trials, the 2008 *Clinical Practice Guideline* [101] recommends that clinicians consider the use of combination pharmacotherapy as a first-line treatment approach for patients during a quit attempt. Combination therapy approaches, which typically include a long-acting formulation (e.g., nicotine patch) in combination with a short-acting formulation (e.g., gum, lozenge, inhaler, or nasal spray) are being increasingly utilized. The long-acting formulation helps to prevent the onset of severe withdrawal symptoms while the short-acting formulation is used as needed to control situational cravings. Furthermore, the optimal combinations, dosages, and duration of dual NRTs are not yet known.

Use of medications in pregnancy

The *Clinical Practice Guideline* [101] states that pregnant smokers should be encouraged to quit without medication, because of insufficient evidence of effectiveness and hypothetical concerns with safety.

Animal data suggest that nicotine is harmful to the developing fetus. As such prescription formulations of NRT are classified by the FDA as pregnancy category D agents. Bupropion and varenicline are classified as a pregnancy category C drug. Correspondingly, the manufacturers recommend that this agent be used during pregnancy only if the potential benefit outweighs the potential risk to the fetus [114, 117].

Summary

Tobacco use remains prevalent among the population and represents a matter of special public health concern. It is the primary risk factor for the development of lung cancer. It has been shown to cause malignancies in other locations, as well as numerous other diseases. The body of knowledge of various aspects of smoking behavior has largely increased over the past several decades. Studies of factors predisposing to smoking initiation among youth may provide important clues for the development of feasible and effective smoking prevention activities. The knowledge of biobehavioral factors leading to development of nicotine dependence may assist in providing more effective treatments to patients who use tobacco products. The 5 A's approach (Ask about tobacco use, Advise patients to quit, Assess readiness to quit, Assist with quitting, and Arrange follow-up) is described in the US Public Health Service *Clinical Practice Guideline for Treating Tobacco Use and Dependence*. Health care providers are encouraged to prevent smoking initiation among youth and implement at least brief interventions (Ask-Advise-Refer) at each encounter with a patient who uses tobacco.

References

1 American Cancer Society (2014) *Cancer Facts and Figures*. American Cancer Society, Atlanta, GA.

2 US Department of Health and Human Services (2012) *Preventing Tobacco Use Among Youth and Young Adults: A Report of the Surgeon General*. US Department of Health

and Human Services, Centers for Disease Control and Prevention, National Center for Chronic Disease Prevention and Health Promotion, Office on Smoking and Health, Atlanta, GA.

3 Pierce JP, White VM, Emery SL (2012) What public health strategies are needed to reduce smoking initiation? *Tob Control*, 21(2): 258–64.

4 CDC (2008) Cigarette smoking among adults and trends in smoking cessation – United States. *MMWR (Morbidity and Mortality Weekly Report)*, 58(44): 1227–32.

5 A Clinical Practice Guideline for Treating Tobacco Use and Dependence: 2008 update. A US Public Health Service report (2008) *Am J Prev Med*, 35(2): 158–76.

6 CDC (2012) Current cigarette smoking among adults – United States, 2011. *MMWR*, 61(44): 889–94.

7 Johnston LD, O'Malley PM, Bachman JG, Schulenberg JE (2012) *Decline in teen smoking continues into 2012*. University of Michigan, Ann Arbor, MI.

8 US Department of Health, Education, and Welfare (1964) *Smoking and Health: Report of the Advisory Committee to the Surgeon General of the Public Health Service*. US Department of Health, Education, and Welfare, Public Health Service, Center for Disease Control, PHS Publication No. 1103, Washington, DC.

9 CDC (2008) Smoking-attributable mortality, years of potential life lost, and productivity losses – United States, 2000–2004. *MMWR*, 57(45): 1226–8.

10 CDC (2002) Annual smoking-attributable mortality, years of potential life lost, and economic costs – United States, 1995–1999. *MMWR*, 51(14): 300–3.

11 US Department of Health and Human Services (2004) *The Health Consequences of Smoking: A Report of the Surgeon General*. US Department of Health and Human Services, Centers for Disease Control and Prevention, National Center for Chronic Disease Prevention and Health Promotion, Office on Smoking and Health.

12 CDC (2003) Cigarette smoking-attributable morbidity – United States, 2000. *MMWR*, 52(35): 842–4.

13 Wingo PA, Ries LA, Giovino GA, Miller DS, Rosenberg HM, Shopland DR, *et al.* (1999) Annual report to the nation on the status of cancer, 1973–1996, with a special section on lung cancer and tobacco smoking. *J Natl Cancer Inst*, 91(8): 675–90.

14 Peto R, Lopez AD, Boreham J, Thun M, Heath C, Jr., Doll R (1996) Mortality from smoking worldwide. *Br Med Bull*, 52(1): 12–21.

15 Doll R, Peto R, Boreham J, Sutherland I (2005) Mortality from cancer in relation to smoking: 50 years observations on British doctors. *Br J Cancer*, 92(3): 426–9.

16 Yoder LH (2006) Lung cancer epidemiology. *Medsurg Nurs*, 15(3): 171–4; quiz 5.

17 Jemal A, Siegel R, Ward E, Murray T, Xu J, Smigal C, *et al.* (2006) Cancer statistics, 2006. *CA Cancer J Clin*. 56(2): 106–30.

18 Spiro SG, Silvestri GA (2005) One hundred years of lung cancer. *Am J Respir Crit Care Med*, 172(5): 523–9.

19 Knop C (2005) Lung cancer. In *Cancer Nursing: Principles and Practice*, Yarbro CH, Frogge MH, Goodman M, eds. Jones and Barlett, Boston, MA.

20 Pastorino U (2006) Early detection of lung cancer. *Thematic Review Series*, 73: 5–13.

21 Rutten LF, Hesse BW, Moser RP, McCaul KD, Rothman AJ (2009) Public perceptions of cancer prevention, screening, and survival: comparison with state-of-science evidence for colon, skin, and lung cancer. *J Cancer Educ*, 24(1): 40–8.

22 IARC (2004) Tobacco smoke and involuntary smoking. IARC Monographs on the Evaluation of Carcinogenic Risks to Humans, Vol. 83. International Agency for Research on Cancer.

23 Anthonisen NR, Connett JE, Murray RP, Grp LHSR (2002) Smoking and lung function of lung health study participants after 11 years. *Am J Respir Crit Care Med* 166(5): 675–9.

24 Kamholz SL (2006) Pulmonary and cardiovascular consequences of smoking. *Clin Occup Environ Med*, 5(1): 157–71, x.

25 Pirie K, Peto R, Reeves GK, Green J, Beral V (2013) The 21st century hazards of smoking and benefits of stopping: a prospective study of one million women in the UK. *Lancet* 381(9861): 133–41.

26 Agudo A, Bonet C, Travier N, Gonzalez CA, Vineis P, Bueno-de-Mesquita HB, *et al.* (2012) Impact of cigarette smoking on cancer risk in the European prospective investigation into cancer and nutrition study. *J Clin Oncol* 30(36): 4550–7.

27 Lee PN, Forey BA, Coombs KJ (2012) Systematic review with meta-analysis of the epidemiological evidence in the 1900s relating smoking to lung cancer. *BMC Cancer* 12: 385.

28 Doll R, Hill AB (1950) Smoking and carcinoma of the lung; preliminary report. *Br Med J* 2(4682): 739–48.

29 Centers for Disease Control and Prevention, Division of Cancer Prevention and Control. Lung Cancer Risk Factors. Atlanta, GA, 2012. Available at: http://www.cdc.gov/cancer/lung/basic_info/risk_factors.htm. Accessed February 20, 2014.

30 Samet JM, Avila-Tang E, Boffetta P, Hannan LM, Olivo-Marston S, Thun MJ, *et al.* (2009) Lung cancer

in never smokers: clinical epidemiology and environmental risk factors. *Clin Cancer Res*, 15(18): 5626–45.

31 Alberg AJ, Nonemaker J (2008) Who is at high risk for lung cancer? Population-level and individual-level perspectives. *Semin Respir Crit Care Med*, 29(3): 223–32.

32 Thomas JL, Guo H, Carmella SG, Balbo S, Han S, Davis A, *et al.* (2011) Metabolites of a tobacco-specific lung carcinogen in children exposed to secondhand or thirdhand tobacco smoke in their homes. *Cancer Epidemiol Biomarkers Prev*, 20(6): 1213–21.

33 US Department of Health and Human Services (2006) *The Health Consequences of Involuntary Exposure to Tobacco Smoke: A Report of the Surgeon General*. US Department of Health and Human Services, Centers for Disease Control and Prevention, Coordinating Center for Health Promotion, National Center for Chronic Disease Prevention and Health Promotion, Office on Smoking and Health.

34 Glantz S, Parmley W (1991) Passive smoking and heart disease: epidemiology, physiology and biochemistry. *Circulation*, 83(1): 1–12.

35 Cox L, Patten C, Ebbert J, Drews A, Croghan G, Clark M, *et al.* (2002) Tobacco use outcomes among patients with lung cancer treated for nicotine dependence. *J Clin Oncol*, 20: 3461–9.

36 van der Bol JM, Mathijssen RH, Loos WJ, Friberg LE, van Schaik RH, de Jonge MJ, *et al.* (2007) Cigarette smoking and irinotecan treatment: pharmacokinetic interaction and effects on neutropenia. *J Clin Oncol*, 1;25(19): 2719–26.

37 Kanai M, Morita S, Matsumoto S, Nishimura T, Hatano E, Yazumi S, *et al.* (2009) A history of smoking is inversely correlated with the incidence of gemcitabine-induced neutropenia. *Ann Oncol*, 20(8): 1397–1401.

38 Parsons A, Daley A, Begh R, Aveyard P (2010) Influence of smoking cessation after diagnosis of early stage lung cancer on prognosis: systematic review of observational studies with meta-analysis. *BMJ*, 340: b5569.

39 Underwood JM, Townsend JS, Tai E, White A, Davis SP, Fairley TL (2012) Persistent cigarette smoking and other tobacco use after a tobacco-related cancer diagnosis. *J Cancer Surviv*, 6(3): 333–44.

40 Underwood JM, Rim SH, Fairley TL, Tai E, Stewart SL (2012) Cervical cancer survivors at increased risk of subsequent tobacco-related malignancies, United States 1992–2008. *Cancer Causes Control*, 23(7): 1009–16.

41 Vander Ark W, DiNardo LJ, Oliver D (1997) Factors affecting smoking cessation in patients with head and neck cancer. *Laryngoscope*, 107: 888–92.

42 Cataldo JK, Dubey S, Prochaska JJ (2010) Smoking cessation: an integral part of lung cancer treatment. *Oncology*, 78(5–6): 289–301.

43 Gritz ER, Fingeret MC, Vidrine DJ, Lazev AB, Mehta NV, Reece GP (2006) Successes and failures of the teachable moment – smoking cessation in cancer patients. *Cancer*, 106(1): 17–27.

44 Garces YI, Yang P, Parkinson J, Zhao X, Wampfler JA, Ebbert JO, *et al.* (2004) The relationship between cigarette smoking and quality of life after lung cancer diagnosis. *Chest*, 126(6): 1733–41.

45 Cooley ME, Sarna L, Kotlerman J, Lukanich JM, Jaklitsch M, Green SB, *et al.* (2009) Smoking cessation is challenging even for patients recovering from lung cancer surgery with curative intent. *Lung Cancer*, 66(2): 218–25.

46 Theadom A, Cropley M (2006) Effects of preoperative smoking cessation on the incidence and risk of intraoperative and postoperative complications in adult smokers: a systematic review. *Tob Control*, 15(5): 352–8.

47 Berg CJ, Carpenter MJ, Jardin B, Ostroff JS (2013) Harm reduction and cessation efforts and interest in cessation resources among survivors of smoking-related cancers. *J Cancer Surviv*, 7(1):44–54.

48 Schnoll R, Malstrom M, James C, *et al.* (2002) Correlates of tobacco use among smokers and recent quitters diagnosed with cancer. *Patient Educ Couns*, 46: 137–45.

49 CDC (2011) Quitting smoking among adults. *MMWR*, 60(44): 1513–19.

50 CDC (2011) Current tobacco use among middle and high school students – United States, 2011. *MMWR*, 61(31): 581–5.

51 Baker F, Ainsworth SR, Dye JT, Crammer C, Thun MJ, Hoffmann D, *et al.* (2000) Health risks associated with cigar smoking. *Jama*, 284(6): 735–40.

52 CDC (2012) Current cigarette smoking among adults – United States, 2011. *MMWR*, 61(44): 889–94.

53 CDC (1999) State-specific prevalence of current cigarette and cigar smoking among adults – United States, 1998. *MMWR*, 48(45): 1034–9.

54 Henningfield JE, Fant R, Radzius A, Frost S (1999) Nicotine concentration, smoke pH and whole tobacco aqueous pH of some cigar brands and types popular in the US. *Nicotine Tob Res*, 1(2): 163–8.

55 Kozlowski LT, Mehta N, Sweeney C, *et al.* (1998) Filter ventilation and nicotine content of tobacco in

cigarettes from Canada, the United Kingdom, and the United States. *Tob Control*, 7(4): 369.

56 Henningfield JE, Hariharan MM, Kozlowski LT (1996) Nicotine content and health risks of cigars. *JAMA*, 276: 1857–8.

57 Nelson DE, Davis RM, Chrismon JH, Giovino GA (1996) Pipe smoking in the United States, 1965–1991: prevalence and attributable mortality. *Prev Med*, 25: 91–9.

58 CDC (1999) Bidi use among urban youth – Massachusetts, March–April 1999. *MMWR*, 48(36): 796–9.

59 Delnevo C, Pevzner E, Hrywna M, *et al.* (2004) Bidi cigarette use among young adults in 15 states. *Prev Med*, 39(1): 207–11.

60 Rickert WS (1999) Determination of yields of "tar," nicotine and carbon monoxide from bidi cigarettes: final report. Ontario, Canada: Labstat International, Inc.

61 Hudmon KS, Kilfoy BA, Prokhorov AV (2006) The epidemiology of tobacco use and dependence. *Crit Care Nurs Clin North Am*, 18(1): 1–11, xi.

62 Substance Abuse and Mental Health Services Administration, Office of Applied Studies (2009). *The NSDUH Report: Smokeless Tobacco Use, Initiation, and Relationship to Cigarette Smoking: 2002 to 2007.* Rockville, MD.

63 US Department of Agriculture (2005) Tobacco Outlook Report (TBS-258), 2005. Available from: http://usda01.library.cornell.edu/usda/ers/TBS/2000s/2005/TBS-04-15-2005.pdf. Accessed February 20, 2014.

64 Delnevo CD, Wackowski OA, Giovenco DP, Manderski MT, Hrywna M, Ling PM (2014) Examining market trends in the United States smokeless tobacco use: 2005–2011. *Tob Control*, 23(2): 107–12.

65 Pederson LL, Nelson DE (2007) Literature review and summary of perceptions, attitudes, beliefs, and marketing of potentially reduced exposure products: communication implications. *Nicotine Tob Res*, 9(5): 525–34.

66 Blank MD, Eissenberg T (2010) Evaluating oral noncombustible potential-reduced exposure products for smokers. *Nicotine Tob Res*, 12(4): 336–43.

67 Parascandola M, Augustson E, O'Connell ME, Marcus S (2009) Consumer awareness and attitudes related to new potential reduced-exposure tobacco product brands. *Nicotine Tob Res*, 11(7): 886–95.

68 American Lung Association (2007) An emerging deadly trend: Waterpipe tobacco use. Washington, DC: American Lung Association. Available from: http://www.lung.org/stop-smoking/tobacco-control-advocacy/reports-resources/tobacco-policy-trend-reports/. Accessed February 20, 2014.

69 Cobb C, Ward KD, Maziak W, Shihadeh AL, Eissenberg T (2010) Waterpipe tobacco smoking: an emerging health crisis in the United States. *Am J Health Behav*, 34(3): 275–85.

70 Eissenberg T, Ward KD, Smith-Simone S, Maziak W (2008) Waterpipe tobacco smoking on a U.S. College campus: prevalence and correlates. *J Adolescent Health*, 42(5): 526–9.

71 Grekin ER, Ayna D (2008) Argileh use among college students in the United States: an emerging trend. *J Stud Alcohol Drugs*, 69(3): 472–5.

72 Smith SY, Curbow B, Stillman FA (2007) Harm perception of nicotine products in college freshmen. *Nicotine Tob Res*, 9(9): 977–82.

73 Martinasek MP, McDermott RJ, Martini L (2011) Waterpipe (hookah) tobacco smoking among youth. *Curr Probl Pediatr Adolesc Health Care*, 41(2): 34–57.

74 Primack B, Shensa A, Kim KH, Carroll M, Hoban M, Leino E, *et al.* (2013) Waterpipe smoking among US university students. *Nicotine Tob Res*, 15(1): 29–35.

75 Sutfin EL, McCoy TP, Reboussin BA, Wagoner KG, Spangler J, Wolfson M (2011) Prevalence and correlates of waterpipe tobacco smoking by college students in North Carolina. *Drug Alcohol Depend.*, May 1; 115(1–2): 131–6.

76 Primack BA, Shensa A, Kim KH, Carroll MV, Hoban MT, Leino EV, *et al.* (2013) Waterpipe smoking among U.S. university students. *Nicotine Tob Res*, Jan;15(1): 29–35.

77 Maziak W (2013) The waterpipe: An emerging global risk for cancer. *Cancer Epidemiol*, 37(1): 1–4.

78 Food and Drug Administration (2009) Electronic cigarettes. Available from: http://www.fda.gov/Safety/MedWatch/SafetyInformation/SafetyAlertsforHumanMedicalProducts/ucm173327.htm. Accessed February 20, 2014.

79 Pearson JL, Richardson A, Niaura RS, Vallone DM, Abrams DB (2012) e-Cigarette awareness, use, and harm perceptions in US adults. *Am J Public Health*, 102(9): 1758–66.

80 Johnston LD, O'Malley PM, Bachman JG, Schulenberg, JE. (2005) Decline in teen smoking appears to be nearing its end. University of Michigan News and Information Services: Ann Arbor, MI. Available from: http://www.monitoringthefuture.org/data/05data.html#2005data-cigs. Accessed February 20, 2014.

81 US Department of Health and Human Services (1994) *Preventing Tobacco Use Among Young People: A Report of the Surgeon General.* Atlanta, GA: US Department of

Health and Human Services, Public Health Service, Centers for Disease Control and Prevention, National Center for Chronic Disease Prevention and Health Promotion, Office on Smoking and Health.

82 Biglan A, Duncan TE, Ary DV, Smolkowski K (1995) Peer and parental influences on adolescent tobacco use. *J Behav Med*, 18(4): 315–30.

83 Gritz ER, Prokhorov AV, Hudmon KS, Mullin Jones M, Rosenblum C, Chang CC, *et al.* (2003) Predictors of susceptibility to smoking and ever smoking: a longitudinal study in a triethnic sample of adolescents. *Nicotine Tob Res*, 5(4): 493–506.

84 Hansen WB (1996) Pilot test results comparing the All Stars program with seventh grade D.A.R.E.: program integrity and mediating variable analysis. *Subst Use Misuse*, 31(10): 1359–77.

85 MacKinnon DP (1994) Analysis of mediating variables in prevention and intervention research. *NIDA Res Monogr*, 139: 127–53.

86 Sargent J (2005) Smoking in movies: Impact on adolescent smoking. *Adoles Med Clin*, 16(2): 345–70.

87 Wahlgren DR, Hovell MF, Slymen DJ, Conway TL, Hofstetter CR, Jones JA (1997) Predictors of tobacco use initiation in adolescents: A two-year prospective study and theoretical discussion. *Tob Control*, 6(2): 95–103.

88 CDC (2006) Youth risk behavior surveillance, United States, 2005. *MMWR*, 55(SS-55): 1–108.

89 Prokhorov AV, Hudmon KS, Marani SK, Bondy ML, Gatus LA, Spitz MR, *et al.* (2013) Eliminating secondhand smoke from Mexican-American households: outcomes from Project Clean Air-Safe Air (CASA). *Addict Behav*, 38(1): 1485–92.

90 Curry SJ, Emery S, Sporer AK, Mermelstein R, Flay BR, Berbaum M, *et al.* (2007) A national survey of tobacco cessation programs for youths. *Am J Public Health*, 97(1): 171–7.

91 Prokhorov AV, Kelder SH, Shegog R, Murray N, Peters R, Jr., Agurcia-Parker C, *et al.* (2008) Impact of A Smoking Prevention Interactive Experience (ASPIRE), an interactive, multimedia smoking prevention and cessation curriculum for culturally diverse high-school students. *Nicotine Tob Res*, 10(9): 1477–85.

92 Joffe A, McNeely C, Colantuoni E, An MW, Wang W, Scharfstein D (2009) Evaluation of school-based smoking-cessation interventions for self-described adolescent smokers. *Pediatrics*, Aug; 124(2): e187–94.

93 Flay BR (2009) The promise of long-term effectiveness of school-based smoking prevention programs: a critical review of reviews. *Tob Induc Dis*, 5(1): 7.

94 Prokhorov AV, Kelder SH, Conroy JL, Shegog R, Murray N, Peters R, Cinciripini PM, de Moor C, Hudmon K (2010) Project ASPIRE: An interactive multimedia smoking prevention and cessation curriculum for culturally diverse high school students. *Subst Use Misuse*, 45(6): 983–1006.

95 Prokhorov AV, Marani SK, Calabro KS, Ford KH (2012) Theory- and technology-driven educational curricula addressing tobacco use. *Procedia – Social and Behavioral Sciences*, 46: 4504–7.

96 Benowitz NL, Hukkanen J, Jacob P, 3rd (2009) Nicotine chemistry, metabolism, kinetics and biomarkers. *Handb Exp Pharmacol*, 192: 29–60.

97 Benowitz NL (2008) Neurobiology of nicotine addiction: implications for smoking cessation treatment. *Am J Med*, 121(4 Suppl 1): S3–10.

98 Benowitz NL (2010) Nicotine addiction. *N Engl J Med*, 362(24): 2295–2303.

99 Benowitz NL (2008) Clinical pharmacology of nicotine: implications for understanding, preventing, and treating tobacco addiction. *Clin Pharmacol Ther*, 83(4): 531–41.

100 Hughes JR (2007) Effects of abstinence from tobacco: valid symptoms and time course. *Nicotine Tob Res*, 9(3): 315–27.

101 Fiore MC, Jaén CR, Baker TB (2008) *Treating Tobacco Use and Dependence: 2008 Update*. Clinical Practice Guideline. Rockville, MD: US Department of Health and Human Services. Public Health Service.

102 CDC (2007) *Best Practices for Comprehensive Tobacco Control Programs – 2007*. National Center for Chronic Disease Prevention and Health Promotion, Office on Smoking and Health, Atlanta, GA, 2007.

103 US Department of Health and Human Services (1990) *The Health Benefits of Smoking Cessation. A Report of the Surgeon General*. US Department of Health and Human Services, Public Health Service, Office on Smoking and Health, Rockville, Maryland, DHHS Publication No. (CDC) 90–8416.

104 Stead LF, Perera R, Lancaster T (2007) A systematic review of interventions for smokers who contact quitlines. *Tob Control*, 16 Suppl 1: i3–8.

105 Zhu S, Melcer T, Sun J, Rosbrook B, Pierce JP (2000) Smoking cessation with and without assistance: a population-based analysis. *Am J Prev Med*, 18(4): 305–11.

106 Smith SS, Keller PA, Kobinsky KH, Baker TB, Fraser DL, Bush T, *et al.* (2013) Enhancing tobacco quitline effectiveness: Identifying a superior pharmacotherapy adjuvant. *Nicotine Tob Res*, 15(3): 718–28.

107 Bonniot Saucedo C, Schroeder SA (2010) Simplicity sells: Making smoking cessation easier. *Am J Prev Med*, 38(3 Suppl): S393–6.

108 *Rx for Change: Clinician-Assisted Tobacco Cessation*. San Francisco, CA: University of California San Francisco, 1999–2014.

109 Choi JH, Dresler CM, Norton MR, Strahs KR (2003) Pharmacokinetics of a nicotine polacrilex lozenge. *Nicotine Tob Res*, 5(5): 635–44.

110 Schneider NG, Olmstead RE, Franzon MA, Lunell E (2001) The nicotine inhaler: clinical pharmacokinetics and comparison with other nicotine treatments. *Clin Pharmacokinet*, 40(9): 661–84.

111 Fant RV, Owen LL, Henningfield JE (1999) Nicotine replacement therapy. *Prim Care*, 26(3): 633–52.

112 Benowitz NL (2009) Pharmacology of nicotine: addiction, smoking-induced disease, and therapeutics. *Annu Rev Pharmacol Toxicol*, 49: 57–71.

113 Slemmer JE, Martin BR, Damaj MI (2000) Bupropion is a nicotinic antagonist. *J Pharmacol Exp Ther*, 295: 321–7.

114 GlaxoSmithKline, Inc. (2012) Zyban package insert. Research Triangle Park, NC.

115 Coe JW, Brooks PR, Vetelino MG, Wirtz MC, Arnold EP, Huang J, *et al*. (2005) Varenicline: an alpha4beta2 nicotinic receptor partial agonist for smoking cessation. *J Med Chem*, 48(10): 3474–7.

116 Foulds J (2006) The neurobiological basis for partial agonist treatment of nicotine dependence: varenicline. *Int J Clin Pract*, 60(5): 571–6.

117 Pfizer, Inc. (2012) Chantix Package Insert. New York, NY.

CHAPTER 2

Lung Cancer Susceptibility and Risk Assessment Models

Xifeng Wu, Xia Pu, and Jie Lin

Department of Epidemiology, The University of Texas MD Anderson Cancer Center, Houston, TX, USA

Introduction

The global incidence of lung cancer (LC) has rapidly increased ever since the beginning of the 20th century. Although the number of new LC cases has steadily decreased among men in the United States during the past two decades, LC is still the number one cause of cancer-related mortality [1]. In 2013, it is estimated that there will be 228 190 new cases of LC and 159 480 LC-related deaths in the USA. These deaths represent 28% of total mortality from all cancers in US men and 26% in US women [1]. While tobacco smoking is the predominant cause of LC, a variety of other exposures, such as family history of LC, various chronic respiratory diseases, and environmental tobacco smoke (ETS), are also linked to elevated LC risk. Host susceptibility may also be involved in LC risk, since only a fraction of smokers develops LC [2–5]. Because carcinogenesis is a multistep process, understanding the multiple components contributing to LC risk can lead to the identification of high-risk subgroups who may benefit from targeted screening or other interventions. Next, we provide a summary of recent advances in the molecular epidemiology of LC.

Epidemiologic risk factors

Smoking is the predominant risk factor for LC. Several additional environmental exposure such as asbestos, arsenic, bischloromethylether, chromium, nickel, polycyclic aromatic compounds, radon, vinyl chloride and air pollution have all been implicated in LC etiology, and have been reviewed extensively in previous chapter. We focus on a few other epidemiological factors that have an established role in the current literature.

Family history

There have been a number of published studies showing familial aggregation of LCs in first-degree relatives of probands with LC [6–12]. Moreover, many association studies have reported an increased risk of LC (1.3 to 6.0 fold) among first-degree relatives [11, 13–15]. In a systematic review and meta-analysis of 53 studies on family history and LC risk, Matakidou *et al.* found a significant increased LC risk among those who have at least one affected relative (RR = 1.84, 95% CI = 1.64–2.05). The association was found

Lung Cancer, Fourth Edition. Edited by Jack A. Roth, Waun Ki Hong and Ritsuko U. Komaki.

stronger in those individuals with early-onset relatives. They also performed a pooled estimate of risk among never-smokers, and identified a similar effect (RR = 1.51, 95% CI = 1.11–2.06), indicating the role of family history on LC independent of smoking [15]. In another meta-analysis of first-degree relatives of 2861 lung cancer cases and 3118 healthy control from 41 studies conducted within the International Agency for Research on Cancer (IARC) multicenter case-control Study, a 1.63 fold increased risk (95% CI = 1.31–2.01) was found in individuals with at least one affected relative. Risk increased to 3.60 fold (95% CI = 1.56–8.31) if the individual has two or more affected relatives. They also found that this risk effect was obvious among squamous cell carcinoma and large cell carcinoma subtype [16].

Prior inflammatory diseases and disorders

COPD

Chronic obstructive pulmonary disease (COPD) occurred in 50–90% of lung cancer cases [17]. Epidemiologic studies have repeatedly shown COPD as a risk factor for LC [18–23]. It has been estimated that the presence of COPD increases the risk of lung cancer by up to 4.5-fold [21] Since lung cancer and COPD are leading causes of morbidity and mortality in the United States and worldwide and they share smoking as the major risk factor, COPD as a comorbidity of lung cancer has received much attention in recent years. The National Heart, Lung, and Blood Institute (NHLBI) and the National Cancer Institute (NCI) held a workshop to expand the collaborative efforts to effectively address the interface of COPD and lung cancer, focusing on identify common epidemiological, genetic and epigenetic risk factors as well as to determine common and disparate pathogenetic mechanisms.

Emphysema

Many studies have identified prior history of emphysema as a risk factor of LC. In a recent meta-analysis of previous lung diseases and lung cancer risk, which included 20 studies with data on emphysema and lung cancer, a twofold increased risk for those with emphysema was reported (relative risk [RR] = 2.04, 95% CI = 1.72–2.41) [24]. Another meta-analysis with 7368 subjects screened with computed tomography revealed that emphysema was associated with 2.11 fold increased risk of LC (95% CI = 1.10–4.04), and that this effect was more obvious in patients with visually detected emphysema (OR = 3.50, 95% CI = 2.71–4.51) [25]. In a pooled analysis of 24 607 cases and 81 829 controls conducted by the International Lung Cancer Consortium, a history of emphysema was found to confer a 2.44-fold increased risk of LC (95% CI = 1.64–3.62) in overall population, and similar increased risk was also observed in never-smokers when stratified by smoking status [26].

Asthma

In a meta-analysis, asthma was a significant risk factor for LC among never-smokers with a pooled relative risk (RR) of 1.9 (95% CI, 1.4–2.5) when adjusted for ETS exposure [27]. Recently, another meta-analysis by the International Lung Cancer Consortium including 585 444 individuals from 16 studies reported a significant association between asthma and LC risk in the overall population (RR = 1.28, 95% CI = 1.16–1.41), and also in squamous cell carcinoma (SCC) subgroup (RR = 1.69, 95% CI = 1.26–2.26) [28].

Hay fever

While no association was observed in early studies (Talbot-Smith *et al.* [29] and Osann *et al.* [10]), prior history of hay fever was found to be associated with reduced risk of LC in a large case-control study (odds ratio [OR] = 0.58; 95% CI, 0.48–0.70) [30]. Consistent with the observation, a significantly lower frequency of hay fever was seen among patients with malignancies of lung, colon, bladder, and prostate as compared to controls [31]. It was suggested that the protective effects were attributed to enhanced immune surveillance resulting in better detection and destruction of malignant cells [10, 29, 31–34]. Alternatively, anti-inflammatory agents used to treat hay fever might contribute to this protection.

Diet and nutritional risk factors

Dietary intakes of fruits and vegetables

Increased vegetable and fruit intake has been associated with reduced risk of LC in several cohort studies [35–38]. In the European Prospective Investigation into Cancer and Nutrition (EPIC) cohort, with data collected from 478 021 subjects, a 40% reduction in LC risk was observed with high fruit consumption after adjusting for smoking and other confounders; however, there was no association with vegetable consumption [38]. In a large prospective Danish cohort study comprising 54 158 participants, with increasing intake of plant food, the age-standardized rate ratio of lung cancer increased significantly from 0.35 (0.27–0.45) to 0.65 (0.45–0.93) after control for smoking [39]. In a pooled analysis of eight prospective studies with a total of 3206 incident LC cases among 430 281 individuals followed for 6–16 years, Neuhouser *et al.* [40] reported that compared to the lowest quintile of consumption, the RRs of the highest quintile consumption for total fruits, total fruits and vegetables, and total vegetables were 0.77 (95% CI, 0.67–0.87; $p < 0.001$), 0.7 (95% CI, 0.69–0.90; $p = 0.001$), and 0.88 (95% CI, 0.78–1.00; $p = 0.12$), respectively. They concluded that higher fruit and vegetable consumption, mostly due to fruit intake, is associated with a modest reduction in LC risk [40]. In a systematic review of epidemiologic studies performed in Japanese populations, it was concluded that fruit intake could possibly decrease lung cancer risk; however, solid data supporting an association between vegetable intake and LC is still lacking [41]. However, data from large prospective studies with extensive adjustment for smoking have revealed nonsignificant associations of fruit and vegetable intake and LC risk [42].

One group of nonnutrient compounds in cruciferous vegetables with anticarcinogenic properties is isothiocyanates (ITCs). One possible mechanism for their anticancer action is through downregulation of cytochrome P-450 biotransformation enzyme levels and induction of phase II enzymes [43, 44]. ITCs can also induce apoptosis, cell cycle arrest, and cell differentiation [45]. Several studies have reported significant associations between low consumption of cruciferous vegetables and increased LC risk, especially within subgroups of population carrying susceptible genetic variants, such as GSTM1 null genotypes [46–48]. In a meta-analysis of LC studies with total cruciferous vegetable consumption (18 studies) or specific cruciferous vegetables (11 studies), cruciferous vegetable intake was associated with slightly decreased LC risk in both case-control (OR = 0.78, 95% CI = 0.70–0.88) and cohort studies (RR = 0.83, 95% CI = 0.62–1.08) and the association was more evident in subjects carrying GSTM1 and GSTT1 double null genotypes (OR = 0.41; 95% CI = 0.26–0.65; P for interaction = 0.01) [49].

Carotenoids

Carotenoids are red and yellow fat-soluble pigments found in fruits and vegetables. In a pooled analysis of seven early cohort studies in North America and Europe based on a follow-up of 7–16 years with 3155 incident LC cases among 399 765 participants, Mannisto *et al.* [50] reported that only β-cryptoxanthin intake was inversely associated with LC risk with a RR of 0.76 (95% CI, 0.67–0.86) after controlling for intake of vitamin C, folate, other carotenoids, multivitamin use, and smoking status. In the Alpha-Tocopherol, β-carotene Cancer Prevention Study (ATBC) [51], a total of 27 084 male smokers who are 50–69 years old have participated with 1644 incident LC cases occurred during 14 years of follow-up, lower risks were observed for the highest versus the lowest quintiles of lycopene (28% reduction), lutein/zeaxanthin (17%), β-cryptoxanthin (15%), total carotenoids (16%), serum β-carotene (19%), and serum retinol (27%), while intakes of β-carotene, α-carotene, and retinol were not associated with significant reduction. In a pooled analysis of the Nurse's Health Study and the Health Professional Follow-up Study (HPFS), Michaud *et al.* [52] reported that only α-carotene and lycopene intakes were significantly associate with lower risk of LC. In overall analyses of all carotenoids combined, LC risk was significantly lower in subjects with high total carotenoid intake (RR = 0.68, 95% CI, 0.49–0.94). Inadequate adjustment for confounding, especially smoking factors, and the lack of consideration of multicollinearity between individual carotenoids may be responsible for inconsistent results across studies. A recent meta-analysis including 25 prospective studies on carotenoids and LC risk reported a pooled RR of 0.79 (95% CI, 0.71–0.87) when comparing the highest and the lowest categories of total carotenoids intake, but no significant reduction in LC risk was observed for high beta-carotene intake [53].

Dietary supplementation of beta-carotene

As data from observational epidemiologic studies accumulated and tended to support an inverse association of LC incidence with beta-carotene intake and with serum concentrations of beta-carotene, several large-scale randomized chemoprevention trials had been initiated to test the hypothesis that beta-carotene supplementation protected against LC. However, data generated by the Beta-Carotene and Retinol Efficacy Trial (CARET) and ATBC trials was disappointing [40, 51]. Contrary to the expectation and observational epidemiologic evidence, supplementation of β-carotene resulted in a surprisingly increased overall LC incidence and higher total mortality among current smokers [54–56]. Debate has been focused on dosage, duration of trials, and the difference between dietary intake and supplement use [57]. Preclinical data provide biologic plausibility for this adverse interaction between cigarette smoking and β-carotene [58, 59]. A recent meta-analysis of six randomized clinical trials comparing beta-carotene supplements with placebo found a pooled RR of 1.10, but not statistically significant, suggesting that beta-carotene supplementation is not associated with reduced risk of LC [53].

Phytoestrogens

Dietary phytoestrogens are plant-derived nonsteroidal compounds with weak estrogen-like activity. A significant reduction in risk of LC with increased phytoestrogen intake was observed [60]. The highest quartile of intake of total phytoestrogens from food sources was associated with a 46% reduction in risk (OR = 0.54, 95% CI 0.42–0.70). Several studies in Asian populations, whose diet contains large quantities of phytoestrogens, also reported reduced risk of LC associated with high intakes of phytoestrogens [61–65]. For example, reduced risk for LC has been observed with high intake of nonfermented soy foods [61] in men and reduce risk of SCC with tofu consumption in women. Soy consumption has also been associated with reduced risk in several studies in China [66, 67].

Folate

Folate deficiency has been implicated in lung carcinogenesis due to its adverse effect on DNA methylation, DNA synthesis, and DNA repair activities [68, 69]; however, observational studies have yielded inconsistent results [69–72]. In a recent large randomized trial with folic acid and vitamin B treatment on cancer incidence and mortality, there was a significant increased risk in the group receiving both folic acid and vitamin B during follow-up as compared to the group receiving neither. Also, a significantly increased risk of LC in the folic acid group was observed (HR = 1.59; 95% CI = 0.92–2.75) as compared to the group who did not receive such treatment.

Genetic susceptibility

Although smoking is the predominant risk factor for LC, only a small fraction of smokers eventually develop the disease, which suggests heritable host factors influencing LC susceptibility. Moreover, evidence from familial clustering has further supported genetic susceptibility to LC [73]. Hence, the elucidation of LC susceptibility genes could help in the understanding of disease mechanism, as well as developing personalized therapeutic and chemoprevention strategies [74].

LC susceptibility genes are generally categorized as having rare high-risk (OR > 10), moderate risk (OR = 2–5), or common low risk variants (OR = 1.2–1.5). Several high risk variants of LC have been identified through linkage analysis studies in members from high-risk families (family with multiple cases). For example, a potential high risk locus on chromosome 6q23–25 has been identified by studying 52 high-risk families with many lung or larynx cancer cases [75]. Follow-up fine-mapping has identified *RGS17* as a potential high risk susceptibility gene [76].

However, most LC susceptibility genes are of moderate or low risk. Individual susceptibility could be modulated by multiple moderate/low risk loci in genes involved in diverse cellular processes such as carcinogen metabolism, DNA repair, cell cycle checkpoint control, apoptosis, telomere integrity and microenvironment control. These moderate/low risk variants are tested by genetic association studies. By comparing the allelic frequencies of genetic loci between cases and healthy controls, population-based association studies are commonly used in susceptibility gene identification. Single nucleotide polymorphism (SNP) is the most commonly investigated form of genetic variation in cancer association studies. Evidence shows that functional SNPs may affect host gene either in terms of gene expression or protein activities, which may impact LC susceptibility [77–79]. In the past few decades, genetic association studies have rapidly evolved from candidate gene-based studies to genome-wide association studies (GWAS). The following section will focus on results from both candidate gene-based studies and GWAS.

Candidate gene approaches

Based on "common variant common disease" hypothesis, candidate gene-based association studies evaluated the association between genetic variations within prespecified genes of interest and cancer risk. Candidate gene study is a hypothesis-driven and largely depends on prior knowledge of the selected gene's known or presumed gene function. Often the selected variants may be functional SNPs in genes with known function relevant to the disease of study. Pathway-based approach is an extension of candidate gene approach. It increases the gene coverage by investigating markers within a whole biological or functional pathway.

Numerous molecular epidemiological studies have used candidate gene- or pathway-based approaches to evaluate the associations of common sequence variants with LC risk. Most efforts have been focused on genetic variants within genes involved in several major cellular processes, mainly carcinogen metabolism, DNA repair, cell cycle regulation pathways, and in some cancer-related genes, such as oncogenes and tumor suppressor genes. However, few studies have included a validation stage, and the results for most polymorphisms are conflicting with a few exceptions [74].

The null genotype of *GSTM1* gene has been repeatedly reported to increase LC risk, likely due to its decreased ability to detoxify carcinogens. Moreover, interactions between nutrition patterns and *GSTM1* genotype have also been identified by various research groups [46–48]. A large meta-analysis of 98 studies including around 45 000 individuals has confirmed the significant association of *GSTM1* null genotype with increased LC risk (OR = 1.22, 95% C = 1.14–1.30). When stratified by ethnicity, the effect was only evident in Asian population (OR = 1.38; 95% CI, 1.24–1.55) [80]. The I157T missense variant in *CHEK2*, a key player in cell-cycle control regulation, is another locus showing consistent association with LC in many reports. This variant is present in 5–7% of northern and central Europe population [81, 82]. Interestingly, the variant allele of this SNP was found to increase susceptibility to several cancers; however, this variant also has been consistently associated with a reduced risk for lung cancer [81–84]. The underlying mechanism of this differential effect has yet to be elucidated.

Genome-wide association studies

With advances in high-throughput genotyping technology, genome-wide association study (GWAS) has emerged as a powerful tool to comprehensively detect genetic susceptibility loci in recent years. As an alternative to candidate gene-based approach, GWAS provides a thorough screening of whole genome by scanning millions of common SNPs across the entire human genome [85]. In order to obtain sufficient statistical power, the GWAS approach usually includes a very large population with multiple phases for validation. A recent report on commercially-available whole-genome SNP panels has claimed that 70–90% of common variants in European population are covered [86]. However, since the panel covers common variants (MAF>1%) in the human genome, the rare variants with low allele frequencies are missed.

Unlike hypothesis-driven candidate gene approach, GWAS is discovery-driven and does not require any prior knowledge of disease processes; therefore, GWAS provides the opportunity to discover novel loci in genes whose function may not be fully understood. In recent years, the GWAS approach has been applied in more than 30 different cancer sites with greater than 230 susceptibility loci being identified. Due to the large number of SNPs tested, the statistical requirement is very stringent (P-value $< 5 \times 10^{-8}$) to account for multiple testing, and multistage validation is usually required to control for false positives [87].

The first GWAS of LC was published in 2007 [88]. An European group performed genome-wide scan using Affymetrix 100K SNP array in a relatively small sample population. A total of 38 significant SNPs were identified, none of which reached genome-wide significance according to current GWAS standard. In the following years, several other groups have conducted large-scale LC GWAS with usually thousands of cases and controls. Moreover, all of these studies included validation stages with thousands of samples. Importantly, the susceptibility regions identified by three earliest GWAS were all mapped to 15q25.1 with similar main effects. These findings confirmed the role of this region in LC susceptibility and provided evidence for the power of the GWAS approach to reproducibly detect cancer associations. Other than 15q25.1, genetic variants on chromosome 5p13 (89), 6p21 (90), and 12p13 (91) were also identified as being associated with LC risk. The results of these studies are detailed below:

15q25.1

In 2008, three separate research groups conducted GWAS of LC risk in populations of European descent: the IARC [92], the University of Texas MD Anderson Cancer Center [75], and Iceland deCODE [93]. Three SNPs (rs10151730, rs8034191, and rs16969968) in *CHRNA5* were identified as being significantly associated with LC risk with similar ORs between 1.30–1.32. The Iceland deCODE study further discovered a significant association between rs1015730 and nicotine dependence. Subsequently, several other studies have replicated the significant association of rs1015730 with LC risk in European populations as well as other ethnicity groups [94–97].

Chromsome 15q25.1 contains three nicotinic-acetylcholine receptor (nAChRs) encoding genes (*CHRNA3*, *CHRNA5*, and *CHRNB4*). NAChRs are ubiquitous cell-surface receptors involved in neurotransmission, which influence smoking behavior. Tobacco-specific carcinogens can bind to nAChRs with a higher affinity than nicotine and induce the flow of cations into the cytoplasm leading to the stimulation of intracellular signaling cascades [98, 99]. These genes are therefore biologically relevant to LC carcinogenesis [75, 92] and nicotine dependence [93]. Although the functional significance of the 15q25 SNPs is unknown, these SNPs could play a role in lung carcinogenesis through modulating host gene functions. This may be especially true for rs16969968, which is a missense SNP (Asp398Arg) causing an amino-acid change in a loop region directly involved in the closure of cation channels (e.g., Ca^{2+}). The underlying mechanisms of how CHRN genes influence LC susceptibility have not yet been completely elucidated. Several hypotheses have been proposed for the impact of CHRN polymorphisms influencing host susceptibility to lung carcinogenesis. Due to the high affinity and sensitivity of nAChRs to nicotine, and taking into account the major risk factor of smoking in LC, it was hypothesized that CHRN genes could modulate a person's LC risk by inducing smoking addiction. Other than nicotine dependence, evidence from studies in never-smokers has shown that CHRN genes also could lead to LC development independent of tobacco smoking [75, 92, 96]. CHRN polymorphisms might affect cell motility of the bronchial epithelium leading to delayed wound healing and persistent tissue damage and inflammation, which provides favorable microenvironment for carcinogenesis and tumor progression [74]. Different expression pattern of genes encoding nAChRs has been identified between smokers and nonsmokers [100]. Hypermethylation of *CHRNA3* and the downregulation of gene expression have been found in cancer cells, while induced expression of *CHRNA3* led to higher apoptotic activity [101]. These studies provided evidence and biological plausibility linking nAChR signaling with lung carcinogenesis [99].

5p15.33

Chromosome 5p15.33 is another region that has been repeatedly identified by GWAS as susceptibility locus for LC [76, 89, 102]. In 2008, two research groups identified rs401681, rs402710 and rs2736100 associated with LC risk; however, only rs401681 reached genome-wide significance [89, 102]. In 2010, an expanded replication was performed through an international consortium effort involving over 20 000 subjects (11 645 cases and 14 954 controls). In this study, rs2736100 and rs402710 both reached genome-wide significance in their association with LC risk [103].

Chromosome 5p15.33, commonly referred as the *TERT-CLPTM1L* locus, contains two genes encoding the telomerase reverse transcriptase (*TERT*) and Cleft Lip and Palate Transmembrane Protein 1-Like protein (*CLPTM1L*). Other than lung cancer, this region has been implicated as susceptibility locus in many other cancers, including bladder, prostate, and cervical cancers [104].

TERT is the protein component of telomerase complex, which is highly conserved among species. It plays a pivotal role in telomerase activation and maintenance. Telomerase is highly active in stem cells and progenitor cells, but is repressed or non-expressed in normal cells. Cancer cell is characterized by its high expression of telomerase to overcome telomere attrition. Although it has not been definitively shown that telomerase activation contributes to lung carcinogenesis, compelling evidence indicated a role of *TERT* in LC development. The human *TERT* gene was either amplified or mutated in LC tissues [105]. Many known oncogenes or tumor suppressor genes (TSG), such as *MYC, RAS* and *p53* have been found to regulate *TERT* transcription. Moreover, the catalytic subunit of TERT was used as a drug target for treatment and prevention in various clinical trials, aiming at stopping cancer cell growth with minimal effect on normal cells [106]. The significant findings in independent GWA studies further highlighted the role of *TERT* in lung carcinogenesis.

CLPTM1L is named after its homolog on chromosome 19p [107]. The role of *CLPTM1L* in cancer was not as extensively investigated as that of *TERT*. The first evidence of *CLPTM1L* in carcinogenesis is the discovery of its overexpression in cisplatin resistant ovarian cancer cell lines [107]. In a recent report, *CLPTM1L* was found to be overexpressed in human lung adenocarcinoma tissues, and was demonstrated to protect from genotoxic stress-induced apoptosis in tumor cells [108].

6p21 and 12p13

6p21 is the third LC susceptibility region identified by several GWAS [102, 109, 110]. A meta-analysis has found 61 candidate LC susceptibility SNPs, most of which are highly linked with rs3117582, with the strongest effect found in SCC [109]. Rs3117582 is mapped 73 bps 5′ to BAG6/BAT3, a gene encoding BCL2-associated athanogene 6 which was known to involve in p53-mediated apoptosis (111). Evidence from animal experiments have supported the critical role of this gene in lung development (112). Another SNP rs3131379, which is highly linked with rs3117582, is located in MSH5, which encodes DNA mismatch repair mutS homolog 5. It is also possible that this region influences host's DNA repair capacity, which may explain the stronger association of this region with SCC since SCC is more closely linked to external carcinogen exposure (109).

The 12p13 region was identified by Shi *et al.* in a pathway-based analysis of nearly 20 000 SNPs in inflammation genes from a GWAS of 5355 lung cancer cases and 4344 controls followed by three validation phases. All the subjects included are European smokers. They identified rs6489769 in RAD52 as a novel susceptibility locus for SCC. RAD52 homolog gene is a key player in DNA double-strand repair and homologous recombination [113,114], therefore biologically supported the role of this region for LC in smokers. In a recent large scale meta-analysis, Timofeeva *et al.* confirmed the significance of this locus in SCC in a recent meta-analysis of GWAS of 14 900 cases and 29 485 controls [109].

Racial subgroups

GWAS of LC were initially focused on subjects of European descent. Because of the racial disparity and genetic heterogeneity in LC, in recent years several research groups have conducted GWAS in specific racial/ethnic subgroups. Several common susceptibility loci have been confirmed of their significance in different racial populations, and a few race-specific susceptibility loci have also been identified. For example, 5p15.33 has been replicated in the Han Chinese population [115]. In addition, several variants of *CHRNA5* in 15q25 were found to be associated with increased LC risk and smoking behavior in African-Americans as well as Chinese population [96,116]. Because the previously identified SNPs (rs1051730, rs8034191 and rs16969968) were identified in European population, which were very rare in Asian population, Wu *et al.* screened this region for other possible candidate SNP in a Chinese population [96]. They identified four novel SNPs (rs2036534, rs667282, rs12910984 and rs6495309) which reached genome-wide significance. Their finding confirmed the importance of this region with LC in Asian population. However, null result was reported for this region in a recent GWAS of lung cancer in Asian women who never smoked, likely due to the tight relationship of this region with smoking behavior [117]. In another large-scale GWAS analysis conducted in Chinese population, Hu *et al.* confirmed association of two identified susceptibility loci (3q28 and 5p15.33) which were previously identified in European population [118]. In addition, they identified two novel loci (13q12.12 and 22q12.2) that appeared specific for Asians, since these two loci were not significant in a large meta-analysis of GWAS of European ancestry population [109]. Table 2.1 summarizes the susceptibility loci in different racial populations.

Tumor histology

Different LC histologies have common and distinct susceptibility loci. Landi *et al.* reported that the association of 5p15 locus with LC was only evident in the adenocarcinoma subgroup, not in the SCC subgroup [119]. In a recent meta-analysis of 14 900 cases and 29 485 controls in the European population, the investigators identified histology-specific effects for the 5p15 (*TERT*: adenocarcinoma; *CLPTM1L*: squamous and large-cell carcinoma), 6p21 (*BAG6/BAT3*: squamous cell carcinoma) and 12p13 (*RAD52*: squamous and small-cell carcinoma), but the 15q25 region was significant for all the histologies [109].

Never-smokers

Approximately 15% of lung cancer cases developed in individuals without any apparent tobacco consumption history [120]. Many hypotheses have been proposed regarding the etiology and environmental exposures of lung cancer in never-smokers (LCINS), such as secondhand smoke, occupational exposure, radon gas, cooking fumes, air pollution, and viral infection. Nevertheless, it is clear that LCINS is characterized by molecular changes and natural history distinct from LC in ever smokers, including the increased frequency of activating mutations in the epidermal growth factor receptor (*EGFR*) gene [121]. The contribution of inherited genetic susceptibility to LCINS has been explored in recent few years. In 2010, the first effort was conducted by Li *et al.* in 377 never-smoker LC cases and equally matched controls, followed by a two validation stages and an expression quantitative trait loci (eQTL) analysis. Two SNPs in 13q31.3 gene were identified as top SNPs associated with risk of LCINS. In addition, these two SNPs were also shown to correlate with the expression of *GPC5* gene [122]. In the following year, a GWAS in Korean population identified another locus on chromosome 18p11.22 [73]. However, the findings from both studies did not reach genome-wide significance, and replication effort with larger sample size is warranted to confirm these two loci. Most recently, Lan *et al.* conducted a GWAS of LC in Asian female never-smokers (5510 cases and 4544 controls) [117] and identified three novel susceptibility loci at 10q25.2, 6q22.2 and 6p21.32 with genome-wide significance. The authors also confirmed previously reported loci at 5p15.33, 3q28 and 17q24.3, which have been previously identified as susceptibility loci in Asian populations [110, 115];

Table 2.1 Summary of susceptibility loci identified from GWAS

Loci	Reported genes	SNPs	Population	Reference
15q25	*PSMA4, CHRNA3, CHRNA5, CHRNB4, LOC123688*	rs1051730/rs8034191 (EUR,AA) rs2036534/rs6495309 (EUR,CN) rs16969968/rs6495308 (EUR) rs10519203/rs2036527/rs684513/rs1696698 (AA) rs667282/rs12910984 (CN)	EUR AA* CN	(75, 92–94, 96, 102, 109)
5p15.33	*TERT/CLPTM1L*	rs2736100 (JPN, AFNS) rs2853677(EUR, JPN) rs10937405/rs4488809 (JPN) rs401681(EUR) rs465498 (CN)	EUR CN JPN AFNS	(102, 109, 110, 115, 117, 205)
12p13.33	*RAD52*	rs6489769 (EUR)	EUR	(91, 109)
6p21	*BAT3/MSH5, HLA-DRA, HLA-DRB5*	rs3117582 (EUR) rs3817963 (JPN) rs2395185 (AFNS)	EUR JPN AFNS	(102, 109) (110, 117)
17q24.3	*BPTF*	rs7216064 (JPN, AFNS)	JPN AFNS	(110, 117)
3q28	*TP63*	rs4488809 (CN, AFNS) rs10937405 (JPN, AFNS) rs10937405 (JPN)	CN JPN AFNS	(110, 115, 117, 205)
13q12.12	*MIPEP-TNFRSF19*	rs753955 (CN)	CN	(115)
22q12.2	*MTMR3-HORMAD2-LIF*	rs17728461/rs36600 (CN)	CN	(115)
9p21	CDKN2A/p16^{INK4},p14^{ARF}, CDKN2B/p15^{INK4B}	rs1333040 (EUR, CN)	EUR CN	(109)
6q22.2	DCBLD1,ROS1	rs9387478 (AFNS)	AFNS	(117)
10q25.2	VTI1A	rs7086803 (AFNS)	AFNS	(117)
18p11.22	*APCDD1, NAPG, FAM38B*	rs11080466/rs11663246 (KNS)	KNS*	(73)

* The reported association did not reach genome-wide significance level of $P < 5 \times 10^{-8}$.
EUR: European; ASN: Asian; AA: African-American; CN: Chinese; JPN: Japan; AFNS: Asian female never-smoker; KNS: Korean never-smoker.

however, 15q25 SNPs were not significant in their population.

Intermediate phenotypic assays in measuring genetic susceptibility

DNA damage and repair phenotypic assays

There were several different phenotypic assays that directly or indirectly measure constitutive DNA damage/repair in peripheral blood lymphocytes (PBLs), include: (a) DNA damage/repair after a chemical or physical mutagen challenge (such as the mutagen sensitivity, comet, and DNA adduct assays); (b) unscheduled DNA synthesis; (c) cellular ability to repair damaged reporter genes (the host–cell reactivation assay); (d) activity of DNA repair enzyme (repair activity assay for 8-OH-Guanine) [123, 124].

Mutagen sensitivity

The mutagen sensitivity assay quantifies chromatid breaks induced by mutagens in cultured PBLs *in vitro* as an indirect measure of DNA repair capacity (DRC) [125, 126]. Different mutagens induce different DNA damage and elicit specific DNA repair pathways. For example, BPDE is a tobacco carcinogen that forms bulky DNA adducts and elicits nucleotide excision repair (NER). Bleomycin is a clastogenic agent that mimics the effects of radiation by generating free oxygen radicals capable of producing DNA single and double-strand breaks (DSB) that initiate base excision repair (BER) and DSB repair [127]. Wu *et al.* showed that higher BPDE and bleomycin sensitivities were independently associated with increased risks of LC, a finding that has been confirmed by other studies [2–4, 128, 129].

Comet assay

The comet assay is a single-cell gel electrophoresis method used to measure DNA damage in individual cells. It is a sensitive and versatile method with high throughout potential [130, 131]. The alkaline version (pH > 13) of the comet assay can detect DNA damage such as single-strand breaks, double-strand breaks, and alkaline labile sites [132]. Common mutagens used in this assay include BPDE, bleomycin, and γ-radiation. Wu *et al.* found that higher γ-radiation- and BPDE-induced olive tail moments, one of the parameters for measuring DNA damage, were significantly associated with 2.32- and 4.49-fold increased risks of LC, respectively [133]. Rajaee-Behbahani *et al.* reported lower repair rate of bleomycin-induced DNA damage using the alkaline comet assay in LC patients compared with controls [134].

DNA adducts

Using phosphorus-32 post-labeling techniques, two studies by the same group reported a significant association between the level of *in vitro* BPDE-induced DNA adducts and risk for LC [135, 136], suggesting suboptimal ability to remove the BPDE-DNA adduct resulted in increased susceptibility to tobacco carcinogen exposure [136].

Host cell reactivation assay

The host cell reactivation assay measures DRC by quantifying the activity of a reporter gene (e.g., luciferase gene) in intact lymphocytes transfected with mutagen-treated, damaged plasmids (137–139). Because a single unrepaired BPDE-induced DNA adduct can block reporter gene transcription [140], the measured reporter gene activity reflects the ability of the transfected cells to remove the adducts from the plasmid. Reduced capacity to repair adducts is observed in cases compared to controls and is associated with an increased risk of LC with evidence of a significant dose–response association between decreased DRC and risk of LC [137–139].

8-OGG assay

The enzyme 8-oxoguanine DNA N-glycosylase is encoded by the OGG1 gene and initiates the BER pathway. The OGG activity assay monitors the ability of OGG to remove an 8-oxoguanine residue from a radiolabeled synthetic DNA oligonucleotide, generating two DNA products that can be distinguished on the basis of size [141]. Paz-Elizur *et al.* showed that OGG activity was significantly lower in peripheral blood mononuclear cells from LC patients than in those from controls. Individuals in the lowest tertile of OGG activity exhibited an increased risk of NSCLC compared with those in the highest tertile (OR = 4.8; 95% CI, 1.5–15.9) [141]. Gackowski *et al.* also reported that the repair activity of OGG was significantly higher in blood leukocytes of healthy volunteers than in LC patients [142].

Gamma-H2AX

It is known that chromatin structure could be modified following DNA damage [143]. Gamma-H2AX (phosphorylation of serine 139 of the histone H2A variant) is rapidly formed on chromatin following double-strand breaks (DSBs) mediated by ATM/ATR/DNA-PK activity [144]. Gamma-H2AX could facilitate DSB repair and amplify DSB signaling [145]. By measuring immunofluorescent foci induced by the reaction of the antibodies against the phosphorylated H2AX C-terminal peptide, the gamma-H2AX cytometry assay can measure DSBs with high accuracy and sensitivity [146, 147]. Gamma-H2AX has been adopted as a biomarker with a wide range of applications [148–150], including lung cancer research [151–153]. Measuring gamma-H2AX signal in peripheral blood leukocytes at baseline and after gamma-irradiation, He *et al.* have found a significantly higher gamma-H2AX ratio in lung cancer cases (1.46 ± 0.14) compared to health subjects (1.41 ± 0.12). They also demonstrated a dose–response relationship between increased gamma-H2AX ratio and escalated lung cancer risk (*P* for trend <0.001) [154].

Cell cycle phenotypic assays

Two types of cell cycle arrest phenotypic assays have been developed to assess LC risk. Using flow cytometry, Zhao *et al.* showed that when compared to control subjects, LC patients exhibited significantly less gamma-radiation-elicited increases in G2/M cell percentages as well as a lower apoptosis rate [155]. Moreover, the change in p53 protein level correlated with the G2/M delay and chromatid breaks upon gamma radiation exposure, indicating that defective cell cycle checkpoint functions in cancer patients might be associated with p53-dependent DNA damage response and DRC. These findings were replicated in a larger case–control study by Wu *et al.* reporting that the gamma-radiation-induced delay of both S and G2/M phases were associated with LC susceptibility [133]. Similarly, Zheng *et al.* reported that less efficient G2/M checkpoint is associated with an increased risk of LC in African Americans [156].

Phenotypic assays in apoptotic pathways

Zhao *et al.* has reported that impaired mutagen induced apoptotic capacity was associated with increased risk of LC using the TUNEL (Terminal transferase dUTP nick end labeling) method [155]. Biros *et al.* [157] reported that in LC patients, individuals with the variant allele of p53 Pro72Arg polymorphism exhibited a lower percentage of apoptotic white blood cells. This finding was consistent with the results from Wu *et al.* [158] who showed that the haplotype containing the wild-type alleles of the three p53 polymorphisms at intron 3, exon 4, and intron 6 was associated with higher apoptotic index than those with at least one variant allele.

Emerging novel biomarkers for LC risk and early detection

Inflammatory biomarkers

Chronic inflammation is well known to be associated with elevated risk of lung cancer; therefore, extensive research has been conducted on identifying novel inflammation-related risk markers with potential clinical application [159]. The level of serum C-reactive protein (CRP), a well-established systematic marker for chronic inflammation, has been consistently reported to be associated with increased lung cancer risk [160–162]. In addition, genetic variations in *CRP* gene have been shown to be correlated with differential blood CRP level and LC risk [160, 163]. Some pro-inflammatory cytokines, such as interleukin 6 (IL-6) and interleukin 8 (IL-8), are also found to be associated with altered LC risk [164, 165]. Other inflammation-related molecules, such as surfactant protein-D [166] and tumor necrosis factor-α [167], have been reported to be associated with altered LC risk. Few of the putative inflammatory biomarkers (except CRP) have been replicated in independent studies.

Circulating MicroRNA (miRNA)

miRNAs are a class of small noncoding RNAs of 18–25 nucleotides, which are highly stable and tissue specific [168]. They regulate an estimated 30% of human genes, and have been extensively investigated for their roles in cancer initiation, progression and prognosis. The expression pattern of miRNAs in normal bronchial tissue has been shown to be altered during LC carcinogenesis [169], and miRNAs could be used as quantitative biomarkers for chemoprevention of high-risk individuals [170]. Moreover, circulating miRNAs are emerging as novel biomarkers for lung cancer risk assessment and early detection [171, 172]. For example, in a phase I/II biomarker study, Hennessey *et al.* reported that a combination of two serum miRNAs miR-15b and miR-27b was able to discriminate NSCLC from healthy controls [184]. In another study, plasma miR-155, miR-182, and miR-197 levels were able to differentiate stage I LC patients from controls [173]. Boeri *et al.* found plasma signature of miRNA ratios was able to predict LC development even prior to detection of clinical disease by computed tomography [174]. Although none of the candidate markers has been validated, these studies provide supportive evidence for circulating miRNAs as potential biomarkers for LC surveillance and early detection.

Circulating DNA and promoter methylation

Lung cancer is a multistep process involving different genetic and epigenetic changes. Turnover of cellular components is associated with shedding of DNA by tumor cells. Circulating, cell-free DNA has been proposed as a promising surrogate noninvasive markers for the detection of these changes, therefore facilitating lung cancer screening and early detection [175]. In a case-control study of NSCLC patients, plasma telomerase reverse transcriptase (hTERT) DNA content was found to be four times higher in cases compared to controls [176]. Belinsky and colleagues reported that gene promoter methylation of cell-free DNA in plasma and sputum DNA was increased with LC risk [177] and that promoter hypermethylation of multiple genes could be detected in the sputum preceding LC incidence [178]. Many other genetic and epigenetic changes were also found in the circulating DNA of LC patients [179]. However, the methods and results described thus far were variable with little data on reproducibility and quality control.

Circulating mRNAs and proteins

hTERT and epidermal growth factor receptor (EGFR) are commonly overexpressed in LC tumors. Using quantitative real-time reverse-transcription polymerase chain reaction (RT-PCR) assay, Miura *et al.* [180] measured serum *hTERT* and *EGFR* transcripts in LC patients and controls and found the two markers have sensitivity of 89% and 73% and specificity of 71% and 80% for *hTERT* and *EGFR*, respectively, which were superior to other tested tumor markers, such as CEA. Moreover, the levels of these transcripts correlated with tumor number and clinical stage, and were prognostic for recurrence and metastasis.

The *CIZ1* gene encodes a cyclin-interacting factor that promotes initiation of DNA replication. A recent study by Higgins *et al.* [181] demonstrated the variant form of Ciz1 protein was detected in the plasma of two sets of early-stage LC patients and could differentiate early stage LC patients from healthy controls with a sensitivity of 95% and a specificity of greater than 70%. Moreover, the authors determined the function of the gene *in vitro* and *in vivo*, providing biological plausibility for it to be used as a promising candidate biomarker for early LC detection.

Telomere length

Telomeres function as protective DNA structures capping the ends of chromosomes and play a key role in maintaining genomic integrity and stability. Shortened telomeres are involved in the initiation and progression of malignancies. Many epidemiological studies have found that short telomeres in PBLs are associated with increased risks of different cancers, including lung cancer [182–184]; however, one study has found opposite result [185]. This discrepancy is likely due to small sample size and different study design. Future large, prospective studies are needed to clarify the associations of telomere length in PBLs with the risk of LC.

LC risk assessment models

An overview of cancer risk prediction models

In the general population, there is a continuous spectrum of risk in cancer development. Because high-risk individuals only represent a small subset of the general population, implementing appropriate surveillance program and developing strategies for intervention trials greatly depend on risk prediction efficiency that can effectively separate those at high risk from those who are not. Statistical models incorporating multiple risk factors is a promising tool to assist identification of high-risk individuals and to assist the development of risk reduction strategies.

Different study designs could be utilized to develop risk model and each study design has strengths and limitations [186]. Cohort studies allow directly obtain baseline hazard rates of incidence, mortality rates from competing risks, and relative risk from the study population but are limited by long follow-up times and imprecise data on competing causes of death. Case-control data can be an efficient approach to use detailed information on covariates in a relatively short time but subject to the usual limitations of case-control study approach such as potential recall bias and the lack of national registry data for many noncancer diseases.

Statistical criteria that are commonly used to assess the performance of risk assessment model include: calibration (reliability), discrimination, and accuracy [186]. Calibration assesses the ability of a model to predict the number of endpoint events in subgroups of the population and is evaluated by using the goodness-of-fit statistic. Discrimination is a measure of a model's ability to distinguish between those who will and will not develop disease, and is quantified by calculating the concordance statistic, or area under a receiver operating characteristic curve (AUC). Accuracy including positive and negative predictive values refers to the model's ability to categorize specific individuals. However, statistical criteria for evaluating the model performance are limited in clinical decision making because the importance of harms and benefits related to treatment decisions should be considered. Two recently proposed methods that put risk model assessment into clinical perspective are decision curve analysis and the relative utility curve methods [187]. In particular, relative utility could assist evaluating the cost-benefit tradeoffs in risk prediction model [187]. To quantify the clinical utility of a model, harms and benefits need to be incorporated into utility formulations to identify a risk threshold. A risk threshold is the absolute risk for lung cancer at which one might choose to initiate screening. One hurdle in risk threshold identification is the complexity to assess multiple levels of harms and benefits associated with lifestyle modification as compared to single test, intervention or treatment.

In the past decade, with the enormous amounts of genomic information being brought to attention and with the rapid advancement in molecular technology, epidemiology has been evolving rapidly from traditional epidemiology to integrative epidemiology [188]. In light of the evolution of epidemiologic approach, cancer risk prediction models have great potential to gain improved model performance by integrating risk factors other than those traditionally obtained from questionnaire data.

Current state of lung cancer risk prediction models

There has been an increasing interest in developing methods of individual risk prediction for lung cancer with the goal to identify high-risk populations for early detection interventions such as computed tomography (CT) screening. Colditz *et al.* [189] postulated number of cigarette per day, lung cancer in first-degree relatives, occupational exposure, air pollution, as exposures with different strength of association with lung cancer risk. This "expert opinion-based" index of cancer risk was the first step toward the development of statistical prediction model.

Bach *et al.* [190] used age, sex, asbestos exposure history, and smoking history to predict LC risk based on data derived from five Carotene and Retinol Efficacy Trial (CARET) study sites and then validated the model in the sixth study site. The model provided strong evidence that LC risk varies greatly among smokers and was validated and well calibrated with a cross-validated concordance index of 0.72. An external validation study [191] in the Alpha-Tocopherol, beta-Carotene Cancer Prevention Study (ATBC) reported that the Bach model slightly underestimated the observed lung cancer incidence over 10 years, which was attributed to the enhanced surveillance of the ATBC population. As limited by the special population (i.e., old heavy smokers), from which the model was derived, Bach's model is most applicable to heavy smokers aged between 50 and 75 years.

Spitz *et al.* [192] developed a set of three lung cancer risk models for never, former, and current smokers, respectively, using data collected in a large case-control study. In addition to age and smoking history, the models included family history, exposure to an array of environmental dusts, and prior lung diseases in the model for smokers. In never-smokers, in addition to family history of lung cancer, exposure to environmental smoke was identified as significant predictor. The models were internally validated with an average cross-validated concordance statistics of 0.60. These models extended the Bach's model by including risk factors other than smoking history. However, as limited by the study design of matching cases and controls by age and smoking status, these models were unable to address the effects of age and smoking status. The same research group expanded their model by adding two DNA repair capacity biomarkers and claimed a modest improvement in discriminative ability [193]. The modest improvement indicated the potential of integrating molecular and clinical markers to risk models, which was evidenced in a bladder cancer risk prediction model [194].

The Liverpool Lung Cancer Project (LLP) model [195] included asbestos exposures, pneumonia, family history of lung cancer and age at onset, and prior malignancy. The model has moderate discrimination power with an AUC statistic of 0.70 [195]. The model was based on case-control design with a smaller number of subjects as compared to the Bach and Spitz models. The LLP model was externally validated in the European Early Lung Cancer (EUELC), Harvard case-control studies and the LLP population-based prospective cohort study (LLPC) with good discrimination accuracy in the Harvard studies and in the LLPC study and a moderate discrimination in the EUELC study [196]. In decision utility analysis, the LLP model was found to have better performance than smoking duration and family history alone in stratifying high-risk patients for LC CT screening [196].

One limitation of the Bach, Spitz, and LLP models is that the models were built using data that were not sampled from the general population. A recently published model built from the general population was the Prostate, Lung, Colorectal, and Ovarian Cancer Screening Trial [181] (PLCO) model which included age, education, body mass index, family history of lung cancer, chronic obstructive disease, recent chest x-ray, smoking status, pack years of smoking, smoking duration, years since quitting (in subgroup of former smokers). The model was based on data collected from the PLCO prospective screening trial which included more than 70 000 subjects and has demonstrated a high discrimination and calibration in external validation.

Another general population-based model was built from the European Prospective Investigation in Cancer and Nutrition (EPIC) cohort. [197]. The EPIC model was developed mainly for former and current smokers using age started smoking, smoking intensity, ten occupational/environmental exposures previously implicated in lung cancer, and SNPs identified from GWAs. Evaluation of model performance suggested that smoking information alone gave good discrimination accuracy with an AUC of 0.84 and that incorporating other risk factors had negligible effects to improve AUC.

As stated earlier, the recent advent of GWAS offers the possibility of integrating panels of genetic variants into existing risk prediction models. However, up to now, challenges have been arising while adding SNPs into risk prediction models [198, 199]. While adding LC GWAS SNPs did not improve model prediction [182], a recent study from the LLP group compared discrimination accuracy between the LLP model and an enhanced model incorporating the seizure 6-like (SEZ6L) SNP(rs663048) identified from high-throughput sequencing revealed a significant improvement as measured by the net reclassification improvements (NRI) [200]. While there is still debate on the value of adding genetic markers into lung cancer risk models, one implication from the enhanced LLP model is that models with genetic markers may be especially applicable to differentiate individuals with intermediate risk, a subgroup whose risk classification is usually ambiguous as defined by models with only traditional epidemiologic model.

In summary, lung cancer risk prediction models hold great promise to improve screening strategies for early detection. CT screening for lung cancer in heavy smokers can reduce lung cancer mortality by 20%, but has a 95% false positive rate [201, 201]. It is imperative to improve risk prediction beyond smoking alone to identify populations suitable for CT screening [203]. Integrating molecular/genetic and other novel risk factors would be a valuable next step to follow.

Concluding remarks

Although smoking is the predominant risk factor in LC etiology, other epidemiological factors and genetic susceptibility markers have been identified as potential risk modifiers for LC. Certain environmental exposures and comorbidities have been consistently associated with elevated LC risk, including various chronic respiratory diseases such as COPD and emphysema. There is also suggestive evidence supporting a link between diet and LC, but the results are less conclusive. Despite the large number of candidate gene studies of LC in literature, the results are often inconsistent and fail to replicate. Limitations in study design, small sample size, lack of control for confounding, selection bias, and multiple testing, may account for the inconsistent results. The transition from candidate gene and pathway-based approaches to GWAS has transformed the landscape of cancer genomics. However, the genetic susceptibility loci identified by GWAS only explained less than 10% of the excess risk for LC. Since GWAS only covers common genetic variants with relatively high frequency (minor allele frequency [MAF] >5%), rare variants (MAF < 1%) with presumably larger effects are missed by the chip design used for GWAS. Given that cancer is a multistep and multifactorial disease, the influence of individual variants on overall cancer risk might be modest. Multigenic models should be developed to integrate the effects of individual genetic loci as well as potential gene–gene and gene–environment interactions. A systematic evaluation of structural variations such as copy number variants, small insertion and deletions, loss of heterozygosity (LOH), and epigenetic alterations also might contribute to an integrative view of LC genetic architecture. Moreover, high-power computational methodologies could be developed to detect the numerous interactions among genetic and environmental factors that are otherwise undetectable by conventional statistical methods. Molecular and cellular functional assays may be carried out to determine the genotype–phenotype correlations and to validate the biological significance of the identified high risk alleles. Genetic determinants of lifestyle factors such as smoking dependence should also be further studied due to the large impact of smoking and other environmental factors on lung cancer carcinogenesis. Furthermore, the implementation of high-throughput next-generation sequencing technologies with high coverage of the whole genome and exome holds great promise to comprehensively detect the "missing heritability" as well as to probe the underlying complexity in LC genomics. Intermediate phenotypic biomarkers, such as DNA repair capacity, telomere length and other phenotypic biomarkers, have high heritability and possibly stronger effects on cancer risk, and are promising biomarkers for risk stratification and prediction. Finally, these environmental, genetic, and phenotypic markers need to be integrated into comprehensive risk prediction models to improve the overall prediction power with careful consideration of cost-benefit tradeoffs, thereby improving screening strategies for LC early detection and prevention.

References

1 Siegel R, Naishadham D, Jemal A (2013) Cancer statistics. *CA: A Cancer Journal for Clinicians*, 63: 11–30.

2 Hsu TC, Spitz MR, Schantz SP (1991) Mutagen sensitivity: a biological marker of cancer susceptibility. *Cancer Epidemiology Biomarkers & Prevention*; 1: 83–9.

3 Spitz MR, Hsu TC, Wu X, Fueger JJ, Amos CI, Roth JA (1995) Mutagen sensitivity as a biological marker of lung cancer risk in African Americans. *Cancer Epidemiology Biomarkers & Prevention*, 4: 99–103.

4 Wu X, Delclos GL, Annegers JF, Bondy ML, Honn SE, Henry B, *et al.* (1995) A case-control study of wood dust exposure, mutagen sensitivity, and lung cancer risk. *Cancer Epidemiology Biomarkers & Prevention*, 4: 583–8.

5 Zheng Y-L, Loffredo CA, Yu Z, Jones RT, Krasna MJ, Alberg AJ, *et al.* (2003) Bleomycin-induced chromosome breaks as a risk marker for lung cancer: a case-control study with population and hospital controls. *Carcinogenesis*, 24: 269–74.

6 Tokuhata GK, Lilienfeld AM (1963) Familial aggregation of lung cancer in humans. *J Natl Cancer Inst*, 30: 289–312.

7 Ooi WL, Elston RC, Chen VW, Bailey-Wilson JE, Rothschild H (1986) Increased familial risk for lung cancer. *J Natl Cancer Inst*, 76: 217–22.

8 Samet JM, Humble CG, Pathak DR (1986) Personal and family history of respiratory disease and lung cancer risk. *Am Rev Respir Dis*, 134: 466–70.

9 Shaw GL, Falk RT, Pickle LW, Mason TT, Buffler PA (1991) Lung cancer risk associated with cancer in relatives. *Journal of Clinical Epidemiology*, 44: 429–37.

10 Osann KE (1991) Lung cancer in women: The importance of smoking, family history of cancer, and medical history of respiratory disease. *Cancer Research*, 51: 4893–7.

11 Schwartz AG, Yang P, Swanson GM (1996) Familial risk of lung cancer among nonsmokers and their relatives. *American Journal of Epidemiology*, 144: 554–62.

12 Mayne ST, Buenconsejo J, Janerich DT (1999) Previous lung disease and risk of lung cancer among men and women nonsmokers. *American Journal of Epidemiology*, 149: 13–20.

13 Bromen K, Pohlabeln H, Jahn I, Ahrens W, Jöckel K-H (2000) Aggregation of lung cancer in families: Results from a population-based case-control study in Germany. *American Journal of Epidemiology*, 152: 497–505.

14 Etzel CJ, Amos CI, Spitz MR (2003) Risk for smoking-related cancer among relatives of lung cancer patients. *Cancer Res*, 63: 8531–5.

15 Matakidou A, Eisen T, Houlston RS (2005) Systematic review of the relationship between family history and lung cancer risk. *Br J Cancer*, 93: 825–33.

16 Lissowska J, Foretova L, Dabek J, Zaridze D, Szeszenia-Dabrowska N, Rudnai P, *et al.* (2010) Family history and lung cancer risk: International multicentre case-control study in Eastern and Central Europe and meta-analyses. *Cancer Causes Control*, 21: 1091–1104.

17 Adcock IM, Caramori G, Barnes PJ (2011) Chronic obstructive pulmonary disease and lung cancer: New molecular insights. *Respiration*, 81: 265–84.

18 Sin DD, Man SF (2007) Systemic inflammation and mortality in chronic obstructive pulmonary disease. *Can J Physiol Pharmacol*, 85: 141–7.

19 Ben-Zaken Cohen S, Pare PD, Man SF, Sin DD (2007) The growing burden of chronic obstructive pulmonary disease and lung cancer in women: examining sex differences in cigarette smoke metabolism. *Am J Respir Crit Care Med*, 176: 113–20.

20 Mannino DM (2005) Epidemiology and global impact of chronic obstructive pulmonary disease. *Semin Respir Crit Care Med*, 26: 204–10.

21 Punturieri A, Szabo E, Croxton TL, Shapiro SD, Dubinett SM (2009) Lung cancer and chronic obstructive pulmonary disease: needs and opportunities for integrated research. *J Natl Cancer Inst*, 101: 554–9.

22 Purdue MP, Gold L, Jarvholm B, Alavanja MC, Ward MH, Vermeulen R (2007) Impaired lung function and lung cancer incidence in a cohort of Swedish construction workers. *Thorax*, 62: 51–6.

23 Tockman MS, Anthonisen NR, Wright EC, Donithan MG (1987) Airways obstruction and the risk for lung cancer. *Ann Intern Med*, 106: 512–18.

24 Brenner DR, McLaughlin JR, Hung RJ (2011) Previous lung diseases and lung cancer risk: a systematic review and meta-analysis. *PLoS One*, 6:e17479.

25 Smith BM, Pinto L, Ezer N, Sverzellati N, Muro S, Schwartzman K (2012) Emphysema detected on computed tomography and risk of lung cancer: A systematic review and meta-analysis. *Lung Cancer*, 77: 58–63.

26 Brenner DR, Boffetta P, Duell EJ, Bickeböller H, Rosenberger A, McCormack V, *et al.* (2012) Previous lung diseases and lung cancer risk: A pooled analysis from the International Lung Cancer Consortium. *American Journal of Epidemiology*, 176: 573–85.

27 Santillan A, Camargo C, Jr., Colditz G (2003) A meta-analysis of asthma and risk of lung cancer (United States). *Cancer Causes & Control*, 14: 327–34.

28 Rosenberger A, Bickeboller H, McCormack V, Brenner DR, Duell EJ, Tjonneland A, *et al.* (2012) Asthma and lung cancer risk: a systematic investigation by the International Lung Cancer Consortium. *Carcinogenesis*, 33: 587–97.

29 Talbot-Smith A, Fritschi L, Divitini ML, Mallon DFJ, Knuiman MW (2003) Allergy, atopy, and cancer: A prospective study of the 1981 Busselton Cohort. *American Journal of Epidemiology*, 157: 606–12.

30 Schabath MB, Delclos GL, Martynowicz MM, Greisinger AJ, Lu C, Wu X, *et al.* (2005) Opposing effects of emphysema, hay fever, and select genetic variants on lung cancer risk. *American Journal of Epidemiology*, 161: 412–22.

31 Cockcroft DW, Klein GJ, Donevan RE, Copland GM (1979) Is there a negative correlation between malignancy and respiratory atopy? *Ann Allergy*, 43: 345–7.

32 Vena JE, Bona JR, Byers TE, Middleton E, Swanson MK, Graham S (1985) Allergy-related diseases and cancer: An inverse association. *American Journal of Epidemiology*, 122: 66–74.

33 Gabriel R, Dudley BM, Alexander WD (1972) Lung cancer and allergy. *Br J Clin Pract*, 26: 202–4.

34 McDuffie HH (1991) Atopy and primary lung cancer: Histology and sex distribution. *CHEST Journal*, 99: 404–7.

35 Feskanich D, Ziegler RG, Michaud DS, Giovannucci EL, Speizer FE, Willett WC, *et al.* (2000) Prospective study of fruit and vegetable consumption and risk of lung cancer among men and women. *Journal of the National Cancer Institute*, 92: 1812–23.

36 Voorrips LE, Goldbohm RA, van Poppel G, Sturmans F, Hermus RJJ, van den Brandt PA (2000) Vegetable and fruit consumption and risks of colon and rectal cancer in a prospective cohort study: The Netherlands Cohort Study on Diet and Cancer. *American Journal of Epidemiology*, 152: 1081–92.

37 Brennan P, Fortes C, Butler J, Agudo A, Benhamou S, Darby S, *et al.* (2000) A multicenter case-control

study of diet and lung cancer among non-smokers. *Cancer Causes & Control*, 11: 49–58.

38 Miller AB, Altenburg H-P, Bueno-de-Mesquita B, Boshuizen HC, Agudo A, Berrino F, *et al.* (2004) Fruits and vegetables and lung cancer: Findings from the European prospective investigation into cancer and nutrition. *International Journal of Cancer*, 108: 269–76.

39 Skuladottir H, Tjoenneland A, Overvad K, Stripp C, Christensen J, Raaschou-Nielsen O, *et al.* (2004) Does insufficient adjustment for smoking explain the preventive effects of fruit and vegetables on lung cancer? *Lung Cancer*, 45: 1–10.

40 Neuhouser ML, Patterson RE, Thornquist MD, Omenn GS, King IB, Goodman GE (2003) Fruits and vegetables are associated with lower lung cancer risk only in the placebo arm of the β-Carotene and Retinol Efficacy Trial (CARET). *Cancer Epidemiology Biomarkers & Prevention*, 12: 350–8.

41 Wakai K, Matsuo K, Nagata C, Mizoue T, Tanaka K, Tsuji I, *et al.* (2011) Lung cancer risk and consumption of vegetables and fruit: An evaluation based on a systematic review of epidemiological evidence from Japan. *Japanese Journal of Clinical Oncology*, 41: 693–708.

42 Key TJ (2011) Fruit and vegetables and cancer risk. *Br J Cancer*, 104: 6–11.

43 Zhang Y, Talalay P (1994) Anticarcinogenic activities of organic isothiocyanates: Chemistry and mechanisms. *Cancer Research*, 54: 1976s–81s.

44 Smith T, Evans K, Lythgoe MF, Anderson PJ, Gordon I (1997) Dosimetry of pediatric radiopharmaceuticals: uniformity of effective dose and a simple aid for its estimation. *Journal of Nuclear Medicine*, 38: 1982–7.

45 Thornalley PJ (2002) Isothiocyanates: mechanism of cancer chemopreventive action. *Anticancer Drugs*, 13: 331–8.

46 Brennan P, Hsu CC, Moullan N, Szeszenia-Dabrowska N, Lissowska J, Zaridze D, *et al.* (2005) Effect of cruciferous vegetables on lung cancer in patients stratified by genetic status: a mendelian randomisation approach. *The Lancet*, 366: 1558–60.

47 Spitz MR, Duphorne CM, Detry MA, Pillow PC, Amos CI, Lei L, *et al.* (2000) Dietary intake of isothiocyanates: evidence of a joint effect with glutathione s-transferase polymorphisms in lung cancer risk. *Cancer Epidemiology Biomarkers & Prevention*, 9: 1017–20.

48 Gao C-m, Tajima K, Kuroishi T, Hirose K, Inoue M (1993) Protective effects of raw vegetables and fruit against lung cancer among smokers and ex-smokers: A case-control study in the Tokai area of Japan. *Cancer Science*, 84: 594–600.

49 Lam TK, Gallicchio L, Lindsley K, Shiels M, Hammond E, Tao X, *et al.* (2009) Cruciferous vegetable consumption and lung cancer risk: A systematic review. *Cancer Epidemiology Biomarkers & Prevention*, 18: 184–95.

50 Männistö S, Smith-Warner SA, Spiegelman D, Albanes D, Anderson K, van den Brandt PA, *et al.* (2004) Dietary carotenoids and risk of lung cancer in a pooled analysis of seven cohort studies. *Cancer Epidemiology Biomarkers & Prevention*, 13: 40–8.

51 Holick CN, Michaud DS, Stolzenberg-Solomon R, Mayne ST, Pietinen P, Taylor PR, *et al.* (2002) Dietary carotenoids, serum β-carotene, and retinol and risk of lung cancer in the alpha-tocopherol, beta-carotene cohort study. *American Journal of Epidemiology*, 156: 536–47.

52 Michaud DS, Feskanich D, Rimm EB, Colditz GA, Speizer FE, Willett WC, *et al.* (2000) Intake of specific carotenoids and risk of lung cancer in 2 prospective US cohorts. *Am J Clin Nutr*, 72: 990–7.

53 Gallicchio L, Boyd K, Matanoski G, Tao X, Chen L, Lam TK, *et al.* (2008) Carotenoids and the risk of developing lung cancer: a systematic review. *American Journal of Clinical Nutrition*, 88: 372–83.

54 The effect of vitamin E and beta carotene on the incidence of lung cancer and other cancers in male smokers. *New England Journal of Medicine*, 330: 1029–35.

55 Hennekens CH, Buring JE, Manson JE, Stampfer M, Rosner B, Cook NR, *et al.* (1996) Lack of effect of long-term supplementation with beta carotene on the incidence of malignant neoplasms and cardiovascular disease. *New England Journal of Medicine*, 334: 1145–9.

56 Omenn GS, Goodman GE, Thornquist MD, Balmes J, Cullen MR, Glass A, *et al.* (1996) Effects of a combination of beta carotene and vitamin A on lung cancer and cardiovascular disease. *New England Journal of Medicine*, 334: 1150–5.

57 Greenwald P (2003) β-carotene and lung cancer: A lesson for future chemoprevention investigations? *Journal of the National Cancer Institute*, 95: E1.

58 Palozza P (1998) Prooxidant actions of carotenoids in biologic systems. *Nutrition Reviews*, 56: 257–65.

59 Touvier M, Kesse E, Clavel-Chapelon F, Boutron-Ruault M-C (2005) Dual association of β-carotene with risk of tobacco-related cancers in a cohort of French women. *Journal of the National Cancer Institute*, 97: 1338–44.

60 Schabath MB, Hernandez L, Wu X, Pillow PC, Spitz MR (2005) Dietary phytoestrogens and lung cancer risk. *JAMA: The Journal of the American Medical Association*, 294: 1493–1504.

61 Wakai K, Egami I, Kato K, Kawamura T, Tamakoshi A, Lin Y, *et al.* (1999) Dietary intake and sources of isoflavones among Japanese. *Nutrition and Cancer*, 33: 139–45.

62 Swanson CA, Mao BL, Li JY, Lubin JH, Yao SX, Wang JZ, *et al.* (1992) Dietary determinants of lung-cancer risk: Results from a case-control study in Yunnan province, China. *International Journal of Cancer*, 50: 876–80.

63 Hu J, Johnson KC, Mao Y, Xu T, Lin Q, Wang C, *et al.* (1997) A case-control study of diet and lung cancer in Northeast China. *International Journal of Cancer*, 71: 924–31.

64 Koo LC (1988) Dietary habits and lung cancer risk among Chinese females in Hong Kong who never smoked. *Nutrition and Cancer*, 11: 155–72.

65 Seow A, Poh W-T, Teh M, Eng P, Wang Y-T, Tan W-C, *et al.* (2002) Diet, reproductive factors and lung cancer risk among Chinese women in Singapore: Evidence for a protective effect of soy in nonsmokers. *International Journal of Cancer*, 97: 365–71.

66 Yang G, Shu XO, Chow WH, Zhang X, Li HL, Ji BT, *et al.* (2012) Soy food intake and risk of lung cancer: evidence from the Shanghai Women's Health Study and a meta-analysis. *Am J Epidemiol*, 176: 846–55.

67 Yang WS, Va P, Wong MY, Zhang HL, Xiang YB (2011) Soy intake is associated with lower lung cancer risk: results from a meta-analysis of epidemiologic studies. *Am J Clin Nutr*, 94: 1575–83.

68 Choi S-W, Mason JB (2000) Folate and carcinogenesis: An integrated scheme. *Journal of Nutrition*, 130: 129–32.

69 Bandera E, Freudenheim J, Marshall J, Zielezny M, Priore R, Brasure J, *et al.* (1997) Diet and alcohol consumption and lung cancer risk in the New York State Cohort (United States). *Cancer Causes & Control*, 8: 828–40.

70 Speizer FE, Colditz GA, Hunter DJ, Rosner B, Hennekens C (1999) Prospective study of smoking, antioxidant intake, and lung cancer in middle-aged women (USA). *Cancer Causes & Control*, 10: 475–82.

71 Voorrips LE, Goldbohm RA, Brants HAM, van Poppel GAFC, Sturmans F, Hermus RJJ, *et al.* (2000) A prospective cohort study on antioxidant and folate intake and male lung cancer risk. *Cancer Epidemiology Biomarkers & Prevention*, 9: 357–65.

72 Shen H, Wei Q, Pillow PC, Amos CI, Hong WK, Spitz MR (2003) Dietary folate intake and lung cancer risk in former smokers. *Cancer Epidemiology Biomarkers & Prevention*, 12: 980–6.

73 Ahn MJ, Won HH, Lee J, Lee ST, Sun JM, Park YH, *et al.* (2012) The 18p11.22 locus is associated with never smoker non-small cell lung cancer susceptibility in Korean populations. *Hum Genet*, 131: 365–72.

74 Brennan P, Hainaut P, Boffetta P (2011) Genetics of lung-cancer susceptibility. *The Lancet Oncology*, 12: 399–408.

75 Amos CI, Wu X, Broderick P, Gorlov IP, Gu J, Eisen T, *et al.* (2008) Genome-wide association scan of tag SNPs identifies a susceptibility locus for lung cancer at 15q25.1. *Nat Genet*, 40: 616–22.

76 Broderick P, Wang Y, Vijayakrishnan J, Matakidou A, Spitz MR, Eisen T, *et al.* (2009) Deciphering the impact of common genetic variation on lung cancer risk: a genome-wide association study. *Cancer Res*, 69: 6633–41.

77 Park JY, Park JM, Jang JS, Choi JE, Kim KM, Cha SI, *et al.* (2006) Caspase 9 promoter polymorphisms and risk of primary lung cancer. *Hum Mol Genet*, 15: 1963–71.

78 Zhang X, Miao X, Sun T, Tan W, Qu S, Xiong P, *et al.* (2005) Functional polymorphisms in cell death pathway genes FAS and FASL contribute to risk of lung cancer. *J Med Genet*, 42: 479–84.

79 Pharoah PD, Dunning AM, Ponder BA, Easton DF (2004) Association studies for finding cancer-susceptibility genetic variants. *Nat Rev Cancer*, 4: 850–60.

80 Carlsten C, Sagoo GS, Frodsham AJ, Burke W, Higgins JPT (2008) Glutathione S-transferase M1 (GSTM1) polymorphisms and lung cancer: A literature-based systematic HuGE review and meta-analysis. *American Journal of Epidemiology*, 167: 759–74.

81 Brennan P, McKay J, Moore L, Zaridze D, Mukeria A, Szeszenia-Dabrowska N, *et al.* (2007) Uncommon CHEK2 mis-sense variant and reduced risk of tobacco-related cancers: Case – control study. *Human Molecular Genetics*, 16: 1794–1801.

82 Cybulski C, Masojć B, Oszutowska D, Jaworowska E, Grodzki T, Waloszczyk P, *et al.* (2008) Constitutional CHEK2 mutations are associated with a decreased risk of lung and laryngeal cancers. *Carcinogenesis*, 29: 762–5.

83 Cybulski C, Górski B, Huzarski T, Masojć B, Mierzejewski M, Dębniak T, *et al.* (2004) CHEK2 is a

multiorgan cancer susceptibility gene. *American Journal of Human Genetics*, 75: 1131–5.

84 Kilpivaara O, Vahteristo P, Falck J, Syrjäkoski K, Eerola H, Easton D, *et al.* (2004) CHEK2 variant I157T may be associated with increased breast cancer risk. *International Journal of Cancer*, 111: 543–7.

85 Bush WS, Moore JH (2012) Chapter 11: Genome-Wide Association Studies. *PLoS Comput Biol.* 8:e1002822.

86 Zhou K, Pearson ER (2013) Insights from genome-wide association studies of drug response. *Annu Rev Pharmacol Toxicol*, 53: 299–310.

87 Pahl R, Schafer H, Muller HH (2009) Optimal multistage designs-a general framework for efficient genome-wide association studies. *Biostatistics*, 10: 297–309.

88 Sugimura H, Tao H, Suzuki M, Mori H, Tsuboi M, Matsuura S, *et al.* (2011) Genetic susceptibility to lung cancer. *Front Biosci (Schol Ed)*, 3: 1463–77.

89 McKay JD, Hung RJ, Gaborieau V, Boffetta P, Chabrier A, Byrnes G, *et al.* (2008) Lung cancer susceptibility locus at 5p15.33. *Nat Genet*, 40: 1404–6.

90 Wang Y, Broderick P, Webb E, Wu X, Vijayakrishnan J, Matakidou A, *et al.* (2008) Common 5p15.33 and 6p21.33 variants influence lung cancer risk. *Nat Genet*, 40: 1407–9.

91 Shi J, Chatterjee N, Rotunno M, Wang Y, Pesatori AC, Consonni D, *et al.* (2011) Inherited variation at chromosome 12p13.33 including RAD52 influences squamous cell lung carcinoma risk. *Cancer Discovery*, 2: 131–9.

92 Hung RJ, McKay JD, Gaborieau V, Boffetta P, Hashibe M, Zaridze D, *et al.* (2008) A susceptibility locus for lung cancer maps to nicotinic acetylcholine receptor subunit genes on 15q25. *Nature*, 452: 633–7.

93 Thorgeirsson TE, Geller F, Sulem P, Rafnar T, Wiste A, Magnusson KP, *et al.* (2008) A variant associated with nicotine dependence, lung cancer and peripheral arterial disease. *Nature*, 452: 638–42.

94 Amos CI, Gorlov IP, Dong Q, Wu X, Zhang H, Lu EY, *et al.* (2010) Nicotinic acetylcholine receptor region on chromosome 15q25 and lung cancer risk among African Americans: a case-control study. *J Natl Cancer Inst* 102: 1199–1205.

95 Truong T, Hung RJ, Amos CI, Wu X, Bickeboller H, Rosenberger A, *et al.* (2010) Replication of lung cancer susceptibility loci at chromosomes 15q25, 5p15, and 6p21: A pooled analysis from the International Lung Cancer Consortium. *J Natl Cancer Inst*, 102: 959–71.

96 Wu C, Hu Z, Yu D, Huang L, Jin G, Liang J, *et al.* (2009) Genetic variants on chromosome 15q25 associated with lung cancer Risk in Chinese populations. *Cancer Research*, 69: 5065–72.

97 Shiraishi K, Kohno T, Kunitoh H, Watanabe S-i, Goto K, Nishiwaki Y, *et al.* (2009) Contribution of nicotine acetylcholine receptor polymorphisms to lung cancer risk in a smoking-independent manner in the Japanese. *Carcinogenesis*, 30: 65–70.

98 Grando SA (2006) Cholinergic control of epidermal cohesion. *Experimental Dermatology*, 15: 265–82.

99 Schuller HM (2009) Is cancer triggered by altered signalling of nicotinic acetylcholine receptors? *Nat Rev Cancer*, 9: 195–205.

100 Al-Wadei HAN, Schuller HM (2009) Nicotinic receptor-associated modulation of stimulatory and inhibitory neurotransmitters in NNK-induced adenocarcinoma of the lungs and pancreas. *Journal of Pathology*, 218: 437–45.

101 Paliwal A, Vaissière T, Krais A, Cuenin C, Cros M-P, Zaridze D, *et al.* (2010) Aberrant DNA methylation links cancer susceptibility locus 15q25.1 to apoptotic regulation and lung cancer. *Cancer Research*, 70: 2779–88.

102 Wang Y, Broderick P, Webb E, Wu X, Vijayakrishnan J, Matakidou A, *et al.* (2008) Common 5p15.33 and 6p21.33 variants influence lung cancer risk. *Nat Genet*, 40: 1407–9.

103 Truong T, Hung RJ, Amos CI, Wu X, Bickeböller H, Rosenberger A, *et al.* (2010) Replication of lung cancer susceptibility loci at chromosomes 15q25, 5p15, and 6p21: A pooled analysis from the International Lung Cancer Consortium. *Journal of the National Cancer Institute*, 102: 959–71.

104 Rafnar T, Sulem P, Stacey SN, Geller F, Gudmundsson J, Sigurdsson A, *et al.* (2009) Sequence variants at the TERT-CLPTM1L locus associate with many cancer types. *Nature Genetics*, 41: 221–7.

105 Fernandez-Garcia I, Ortiz-De-Solorzano C, Montuenga LM (2008) Telomeres and telomerase in lung cancer. *Journal of Thoracic Oncology*, 3: 1085–8.

106 Chen H, Li Y, Tollefsbol TO (2009) Strategies targeting telomerase inhibition. *Molecular Biotechnology*, 41: 194–9.

107 Yoshiura K-i, Machida J, Daack-Hirsch S, Patil SR, Ashworth LK, Hecht JT, *et al.* (1998) Characterization of a novel gene disrupted by a balanced chromosomal translocation t(2;19)(q11.2;q13.3) in a family with cleft lip and palate. *Genomics*, 54: 231–40.

108 James MA, Wen W, Wang Y, Byers LA, Heymach JV, Coombes KR, *et al.* (2012) Functional characterization of CLPTM1L as a lung cancer risk candidate gene in the 5p15.33 Locus. *PLoS One*, 7: e36116.

109 Timofeeva MN, Hung RJ, Rafnar T, Christiani DC, Field JK, Bickeböller H, *et al.* (2012) Influence of common genetic variation on lung cancer risk: meta-analysis of 14 900 cases and 29 485 controls. *Human Molecular Genetics*, 21:4980–95.

110 Shiraishi K, Kunitoh H, Daigo Y, Takahashi A, Goto K, Sakamoto H, *et al.* (2012) A genome-wide association study identifies two new susceptibility loci for lung adenocarcinoma in the Japanese population. *Nat Genet*, 44: 900–3.

111 Sasaki T, Gan EC, Wakeham A, Kornbluth S, Mak TW, Okada H (2007) HLA-B-associated transcript 3 (Bat3)/Scythe is essential for p300-mediated acetylation of p53. *Genes & Development*, 21: 848–61.

112 Desmots F, Russell HR, Lee Y, Boyd K, McKinnon PJ (2005) The reaper-binding protein scythe modulates apoptosis and proliferation during mammalian development. *Molecular and Cellular Biology*, 25: 10329–37.

113 Mortensen UH, Lisby M, Rothstein R (2009) Rad52. *Current Biology*, 19: R676–R7.

114 Khanna KK, Jackson SP (2001) DNA double-strand breaks: signaling, repair and the cancer connection. *Nat Genet*, 27: 247–54.

115 Hu Z, Wu C, Shi Y, Guo H, Zhao X, Yin Z, *et al.* (2011) A genome-wide association study identifies two new lung cancer susceptibility loci at 13q12.12 and 22q12.2 in Han Chinese. *Nat Genet*, 43: 792–6.

116 Amos CI, Gorlov IP, Dong Q, Wu X, Zhang H, Lu EY, *et al.* (2010) Nicotinic acetylcholine receptor region on chromosome 15q25 and lung cancer risk among African Americans: A case-control study. *Journal of the National Cancer Institute*, 102: 1199–1205.

117 Lan Q, Hsiung CA, Matsuo K, Hong YC, Seow A, Wang Z, *et al.* (2012) Genome-wide association analysis identifies new lung cancer susceptibility loci in never-smoking women in Asia. *Nat Genet*, 44: 1330–5.

118 Hu L, Wu C, Zhao X, Heist R, Su L, Zhao Y, *et al.* (2012) Genome-wide association study of prognosis in advanced non-small cell lung cancer patients receiving platinum-based chemotherapy. *Clin Cancer Res*, 18: 5507–14.

119 Landi MT, Chatterjee N, Yu K, Goldin LR, Goldstein AM, Rotunno M, *et al.* (2009) A genome-wide association study of lung cancer identifies a region of chromosome 5p15 associated with risk for adenocarcinoma. *American Journal of Human Genetics*, 85: 679–91.

120 Torok S, Hegedus B, Laszlo V, Hoda MA, Ghanim B, Berger W, *et al.* (2011) Lung cancer in never smokers. *Future Oncol*, 7: 1195–1211.

121 Subramanian J, Govindan R (2007) Lung cancer in never smokers: a review. *J Clin Oncol*, 25: 561–70.

122 Li Y, Sheu CC, Ye Y, de Andrade M, Wang L, Chang SC, *et al.* (2010) Genetic variants and risk of lung cancer in never smokers: a genome-wide association study. *Lancet Oncol*, 11: 321–30.

123 Potter JD, Goode E, Morimoto L (2003) AACR Special Conference: The molecular and genetic epidemiology of cancer. *Cancer Epidemiol Biomarkers Prev*, 12: 803–5.

124 Spitz MR, Wei Q, Dong Q, Amos CI, Wu X (2003) Genetic susceptibility to lung cancer: the role of DNA damage and repair. *Cancer Epidemiol Biomarkers Prev*, 12: 689–98.

125 Hsu TC, Johnston DA, Cherry LM, Ramkissoon D, Schantz SP, Jessup JM, *et al.* (1989) Sensitivity to genotoxic effects of bleomycin in humans: Possible relationship to environmental carcinogenesis. *International Journal of Cancer*, 43: 403–9.

126 Wu X, Gu J, Amos CI, Jiang H, Hong WK, Spitz MR (1998) A parallel study of in vitro sensitivity to benzo[a]pyrene diol epoxide and bleomycin in lung carcinoma cases and controls. *Cancer*, 83: 1118–27.

127 Burger RM, Peisach J, Band Horwitz S (1981) Mechanism of bleomycin action: In vitro studies. *Life Sciences*, 28: 715–27.

128 Wei Q, Gu J, Cheng L, Bondy ML, Jiang H, Hong WK, *et al.* (1996) Benzo(a)pyrene diol epoxide-induced chromosomal aberrations and risk of lung cancer. *Cancer Res*, 56: 3975–9.

129 Strom SS, Wu S, Sigurdson AJ, Hsu TC, Fueger JJ, Lopez J, *et al.* (1995) Lung cancer, smoking patterns, and mutagen sensitivity in Mexican-Americans. *J Natl Cancer Inst Monogr*, 18: 29–33.

130 Kassie F, Parzefall W, Knasmüller S (2000) Single cell gel electrophoresis assay: a new technique for human biomonitoring studies. *Mutation Research/Reviews in Mutation Research*, 463: 13–31.

131 Tice RR, Agurell E, Anderson D, Burlinson B, Hartmann A, Kobayashi H, *et al.* (2000) Single cell gel/comet assay: Guidelines for in vitro and in vivo genetic toxicology testing. *Environmental and Molecular Mutagenesis*, 35: 206–21.

132 Moller P, Knudsen LE, Loft S, Wallin H (2000) The comet assay as a rapid test in biomonitoring occupational exposure to DNA-damaging agents and effect

of confounding factors. *Cancer Epidemiol Biomarkers Prev*, 9: 1005–15.

133 Wu X, Roth JA, Zhao H, Luo S, Zheng YL, Chiang S, *et al.* (2005) Cell cycle checkpoints, DNA damage/repair, and lung cancer risk. *Cancer Res*, 65: 349–57.

134 Rajaee-Behbahani N, Schmezer P, Risch A, Rittgen W, Kayser KW, Dienemann H, *et al.* (2001) Altered DNA repair capacity and bleomycin sensitivity as risk markers for non-small cell lung cancer. *International Journal of Cancer*, 95: 86–91.

135 Li D, Wang M, Cheng L, Spitz MR, Hittelman WN, Wei Q (1996) In vitro induction of benzo(a)pyrene diol epoxide-DNA adducts in peripheral lymphocytes as a susceptibility marker for human lung cancer. *Cancer Res*, 56: 3638–41.

136 Li D, Firozi PF, Wang LE, Bosken CH, Spitz MR, Hong WK, *et al.* (2001) Sensitivity to DNA damage induced by benzo(a)pyrene diol epoxide and risk of lung cancer: a case-control analysis. *Cancer Res*, 61: 1445–50.

137 Shen H, Spitz MR, Qiao Y, Guo Z, Wang L-E, Bosken CH, *et al.* (2003) Smoking, DNA repair capacity and risk of nonsmall cell lung cancer. *International Journal of Cancer*, 107: 84–8.

138 Wei Q, Cheng L, Amos CI, Wang L-E, Guo Z, Hong WK, *et al.* (2000) Repair of tobacco carcinogen-induced DNA adducts and lung cancer risk: A molecular epidemiologic study. *Journal of the National Cancer Institute*, 92: 1764–72.

139 Wei Q, Cheng L, Hong WK, Spitz MR (1996) Reduced DNA repair capacity in lung cancer patients. *Cancer Res*, 56: 4103–7.

140 Koch KS, Fletcher RG, Grond MP, Inyang AI, Lu XP, Brenner DA, *et al.* (1993) Inactivation of plasmid reporter gene expression by one benzo(a)pyrene diol-epoxide DNA adduct in adult rat hepatocytes. *Cancer Res*, 53: 2279–86.

141 Paz-Elizur T, Krupsky M, Blumenstein S, Elinger D, Schechtman E, Livneh Z (2003) DNA repair activity for oxidative damage and risk of lung cancer. *Journal of the National Cancer Institute*, 95: 1312–19.

142 Gackowski D, Speina E, Zielinska M, Kowalewski J, Rozalski R, Siomek A, *et al.* (2003) Products of oxidative DNA damage and repair as possible biomarkers of susceptibility to lung cancer. *Cancer Res*, 63: 4899–4902.

143 Misteli T, Soutoglou E (2009) The emerging role of nuclear architecture in DNA repair and genome maintenance. *Nat Rev Mol Cell Biol*, 10: 243–54.

144 Redon C, Pilch D, Rogakou E, Sedelnikova O, Newrock K, Bonner W (2012) Histone H2A variants H2AX and H2AZ. *Curr Opin Genet Dev*, 12: 162–9.

145 Huen MS, Chen J (2008) The DNA damage response pathways: at the crossroad of protein modifications. *Cell Res*, 18: 8–16.

146 Rothkamm K, Lobrich M (2003) Evidence for a lack of DNA double-strand break repair in human cells exposed to very low x-ray doses. *Proc Natl Acad Sci USA*, 100: 5057–62.

147 Ismail IH, Wadhra TI, Hammarsten O (2007) An optimized method for detecting gamma-H2AX in blood cells reveals a significant interindividual variation in the gamma-H2AX response among humans. *Nucleic Acids Research*, 35:e36.

148 Lobrich M, Rief N, Kuhne M, Heckmann M, Fleckenstein J, Rube C, *et al.* (2005) In vivo formation and repair of DNA double-strand breaks after computed tomography examinations. *Proc Natl Acad Sci USA*, 102: 8984–9.

149 Sedelnikova OA, Horikawa I, Redon C, Nakamura A, Zimonjic DB, Popescu NC, *et al.* (2008) Delayed kinetics of DNA double-strand break processing in normal and pathological aging. *Aging Cell*, 7: 89–100.

150 Redon CE, Nakamura AJ, Zhang YW, Ji JJ, Bonner WM, Kinders RJ, *et al.* (2010) Histone gammaH2AX and poly(ADP-ribose) as clinical pharmacodynamic biomarkers. *Clin Cancer Res*, 16: 4532–42.

151 Postel-Vinay S, Vanhecke E, Olaussen KA, Lord CJ, Ashworth A, Soria J-C (2012) The potential of exploiting DNA-repair defects for optimizing lung cancer treatment. *Nat Rev Clin Oncol*, 9: 144–55.

152 Gazdar AF (2007) DNA repair and survival in lung cancer – the two faces of Janus. *New England Journal of Medicine*, 356: 771–3.

153 Matthaios D, Bouros D, Kakolyris S (2013) H2AX and lung cancer: Is it the Ariadne's thread? *DNA Repair*, 12: 90–1.

154 He Y, Gong Y, Lin J, Chang DW, Gu J, Roth JA, *et al.* (2013) Ionizing radiation-induced γ-H2AX activity in whole blood culture and the risk of lung cancer. *Cancer Epidemiology Biomarkers & Prevention*, 22: 443–51.

155 Zhao H, Spitz MR, Tomlinson GE, Zhang H, Minna JD, Wu X (2001) Gamma-radiation-induced G2 delay, apoptosis, and p53 response as potential susceptibility markers for lung cancer. *Cancer Res*, 61: 7819–24.

156 Zheng Y-L, Loffredo CA, Alberg AJ, Yu Z, Jones RT, Perlmutter D, *et al.* (2005) Less efficient G2-M checkpoint is associated with an increased risk of lung cancer in African Americans. *Cancer Research*, 65: 9566–73.

157 Biroš E, Kohút A, Biroš I, Kalina I, Bogyiová E, Štubňa J (2002) A link between the p53 germ line

polymorphisms and white blood cells apoptosis in lung cancer patients. *Lung Cancer*, 35: 231–5.

158 Wu X, Zhao H, Amos CI, Shete S, Makan N, Hong WK, *et al.* (2002) p53 genotypes and haplotypes associated with lung cancer susceptibility and ethnicity. *Journal of the National Cancer Institute*, 94: 681–90.

159 Grivennikov SI, Greten FR, Karin M (2011) Immunity, inflammation, and cancer. *Cell*, 140: 883–99.

160 Siemes C, Visser LE, Coebergh JW, Splinter TA, Witteman JC, Uitterlinden AG, *et al.* (2006) C-reactive protein levels, variation in the C-reactive protein gene, and cancer risk: the Rotterdam Study. *J Clin Oncol*, 24: 5216–22.

161 Trichopoulos D, Psaltopoulou T, Orfanos P, Trichopoulou A, Boffetta P (2006) Plasma C-reactive protein and risk of cancer: a prospective study from Greece. *Cancer Epidemiol Biomarkers Prev*, 15: 381–4.

162 Heikkila K, Ebrahim S, Lawlor DA (2007) A systematic review of the association between circulating concentrations of C reactive protein and cancer. *J Epidemiol Community Health.*, 61: 824–33.

163 Szalai AJ, Wu J, Lange EM, McCrory MA, Langefeld CD, Williams A, *et al.* (2005) Single-nucleotide polymorphisms in the C-reactive protein (CRP) gene promoter that affect transcription factor binding, alter transcriptional activity, and associate with differences in baseline serum CRP level. *J Mol Med (Berl)*, 83: 440–7.

164 Orditura M, De Vita F, Catalano G, Infusino S, Lieto E, Martinelli E, *et al.* (2002) Elevated serum levels of interleukin-8 in advanced non-small cell lung cancer patients: relationship with prognosis. *J Interferon Cytokine Res*, 22: 1129–35.

165 Yanagawa H, Sone S, Takahashi Y, Haku T, Yano S, Shinohara T, *et al.* (1995) Serum levels of interleukin 6 in patients with lung cancer. *Br J Cancer*, 71: 1095–8.

166 Shiels MS, Chaturvedi AK, Katki HA, Gochuico BR, Caporaso NE, Engels EA (2011) Circulating markers of interstitial lung disease and subsequent risk of lung cancer. *Cancer Epidemiology Biomarkers & Prevention*, 20: 2262–72.

167 Il'yasova D, Colbert LH, Harris TB, Newman AB, Bauer DC, Satterfield S, *et al.* (2005) Circulating levels of inflammatory markers and cancer risk in the health aging and body composition cohort. *Cancer Epidemiology Biomarkers & Prevention*, 14: 2413–18.

168 Mitchell PS, Parkin RK, Kroh EM, Fritz BR, Wyman SK, Pogosova-Agadjanyan EL, *et al.* (2008) Circulating microRNAs as stable blood-based markers for cancer detection. *Proc Natl Acad Sci USA*, 105: 10513–18.

169 Mascaux C, Laes JF, Anthoine G, Haller A, Ninane V, Burny A, *et al.* (2009) Evolution of microRNA expression during human bronchial squamous carcinogenesis. *Eur Respir J*, 33: 352–9.

170 Mascaux C, Feser WJ, Lewis MT, Baron AE, Coldren CD, Merrick DT, *et al.* (2012) Endobronchial miRNAs as biomarkers in lung cancer chemoprevention. *Cancer Prev Res (Phila)*, 100–8.

171 Bianchi F, Nicassio F, Veronesi G, di Fiore PP (2012) Circulating microRNAs: next-generation biomarkers for early lung cancer detection. *Ecancermedicalscience*, 6: 246.

172 Hennessey PT, Sanford T, Choudhary A, Mydlarz WW, Brown D, Adai AT, *et al.* (2012) Serum microRNA biomarkers for detection of non-small cell lung cancer. *PLoS One*, 7: e32307.

173 Zheng D, Haddadin S, Wang Y, Gu LQ, Perry MC, Freter CE, *et al.* (2011) Plasma microRNAs as novel biomarkers for early detection of lung cancer. *Int J Clin Exp Pathol*, 4: 575–86.

174 Boeri M, Verri C, Conte D, Roz L, Modena P, Facchinetti F, *et al.* (2011) MicroRNA signatures in tissues and plasma predict development and prognosis of computed tomography detected lung cancer. *Proc Natl Acad Sci USA*, 108: 3713–18.

175 Pathak AK, Bhutani M, Kumar S, Mohan A, Guleria R (2006) Circulating cell-free DNA in plasma/serum of lung cancer patients as a potential screening and prognostic tool. *Clinical Chemistry*, 52: 1833–42.

176 Paci M, Maramotti S, Bellesia E, Formisano D, Albertazzi L, Ricchetti T, *et al.* (2009) Circulating plasma DNA as diagnostic biomarker in non-small cell lung cancer. *Lung Cancer*, 64: 92–7.

177 Belinsky SA, Klinge DM, Dekker JD, Smith MW, Bocklage TJ, Gilliland FD, *et al.* (2005) Gene promoter methylation in plasma and sputum increases with lung cancer risk. *Clin Cancer Res*, 11: 6505–11.

178 Belinsky SA, Liechty KC, Gentry FD, Wolf HJ, Rogers J, Vu K, *et al.* (2006) Promoter hypermethylation of multiple genes in sputum precedes lung cancer incidence in a high-risk cohort. *Cancer Res*, 66: 3338–44.

179 Xue X, Zhu YM, Woll PJ (2006) Circulating DNA and lung cancer. *Annals of the New York Academy of Sciences*, 1075: 154–64.

180 Miura N, Nakamura H, Sato R, Tsukamoto T, Harada T, Takahashi S, *et al.* (2006) Clinical usefulness of serum telomerase reverse transcriptase (hTERT) mRNA and epidermal growth factor receptor (EGFR)

mRNA as a novel tumor marker for lung cancer. *Cancer Sci*, 97: 1366–73.

181 Higgins G, Roper KM, Watson IJ, Blackhall FH, Rom WN, Pass HI, *et al.* (2012) Variant Ciz1 is a circulating biomarker for early-stage lung cancer. *Proc Natl Acad Sci USA*, 109: E3128–35.

182 Wu X, Amos CI, Zhu Y, Zhao H, Grossman BH, Shay JW, *et al.* (2003) Telomere dysfunction: a potential cancer predisposition factor. *J Natl Cancer Inst*, 95: 1211–18.

183 Jang JS, Choi YY, Lee WK, Choi JE, Cha SI, Kim YJ, *et al.* (2008) Telomere length and the risk of lung cancer. *Cancer Sci.*, 99: 1385–9.

184 Wentzensen IM, Mirabello L, Pfeiffer RM, Savage SA (2011) The association of telomere length and cancer: a meta-analysis. *Cancer Epidemiol Biomarkers Prev*, 20: 1238–50.

185 Shen M, Cawthon R, Rothman N, Weinstein SJ, Virtamo J, Hosgood HD, 3rd, *et al.* (2011) A prospective study of telomere length measured by monochrome multiplex quantitative PCR and risk of lung cancer. *Lung Cancer*, 73: 133–7.

186 Freedman AN, Seminara D, Gail MH, Hartge P, Colditz GA, Ballard-Barbash R, *et al.* (2005) Cancer risk prediction models: A workshop on development, evaluation, and application. *Journal of the National Cancer Institute*, 97: 715–23.

187 Baker SG (2009) Putting risk prediction in perspective: relative utility curves. *J Natl Cancer Inst*, 101: 1538–42.

188 Spitz MR, Caporaso NE, Sellers TA (2012) Integrative cancer epidemiology – the next generation. *Cancer Discov*, 2: 1087–90.

189 Colditz GA, Atwood KA, Emmons K, Monson RR, Willett WC, Trichopoulos D, *et al.* (2000) *Harvard Report on Cancer Prevention Volume 4: Harvard Cancer Risk Index*. Risk Index Working Group, Harvard Center for Cancer Prevention. *Cancer Causes Control*, 2000;11:477–88.

190 Bach PB, Kattan MW, Thornquist MD, Kris MG, Tate RC, Barnett MJ, *et al.* (2003) Variations in lung cancer risk among smokers. *Journal of the National Cancer Institute*, 95: 470–8.

191 Cronin KA, Gail MH, Zou Z, Bach PB, Virtamo J, Albanes D (2006) Validation of a model of lung cancer risk prediction among smokers. *J Natl Cancer Inst*, 98: 637–40.

192 Spitz MR, Hong WK, Amos CI, Wu X, Schabath MB, Dong Q, *et al.* (2007) A risk model for prediction of lung cancer. *Journal of the National Cancer Institute*, 99: 715–26.

193 Spitz MR, Etzel CJ, Dong Q, Amos CI, Wei Q, Wu X, *et al.* (2008) An expanded risk prediction model for lung cancer. *Cancer Prevention Research*, 1: 250–4.

194 Wu X, Lin J, Grossman HB, Huang M, Gu J, Etzel CJ, *et al.* (2007) Projecting individualized probabilities of developing bladder cancer in white individuals. *J Clin Oncol*, 25: 4974–81.

195 Cassidy A, Myles JP, van Tongeren M, Page RD, Liloglou T, Duffy SW, *et al.* (2008) The LLP risk model: an individual risk prediction model for lung cancer. *Br J Cancer*, 98: 270–6.

196 Raji OY, Duffy SW, Agbaje OF, Baker SG, Christiani DC, Cassidy A, *et al.* (2012) Predictive accuracy of the Liverpool Lung Project risk model for stratifying patients for computed tomography screening for lung cancer: a case-control and cohort validation study. *Ann Intern Med*, 157: 242–50.

197 Hoggart C, Brennan P, Tjonneland A, Vogel U, Overvad K, Østergaard JN, *et al.* (2012) A risk model for lung cancer incidence. *Cancer Prevention Research*, 5: 834–46.

198 Gail MH (2008) Discriminatory accuracy from single-nucleotide polymorphisms in models to predict breast cancer risk. *J Natl Cancer Inst*, 100: 1037–41.

199 Gail MH (2009) Value of adding single-nucleotide polymorphism genotypes to a breast cancer risk model. *J Natl Cancer Inst*, 101: 959–63.

200 Raji OY, Agbaje OF, Duffy SW, Cassidy A, Field JK (2010) Incorporation of a genetic factor into an epidemiologic model for prediction of individual risk of lung cancer: the Liverpool Lung Project. *Cancer Prev Res (Phila)*, 3: 664–9.

201 Bach PB, Mirkin JN, Oliver TK, Azzoli CG, Berry DA, Brawley OW, Byers T, Colditz GA, Gould MK, Jett JR, Sabichi AL, Smith-Bindman R, *et al.* (2012) Benefits and harms of ct screening for lung cancer: A systematic review. *JAMA*, 307: 2418–29.

202 Aberle DR, Adams AM, Berg CD, Black WC, Clapp JD, Fagerstrom RM, *et al.* (2011) Reduced lung-cancer mortality with low-dose computed tomographic screening. *N Engl J Med*, 365: 395–409.

203 Duffy SW, Raji OY, Agbaje OF, Allgood PC, Cassidy A, Field JK (2009) Use of lung cancer risk models in planning research and service programs in CT screening for lung cancer. *Expert Rev Anticancer Ther*, 9: 1467–72.

204 Miki D, Kubo M, Takahashi A, Yoon KA, Kim J, Lee GK, *et al.* (2010) Variation in TP63 is associated with lung adenocarcinoma susceptibility in Japanese and Korean populations. *Nat Genet*, 42: 893–6.

CHAPTER 3
Molecular Profiling

Lauren Averett Byers
Department of Thoracic/Head and Neck Medical Oncology, The University of Texas MD Anderson Cancer Center, Houston, TX, USA

Introduction

In 2001, drafts of the first two human genomes were published, marking a landmark advance in molecular profiling [1, 2]. Since that time, rapid progress in technologies and new discoveries in biology, such as the identification of microRNAs (miRNAs), have contributed to a growing body of molecular information about many diseases, including lung cancer. Although there are 20 000–25 000 protein-coding genes, only a fraction of these are expressed within a cell at any given time. Understanding the genes that are active within a patient's lung cancer cells; how these genes are regulated; their impact on cancer growth, invasion, and metastasis; and how these molecular characteristics are associated with specific clinical outcomes (e.g., response to therapy) are some of the key goals of molecular profiling.

In the previous decade, two major advances in lung cancer have been directly tied to molecular profiling: the discoveries that non-small cell lung cancers (NSCLCs) harboring an Epidermal Growth Factor Receptor (EGFR) mutation or echinoderm microtubule-associated protein-like 4-Anaplastic lymphoma kinase (EML4-ALK) fusion are highly sensitive to, respectively, EGFR inhibitors (e.g., erlotinib, gefitinib) and ALK inhibitors (e.g., crizotinib) [3–7]. These discoveries have led to routine tumor testing for these genetic abnormalities to guide drug selection in the frontline treatment of metastatic, non-squamous NSCLC [8]. ROS1 fusions and DDR1 mutations are examples of some of the newly recognized molecular drivers that may also predict response to targeted therapies [9, 10]. The roles of these and other gene mutations as potential predictive markers of drug response are being actively investigated in several ongoing clinical trials.

Nevertheless, for a majority of lung cancers, the critical genes or pathways driving tumorigenic behavior are not yet fully known or understood. NSCLC and small cell lung cancer (SCLC) are complex diseases with a great deal of heterogeneity both between tumors (i.e., many molecular subtypes of these cancers) and within tumors or patients (i.e., different clonal populations of cancer cells with distinct mutations or molecular profiles within an individual patient). The ability to reliably measure and analyze key features of DNA, RNA, and protein (the "molecular profile") across a large number of lung cancers will allow us to better understand lung cancer biology and, in turn, will be applied to critical aspects of patient care. The clinical goals of molecular profiling include (1) selection of the most effective treatment for an individual patient, (2) development of new biomarkers for early cancer detection or treatment selection, and (3) identification of drug targets. Already, there is a growing body of molecular data on thousands of lung

Lung Cancer, Fourth Edition. Edited by Jack A. Roth, Waun Ki Hong and Ritsuko U. Komaki.

cancers, as well as new tools to mine these data and put them into clinical context. These resources include major publicly funded efforts such as The Cancer Genome Atlas (TCGA), which has profiled more than 400 squamous and adenocarcinoma lung cancers [11], and efforts by individual investigators and research consortiums [12, 13] (e.g., the Lung Cancer Mutation Consortium, http://www.golcmc.com). Much of the molecular information, especially mRNA gene expression data, is made publicly available when the primary research paper is published, as required by many top peer-reviewed journals and by the US National Institutes of Health (NIH) for research that it funds. These data can be accessed through online repositories such as the Gene Expression Omnibus (GEO) [14], Oncomine [15], or the cBio Cancer Genomics Portal [16].

Finally, in the face of growing information about how mutations and other molecular markers may be used to direct patient care, additional resources are being developed to connect health care providers and patients with evidence-based information about potential clinical applications of molecular test results, including ongoing clinical trials for patients with specific mutations or biomarkers. One example of this is the website www.mycancergenome.org, which was developed by translational investigators at Vanderbilt University and provides information about specific mutations, primary references, and links to relevant trials.

Molecular profiling encompasses experiments in which the expression of hundreds or thousands of unique molecules (e.g., mRNA, genomic DNA, proteins) is measured within a single sample (Figure 3.1). For example, investigators might analyze DNA from a set of tumors to assess the frequency of specific gene mutations, changes in gene copy number (e.g., amplifications, deletions), or patterns of gene methylation (i.e., epigenetic regulation). Likewise, RNA extracted from lung tumors could be analyzed for the levels of several thousand messenger RNAs (mRNAs) or miRNAs within each tumor.

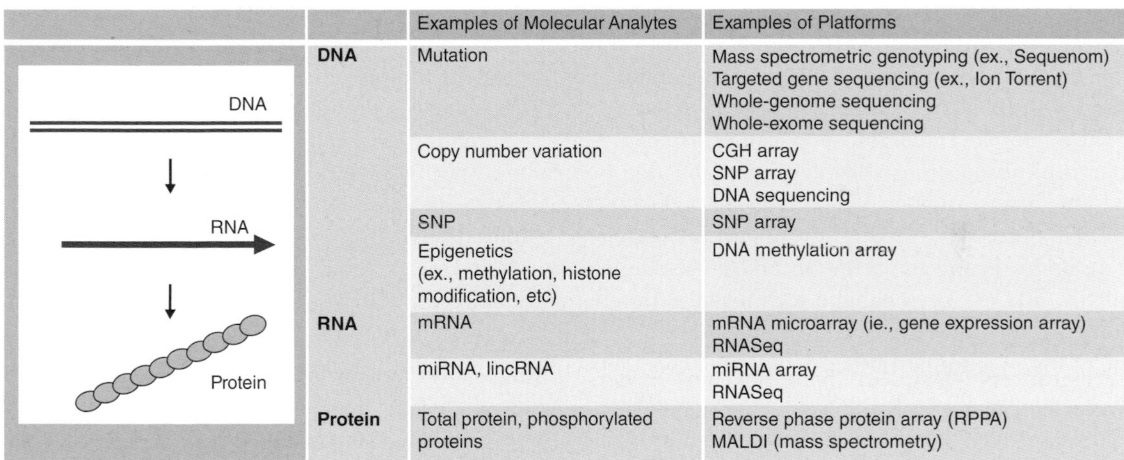

	Examples of Molecular Analytes	Examples of Platforms
DNA	Mutation	Mass spectrometric genotyping (ex., Sequenom) Targeted gene sequencing (ex., Ion Torrent) Whole-genome sequencing Whole-exome sequencing
	Copy number variation	CGH array SNP array DNA sequencing
	SNP	SNP array
	Epigenetics (ex., methylation, histone modification, etc)	DNA methylation array
RNA	mRNA	mRNA microarray (ie., gene expression array) RNASeq
	miRNA, lincRNA	miRNA array RNASeq
Protein	Total protein, phosphorylated proteins	Reverse phase protein array (RPPA) MALDI (mass spectrometry)

Figure 3.1 Modes of analysis for DNA, RNA, and protein profiling. Various genotyping and sequencing platforms are available to profile molecular changes at the DNA, RNA, and protein level. DNA mutations can be identified by numerous sequencing or genotyping techniques. Copy number variations in DNA are commonly analyzed with DNA sequencing, CGH, or SNP arrays. SNP arrays, along with methylation arrays, can also detect variations in DNA methylation. Gene expression arrays are frequently used to detect changes at the mRNA level, while RNA-Seq can determine alterations in mRNA, miRNA, or lincRNA. Proteins are most often profiled with reverse phase protein array or mass spectrometry techniques. CGH: comparative genomic hybridization; SNP: single nucleotide polymorphism; miRNA: microRNA; lincRNA: large intergenic noncoding RNAs; MALDI: matrix-assisted laser desorption/ionization.

The resulting sets of measurements can be compared over a large collection of patient samples using a variety of statistical techniques to identify molecular features or "profiles" that underlie specific disease behavior. Relationships between the expression pattern and the disease behavior are first developed based on analysis of a "training set" of samples. The training set conclusions are then validated in a new set (or sets) of samples (the "testing set") to determine whether the relationships observed in the training set hold up in an independent set of samples [17]. Molecular profiling is a dynamic concept – theoretically, it can be used to investigate and define relationships between any measurable set of analytes and any phenotype associated with a specific variable (e.g., disease stage, drug response, mutation status), provided each is adequately described and reliably measured.

Techniques used in molecular profiling

Molecular profiling experiments can be used to investigate relationships between any clinical variable and any type of analyte. Thus, any technique that measures a large number of distinct molecules from a sample could find application for particular clinical questions. However, partially due to (1) the diverse actions of proteins in regulating cellular processes, (2) the dependence of protein translation on the transcription and processing of mRNA, and (3) key enabling technological developments, the best developed techniques are profiling of DNA (genomics), RNA (e.g., gene expression profiling), and proteins (proteomics); these are the current forerunners in advancing our understanding of human disease.

Genomics and proteomics are complementary modes of investigation. Genomics is currently more widely used and more developmentally mature. The physical properties of DNA and RNA that allow complementary base pairing simplify their analysis. Proteins are, by virtue of their heterogeneity, more difficult to characterize. However, proteins have more direct impact on pathological behavior, and many complexities of their regulation and/or function are not captured by studies of gene expression levels. For these reasons, integrated analyses of DNA, RNA, and protein expression will be key to understanding the complex biology and heterogeneity underlying lung cancer.

The technologies available to measure specific characteristics of tumor DNA, RNA, and protein – often on a genome-wide scale – have rapidly evolved over the past several years and continue to rapidly expand. Here, we will review some of the key platforms that are currently being used.

DNA sequencing

As described above, an area of great success in the treatment of lung cancer has been the identification of druggable driver mutations, such as EGFR and ALK. Recent studies such as one by the Lung Cancer Mutation Consortium [18] have added to the body of knowledge regarding the frequency of these and other mutations in NSCLC. With the growing availability of targeted drugs (>800 currently in development), there is interest in profiling larger numbers of potentially actionable genetic alterations in patient tumors. These alterations include mutations, gene copy number alterations (e.g., deletions or amplifications), and gene fusions. Information about specific mutations or alterations can then be used to direct patients to standard treatments or clinical trials.

Discovery efforts involving more extensive genomic analysis continue to grow as the cost of DNA sequencing falls. One approach that is being used frequently in research and clinical application involves targeted sequencing of individual cancer genes (e.g., EGFR, KRAS, BRAF) or gene panels (~50–400 genes) that can be used for drug selection or other potential clinical application. Methods for this type of directed sequencing are evolving rapidly. Previous approaches have focused on assaying only mutation hot spots [19], but many molecular pathology labs are transitioning to targeted deep sequencing of entire gene exons (protein-coding regions) as the associated costs and required labor rapidly decrease. These types of analyses are being done in many academic centers and are also commercially available through companies such as Foundation Medicine (Cambridge, MA) or Knight Diagnostic Laboratories (Oregon Health & Science University, Portland, Oregon).

Beyond targeted analysis of a select group of cancer genes, whole-exome sequencing and whole-genome sequencing are increasingly employed as a way of investigating DNA alterations that may be contributing to cancer behavior and/or that represent potential therapeutic targets. Since the first human genomes were published in 2001 [1, 2], next-generation sequencing technology has allowed for faster and cheaper whole-genome analyses. In 2008, the first complete human genome sequenced using this technology was published [20]. Recently, we have seen a growing number of publications of complete lung cancer genomes [10, 12, 13].

Whole-exome sequencing (in contrast to whole genome sequencing) provides a less expensive approach to sequencing by focusing just on the exons. This represents roughly 3% of the total DNA content and is the part of the genome transcribed into mRNA. In contrast, whole-genome sequencing provides information about both the protein-coding and noncoding regions. Advantages of whole-genome sequencing include better detection of copy number variants, the ability to detect fusion events (e.g., EML4-ALK, Kif5b/RET) [21, 22], and the inclusion of noncoding DNA regions (such as miRNAs and large intergenic noncoding RNAs [lincRNAs]), which play important roles in regulating mRNA and protein expression – and, thus, cancer cell behavior.

Nevertheless, as with any new technology, there are challenges associated with DNA sequencing. These include the need to process, analyze, and store massive quantities of data. Interpretation of the results is further complicated by incomplete information – so far – on which DNA alternations are normal variants and which may be contributing to disease behavior. For example, despite a majority of DNA sequences being conserved between humans and even across species, out of 6 billion base pairs (bp) in the human genome (in each cell), approximately 24 million bp (<1%) would be expected to vary between individuals due to normal person-to-person variation [23].

Finally, even with highly accurate sequencing techniques, a large number of variant calls will be false positives (up to 6000 per genome) [23]. Although most whole-exome and whole-genome sequencing is currently done in the context of research, decreases in cost, more rapid turnaround time, and direct-to-consumer marketing will likely bring this type of sequence data into the clinic with increasing frequency in the near future. Sorting out the true mutations or other alterations from the background "noise" represents a major challenge facing molecular biologists, bioinformaticians, and physicians.

Other types of DNA analyses, such as single-nucleotide polymorphism (SNP) array, copy number assessment, and methylation profiling can give information about the genome and may be complementary to mRNA expression levels (described below) [24–29]. Comparative genomic hybridization allows a rapid means of determining changes in gene copy number across the genome relative to that in normal tissues. This technique can be performed with gene arrays similar to those used for profiling mRNA. Specific gene amplifications can also be assessed in tumor tissues using fluorescent in situ hybridization (FISH), frequently used to assess Her2 copy number in breast cancer tumors. Profiling of large numbers of SNPs allows linkage of phenotype inheritance with specific chromosomal regions in populations as well as uncovering losses of heterozygosity in tumor samples that may be related to malignant transformation and disease phenotype.

RNA profiling

Two types of RNA that are commonly measured in molecular profiling studies are mRNA and miRNA. mRNA is transcribed from protein-coding genes contained within a cell's DNA and, in turn, can be translated into proteins. In any given cell, only 3–5% of genes are actively transcribed into mRNA, despite all cells having the same DNA content. mRNA has been used extensively in molecular profiling studies to give a picture of what genes are "turned on" or expressed within a cell, which is frequently referred to as gene expression profiling. Different patterns of mRNA expression have been shown in lung cancer to correspond to differences in tumor types (e.g., NSCLC versus SCLC) and may correspond to differences in drug sensitivity.

Like mRNA, miRNA can also be measured using array technologies. miRNA are short, noncoding RNA (usually 22 nucleotides long) that can regulate cell behavior by inhibiting multiple mRNAs. Because a single miRNA can regulate many targets, they can act as a switch turning "on" or "off" complex biological processes [23, 30, 31]. In lung cancer, differences in miRNA have been associated with differences in survival, NSCLC subtypes [32–34], and key biological programs such as epithelial-to-mesenchymal transition [35]. More recently, a new class of RNA called lincRNA has been described [36] that can be measured with whole-genome sequencing.

Three approaches are commonly used today to measure mRNA expression levels. These include [1] oligonucleotide arrays (microarrays), [2] transcriptome sequencing (or "RNA-Seq"), and [3] reverse-transcription quantitative polymerase chain reaction (RT-PCR). Early microarray studies used fewer than 10 000 oligomer probes mounted on in-house-produced chips [37, 38]. The potential power of microarray technology was readily apparent, and the technique was featured on the cover of the journal *Science* in 1991 [39], 3 years after the first prototype was manufactured. With the dramatic increase in interest and use, chips are now commercially manufactured, and the number of oligomer probes represented on a chip has also greatly increased (>1 million per array). Landmark studies using the early microarrays included the description of distinct molecular subsets in breast cancer and lymphomas associated with differences in clinical outcome [40, 41].

Oligonucleotide arrays (microarrays) are the contemporary version of spotted cDNA arrays, which were used in many of the early, high-impact microarray experiments [42, 43]. In contrast to spotted cDNA arrays, where cDNA probes representing genes of interest were printed onto glass slides, for oligonucleotide arrays, short probes measuring 20–60 bp are synthesized directly on each array. mRNA is then isolated from the cells or tissue of interest, reverse-transcribed into cDNA, and converted into biotin-labeled cRNA. cRNA representing all of the mRNA expressed in the experimental sample (e.g., cell line, tumor) is then hybridized with the array and binds probes with complementary sequences. To quantify the level of each cRNA present in the sample, it is labeled with a fluorophore that emits light when exposed to a laser scanner. The intensity of fluorescent signal that is bound to that probe mounted on the array reflects the amount of cRNA (and therefore mRNA) present in the original sample. Commercially available mRNA arrays that are frequently used include those made by Affymetrix (Santa Clara, CA) and Illumina (San Diego, CA). miRNA arrays are also available; they use a similar approach to assess the levels of >1000 miRNAs within a sample.

A newer approach to measuring RNA expression levels within cancer cells is transcriptome sequencing (RNA-Seq). In this method, the expression levels of mRNA are quantified using direct sequencing of the RNA. In addition to providing information about the level of mRNA expression, this technique has the potential to identify other genomic characteristics of the sample, such as the detection of mutations or polymorphisms within a transcript [44].

Finally, RT-PCR may be used to measure RNA expression in a smaller set of genes (whereas in a microarray or RNA-Seq, all protein-coding genes are routinely measured). RT-PCR is in routine use for certain clinical applications of RNA expression analysis; for example, Oncotype DX (Genomic Health, Redwood City, CA), a RT-PCR-based test to determine a breast cancer patient's risk of relapse, is used to guide decisions about adjuvant chemotherapy.

With the rapid adoption of expression arrays into biomedical research, top peer-reviewed journals and the NIH (for NIH-funded research) mandate the publication of full expression data from their experiments at the time the primary research paper is published. The publication of array data allows for scientific transparency in providing the full gene expression results (in addition to the summary analysis of key findings) and also makes these datasets readily available for other investigators to use as independent sets for hypothesis testing or validation. Expression array data are maintained in the online Gene Expression Omnibus (GEO, http://www.ncbi.nlm.nih.gov/geo/), an open-access database run by the NIH/National Center for Biotechnology Information [14].

Proteomics

Proteomics encompasses the study of protein expression, including spatial and temporal profiles, posttranslational modifications, and interactions with other molecules. Protein function is often dysregulated in lung cancers, and sometimes these alterations are not visible at the level of the RNA or DNA. For example, proteins are frequently modified after their translation from mRNA in important ways that affect their activity and function (e.g., phosphorylation or cleavage). Therefore, these posttranslational modifications need to be reflected in proteomic profiles for the protein data to be useful. Furthermore, studies comparing genomic and proteomic data have shown that there may be important differences between gene and protein levels and that changes in expression level may occur discordantly [24, 25, 45].

Characterization of the expression and activation of particular signaling proteins within a tumor can enable the physician to identify the best therapeutic for a patient. Several important analytical tools and methodologies have been used extensively in proteomic research. These include reverse phase protein array (RPPA), mass spectrometry (MS), forward phase arrays (e.g., receptor tyrosine kinase arrays), ELISA for single-analyte analysis, bead-based assays for multi-analyte testing, and analysis of circulating tumor cells.

Antibody microarrays are an extremely valuable technique for assaying protein expression and activation. RPPAs are fundamentally similar to mRNA microarrays in that very small quantities of samples, in this case protein lysates, are spotted onto an inert substrate, often a glass slide. It is imperative that lysates are diluted to equal concentrations prior to their application and spotted in multiple dilutions. The slide is then incubated with an antibody against one or more known proteins. RPPAs will often test nearly 200 antibodies, allowing the user to simultaneously examine changes in numerous proteins that may belong to the same or complementary signaling pathways or networks. Either fluorescent or chemiluminescent detection methods will then determine the relative expression of the corresponding target protein. Because antibodies that target both total and phosphoproteins are used, RPPAs reveal changes in the activation status of proteins, which often correspond to a phosphorylated form of the protein. As with genomic profiling techniques, RPPAs can be used to examine proteins related to lung cancer phenotypes and underlying similarities between samples. For example, RPPA experiments recently revealed distinct protein signaling differences between NSCLC and SCLC [46, 47]. Additionally, RPPAs may allow development of practical clinical assays for multifactor predictive markers derived using other technologies.

RPPAs are highly sensitive, but they have some limitations. Because each antibody may have slightly different optimal binding conditions, it can be difficult to both obtain antibodies that are suitable for RPPA and determine their ideal experimental conditions. When selecting antibodies to use for this method, it is therefore important to consider the experimental questions at hand and tailor the selection of antibodies accordingly. Using antibodies that recognize proteins involved in key cell signaling pathways with known biological relevance will likely yield better results than those targeting an unbiased list of proteins. Additional considerations should be made when using clinical tissue specimens. Although RPPAs are highly sensitive and reliable when using lysates derived from cell lines or snap-frozen tissue, when formalin-fixed, paraffin-embedded tissues are used, detection of phosphoproteins may be problematic.

MS is an accurate means of determining the molecular weight of proteins and is sensitive in detecting proteins in low concentrations. MS can be coupled with a variety of protein separation techniques, including gel and column separations, and can also be used directly (without a separation step) to assay protein profiles in tissues or blood. The mass spectrometer ionizes molecules from a sample and measures the abundance and the ratio of molecular mass to unit charge (m/z) for all ions produced above a certain sensitivity threshold. A sample is ionized in a vacuum, and the m/z ratios of each ionized species are distinguished by different physical properties depending on the type of detector: time-of-flight (TOF), Fourier-transform (FT), quadrupole, etc. Two methods of ionization are generally employed: matrix-assisted laser desorption/ionization (MALDI) and electrospray ionization (ESI). The important distinction between MALDI and ESI is that MALDI produces ions by laser irradiation of samples fixed to a solid conductive plate coated with a crystalline layer of organic acid, whereas ESI produces ions from a sample in solution as it passes through a small-bore highly charged capillary. MALDI can be used to produce protein profiles from frozen tissue sections or whole-cell cytological preparations; unfortunately, with limited exceptions, paraffin-embedded tissue cannot be used. Multiple protein mass spectra can be obtained from different positions on a frozen tissue section, allowing analysis of a protein's spatial distribution and production of two-dimensional images of protein location and abundance. Thus, MALDI is useful for discerning field effects or distinguishing protein expression in tumor from that in surrounding stroma or lymphocytic infiltrate. MALDI can also be used to analyze dried droplets of biologic samples, such as blood, serum, or plasma, pleural or ascitic fluid, or fractions collected from column separations or extracted proteins from one-dimensional or two-dimensional gel separations. ESI requires samples to be in solution and has been particularly useful for online analysis of proteins and peptides in the eluate of column separations. MALDI experiments have been used in profiling studies of rescued lung tumors and patient serum.

More recently, the technique of tandem mass spectrometry, also called MS/MS, has enabled direct sequencing of peptides in a mixture. Intact peptide ions are separated in one stage of the mass spectrometer; next, a collision gas is introduced into the vacuum, which causes the ions to fragment, producing characteristic fragment ions resulting from cleavage of the carbon–carbon and carbon–nitrogen bonds of the polypeptide backbone. These fragments are then separated and detected in the second stage of the mass spectrometer. This fragmentation does not occur efficiently with full-length proteins, which must first be digested into smaller peptides by proteolytic enzymes such as trypsin. For each peptide undergoing MS/MS analysis, a new mass spectrum is recorded that measures the m/z ratios of the fragment ions, and the identity of the parent ion is established by matching to the predicted fragmentation patterns of peptides in a human protein database. These fragmentation patterns can also be used to study post-translational modifications.

Enzyme-linked immunosorbent assay (ELISA) is a commonly used laboratory technique that detects secreted proteins, such as cytokines, chemokines, and angiogenic and growth factors. These assays are run in a 96-well plate format and can often be purchased commercially. In general, the 96-well plates are pre-coated with the antibody of interest. Samples are then applied to the wells of each plate and allowed to incubate, and a colorimetric change indicates the detection of proteins. Clinically, ELISAs can be used for profiling of circulating proteins using blood or other biological fluids from patients. One disadvantage to an ELISA is that it can only test one secreted protein or analyte at a time. Although the sample size required for each ELISA is quite small (on the order of 50–100 μL), multiple ELISAs must be run to examine a number of proteins.

Multiplex bead-based technology is similar to an ELISA assay in that it can detect small quantities of secreted proteins; however, it has one major advantage over an ELISA in that it enables the simultaneous quantitation of up to 100 analytes. This technology uses polystyrene beads internally dyed with differing ratios of two spectrally distinct fluorophores. Each fluorophore can have any of 10 possible levels of fluorescent intensity; thereby creating a family of 100 spectrally addressed bead sets. These assays contain dyed beads conjugated with monoclonal antibodies specific for a target protein or peptide, such as a cytokine or a phosphoprotein. Each of the 100 spectrally addressed bead sets can contain a capture antibody specific for a unique target protein. The antibody-conjugated beads are allowed to react with sample and a secondary, or detection, antibody in a microplate well to form a capture sandwich immunoassay. Multiplex assays can be created by mixing bead sets with different conjugated antibodies to simultaneously test for many analytes in a single sample. The use of this technique has been well documented in the literature, and results are comparable to that of ELISA [48–50].

Proteomic profiling of blood-based markers has one important advantage over other types of testing in that samples are readily available, simple to prepare and store, and can be taken prior to, during, or after treatment. The resulting proteomic profiles can then be used to identify patients likely to benefit from anticancer treatments, select the dose, and understand mechanisms of resistance. This allows for the assessment of predictive markers based on the baseline evaluation as well as markers of activity and resistance based on changes that occur during treatment [51–53].

The identification, isolation, and analysis of circulating tumor cells (CTCs) holds promise for early detection of cancer, rapid monitoring of tumor response and drug efficacy, serial noninvasive analysis of tumor genotypes, and eventual characterization of "metastasis precursors," a currently poorly understood tumor cell subpopulation whose targeting with novel therapies may provide effective prevention of cancer metastasis [54, 55]. However to date, technological limitations in rare cell detection have prevented successful application of either diagnostic or therapeutic approaches based on CTC analysis [56, 57]. The current state-of-the-art commercial technology is the CellSearch assay (Veridex Co.), involving multistep batch purification of fixed cells, using antibodies against the ubiquitous epithelial adhesion marker EpCAM conjugated to magnetic beads, which are then used to separate cells in a magnetic field [58–61]. While elegant in design, this assay can only identify CTCs in ~50% of patients with known metastatic disease, with an average yield of 1 CTC/mL (cut-off 5 cells/7.5 mL), and a final purity of 1 CTC/1000 leukocytes (0.1%). While this is a considerable achievement, given that the prevalence of CTCs is estimated to be 1 CTC/1 billion blood cells, the yield and purity of CTCs isolated using this approach are not sensitive enough for clinically useful dynamic monitoring and are too low for detailed molecular analyses. Hence, presence of CTCs has been proposed as a general prognostic marker, rather than being of direct utility in monitoring or designing cancer treatments [62].

Data analysis and statistics

Each molecular profiling experiment yields data on the relative abundances of large numbers of mRNA species or proteins in a number of different samples. Statistical algorithms have been developed that allow clustering of different samples with similar expression profiles. When coupled with biologic or clinical data for each sample – response to chemotherapy, metastatic patterns, or survival, for example – statistical correlations between molecular profile clusters and clinical outcome can be made. Although different profiling techniques vary in the type and quantity of molecular analytes measured, the statistical methods used to analyze the data are quite similar. A first step may include removing low-quality samples or data values from the analysis and filtering out molecular variables that are either expressed only sporadically or expressed with low variance across samples. Sophisticated statistical techniques are then required to discover statistically meaningful classifications of samples or relationships between clinical parameters and measured molecular variables. Most studies use a training–testing approach to developing these relationships. A sufficiently large training set is used to define a set of predictive genes or proteins, and the accuracy of this model is then assessed in an independent testing set, with no samples overlapping between the training and testing sets [17].

Once samples and genes are selected, a number of statistical techniques are applied to discover patterns of gene or protein expression that underlie tumor biology or phenotype. These techniques can be broadly classified as either "supervised" or "unsupervised." Unsupervised techniques use gene expression data without input of nongenetic descriptors to discover subgroups whose members share genetic similarities. Supervised techniques, on the other hand, include one or more clinical covariates such as histological type, presence of distant metastasis, or clinical outcome data, and use gene expression data to discover relationships that specifically pertain to a clinical question of interest.

Unsupervised clustering is based on the hypothesis that there may exist subgroups that can be discerned solely on the basis of shared gene expression profiles, and that these clusters may exhibit distinct clinical behaviors not previously appreciated without the profiling data. Hierarchical clustering is a common means of defining genetic clusters in which correlations of gene expression between two samples are calculated and a clustering diagram is produced that visually represents underlying similarity of gene expression. Researchers define some number of subgroups based on the clustering results and attempt to discern whether any of these apparent genetic groupings has significance with regard to clinically relevant variables. A common method is to produce Kaplan–Meier survival curves comparing overall or disease-free survival for members of one subgroup against all nonmembers. Any number of subgroups can be defined from the results of a given clustering experiment, depending on the cutoff used to define two tumor samples as similar or dissimilar. A given cutoff may define two patient groups but may fail to adequately capture the genetic complexities of the sample set. A more stringent similarity cutoff can define a larger number of subgroups, each composed of samples that have more uniform gene expression profiles; however, this makes it more difficult for observed differences (e.g., in survival) to reach statistical significance, because of the shrinking number of patients in each group, and increases the likelihood of arriving at false conclusions due to multiple subgroup analysis. On the other hand, if newly discovered clinical correlations are statistically robust, the information may be further validated in prospective studies and be applied in individualizing treatment decisions.

Supervised classification schemes start with two or more clinically or biologically defined groups – for instance, node negative versus node positive, responders versus nonresponders, or tumors that harbor a mutation versus those that do not – and attempt to determine genetic profiles capable of predicting to which group an unknown sample belongs. One can perform a clustering approach similar to that described earlier but with the constraint that the two dominant clusters must differ by the clinical variable of interest. Alternatively, one can use statistical tests (e.g., *t*-test, analysis of variance (ANOVA)) to determine individual genes or proteins that may correlate with the clinical variable of interest and then construct a model using weighted linear combinations of these features to make predictions on unknown samples.

One important consideration is the impact of repeat testing on the significance of a finding. When comparing thousands of variables between two groups, some of the observed differences will be false positives. Various analytical approaches can be applied that correct for "multiple comparison testing" and will give an estimate of the p-value (or level of significance) at which an observation is likely to be real. For example, one method commonly used is the Bonferroni correction, in which the desired p-value (commonly set at $p = 0.05$, meaning there is a 1 in 20 chance of detecting a difference between two groups when none actually exists) is divided by the number of variables being tested. In other words, if the mRNA expression of 10 000 genes were being compared between patients in two groups, those differences with p-values less than 0.05/10 000 (i.e., $p = 5 \times 10^{-6}$) would be considered significant. This approach minimizes the number of false positives, but at the risk of throwing out some results that may be real but fall below the strict p-value cutoff. Another approach is to set an acceptable false discovery rate (FDR) using the Benjamini-Hochberg method, which can be adjusted to be more or less strict [63, 64]. The acceptable FDR (or percentage of genes or observations that are allowed to be falsely positive) is then used to determine the p-value cutoff. For example, if 5000 genes are below a certain p-value determined to correspond to an FDR of 0.05 (or 5%), then 250 of those can be expected to be false positives. This approach allows for greater flexibility to scale how many false positives would be acceptable, depending on the goals and design of the experiment.

Both supervised and unsupervised techniques have the potential to "overtrain" the data, yielding models that perform well on the sample set from which they were derived, but with poor accuracy on independent testing cohorts. Validation of results is thus the most important step in any molecular profiling experiment, since even relationships that appear convincing may fail to have significance when applied to an independent set of samples.

It is often underappreciated that high-quality clinical samples are difficult to obtain and costly to collect and store, and maintaining accurate and complete clinical follow-up is labor-intensive. Thus, the limited size of many studies necessitates the most efficient possible use of samples, and setting aside a large number of samples for adequate validation leaves fewer samples for training and less robust predictive models. Furthermore, the genes picked as predictive are very dependent on the patients included in the training set [65]. Cross-validation is an approach that maximizes the size of the training set while still allowing validation of results on a sufficiently large testing set [66, 67]. In this method, a single sample or a small number of samples is removed from a set, and the remaining samples are used to construct a predictive model. The model is applied to the sample or samples that were left out of the model-building process, and its accuracy in predicting the feature of interest is recorded. This is then repeated a large number of times, and the combined accuracy over all the left-out samples is reported as an estimate of the classification accuracy rate of the model.

Another method to minimize the necessary number of precious samples required for validating results is to use online databases of previously published gene expression profiles as independent test sets, as described above. This is an attractive method made possible by the increasing standardization of some of the technologies [68–72], but there are challenges in integrating data sets from different experiments. There may be substantial differences in the methods used to obtain the expression profiles; for instance, studies use microarray chips from different manufacturers and even arrays produced at in-house microarray facilities. Even data obtained for the same genes from newer versions of chips from a given manufacturer may not be directly comparable to data obtained from earlier versions. Also, compared with older versions, newer microarrays typically have more probes spanning more genetic elements. Thus, many genes may not be represented in both data sets, and it may be difficult to translate expression data from one set to another. With the advent of exon arrays, it has become clear that the location of the oligonucleotide within the putative transcript yields different measurement results. Furthermore, idiosyncratic differences in sample handling and experimental protocol can lead to other systematic differences between gene expression sets.

Despite these challenges, many studies have shown that relationships observed in one data set can be successfully and convincingly demonstrated to hold true in large independent sets. When efforts are taken to standardize procedures, interlaboratory reproducibility has been shown to be quite good [68–71, 73]. Current microarray-based profiling will likely benefit from such increased standardization across laboratories, careful attention to sources of error or variation that can be controlled (such as batch effect), and the ongoing development of bioinformatics tools that permit sharing of large data sets and integrating data optimally despite lab-to-lab differences. These advances not only will lead to more effective validation of models but also will allow large-scale meta-analyses to look for important molecular–clinical relationships in much larger sample sets, with better statistical power for developing robust molecular signatures. Of course, regardless of its reproducibility in training and validation sets, the real rubric of success for any molecular classification scheme will be its performance in prospective clinical trials that determine whether its clinical use improves patient outcomes.

Clinical applications

Data being generated now will change the treatment of lung cancer significantly over the next 5, 10, and 20 years in ways that we cannot fully predict today. Currently, the most widespread type of molecular profiling within the clinic – and, therefore, the one likely to have the most immediate impact on clinical decision making – is the DNA testing of lung tumors (usually formalin-fixed, paraffin-embedded tissue from diagnostic biopsies) for panels of mutations and/or fusions. The introduction of technologies that allow several genes to be tested in parallel in a single reaction (i.e., multiplexed) is making it possible for an expanding number of genes to be profiled on relatively small amounts of tissue and without significant increases in cost. Cancer gene panels are being run routinely in many academic centers and by community-based oncologists using commercially available profiling. Increasingly, patient tumors are also being assessed for mRNA and protein expression levels that may predict response to certain treatments. While the clinical utility of many of these is not yet clear, it is likely that some of these will become the standard of care in the management of lung cancer patients based on the results of ongoing clinical trials that are investigating targeted drugs in molecularly defined subsets of patients. In addition to predictive biomarkers for drug selection, other areas in which molecular profiling will likely affect clinical care include early detection and diagnosis, subclassification and staging, and surveillance. Finally, advances in molecular testing technologies are likely to expand the availability of molecular profiling in blood, saliva, urine, or other samples that can be collected in minimally invasive ways. The further development of nontumor (e.g., blood-based) biomarkers will also help facilitate broader implementation of molecular testing in patients for whom available tumor tissue is limited or cannot be safely obtained, or when repeat testing would be informative (e.g., at the time of progression or after acquisition of drug resistance).

Early detection and diagnosis

The peripheral blood is clearly the most readily available and clinically practical biospecimen source for early detection and diagnosis. Pathological states can cause disease-related changes in molecules circulating in the blood, due to altered cellular expression of secreted proteins, proteins being directly released into extracellular fluid after cell death, posttranslational modification by cleavage, glycosylation, or other processes, or as a result of the host's response to the disease. If a change in blood protein composition occurs reproducibly in the presence of a disease, then such a change may be useful for disease detection and diagnosis. For example, the detection of troponins and other proteins leaked from damaged cardiac myocytes has become the gold standard for detection of myocardial infarction, even though they are not themselves causal.

One reason for the abysmal survival rates in lung cancer may be the absence of effective screening for early detection. Previously, a variety of screening tests for lung cancer in patients at high risk failed to show any impact on survival, including yearly chest X-rays, sputum cytologies, and bronchoscopic screening. However, a large randomized study recently demonstrated that spiral CT scans could detect early lung cancers in high-risk patients with strong smoking histories and that this early detection of lung cancers translated into an improvement in overall survival [74].

Molecular profiling studies of blood and/or sputum samples obtained from patients on this trial are planned and may provide markers that could be used in molecular tests to identify patients at highest risk for lung cancer or, as a companion to imaging studies, to aid in early detection of lung cancer, when it is most treatable. These types of noninvasive tests would be particularly attractive for nonsmoking patients, for whom incidence of lung cancer is relatively lower and, therefore, the benefits of CT screening are currently outweighed by the risk associated with repeated exposure to radiation from CT screening.

Molecular subclassification and staging

Treatment decisions in lung cancer are based largely on the extent of disease as determined by staging criteria and generalizations on disease behavior associated with histological distinctions. Stage has a strong impact on determining which patients are most likely to benefit from different types of treatment. However, there is significant variability in the clinical outcome of individual patients within each stage classification or histological subgroup, with some lung cancers showing more aggressive behavior in terms of metastatic potential, pace of disease progression, or resistance to chemotherapy. The ability to elucidate factors predicting individual prognosis and response to therapy will be invaluable clinically by helping to identify patients most likely to benefit from more (or less) aggressive therapy, such as adjuvant chemotherapy.

The most important pathologic distinction described so far is that between SCLC and NSCLC. These are readily apparent by histological and immunohistochemical evaluation and have fundamental differences in probable cell of origin, natural history, and response to chemotherapy. Subtype classification of NSCLC has minimal impact on patient care, with a few notable exceptions: e.g., enrichment of EGFR mutations and ALK fusions in non-squamous tumors, greater response of non-squamous cancers to pemetrexed relative to gemcitabine chemotherapy. Unfortunately, the behavioral features that most likely affect clinical outcome – aggressiveness, likelihood of metastasis, resistance to apoptosis, and response to therapy – are indistinguishable with conventional microscopic evaluation. However, these features clearly have underlying genetic determinants, and uncovering these with molecular profiling may lead to dramatic changes in the management of lung cancer.

Gene profiling experiments in other cancer disciplines have uncovered such determinants. For example, five reproducible genetic clusters within breast cancer have been disclosed by mRNA expression profiling, with corresponding differences in prognosis and response to therapy; the basal-like, or "triple-negative," subtype in particular has a distinctly worse prognosis [75–78]. Other expression studies have uncovered independent sets of genes capable of reliably distinguishing good-prognosis from poor-prognosis patients among women with node-negative, estrogen receptor-positive breast cancer treated with tamoxifen. In the clinic, the Oncotype DX assay is a commonly used 21-gene marker set that uses RT-PCR to profile expression and predict those patients most likely to benefit from the addition of chemotherapy to their treatment [79, 80].

Efforts to uncover useful predictive classifiers in lung cancer have also been fruitful. Many studies [24, 26, 27, 46, 47, 81–94] have identified subtypes of lung cancer based on overall similarities in gene and protein expression profiles using approaches comparable to those successfully employed in breast and other cancers. The numbers of patients enrolled in these studies have ranged from approximately 50 to >200, and the number of RNA probes has increased in recent studies as commercial chip technology has advanced.

Early studies such as those by Bhattacharjee *et al.* demonstrated that many clinical or histological groups clustered together by their natural genetic similarity [82]. Normal lung could be distinguished from tumor, NSCLC from SCLC, and adenocarcinomas, squamous cell carcinomas, and large cell carcinomas largely segregated into their respective groups. The ability to differentiate samples with obvious histological differences was not a step forward in itself but proved the concept that gene profiling experiments could lead to meaningful classifications. Several studies have demonstrated clustering of samples within one or more histological subtypes [24, 83, 85, 88–90, 95–100]. These results suggest that there may be genetic subgroups within the main histological subtypes, with possible different biologic implications. This likelihood is supported by more recent studies such as the molecular profiling of squamous lung tumors by TCGA [11].

Some signatures or molecular profiles may also be prognostic in lung cancer [22, 101]. These can be single biomarkers (such as EGFR mutation, which is associated with longer overall survival) or marker signatures. For example, Beer *et al.* used microarray profiling to study 86 patients with adenocarcinoma and described three dominant clusters within this cohort, one of which differed significantly from the others prognostically [83]. Other signatures that are prognostic in specific patient populations, such as those receiving adjuvant chemotherapy, have also been published and could have future applications for selecting patients with the greatest chance of benefiting from existing therapies [102]. Alternatively, results from recent studies have shown that these molecular differences may be associated with expression of novel druggable targets such as DDR2 mutations and FGFR1 alterations in squamous lung cancers or PARP1 in SCLC [10, 46, 103]. Finally, integrated analyses linking differences in mRNA or protein expression with alterations at the DNA level are advancing our understanding of the biology underlying specific molecular subgroups such as LKB1- and KRAS-mutated NSCLC and will help guide the development of new therapies for patients with these common genetic alterations [104, 105].

Selection of therapy

Although numerous chemotherapy regimens and/or targeted drugs have clear clinical activity in the treatment of lung cancer, their observed effectiveness in individual patients varies greatly. The ability to select the most active regimen for a specific patient is a key goal of molecular profiling, especially considering the substantial treatment-related morbidity and opportunity cost associated with ineffective therapy. The ability of molecular profiling to effectively predict the clinical efficacy of different therapies against a particular tumor has already had a profound impact on patient care. The best examples of these currently are the use of EGFR mutations and ALK fusions to identify those patients most likely to respond to FDA-approved, oral targeted drugs (erlotinib and crizotinib, respectively), which became part of the NCCN guidelines for management of metastatic NSCLC in 2012. The discovery of these predictive biomarkers and their use in clinical practice are described in greater detail in subsequent chapters.

In addition to alterations in EGFR and ALK, a growing number of new driver genes have been identified in lung cancer, including BRAF, PIK3CA, ROS1, RET, and HER2 (Figure 3.2). Drugs capable

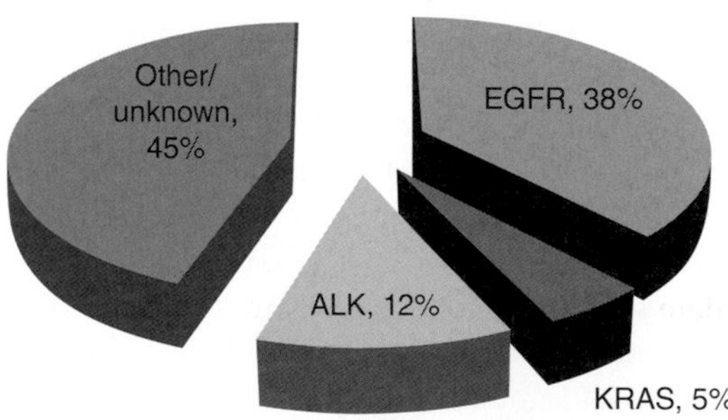

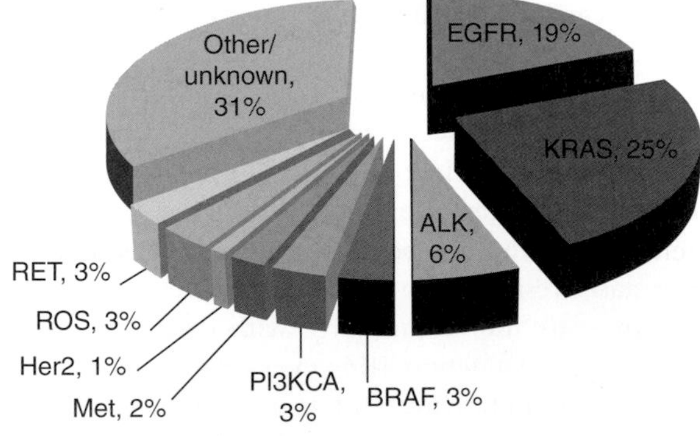

Figure 3.2 Different mutation spectrums in lung adenocarcinomas in never-smokers and current/former smokers. EGFR mutations and other targetable mutations (e.g., ALK fusions) are more common in never-smokers vs. current/former smokers. However, the driver mutations have not been identified in 45% of never-smokers.
Source: Adapted from Paik *et al.* [108]. Reproduced with permission of John Wiley and Sons, Inc.

of inhibiting these targets may have clinical benefit for molecularly defined subsets of patients (such as those whose tumors carry a mutation, fusion, or amplification in one of these genes). However, because each driver may be present in only a fraction of NSCLC patients (e.g., 1–5%), even a drug that has a major impact in some patients could fail in clinical trials if its activity is not evaluated (at least in part) in a molecularly defined subset of patients. An example of this is HER2 inhibitors (e.g., traztuzumab, lapatinib), which are highly active in and a standard of care for HER2-amplified breast cancer. However, had the activity of these drugs been studied exclusively in an unselected population of breast cancer patients, their substantial benefit would have been missed.

Conversely, some number of patients without recognized driver mutations may still benefit from a targeted drug, and our hypothesis about the biomarkers likely to predict response may be inaccurate or incomplete. For example, a recent study of NSCLC patients with recurrent, refractory disease demonstrated that epithelial-to-mesenchymal transition may predict response to the EGFR inhibitor erlotinib in patients with normal (nonmutated) EGFR [47]. For these reasons, thoughtful clinical trial design – with carefully planned correlative biomarker studies – is critical for making sure we do not dismiss potentially active drugs or patient populations that could benefit from them. Key challenges to routine molecular testing in standard practice and in clinical trials include the need for adequate amounts of tumor tissue and the type of tissue available. For example, most diagnostic biopsy samples are formalin fixed and paraffin embedded. Although this is not an issue for many DNA analyses, such tissues are currently limited in their utility for other types of profiling, such as gene expression arrays and proteomic profiling. Furthermore, several studies have documented that cancers change at the molecular level over time, especially in response to therapies. For example, a study by Sequist *et al.* demonstrated that patients with EGFR-mutated cancers who became resistant to EGFR inhibitors had a variety of histological or molecular changes that contributed to resistance. Repeat biopsies to identify the features contributing to drug resistance (e.g., the appearance of resistance mutations, such as T790M, in the EGFR gene or expression of EMT markers [106, 107]) are likely to have important implications for selecting second-line and subsequent therapies. Thus, repeat molecular testing of a patient's cancer cells (or other biospecimen, such as blood) at the time of disease progression or acquired drug resistance to document the current tumor biology or profile will have important clinical applications.

Future directions and conclusions

Many challenges must be met before profiling techniques can reach their full potential. A major limitation of many lung cancer studies in the past has been that the number of patient samples investigated has been too small to draw meaningful conclusions. However, with the growth of publicly available biomarker databases, decreased cost associated with molecular profiling, and technologies to analyze smaller and smaller tissue samples, this landscape is changing. Given the growing use of DNA sequencing and other high-throughput platforms, continuing advances in bioinformatics and computational tools will also be essential to efficiently utilize the large quantities of data, to adjust for variability between labs, and to integrate different types of molecular data (e.g., proteomic and genomic studies).

Once a predictive profile has been described and validated, an additional challenge is posed in developing a suitable clinical assay. This may pose a particular challenge for profiles derived from cell lines or animal models or from highly technical, limited-availability platforms. Once assays are developed, clinical utility will be aided by efforts to accommodate smaller samples and to get accurate results from potentially lower quality real-world clinical samples. For mRNA markers, quantitative real-time PCR is highly sensitive and can be used clinically to measure expression levels of each gene used in a profile. Furthermore, this technique can be applied to fixed tissue embedded in paraffin, rather than the fresh-frozen samples required for full microarray analysis. For protein markers identified in high-throughput platforms, immunohistochemistry and

ELISA are potential options for rapidly translating these markers into the clinic.

Although many challenges remain, molecular profiling experiments have already produced exciting results in lung cancer and are changing treatment for lung cancer patients. These early successes attest to the potential of profiling experiments to improve patient outcome through individualized risk assessment and optimal selection of therapy options. As proteomic and genomic technology and methodology continue to mature, they will without doubt become more and more integral to research and patient care. The level of information and understanding that can be attained from molecular profiling and the speed at which these technologies are evolving are revolutionizing the study of cancer biology and the practice of clinical oncology.

Acknowledgments

L.A.B. acknowledges Emily B. Roarty for scientific review and editing of this chapter as well as the contributions of the authors of the previous edition, Jacob M. Kaufman and David P Carbone.

References

1 Lander ES, Linton LM, Birren B, Nusbaum C, Zody MC, Baldwin J, *et al.* (2001) Initial sequencing and analysis of the human genome. *Nature*, Feb 15; 409(6822): 860–921.

2 Venter JC, Adams MD, Myers EW, Li PW, Mural RJ, Sutton GG, *et al.* (2001) The sequence of the human genome. *Science*, Feb 16; 291(5507): 1304–51.

3 Lynch TJ, Bell DW, Sordella R, Gurubhagavatula S, Okimoto RA, Brannigan BW, *et al.* (2004) Activating mutations in the epidermal growth factor receptor underlying responsiveness of non-small-cell lung cancer to gefitinib. *N Engl J Med*, May 20; 350(21): 2129–39.

4 Paez JG, Janne PA, Lee JC, Tracy S, Greulich H, Gabriel S, *et al.* (2004) EGFR mutations in lung cancer: correlation with clinical response to gefitinib therapy. *Science*, Jun 4; 304(5676): 1497–1500.

5 Fukuoka M, Yano S, Giaccone G, Tamura T, Nakagawa K, Douillard JY, *et al.* (2003) Multi-institutional randomized phase II trial of gefitinib for previously treated patients with advanced non-small-cell lung cancer (The IDEAL 1 Trial) [corrected]. *J Clin Oncol*, Jun 15; 21(12): 2237–46.

6 Inamura K, Takeuchi K, Togashi Y, Hatano S, Ninomiya H, Motoi N, *et al.* (2009) EML4-ALK lung cancers are characterized by rare other mutations, a TTF-1 cell lineage, an acinar histology, and young onset. *Mod Pathol*, Apr; 22(4): 508–15.

7 Kwak EL, Bang YJ, Camidge DR, Shaw AT, Solomon B, Maki RG, *et al.* (2010) Anaplastic lymphoma kinase inhibition in non-small-cell lung cancer. *N Engl J Med*, Oct 28; 363(18): 1693–1703.

8 National Comprehensive Cancer Network. NCCN Guidelines on Non-Small Cell Lung Cancer V, accessed 2/03/2013, www.nccn.org.

9 Bergethon K, Shaw AT, Ou SH, Katayama R, Lovly CM, McDonald NT, *et al.* (2012) ROS1 rearrangements define a unique molecular class of lung cancers. *J Clin Oncol*, Mar 10; 30(8): 863–70.

10 Hammerman PS, Sos ML, Ramos AH, Xu C, Dutt A, Zhou W, *et al.* (2011) Mutations in the DDR2 kinase gene identify a novel therapeutic target in squamous cell lung cancer. *Cancer Discov*, Jun; 1(1): 78–89.

11 Comprehensive genomic characterization of squamous cell lung cancers. *Nature*, Sep 27; 489(7417): 519–25.

12 Imielinski M, Berger AH, Hammerman PS, Hernandez B, Pugh TJ, Hodis E, *et al.* (2012) Mapping the hallmarks of lung adenocarcinoma with massively parallel sequencing. *Cell*, Sep 14; 150(6): 1107–20.

13 Rudin CM, Durinck S, Stawiski EW, Poirier JT, Modrusan Z, Shames DS, *et al.* (2012) Comprehensive genomic analysis identifies SOX2 as a frequently amplified gene in small-cell lung cancer. *Nat Genet*, Oct; 44(10): 1111–16.

14 NCBI (2012) Gene Expression Omnibus. Available from: http://www.ncbi.nlm.nih.gov/geo/.

15 Bioscience C (2012) Oncomine. Available from: https://www.oncomine.org/resource/login.html.

16 Cerami E, Gao J, Dogrusoz U, Gross BE, Sumer SO, Aksoy BA, *et al.* (2012) The cBio cancer genomics portal: an open platform for exploring multidimensional cancer genomics data. *Cancer Discov*, May; 2(5): 401–4.

17 Ransohoff DF (2004) Rules of evidence for cancer molecular-marker discovery and validation. *Nat Rev Cancer*, Apr; 4(4): 309–14.

18 Kris MG, Johnson BE, Kwiatkowski DG, lafrate AJ, Wistuba II, Aronson SL, *et al.* (2011) Identification of driver mutations in tumor specimens from 1,000

patients with lung adenocarcinoma: The NCI's Lung Cancer Mutation Consortium (LCMC). *J Clin Oncol*. [Abstract]. 29(suppl): abstr CRA7506.

19 Thomas RK, Baker AC, Debiasi RM, Winckler W, Laframboise T, Lin WM, *et al.* (2007) High-throughput oncogene mutation profiling in human cancer. *Nat Genet*, Mar; 39(3): 347–51.

20 Wheeler DA, Srinivasan M, Egholm M, Shen Y, Chen L, McGuire A, *et al.* (2008) The complete genome of an individual by massively parallel DNA sequencing. *Nature*, Apr 17; 452(7189): 872–6.

21 Kohno T, Ichikawa H, Totoki Y, Yasuda K, Hiramoto M, Nammo T, *et al.* (2012) KIF5B-RET fusions in lung adenocarcinoma. *Nat Med*, Mar; 18(3): 375–7.

22 Lipson D, Capelletti M, Yelensky R, Otto G, Parker A, Jarosz M, *et al.* (2012) Identification of new ALK and RET gene fusions from colorectal and lung cancer biopsies. *Nat Med*, Mar; 18(3): 382–4.

23 Feero WG, Guttmacher AE, Collins FS (2010) Genomic medicine-an updated primer. *N Engl J Med*, May 27; 362(21): 2001–11.

24 Chen G, Gharib TG, Wang H, Huang CC, Kuick R, Thomas DG, *et al.* (2003) Protein profiles associated with survival in lung adenocarcinoma. *Proc Natl Acad Sci USA*, Nov 11; 100(23): 13537–42.

25 Chen G, Gharib TG, Huang CC, Taylor JM, Misek DE, Kardia SL, *et al.* (2002) Discordant protein and mRNA expression in lung adenocarcinomas. *Mol Cell Proteomics*, Apr; 1(4): 304–13.

26 Shibata T, Uryu S, Kokubu A, Hosoda F, Ohki M, Sakiyama T, *et al.* (2005) Genetic classification of lung adenocarcinoma based on array-based comparative genomic hybridization analysis: its association with clinicopathologic features. *Clin Cancer Res*, 2005 Sep 1; 11(17): 6177–85.

27 Li R, Wang H, Bekele BN, Yin Z, Caraway NP, Katz RL, *et al.* (2006) Identification of putative oncogenes in lung adenocarcinoma by a comprehensive functional genomic approach. *Oncogene*, Apr 27; 25(18): 2628–35.

28 Massion PP, Kuo WL, Stokoe D, Olshen AB, Treseler PA, Chin K, *et al.* (2002) Genomic copy number analysis of non-small cell lung cancer using array comparative genomic hybridization: implications of the phosphatidylinositol 3-kinase pathway. *Cancer Res*, Jul 1; 62(13): 3636–40.

29 Weir BA, Woo MS, Getz G, Perner S, Ding L, Beroukhim R, *et al.* (2007) Characterizing the cancer genome in lung adenocarcinoma. *Nature*, Dec 6; 450(7171): 893–8.

30 Carthew RW, Sontheimer EJ (2009) Origins and mechanisms of miRNAs and siRNAs. *Cell*, Feb 20; 136(4): 642–55.

31 Bartels CL, Tsongalis GJ (2009) MicroRNAs: novel biomarkers for human cancer. *Clin Chem*, Apr; 55(4): 623–31.

32 Yanaihara N, Caplen N, Bowman E, Seike M, Kumamoto K, Yi M, *et al.* (2006) Unique microRNA molecular profiles in lung cancer diagnosis and prognosis. *Cancer Cell*, Mar; 9(3): 189–98.

33 Takamizawa J, Konishi H, Yanagisawa K, Tomida S, Osada H, Endoh H, *et al.* (2004) Reduced expression of the let-7 microRNAs in human lung cancers in association with shortened postoperative survival. *Cancer Res*, Jun 1; 64(11): 3753–6.

34 Lebanony D, Benjamin H, Gilad S, Ezagouri M, Dov A, Ashkenazi K, *et al.* (2009) Diagnostic assay based on hsa-miR-205 expression distinguishes squamous from nonsquamous non-small-cell lung carcinoma. *J Clin Oncol*, Apr 20; 27(12): 2030–7.

35 Gibbons DL, Lin W, Creighton CJ, Rizvi ZH, Gregory PA, Goodall GJ, *et al.* (2009) Contextual extracellular cues promote tumor cell EMT and metastasis by regulating miR-200 family expression. *Genes Dev*, Sep 15; 23(18): 2140–51.

36 Birney E, Stamatoyannopoulos JA, Dutta A, Guigo R, Gingeras TR, Margulies EH, *et al.* (2007) Identification and analysis of functional elements in 1% of the human genome by the ENCODE pilot project. *Nature*, Jun 14; 447(7146): 799–816.

37 Schena M, Shalon D, Davis RW, Brown PO (1995) Quantitative monitoring of gene expression patterns with a complementary DNA microarray. *Science*, Oct 20; 270(5235): 467–70.

38 Churchill GA (2002) Fundamentals of experimental design for cDNA microarrays. *Nat Genet*, Dec; 32 Suppl: 490–5.

39 Fodor SP, Read JL, Pirrung MC, Stryer L, Lu AT, Solas D (1991) Light-directed, spatially addressable parallel chemical synthesis. *Science*, Feb 15; 251(4995): 767–73.

40 van 't Veer LJ, Dai H, van de Vijver MJ, He YD, Hart AA, Mao M, *et al.* (2002) Gene expression profiling predicts clinical outcome of breast cancer. *Nature*, Jan 31; 415(6871): 530–6.

41 Alizadeh AA, Eisen MB, Davis RE, Ma C, Lossos IS, Rosenwald A, *et al.* (2000) Distinct types of diffuse large B-cell lymphoma identified by gene expression profiling. *Nature*, Feb 3; 403(6769): 503–11.

42 DeRisi J, Penland L, Brown PO, Bittner ML, Meltzer PS, Ray M, *et al.* (1996) Use of a cDNA microarray to

analyse gene expression patterns in human cancer. *Nat Genet*, Dec; 14(4): 457–60.

43 Wang SM, Rowley JD (1998) A strategy for genome-wide gene analysis: integrated procedure for gene identification. *Proc Natl Acad Sci USA*, Sep 29; 95(20): 11909–14.

44 Wang Z, Gerstein M, Snyder M (2009) RNA-Seq: a revolutionary tool for transcriptomics. *Nat Rev Genet*, Jan; 10(1): 57–63.

45 Nishizuka S, Charboneau L, Young L, Major S, Reinhold WC, Waltham M, *et al.* (2003) Proteomic profiling of the NCI-60 cancer cell lines using new high-density reverse-phase lysate microarrays. *Proc Natl Acad Sci USA*, Nov 25; 100(24): 14229–34.

46 Byers LA, Wang J, Nilsson MB, Fujimoto J, Saintigny P, Yordy J, *et al.* (2012) Proteomic profiling identifies dysregulated pathways in small cell lung cancer and novel therapeutic targets including PARP1. *Cancer Discov*, Sep; 2(9): 798–811.

47 Byers LA, Diao L, Wang J, Saintigny P, Girard L, Peyton M, *et al.* (2013) An epithelial-mesenchymal transition gene signature predicts resistance to EGFR and PI3K inhibitors and identifies axl as a therapeutic target for overcoming EGFR Inhibitor resistance. *Clin Cancer Res*, Jan 1; 19(1): 279–90.

48 Skogstrand K, Thorsen P, Norgaard-Pedersen B, Schendel DE, Sorensen LC, Hougaard DM (2005) Simultaneous measurement of 25 inflammatory markers and neurotrophins in neonatal dried blood spots by immunoassay with xMAP technology. *Clin Chem*, Oct; 51(10): 1854–66.

49 Giavedoni LD (2005) Simultaneous detection of multiple cytokines and chemokines from nonhuman primates using luminex technology. *J Immunol Methods*, Jun; 301(1–2): 89–101.

50 Dupont NC, Wang K, Wadhwa PD, Culhane JF, Nelson EL (2005) Validation and comparison of luminex multiplex cytokine analysis kits with ELISA: Determinations of a panel of nine cytokines in clinical sample culture supernatants. *J Reprod Immunol*, Aug; 66(2): 175–91.

51 Hanrahan EO, Heymach JV (2007) Vascular endothelial growth factor receptor tyrosine kinase inhibitors vandetanib (ZD6474) and AZD2171 in lung cancer. *Clin Cancer Res*, Aug 1; 13(15 Pt 2): s4617–22.

52 Norden-Zfoni A, Desai J, Manola J, Beaudry P, Force J, Maki R, *et al.* (2007) Blood-based biomarkers of SU11248 activity and clinical outcome in patients with metastatic imatinib-resistant gastrointestinal stromal tumor. *Clin Cancer Res*, May 1; 13(9): 2643–50.

53 Nikolinakos PG, Altorki N, Yankelevitz D, Tran HT, Yan S, Rajagopalan D, *et al.* (2010) Plasma cytokine and angiogenic factor profiling identifies markers associated with tumor shrinkage in early-stage non-small cell lung cancer patients treated with pazopanib. *Cancer Res*, Mar 15; 70(6): 2171–9.

54 Papadopoulos N, Kinzler KW, Vogelstein B (2006) The role of companion diagnostics in the development and use of mutation-targeted cancer therapies. *Nat Biotechnol*, Aug; 24(8): 985–95.

55 Greenman C, Stephens P, Smith R, Dalgliesh GL, Hunter C, Bignell G, *et al.* (2007) Patterns of somatic mutation in human cancer genomes. *Nature*, Mar 8; 446(7132): 153–8.

56 Allard WJ, Matera J, Miller MC, Repollet M, Connelly MC, Rao C, *et al.* (2004) Tumor cells circulate in the peripheral blood of all major carcinomas but not in healthy subjects or patients with nonmalignant diseases. *Clin Cancer Res*, Oct 15; 10(20): 6897–6904.

57 Zieglschmid V, Hollmann C, Bocher O (2005) Detection of disseminated tumor cells in peripheral blood. *Crit Rev Clin Lab Sci*, 42(2): 155–96.

58 Braun S, Marth C (2004) Circulating tumor cells in metastatic breast cancer-toward individualized treatment? *N Engl J Med*, Aug 19; 351(8): 824–6.

59 Cristofanilli M, Budd GT, Ellis MJ, Stopeck A, Matera J, Miller MC, *et al.* (2004) Circulating tumor cells, disease progression, and survival in metastatic breast cancer. *N Engl J Med*, Aug 19; 351(8): 781–91.

60 Cristofanilli M, Hayes DF, Budd GT, Ellis MJ, Stopeck A, Reuben JM, *et al.* (2005) Circulating tumor cells: a novel prognostic factor for newly diagnosed metastatic breast cancer. *J Clin Oncol*, Mar 1; 23(7): 1420–30.

61 Smerage JB, Hayes DF (2006) The measurement and therapeutic implications of circulating tumour cells in breast cancer. *Br J Cancer*, Jan 16; 94(1): 8–12.

62 Smirnov DA, Zweitzig DR, Foulk BW, Miller MC, Doyle GV, Pienta KJ, *et al.* (2005) Global gene expression profiling of circulating tumor cells. *Cancer Res*, Jun 15; 65(12): 4993–7.

63 Storey JD, Tibshirani R (2003) Statistical significance for genomewide studies. *Proc Natl Acad Sci USA*, Aug 5; 100(16): 9440–5.

64 Benjamini Y, Hochberg Y (1995) Controlling the false discovery rate: A practical and powerful approach to multiple testing. *Journal of the Royal Statistical Society Series B (Methodological)*, 57(1): 289–300.

65 Michiels S, Koscielny S, Hill C (2005) Prediction of cancer outcome with microarrays: A multiple random validation strategy. *Lancet*, Feb 5–11; 365(9458): 488–92.

66 Braga-Neto UM, Dougherty ER (2004) Is cross-validation valid for small-sample microarray classification? *Bioinformatics*, Feb 12; 20(3): 374–80.

67 Simon R, Radmacher MD, Dobbin K, McShane LM (2003) Pitfalls in the use of DNA microarray data for diagnostic and prognostic classification. *J Natl Cancer Inst*, Jan 1; 95(1): 14–18.

68 Canales RD, Luo Y, Willey JC, Austermiller B, Barbacioru CC, Boysen C, *et al.* (2006) Evaluation of DNA microarray results with quantitative gene expression platforms. *Nat Biotechnol*, Sep; 24(9): 1115–22.

69 Guo L, Lobenhofer EK, Wang C, Shippy R, Harris SC, Zhang L, *et al.* (2006) Rat toxicogenomic study reveals analytical consistency across microarray platforms. *Nat Biotechnol*, Sep; 24(9): 1162–9.

70 Shi L, Reid LH, Jones WD, Shippy R, Warrington JA, Baker SC, *et al.* (2006) The MicroArray Quality Control (MAQC) project shows inter- and intraplatform reproducibility of gene expression measurements. *Nat Biotechnol*, Sep; 24(9): 1151–61.

71 Shippy R, Fulmer-Smentek S, Jensen RV, Jones WD, Wolber PK, Johnson CD, *et al.* (2006) Using RNA sample titrations to assess microarray platform performance and normalization techniques. *Nat Biotechnol*, Sep; 24(9): 1123–31.

72 Tong W, Lucas AB, Shippy R, Fan X, Fang H, Hong H, *et al.* (2006) Evaluation of external RNA controls for the assessment of microarray performance. *Nat Biotechnol*, Sep; 24(9): 1132–9.

73 Dobbin KK, Beer DG, Meyerson M, Yeatman TJ, Gerald WL, Jacobson JW, *et al.* (2005) Interlaboratory comparability study of cancer gene expression analysis using oligonucleotide microarrays. *Clin Cancer Res*, Jan 15; 11(2 Pt 1): 565–72.

74 Aberle DR, Adams AM, Berg CD, Black WC, Clapp JD, Fagerstrom RM, *et al.* (2011) Reduced lung-cancer mortality with low-dose computed tomographic screening. *N Engl J Med*, Aug 4; 365(5): 395–409.

75 Hu Z, Fan C, Oh DS, Marron JS, He X, Qaqish BF, *et al.* (2006) The molecular portraits of breast tumors are conserved across microarray platforms. *BMC Genomics*, 7: 96.

76 Perou CM, Sorlie T, Eisen MB, van de Rijn M, Jeffrey SS, Rees CA, *et al.* (2000) Molecular portraits of human breast tumours. *Nature*, Aug 17; 406(6797): 747–52.

77 Sorlie T, Perou CM, Tibshirani R, Aas T, Geisler S, Johnsen H, *et al.* (2001) Gene expression patterns of breast carcinomas distinguish tumor subclasses with clinical implications. *Proc Natl Acad Sci USA*, Sep 11; 98(19): 10869–74.

78 Sorlie T, Tibshirani R, Parker J, Hastie T, Marron JS, Nobel A, *et al.* (2003) Repeated observation of breast tumor subtypes in independent gene expression data sets. *Proc Natl Acad Sci USA*, Jul 8; 100(14): 8418–23.

79 Paik S, Shak S, Tang G, Kim C, Baker J, Cronin M, *et al.* (2004) A multigene assay to predict recurrence of tamoxifen-treated, node-negative breast cancer. *N Engl J Med*, Dec 30; 351(27): 2817–26.

80 Paik S, Tang G, Shak S, Kim C, Baker J, Kim W, *et al.* (2006) Gene expression and benefit of chemotherapy in women with node-negative, estrogen receptor-positive breast cancer. *J Clin Oncol*, Aug 10; 24(23): 3726–34.

81 Guo L, Ma Y, Ward R, Castranova V, Shi X, Qian Y (2006) Constructing molecular classifiers for the accurate prognosis of lung adenocarcinoma. *Clin Cancer Res*, Jun 1; 12(11 Pt 1): 3344–54.

82 Bhattacharjee A, Richards WG, Staunton J, Li C, Monti S, Vasa P, *et al.* (2001) Classification of human lung carcinomas by mRNA expression profiling reveals distinct adenocarcinoma subclasses. *Proc Natl Acad Sci USA*, Nov 20; 98(24): 13790–5.

83 Beer DG, Kardia SL, Huang CC, Giordano TJ, Levin AM, Misek DE, *et al.* (2002) Gene-expression profiles predict survival of patients with lung adenocarcinoma. *Nat Med*, Aug; 8(8): 816–24.

84 Creighton C, Hanash S, Beer D (2003) Gene expression patterns define pathways correlated with loss of differentiation in lung adenocarcinomas. *FEBS Lett*, Apr 10; 540(1–3): 167–70.

85 Endoh H, Tomida S, Yatabe Y, Konishi H, Osada H, Tajima K, *et al.* (2004) Prognostic model of pulmonary adenocarcinoma by expression profiling of eight genes as determined by quantitative real-time reverse transcriptase polymerase chain reaction. *J Clin Oncol*, Mar 1; 22(5): 811–19.

86 Garber ME, Troyanskaya OG, Schluens K, Petersen S, Thaesler Z, Pacyna-Gengelbach M, *et al.* (2001) Diversity of gene expression in adenocarcinoma of the lung. *Proc Natl Acad Sci USA*, Nov 20; 98(24): 13784–9.

87 Hayes DN, Monti S, Parmigiani G, Gilks CB, Naoki K, Bhattacharjee A, *et al.* (2006) Gene expression profiling reveals reproducible human lung adenocarcinoma subtypes in multiple independent patient cohorts. *J Clin Oncol*, Nov 1; 24(31): 5079–90.

88 Takeuchi T, Tomida S, Yatabe Y, Kosaka T, Osada H, Yanagisawa K, *et al.* (2006) Expression profile-defined classification of lung adenocarcinoma shows close relationship with underlying major genetic changes and clinicopathologic behaviors. *J Clin Oncol*, Apr 10; 24(11): 1679–88.

89 Talbot SG, Estilo C, Maghami E, Sarkaria IS, Pham DK, P Oc, *et al.* (2005) Gene expression profiling allows distinction between primary and metastatic squamous cell carcinomas in the lung. *Cancer Res*, Apr 15; 65(8): 3063–71.

90 Tomida S, Koshikawa K, Yatabe Y, Harano T, Ogura N, Mitsudomi T, *et al.* (2004) Gene expression-based, individualized outcome prediction for surgically treated lung cancer patients. *Oncogene*, Jul 8; 23(31): 5360–70.

91 Yanagisawa K, Shyr Y, Xu BJ, Massion PP, Larsen PH, White BC, *et al.* (2003) Proteomic patterns of tumour subsets in non-small-cell lung cancer. *Lancet*, Aug 9; 362(9382): 433–9.

92 Nanjundan M, Byers LA, Carey MS, Siwak DR, Raso MG, Diao L, *et al.* (2010) Proteomic profiling identifies pathways dysregulated in non-small cell lung cancer and an inverse association of AMPK and adhesion pathways with recurrence. *J Thorac Oncol*, Dec; 5(12): 1894–1904.

93 Wilkerson MD, Yin X, Walter V, Zhao N, Cabanski CR, Hayward MC, *et al.* (2012) Differential pathogenesis of lung adenocarcinoma subtypes involving sequence mutations, copy number, chromosomal instability, and methylation. *PLoS One*, 7(5): e36530.

94 Wilkerson MD, Yin X, Hoadley KA, Liu Y, Hayward MC, Cabanski CR, *et al.* (2010) Lung squamous cell carcinoma mRNA expression subtypes are reproducible, clinically important, and correspond to normal cell types. *Clin Cancer Res*, Oct 1; 16(19): 4864–75.

95 Blackhall FH, Wigle DA, Jurisica I, Pintilie M, Liu N, Darling G, *et al.* (2004) Validating the prognostic value of marker genes derived from a non-small cell lung cancer microarray study. *Lung Cancer*, Nov; 46(2): 197–204.

96 Wigle DA, Jurisica I, Radulovich N, Pintilie M, Rossant J, Liu N, *et al.* (2002) Molecular profiling of non-small cell lung cancer and correlation with disease-free survival. *Cancer Res*, Jun 1; 62(11): 3005–8.

97 Borczuk AC, Gorenstein L, Walter KL, Assaad AA, Wang L, Powell CA (2003) Non-small-cell lung cancer molecular signatures recapitulate lung developmental pathways. *Am J Pathol*, Nov; 163(5): 1949–60.

98 Larsen JE, Pavey SJ, Passmore LH, Bowman R, Clarke BE, Hayward NK, *et al.* (2007) Expression profiling defines a recurrence signature in lung squamous cell carcinoma. *Carcinogenesis*, Mar; 28(3): 760–6.

99 Raponi M, Zhang Y, Yu J, Chen G, Lee G, Taylor JM, *et al.* (2006) Gene expression signatures for predicting prognosis of squamous cell and adenocarcinomas of the lung. *Cancer Res*, Aug 1; 66(15): 7466–72.

100 Yamagata N, Shyr Y, Yanagisawa K, Edgerton M, Dang TP, Gonzalez A, *et al.* (2003) A training-testing approach to the molecular classification of resected non-small cell lung cancer. *Clin Cancer Res*, Oct 15; 9(13): 4695–4704.

101 Xie Y, Xiao G, Coombes KR, Behrens C, Solis LM, Raso G, *et al.* (2011) Robust gene expression signature from formalin-fixed paraffin-embedded samples predicts prognosis of non-small-cell lung cancer patients. *Clin Cancer Res*, Sep 1; 17(17): 5705–14.

102 Zhu CQ, Ding K, Strumpf D, Weir BA, Meyerson M, Pennell N, *et al.* (2010) Prognostic and predictive gene signature for adjuvant chemotherapy in resected non-small-cell lung cancer. *J Clin Oncol*, Oct 10; 28(29): 4417–24.

103 Weiss J, Sos ML, Seidel D, Peifer M, Zander T, Heuckmann JM, *et al.* (2010) Frequent and focal FGFR1 amplification associates with therapeutically tractable FGFR1 dependency in squamous cell lung cancer. *Sci Transl Med*, Dec 15; 2(62): 62ra93.

104 Fernandez P, Carretero J, Medina PP, Jimenez AI, Rodriguez-Perales S, Paz MF, *et al.* (2004) Distinctive gene expression of human lung adenocarcinomas carrying LKB1 mutations. *Oncogene*, Jun 24; 23(29): 5084–91.

105 Sanchez-Cespedes M, Parrella P, Esteller M, Nomoto S, Trink B, Engles JM, *et al.* (2002) Inactivation of LKB1/STK11 is a common event in adenocarcinomas of the lung. *Cancer Res*, Jul 1; 62(13): 3659–62.

106 Sequist LV, Waltman BA, Dias-Santagata D, Digumarthy S, Turke AB, Fidias P, *et al.* (2011) Genotypic and histological evolution of lung cancers acquiring resistance to EGFR inhibitors. *Sci Transl Med*, Mar 23; 3(75): 75ra26.

107 Zhang Z, Lee JC, Lin L, Olivas V, Au V, LaFramboise T, *et al.* (2012) Activation of the AXL kinase causes resistance to EGFR-targeted therapy in lung cancer. *Nat Genet*, Aug; 44(8): 852–60.

108 Paik PK, Johnson ML, D'Angelo SP, Sima CS, Ang D, Dogan S, *et al.* (2012) Driver mutations determine survival in smokers and never-smokers with stage IIIB/IV lung adenocarcinomas. *Cancer*, Dec 1; 118(23): 5840–7.

CHAPTER 4

Somatic Genome Alterations in Human Lung Cancers

Marcin Imielinski,[1] Peter S. Hammerman,[1] Roman Thomas,[2] and Matthew Meyerson[1]
[1]Broad Institute of Harvard and MIT, Cambridge, MA, USA
[2]Department of Translational Genomics, Center of Integrated Oncology Köln – Bonn, University of Köln, Köln, Germany

Lung cancer genetics overview

While this chapter will review the unique genomic alterations found in lung adenocarcinomas, lung squamous cell carcinomas and small cell lung carcinomas, respectively, we begin by discussing some general features that are common to the genomes of lung cancers – notably the high somatic mutation rates, the relative rarity of familial or germline causation, and the identification of oncogenic driver mutations that provide targets for genome-directed therapies.

Lung cancers are characterized by unusually high rates of somatic mutation (those mutations found only in the tumor cells and not in the germline or other cells or tissues), high levels of inter- and intra-chromosomal rearrangement, and frequent chromosome arm level and focal copy number alterations [1–5]. Along with melanomas, lung cancers exhibit the highest frequency of somatic mutations [5, 6] – these two cancer types are those most clearly caused by DNA-damaging mutagens, ultraviolet radiation in the case of melanoma and tobacco-smoke derived carcinogens in the case of lung cancer.

In addition, lung carcinomas have been at the heart of the revolution in genomically targeted therapies for cancer. For lung adenocarcinoma, therapies that target tumors with mutations in the epidermal growth factor receptor tyrosine kinase gene, *EGFR* [7–9], and the anaplastic lymphoma kinase gene, *ALK* [10–12], have proven highly effective. For lung squamous cell carcinoma, the identification of multiple targetable alterations now promises the potential of direct therapeutic targeting as well. Finally, for small cell lung carcinoma, comprehensive profiling has identified a number of recurrent genomic alterations, but clear paths to targeted tharpy are less apparent in most cases.

For all types of lung carcinoma, systematic genomic studies have been both confirming known genomic alterations and revealing new ones. Beyond the protein kinase signal transduction pathways and common *TP53* mutations and aneuploidy, these include recurrent mutations in cell cycle genes and in chromatin modifiers and splicing factors. Understanding the role of each of these types of pathways in lung cancers will be important for the development of future targeted therapies, while the understanding of the high mutational burden of lung carcinomas may contribute to the development of immune-modulatory therapies.

Lung Cancer, Fourth Edition. Edited by Jack A. Roth, Waun Ki Hong and Ritsuko U. Komaki.

Lung adenocarcinoma genomics

Lung adenocarcinoma is the most common subtype of lung cancer and ranks as one of the best genetically characterized human epithelial malignancies. In recent years, discoveries regarding the somatic genetic features of lung adenocarcinoma have been translated into targeted therapies that routinely impact patient care.

The characterization of somatic alterations in lung cancer, as in other tumor types, has proceeded in roughly three historical phases. The first phase leveraged insight from cytogenetics, tumor virology, and pedigree analysis. These early studies employed transformation, cloning, and targeted sequencing approaches to implicate specific genetic alterations in lung tumorigenesis, including mutations in Ras family genes (*KRAS, NRAS, HRAS*), *TP53,* and *CDKN2A,* among others [13–21]. The sequencing of the human genome in 2001 [22, 23] greatly improved the feasibility of targeted molecular genetic analyses, heralding a second wave of discoveries, including therapy-sensitizing mutations in *EGFR* [24–26], oncogenic *ERBB2* [27] and *BRAF* [28–30] mutations, *ALK* fusions [31, 32], and truncating mutations in *STK11* [33] and *SMARCA4* [34, 35].

During the past decade, the advent of high-throughput molecular genetic technologies, including microarrays and massively parallel sequencing, has revolutionized cancer genomics [36–40]. This third phase of investigation has involved large-scale surveys of somatic alterations that yield global spectra of gene expression, copy number alteration, rearrangement, and/or mutation across many lung adenocarcinoma tumor samples [41–47]. This is highlighted most recently by studies employing massively parallel sequencing to analyze the exomes, genomes, and transcriptomes of lung adenocarcinoma tumor-normal pairs [2, 3, 44, 48–52].

Genome-wide studies provide compendia of molecular features for pathological tumor classification and serve as unbiased screens for recurrent alterations that have previously evaded hypothesis-based investigation. Discoveries made during this third phase include focal amplifications in the lineage-specific transcription factor gene *NKX2–1* [45, 47, 53, 54], recurrent fusions involving the receptor tyrosine kinase genes *RET* and *ROS1* [31, 48, 55–58], and the discovery of genetic alterations in genes and pathways not previously known to be mutated in cancer (*U2AF1, RBM10, ARID1A, SETD2*) [3, 49].

Molecular alteration spectra of lung adenocarcinoma

The molecular alteration burden in lung adenocarcinomas is among the highest found in human cancer. This is apparent whether one examines the frequency of somatic mutations, broad and focal copy number alterations, rearrangements, or gene expression changes. Lung adenocarcinomas harbor on average 12 somatic mutations (substitutions or small insertions/deletions) per exonic megabase [2, 3, 50], an estimated 26 regions of recurrent arm level amplification or deletion (spanning over half of the genome) and an estimated 31 regions of recurrent focal copy gain or loss [47], and 98 detectable rearrangement breakpoints.

This genetic complexity of lung adenocarcinoma poses a challenge in differentiating between alterations that are causal for carcinogenesis (i.e., "drivers") and those that are bystanders to the underlying alteration mechanism (i.e., "passengers"). Virtually all known mechanisms of cancer gene activation and inactivation have been shown to play a role in lung adenocarcinoma: Lung adenocarcinoma genes may accumulate abnormal numbers of truncating mutations (e.g., *NF1*) [44] or hotspots of mutation around particular codons (e.g., *KRAS G12V*) [59]. They may be often focally amplified to a high copy number (e.g., *NKX2–1*) [45, 47, 53, 54] or frequently homozygously deleted (e.g., *PTEN*) [47, 60]. They may undergo recurrent genetic fusions that retain an important catalytic domain of the encoded protein (e.g., *ALK*) [31, 32]. They may be transcriptionally silenced through promoter methylation (e.g., *CDKN2A*), alternatively spliced (e.g., *MET*), or upregulated through the aberrant activity of a transcription factor (e.g., *MYC*). Notwithstanding these important examples, the majority of genetic alterations in lung adenocarcinoma, particularly those at the DNA level, are thought to be neutral. Statistical analyses of genome-wide data must be exquisitely calibrated to differentiate between these neutral changes and those that undergo somatic selection in the tumor [3].

Global molecular spectra can be used to group lung adenocarcinoma cases into subtypes and generate complex signatures that predict patient outcome. This approach has been pioneered with microarray-based gene expression profiling. The earliest such analyses employed unsupervised clustering to group lung adenocarcinoma cases into subsets, with the observation that the resulting clusters displayed distinct survival and histopathological features [41, 43, 61]. A comprehensive analysis grouped lung adenocarcinoma into three reproducible gene-expression based groups: bronchioid, squamoid, and magnoid [62]. Additional studies have employed supervised approaches to define gene-expression based prognostic classifiers. Among these, Shedden *et al.*, used a multisite blinded retrospective analysis of 442 cases to identify a robust gene-expression based predictor of patient overall-survival [46]. This signature employed the expression of hundreds of genes involved in pathways mediating cellular proliferation, differentiation, and immunologic function to differentiate between aggressive and indolent lung adenocarcinoma cases. The signature was most effective when used in tandem with clinical and pathological covariates.

Similar approaches have been applied to group lung adenocarcinoma cases with respect to DNA alteration-based features, such as point mutations. For example, smokers and never-smokers are readily distinguished on the basis of total or context-specific mutation somatic substitution rates. On average, lung adenocarcinomas arising in never-smokers harbor an order of magnitude fewer mutations than those in smokers, the majority of which cytosine deaminations at CpG dinucleotides (C[pG]→T). In contrast, tumors arising in heavy smokers preferentially contain C→A transversions, both in and outside of the CpG context [2, 3]. C→A are thought to arise from polycycline amine hydrocarbon adducts in tobacco smoke [63]. Smokers and never-smokers also differ distinctly with regard to the pattern of "driver" sequence alterations (discussed below), leading some to posit that these represent distinct disease entities [64]. Lung adenocarcinomas from never-smokers preferentially harbor kinase domain mutations in *EGFR* and *ERBB2* and rearrangements in *ALK, RET,* and *ROS1,* while lung adenocarcinomas from smokers often harbor *KRAS, TP53,* and *STK11* mutations.

Key genetic alterations in lung adenocarcinoma in a few selected pathways

The key genetic alterations in lung adenocarcinoma (and other tumor types) have been identified on the basis of their recurrence in clinical patient samples and (for most) a demonstrated role in experimental models of cancer [36, 37, 65–67]. Such models include benign and malignant cell lines that are engineered to over-express the mutant form of a gene or undergo knockdown, and assayed for proliferation or anchorage independent growth in cell culture or xenograft formation in nude mice. These models also include genetically engineered mice in which mutated genes are stably integrated into the germline genome and expressed constitutively, inducibly, or under the guidance of tissue specific promoters, following which specific phenotypes (e.g., decreased tumor latency) are observed. For many of these key alterations, pathways have been elucidated that mechanistically link specific genetic perturbations to biochemical models of cellular processes, such as growth, motility, and apoptosis. In a subset of cases, therapies have been developed that target these altered pathways and yield significant clinical response in lung adenocarcinoma patients – most notably inhibitors of mutated EGFR [7, 8, 68] and translocated ALK [10–12].

Proliferation circuits

Growth and proliferation are exquisitely regulated cellular processes that are constitutively activated in malignancy [36, 37, 65–67]. Lung adenocarcinomas activate these circuits through the mitogen activated kinase pathway (MAPK), the PI(3)-K / mTOR pathway, and through the amplification of c-Myc. These pathways have been of considerable interest as therapeutic targets in lung adenocarcinoma, where a few have met significant success [69–71].

The MAPK pathway regulates proliferation in benign cells in response to extracellular ligand binding, which causes homo- or hetero- dimerization of receptor tyrosine kinase monomers. This triggers a signaling cascade through the small G-protein Ras and the Raf, Mek, and Erk serine-threonine kinases.

In North America 10–20% of lung adenocarcinoma cases (and 30–50% of cases in Asia) harbor kinase domain somatic mutations in the receptor tyrosine kinase gene *EGFR* (epidermal growth factor receptor) [24–26,72]. The vast majority of these comprise exon 18 nucleotide binding loop mutations (G719A), frame-preserving exon 19 deletions near the ELREA motif at amino acid 746, frame-preserving exon 20 insertions, and exon 21 activation loop point mutations (L858R), most of which result in increased or constitutive kinase activation. These *EGFR* mutations correlate exquisitely with sensitivity to targeted EGFR inhibition through the small-molecules erlotinib and gefitinib [24–26], with the exception of the exon 20 insertion mutations [73]. Focal amplification of *EGFR* is often seen both in conjunction and in the absence of EGFR kinase domain mutations; however, amplification does not correlate with sensitivity to either small molecule (e.g., erlotinib) or antibody-based (e.g., cetuximab) anti-EGFR therapy.

The related tyrosine kinase genes *ERBB2* (v-erb-b2 erythroblastic leukemia viral oncogene homolog 2), also harbors point mutations and frame-preserving deletions in its extracellular and kinase domains in another 2–3% of lung adenocarcinoma cases [27, 44, 74]. There has not yet been any clinical correlation between the status of these mutations and response to anti-Erbb2 antibodies (trastuzumab) or small molecule Erbb2 inhibition (lapatanib, neratinib, or afatinib), though initial cell line evidence has demonstrated response [74–77].

Receptor tyrosine kinase gene rearrangements affect 3–8% of lung adenocarcinoma patients, primarily never-smokers [31, 32, 48, 55–58]. The 3′ regions of tyrosine kinases *ALK* (anaplastic lymphoma kinase), *RET* (ret proto-oncogene), and *ROS1* undergo recurrent rearrangements that preserve the kinase domain and fuse to at least 6 different genes as their 5′ binding partners, including *EML4, CCD6,* and *KIF5B* [31,32,48,55–58]. The proteins encoded by the 5′ fusion partners of these genes engage in spontaneous homo-dimerization as part of their normal cellular function, which implies a mechanism for the oncogenicity of their fusion protein product. Patients whose tumors harbor *ALK* fusions show a dramatic response to ALK inhibition via crizotinib [11], which has also been shown to have preliminary efficacy in patients harboring *ROS1* rearrangements [55]. Preliminary studies of *RET1* fusions in lung cancer cell lines have demonstrated sensitivity to several kinase inhibitors, including the RET specific small-molecule vandetanib [57].

The most common mechanism for MAPK pathway activation in lung adenocarcinoma from smokers is through substitution mutations in 12th, 13th, and 61st amino acids of the Ras family gene [14, 16, 17, 78, 79]. This occurs predominantly through *KRAS* (20–30%) but also through *NRAS* and *HRAS* (<1–2%). Ras proteins are cellular switches that exist in the inactive GDP-bound and the active GTP-bound state, the latter which is stabilized through hotspot mutations that abolish Ras's intrinsic GTP-ase activity. There are no current targeted therapies that are clinically effective against mutated Ras, despite initial attempts using farnesyltransferase inhibitors and ongoing trials involving small molecule inhibition of the downstream protein Mek [80].

Constitutive Ras activation in lung adenocarcinoma can occur through the mutational inactivation or deletion of *NF1*. *NF1* encodes one of the key GTP-ase activating proteins that converts Ras into its inactive GDP bound state [81]. Deletions and truncating mutations in *NF1* occur in 10–20% of lung adenocarcinoma cases, and predominantly in smokers [3, 44, 49].

BRAF encodes the first direct effector of Ras in the MAPK pathway and is mutated in 5–10% of lung adenocarcinoma at two hotspots encoding the glycine-rich loop near residue 469 (G469) and the activation segment near residue 600 (V600E) [3, 28, 30, 44, 49]. Though V600E mutations have been associated with therapeutic sensitivity to the mutant-specific B-raf inhibitor vemurafenib in melanoma [82,83], such a response has yet to be clinically demonstrated in *BRAF* mutant lung adenocarcinomas. The remaining two kinases in the core MAPK signaling cascade are rarely mutated in lung adenocarcinoma, though activating *MEK* mutations (p.K57N) have been previously described in this disease (<1%) [84] Other recurrent MAPK pathway mutations that have been reported include splicing mutations in *MET* [52,85], point mutations in the Ntrk gene family (*NTRK1*, *NTRK2*, *NTRK3*), and point mutations in *PTPN11* [44,52,86].

Receptor tyrosine kinases activate a second intracellular signaling pathway mediated by the lipid kinase PI(3)-K [87, 88]. This pathway comprises a highly conserved eukaryotic mechanism for growth control under fluctuating nutrient conditions, which synapses on the mammalian target of rapamycin (mTOR) [89]. *PIK3CA*, which encodes the 110-kD catalytic subunit of PI(3)-K, is mutated or focally amplified in 5–10% of lung adenocarcinomas [3,44,49]. The majority of mutations cluster at two hotspots in exon 9 and exon 20, causing constitutive kinase activity and production of second messenger molecules PtdIns(3,4,5)P_3, which activate downstream effector, Akt.

A second mechanism of PI(3)-K pathway activation in lung adenocarcinomas is through the deletion or mutational inactivation of the phosphatase and tensin homologue Pten [3, 44, 47, 49]. Pten is a lipid phosphatase that results in PtdIns(3,4,5)P_3 hydrolysis, reversing the reaction catalyzed by PI(3)K. *PTEN* deletion or mutational inactivation is seen in 2–8% of lung adenocarcinomas. Akt, the downstream effector of PI(3)-K, harbors rare constitutively activating N-terminal mutations at a hotspot around Glutamic Acid 17 (E17K) in <1% of lung adenocarcinoma cases [44,49]. The oncogenic effect of Akt activation is thought to be mediated through mTOR, whose activity is antagonized through the drug rapamycin and its chemical derivatives. Clinical trials employing pharmaceutical inhibition of *PIK3CA* and *PTEN* mutant lung adenocarcinomas using small molecular inhibitors against PI(3)K, Akt, or mTOR, are currently in progress [90].

Of lung adenocarcinomas 5–15% harbor focal or high level amplification of *MYC* [3, 47, 91]. *MYC* encodes a transcription factor, c-Myc, classically associated with the initiation of cellular proliferation and survival programs immediately following serum reconstitution in cell culture [65, 66]. The biological role of c-Myc has since been demonstrated to be much broader: it is implicated in the direct regulation of as many as 15% of all human genes and recently suggested to be a "global amplifier" of transcription [92]. c-Myc is also one of the key transcriptional effectors downstream of the MAPK pathway, though *MYC* amplifications are not mutually exclusive with MAPK pathway mutations [3].

Cell cycle and *TP53* circuits

The most frequently mutated gene in lung adenocarcinoma (and in human cancer) is *TP53* [3,44,49]. *TP53* encodes a transcription factor that promotes cell death and cell cycle arrest in response to DNA damage, hypoxia, and metabolic stress [93]. Genes upregulated by TP53 also catalyze DNA repair, promote autophagy, block glycolysis, promote mitochondrial respiration, reduces levels of reactive oxygen species, and promotes stem cell differentiation. Over 50% of lung adenocarcinoma harbor truncating, splice site, or missense mutations in *TP53* [3, 44, 49]. Lung adenocarcinomas lacking *TP53* mutations often harbor alterations in proteins that directly engage TP53: 7–10% of lung adenocarcinomas harbor mutations of *ATM* [3, 44, 49], which encodes a DNA damage sensor and cell cycle checkpoint kinase that activates TP53 through phosphorylation; 6–8% of cases harbor focal or high level amplifications in *MDM2* [47], which encodes an E3 ubiquitin ligase that targets *TP53* for degradation. Though the ubiquity of direct or indirect genetic lesions of *TP53* in lung adenocarcinoma makes it an attractive therapeutic target, the development of drugs directed against this pathway has been challenging. Efforts to either restore *TP53* function (through gene reconstitution or native protein conformation stabilization) or target synthetic lethal vulnerabilities (e.g., G2 checkpoint abrogation) in *TP53* mutant tumors have not met widespread clinical success.

The cell cycle machinery upon which TP53 synapses is often dysregulated by somatic genetic alterations that inhibit the protein Rb. In its unphosphorylated state, Rb is a transcriptional repressor of genes that mediate G1 cell cycle progression [65–67]. *RB1,* the gene encoding Rb is mutated in 3–4% of lung adenocarcinomas and a target of copy number loss in another 10–20% of cases [3, 44, 47]. More frequently, Rb is inactivated through the genetic loss of p16/CDKN2A, which promotes G1 cell cycle arrest by inhibiting Rb phosphorylation. *CDKN2A* is lost or mutationally inactivated in 10–30% of lung adenocarcinomas, including via truncating or missense mutations in 5% of cases [3, 18, 19, 44, 47]. Conversely, the amplification of *CDK4, CCND1,* and *CCNE1* (10–20% of cases) [47] promote Rb phosphorylation and G1 cell cycle progression. Rb is also believed to integrate upstream extracellular growth suppression signals from the TGF-Beta pathway, which are genetically silenced through the mutation of *SMAD4* in 2–4% of lung adenocarcinoma cases [3].

Viability circuits

The most frequent focal copy number alteration in lung adenocarcinoma is the amplification of *NKX2–1* (10–20% of cases) [45, 47, 53, 54]. *NKX2–1* (also referred to as *TITF1*) resides on chr 14q13.3 and encodes a transcription factor that is essential for the development of type II pneumocytes, which line alveoli of the lung. These features suggest that *NKX2–1* may be a lineage-specific survival factor. Initial cell-line experiments implicated *NKX2–1* as necessary for anchorage independent growth in lung cancer cell lines expressing *NKX2–1,* supporting its putative role as an oncogene. However, recent data from a transgenic mouse model suggests that in certain contexts *NKX2–1* may behave as a lung cancer tumor suppressor gene [94].

Another viability circuit that is genetically activated in lung adenocarcinoma mediates survival under oxidative stress. *KEAP1* encodes a cysteine-rich redox sensor protein that binds the transcription factor NRF2 and targets it for proteosomal degradation [95]. Oxidative stress disrupts KEAP1-NRF2 binding, resulting in NRF2 translocation to the nucleus and transcription of genes promoting survival under stress. *KEAP1* mutations are frequent in lung adenocarcinoma (11% of cases) [3, 49, 96], and presumably disrupt the KEAP1-NRF2 complex and promote survival under conditions of oxidative stress. Mutations in *KEAP1* and the *NFE2L2* gene are even more common in squamous cell lung carcinomas, as described below [1, 97]. Despite the extensive evidence showing *KEAP1* to be a mutational target in lung cancer and other tumor types, the tumorigenicity of *KEAP1* variants remain to be demonstrated in cellular or animal cancer models.

Motility circuits

One of the more common sequence alterations in lung adenocarcinoma is mutational loss of serine-threonine protein kinase 11 (also known as Lkb1) [33]. Truncating mutations and deletions targeting *STK11* occur in 15–35% of lung adenocarcinomas, and are predominantly found in smokers [3, 49]. STK11 is necessary for the catalytic activity of a family of 14 structurally related Lkb1-dependent kinases that mediate cell metabolism, growth, and polarity [98]. These targets include AMPK, a multi-functional protein kinase that inhibits mTOR, and SIK1, which mediates anoikis (apoptosis by cell detachment) through TP53 dependent pathways. *STK11* knockdown accelerates tumorigenesis and metastasis in *KRAS* mutant mouse models of NSCLC [99]. These results suggest that *STK11* loss acts in concert with other genetic lesions to modulate invasion, metastasis, and differentiation programs at various stages of lung tumorigenesis.

The APC pathway links cellular adhesion signals to growth and proliferation [100]. This pathway is targeted in lung adenocarcinoma through activating mutations in *CTNNB1* (encoding beta-catenin) and truncating mutations and deletions in *APC* (adenomatous polyposis coli). Beta-catenin is normally sequestered at adhesion junctions or targeted for degradation by an APC-containing "destruction complex" through phosphorylation at four N-terminal serine/threonine residues. *CTNNB1* mutations (1–2% of cases) at one of these residues (e.g., p.S37) or loss-of-function alterations in APC (3–5% of cases) are recurrently found in lung adenocarcinoma [3, 44, 49]. These alterations are predicted to enable beta-catenin translocation into the nucleus and activation of transcriptional programs promoting invasion, metastasis, and proliferation.

Epigenetic modifier pathways

Epigenetic modifiers, as a gene class, have recently been shown to be recurrently mutated in lung adenocarcinoma and other tumor types [101, 102]. 10% of lung adenocarcinomas harbor truncating and/or missense mutations in *SMARCA4*, which encodes an ATPase subunit of the SWI / SNF complex (also called BRG1) [34, 35]. SWI/SNF complexes contribute to both silencing and activation of target genes, including genes in pathways mediating cell cycle checkpoint control, cell migration, proliferation, and embryonic stem cell programs. *SMARCA4* knockout increases the number and size of tumors in a carcinogen-induced mouse model of lung cancer [103]. Recently, lung adenocarcinomas have been shown to harbor truncating or missense mutations in another SWI/SNF complex gene *ARID1A* (10%) and the histone demethylase gene *SETD2* (13%) [3]. RNA binding proteins are another gene class to recently emerge as significantly mutated in genome-wide somatic mutation scans. *U2AF1* encodes a core member of the U2 spliceosome and is recurrently mutated at a single codon (p.S34F) in 3–5% of lung adenocarcinomas [3] as well as over 50% of certain myelodysplastic syndrome subtypes [104]. *RBM10* is a less well characterized RNA binding protein targeted by truncating and missense mutations in 7% of lung adenocarcinomas. *RBM10, U2AF1, SETD2,* and *ARID1A* variants have yet to be validated in a cell-line or animal model of cancer. Furthermore, the biochemical mechanism through which these epigenetic and splicing modifiers impact carcinogenesis remains to be fully elucidated.

Genetic correlates of sensitivity and resistance

The era of targeted therapy in lung adenocarcinoma was instantiated in 2004 following the correlation of *EGFR* mutations with erlotinib sensitivity [24, 26, 105]. The subsequent link between *ALK* fusions and crizotinib sensitivity in 2010 gave additional momentum to the targeted treatment paradigm [10–12]. Ongoing trials employing agents targeted against BRAF, HER2, PI3 Kinase, AKT, MEK, and MET (among others) are imminently poised to extend this approach to additional patient subgroups [106].

A key caveat in the widespread application of targeted therapy in cancer is drug resistance [69]. Patients receiving EGFR inhibitors receive an indisputable survival benefit, however their tumor invariably returns, often harboring a novel change in somatic genotype and/or histology [107]. In about half of patients, this relapsed tumor harbors a second site mutation in *EGFR* converting the "gatekeeper" residue p.T790 to a methionine and inhibiting drug binding [108, 109]. Smaller subsets of patients acquire novel alterations, including *MET* amplifications [110]. An intriguing subset of patients (14%) show conversion to a small-cell lung cancer phenotype, which reverts to lung adenocarcinoma histology following small-cell chemotherapy [107]. A similar phenomenon has been observed with second site mutations in the ALK gene following crizotinib therapy (p.C1196M, C1156Y), however the spectrum of resistance alterations in the ALK / crizotinib setting has yet to be fully explored [111–113].

These examples suggest that the next era in cancer molecular genetics (and targeted therapy) may involve multiple snapshots of a "dynamic genotype" that evolves through several treatment cycles. Tumor genomes subjected to novel selective pressures induced by targeted agents will evolve novel (and possibly recurrent) patterns of alteration that may require treatment with alternate classes of drugs. Lung adenocarcinoma patients of the future may expect to receive multiple longitudinal biopsies and complex cocktails of targeted agents specifically designed to prevent the emergence of resistance. Clinical cancer genetics, which has been mostly a static and observational science, will need to evolve dynamic predictive models to account for the somatic evolutionary consequences of tailored drug treatments [114].

Germline predisposition

The discussion of lung cancer genetics is primarily focused on somatic genetic alterations that develop during a patient's lifetime. Until recently, not much was known regarding genetic mediators of inherited lung cancer risk. Genome wide association studies (GWAS) employing high density single nucleotide polymorphism (SNP) arrays on large retrospective series of cases and controls have been recently used to probe the common variant inheritance of many complex inherited diseases, including many cancer types [115, 116].

GWAS's performed on European populations have yielded three loci (15q25.1, 5p15.33, and 6p21.33) demonstrating reproducible clusters of association across multiple independent cohorts. The genes associated with these loci include *CHRNA5, CHRNA3,* and *CHRNB4* (15q25.1), *TERT* and *CLPTM1L* (5p15.33), and *BAT3-MSH5* (6p21.33) [117–122]. Genes associated with 15q25.1 encode nicotinic acetylcholine receptor subunits that are expressed in neuronal and alveolar cells and known to bind nicotine and its derivatives. Variants in this region were previously associated with nicotine addiction, though the impact of these variants on lung cancer susceptibility were shown to be independent of smoking behavior.

GWAS's performed on East Asian populations have identified additional population specific risk loci in addition to those susceptibility regions found in European populations: GWAS's in Korean and Japanese populations have associated three loci: 3q28 (near *TP63*), 17q24 (near *BPTF*), and 6p21.3 (near *BTNL2*), that appear to be population specific [123, 124]. GWAS's in Han Chinese population have identified additional loci at 13q12.12 (near *MIPEP* and *TNFRSF19*) and 22q12.2 (near *MTMR3, HORMAD2, LIF*) [125]. One of the most compelling phenomena in lung cancer genetics is the increased risk of east Asian never-smokers, in particular females, to develop lung adenocarcinomas, in particular those harboring activating somatic *EGFR* mutations. The contrasting landscape of genetic lung cancer susceptibility between European and East Asian populations suggests that a complex and yet uncharacterized interplay between the germline and somatic genome may play a role in this phenomenon.

Unlike Mendelian predisposition alleles, common variants nominated by GWAS studies tend to have a weak prognostic effects and in many cases are only correlated to a causal (and likely rare) inherited allele. Further fine-mapping around existing loci and next-generation sequencing based GWAS's will further expand the knowledge of germline lung adenocarcinoma predisposition.

Future directions

The age of next-generation sequencing and large statistically powered case-series is poised to greatly illuminate the understanding of lung adenocarcinoma genetics. Increased power to detect rare "driver" alterations through the analysis of large clinically annotated sample sets and correlations of alteration patterns across many tumor types will greatly enrich this knowledge. The correlation and mutual exclusivity of DNA-based alterations with each other in large sample sets will provide an important signal to untangle cooperating and redundant cancer pathways. Large scale analyses of methylation, histone modification, and mRNA and microRNA expression, such as those carried out by The Cancer Genome Atlas in conjunction with sequencing studies [1, 126–128], will shed light on the role of these additional sources of somatic genetic variation in lung adenocarcinomagenesis. The correlation of molecular features with the recently revised histopathological subclassification of lung adenocarcinoma [129] will improve diagnostic paradigms and generate important biological insight. Longitudinal analyses of molecular genetic changes in the context of multiple rounds of novel targeted therapeutics will impact the understanding of treatment resistance and somatic evolution. Next-generation sequencing based germline association studies may yield further insight into the inherited susceptibility of lung adenocarcinoma. These insights will be bolstered through the development of novel targeted therapeutics and more efficient approaches for screening variants in cellular and animal models of cancers.

Lung squamous cell carcinoma genomics

Introduction and overview of genomic alterations of lung SqCCs

Lung squamous cell carcinoma (lung SqCC) is the second most commonly diagnosed subtype of non-small cell lung cancer (NSCLC). It is thought to originate in the proximal airways through a process of squamous metaplasia secondary to chronic airway injury, typically the result of tobacco smoke [130]. Squamous epithelial cells are not normally resident in the adult lung and the molecular events which drive metaplasia are only recently beginning to be described [130, 131]. Lung SqCC can be distinguished from other subtypes of NSCLC by a combination of morphology and immunohistochemical analysis with a typical staining pattern of TTF1 negativity and p40/p63 positivity. Until recently it was unclear whether specific molecular features distinguished lung SqCCs from other lung cancer subtypes; however, several studies have now provided definitive evidence that squamous cell carcinoma is a distinct entity from lung adenocarcinoma and small cell carcinoma and more closely resembles squamous cell carcinomas of the head and neck than other lung cancer subtypes [1]. While the use of targeted therapeutic agents has not been as successful in lung SqCC as compared to lung adenocarcinoma, the recent comprehensive description of the molecular features of lung SqCCs provides hope that personalized treatment of this disease will be achievable in the near future.

Squamous cell carcinoma, like other subtypes of lung cancer, is strongly associated with tobacco exposure. Prior studies of cohorts of lung SqCC patients have reported rates of smoking in patients with this disease in excess of 90% [132]. In contrast to lung adenocarcinoma, no large studies of non-smokers with lung SqCCs have been reported and it is not known whether there are specific genomic alterations found in nonsmokers with this disease. Furthermore, large studies comparing patients from different ethnic backgrounds with lung SqCCs have not been published, and it is not clear if there will be significant differences in molecular features based on ethnic background in lung SqCCs as there are in adenocarcinoma.

Lung SqCCs are defined by a substantial degree of genomic complexity. The Cancer Genome Atlas Network (TCGA) reported that lung SqCCs display among the highest rates of somatic mutation, copy number alteration and gene rearrangements of all epithelial tumor types [1]. This observation presents a challenge to identification of which alterations described in lung SqCCs are the most critical for cancer development and therapeutics.

Gene expression

Microarray profiling of cohorts of non-small cell lung cancers by several groups demonstrated that gene expression profiles of lung SqCCs are distinct from lung adenocarcinoma [43, 46, 61, 133]. Furthermore, lung SqCCs could be separated by gene expression profiles into distinct subtypes with different biologic and clinical characteristics and which represent different cell types and differentiation states of the normal lung [134]. These subtypes have been reproduced in more recent studies using RNA sequencing and are associated with specific genomic alterations. For example, the most common expression subtype, the "classical" type, is associated with amplification of chromosome 3q26 (including *SOX2*, *PIK3CA* and *TP63)*, mutation of *NFE2L2* and *KEAP1* and a high degree of CpG promoter methylation when compared to the other three expression subtypes [1]. In contrast, alterations of *FGFR* family kinases, *RB1* and *PTEN* were more associated with other expression subtypes. Several studies have reported gene expression signatures associated with patient outcome in lung SqCCs; however, validation of these data by independent groups has demonstrated that developing clinical predictors with gene expression data alone remains challenging.

Somatic copy number alterations

SNP array and aCGH analysis of lung SqCCs has demonstrated that SqCCs harbor complex and distinct copy number profiles when compared to lung adenocarcinomas. Lung SqCCs also share recurrent regions of gene amplification and deletion with squamous cell carcinomas from other tissue types such as the skin and cervix [42]. Lung SqCCs are characterized and distinct from lung adenocarcinomas in amplification of 3q26, where the transcription factor *SOX2* has been shown to play a critical role in squamous differentiation, 8p11–12, a region containing *FGFR1* and *WHSC1L1* and 7p11, where the *EGFR* gene is located [135–140]. [135–140]*SOX2* and *FGFR1* are essential genes in a subset of lung SqCC cell lines [135, 136, 140] and anti-*FGFR1* therapies are being pursued clinically [141]. Other regions of gene amplification in lung SqCCs include the *PDGFRA, CCND1, MYC, CDK6, BCL2L1, MDM2* and *NFE2L2* loci [1]. *CDKN2A* and *PTEN* deletion have been commonly observed [1].

Somatic mutations

Early Sanger sequencing studies of lung SqCCs identified recurrent mutations in the tumor suppressor TP53 [21, 142] and the oncogene NFE2L2 [97]. In addition, focused seqeuncing studies suggested a lack of frequent mutations in lung SqCC in EGFR or KRAS [143], which are commonly observed events in lung adenocarcinoma [14, 24–26, 59]. More comprehensive profiling by Sanger sequencing of all tyrosine kinases demonstrated that the DDR2 kinase is mutated in 3–4% of lung SqCCs [144]. DDR2 is known to be the target of several kinase inhibitors and trials of anti-DDR2 therapy are ongoing. Sequencing of lung SqCCs by DNA mismatch repair technology identified recurrent mutations of TP53, NFE2L2, KEAP1, BAI3, FBXW7, GRM8, MUC16, RUNX1T1, STK11 and ERBB4, several of which demonstrated statistical evidence of mutational enrichment in lung SqCCs [49].

Whole-exome and whole genome sequencing studies of lung SqCCs have only recently begun to be reported. The Cancer Genome Atlas Research Network (TCGA) completed whole-exome sequencing of 178 lung SqCCs and whole-genome sequencing of 19 tumor/normal pairs [1]. The analysis revealed that lung SqCCs display a high rate of somatic mutations with a median rate of 8.4 mutations per sequenced megabase (Mb). Mutations were most commonly observed at CpG sites (20.6/Mb) as compared to non-CpG sites and there was an enrichment for transversion mutations, as has been reported for tobacco-associated lung adenocarcinomas [2, 3] and small cell lung carcinomas [4, 5, 145] as well.

As in lung adenocarcinoma, the majority of genes in the genome were found to be mutated in one or more cases in this study of lung SqCC, presenting a challenge for discovery of genes which are the most important in the biology of lung SqCCs. To this end, statistical analysis was applied to the dataset to identify genes displaying rates of mutation above which would be expected by chance given the background mutation rate of a gene. This analysis identified 10 genes which displayed statistical enrichment for mutation and clear evidence of expression in the studied tumors: *TP53, CDKN2A, PTEN, PIK3CA, KEAP1, MLL2, HLA-A, NFE2L2, NOTCH1* and *RB1* [1]. Additional statistical analysis demonstrated that other genes also displayed enrichment for mutation and included *FAM123B (WTX), HRAS, FBXW7, SMARCA4, NF1, SMAD4, EGFR, APC, TSC1, BRAF, TNFAIP3* and *CREBBP*. Importantly, no instances of *EGFR* L858R or exon 19 deletion mutations were identified though the report documented two cases of *EGFR* L861Q mutations. *KRAS* mutations were notably rare as well. Mutations in *BRAF* did reach statistical significance though no position 600 mutations were identified, raising the issue of whether these mutations are therapeutically important [1].

Whole genome sequencing confirmed the high degree of genomic complexity of lung SqCCs and documented a high rate of genomic rearrangements with an average of 165 per studied tumor, a number comparable to the rate in smokers with lung adenocarcinoma. No recurrent fusion events involving kinases were identified in this relatively small number of studied tumors, though an intriguing finding was the observation of a number of tumor suppressor gene disruptions (*CDKN2A, RB1, NF1)* by rearrangements [1].

Pathway alterations

The genomic alterations of lung SqCCs suggest that a number of key cellular pathways are commonly altered in this disease. Two of the most significantly mutated genes in lung SqCC, *NFE2L2* and *KEAP1*, encode binding partners with a well-established role in the regulation of transcription of genes involved in the cellular response to oxidative stress [96, 97, 146]. It has been hypothesized that alterations in *NFE2L2* and *KEAP1* may confer a survival advantage to airway cells chronically exposed to carcinogens from tobacco smoke by constitutive activation of a cytoprotective transcriptional program [147–149]. However, in the setting of cancer, activation of this pathway has been shown to promote chemo- and radioresistance in tumor cells

[150–155]. Mutated *NF2L2* and *KEAP1* have been shown to cooperative with mutated *KRAS* in driving lung carcinomas in mouse models, suggesting that this pathway may regulate processes in addition to the cellular response to oxidative damage [156].

Loss-of-function *NOTCH1* mutations have been described in squamous cell carcinomas of the head and neck and skin [157–159]. *NOTCH* genes have a documented role in squamous metaplasia, suggesting that genes involved in the normal development of squamous epithelium may be dysregulated in SqCCs. *NOTCH1* is also subject to loss-of-function mutations in lung SqCCs; other genes implicated in differentiation such as *SOX2* and *TP63* are also commonly altered in SqCCs and largely exclusive with mutations of *NOTCH1* [1]. Given that squamous epithelial cells are not resident in the normal human airway, it is likely that an alteration of a gene or genes involved in squamous differentiation would be required for the development of a lung SqCC.

In addition to deregulation of redox response genes and genes involved in squamous differentiation, mitogenic and pro-survival kinases are commonly altered in lung SqCCs. The most commonly altered kinase pathway in lung SqCC is PI3K/AKT [1]. Approximately half of lung SqCCs in the TCGA cohort had a documented mutation, somatic copy number alteration or significant up- or down-regulation of expression of a Pi3K/AKT pathway gene, most commonly *PIK3CA* or *PTEN* [1]. Other frequently altered kinase families are *FGFR* genes which display copy number alteration or mutation in 10–20% of cases [1]. *EGFR* and other *ERBB* kinases are also commonly altered by amplification or mis-expression, though the significance of these alterations is less clear than in lung adenocarcinoma. Other kinase families also display recurrent evidence of alteration such as *DDR2*, *BRAF* and *JAK* kinases which may also be important therapeutic biomarkers [1].

A surprising result from the TCGA survey of lung SqCC was the identification of recurrent loss-of-function mutations in the *HLA-A* gene [1]. These alterations would be predicted to decrease the ability of the tumor to present immunogenic peptides to the immune system and could enable the tumor to escape some degree of immuno-surveillance. Somatic alterations of genes involved in the recognition of a lung SqCC by the host immune system are encountered frequently in this disease and may explain the efficacy of immune checkpoint inhibitors in preliminary clinical studies [160, 161], that could help restore the ability of the immune system to recognize and respond to the tumor.

In summary, squamous cell lung cancers have high levels of targetable genomic alterations, suggesting that targeted therapies are likely to play a large role in this disease. Furthermore, lung SqCCs have mutational signatures of immune evasion, supporting the potential of immune modulatory therapies.

Genomic features of small cell lung cancers

Small cell lung cancer (SCLC) is a highly malignant tumor of the lung, which belongs to the family of pulmonary neuroendocrine tumors. In addition to SCLC this tumor entity includes the histological subtypes of large-cell neuroendocrine lung cancer (LCNEC), and the clinically benign lung carcinoids. SCLC is the most common tumor type within this group of neuroendocrine tumors accounting for approximately 80% of the cases, followed by LCNECs with 12% [162]. Combined, SCLC and LCNEC are responsible for approximately 20–25% of all lung cancer cases in humans [163].

Previous molecular findings in SCLC

SCLC and LCNEC are characterized by a high load of genetic alterations with frequent losses on 3p, which is invariably lost in SCLC, 13q, 9p, and 17p [164–166]. Furthermore, *TP53* mutations are frequently found in LCNECs (59%) and SCLC (71%) tumors [21, 167, 168]. Carcinoids are shown to have G:C > A:T transition or non-sense mutations, whereas SCLC and LCNEC tumors mainly bear G:C > T:A transversions [5]. This fact supports the finding that in contrast to carcinoids, smoking is involved in the pathogenesis of SCLC and LCNEC tumors [169]. Genetic changes in the p16INK4 / Cyclin D1 / Rb pathway play a decisive role in deregulating the cell cycle of neuroendocrine lung tumors. The loss of *RB1* is a common event in SCLC and LCNEC [18, 170–172], but is rare in carcinoids [170]. According to the COSMIC database of somatic mutations found in cancer (www.sanger.ac.uk/genetics/CGP/cosmic/), the most frequent mutations in SCLC are in *TP53* (90% of the cases tested), *RB1* (57%), *PTEN* (15%), *PIK3CA* (10%), and *EGFR* (5%).

In traditional genetic studies, the hallmark alterations of SCLC and LCNECs were both mutations in *TP53* and *RB1*. Loss of *RB1* is by far more frequent in these tumors than in any of the other lung tumor types. Furthermore, while combined lung-specific inactivation of *TP53* and *KRAS* give rise to adenocarcinomas in genetically manipulated mice [173], lung epithelial cells deficient of *TP53* and *RB1* give rise to small cell carcinomas in mice [174]. Thus, loss of *RB1* appears to be a critical event in the pathogenesis of the SCLC tumor type. There is increasing evidence proving that beyond its role in cell cycle control, Rb1 is also are involved in many other cellular pathways which impact on tumor initiation and progression (see below).

Large-scale genome analysis studies of SCLC

Unfortunately, comprehensive genomic analyses in neuroendocrine cancers are notoriously difficult because of limiting amounts of tissue available. SCLC is usually diagnosed by small biopsies, which are not suitable for comprehensive genomic analyses. Only in extremely rare cases SCLC is treated by surgical resection yielding samples that are suitable for in-depth genomic studies. Thus, despite their relatively high frequency in the population, obtaining large numbers of adequate tumor specimens is difficult.

Recently, two studies have addressed the need for comprehensive genomic characterization of small cell lung cancer [4, 145]. In total, over 100 SCLC specimens were analyzed by exome sequencing in addition to copy number arrays and transcriptome sequencing. One of the most striking observations was the extremely high background mutation rate of up to 7.4 somatic mutations per megabase of sequence. C:G>A:T transversions, which are typically caused by tobacco-associated carcinogens, were frequently detected in SCLC, thus confirming the association with heavy smoking. The high mutation rate in SCLC tumors poses a major challenge in identifying biologically relevant gene mutations, as for lung adenocarcinoma and lung SqCC. In order to address this need, analytical approaches are required to assign significance to recurrently mutated genes. These filters correct for gene size, gene-specific background mutation rate, determine, whether a given gene is also expressed, analyze if the pattern of mutations is reminiscent of tumor suppressor genes (out-of-frame insertions or deletions, mutations introducing stop codons) or oncogenes (in-frame insertions or deletions), furthermore local clustering of mutations is assigned to a given gene. When applying these approaches, the authors found almost universal mutations of *TP53* as well as frequent mutations of *RB1* [4,145]. Furthermore, both studies identified mutations in *PTEN* and in histone modifying genes, such as *EP300* and *MLL2*. Another histone acetyl transferase, *CREBBP*, was also recurrently mutated in one of these studies [4]. The mutations in *CREBBP* and in *EP300* occurred in mutually exclusive fashion suggesting that the inactivation of both genes may fulfill overlapping functions. Furthermore, mutations in *CREBBP* and *EP300* clustered around the histone acetyl transferase domain. Altogether, genomic events affecting either of these two genes occurred in 18% of all SCLC cases. Thus, next to *TP53* and *RB1*, the two histone acetyltransferase genes *EP300* and *CREBBP* were identified as the third most frequently mutated class of genes in this tumor type. Several of the additional gene mutations detected in SCLC affect kinases which in some instances are involved in the PI3-kinase pathway [145].

Detailed analyses of chromosomal gene copy number have revealed a remarkable pattern of somatic copy number alterations (SCNAs) [4, 145, 175]. Predominantly, large chromosome-level events are detectable, whereas highly focal amplifications and deletions are typically rare. These events include hemizygous losses affecting the short arm of chromosome 3, gains of 5p (possibly targeting the telomerase gene *TERT*), losses of *RB1* (13q) and *TP53* (17p), amplifications of all three MYC family members (*MYCL1, MYCN, MYC*), and finally *FGFR1* (8p) amplifications detected in approximately 6% of the cases [4, 145]. At least one *FGFR1*-amplified cell line was found to be highly sensitive to FGFR inhibition [140, 176], suggesting that treatment with FGFR inhibitors may be beneficial in *FGFR1*-amplified SCLC. The *SOX2* gene was also found to be amplified at high levels in approximately 25% of the cases [145]. *SOX2* is a lineage transcription factor that was identified to be amplified in a large proportion of squamous cell lung cancers [135]. Consistent with the notion that *SOX2* amplifications may contribute to the oncogenic phenotype in SCLC as well, two *SOX2*-amplified SCLC cell lines showed a decrease in proliferation upon knockdown of *SOX2* [145]. It is currently unclear whether amplifications of 3q have the same biological effects in SCLC as they have in lung squamous cell carcinomas.

Biological and clinical implications of SCLC genome alterations

Despite the fact that several novel mutations have been characterized in SCLC, none of the recent studies provide a plausible explanation for the characteristic clinical features of this tumor type; namely, the extremely high proliferation rate, the tendency to early metastasis, the high sensitivity to chemotherapy treatment, and the rapid relapse.

One intriguing possibility for explaining the high sensitivity to chemotherapy is the almost universal loss of *RB1* itself. *RB1* is involved in DNA damage repair partly through the interaction with E2F1 and its pro-apoptotic target genes [177]. Consequently, loss of *RB1* may enhance chemosensitivity by inhibiting DNA damage repair. This notion is supported by a recent study in which SCLC cell lines were shown to be highly sensitive to PARP1 inhibition [178]. PARP1 is involved in DNA damage repair, and acts as a transcriptional co-activator of the transcription factor E2F1, which itself is repressed by RB1. PARP inhibition may therefore repress E2F1 target genes involved in the DNA damage response. Furthermore, the large amount of somatic mutations in SCLC points to an intrinsic DNA damage repair deficiency in these cells [4, 145]. In the context of a constant rate of background mutations, inhibition of both, the DNA double-strand repair machinery (by PARP itself) and other mechanisms involved in the repair of single base substitution, may synergistically aid in suppressing the growth of SCLC tumors.

Furthermore, genetic defects in SCLC are repeatedly found to impact histone modifying genes. At this point it is unclear how the inactivation of the histone acetyl transferases, *CREBBP* or *EP300*, or the histone methyl transferase *MLL*, may contribute to the tumorigenesis in SCLC. In addition to histone modifications, these histone acetyl transferases have been reported to directly acetylate other proteins that may be centrally involved in protecting cells from oncogenic transformation. Alternatively, inactivation of the *EP300, CREBBP*, and *MLL* genes could also alter the pattern of histone acetylation, which may consequently lead to a global change in gene expression. The primary target of CBP and p300 is histone H3; where in particular acetylation occurs on the lysine residues K18 and K27 [179]. Since hypoacetylation of H3K18 is associated with oncogenic transformation [180–182], it is tempting to speculate that this histone mark is also the functional consequence of *CREBBP* and *EP300* inactivation in SCLC.

As mentioned above, only a few candidate alterations were found that could serve as therapeutic targets in SCLC. Among these, *FGFR1* amplifications may point to a therapeutic opportunity for *FGFR1*-amplified SCLC [140, 176]. Furthermore, tumors with inactivation of PTEN may be susceptible to inhibition of PI3-kinase, AKT, or HSP90 [176]. Additionally, cancers bearing EPHA kinase fusions [145] could be treated with EPHA kinase inhibitors. However, the number of preclinical models harboring these respective genetic alterations is currently limited. Furthermore, the molecular epidemiology of most of these genetic lesions is at this point in time not fully explored. Therefore, the degree of preclinical validation of these possible targets needs to be further investigated.

A recent report provided preclinical evidence that the Hedgehog signaling pathway is activated in

SCLC [183]. It was found that SCLC tumors in mice were sensitive to a combination of chemotherapy with the Hedgehog pathway inhibitor NVP-LDE225, which is currently in Phase-II clinical trials. The mechanistic basis of the observed dependency on the Hedgehog pathway remains at this point unclear. While somatic mutations are found to cause the activation of the Hedgehog pathway in medulloblastoma and basal cell carcinoma of the skin [184], no such mutations have been observed in SCLC [4, 145].

In summary, multiple novel genome alterations have recently been discovered in SCLC, several of which occur at high frequency (e.g., *CREBBP, EP300* mutations). Detailed mechanistic studies in cells and mice are needed to provide explanations as to how these novel alterations cause SCLC, and if they associate with therapeutically tractable pathway activation.

References

1 Cancer Genome Atlas Research N. (2012) Comprehensive genomic characterization of squamous cell lung cancers. *Nature*, Sep 27; 489(7417): 519–25. PubMed PMID: 22960745. Pubmed Central PMCID: 3466113.

2 Govindan R, Ding L, Griffith M, Subramanian J, Dees ND, Kanchi KL, *et al.* (2012) Genomic landscape of non-small cell lung cancer in smokers and never-smokers. *Cell*. Sep 14; 150(6): 1121–34. PubMed PMID: 22980976.

3 Imielinski M, Berger AH, Hammerman PS, Hernandez B, Pugh TJ, Hodis E, *et al.* (2012) Mapping the hallmarks of lung adenocarcinoma with massively parallel sequencing. *Cell*, Sep 14; 150(6): 1107–20. PubMed PMID: 22980975. Pubmed Central PMCID: 3557932.

4 Peifer M, Fernandez-Cuesta L, Sos ML, George J, Seidel D, Kasper LH, *et al.* (2012) Integrative genome analyses identify key somatic driver mutations of small-cell lung cancer. *Nat Genet*, Oct; 44(10): 1104–10. PubMed PMID: 22941188.

5 Pleasance ED, Stephens PJ, O'Meara S, McBride DJ, Meynert A, Jones D, *et al.* (2010) A small-cell lung cancer genome with complex signatures of tobacco exposure. *Nature*, Jan 14; 463(7278): 184–90. PubMed PMID: 20016488. Epub 2009/12/18. eng.

6 Pleasance ED, Cheetham RK, Stephens PJ, McBride DJ, Humphray SJ, Greenman CD, *et al.* (2010) A comprehensive catalogue of somatic mutations from a human cancer genome. *Nature*, Jan 14; 463(7278): 191–6. PubMed PMID: 20016485. Epub 2009/12/18. eng.

7 Mitsudomi T, Morita S, Yatabe Y, Negoro S, Okamoto I, Tsurutani J, *et al.* (2009) Gefitinib versus cisplatin plus docetaxel in patients with non-small-cell lung cancer harbouring mutations of the epidermal growth factor receptor (WJTOG3405): an open label, randomised phase 3 trial. *Lancet Oncol*, Dec 18. PubMed PMID: 20022809. Epub 2009/12/22. Eng.

8 Mok TS, Wu YL, Thongprasert S, Yang CH, Chu DT, Saijo N, *et al.* (2009) Gefitinib or carboplatin-paclitaxel in pulmonary adenocarcinoma. *N Engl J Med*, Sep 3; 361(10): 947–57. PubMed PMID: 19692680. Epub 2009/08/21. eng.

9 Rosell R, Moran T, Queralt C, Porta R, Cardenal F, Camps C, *et al.* (2009) Screening for epidermal growth factor receptor mutations in lung cancer. *N Engl J Med*, Sep 3; 361(10): 958–67. PubMed PMID: 19692684. Epub 2009/08/21. eng.

10 Camidge DR, Bang YJ, Kwak EL, Iafrate AJ, Varella-Garcia M, Fox SB, *et al.* (2012) Activity and safety of crizotinib in patients with ALK-positive non-small-cell lung cancer: updated results from a phase 1 study. *Lancet Oncol*, Oct; 13(10): 1011–19. PubMed PMID: 22954507.

11 Kwak EL, Bang YJ, Camidge DR, Shaw AT, Solomon B, Maki RG, *et al.* (2010) Anaplastic lymphoma kinase inhibition in non-small-cell lung cancer. *N Engl J Med*, Oct 28; 363(18): 1693–703. PubMed PMID: 20979469. Epub 2010/10/29. eng.

12 Shaw AT, Yeap BY, Solomon BJ, Riely GJ, Gainor J, Engelman JA, *et al.* (2011) Effect of crizotinib on overall survival in patients with advanced non-small-cell lung cancer harbouring ALK gene rearrangement: a retrospective analysis. *Lancet Oncol*, Oct; 12(11): 1004–12. PubMed PMID: 21933749. Pubmed Central PMCID: 3328296.

13 Cairns P, Mao L, Merlo A, Lee DJ, Schwab D, Eby Y, *et al.* (1994) Rates of p16 (MTS1) mutations in primary tumors with 9p loss. *Science*, Jul 15; 265(5170): 415–17. PubMed PMID: 8023167.

14 Capon DJ, Seeburg PH, McGrath JP, Hayflick JS, Edman U, Levinson AD, *et al.* (1983) Activation of Ki-ras2 gene in human colon and lung carcinomas by two different point mutations. *Nature*, Aug 11–17; 304(5926): 507–13. PubMed PMID: 6308467.

15 Kamb A, Gruis NA, Weaver-Feldhaus J, Liu Q, Harshman K, Tavtigian SV, *et al.* (1994) A cell cycle regulator potentially involved in genesis of many tumor types. *Science*, 264(5157): 436–40.
16 McCoy MS, Toole JJ, Cunningham JM, Chang EH, Lowy DR, Weinberg RA (1983) Characterization of a human colon/lung carcinoma oncogene. *Nature*, Mar 3; 302(5903): 79–81. PubMed PMID: 6298638.
17 Sakaguchi AY, Naylor SL, Shows TB, Toole JJ, McCoy M, Weinberg RA (1983) Human c-Ki-ras2 proto-oncogene on chromosome 12. *Science*, Mar 4; 219(4588): 1081–3. PubMed PMID: 6823569.
18 Shapiro GI, Edwards CD, Kobzik L, Godleski J, Richards W, Sugarbaker DJ, *et al.* (1995) Reciprocal Rb inactivation and p16INK4 expression in primary lung cancers and cell lines. *Cancer Res*, 55(3): 505–9.
19 Shapiro GI, Park JE, Edwards CD, Mao L, Merlo A, Sidransky D, *et al.* (1995) Multiple mechanisms of p16INK4A inactivation in non-small cell lung cancer cell lines. *Cancer Res*, 55(24): 6200–9.
20 Shiraishi M, Noguchi M, Shimosato Y, Sekiya T (1989) Amplification of protooncogenes in surgical specimens of human lung carcinomas. *Cancer Res*, Dec 1; 49(23): 6474–9. PubMed PMID: 2573414.
21 Takahashi T, Nau MM, Chiba I, Birrer MJ, Rosenberg RK, Vinocour M, *et al.* (1989) p53: a frequent target for genetic abnormalities in lung cancer. *Science*, 246(4929): 491–4.
22 Lander ES, Linton LM, Birren B, Nusbaum C, Zody MC, Baldwin J, *et al.* (2001) Initial sequencing and analysis of the human genome. *Nature*, 409(6822): 860–921. PubMed PMID: 11237011.
23 Venter JC, Adams MD, Myers EW, Li PW, Mural RJ, Sutton GG, *et al.* (2001) The sequence of the human genome. *Science*. 291(5507): 1304–51. PubMed PMID: 11181995.
24 Lynch TJ, Bell DW, Sordella R, Gurubhagavatula S, Okimoto RA, Brannigan BW, *et al.* (2004) Activating mutations in the epidermal growth factor receptor underlying responsiveness of non-small-cell lung cancer to gefitinib. *N Engl J Med*, May 20; 350(21): 2129–39. PubMed PMID: 15118073.
25 Paez JG, Janne PA, Lee JC, Tracy S, Greulich H, Gabriel S, *et al.* (2004) EGFR mutations in lung cancer: correlation with clinical response to gefitinib therapy. *Science*, Jun 4; 304(5676): 1497–1500. PubMed PMID: 15118125.
26 Pao W, Miller V, Zakowski M, Doherty J, Politi K, Sarkaria I, *et al.* (2004) EGF receptor gene mutations are common in lung cancers from "never smokers" and are associated with sensitivity of tumors to gefitinib and erlotinib. *Proc Natl Acad Sci USA*, 2004 Sep 7; 101(36): 13306–11. PubMed PMID: 15329413.
27 Stephens P, Hunter C, Bignell G, Edkins S, Davies H, Teague J, *et al.* (2004) Lung cancer: intragenic ERBB2 kinase mutations in tumours. *Nature*, Sep 30; 431(7008): 525–6. PubMed PMID: 15457249.
28 Brose MS, Volpe P, Feldman M, Kumar M, Rishi I, Gerrero R, *et al.* (2002) BRAF and RAS mutations in human lung cancer and melanoma. *Cancer Res*, Dec 1; 62(23): 6997–7000. PubMed PMID: 12460918.
29 Davies H, Bignell GR, Cox C, Stephens P, Edkins S, Clegg S, *et al.* (2002) Mutations of the BRAF gene in human cancer. *Nature*, Jun 27; 417(6892): 949–54. PubMed PMID: 12068308.
30 Naoki K, Chen TH, Richards WG, Sugarbaker DJ, Meyerson M (2002) Missense mutations of the BRAF gene in human lung adenocarcinoma. *Cancer Res*, Dec 1; 62(23): 7001–3. PubMed PMID: 12460919.
31 Rikova K, Guo A, Zeng Q, Possemato A, Yu J, Haack H, *et al.* (2007) Global survey of phosphotyrosine signaling identifies oncogenic kinases in lung cancer. *Cell*, Dec 14; 131(6): 1190–1203. PubMed PMID: 18083107. Epub 2007/12/18. eng.
32 Soda M, Choi YL, Enomoto M, Takada S, Yamashita Y, Ishikawa S, *et al.* (2007) Identification of the transforming EML4-ALK fusion gene in non-small-cell lung cancer. *Nature*, Aug 2; 448(7153): 561–6. PubMed PMID: 17625570.eng.
33 Sanchez-Cespedes M, Parrella P, Esteller M, Nomoto S, Trink B, Engles JM, *et al.* (2002) Inactivation of LKB1/STK11 is a common event in adenocarcinomas of the lung. *Cancer Res*, Jul 1; 62(13): 3659–62. PubMed PMID: 12097271.
34 Medina PP, Carretero J, Fraga MF, Esteller M, Sidransky D, Sanchez-Cespedes M (2004) Genetic and epigenetic screening for gene alterations of the chromatin-remodeling factor, SMARCA4/BRG1, in lung tumors. *Genes Chromosomes Cancer*, Oct; 41(2): 170–7. PubMed PMID: 15287030.
35 Medina PP, Romero OA, Kohno T, Montuenga LM, Pio R, Yokota J, *et al.* (2008) Frequent BRG1/SMARCA4-inactivating mutations in human lung cancer cell lines. *Hum Mutat*, May; 29(5): 617–22. PubMed PMID: 18386774.
36 Futreal PA, Coin L, Marshall M, Down T, Hubbard T, Wooster R, *et al.* (2004) A census of human cancer genes. *Nat Rev Cancer*, Mar; 4(3): 177–83. PubMed PMID: 14993899. Pubmed Central PMCID: 2665285.
37 Futreal PA, Kasprzyk A, Birney E, Mullikin JC, Wooster R, Stratton MR (2001) Cancer and

genomics. *Nature*, Feb 15; 409(6822): 850–2. PubMed PMID: 11237008.
38 Meyerson M, Gabriel S, Getz G (2010) Advances in understanding cancer genomes through second-generation sequencing. *Nat Rev Genet*, Oct; 11(10): 685–96. PubMed PMID: 20847746. Epub 2010/09/18. eng.
39 Stratton MR, Campbell PJ, Futreal PA (2009) The cancer genome. *Nature*, Apr 9; 458(7239): 719–24. PubMed PMID: 19360079. Pubmed Central PMCID: 2821689. Epub 2009/04/11. eng.
40 Weir B, Zhao X, Meyerson M (2004) Somatic alterations in the human cancer genome. *Cancer Cell*, Nov; 6(5): 433–8. PubMed PMID: 15542426.
41 Beer DG, Kardia SL, Huang CC, Giordano TJ, Levin AM, Misek DE, *et al.* (2002) Gene-expression profiles predict survival of patients with lung adenocarcinoma. *Nat Med*, Jul 15. PubMed PMID: 12118244.
42 Beroukhim R, Mermel CH, Porter D, Wei G, Raychaudhuri S, Donovan J, *et al.* (2010) The landscape of somatic copy-number alteration across human cancers. *Nature*, Feb 18; 463(7283): 899–905. PubMed PMID: 20164920. Pubmed Central PMCID: 2826709. Epub 2010/02/19. eng.
43 Bhattacharjee A, Richards WG, Staunton J, Li C, Monti S, Vasa P, *et al.* (2001) Classification of human lung carcinomas by mRNA expression profiling reveals distinct adenocarcinoma subclasses. *Proc Natl Acad Sci USA*, 98(24): 13790–5. PubMed PMID: 11707567.
44 Ding L, Getz G, Wheeler DA, Mardis ER, McLellan MD, Cibulskis K, *et al.* (2008) Somatic mutations affect key pathways in lung adenocarcinoma. *Nature*, Oct 23; 455(7216): 1069–75. PubMed PMID: 18948947. eng.
45 Kendall J, Liu Q, Bakleh A, Krasnitz A, Nguyen KC, Lakshmi B, *et al.* (2007) Oncogenic cooperation and coamplification of developmental transcription factor genes in lung cancer. *Proc Natl Acad Sci USA*, Oct 16; 104(42): 16663–8. PubMed PMID: 17925434. eng.
46 Shedden K, Taylor JM, Enkemann SA, Tsao MS, Yeatman TJ, Gerald WL, *et al.* (2008) Gene expression-based survival prediction in lung adenocarcinoma: a multi-site, blinded validation study. *Nat Med*, Aug; 14(8): 822–7. PubMed PMID: 18641660. eng.
47 Weir BA, Woo MS, Getz G, Perner S, Ding L, Beroukhim R, *et al.* (2007) Characterizing the cancer genome in lung adenocarcinoma. *Nature*, Dec 6; 450(7171): 893–8. PubMed PMID: 17982442. eng.
48 Ju YS, Lee WC, Shin JY, Lee S, Bleazard T, Won JK, *et al.* (2012) A transforming KIF5B and RET gene fusion in lung adenocarcinoma revealed from whole-genome and transcriptome sequencing. *Genome Research*, Mar; 22(3): 436–45. PubMed PMID: 22194472. Pubmed Central PMCID: 3290779. Epub 2011/12/24. eng.
49 Kan Z, Jaiswal BS, Stinson J, Janakiraman V, Bhatt D, Stern HM, *et al.* (2010) Diverse somatic mutation patterns and pathway alterations in human cancers. *Nature*, Aug 12; 466(7308): 869–73. PubMed PMID: 20668451.
50 Lee W, Jiang Z, Liu J, Haverty PM, Guan Y, Stinson J, *et al.* (2010) The mutation spectrum revealed by paired genome sequences from a lung cancer patient. *Nature*, May 27; 465(7297): 473–7. PubMed PMID: 20505728. Epub 2010/05/28. eng.
51 Liu J, Lee W, Jiang Z, Chen Z, Jhunjhunwala S, Haverty PM, *et al.* (2012) Genome and transcriptome sequencing of lung cancers reveal diverse mutational and splicing events. *Genome Res*, Dec; 22(12): 2315–27. PubMed PMID: 23033341. Pubmed Central PMCID: 3514662.
52 Seo JS, Ju YS, Lee WC, Shin JY, Lee JK, Bleazard T, *et al.* (2012) The transcriptional landscape and mutational profile of lung adenocarcinoma. *Genome Res*, Nov; 22(11): 2109–19. PubMed PMID: 22975805. Pubmed Central PMCID: 3483540.
53 Kwei KA, Kim YH, Girard L, Kao J, Pacyna-Gengelbach M, Salari K, *et al.* (2008) Genomic profiling identifies TITF1 as a lineage-specific oncogene amplified in lung cancer. *Oncogene*, Jun 5; 27(25): 3635–40. PubMed PMID: 18212743. eng.
54 Tanaka H, Yanagisawa K, Shinjo K, Taguchi A, Maeno K, Tomida S, *et al.* (2007) Lineage-specific dependency of lung adenocarcinomas on the lung development regulator TTF-1. *Cancer Res*, Jul 1; 67(13): 6007–11. PubMed PMID: 17616654. eng.
55 Bergethon K, Shaw AT, Ou SH, Katayama R, Lovly CM, McDonald NT, *et al.* (2012) ROS1 rearrangements define a unique molecular class of lung cancers. *Journal of Clinical Oncology*, Mar 10; 30(8): 863–70. PubMed PMID: 22215748. Pubmed Central PMCID: 3295572. Epub 2012/01/05. eng.
56 Kohno T, Ichikawa H, Totoki Y, Yasuda K, Hiramoto M, Nammo T, *et al.* (2012) KIF5B-RET fusions in lung adenocarcinoma. *Nature Medicine*, Mar; 18(3): 375–7. PubMed PMID: 22327624. Epub 2012/02/14. eng.
57 Lipson D, Capelletti M, Yelensky R, Otto G, Parker A, Jarosz M, *et al.* (2012) Identification of new ALK and RET gene fusions from colorectal and lung cancer

biopsies. *Nature Medicine*, Mar; 18(3): 382–4. PubMed PMID: 22327622. Epub 2012/02/14. eng.

58 Takeuchi K, Soda M, Togashi Y, Suzuki R, Sakata S, Hatano S, *et al.* (2012) RET, ROS1 and ALK fusions in lung cancer. *Nature Medicine*, Mar; 18(3): 378–81. PubMed PMID: 22327623. Epub 2012/02/14. eng.

59 Rodenhuis S, van de Wetering ML, Mooi WJ, Evers SG, van Zandwijk N, Bos JL (1987) Mutational activation of the K-ras oncogene. A possible pathogenetic factor in adenocarcinoma of the lung. *N Engl J Med*, 317(15): 929–35.

60 Forgacs E, Biesterveld EJ, Sekido Y, Fong K, Muneer S, Wistuba, II, *et al.* (1998) Mutation analysis of the PTEN/MMAC1 gene in lung cancer. *Oncogene*, 17(12): 1557–65.

61 Garber ME, Troyanskaya OG, Schluens K, Petersen S, Thaesler Z, Pacyna-Gengelbach M, *et al.* (2001) Diversity of gene expression in adenocarcinoma of the lung. *Proc Natl Acad Sci USA*, 98(24): 13784–9. PubMed PMID: 11707590.

62 Hayes DN, Monti S, Parmigiani G, Gilks CB, Naoki K, Bhattacharjee A, *et al.* (2006) Gene expression profiling reveals reproducible human lung adenocarcinoma subtypes in multiple independent patient cohorts. *J Clin Oncol*, Nov 1; 24(31): 5079–90. PubMed PMID: 17075127. eng.

63 Hainaut P, Olivier M, Pfeifer GP (2001) TP53 mutation spectrum in lung cancers and mutagenic signature of components of tobacco smoke: lessons from the IARC TP53 mutation database. *Mutagenesis*, 16(6): 551–3. PubMed PMID: 11682648.

64 Sun S, Schiller JH, Gazdar AF (2007) Lung cancer in never smokers – a different disease. *Nat Rev Cancer*, Oct; 7(10): 778–90. PubMed PMID: 17882278.

65 Hanahan D, Weinberg RA (2000) The hallmarks of cancer. *Cell*, Jan 7; 100(1): 57–70. PubMed PMID: 10647931.

66 Hanahan D, Weinberg RA (2011) Hallmarks of cancer: the next generation. *Cell*, Mar 4; 144(5): 646–74. PubMed PMID: 21376230.

67 Vogelstein B, Kinzler KW (2004) Cancer genes and the pathways they control. *Nat Med*, Aug; 10(8): 789–99. PubMed PMID: 15286780.

68 Maemondo M, Inoue A, Kobayashi K, Sugawara S, Oizumi S, Isobe H, *et al.* (2010) Gefitinib or chemotherapy for non-small-cell lung cancer with mutated EGFR. *N Engl J Med*, Jun 24; 362(25): 2380–8. PubMed PMID: 20573926. Epub 2010/06/25. eng.

69 Pao W, Chmielecki J (2010) Rational, biologically based treatment of EGFR-mutant non-small-cell lung cancer. *Nat Rev Cancer*, Nov; 10(11): 760–74. PubMed PMID: 20966921. Pubmed Central PMCID: 3072803.

70 Sebolt-Leopold JS, Herrera R (2004) Targeting the mitogen-activated protein kinase cascade to treat cancer. *Nat Rev Cancer*, Dec; 4(12): 937–47. PubMed PMID: 15573115.

71 Zhang J, Yang PL, Gray NS (2009) Targeting cancer with small molecule kinase inhibitors. *Nat Rev Cancer*, Jan; 9(1): 28–39. PubMed PMID: 19104514.

72 Sharma SV, Bell DW, Settleman J, Haber DA (2007) Epidermal growth factor receptor mutations in lung cancer. *Nat Rev Cancer*, Mar; 7(3): 169–81. PubMed PMID: 17318210.

73 Greulich H, Chen TH, Feng W, Janne PA, Alvarez JV, Zappaterra M, *et al.* (2005) Oncogenic transformation by inhibitor-sensitive and -resistant EGFR mutants. *PLoS Med*, Nov; 2(11): e313. PubMed PMID: 16187797. eng.

74 Greulich H, Kaplan B, Mertins P, Chen TH, Tanaka KE, Yun CH, *et al.* (2012) Functional analysis of receptor tyrosine kinase mutations in lung cancer identifies oncogenic extracellular domain mutations of ERBB2. *Proc Natl Acad Sci USA*, Sep 4; 109(36): 14476–81. PubMed PMID: 22908275. Pubmed Central PMCID: 3437859.

75 Engelman JA, Zejnullahu K, Gale CM, Lifshits E, Gonzales AJ, Shimamura T, *et al.* (2007) PF00299804, an irreversible pan-ERBB inhibitor, is effective in lung cancer models with EGFR and ERBB2 mutations that are resistant to gefitinib. *Cancer Res*, Dec 15; 67(24): 11924–32. PubMed PMID: 18089823. eng.

76 Minami Y, Shimamura T, Shah K, LaFramboise T, Glatt KA, Liniker E, *et al.* (2007) The major lung cancer-derived mutants of ERBB2 are oncogenic and are associated with sensitivity to the irreversible EGFR/ERBB2 inhibitor HKI-272. *Oncogene*, Jul 26; 26(34): 5023–7. PubMed PMID: 17311002. eng.

77 Shimamura T, Ji H, Minami Y, Thomas RK, Lowell AM, Shah K, *et al.* (2006) Non-small-cell lung cancer and Ba/F3 transformed cells harboring the ERBB2 G776insV_G/C mutation are sensitive to the dual-specific epidermal growth factor receptor and ERBB2 inhibitor HKI-272. *Cancer Res*, Jul 1; 66(13): 6487–91. PubMed PMID: 16818618. eng.

78 Feinberg AP, Vogelstein B, Droller MJ, Baylin SB, Nelkin BD (1983) Mutation affecting the 12th amino acid of the c-Ha-ras oncogene product occurs infrequently in human cancer. *Science*, Jun 10; 220(4602): 1175–7. PubMed PMID: 6304875.

79 Shimizu K, Goldfarb M, Suard Y, Perucho M, Li Y, Kamata T, *et al.* (1983) Three human transforming genes are related to the viral ras oncogenes. *Proc Natl Acad Sci USA*, Apr; 80(8): 2112–6. PubMed PMID: 6572964. Pubmed Central PMCID: 393767. Epub 1983/04/01. eng.

80 Greulich H (2010) The genomics of lung adenocarcinoma: opportunities for targeted therapies. *Genes & Cancer*, Dec; 1(12): 1200–10. PubMed PMID: 21779443. Pubmed Central PMCID: 3092285.

81 Ballester R, Marchuk D, Boguski M, Saulino A, Letcher R, Wigler M, *et al.* (1990) The NF1 locus encodes a protein functionally related to mammalian GAP and yeast IRA proteins. *Cell*, Nov 16; 63(4): 851–9. PubMed PMID: 2121371.

82 Chapman PB, Hauschild A, Robert C, Haanen JB, Ascierto P, Larkin J, *et al.* (2011) Improved survival with vemurafenib in melanoma with BRAF V600E mutation. *N Engl J Med*, Jun 30; 364(26): 2507–16. PubMed PMID: 21639808. Pubmed Central PMCID: 3549296.

83 Sosman JA, Kim KB, Schuchter L, Gonzalez R, Pavlick AC, Weber JS, *et al.* (2012) Survival in BRAF V600-mutant advanced melanoma treated with vemurafenib. *N Engl J Med*, Feb 23; 366(8): 707–14. PubMed PMID: 22356324.

84 Marks JL, Gong Y, Chitale D, Golas B, McLellan MD, Kasai Y, *et al.* (2008) Novel MEK1 mutation identified by mutational analysis of epidermal growth factor receptor signaling pathway genes in lung adenocarcinoma. *Cancer Res*, Jul 15; 68(14): 5524–8. PubMed PMID: 18632602. Pubmed Central PMCID: 2586155.

85 Kong-Beltran M, Seshagiri S, Zha J, Zhu W, Bhawe K, Mendoza N, *et al.* (2006) Somatic mutations lead to an oncogenic deletion of met in lung cancer. *Cancer Res*, Jan 1; 66(1): 283–9. PubMed PMID: 16397241.

86 Bentires-Alj M, Paez JG, David FS, Keilhack H, Halmos B, Naoki K, *et al.* (2004) Activating mutations of the noonan syndrome-associated SHP2/PTPN11 gene in human solid tumors and adult acute myelogenous leukemia. *Cancer Res*, Dec 15; 64(24): 8816–20. PubMed PMID: 15604238.

87 Samuels Y, Wang Z, Bardelli A, Silliman N, Ptak J, Szabo S, *et al.* (2004) High frequency of mutations of the PIK3CA gene in human cancers. *Science*, Apr 23; 304(5670): 554. PubMed PMID: 15016963.

88 Yamamoto H, Shigematsu H, Nomura M, Lockwood WW, Sato M, Okumura N, *et al.* (2008) PIK3CA mutations and copy number gains in human lung cancers. *Cancer Res*, Sep 1; 68(17): 6913–21. PubMed PMID: 18757405. Pubmed Central PMCID: 2874836.

89 Shaw RJ, Cantley LC (2006) Ras, PI(3)K and mTOR signalling controls tumour cell growth. *Nature*, May 25; 441(7092): 424–30. PubMed PMID: 16724053.

90 Liu P, Cheng H, Roberts TM, Zhao JJ (2009) Targeting the phosphoinositide 3-kinase pathway in cancer. *Nature Reviews Drug Discovery*, Aug; 8(8): 627–44. PubMed PMID: 19644473. Pubmed Central PMCID: 3142564.

91 Little CD, Nau MM, Carney DN, Gazdar AF, Minna JD (1983) Amplification and expression of the c-myc oncogene in human lung cancer cell lines. *Nature*, 306(5939): 194–6.

92 Nie Z, Hu G, Wei G, Cui K, Yamane A, Resch W, *et al.* (2012) c-Myc is a universal amplifier of expressed genes in lymphocytes and embryonic stem cells. *Cell*, Sep 28; 151(1): 68–79. PubMed PMID: 23021216. Pubmed Central PMCID: 3471363.

93 Whibley C, Pharoah PD, Hollstein M (2009) p53 polymorphisms: cancer implications. *Nat Rev Cancer*, Feb; 9(2): 95–107. PubMed PMID: 19165225.

94 Winslow MM, Dayton TL, Verhaak RG, Kim-Kiselak C, Snyder EL, Feldser DM, *et al.* (2011) Suppression of lung adenocarcinoma progression by Nkx2–1. *Nature*, May 5; 473(7345): 101–4. PubMed PMID: 21471965. Pubmed Central PMCID: 3088778. Epub 2011/04/08. eng.

95 Sporn MB, Liby KT (2012) NRF2 and cancer: The good, the bad and the importance of context. *Nat Rev Cancer*, Aug; 12(8): 564–71. PubMed PMID: 22810811.

96 Singh A, Misra V, Thimmulappa RK, Lee H, Ames S, Hoque MO, *et al.* (2006) Dysfunctional KEAP1-NRF2 interaction in non-small-cell lung cancer. *PLoS Med*, Oct; 3(10): e420. PubMed PMID: 17020408. Pubmed Central PMCID: 1584412.

97 Shibata T, Ohta T, Tong KI, Kokubu A, Odogawa R, Tsuta K, *et al.* (2008) Cancer related mutations in NRF2 impair its recognition by Keap1-Cul3 E3 ligase and promote malignancy. *Proc Natl Acad Sci USA*, Sep 9; 105(36): 13568–73. PubMed PMID: 18757741. Pubmed Central PMCID: 2533230. Epub 2008/09/02. eng.

98 Shaw RJ (2009) Tumor suppression by LKB1: SIKness prevents metastasis. *Sci Signal*, 2(86): pe55. PubMed PMID: 19724060.

99 Ji H, Ramsey MR, Hayes DN, Fan C, McNamara K, Kozlowski P, *et al.* (2007) LKB1 modulates lung cancer differentiation and metastasis. *Nature*, Aug 16; 448(7155): 807–10. PubMed PMID: 17676035. eng.

100 Fodde R, Smits R, Clevers H (2001) APC, signal transduction and genetic instability in colorectal

cancer. *Nat Rev Cancer,* Oct; 1(1): 55–67. PubMed PMID: 11900252.

101 Baylin SB, Jones PA (2011) A decade of exploring the cancer epigenome – biological and translational implications. *Nat Rev Cancer,* Oct; 11(10): 726–34. PubMed PMID: 21941284. Pubmed Central PMCID: 3307543.

102 Ryan RJ, Bernstein BE (2012) Molecular biology. Genetic events that shape the cancer epigenome. *Science,* Jun 22; 336(6088): 1513–14. PubMed PMID: 22723401.

103 Glaros S, Cirrincione GM, Palanca A, Metzger D, Reisman D (2008) Targeted knockout of BRG1 potentiates lung cancer development. *Cancer Res,* May 15; 68(10): 3689–96. PubMed PMID: 18483251.

104 Yoshida K, Sanada M, Shiraishi Y, Nowak D, Nagata Y, Yamamoto R, *et al.* (2011) Frequent pathway mutations of splicing machinery in myelodysplasia. *Nature,* Oct 6; 478(7367): 64–9. PubMed PMID: 21909114.

105 Paez JG, Lin M, Beroukhim R, Lee JC, Zhao X, Richter DJ, *et al.* (2004) Genome coverage and sequence fidelity of phi29 polymerase-based multiple strand displacement whole genome amplification. *Nucleic Acids Res,* May; 32(9): e71. PubMed PMID: 15150323.

106 Pao W, Girard N (2011) New driver mutations in non-small-cell lung cancer. *Lancet Oncol,* Feb; 12(2): 175–80. PubMed PMID: 21277552.

107 Sequist LV, Waltman BA, Dias-Santagata D, Digumarthy S, Turke AB, Fidias P, *et al.* (2011) Genotypic and histological evolution of lung cancers acquiring resistance to EGFR inhibitors. *Science Translational Medicin,* Mar 23; 3(75): 75ra26. PubMed PMID: 21430269. Epub 2011/03/25. eng.

108 Kobayashi S, Boggon TJ, Dayaram T, Janne PA, Kocher O, Meyerson M, *et al.* (2005) EGFR mutation and resistance of non-small-cell lung cancer to gefitinib. *N Engl J Med,* Feb 24; 352(8): 786–92. PubMed PMID: 15728811.

109 Pao W, Miller VA, Politi KA, Riely GJ, Somwar R, Zakowski MF, *et al.* (2005) Acquired resistance of lung adenocarcinomas to gefitinib or erlotinib is associated with a second mutation in the EGFR kinase domain. *PLoS Med,* Mar; 2(3): e73. PubMed PMID: 15737014.

110 Engelman JA, Zejnullahu K, Mitsudomi T, Song Y, Hyland C, Park JO, *et al.* (2007) MET amplification leads to gefitinib resistance in lung cancer by activating ERBB3 signaling. *Science,* May 18; 316(5827): 1039–43. PubMed PMID: 17463250. Epub 2007/04/28. eng.

111 Choi YL, Soda M, Yamashita Y, Ueno T, Takashima J, Nakajima T, *et al.* (2010) EML4-ALK mutations in lung cancer that confer resistance to ALK inhibitors. *N Engl J Med,* Oct 28; 363(18): 1734–9. PubMed PMID: 20979473.

112 Heuckmann JM, Balke-Want H, Malchers F, Peifer M, Sos ML, Koker M, *et al.* (2012) Differential protein stability and ALK inhibitor sensitivity of EML4-ALK fusion variants. *Clin Cancer Res,* Sep 1; 18(17): 4682–90. PubMed PMID: 22912387.

113 Tanizaki J, Okamoto I, Okabe T, Sakai K, Tanaka K, Hayashi H, *et al.* (2012) Activation of HER family signaling as a mechanism of acquired resistance to ALK inhibitors in EML4-ALK-positive non-small cell lung cancer. *Clin Cancer Res,* Nov 15; 18(22): 6219–26. PubMed PMID: 22843788.

114 Michor F, Liphardt J, Ferrari M, Widom J (2011) What does physics have to do with cancer? *Nat Rev Cancer,* Sep; 11(9): 657–70. PubMed PMID: 21850037.

115 Fletcher O, Houlston RS (2010) Architecture of inherited susceptibility to common cancer. *Nat Rev Cancer,* May; 10(5): 353–61. PubMed PMID: 20414203.

116 Pharoah PD, Dunning AM, Ponder BA, Easton DF (2004) Association studies for finding cancer-susceptibility genetic variants. *Nat Rev Cancer,* Nov; 4(11): 850–60. PubMed PMID: 15516958.

117 Amos CI, Pinney SM, Li Y, Kupert E, Lee J, de Andrade MA, *et al.* (2010) A susceptibility locus on chromosome 6q greatly increases lung cancer risk among light and never smokers. *Cancer Res,* Mar 15; 70(6): 2359–67. PubMed PMID: 20215501. Pubmed Central PMCID: 2855643.

118 Amos CI, Wu X, Broderick P, Gorlov IP, Gu J, Eisen T, *et al.* (2008) Genome-wide association scan of tag SNPs identifies a susceptibility locus for lung cancer at 15q25.1. *Nat Genet,* May; 40(5): 616–22. PubMed PMID: 18385676. Pubmed Central PMCID: 2713680.

119 Hung RJ, McKay JD, Gaborieau V, Boffetta P, Hashibe M, Zaridze D, *et al.* (2008) A susceptibility locus for lung cancer maps to nicotinic acetylcholine receptor subunit genes on 15q25. *Nature,* Apr 3; 452(7187): 633–7. PubMed PMID: 18385738.

120 Landi MT, Chatterjee N, Yu K, Goldin LR, Goldstein AM, Rotunno M, *et al.* (2009) A genome-wide association study of lung cancer identifies a region of chromosome 5p15 associated with risk for adenocarcinoma. *Am J Hum Genet,* Nov; 85(5): 679–91. PubMed PMID: 19836008. Pubmed Central PMCID: 2775843.

121 Liu P, Vikis HG, Wang D, Lu Y, Wang Y, Schwartz AG, *et al.* (2008) Familial aggregation of common sequence variants on 15q24–25.1 in lung cancer. *J Natl Cancer Inst*, Sep 17; 100(18): 1326–30. PubMed PMID: 18780872. Pubmed Central PMCID: 2538550.
122 Wang Y, Broderick P, Webb E, Wu X, Vijayakrishnan J, Matakidou A, *et al.* (2008) Common 5p15.33 and 6p21.33 variants influence lung cancer risk. *Nat Genet*, Dec; 40(12): 1407–9. PubMed PMID: 18978787. Pubmed Central PMCID: 2695928.
123 Miki D, Kubo M, Takahashi A, Yoon KA, Kim J, Lee GK, *et al.* (2010) Variation in TP63 is associated with lung adenocarcinoma susceptibility in Japanese and Korean populations. *Nat Genet*, Oct; 42(10): 893–6. PubMed PMID: 20871597.
124 Yoon KA, Park JH, Han J, Park S, Lee GK, Han JY, *et al.* (2010) A genome-wide association study reveals susceptibility variants for non-small cell lung cancer in the Korean population. *Hum Mol Genet*, Dec 15; 19(24): 4948–54. PubMed PMID: 20876614.
125 Hu Z, Wu C, Shi Y, Guo H, Zhao X, Yin Z, *et al.* (2011) A genome-wide association study identifies two new lung cancer susceptibility loci at 13q12.12 and 22q12.2 in Han Chinese. *Nat Genet*, Aug; 43(8): 792–6. PubMed PMID: 21725308.
126 Cancer Genome Atlas N. (2012) Comprehensive molecular portraits of human breast tumours. *Nature*, Oct 4; 490(7418): 61–70. PubMed PMID: 23000897. Pubmed Central PMCID: 3465532.
127 Cancer Genome Atlas N. (2012) Comprehensive molecular characterization of human colon and rectal cancer. *Nature*, Jul 19; 487(7407): 330–7. PubMed PMID: 22810696. Pubmed Central PMCID: 3401966.
128 Cancer Genome Atlas Research N. (2011) Integrated genomic analyses of ovarian carcinoma. *Nature*, Jun 30; 474(7353): 609–15. PubMed PMID: 21720365. Pubmed Central PMCID: 3163504.
129 Travis WD, Brambilla E, Noguchi M, Nicholson AG, Geisinger KR, Yatabe Y, *et al.* (2011) International Association for the Study of Lung Cancer/American Thoracic Society/European Respiratory Society International Multidisciplinary Classification of Lung Adenocarcinoma. *J Thorac Oncol*, Feb; 6(2): 244–85. PubMed PMID: 21252716.
130 Rock JR, Onaitis MW, Rawlins EL, Lu Y, Clark CP, Xue Y, *et al.* (2009) Basal cells as stem cells of the mouse trachea and human airway epithelium. *Proc Natl Acad Sci USA*, Aug 4; 106(31): 12771–5. PubMed PMID: 19625615. Pubmed Central PMCID: 2714281. Epub 2009/07/25. eng.
131 Guseh JS, Bores SA, Stanger BZ, Zhou Q, Anderson WJ, Melton DA, *et al.* (2009) Notch signaling promotes airway mucous metaplasia and inhibits alveolar development. *Development*, May; 136(10): 1751–9. PubMed PMID: 19369400. Pubmed Central PMCID: 2673763.
132 Kenfield SA, Wei EK, Stampfer MJ, Rosner BA, Colditz GA (2008) Comparison of aspects of smoking among the four histological types of lung cancer. *Tobacco Control*, Jun; 17(3): 198–204. PubMed PMID: 18390646. Pubmed Central PMCID: 3044470.
133 Raponi M, Zhang Y, Yu J, Chen G, Lee G, Taylor JM, *et al.* (2006) Gene expression signatures for predicting prognosis of squamous cell and adenocarcinomas of the lung. *Cancer Res*, Aug 1; 66(15): 7466–72. PubMed PMID: 16885343.
134 Wilkerson MD, Yin X, Hoadley KA, Liu Y, Hayward MC, Cabanski CR, *et al.* (2010) Lung squamous cell carcinoma mRNA expression subtypes are reproducible, clinically important, and correspond to normal cell types. *Clin Cancer Res*, Oct 1; 16(19): 4864–75. PubMed PMID: 20643781. Pubmed Central PMCID: 2953768.
135 Bass AJ, Watanabe H, Mermel CH, Yu S, Perner S, Verhaak RG, *et al.* (2009) SOX2 is an amplified lineage-survival oncogene in lung and esophageal squamous cell carcinomas. *Nat Genet*, Nov; 41(11): 1238–42. PubMed PMID: 19801978. Pubmed Central PMCID: 2783775. Epub 2009/10/06. eng.
136 Dutt A, Ramos AH, Hammerman PS, Mermel C, Cho J, Sharifnia T, *et al.* (2011) Inhibitor-sensitive FGFR1 amplification in human non-small cell lung cancer. *PLoS ONE*, 6(6): e20351. PubMed PMID: 21666749. Pubmed Central PMCID: 3110189. Epub 2011/06/15. eng.
137 Lockwood WW, Chari R, Coe BP, Thu KL, Garnis C, Malloff CA, *et al.* (2010) Integrative genomic analyses identify BRF2 as a novel lineage-specific oncogene in lung squamous cell carcinoma. *PLoS Med*, Jul; 7(7): e1000315. PubMed PMID: 20668658. Pubmed Central PMCID: 2910599.
138 Ramos AH, Dutt A, Mermel C, Perner S, Cho J, Lafargue CJ, *et al.* (2009) Amplification of chromosomal segment 4q12 in non-small cell lung cancer. *Cancer Biology & Therapy*, Nov; 8(21): 2042–50. PubMed PMID: 19755855. Epub 2009/09/17. eng.
139 Tonon G, Wong KK, Maulik G, Brennan C, Feng B, Zhang Y, *et al.* (2005) High-resolution genomic profiles of human lung cancer. *Proc Natl Acad Sci USA*, Jul 5; 102(27): 9625–30. PubMed PMID:

15983384. Pubmed Central PMCID: 1160520. Epub 2005/06/29. eng.

140 Weiss J, Sos ML, Seidel D, Peifer M, Zander T, Heuckmann JM, *et al.* (2010) Frequent and focal FGFR1 amplification associates with therapeutically tractable FGFR1 dependency in squamous cell lung cancer. *Sci Transl Med*, Dec 15; 2(62): 62ra93. PubMed PMID: 21160078. Epub 2010/12/17. eng.

141 Guagnano V, Kauffmann A, Wohrle S, Stamm C, Ito M, Barys L, *et al.* (2012) FGFR genetic alterations predict for sensitivity to NVP-BGJ398, a selective pan-FGFR inhibitor. *Cancer Discov*, Dec; 2(12): 1118–33. PubMed PMID: 23002168.

142 Chiba I, Takahashi T, Nau MM, D'Amico D, Curiel DT, Mitsudomi T, *et al.* (1990) Mutations in the p53 gene are frequent in primary, resected non-small cell lung cancer. Lung Cancer Study Group. *Oncogene*, 5(10): 1603–10.

143 Rekhtman N, Paik PK, Arcila ME, Tafe LJ, Oxnard GR, Moreira AL, *et al.* (2012) Clarifying the spectrum of driver oncogene mutations in biomarker-verified squamous carcinoma of lung: lack of EGFR/KRAS and presence of PIK3CA/AKT1 mutations. *Clin Cancer Res*, Feb 15; 18(4): 1167–76. PubMed PMID: 22228640. Pubmed Central PMCID: 3487403.

144 Hammerman PS, Sos ML, Ramos AH, Xu C, Dutt A, Zhou W, *et al.* (2011) Mutations in the DDR2 kinase gene identify a novel therapeutic target in squamous cell lung cancer. *Cancer Discov*, Jun; 1(1): 78–89. PubMed PMID: 22328973. Pubmed Central PMCID: 3274752. Epub 2012/02/14. eng.

145 Rudin CM, Durinck S, Stawiski EW, Poirier JT, Modrusan Z, Shames DS, *et al.* (2012) Comprehensive genomic analysis identifies SOX2 as a frequently amplified gene in small-cell lung cancer. *Nat Genet*, Oct; 44(10): 1111–16. PubMed PMID: 22941189. Pubmed Central PMCID: 3557461.

146 Shibata T, Kokubu A, Gotoh M, Ojima H, Ohta T, Yamamoto M, *et al.* (2008) Genetic alteration of Keap1 confers constitutive Nrf2 activation and resistance to chemotherapy in gallbladder cancer. *Gastroenterology*, Oct; 135(4): 1358–68, 68 e1-4. PubMed PMID: 18692501.

147 Frohlich DA, McCabe MT, Arnold RS, Day ML (2008) The role of Nrf2 in increased reactive oxygen species and DNA damage in prostate tumorigenesis. *Oncogene*, Jul 17; 27(31): 4353–62. PubMed PMID: 18372916.

148 Itoh K, Mochizuki M, Ishii Y, Ishii T, Shibata T, Kawamoto Y, *et al.* (2004) Transcription factor Nrf2 regulates inflammation by mediating the effect of 15-deoxy-Delta(12,14)-prostaglandin j(2). *Mol Cell Biol*, Jan; 24(1): 36–45. PubMed PMID: 14673141. Pubmed Central PMCID: 303336.

149 Osburn WO, Wakabayashi N, Misra V, Nilles T, Biswal S, Trush MA, *et al.* (2006) Nrf2 regulates an adaptive response protecting against oxidative damage following diquat-mediated formation of superoxide anion. *Archives of Biochemistry and Biophysics*, Oct 1; 454(1): 7–15. PubMed PMID: 16962985. Pubmed Central PMCID: 1851923.

150 Kobayashi A, Kang MI, Watai Y, Tong KI, Shibata T, Uchida K, *et al.* (2006) Oxidative and electrophilic stresses activate Nrf2 through inhibition of ubiquitination activity of Keap1. *Mol Cell Biol*, Jan; 26(1): 221–9. PubMed PMID: 16354693. Pubmed Central PMCID: 1317630.

151 Li QK, Singh A, Biswal S, Askin F, Gabrielson E (2011) KEAP1 gene mutations and NRF2 activation are common in pulmonary papillary adenocarcinoma. *Journal of Human Genetics*, Mar; 56(3): 230–4. PubMed PMID: 21248763. Pubmed Central PMCID: 3268659.

152 Ohta T, Iijima K, Miyamoto M, Nakahara I, Tanaka H, Ohtsuji M, *et al.* (2008) Loss of Keap1 function activates Nrf2 and provides advantages for lung cancer cell growth. *Cancer Res*, Mar 1; 68(5): 1303–9. PubMed PMID: 18316592.

153 Shibata T, Kokubu A, Saito S, Narisawa-Saito M, Sasaki H, Aoyagi K, *et al.* (2011) NRF2 mutation confers malignant potential and resistance to chemoradiation therapy in advanced esophageal squamous cancer. *Neoplasia*, Sep; 13(9): 864–73. PubMed PMID: 21969819. Pubmed Central PMCID: 3182278.

154 Singh A, Bodas M, Wakabayashi N, Bunz F, Biswal S (2010) Gain of Nrf2 function in non-small-cell lung cancer cells confers radioresistance. *Antioxidants & Redox Signaling*, Dec 1; 13(11): 1627–37. PubMed PMID: 20446773. Pubmed Central PMCID: 3541552.

155 Solis LM, Behrens C, Dong W, Suraokar M, Ozburn NC, Moran CA, *et al.* (2010) Nrf2 and Keap1 abnormalities in non-small cell lung carcinoma and association with clinicopathologic features. *Clin Cancer Res*, Jul 15; 16(14): 3743–53. PubMed PMID: 20534738. Pubmed Central PMCID: 2920733.

156 Bauer AK, Cho HY, Miller-Degraff L, Walker C, Helms K, Fostel J, *et al.* (2011) Targeted deletion of Nrf2 reduces urethane-induced lung tumor development in mice. *PLoS ONE*, 6(10): e26590. PubMed PMID: 22039513. Pubmed Central PMCID: 3198791.

157 Agrawal N, Frederick MJ, Pickering CR, Bettegowda C, Chang K, Li RJ, *et al.* (2011) Exome sequencing

of head and neck squamous cell carcinoma reveals inactivating mutations in NOTCH1. *Science*, Aug 26; 333(6046): 1154–7. PubMed PMID: 21798897. Pubmed Central PMCID: 3162986.

158 Stransky N, Egloff AM, Tward AD, Kostic AD, Cibulskis K, Sivachenko A, *et al.* (2011) The mutational landscape of head and neck squamous cell carcinoma. *Science*, Aug 26; 333(6046): 1157–60. PubMed PMID: 21798893. Epub 2011/07/30. eng.

159 Wang NJ, Sanborn Z, Arnett KL, Bayston LJ, Liao W, Proby CM, *et al.* (2011) Loss-of-function mutations in Notch receptors in cutaneous and lung squamous cell carcinoma. *Proc Natl Acad Sci USA*, Oct 25; 108(43): 17761–6. PubMed PMID: 22006338. Pubmed Central PMCID: 3203814.

160 Brahmer JR, Tykodi SS, Chow LQ, Hwu WJ, Topalian SL, Hwu P, *et al.* (2012) Safety and activity of anti-PD-L1 antibody in patients with advanced cancer. *N Engl J Med*, Jun 28; 366(26): 2455–65. PubMed PMID: 22658128. Pubmed Central PMCID: 3563263.

161 Topalian SL, Hodi FS, Brahmer JR, Gettinger SN, Smith DC, McDermott DF, *et al.* (2012) Safety, activity, and immune correlates of anti-PD-1 antibody in cancer. *N Engl J Med*, Jun 28; 366(26): 2443–54. PubMed PMID: 22658127. Pubmed Central PMCID: 3544539.

162 Chen LC, Travis WD, Krug LM (2006) Pulmonary neuroendocrine tumors: What (little) do we know? *Journal of the National Comprehensive Cancer Network: JNCCN*, Jul; 4(6): 623–30. PubMed PMID: 16813729.

163 Travis WD (2009) Lung tumours with neuroendocrine differentiation. *Eur J Cancer*, Sep; 45 Suppl 1: 251–66. PubMed PMID: 19775623.

164 Whang-Peng J, Kao-Shan CS, Lee EC, Bunn PA, Carney DN, Gazdar AF, *et al.* (1982) Specific chromosome defect associated with human small-cell lung cancer; deletion 3p(14-23). *Science*, 215(4529): 181–2.

165 Naylor SL, Johnson BE, Minna JD, Sakaguchi AY (1987) Loss of heterozygosity of chromosome 3p markers in small-cell lung cancer. *Nature*, 329(6138): 451–4.

166 Mori N, Yokota J, Oshimura M, Cavenee WK, Mizoguchi H, Noguchi M, *et al.* (1989) Concordant deletions of chromosome 3p and loss of heterozygosity for chromosomes 13 and 17 in small cell lung carcinoma. *Cancer Res*, 49(18): 5130–5.

167 Takahashi T, Takahashi T, Suzuki H, Hida T, Sekido Y, Ariyoshi Y, *et al.* (1991) The p53 gene is very frequently mutated in small-cell lung cancer with a distinct nucleotide substitution pattern. *Oncogene*, 6(10): 1775–8.

168 Sameshima Y, Matsuno Y, Hirohashi S, Shimosato Y, Mizoguchi H, Sugimura T, *et al.* (1992) Alterations of the p53 gene are common and critical events for the maintenance of malignant phenotypes in small-cell lung carcinoma. *Oncogene*, 7(3): 451–7.

169 Onuki N, Wistuba, II, Travis WD, Virmani AK, Yashima K, Brambilla E, *et al.* (1999) Genetic changes in the spectrum of neuroendocrine lung tumors. *Cancer*, Feb 1; 85(3): 600–7. PubMed PMID: 10091733.

170 Beasley MB, Lantuejoul S, Abbondanzo S, Chu WS, Hasleton PS, Travis WD, *et al.* (2003) The P16/cyclin D1/Rb pathway in neuroendocrine tumors of the lung. *Hum Pathol*, Feb; 34(2): 136–42. PubMed PMID: 12612881.

171 Kelley MJ, Nakagawa K, Steinberg SM, Mulshine JL, Kamb A, Johnson BE (1995) Differential inactivation of CDKN2 and Rb protein in non-small-cell and small-cell lung cancer cell lines. *J Natl Cancer Inst*, 87(10): 756–61.

172 Yokota J, Akiyama T, Fung YK, Benedict WF, Namba Y, Hanaoka M, *et al.* (1988) Altered expression of the retinoblastoma (RB) gene in small-cell carcinoma of the lung. *Oncogene*, 3(4): 471–5.

173 Zheng S, El-Naggar AK, Kim ES, Kurie JM, Lozano G (2007) A genetic mouse model for metastatic lung cancer with gender differences in survival. *Oncogene*, Oct 18; 26(48): 6896–6904. PubMed PMID: 17486075.

174 Meuwissen R, Linn SC, Linnoila RI, Zevenhoven J, Mooi WJ, Berns A (2003) Induction of small cell lung cancer by somatic inactivation of both Trp53 and Rb1 in a conditional mouse model. *Cancer Cell*, Sep;4(3):181–9. PubMed PMID: 14522252. Epub 2003/10/03. eng.

175 Voortman J, Lee JH, Killian JK, Suuriniemi M, Wang Y, Lucchi M, *et al.* (2010) Array comparative genomic hybridization-based characterization of genetic alterations in pulmonary neuroendocrine tumors. *Proc Natl Acad Sci USA*, Jul 20; 107(29): 13040–5. PubMed PMID: 20615970. Pubmed Central PMCID: 2919980.

176 Sos ML, Dietlein F, Peifer M, Schottle J, Balke-Want H, Muller C, *et al.* (2012) A framework for identification of actionable cancer genome dependencies in small cell lung cancer. *Proc Natl Acad Sci USA*, Oct 16; 109(42): 17034–9. PubMed PMID: 23035247. Pubmed Central PMCID: 3479457.

177 Burkhart DL, Sage J (2008) Cellular mechanisms of tumour suppression by the retinoblastoma gene.

Nat Rev Cancer, Sep; 8(9): 671–82. PubMed PMID: 18650841.

178 Byers LA, Wang J, Nilsson MB, Fujimoto J, Saintigny P, Yordy J, *et al.* (2012) Proteomic profiling identifies dysregulated pathways in small cell lung cancer and novel therapeutic targets including PARP1. *Cancer Discov*, Sep; 2(9): 798–811. PubMed PMID: 22961666. Pubmed Central PMCID: 3567922.

179 Bedford DC, Brindle PK (2012) Is histone acetylation the most important physiological function for CBP and p300? *Aging*, 4(4): 247–55. PubMed PMID: 22511639. Pubmed Central PMCID: 3371760.

180 Barber MF, Michishita-Kioi E, Xi Y, Tasselli L, Kioi M, Moqtaderi Z, *et al.* (2012) SIRT7 links H3K18 deacetylation to maintenance of oncogenic transformation. *Nature*, Jul 5; 487(7405): 114–18. PubMed PMID: 22722849. Pubmed Central PMCID: 3412143.

181 Ferrari E, Lucca C, Foiani M (2010) A lethal combination for cancer cells: synthetic lethality screenings for drug discovery. *Eur J Cancer*, Nov; 46(16): 2889–95. PubMed PMID: 20724143.

182 Horwitz GA, Zhang K, McBrian MA, Grunstein M, Kurdistani SK, Berk AJ (2008) Adenovirus small e1a alters global patterns of histone modification. *Science*, Aug 22; 321(5892): 1084–5. PubMed PMID: 18719283. Pubmed Central PMCID: 2756290.

183 Park KS, Martelotto LG, Peifer M, Sos ML, Karnezis AN, Mahjoub MR, *et al.* (2011) A crucial requirement for Hedgehog signaling in small cell lung cancer. *Nat Med*, 17(11): 1504–8. PubMed PMID: 21983857. Pubmed Central PMCID: 3380617.

184 Teglund S, Toftgard R (2010) Hedgehog beyond medulloblastoma and basal cell carcinoma. *Biochimica et biophysica acta*, Apr; 1805(2): 181–208. PubMed PMID: 20085802.

CHAPTER 5
Serum Proteomic Biomarkers

Mohamed Hassanein[1] *and David P. Carbone*[2]
[1]Division of Allergy, Pulmonary and Critical Care Medicine, Vanderbilt University Medical Center, Nashville, TN, USA
[2]James Comprehensive Cancer Center, Ohio State University Medical Center, Columbus, OH, USA

Natural history of lung cancer progression and potential utility for biomarkers in the clinic

Lung cancer represents a spectrum of diseases with tremendous heterogeneity both at the pathological and molecular levels [1–4] that is strongly associated with smoking as a risk factor. With about 20% of the US adult population smoking and 1 billion people worldwide, lung cancer claims more lives than breast, prostate, colon, liver, kidney and melanoma cancers combined [5, 6]. Despite the recent improvements of bronchoscopic and surgical techniques as well as advances in chemotherapy, targeted therapies, and radiation therapy treatments, attempts to improve patient outcomes by targeting patients with advanced disease are faced with immense challenges. In order to detect cancer earlier, when it is most curable, several noninvasive detection technologies have been investigated. Imaging techniques such as chest X-ray, low-dose spiral computed tomography (CT), sputum cytology and molecular biomarkers in various biological samples have been tested for their diagnostic value for early detection for lung cancer [7, 8]. Although these tests vary in their sensitivity and specificity, only low dose chest CT was shown to reduce lung cancer specific mortality [9–11]. This very encouraging finding increases the importance of finding new molecular biomarkers for risk assessment and noninvasive diagnosis, and potentially to identify the patient population that can most benefit from specific targeted chemopreventive or therapeutic strategies. These molecular biomarkers will have to be rigorously tested to demonstrate their clinical utility and complement currently used strategies.

Lung cancer in smokers can be considered to result from a long history of repeated airway damage and repair cycles. This disease process develops over the course of many years before coming to clinical attention. This rather long disease process (Figure 5.1) represents a window of opportunity during which intervention could take place with the potential for preventing the development of disease (e.g., primary prevention-smoking cessation or chemoprevention). While only about 20% of high risk individuals develop lung cancer [12], some of the key unanswered questions remaining include: who will develop a malignancy (who might benefit from screening or preventive strategies), at what rate will the disease progress when it develops (is the detected disease "clinically significant"), and what patient population will benefit most from specific targeted therapies (therapy selection)? To this aim, the search for lung cancer specific biomarkers has been intensified; however, no biomarker has been proven clinically useful or widely applied to the diagnosis of lung cancer [13].

Lung Cancer, Fourth Edition. Edited by Jack A. Roth, Waun Ki Hong and Ritsuko U. Komaki.

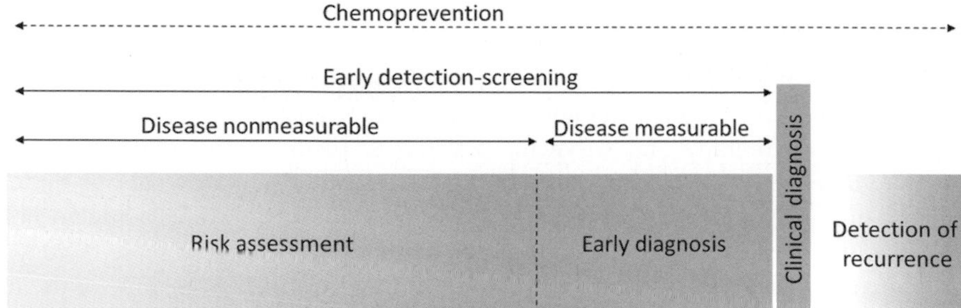

Figure 5.1 Clinical contexts for biomarker utility during lung cancer progression. This diagram illustrates four clinical contexts within four windows of time. The period during which lung cancer is nonmeasurable and precedes the diagnosis characterizes the context of *risk assessment*. It represents a long window of time during which the disease develops and corresponds to an opportunity for chemoprevention. When the disease becomes measurable but remains asymptomatic, we enter the context of *early diagnosis*. Two other clinical contexts relate to *clinical diagnosis*, i.e., when the disease is measurable and patients symptomatic, and to *detection of recurrence*. These windows of time correspond to the different contexts during which different biomarker targets can be developed.
Source: Adapted from Hassanein *et al.* [94]. Reprinted with permission of the American Thoracic Society. Copyright © 2012 American Thoracic Society. This modified figure is based on the original figure available from www.atsjournals.org.

The blood proteome

Blood is a complex and dynamic medium whose components can reflect various physiological or pathological states throughout the body, including the presence of some cancers. Blood proteome analysis assumes that tissue perfusion of tumors or host responses contribute to novel or modified circulating proteins or peptides (Figure 5.2). Proteomic analysis of blood represents an appealing choice to researchers addressing the discovery of biomarkers since it can be quickly and easily

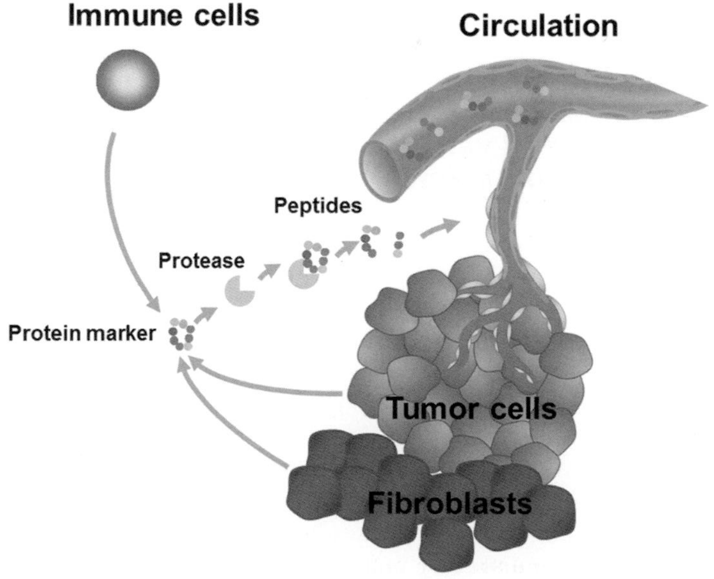

Figure 5.2 Origins of serum protein and peptide biomarkers. Tumor associated proteins can be generated by tumor cells directly or as host response to carcinogenesis by surrounding cells of microenvironment including fibroblasts and immune cells. Proteolytic cascades within the tissue (a product of the interacting cellular ecology such as stromal epithelial interactions), immune cell MHC presentation, or apoptosis generate protein fragments (peptides) that passively diffuse into the circulation.

obtained in a noninvasive manner and in adequate quantities over time. These features can potentially allow for early diagnosis of cancer, monitoring of disease status, development of targeted therapies, evaluation of response to therapy and survival. Given the low abundance of known cancer markers in serum or plasma, it is critical to select proteomic technologies that provide sufficient depth of analysis for biomarker discovery. Several recent studies have investigated the extent to which proteomic technologies can unravel the complexity of the plasma proteome, and the Human Proteome Organization published a comprehensive collaborative study that characterized the human serum and plasma proteomes [14].

Proteomic discovery platforms

Several analytical approaches have been adopted to identify novel proteins and understand their structure, function and interaction with proteins and other molecules. There have been attempts to bring this knowledge to the clinic by means of new diagnostic and predictive biomarkers as well as the identification of therapeutic targets. A list of the most common proteomic approaches is summarized in Table 5.1. These were reviewed in detail elsewhere [15–17].

Proteomic approaches for discovery and validation of blood biomarkers

Considerable progress has been made in the past decade in identifying tumor characteristics through advances of molecular biology technologies. Much of this progress was driven by increasing knowledge of tumor related aberrations that affect nucleic acids both at genomic, transcriptional, and post-transcriptional levels. Proteins are the functional end product of genes that ultimately control vital biological processes via their expression level, posttranslational modifications, and function. Moreover, the number of proteins produced by cells far exceeds the number of genes because proteins vary in their stability compared to mRNA, and are subjected to many levels of post transcriptional and post translational regulation such as splicing variants, fusions, and posttranslational modifications. Therefore, to advance our understanding of the biology of lung cancer and to obtain a more integrated view of the disease biology, it is critical to capture as much as possible of the full spectrum of the variations in protein expression patterns, their post translational modifications and functions in cancer cells. This information can thus provide a more comprehensive understanding of the disease when integrated into comprehensive genomic and transcriptomic analysis. Table 5.2 summarizes the results of several published studies of proteomic lung cancer diagnostic markers.

MALDI-TOF MS serum analysis for diagnosis

Among proteomic technologies, matrix assisted laser desorption ionization time-of-flight mass spectrometry (MALDI-TOF MS) is a technique that has allowed rapid progress in cancer biology. It is a simple and high-throughput technique that analyzes with modest sensitivity but higher specificity proteins expressed in complex biological mixtures, such as serum, urine and tissues. This technique requires sample co-crystallization of the biospecimen with a matrix that absorbs laser energy and subsequently ejects and ionizes molecules into the gas phase (Figure 5.3). Ions are then accelerated in the ion source by a fixed potential difference and travel a fixed distance before reaching the detector time of flight (TOF), inversely proportional to their m/z ratios (lighter ions are faster to reach the detector than heavier ions for a same charge). The time it takes for each ion to hit the detector creates a signal, which indicates m/z ratio in the X axis and ion intensity in the Y axis. Because the MALDI process essentially favors the production of singly charged molecular ions, it allows the analysis of complex protein mixtures with or without fractionation [18]. Molecular masses from 1 to >100 kDa can be determined with high accuracy.

Table 5.1 Comparison of proteomic approaches in cancer biomarker discovery research

	2-D gel separation	MALDI MS	LC-MS/MS	LC-MRM MS	Protein/antibody arrays
Purpose	Profiling, separation and identification	Profiling	Inventory and identification	Targeted protein quantitation	Targeted protein detection
Protein detection and identification	Protein pI and MW. Identification by peptide mapping and sequencing	Detection of intact peptides and proteins	Identification via peptide sequences	Peptide specific MS/MS transitions	Detection using antibodies or ligands
Quantitation	Semi-quantitative	Semi-quantitative	Semi-quantitative	Quantitative, labeled reference peptides. Label free techniques	Not quantitative
PTM detection	Yes	No	Yes	Yes	Yes
Throughput	Low	High	High	Low	High
Reproducibility	High	High	High	High	High
Sensitivity	Moderate	low	High	High	High
Depth of analysis	100–1000 proteins	100–300 peaks	500–4000 proteins	1–100 proteins	50–500 proteins
Major disadvantages	pI and MW range limitations. Contamination by polysaccharides and nucleic acids	Detection of abundant proteins. Limited MW range (2–30 kDa). No identification	High false discovery rate	Cost of labeled peptides for absolute quantitation	Antibody specificity and availability. Only known proteins can be detected

Abbreviations: 2-D: 2 dimensional; LC: liquid chromatography; MALDI MS: matrix assisted laser desorption ionization mass spectrometry; MRM: multiple reaction monitoring; MW: molecular weight; pI: isoelectric point; PTM: posttranslational modification.

Several characteristics of MALDI-TOF MS makes it a widely used technique for analysis of complex biological samples (such as tissues, whole cells, laser-captured microdissected cells, blood, serum, urine) with high mass accuracy (far better than any gel system), high-throughput capability (sample analysis in seconds), small required sample size (possible analysis of just a few cells) and higher tolerance for salts, buffers, or biological contaminants. When used in combination with surface chromatography, this method is also known as surface-enhanced laser desorption/ionization time-of-flight mass spectrometry (SELDI-TOF MS). It uses chromatographic chip arrays to selectively bind subsets of proteins from complex samples. The surfaces can be washed to remove nonspecifically bound proteins and substances that can interfere with the ionization process. Then, matrix solution is applied to the array binding the proteins and MALDI-TOF MS is performed.

The rapid proteomic profiling of blood, tissue, or urine with minimal sample preparation, using the peak pattern as a diagnostic tool, has generated great enthusiasm, but has yet to be minimally

Table 5.2 Characteristics and performance of the most recent blood-based biomarkers for the early detection of lung cancer

References	Specimen	Marker type	Analyte	# markers	Pathological subtype	Assay platform	Preclinical samples	BM Dev. phase	Training set	Validation set	Sensitivity	Specificity	AUC
Zhong, 2006 [66]	Serum	AutoAB	phage peptide clones	5	Lung cancer	ELISA	n/a	II	46	56	91*	91*	99*
Chapman, 2008 [72]	Serum	AutoAB	p53, cmyc, *HER2*, *NY-ESO-1*, *CAGE*, *MUC1*,*GBU4-5*	7	Lung cancer	ELISA	n/a	I	154	n/a	n/a	n/a	n/a
Qiu, 2008 [84]	Serum	AutoAB	annexin I, 14-3-3 theta, LAMR1	3	NSCLC	Protein-array	170	III		170	51	82	73
Wu, 2010 [85]	Serum	AutoAB	phage peptide clones	6	NSCLC	ELISA	n/a	II	20	180	92	92	96
Farlow, 2010 [86]	Serum	AutoAB	*IMPDH*, *PGAM1*, ubiquillin, *ANXA1*, *ANXA2*, *HSP70-9B*	6	NSCLC	ELISA	n/a	II	196	n/a	94.8*	91.1*	96.4*
Boyle, 2010 [87]	Serum	AutoAB	*p53*, *NY-ESO-1*, *CAGE*, *GBU4-5*, *Annexin 1* and *SOX2*	6	NSCLC	ELISA	n/a	II	241	255	32	91	64
Kulpa, 2002 [88]	Serum	Protein	CEA, CYFRA 21-1, SCC-Ag, NSE	4	SCC	ELISA	n/a	II		420	20–62	95	71–90
Patz, 2007 [21]	Serum	Protein	CEA,RBP4, hAAT, SCCA	4	LC	ELISA	n/a	II	100	97	78	75	n/a
Takano, 2009 [89]	Serum	Protein	Nectin-4	1	NSCLC	ELISA	n/a	II		295	54	98	n/a

Yildiz, 2007 [20]	Serum	Protein	MALDI MS signature	7	NSCLC	MALDI MS	n/a	II	185	105	58	85.7	82
Pecot, 2012 [90]	Serum	Protein	Model: MALDI MS signature + clinical and imaging data	7	Indeterm. Lung nodule	MALDI MS	n/a	II		100	n/a	n/a	72
Diamandis, 2011 [91]	Serum	Protein	Penatraxin-3	1	LC	ELISA	n/a	I		426	37–48	80–90	60–74
Ostroff, 2010 [92]	Serum	Aptamers	*cadherin-1, CD30 ligand, endostatin, HSP90a, LRIG3, MIP-4, pleiotrophin, PRKCI, RGM-C, SCF-sR, sL-selectin, and YES*	6	NSCLC	Aptamers	n/a	II	985	341	89	83	90
Zhong, 2005 [67]	Plasma	AutoAB	TAA signature	5	NSCLC	Protein microarray	5	I	81	n/a	90*	95*	n/a
Taguchi, 2011 [93]	Plasma	Protein	*EGFR, SFTPB, WFDC2, ANGPTL3, ANXA1, YWHAQ, Lmr1*	7	NSLCL	ELISA	52	III		n/a	n/a	n/a	89

AUC: area under the curve, note*= values derived from training set only; BM Dev Phase: biomarker development phase, n/a= not available.
LC: lung cancer.
Source: Adapted from Hassanein *et al.*, 2012 [78].

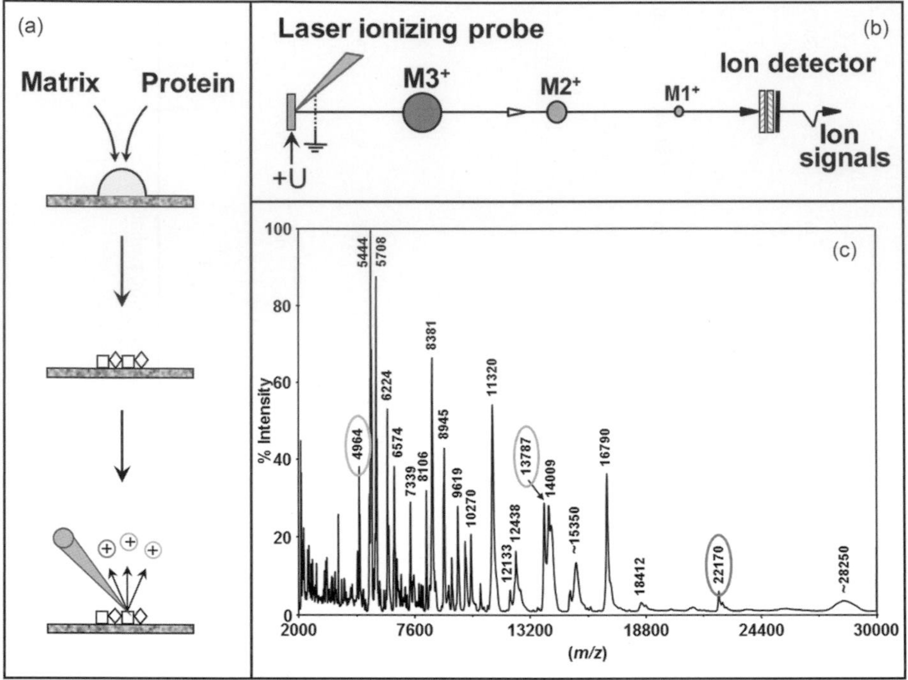

Figure 5.3 Principle of matrix-assisted laser desorption/ionization (MALDI) time-of-flight mass spectrometry. a: Analyte molecules are first mixed with matrix molecules in a ratio ~1 to 5000. Upon solvent evaporation, matrix-analyte co-crystals form. In the ion source of the instrument, irradiation of these with a brief laser pulse initiates the desorption-ionization events. b: The newly formed molecular ions are accelerated in the source of the instrument by a constant potential difference, giving all of the ions of the same charge the same energy. Ions are therefore separated in time according to their mass as they travel the length of the time-of-flight. c: MALDI time-of-flight mass spectrum obtained in the positive ionization mode from a complex protein mixture.
Source: Adapted from Ocak *et al.* [15]. Reprinted with permission of the American Thoracic Society. Copyright © 2013 American Thoracic Society. This modified figure is based on the original figure available from www.atsjournals.org.

successful in providing robust signatures to translate to the clinic for diagnostic/early detection purposes. One application of MALDI TOF MS is to detect patterns of abundant proteins or peptide fragments diagnostic of cancer. In this application, detected MS peaks are typically abundant proteins or peptide fragments that correlate with the disease state but are usually not readily connected with the disease mechanistically (Figure 5.4). Several studies have utilized MALDI MS to develop diagnostic signatures of proteins/peptides in serum [19, 20]. For example, we previously identified a seven signal proteomic signature diagnostic of stage I NSCLC (non-small cell lung cancer) using MALDI MS analysis of undepleted and unfractionated serum with an overall accuracy of 78% and a sensitivity of 67.4% [20]. Patz and colleagues were also able to identify four differentially expressed serum proteins (transferrin, retinol-binding protein [RBP], antitrypsin and haptoglobin) that discriminate between NSCLC and controls [21]. Using the same MALDI MS approaches, several other groups have reported serum protein expression profiles that distinguish patients with various cancers from control subjects [15].

Han *et al.*, used SELDI-TOF MS to analyze the serum of 253 individuals split into a training set (89 NSCLC, 68 controls) and a validation set

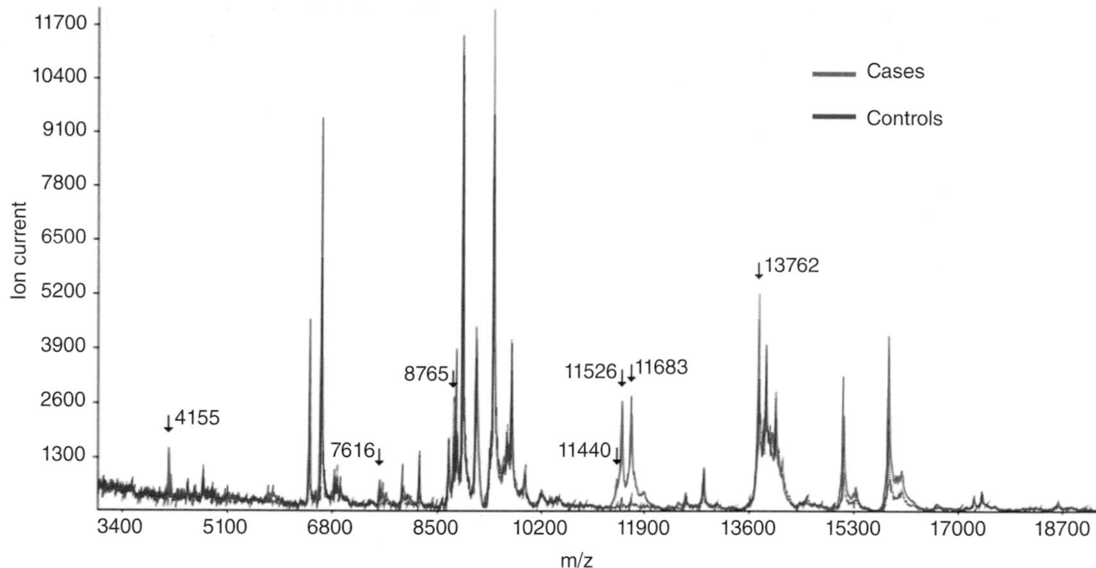

Figure 5.4 MALDI MS serum spectra from individuals with lung cancer and matched controls. Average intensity of spectrum analysis between matched cases (red, plain line) and controls (blue dotted line) are presented. Arrows point to *m/z* values of discriminatory features. *Source*: Adapted from Ocak *et al.* [15]. Reprinted with permission of the American Thoracic Society. Copyright © 2013 American Thoracic Society. This modified figure is based on the original figure available from www.atsjournals.org.

(62 NSCLC, 34 controls) [22]. From the proteomic spectra of serum samples obtained from the training set, using Biomarker Pattern software, they generated a classification tree with 3 different protein masses that effectively identified lung cancer patients from controls with 94% accuracy, 91% sensitivity and 97% specificity. When applied to the validation test, the classification tree allowed 89% sensitivity, 91% specificity and 90% positive predictive value. The authors also used electrochemiluminescent immunoassay to detect CEA and Cyfra21-1 serum levels, and showed that the specificity and sensitivity of these biomarkers taken individually or in combination were significantly lower compared to the SELDI proteomic profile (42% sensitivity and 72% specificity for Cyfra21-1; 46% sensitivity and 76% specificity for CEA). Using SELDI-TOF MS on serum samples from 158 lung cancer patients and 50 controls, Yang *et al.* [23] reported a 5-signal protein signature distinguishing lung cancer cases from controls with 86.9% sensitivity and 80.0% specificity in the validation set.

Despite the technical advantages of SELDI-TOF MS and MALDI-TOF MS technologies, several pre-analytical and analytical limitations still hinder wider applications and implementation of this approach in the clinical setting. The major pre-analytical challenges are related to variability in collection and preparation techniques, leading to the introduction of analytical bias and lack of reproducibility. Analytically, it has been proven challenging to detect low-abundance/high molecular weight proteins and to develop a robust signal analytic algorithm for single patient classification.

The extreme complexity of biofluids such as blood, serum, or plasma and the low abundance of most of the specific protein markers are among other factors that reduce the sensitivity of detection by MS technologies. In fact, the sensitivity of MALDI MS and most other MS technologies is limited to the most abundant proteins, typically within the 1 μg/ml range, while most of the known serum biomarkers are present at 1000-fold lower concentrations. Finally, while implementation of MALDI

MS techniques to fresh tissue or blood samples may provide a large number of discriminatory peaks, direct identification of the corresponding proteins has been proven challenging [15].

An alternative approach to direct analysis of serum by MS is to separate serum samples in 1 or 2 dimensional gels, subject excise bands of interest to tryptic digestion, then identify proteins of interest by mass spectrometry (Table 5.1). *Patz et al.* used 2D difference gel electrophoresis (DIGE) and MALDI-TOF MS. They identified 3 differentially expressed serum proteins by 2D DIGE (transferrin, retinol binding protein (RBP) and haptoglobin) and 1 by MALDI-TOF MS (α1-antitrypsin)[21]. They assayed these 4 proteins as well as 2 others previously known to be cancer associated (SCC (squamous cell carcinoma) antigen, CEA) on a training set of sera from 100 patients (50 lung cancers, 50 controls). Using Classification and Regression Tree (CART) analysis, they found that 4 of these proteins (CEA, RBP, α1-antitrypsin and SCC antigen) were able to distinguish lung cancer cases from controls with 89.3% sensitivity and 84.7% specificity in the training set. When applied to the independent validation set, these markers displayed 77.8% sensitivity and 75.4% specificity. Using the classification scheme produced by CART analysis, the probability of lung cancer for each patient was determined based on the terminal node into which they fell. For patients assigned to 3 of the different terminal nodes, the probability of having cancer was 92% in the training set and 90% in the validation set. When used alone, none of these 4 markers had sufficient diagnostic power, but when combined, they appeared to have value in suggesting lung cancer diagnosis and may be helpful for clinical management at different levels.

Serum proteomics for response to therapy

To identify NSCLC patients who are likely to benefit from treatment with epidermal growth factor receptor (EGFR) tyrosine kinase inhibitors (TKIs), Taguchi *et al.* [24] used MALDI MS on pretreatment serum of 302 patients treated with gefitinib or erlotinib, 139 of them assigned to a training set (from 3 cohorts) and 163 into a validation set (from 2 independent cohorts). Sera from 158 NSCLC patients not treated with EGFR TKIs (from 3 cohorts) were also tested. Based on survival and time to progression after EGFR TKIs treatment, an algorithm based on 8 mass spectrometry signals was developed in the training set. The classification algorithm was then applied to the validation set, successfully identifying patients with improved outcome after EGFR TKIs treatment. Indeed, the median survival of patients in the predicted "good" and "poor" groups was 207 and 92 days, respectively, (HR of death in the good versus poor groups = 0.50, 95% CI = 0.24 to 0.78) in the first cohort, and 306 and 107 days respectively (HR = 0.41, 95% CI = 0.17 to 0.63) in the second cohort. The algorithm kept its predictive value independent of clinical factors associated with sensitivity to EGFR TKIs, such as gender, smoking history and histology. The algorithm identified subgroups of smokers with favorable outcome after EGFR TKIs treatment, showing its benefit even in patients with clinical characteristics associated with low sensitivity to these drugs. For patients not treated with chemotherapy and not EGFR TKIs, the classification algorithm did not classify patients for survival. This classifier was applied to the available samples from BR.21, a randomized trial of erlotinib vs. placebo in second and third line therapy of patients felt to be unfit for chemotherapy [25]. This classifier was highly predictive of response to erlotinib and 18 of 19 responders were identified as proteomics "good". Patients on erlotinib who were proteomics "good" lived significantly longer than patients who were proteomics "poor" (median survivals of 10.5 vs 6.6 months), but patients in the placebo arm also had a not significant difference in survival (4 vs. 3.4 months), and the interaction test was not significant. This signature was recently reported to be statistically significantly predictive of survival in a prospective randomized trial (PROSE) and is currently being tested in another large randomized trials in squamous cancer patients [26].

In a separate study using candidate protein markers, the prognostic and predictive value of the plasma levels of two adhesion molecules, soluble intercellular adhesion molecule (ICAM) and E-selectin, and two angiogenic factors vascular endothelial growth factor (VEGF) and basic fibroblast growth factor (bFGF) were evaluated in E4599 phase II/phase III clinical trial cohorts, in which 878 patients with advanced NSCLC were randomized to carboplatin + paclitaxel (PC arm) or PC + bevacizumab (BPC arm). Only ICAM levels were prognostic for survival and predictive of response to chemotherapy with or without bevacizumab, while VEGF levels were predictive of response to bevacizumab but not survival [27]. Another report also showed that the plasma level of a panel of 8 cytokine and angiogenic factors (CAFs) measured by multiplex assays or ELISA (enzyme linked immunosorbant assay) can accurately predict the response to pazopanib, an oral angiogenesis inhibitor targeting VEGFR, platelet-derived growth factor receptor, and c-kit in 33 patients with early-stage NSCLC participating in a single-arm phase II trial [28].

Recently, an automated technology has been developed for the simultaneous measurement of serum peptides. In this approach, peptides are captured and concentrated using reversed-phase batch processing in a magnetic particle-based format, automated on a liquid handling robot, followed by MALDI-TOF MS. This technique is simple, scalable and may provide better reproducibility, multidimensionality and high throughput [29], but must be validated in larger populations and from several institutions.

Strategies to address serum proteome complexity

The enormous complexity of the serum proteome with tens of thousands of different protein species [30], a wide range of concentrations, a large number of peptides generated from each protein, their posttranslational modifications [30] and isoforms variations among individuals [31] present current proteomic technologies with unlimited challenges. To overcome some these challenges, different complexity reduction strategies have been implemented. In one strategy, affinity depletion removes the most abundant serum proteins such as albumin [32–35] and detects lower-abundance proteins, which are more informative as tumor-specific biomarkers but otherwise are obscured by high-abundance proteins. Depletion procedures are limited by difficulties in standardization and of reproducibility. In a second strategy, proteins or peptides are fractionated using physicochemical properties such as size, residue charge, and hydropathy before analysis by MS [34, 36, 37]. This fractionation has several limitations as it requires large sample amounts, is more expensive and time-consuming, and increases the risk of variability within and between samples.

Liquid chromatography (LC) tandem mass spectrometry (MS/MS)

LC MS/MS is a powerful tool for the separation and identification of peptides and proteins in a complex mixture, this technique directly couples liquid chromatography (HPLC) with ESI MS and has a profound impact on tumor protein profiling [38]. This fully automated platform follows a "bottom-up" approach (as opposed to "top down" approach where intact proteins are ionized and fragmented to peptide fragments). In the bottom-up (also referred to as "shotgun") proteomic approach, proteins are first digested with site-specific proteases, and the resulting peptides are separated by LC and analyzed online by ESI MS and MS/MS (Figure 5.5) [15, 39]. In the first MS, charged peptides are measured according to their m/z ratios. The most abundant of these are sequentially selected for MS/MS analyses. The resulting fragment ions are then analyzed in a second MS scan according to their m/z ratios. Based on our understanding of the fragments produced in the collision cell and their precise molecular weight, the peptide sequence can be deduced. Through comparisons of predicted sequences with the same nominal mass in databases, peptides are identified and proteins from which they came are deduced. However, with extremely complex protein mixtures, confident and reproducible identification by MS/MS sequencing becomes difficult. Also, high abundance proteins may obscure low abundance ones. To overcome these problems, different separation methods are

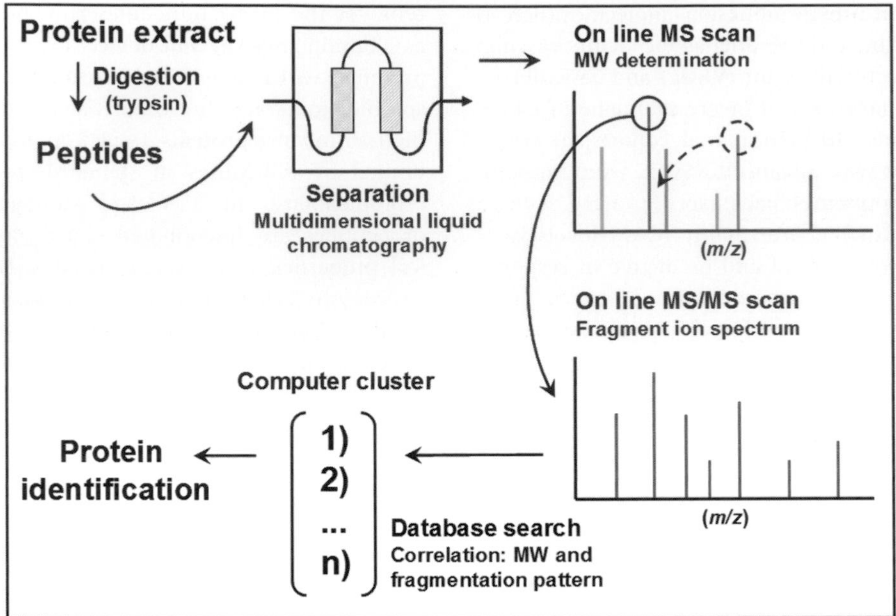

Figure 5.5 Shotgun protein identification by liquid chromatography (LC)-mass spectrometry (MS)/MS from a complex protein mixture. a: the protein mixture is first digested (by trypsin) and the resulting peptides are separated by multidimensional liquid chromatography (typically strong cation exchange followed by reverse-phase separation) coupled online to the mass spectrometer. As they elute, the *m/z* ratios of the peptides are first determined followed by one or several MS/MS scans from the most abundant peptide signals. This cycle is repeated until all of the peptides have eluted from the chromatography column. For each precursor peptide selected for MS/MS, peptides of similar nominal mass are extracted from sequence databases and predicted fragmentation patterns are derived *in silico*. These patterns are then compared to the experimental fragmentation spectrum to generate correlation scores. Positive identification of a protein is based on the observation of two or more peptides issued from its sequence.
Source: Adapted from Ocak *et al.* [15]. Reprinted with permission of the American Thoracic Society. Copyright © 2013 American Thoracic Society. This modified figure is based on the original figure available from www.atsjournals.org.

combined with MS analysis, such as size exclusion, anion exchange, strong cation exchange, isoelectric focusing and reverse phase chromatography. In particular, multidimensional protein identification technology (MudPIT), a combination of strong cation exchange and reverse phase columns can be adapted to a shotgun MS proteomics platform [40–42] taking advantage of ion exchange and reverse phase separations, data-independent scanning [43] and a reduced total analysis time. Using shotgun proteomics combined with MudPIT [42,44,45] on the plasma of patients with lung cancer, 120 proteins have been shown to be exclusively expressed in the plasma of lung ADC patients [46].

In the last strategy, specific chemical probes are used to tag and facilitate isolation of a target peptide. After digestion of proteins with trypsin in the shotgun approach, analyses are complicated by the large number of redundant peptides from each protein. By targeting peptides containing unique or rare amino acids or posttranslational modifications such as phosphorylation or glycosylation [47], we can reduce the complexity of the biological samples and analyze subproteomes. For example, Zhou *et al.* [48] developed a method for high-throughput analysis of serum glycoproteins using solid-phase extraction of N-linked glycopeptides from glycoproteins (SPEG). Glycoproteins are conjugated to a solid support using hydrazide chemistry, nonglycosylated proteins are removed by trypsin digestion, and N-glycopeptides are specifically released via peptide-N-glycosidase F before finally being identified and quantified by tandem MS [49]. Although quite appealing these subproteomic strategies are early in development and require methodological standardization.

Targeted proteomics using multiple reaction monitoring (LC MRM MS)

MRM MS (multiple reaction monitoring: molecular weight) allows for the verification of candidate biomarkers by accurate quantitation of proteins/peptides. In this strategy, which requires a triple quadrupole-class tandem MS [50], there are two stages of mass selection: the first stage (MS1) selects a limited number of precursor ions with prespecified *m/z* values that will undergo fragmentation, while the second stage (MS2) gives spectra only for a specific pre-identified fragment ion associated with a given precursor. The association of two mass filters leads to a very specific and sensitive identification. Several "precursor ion/fragment ion" pairs can be specified in a single LC-MS/MS (liquid chromatography coupled to tandem mass spectrometry) run, allowing parallel quantification of several proteins/peptides. Improved quantification can be achieved by iTRAQ (isobaric Tags for Relative and Absolute Quantification; covalent linkage to lysines, -NH_2 termini) [51] at the MS2 level or by label-free methodology at the MS1 level. C-reactive protein [52], apolipoprotein A-I [53], human growth hormone [54] and prostate-specific antigen [55] have been measured in plasma or serum using the MRM approach.

Bio-analytical validation of serum protein biomarkers

Following the discovery of new biomarkers, the next critical steps are to validate and evaluate their performance in clinically relevant patient populations [56]. Multiple levels of validation have to take place before confirming the clinical utility of the biomarkers [57, 58]. This includes confirmation of detected changes in protein level by different techniques, correlation with biological outcomes of lung cancer such as early detection, chemosensitivity, or survival. These phases of clinical validation will evaluate the biomarkers performance in relevant clinical context and how they may impact clinical management of risk or disease [59] (see "Clinical validation of serum biomarkers" section below).

Biochemical methods for protein markers validation have been dominated by immuno-based assays. Although immune-based detection assays have been the most trusted and reliable method for biomarker validation, they rely on the tight and specific binding of the antibodies against the targeted molecule but are limited by the quality of antibodies, high labor intensity and relatively low-throughput [60]. Recently, Kuhn *et al.* used MRM to identify a panel of serum biomarkers from rheumatoid arthritis patients [61]. Another novel technology that combines the specificity of immune assays with the sensitivity of mass spectrometry, denoted by stable isotope standards and capture by anti-peptide antibodies or SISCAPA, was developed to quantify peptides in complex digests [62]. In this method, anti-peptide antibodies immobilized on nano affinity columns are used to enrich specific peptides along with spiked stable-isotope-labeled internal standards of the same sequence. Upon elution from the anti-peptide antibody supports, electrospray mass spectrometry is used to quantify the peptides (natural and labeled). SISCAPA is thus limited to sequence-defined (predetermined) analytes, but offers the possibility of significantly increased sensitivity by removing unwanted peptides from the set delivered to the MS. No blood-based biomarker for lung cancer has yet been validated using these techniques, although ongoing technical improvements of protein separation and detection may allow for applications of these approaches as validation platforms in the near future. Blood samples repositories were recently developed in the context of a joint NCI/SPORE/EDRN effort and are now available for phase II validation of candidate biomarkers (http://edrn.nci.nih.gov/resources/sample-reference-sets).

Circulating autoantibodies

Tumor associated antigens or TAA are proteins that are altered in a variety of ways in cancer cells that render them immunogenic. These include overexpression, mutations, misfolding, truncation, and degradation [63]. A large number of TAA targets have been identified from patient sera in several immunological diseases and malignancies using various high throughput screening platforms such as cDNA expression phage display libraries and protein microarrays [64]. In lung cancer, autoantibodies against the protein gene product 9.5 (PGP 9.5) have been identified as a potential lung cancer TAA using immunoreactivity of patients sera against tumor proteins isolated by two dimensional proteomics [65]. Interestingly, using phage display libraries, TAAs have been detected in the blood of patients who developed lung cancer up to 5 years before any tumor were detected with spiral computed tomography using screening [66]. Therefore, monitoring these autoantibodies in serum from individuals at high risk for lung cancer represents an attractive option for developing a screening test.

Using these approaches, several groups reported the identification of large numbers of immunogenic peptides that are potential targets for autoantibodies. For example, two separate groups identified several potential immunoreactive peptides for autoantibodies using the T-7 cDNA-based phage library as a screen from sera of NSCLC patients [66–68]. Using similar techniques, Chen *et al.* also identified and validated ubiquitin 1 amongst several other peptides as a potential autoantibody target in lung adenocarcinoma from sera of patients with early stage disease [69]. Also recently, a study by Wu *et al.* reported the identification of 6 peptide clones discriminatory of NSCLC using phage display techniques, but only one protein identity has been confirmed [70]. However, most of the identified antigens were found to elicit antibodies in a relatively small proportion of patients, yielding a test of high specificity but very low sensitivity.

One other common challenge to these phage display techniques is the inability to detect post-translational modifications. Recently this obstacle was overcome by the development of a multidimensional fractionation technique using liquid chromatography (LC) to isolate a mixture of native proteins extracted from cancer cell lines. Using this method, antibodies directed against C-terminal hydrolase L3 ubiquitin were identified in the sera of patients with colon cancer and, more recently, in the blood of patients with lung adenocarcinoma [71]. The validation of these novel lung cancer autoantibodies mandated the development of robust detection assays that are sensitive, reproducible, and high-throughput.

To test the utility of autoantibodies as a diagnostic tool for lung cancer, indirect ELISA tests were developed and validated for a panel of 6 known lung cancer TAAs (p53, NY-ESO-1, cancer-associated antigen (CAGE), GBU4-5, Annexin 1 and SOX2) [72, 73]. These efforts yielded an assay with high reproducibility, precision, and linearity that was able to identify nearly 40% of primary lung cancers via a peripheral blood test. This approach promises to address the need for early diagnosis (Figure 5.2) particularly for presymptomatic, curable disease. These assays will also need further clinical validation in large cohorts of high-risk patients, both retrospectively and prospectively before moving to the clinical practice.

Clinical validation of serum biomarkers

Appropriate study design is critical for the successful validation of a promising biomarker for clinical use. Validation of a biomarker useful for lung cancer diagnosis or early screening should be conducted using a nested case-control study design within a prospective longitudinal cohort following the PRoBE design [74]. Specifically, random sampling of cases and controls identified from within a well-defined cohort population allows both cases and controls to be sampled from the same source population, thus providing validity to the case-control design. Matching strategies may be considered, such as using incidence density sampling to sample controls at the same time each case occurs so that cases and controls are matched on time. While there are advantages to matching the potential pitfalls of matching should be carefully considered prior to implementation [74, 75].

Assessment of the generalizability of biomarkers in different clinical settings and populations is necessary for a clinically useful biomarker. In biomarker discovery, the prospective cohort from which the cases and controls are sampled must be representative of the targeted clinical population to which the biomarker will be applied. Thus the cohort study population should comprise individuals with conditions found in the target population, such as inflammatory disease, granulomas, or benign tumors so that false positives can be minimized and individuals developing lung cancer can be differentiated from those not developing the disease [76].

Biospecimens necessary for biomarker development should be collected at the initiation of the prospective cohort study, prior to ascertainment of lung cancer status [74], and potentially over multiple time points if the biomarker changes with age and with progression to disease [76]. These biospecimens are then evaluated in patients who develop biopsy proven cancer (cases) and those who do not (controls) to develop a biomarker for clinical use as a cost efficient approach. Importantly, the outcome should be clearly defined [77] and the biomarker assay development should be blinded to case-control status to avoid information bias [74]. To validate the usefulness of a biomarker for early detection of lung cancer, diagnostic validation of the biomarker should be conducted in different, potentially confounding, populations other than the one in which the biomarker was developed to test specificity for lung cancer [78]. Finally, this should be followed by early diagnostic validation using a screening trial with lung cancer mortality as the endpoint [79].

Assessing whether a biomarker has clinical validity requires estimation of sensitivity and specificity, which can be summarized with the receiver operator characteristic curve (ROC) [80]. Two additional clinically relevant measures that can be measured by ROC include negative predictive value (NPV) and positive predictive value (PPV), which are estimated using sensitivity and specificity. These clinically important indices describe the probability of developing or having disease given a positive test and the probability of not having the disease given a negative test. Estimates of PPV and NPV are influenced by the prevalence of the disease and consequently will vary by patient age, target population, and disease stage. Merely targeting the screening to a high-risk population based on demographic factors can alter the screening test performance characteristics [81]. Thus for a biomarker to be clinically valid and generalizable, the biomarker validation process must be applied to multiple populations having different demographic characteristics for determining the clinical validity and utility of a biomarker, and each population may have different requirements for biomarker clinical utility.

Current challenges in lung cancer biomarker development and implementation

One of the main objectives of molecular medicine in lung cancer is to identify biomarkers that discriminate between low and high risk individuals and between benign and malignant lung tumors. Ultimately these biomarkers can potentially be translated to noninvasive, simple, and reliable diagnostic tests for early detection of the disease. The underlying assumption behind these efforts is that tumor-specific or overexpressed proteins can be detected simply and accurately in complex clinical samples such as surrogate tissues and biofluids. The intensive research in genomics and proteomics aimed at identifying these biomarkers has yielded a large number of potential diagnostic biomarkers, although few have progressed to the level of FDA-approval for diagnostics [82]. A list of several recent diagnostic serum protein biomarker studies is summarized in Table 5.2. These biomarkers were selected based on two main criteria. First, the proposed marker, or panel of markers must be quantitatively measurable and its performance tested in at least one sample set of clinically relevant specimens. Second, the report must adhered to the rigorous clinical validation guidelines discussed above ("Clinical validation of serum biomarkers" section). The validation sets reported in the tables correspond to an attempt to test the biomarker (or signature) in a true independent population, also described as clinical validation [83], to evaluate the performance of the test in an independent cohort.

This disappointingly slow pace of lung cancer biomarkers discovery and validation is attributed to a host of technological and methodological factors. The gap between promise and product can partially be explained by the fact that current discovery methods are neither reliable nor efficient. One reason is that the current analytical technologies still suffer from the limited power to detect low-abundant cancer markers against a high background of high-abundance molecular species such as proteins in very complex matrices such as plasma or serum. These low-abundance markers in biofluids such as serum may be the most promising cancer biomarkers. Consequently, many of the best candidates may be missed during the discovery phase.

Another quandary is the limited capacity to verify and validate analytically existing candidate markers in a high-throughput manner. This is particularly true in proteomics research. The lack of available quality reagents such as antibodies, or methodologies to translate the discovery of candidates in tissue specimens and measure their concentration in the circulation remains an enormous challenge. Therefore it is possible that biomarkers have already been "discovered," but not yet validated. Furthermore, once a long list of candidate biomarkers is compiled, no current standardized method exists for selecting those that are most promising for systematic validation. In addition, the reproducibility of biomarker data has been flawed because of the poor design (e.g., underrepresentation of studies using a nested case-control design [74]), model over-fitting, and the lack of cross-validation and independent validation. Changing technology, low concentration of signals combined with very few prospective studies, and a low incidence disease, make the area of biomarker research challenging.

Conclusions and future clinical implications

The molecular analysis of a variety of biospecimens has allowed the discovery of relevant candidate biomarkers and consequently the identification of novel proteins that may have a role in the development of lung cancer. High volume of data from multiple high-throughput biochemical analyses of clinical material from "Omics" sources has been accumulating at an exponential rate in the last few years, generating large number of biomarker candidates. None of the published candidate biomarkers of risk or of lung cancer diagnosis is ready for clinical use, and few have moved to phase III biomarker development. Lung cancer is recognized as a complex and heterogeneous disease, not only at the biochemical level (genes, proteins, metabolites), but also at the tissue, organism, and population level. There is a need for incorporating findings from multiple discovery platforms into a mathematical framework that can improve our level of understanding of the disease process. A biofluids-based molecular test may improve the selection of high risk individuals for CT screening, distinguish those with malignant nodules from benign lesions, and identify patients with particularly aggressive cancer. Clinical benefit could include further reductions in mortality and thus provide significant cost-savings to the healthcare system.

The importance of serum biomarkers also arises from its potential impact on our understanding of pathogenesis and progression of complex disease such as lung cancer, and will offer new opportunities in the early detection, prognosis, and therapeutic management of the disease. In this chapter we attempted to provide an up-to-date overview of the recent progress in serum proteomics technologies and their wide range of applications in lung cancer, with a main emphasis on early detection. The rapid development of proteomic technologies has led to the assembly of large protein and peptide inventories and to a better understanding of how they interact, of the role of specific posttranslational modifications, and to addressing some of their biological functions. Although proteomic profiling of lung cancer sera and related biological specimens have yet to demonstrate clinical utility, it has the potential to highlight differences between lung cancer and nonmalignant lesions, and between different levels of risks as well as stages and histology subtypes. Molecular profiling may assist with identifying high-risk populations, offering a unique opportunity to study early carcinogenesis or aid with identifying patient populations that can benefit from specific targeted therapy. Integrating the findings from different scales of biological organization from gene to protein to cell using systems biology approaches will provide a global view of the key molecular changes associated with tumor progression. Therefore, systems biology can potentially expedite the translation of "Omics" to personalized molecular medicine in the foreseeable future.

The development of specific and sensitive diagnostic biomarkers from biological fluids, such as sputum, blood, or exhaled breath, should improve early detection strategies, monitoring of disease progression, treatment response, and surveillance for recurrence. There is a need for extensive validation using novel proteomics research platforms and demonstration of clinical utility.

References

1 Bhattacharjee A, Richards WG, Staunton J, Li C, Monti S, Vasa P, *et al.* (2001) Classification of human lung carcinomas by mRNA expression profiling reveals distinct adenocarcinoma subclasses. *Proc Natl Acad Sci USA*, 98(24): 13790–5.

2 Brambilla E, Travis WD, Colby TV, Corrin B, Shimosato Y (2001) The new World Health Organization classification of lung tumours. *European Respiratory Journal*, 18(6): 1059–68.

3 Beer DG, Kardia SL, Huang CC, Giordano TJ, Levin AM, Misek DE, *et al.* (2002) Gene-expression profiles predict survival of patients with lung adenocarcinoma. *Nature Medicine*, 8(8): 816–24.

4 Garber ME, Troyanskaya OG, Schluens K, Petersen S, Thaesler Z, Pacyna-Gengelbach M, *et al.* (2001) Diversity of gene expression in adenocarcinoma of the lung. *Proc Natl Acad Sci USA*, 98(24): 13784–9.

5 Siegel R, Naishadham D, Jemal A (2012) Cancer statistics, 2012. *CA: A Cancer Journal for Clinicians*, 62(1): 10–29. Epub 2012/01/13.

6 Zhu L, Pickle LW, Ghosh K, Naishadham D, Portier K, Chen HS, *et al.* (2012) Predicting US- and state-level cancer counts for the current calendar year: Part II: evaluation of spatiotemporal projection methods for incidence. *Cancer*, 118(4): 1100–9. Epub 2012/01/10.

7 Hoffman PC, Mauer AM, Vokes EE (2000) Lung cancer. *Lancet*, 355(9202): 479–85.

8 Patz EF, Jr., Caporaso NE, Dubinett SM, Massion PP, Hirsch FR, Minna JD, *et al.* (2010) National Lung Cancer Screening Trial American College of Radiology Imaging Network Specimen Biorepository originating from the Contemporary Screening for the Detection of Lung Cancer Trial (NLST, ACRIN 6654): design, intent, and availability of specimens for validation of lung cancer biomarkers. *J Thorac Oncol*, 5(10): 1502–6. Epub 2010/09/28.

9 Manser RL, Irving LB, Byrnes G, Abramson MJ, Stone CA, Campbell DA (2003) Screening for lung cancer: a systematic review and meta-analysis of controlled trials. *Thorax*, 58(9): 784–9.

10 Manser R. Screening for lung cancer: a review. *Curr Opin Pulm Med*, 10(4): 266–71. Epub 2004/06/29.

11 Pastorino U (2010) Lung cancer screening. *Br J Cancer*, 102(12): 1681–6. Epub 2010/04/29.

12 National Institute of Health NCIN, NCI Office of Media Relations (2010) Twenty percent fewer lung cancer deaths seen among those who were screened with low-dose spiral CT than with chest X-ray. *US NIH News*.

13 Ludwig JA, Weinstein JN (2005) Biomarkers in cancer staging, prognosis and treatment selection. *Nat Rev Cancer*, 5(11): 845–56.

14 Anderson L, Hunter CL (2006) Quantitative mass spectrometric multiple reaction monitoring assays for major plasma proteins. *Mol Cell Proteomics*, 5(4): 573–88. Epub 2005/12/08.

15 Ocak S, Chaurand P, Massion PP (2009) Mass spectrometry-based proteomic profiling of lung cancer. *Proceedings of the American Thoracic Society*, 6(2): 159–70. Epub 2009/04/08.

16 Addona TA, Abbatiello SE, Schilling B, Skates SJ, Mani DR, Bunk DM, *et al.* (2009) Multi-site assessment of the precision and reproducibility of multiple reaction monitoring-based measurements of proteins in plasma. *Nat Biotechnol*, 27(7): 633–41. Epub 2009/06/30.

17 Gonzalez-Angulo AM, Hennessy BT, Mills GB. Future of personalized medicine in oncology: a systems biology approach. *J Clin Oncol*, 28(16): 2777–83. Epub 2010/04/22.

18 Beavis RC, Chait BT (1990) Rapid, sensitive analysis of protein mixtures by mass spectrometry. *Proc Natl Acad Sci USA*, 87(17): 6873–7.

19 Sidransky D, Irizarry R, Califano JA, Li X, Ren H, Benoit N, *et al.* (2003) Serum protein MALDI profiling to distinguish upper aerodigestive tract cancer patients from control subjects. *J Natl Cancer Inst*, 95(22): 1711–17.

20 Yildiz PB, Shyr Y, Rahman JS, Wardwell NR, Zimmerman LJ, Shakhtour B, *et al.* (2007) Diagnostic accuracy of MALDI mass spectrometric analysis of unfractionated serum in lung cancer. *J Thorac* Oncol, 2(10): 893–901. Epub 2007/10/03.

21 Patz EF, Jr., Campa MJ, Gottlin EB, Kusmartseva I, Guan XR, Herndon JE, 2nd (2007) Panel of serum biomarkers for the diagnosis of lung cancer. *J Clin Oncol*, 25(35): 5578–83.

22 Han KQ, Huang G, Gao CF, Wang XL, Ma B, Sun LQ, *et al.* (2008) Identification of lung cancer patients by serum protein profiling using surface-enhanced laser desorption/ionization time-of-flight mass spectrometry. *Am J Clin Oncol*, 31(2): 133–9.

23 Yang SY, Xiao XY, Zhang WG, Zhang LJ, Zhang W, Zhou B, *et al.* (2005) Application of serum SELDI proteomic patterns in diagnosis of lung cancer. *BMC Cancer*, 5: 83.

24 Taguchi F, Solomon B, Gregorc V, Roder H, Gray R, Kasahara K, *et al.* (2007) Mass spectrometry to classify non-small-cell lung cancer patients for clinical outcome after treatment with epidermal growth factor receptor tyrosine kinase inhibitors: a multicohort cross-institutional study. *J Natl Cancer Inst*, 99(11): 838–46.

25 Carbone DP, Ding K, Roder H, Grigorieva J, Roder J, Tsao MS, *et al.* (2012) Prognostic and predictive role of the VeriStrat plasma test in patients with advanced non-small-cell lung cancer treated with erlotinib or placebo in the NCIC Clinical Trials Group BR.21 trial. *J Thorac Oncol*, 7(11): 1653–60. Epub 2012/10/13.

26 Lazzari C, Novello S, Barni S, Aieta M, Marinis FD, Pas TD, *et al.* (2013) Randomized proteomic stratified phase III study of second-line erlotinib (E) versus chemotherapy (CT) in patients with inoperable non-small cell lung cancer (PROSE). *J Clin Oncol*, 31:(suppl; abstr LBA8005).

27 Dowlati A, Gray R, Sandler AB, Schiller JH, Johnson DH (2008) Cell adhesion molecules, vascular endothelial growth factor, and basic fibroblast growth factor in patients with non-small cell lung cancer treated with chemotherapy with or without bevacizumab-an Eastern Cooperative Oncology Group Study. *Clin Cancer Res*, 14(5): 1407–12. Epub 2008/03/05.

28 Nikolinakos PG, Altorki N, Yankelevitz D, Tran HT, Yan S, Rajagopalan D, *et al.* (2010) Plasma cytokine and angiogenic factor profiling identifies markers associated with tumor shrinkage in early-stage non-small cell lung cancer patients treated with pazopanib. *Cancer Res*, 70(6): 2171–9.

29 Villanueva J, Philip J, Entenberg D, Chaparro CA, Tanwar MK, Holland EC, *et al.* (2004) Serum peptide profiling by magnetic particle-assisted, automated sample processing and MALDI-TOF mass spectrometry. *Anal Chem*, 76(6): 1560–70.

30 Anderson NL, Anderson NG (2002) The human plasma proteome: history, character, and diagnostic prospects. *Mol Cell Proteomic*, 1(11): 845–67.

31 Nedelkov D, Kiernan UA, Niederkofler EE, Tubbs KA, Nelson RW (2005) Investigating diversity in human plasma proteins. *Proc Natl Acad Sci USA*, 102(31): 10852–7.

32 Pieper R, Gatlin CL, Makusky AJ, Russo PS, Schatz CR, Miller SS, *et al.* (2003) The human serum proteome: display of nearly 3700 chromatographically separated protein spots on two-dimensional electrophoresis gels and identification of 325 distinct proteins. *Proteomics*, 3(7): 1345–64.

33 Pieper R, Su Q, Gatlin CL, Huang ST, Anderson NL, Steiner S (2003) Multi-component immunoaffinity subtraction chromatography: an innovative step towards a comprehensive survey of the human plasma proteome. *Proteomics*, 3(4): 422–32.

34 Adkins JN, Varnum SM, Auberry KJ, Moore RJ, Angell NH, Smith RD, *et al.* (2002) Toward a human blood serum proteome: analysis by multidimensional separation coupled with mass spectrometry. *Mol Cell Proteomics*, 1(12): 947–55.

35 Liu T, Qian WJ, Chen WN, Jacobs JM, Moore RJ, Anderson DJ, *et al.* (2005) Improved proteome coverage by using high efficiency cysteinyl peptide enrichment: the human mammary epithelial cell proteome. *Proteomics*, 5(5): 1263–73.

36 Shen Y, Jacobs JM, Camp DG, 2nd, Fang R, Moore RJ, Smith RD, *et al.* (2004) Ultra-high-efficiency strong cation exchange LC/RPLC/MS/MS for high dynamic range characterization of the human plasma proteome. *Anal Chem*, 76(4): 1134–44.

37 Tirumalai RS, Chan KC, Prieto DA, Issaq HJ, Conrads TP, Veenstra TD (2003) Characterization of the low molecular weight human serum proteome. *Mol Cell Proteomics*, 2(10): 1096–1103.

38 McCormack AL, Schieltz DM, Goode B, Yang S, Barnes G, Drubin D, *et al.* (1997) Direct analysis and identification of proteins in mixtures by LC/MS/MS and database searching at the low-femtomole level. *Anal Chem*, 69(4): 767–76.

39 Ocak S, Sos ML, Thomas RK, Massion PP (2009) High-throughput molecular analysis in lung cancer: insights into biology and potential clinical applications.

European Respiratory Journal, 34(2): 489–506. Epub 2009/08/04.

40 Link AJ, Eng J, Schieltz DM, Carmack E, Mize GJ, Morris DR, *et al.* (1999) Direct analysis of protein complexes using mass spectrometry. *NatBiotechnol*, 17(7): 676–82.

41 Wolters DA, Washburn MP, Yates JR, 3rd (2001) An automated multidimensional protein identification technology for shotgun proteomics. *Anal Chem*, 73(23): 5683–90. Epub 2002/01/05.

42 Washburn MP, Wolters D, Yates JR (2001) Large-scale analysis of the yeast proteome by multidimensional protein identification technology. *NatBiotechnol*, 19(3): 242–7.

43 Liebler DC (2004) Shotgun mass spec goes independent. *Nat Methods*, 1(1): 16–17. Epub 2005/03/23.

44 Chen EI, Hewel J, Felding-Habermann B, Yates JR, 3rd (2006) Large scale protein profiling by combination of protein fractionation and multidimensional protein identification technology (MudPIT). *Mol Cell Proteomics*, 5(1): 53–6.

45 Jessani N, Niessen S, Wei BQ, Nicolau M, Humphrey M, Ji Y, *et al.* (2005) A streamlined platform for high-content functional proteomics of primary human specimens. *Nat Methods*, 2(9): 691–7.

46 Fujii K, Nakano T, Kanazawa M, Akimoto S, Hirano T, Kato H, *et al.* (2005) Clinical-scale high-throughput human plasma proteome analysis: lung adenocarcinoma. *Proteomics*, 5(4): 1150–9.

47 Zhang Z, Bast RC, Jr., Yu Y, Li J, Sokoll LJ, Rai AJ, *et al.* (2004) Three biomarkers identified from serum proteomic analysis for the detection of early stage ovarian cancer. *Cancer Res*, 64(16): 5882–90.

48 Zhou Y, Aebersold R, Zhang H (2007) Isolation of N-linked glycopeptides from plasma. *Anal Chem*, 79(15): 5826–37.

49 Zhang H, Li XJ, Martin DB, Aebersold R (2003) Identification and quantification of N-linked glycoproteins using hydrazide chemistry, stable isotope labeling and mass spectrometry. *Nat Biotechnol*, 21(6): 660–6.

50 Domon B, Aebersold R (2006) Mass spectrometry and protein analysis. *Science*, 312(5771): 212–17.

51 Wolf-Yadlin A, Hautaniemi S, Lauffenburger DA, White FM (2007) Multiple reaction monitoring for robust quantitative proteomic analysis of cellular signaling networks. *Proc Natl Acad Sci USA*, 104(14): 5860–5.

52 Kuhn E, Wu J, Karl J, Liao H, Zolg W, Guild B (2004) Quantification of C-reactive protein in the serum of patients with rheumatoid arthritis using multiple reaction monitoring mass spectrometry and 13C-labeled peptide standards. *Proteomics*, 4(4): 1175–86.

53 Barr JR, Maggio VL, Patterson DG, Jr., Cooper GR, Henderson LO, Turner WE, *et al.* (1996) Isotope dilution-mass spectrometric quantification of specific proteins: model application with apolipoprotein A-I. *Clin Chem*, 42(10): 1676–82.

54 Wu CC, MacCoss MJ (2002) Shotgun proteomics: tools for the analysis of complex biological systems. *Curr Opin Mol Ther*, 4(3): 242–50. Epub 2002/07/26.

55 Barnidge DR, Goodmanson MK, Klee GG, Muddiman DC (2004) Absolute quantification of the model biomarker prostate-specific antigen in serum by LC-Ms/MS using protein cleavage and isotope dilution mass spectrometry. *J Proteome Res*, 3(3): 644–52.

56 George SL (2008) Statistical issues in translational cancer research. *Clin Cancer Res*, 14(19): 5954–8. Epub 2008/10/03.

57 Pepe MS, Etzioni R, Feng Z, Potter JD, Thompson ML, Thornquist M, *et al.* (2001) Phases of biomarker development for early detection of cancer. *J Natl Cancer Inst*, 93(14): 1054–61.

58 Srivastava S, Gopal-Srivastava R (2002) Biomarkers in cancer screening: a public health perspective. *J Nutr*, 132(8 Suppl): 2471S–5S.

59 Moons KG (2010) Criteria for scientific evaluation of novel markers: a perspective. *Clin Chem*, 56(4): 537–41. Epub 2010/02/06.

60 Huang SN, Minassian H, More JD (1976) Application of immunofluorescent staining on paraffin sections improved by trypsin digestion. *Lab Invest*, 35(4): 383–90. Epub 1976/10/01.

61 Kuhn E, Wu J, Karl J, Liao H, Zolg W, Guild B (2004) Quantification of C-reactive protein in the serum of patients with rheumatoid arthritis using multiple reaction monitoring mass spectrometry and C-13-labeled peptide standards. *Proteomics*, 4(4): 1175–86.

62 Anderson NL, Polanski M, Pieper R, Gatlin T, Tirumalai RS, Conrads TP, *et al.* (2004) The human plasma proteome: a nonredundant list developed by combination of four separate sources. *Mol Cell Proteomics*, 3(4): 311–26.

63 Caron M, Choquet-Kastylevsky G, Joubert-Caron R (2007) Cancer immunomics using autoantibody signatures for biomarker discovery. *Mol Cell Proteomics*, 6(7): 1115–22. Epub 2007/03/23.

64 Feng Z, Prentice R, Srivastava S (2004) Research issues and strategies for genomic and proteomic biomarker discovery and validation: a statistical perspective. *Pharmacogenomics*, 5(6): 709–19.

65 Brichory F, Beer D, Le Naour F, Giordano T, Hanash S (2001) Proteomics-based identification of protein gene product 9.5 as a tumor antigen that induces a humoral immune response in lung cancer. *Cancer Res*, 61(21): 7908–12.

66 Zhong L, Coe SP, Stromberg AJ, Khattar NH, Jett JR, Hirschowitz EA (2006) Profiling tumor-associated antibodies for early detection of non-small cell lung cancer. *J Thorac Oncol*, 1(6): 513–19. Epub 2007/04/06.

67 Zhong L, Hidalgo GE, Stromberg AJ, Khattar NH, Jett JR, Hirschowitz EA (2005) Using protein microarray as a diagnostic assay for non-small cell lung cancer. *Am J Respir Crit Care Med*, 172(10): 1308–14.

68 Khattar NH, Coe-Atkinson SP, Stromberg AJ, Jett JR, Hirschowitz EA (2010) Lung cancer-associated autoantibodies measured using seven amino acid peptides in a diagnostic blood test for lung cancer. *Cancer Biology & Therapy*, 10(3). Epub 2010/06/15.

69 Chen EI, Cociorva D, Norris JL, Yates JR, 3rd (2007) Optimization of mass spectrometry-compatible surfactants for shotgun proteomics. *J Proteome Res*, 6(7): 2529–38. Epub 2007/05/29.

70 Wu D, Gao Y, Chen L, Qi Y, Kang Q, Wang H, *et al.* (2010) Anti-tumor effects of a novel chimeric peptide on S180 and H22 xenografts bearing nude mice. *Peptides*, 31(5): 850–64. Epub 2010/02/06.

71 Hanash S (2003) Harnessing immunity for cancer marker discovery. *Nat Biotechnol*, 21(1): 37–8.

72 Chapman CJ, Murray A, McElveen JE, Sahin U, Luxemburger U, Tureci O, *et al.* (2008) Autoantibodies in lung cancer: possibilities for early detection and subsequent cure. *Thorax*, 63(3): 228–33. Epub 2007/10/13.

73 Murray A, Chapman CJ, Healey G, Peek LJ, Parsons G, Baldwin D, *et al.* (2010) Technical validation of an autoantibody test for lung cancer. *Ann Oncol*, 21(8): 1687–93. Epub 2010/02/04.

74 Pepe MS, Feng Z, Janes H, Bossuyt PM, Potter JD (2008) Pivotal evaluation of the accuracy of a biomarker used for classification or prediction: standards for study design. *J Natl Cancer Inst*, 100(20): 1432–8. Epub 2008/10/09.

75 Janes H, Pepe MS (2008) Matching in studies of classification accuracy: implications for analysis, efficiency, and assessment of incremental value. *Biometrics*, 64(1): 1–9. Epub 2007/05/16.

76 Baker SG, Kramer BS, Srivastava S (2002) Markers for early detection of cancer: Statistical guidelines for nested case-control studies. *BMC Med Res Methodol*, 2(1): 4.

77 Moons KG, Altman DG, Vergouwe Y, Royston P (2009) Prognosis and prognostic research: application and impact of prognostic models in clinical practice. *BMJ*, 338: b606. Epub 2009/06/09.

78 Hassanein M, Callison JC, Callaway-Lane C, Aldrich MC, Grogan EL, Massion PP (2012) The state of molecular biomarkers for the early detection of lung cancer. *Cancer Prev Res (Phila)*, Aug; 5(8): 992–1006. doi: 10.1158/1940-6207.CAPR-11-0441. Epub 2012 Jun 11.

79 Baker SG (2009) Improving the biomarker pipeline to develop and evaluate cancer screening tests. *J Natl Cancer Inst*, 101(16): 1116–19. Epub 2009/07/04.

80 Taylor JM, Ankerst DP, Andridge RR (2008) Validation of biomarker-based risk prediction models. *Clin Cancer Res*, 14(19): 5977–83. Epub 2008/10/03.

81 Moons KG, Biesheuvel CJ, Grobbee DE (2004) Test research versus diagnostic research. *Clin Chem*, 50(3): 473–6.

82 Anderson JE, Hansen LL, Mooren FC, Post M, Hug H, Zuse A, *et al.* (2006) Methods and biomarkers for the diagnosis and prognosis of cancer and other diseases: towards personalized medicine. *Drug Resist Updat*, 9(4–5): 198–210. Epub 2006/10/03.

83 Brenner DE, Normolle DP (2007) Biomarkers for cancer risk, early detection, and prognosis: the validation conundrum. *Cancer Epidemiol Biomarkers Prev*, 16(10): 1918–20. Epub 2007/10/13.

84 Qiu J, Choi G, Li L, Wang H, Pitteri SJ, Pereira-Faca SR, *et al.* (2008) Occurrence of autoantibodies to annexin I, 14-3-3 theta and LAMR1 in prediagnostic lung cancer sera. *J Clin Oncol*, 26(31): 5060–6. Epub 2008/09/17.

85 Wu L, Chang W, Zhao J, Yu Y, Tan X, Su T, *et al.* (2010) Development of autoantibody signatures as novel diagnostic biomarkers of non-small cell lung cancer. *Clinical Cancer Research*, 16(14): 3760–8. Epub 2010/05/27.

86 Farlow EC, Patel K, Basu S, Lee BS, Kim AW, Coon JS, *et al.* (2010) Development of a multiplexed tumor-associated autoantibody-based blood test for the detection of non-small cell lung cancer. *Clin Cancer Res*, 16(13): 3452–62. Epub 2010/06/24.

87 Boyle P, Chapman CJ, Holdenrieder S, Murray A, Robertson C, Wood WC, *et al.* (2011) Clinical validation of an autoantibody test for lung cancer. *Ann Oncol*, 22(2): 383–9. Epub 2010/08/03.

88 Kulpa J, Wojcik E, Reinfuss M, Kolodziejski L (2002) Carcinoembryonic antigen, squamous cell carcinoma antigen, CYFRA 21-1, and neuron-specific enolase in squamous cell lung cancer patients. *Clin Chem*, 48(11): 1931–7.

89 Takano A, Ishikawa N, Nishino R, Masuda K, Yasui W, Inai K, *et al.* (2009) Identification of Nectin-4 oncoprotein as a diagnostic and therapeutic target for lung cancer. *Cancer Res,* 69(16): 6694–6703.

90 Pecot CV, Li M, Zhang XJ, Rajanbabu R, Calitri C, Bungum A, *et al.* (2012) Added value of a serum proteomic signature in the diagnostic evaluation of lung nodules. *Cancer Epidemiol Biomarkers Prev,* May; 21(5): 786–92. doi: 10.1158/1055-9965.EPI-11-0932. Epub 2012 Feb 28.

91 Diamandis EP, Goodglick L, Planque C, Thornquist MD (2011) Pentraxin-3 is a novel biomarker of lung carcinoma. *Clinical Cancer Research,* 17(8): 2395–9.

92 Ostroff RM, Bigbee WL, Franklin W, Gold L, Mehan M, Miller YE, *et al.* (2010) Unlocking biomarker discovery: large scale application of aptamer proteomic technology for early detection of lung cancer. *PLoS ONE,* 5(12): e15003. Epub 2010/12/21.

93 Taguchi A, Politi K, Pitteri SJ, Lockwood WW, Faca VM, Kelly-Spratt K, *et al.* (2011) Lung cancer signatures in plasma based on proteome profiling of mouse tumor models. *Cancer Cell,* 20(3): 289–99. Epub 2011/09/13.

94 Hassanein M, Rahman JS, Chaurand P, Massion PP (2011) Advances in proteomic strategies toward the early detection of lung cancer. *Proc Am Thorac Soc,* 8(2): 183–8. Epub 2011/05/06.

CHAPTER 6

Molecular Biology of Lung Preneoplasia

Humam Kadara and Ignacio I. Wistuba
Department of Translational Molecular Pathology, Division of Pathology and Laboratory Medicine, The University of Texas MD Anderson Cancer Center, Houston, TX, USA

Introduction

From histopathological and biological perspectives, lung cancer is a highly complex set of different but related neoplasms [1], probably having multiple preneoplastic pathways. Lung cancer consists of several histological types, including small cell lung carcinoma (SCLC) and non-small cell lung carcinoma (NSCLC) types of squamous cell carcinoma, adenocarcinoma (including the noninvasive type of bronchioloalveolar carcinoma, BAC), and large cell carcinoma [2]. Lung cancers may arise from the major bronchi (central tumors) or small bronchi, bronchioles, or alveoli (peripheral tumors) of the distant airway of the lung. Squamous cell carcinomas and SCLCs usually arise centrally, whereas adenocarcinomas and large cell carcinomas usually arise peripherally [2]. However, the specific respiratory epithelial cell type from which each lung cancer type develops has not been established. As with other epithelial malignancies, it is believed that lung cancers arise after a series of progressive pathological changes, known as preneoplastic or premalignant lesions [3, 4]. Although the sequential preneoplastic changes have been defined for centrally arising squamous carcinomas of the lung [2], they have been poorly documented for the other major forms of lung cancers [3, 4].

Several studies have provided information regarding the molecular characterization of the preneoplastic changes involved in the pathogenesis of lung cancer, especially squamous cell carcinoma and adenocarcinoma [5–8]. Moreover, earlier studies have demonstrated that lung cancer displays a field cancerization phenomenon in which molecular abnormalities (e.g., loss of heterozygosity) are shared between lung tumors and adjacent histologically normal-appearing tissue [2, 9, 10]. Many of these molecular changes have been detected in the histologically normal respiratory mucosa of smokers [9–12]. The high-risk population targeted for early detection efforts are heavy smokers and patients who have survived a cancer of the upper aerodigestive tract suggesting that further understanding the field cancerization phenomenon would have favorable impact on earlier diagnosis of lung cancer [9, 13]. It is important to mention that conventional morphologic methods for the identification of premalignant cell populations in the lung airways have important limitations. This has

Lung Cancer, Fourth Edition. Edited by Jack A. Roth, Waun Ki Hong and Ritsuko U. Komaki.

led to research in biological properties, including molecular and genetic changes, of the respiratory epithelium and its corresponding preneoplastic cells and lesions.

Compared to the molecular pathology of overt or clinically evident lung tumors [1, 2, 14, 15], relatively little is known about the molecular events preceding the development of lung carcinomas and the underlying genetic basis of lung carcinogenesis. Thus, our current state of knowledge is not sufficient to identify with certainty molecular markers useful for risks assessment, targeted chemoprevention or treatment, and early detection of lung premalignant lesions. Moreover, attempts to better define the pathogenesis of lung premalignancy have been thwarted by the relative invisibility of the cellular lesions and their random distribution throughout the respiratory airway field. Moreover, despite recent encouraging findings from the National Lung Screening Trial (NLST) [16], early detection and prevention of lung cancer is challenging due to the lack of biomarkers for early diagnosis of the disease and to the presence of multiple neoplastic molecular pathways that mediate lung carcinogenesis. It is plausible to assume that further research in this area and increasing our understanding of early phases in lung tumor development including those that commence in normal epithelia would pave the way for unmet and effective early detection and prevention strategies.

In this chapter we summarize the current information on lung cancer molecular and histopathologic pathogenesis and discuss the complexity of the identification of novel molecular mechanisms involved in the development of the lung premalignant disease, and their relevance to the development of new strategies for early detection and chemoprevention. In addition, we describe the recognized preneoplastic lesions for major types of lung cancers and review the current concepts of early pathogenesis and the progression of the most important histologic types of lung cancer. Furthermore, we summarize recent advances in understanding the field cancerization phenomenon and the potential relevance of this knowledge to gain important and novel insights into the molecular pathogenesis of lung cancer.

Pathology of lung cancer preneoplastic lesions

Lung cancers are believed to arise after a series of progressive pathological changes (preneoplastic or precursor lesions) in the respiratory mucosa [2, 5]. The International Association for the Study of Lung Cancer (IASLC) histological classification of preinvasive lesions of the lung lists three main morphologic forms of preneoplastic lesions in the lung [17]. (a) squamous dysplasia and carcinoma *in situ* (CIS); (b) atypical adenomatous hyperplasia (AAH); and (c) diffuse idiopathic pulmonary neuroendocrine cell hyperplasia (DIPNECH). While the sequential preneoplastic changes have been defined for centrally arising squamous carcinomas, they have been poorly documented for large cell carcinomas, adenocarcinomas and SCLCs [3, 4, 15]. Changes in airways that precede invasive squamous cell carcinoma include squamous dysplasia and CIS [3, 4]. Adenocarcinomas may be preceded by morphological changes including AAH in peripheral airway cells [3, 18] While DIPNECH are thought to be precursors lesions for carcinoids of the lung. For SCLC, there are no specific preneoplastic changes that have been identified.

Squamous cell carcinoma preneoplasia

Hyperplasia, squamous metaplasia, squamous dysplasia and CIS [2–4, 8] comprise changes in the large airways that precede or accompany invasive squamous cell carcinoma (Figure 6.1). It is important to note that there are no squamous cells in the normal airways. Moreover, progenitor or stem cells for squamous metaplastic epithelium have not been identified. It has been postulated that the basal cells in the large airways exhibit pluripotent capacity following cigarette smoke exposure giving rise to metaplastic and dysplastic squamous cells, which in turn function as precursors of squamous cell carcinomas.

Dysplastic squamous lesions are typically categorized in different intensities; (mild, moderate and severe); however, these lesions represent a continuum of cytologic and histologic atypical

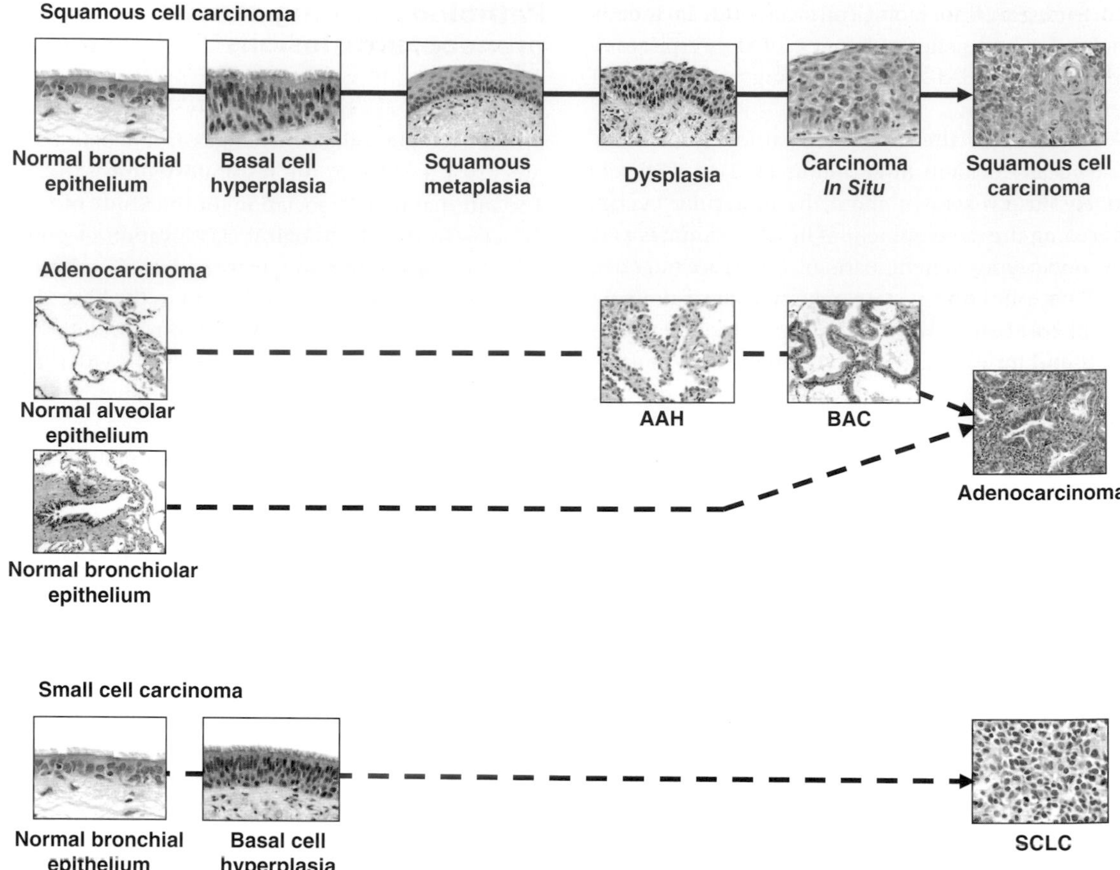

Figure 6.1 Summary of histopatholologic changes involved in the pathogenesis of lung cancer. The sequence of preneoplastic lesions involved in the development of squamous cell carcinoma of the lung has been elucidated. For adenocarcinoma histology, the only known preneoplastic lesion is AAH (atypical adenomatous hyperplasia), which seems to be the precursor for a subset of lung adenocarcinomas. No preneoplastic lesion has been recognized for SCLC (microphotographs of histological tissue sections stained with hematoxylin and eosin). (For a color version, see the color plate section.)

changes that may show some overlap between categories. Mild squamous dysplasias are characterized by minimal architectural and cytological disturbance, moderate dysplasias exhibit more cytological irregularity, and severe dysplasias display further irregular cytology as well as substantial cellular polymorphism. In addition and in a subset of dysplastic lesions, termed angiogenic squamous dysplasias, the basal membrane thickens and there is vascular budding in the subepithelial tissue that results in papillary protrusions of the epithelium [19]. These lesions highly suggest that angiogenesis, a hallmark of overt tumors [20], commences at a relatively early preneoplastic stage. CIS demonstrates extreme cytological aberrations with almost complete architectural disarray, but with an intact basement membrane and absence of stromal invasion. Foci of CIS usually arise near bifurcations in the segmental bronchi, subsequently extending proximally into the adjacent lobar bronchus and distally into subsegmental branches. These lesions are often not detected by conventional white-light bronchoscopy or gross examination. However, the utilization of fluorescent bronchoscopy, such as lung-imaging fluorescent endoscopy (LIFE), greatly increases the sensitivity for detection of squamous dysplastic and CIS lesions [21].

Adenocarcinoma precursor lesions

Clara cells and the type II pneumocytes are believed to be the progenitor cells of the peripheral airways, and peripherally arising adenocarcinomas often express markers of these cell types [22–24]. AAHs are considered to be a precursor lesion for peripheral lung adenocarcinomas [2, 3, 18]. However and until now, AAH is the only sequence of morphologic change identified so far for the development of invasive lung adenocarcinomas and there is consensus that the pathogenesis of many adenocarcinomas is largely unknown. The postulated progression of AAHs to adenocarcinomas *in situ*, which is characterized by the growth of neoplastic cells along pre-existing alveolar structures without invasion, is supported by molecular studies [4, 18]. Distinction between highly atypical AAH and what was known as bronchioalveolar carcinoma (BAC) is sometimes difficult. Notably, the ERS, IASLC and ATS sponsored a new classification of lung adenocarcinoma that presented several modifications to the WHO 2004 criteria for diagnosis of resected adenocarcinoma specimens. The term BAC was suggested to be discontinued and replaced with adenocarcinoma *in situ* and minimally invasive adenocarcinoma used for small adenocarcinomas with either pure lepidic growth or predominant lepidic growth with less than 5 mm invasion, respectively. Importantly, the clinical features of both adenocarcinoma progression types are unique as patients with adenocarcinoma *in situ* or minimally invasive adenocarcinoma have a 100% 5 year survival rate after definitive surgery [17].

The differentiation phenotype derived from immunohistochemical and ultrastructural features indicates that AAHs originate from the progenitor cells of the peripheral airways [2, 15, 22–24]. Surfactant apoprotein and Clara cell–specific 10-kDd protein are expressed in almost all AAHs. In addition, an increasing body of evidence suggests that AAH is the precursor of at least a subset of adenocarcinomas. For example, AAH is most frequently detected in lungs of patients bearing lung cancers (9–20%), especially adenocarcinomas (as many as 40%), compared with lung SCCs (11%) [25]. It is important to note that AAH is detected more frequently in East Asian patients relative to Western patients. In such studies, it has been suggested that AAH is involved in the linear progression of cells of the "terminal respiratory unit" (TRU) to adenocarcinoma *in situ* and subsequently invasive adenocarcinomas [24, 26, 27] due to the expression of common genes between the TRU and AAH. Such studies have postulated that most if not all peripheral lung adenocarcinomas progress from alveoli through AAH as a preneoplastic lesion. As will be discussed further below, we have noted similar molecular abnormalities (e.g., epidermal growth factor receptor mutations) between adenocarcinomas arising in never-smokers and small bronchioles within the localized and adjacent fields of the adenocarcinomas suggesting that lung adenocarcinomas may arise from bronchiolar epithelium and small bronchi and not only from alveoli [28, 29]. In a recent review by Yatabe *et al.*, a nonlinear progression schema for lung adenocarcinomas was suggested [26]. In this nonlinear schema, Yatabe *et al.* postulated that lung adenocarcinomas of the TRU subtype, as named by the authors, develop through AAH. On the other hand and according to the same non-linear progression hypothesis, some lung adenocarcinomas arise through unknown preneoplastic precursors from other cells besides the TRU, which we believe, may as well be the bronchiolar epithelium [15, 28, 29].

Precursor lesions of neuroendocrine tumors

As stated above, the precursor lesions for the most common type of neuroendocrine carcinoma of the lung, the SCLC, are unknown [2–4] (Figure 6.1). However, a rare lesion called DIPENECH has been associated with the development of other neuroendocrine tumors of the lung, typical and atypical carcinoids [3, 30]. DIPENECH lesions include local extraluminal proliferations in the form of tumorlets. Carcinoid tumors are arbitrarily separated from tumorlets if the neuroendocrine proliferation is 0.5 cm or larger.

Molecular pathogenesis of lung cancer

Previous studies have shed light on important vignettes in the molecular pathogenesis of lung cancer, including the following: (a) There are several histopathologic and molecular pathways associated with the development of the major types of NSCLC [2]. (b) Lung adenocarcinomas and SCCs exhibit differential expression of cell-lineage genes that play important roles in the pathogenesis of the diseases [15]. (c) Although there is a field effect phenomenon for lung preneoplastic lesions, recent data suggest that there are at least two distinct lung airways compartments (central and peripheral) for lung cancer pathogenesis [9]. (d) Inflammation may play an important role in lung cancer development and it could be an important component of the field effect phenomenon [2, 10]. (e) For lung adenocarcinoma, at least two smoking and nonsmoking-related pathways have been identified mediated by the Kirsten rat sarcoma viral oncogene (*KRAS*) and epidermal growth factor receptor (*EGFR*) oncogenes, respectively [14, 31–38].

Several studies have revealed that multiple genetic changes are found in clinically evident lung cancers, and involve known and putative tumor suppressor genes as well as several dominant oncogenes [1, 14]. Lung cancers arise after a series of molecular changes that commence in histologically normal epithelium and demonstrate a specific sequence [5, 8]. There is a preferred order of these allele loss changes with 3p allele loss (several 3p sites) followed by 9p ($p16^{INK4a}$ locus) as the earliest changes occurring in histologically normal epithelium [5, 6, 39] (Table 6.1). Various 3p genes are involved in lung cancer pathogenesis including *RARβ* at 3p24, *FHIT* at 3p14.2, *RASSF1A, BLU, FUS1*, and *SEMA3B* located at 3p21.3, and potentially *ROBO1* at 3p12 [6, 40, 41].

Telomerase activation has been also implicated as an early event in lung cancer pathogenesis [42, 43]. Telomerase shortening represents an early genetic abnormality in bronchial carcinogenesis, preceding telomerase expression and p53/Rb inactivation, which predominate in high-grade squamous preinvasive lesions [44]. Precise microscopic based microdissection of epithelial tissue followed by allelotyping of smoking damaged lung from lung cancer patients or current or former smokers without lung cancer revealed multiple lesions containing clonal abnormalities of allele loss, occurring in both histologically normal as well as mildly abnormal (hyperplasia and squamous metaplasia) and preneoplastic (dysplasia) respiratory epithelium [45]. While those changes are found in the lungs

Table 6.1 Histopathological and molecular abnormalities of lung cancer precursor lesions

Abnormality	NSCLC Adenocarcinoma	NSCLC Squamous cell carcinoma	SCLC
Histopathology			
Precursor	Probable	Known	Unknown
Lesion	AAH?	Squamous dysplasia and carcinoma in situ	Normal epithelium and hyperplasia?
Molecular			
Gene abnormalities	*KRAS* mutation *EGFR* mutation	*TP53* LOH and mutation *SOX2* amplification	*MYC* overexpression *TP53* LOH and mutation
Genetic instability	Low	Intermediate	High
Frequency	13%	10%	68%
LOH	Low	Intermediate	High
Frequency	10%	54%	90%
Chromosomal regions	9p21, 17p/*TP53*	8p21–23, 9p21, 17p/*TP53*	5q21, 8p21–23, 9p21, 17p/*TP53*

LOH: loss of heterozygosity.

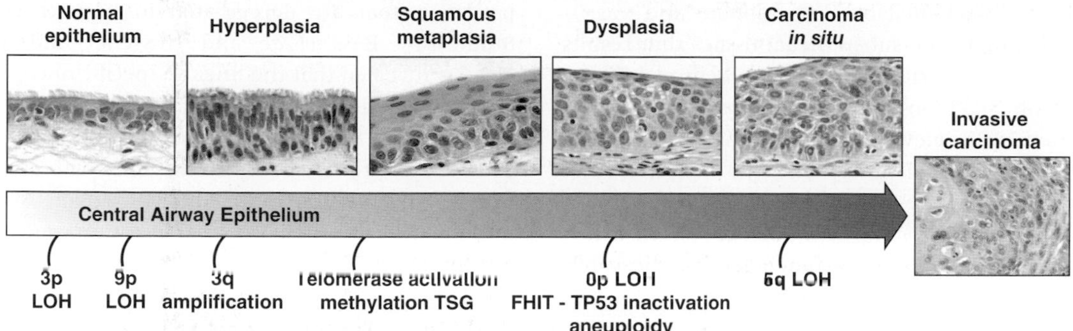

Figure 6.2 Molecular pathogenesis of squamous cell carcinoma of the lung. Several sequential molecular abnormalities have been recognized in the multistep pathogenesis of squamous cell carcinoma of the lung and have been detected in high-risk individuals. (For a color version, see the color plate section.)

of current and former smokers without lung cancer they are almost never found in lifetime never-smokers [11,12]. Interestingly, these clonal changes persist for decades after smoking cessation [11]. These previous findings pinpoint to a multistage and multistep fashion of lung cancer development.

It important to mention that one cannot neglect the alternative hypothesis that the sequence of molecular and genetic changes is irrelevant to lung cancer pathogenesis but rather the accumulation of molecular aberrations. For example, mutations in *KRAS* have been shown to be more frequent in AAHs than in invasive adenocarcinomas [24, 26]. Conversely, our group revealed that *EGFR* mutations, which commence in normal bronchial or bronchiolar epithelia, precede copy number gains of the oncogene in the course of the pathogenesis of adenocarcinomas [29]. It is plausible to suggest that increasing our understanding of lung cancer molecular pathogenesis would help to determine the nature (sequential vs nonsequential) of the development of the disease, and for now, it is not counterintuitive to suggest that lung cancer pathogenesis is due to both stepwise and sequence-specific changes as well as accumulation of genetic molecular abnormalities [9].

Pathogenesis of squamous cell carcinoma.

The current working model of the sequential molecular abnormalities in the pathogenesis of squamous cell lung carcinoma indicates that genetic abnormalities commence in histologically normal epithelium and increase with increasing severity of histologic changes [45] (Figure 6.2). Moreover, molecular changes in the respiratory epithelium are extensive and multifocal throughout the bronchial tree of smokers and lung cancer patients, indicating a field effect or field cancerization [5, 6, 11, 12]. It is important to note that mutations follow a sequence, with progressive allelic losses at multiple 3p (3p21, 3p14, 3p22–24 and 3p12) chromosome sites and 9p21 ($p16^{INK4a}$) as the earliest detected changes. Later changes include 8p21–23, 13q14 (*RB*) and 17p13 (*TP53*) [5, 6, 39]. $p16^{INK4a}$ methylation has been also detected at an early stage of squamous preinvasive lesions with a frequency that increases during histopathologic progression (24% in squamous metaplasia and 50% in CIS) [46]. Multiple clonal and subclonal patches of molecular abnormalities not much larger in size than the average bronchial biopsy obtained by fluorescent bronchoscopy, estimated to be approximately 40 000 to 360 000 cells, can be detected in the normal and slightly abnormal bronchial epithelium of patients with lung cancer [45]. Despite encouraging results from isolated studies [47], most of these findings have not been useful for the development of successful strategies for lung cancer risk assessment, early detection and chemoprevention.

As mentioned before, angiogenic squamous dysplasias (ASDs), a subset of squamous dysplasias, exhibit a thickened basal membrane and vascular budding in the subepithelial tissues that results in papillary protrusions of the epithelium [19]. In the bronchial biopsies with these lesions microvessel density is elevated in comparison to normal mucosa but not in comparison to other forms of hyperplasia or dysplasia. ASD thus represents a qualitatively distinct form of angiogenesis in which there is architectural rearrangement of the capillary microvasculature. Genetic analysis of surface epithelium in a subset of lesions revealed loss of heterozygosity (LOH) at chromosome 3p in 53% of lesions, and compared with normal epithelium, proliferative activity was markedly elevated in ASD lesions. ASD was found to occur in approximately 19% of high-risk smokers without carcinoma who underwent fluorescence bronchoscopy [48] and was not present in biopsies from 16 normal nonsmoker control subjects [19]. The presence of this lesion in high-risk smokers suggests that aberrant patterns of microvascularization may occur at an early stage of bronchial carcinogenesis. The finding of vascular endothelial growth factor (VEGF) isoforms and VEGF receptors (VEGFR) by semiquantitative reverse transcriptase-PCR confirmed by immunohistochemistry in bronchial squamous dysplastic compared to normal bronchial epithelia [49] supports the notion that angiogenesis develops early in lung carcinogenesis and that these abnormalities provide rationale for the development of targeted antiangiogenic chemoprevention strategies. Of interest, most important signaling pathways that are being targeted in lung cancer have been shown to be also deregulated in lung cancer preneoplastic lesions, mostly in the squamous cell carcinoma pathway, including, among others, the inflammation-related polyunsaturated fatty acid metabolic pathways [50], retinoic acid signaling [51], and pathways involving Ras [14,18], EGFR [52], phosphoinositide 3-kinase (PI3K)/AKT [53], insulin-like growth (IGF) factor axis [54] and mTOR [55]. Thus, the possible activation of therapeutically pliable signaling pathways early in the pathogenesis of lung cancer creates an opportunity for the design of targeted chemoprevention strategies [56].

The recent developments in molecular biology have increased our knowledge of critical biological pathways that are deregulated in lung cancers. Studies by Bass *et al.* and Hussenet and colleagues revealed that the lineage-specific oncogene *SOX2* is amplified in the 3q (3q26.3) chromosomal region in lung SCC and squamous esophageal cancers and promotes survival of SCCs with amplification of this gene [57, 58]. Moreover, SOX2 immunohistochemical protein expression was completely absent in lung adenocarcinoma pathogenesis, highly expressed in SCC development and significantly elevated in lung SCCs relative to adenocarcinomas [59]. In addition, various studies have highlighted tumor promoting roles for this lineage-specific oncogene in lung cancer [57, 60, 61]. Later, McCaughan and colleagues specifically analyzed 3q copy number alteration in bronchial dysplasia of varying grades and severity and demonstrated that *SOX2* amplification, found in overt SCCs, was also present in high-grade bronchial dysplasias but not in low grade lesions and, importantly, was associated with clinical progression of high-grade preinvasive squamous lesions [62]. It is important to mention that Yuan *et al.* had found relatively high SOX2 immunohistochemical protein expression in normal bronchial epithelia and alveolar bronchiolarization structures [59]. The studies by both Yuan *et al.* and McCaughan and colleagues demonstrate the implication of *SOX2* in the early pathogenesis of lung SCCs [59, 62].

Pathogenesis of lung adenocarcinoma

Several molecular changes frequently present in lung adenocarcinomas are also present in AAH lesions, and they are further evidence that AAH may represent true preneoplastic lesions [22] (Figure 6.3). The most important finding is the presence of *KRAS* (codon 12) mutations in as many as 39% of AAHs, which are also a relatively frequent alteration in lung adenocarcinomas [2, 63]. Other molecular aberrations that were identified in AAH are overexpression of Cyclin D1 (70%), survivin (48%), and HER2/neu (7%) proteins [2]. Moreover, and as mentioned in the review by Wistuba and Gazdar, some AAH lesions were found to exhibit LOH in chromosomes 3p (18%), 9p ($p16^{INK4a}$, 13%), 9q (53%), 17q, and 17p (*TP53*, 6%) [2]. It is noteworthy that most if not all of the

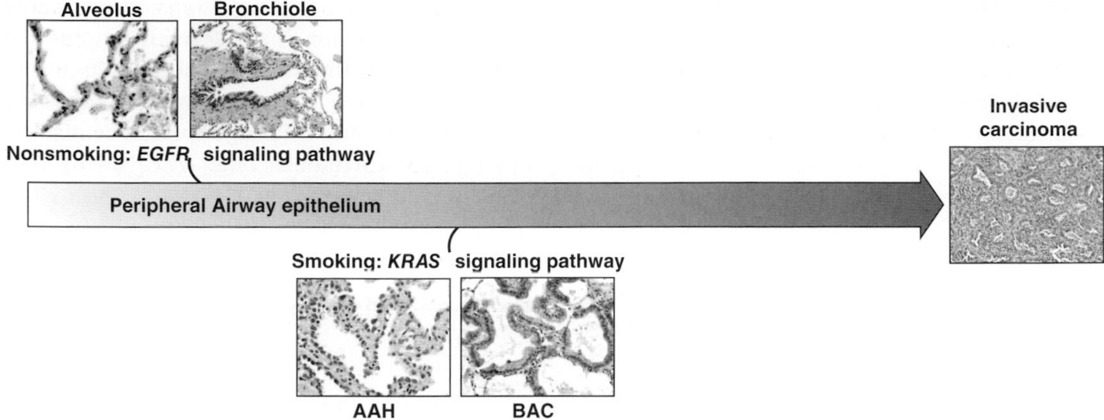

Figure 6.3 Molecular pathogenesis of adenocarcinoma of the lung. At least two molecular pathways have been identified in the development of lung adenocarcinoma, smoking and nonsmoking-related (AAH, atypical adenomatous hyperplasia; BAC, bronchioloalveolar carcinoma). (For a color version, see the color plate section.)

aforementioned changes identified in AAH lesions are also frequently detected in lung adenocarcinomas. Later, AAH lesions were shown to exhibit LOH of tuberous sclerosis complex (TSC)-associated regions, activation of telomerase, loss of *LKB1*, overexpression of DICER, a key effector protein for small interfering RNA and miRNA function, and DNA methylation of *CDKN2A* and *PTPRN2* [2, 64, 65]. It is important to note that several studies have attempted to globally comprehend differential gene expression patterns and copy number alterations between low-grade lesions (e.g., precursor lesions) or *in situ* adenocarcinomas and invasive tumors and found that amplification of the *EGFR* oncogene was the predominant differential molecular feature between the two different adenocarcinoma grade classes and occurred after mutations in the gene [26].

A large body of evidence suggests that at least two molecular pathways are involved, the *KRAS* and *EGFR* pathways in smoker and never-smoker adenocarcinoma subpopulations, respectively [14, 31–38]. Mutations in *EGFR*, in particular in-frame deletions of exon 19 and L858R and L861Q of exon 21, are strongly associated with never-smoking status, female gender and East Asian ethnicity as well as predict favorable response to *EGFR* TKIs [14, 33, 36, 37, 66, 67]. On the other hand, mutations in *KRAS*, are strongly associated with development of adenocarcinomas linked to tobacco consumption [14, 32–35, 37].

It has been suggested that the vast majority of AAH precursor lesions and adenocarcinomas *in situ* are associated with the "terminal respiratory unit" adenocarcinoma subtype that were found to express high levels of *TITF-1* and surfactant proteins leading to the conclusion that such adenocarcinomas are of the same lineage as terminal airway epithelial cells [27]. In addition, it has been postulated that *EGFR* mutations are predominant in or specific to peripheral lung adenocarcinomas of the TRU subtype, that were suggested to arise from AAH lesions [24, 27, 68], since 90 of 97 *EGFR* mutant adenocarcinomas were positive for *TITF-1* and 91 of the 97 tumors were of the TRU subtype [68]. In addition, the hypothesis put forward that *EGFR* mutations are associated with or specific to the TRU subtype of lung adenocarcinomas is also in part due to the observation that the frequency of *EGFR* and *KRAS* mutations among AAH lesions, adenocarcinomas *in situ* and invasive adenocarcinomas is significantly different [24, 26]. It was determined that whereas *KRAS* mutations decreased along adenocarcinoma progression, from 33% in AAH to 8% in adenocarcinomas, *EGFR* mutations were evenly distributed suggesting that

KRAS-mutated AAH lesions rarely progress to adenocarcinomas.

Mutations in the tyrosine kinase domain of *EGFR* mutations were shown to be involved in the early pathogenesis of lung cancer, being identified in histologically normal epithelium of small bronchi and bronchioles adjacent to *EGFR* mutant adenocarcinomas [28]. *EGFR* mutations were detected in normal-appearing peripheral respiratory epithelium in adenocarcinoma patients [28], but not in patients without mutation in the tumor [28]. These findings may signify different cell types comprising the examined epithelia, which could represent sites of the cells of origin for *EGFR* mutant adenocarcinomas of the lung. Although the cell type having those mutations is unknown, our group has hypothesized that stem or progenitor cells of the bronchial and bronchiolar epithelium bear such mutations. It is also noteworthy that *EGFR* mutations were identified in only 3 of 40 AAH lesions examined [68, 69] and were shown to be absent [36] or relatively infrequent in what was previously known as BACs of the lung [69]. These earlier observations support the argument that abnormalities of *EGFR* are not only relevant to the pathogenesis of alveolar-type lung neoplasia but also may drive the development of peripheral lung adenocarcinoma from bronchiolar epithelium cells that are distinct from terminal respiratory and alveolar cells [2, 15, 24].

TITF-1 is a homeodomain-containing transactivating factor predominantly expressed in the terminal lung bronchioles and lung periphery in the developing and adult mouse [70, 71]. In addition, *TITF-1* is crucial for branching morphogenesis during normal lung development [70–72] and transactivates the expression of the surfactant proteins (*SP*s) such as *SP*s-*A*, -*B* and –*C* which are in turn typically expressed in the Clara cells and are important for the differentiation of alveolar type II pneumocyte cells in the peripheral lung [73]. Several studies have demonstrated increased copy number and amplification of the 14q13.3 locus that harbors the *TITF-1* gene [74, 75] pinpointing to cell-lineage specific oncogenic function to this transcriptional factor in lung adenocarcinomas. It is postulated that *TITF-1* functions as a lineage-specific oncogene in lung adenocarcinoma as knockdown of *TITF-1* expression, in cells with amplification of the gene, by RNA interference results in lung adenocarcinoma cell growth inhibition and apoptosis demonstrating a lineage-specific dependency of lung adenocarcinomas on *TITF-1* [74–76]. However, recently in Kras(LSL-G12D/+);p53(flox/flox) mice, *TITF-1* was shown to suppress tumorigenesis and limit metastatic potential *in vivo* [77].

Pathogenesis of SCLC

As stated before, no phenotypically identifiable epithelial lesion has been identified as a precursor for SCLC (Figure 6.1). A study comparing the molecular changes (LOH at several chromosomal sites and microsatellite instability) occurring in histologically normal and mildly abnormal (hyperplastic) centrally located bronchial epithelia accompanying SCLCs and NSCLCs tumors demonstrated a significantly higher incidence of genetic abnormalities in bronchial epithelia accompanying SCLC than those adjacent to NSCLC (squamous cell carcinoma and adenocarcinoma) [7]. These findings indicate that more widespread and more extensive genetic damage is present in bronchial epithelium in patients with SCLC. The finding that some specimens of normal or mildly abnormal epithelia accompanying SCLCs have a high incidence of genetic changes suggests that SCLC may arise directly from histologically normal or mildly abnormal epithelium, without passing through a more complex histologic sequence. Animal model studies have shown that SCLC development is driven by inactivation of *TP53* and *RB* [78] and activation of the hedgehog pathway [79, 80]. Recently, integrative genomic analyses of SCLCs confirmed known inactivation of *TP53* and *RB1* and identified recurrent mutations in the histone modifiers *CREBBP*, *EP300* and *MLL*, mutations in *PTEN*, *SLIT2* and *EPHA7*, and *FGFR1* amplifications [81].

Field cancerization in lung cancer pathogenesis

Earlier work by Danely Slaughter in patients with oral cancer and oral premalignant lesions has suggested that histologically normal-appearing tissue adjacent to neoplastic and preneoplastic lesions display molecular abnormalities some of which are in common with those in the tumors [82]. In 1961, a seminal report by Auerbach *et al.* suggested that cigarette smoke induces extensive histological changes in the bronchial epithelia in the lungs of smokers and that premalignant lesions are widespread and multifocal throughout the respiratory epithelium, suggestive of a field effect [83]. This phenomenon, coined "field of cancerization," was later shown to be evident in various epithelial cell malignancies including lung cancer. Some degree of inflammation and inflammatory-related damage is almost invariably present in the central and peripheral airways of smokers and may precede the development of lung cancer [2, 9]. Thus, the field of cancerization may also be explained by both direct effect of tobacco carcinogens and initiation of inflammatory response. In this context, different theories for the origin of the field cancerization or smoking related field of injury have been put forward and extensively reviewed elsewhere by Steiling *et al.* [10].

Smoking damaged epithelium and lung field cancerization

Multiple altered foci of bronchial epithelium are present throughout the airway in lung cancer patients and smokers [5–7]. Detailed analysis of histologically normal epithelium, premalignant and malignant epithelia from lung SCC patients indicated that multiple, sequentially occurring allele-specific chromosomal deletions of LOH commence in clonally independent foci early in the multistage pathogenesis of SCCs [5,6]. Notably, 31% percent of histologically normal epithelium and 42% of mildly abnormal (hyperplasia/metaplasia) specimens had clones of cells with allelic loss at one or more regions examined. Nelson *et al.* demonstrated that *KRAS* is also mutated in histologically normal lung tissue adjacent to lung tumors [84]. In addition, similar epigenetic and gene methylation patterns between tumors and adjacent histologically normal epithelia were described. Belinsky *et al* reported aberrant promoter methylation of *p16*, which was described to be commonly methylated in lung tumors [46], in at least one bronchial epithelial site from 44% of lung cancer cases examined [85]. Moreover, *p16* and death associated protein kinase (*DAPK*) promoter methylation were frequently observed in bronchial epithelium from smoker but not from never-smoker lung cancer patients and persisted after smoking cessation [85].

The aforementioned molecular abnormalities were detected in histologically normal epithelia adjacent to archival surgically resected tumors from primary lung cancer patients. LOH and microsatellite alterations in multiple foci were also detected in distal histological normal bronchial epithelia of smokers without cancer [11, 12]. Moreover and importantly, these molecular abnormalities were detected in bronchial epithelia of cancer-free former smokers that appeared to have persisted for many years after smoking cessation. In addition, LOH was detected in DNA obtained from bronchial brushings of normal and abnormal lungs from patients undergoing diagnostic bronchoscopy and was detected in cells from the ipsilateral and contralateral lung [86]. Mutations in *TP53* were also described to occur in bronchial epithelia of cancer-free smokers in a widely dispersed manner [87]. Similar evidence also exists for promoter methylation and epigenetic changes in smoking-damaged lung epithelium of cancer-free patients. Methylation of various genes, including retinoic acid receptor 2 beta (*RAR-β2*), H-cadherin (*CDH13*), adenomatous polyposis coli (*APC*), *p16* and Ras association (RalGDS/AF-6) domain family member 1 (*RASSFF1A*) has been described in bronchial epithelial cells of heavy smokers [88]. Moreover, methylation of *p16*, glutathione S-transferase pi 1 (*GSTP1*) and *DAPK* was reported to be evident in bronchial brushings of one third of cancer-free smokers examined [89]. A more detailed list of aberrant gene promoter methylation in lung cancer patients and cancer-free smokers is well summarized and explained in the review by Heller *et al.* [90].

Field cancerization transcriptome

High-throughput microarray profiling was shown to be useful to study the transcriptome of lung airways. Hackett *et al.* studied the expression of 44 anti-oxidant related genes using bronchial brushings from cancer-free current smokers and never-smokers littand found significant up-regulation of 16 of the antioxidant genes in the airways of smokers compared to nonsmokers [91]. Later, Spira *et al.* described global alterations in gene expression between normal-appearing bronchial epithelium of healthy cancer-free smokers and that of nonsmokers [92]. Importantly, irreversible changes in expression in airways of former smokers after years of smoking cessation were described that were thought to underlie the increased risk former smokers exhibit for developing lung cancer [92, 93]. Alterations in the expression of microRNAs (miRNAs) were also demonstrated between large airways of current and never-smokers [94]. Notably, an 80-gene signature was derived from the transcriptome of large airway epithelial cells that can distinguish smokers without overt cancer from smokers with lung cancer despite originating from normal bronchial epithelia [95]. More recently, Gustafson *et al.* derived a phosphoinositide-3-kinase (*PI3K*) pathway activation signature by using recombinant adenoviruses to express the 110α subunit of *PI3K* in primary human epithelial cells [96]. The *PI3K* pathway activation signature was elevated in cytologically normal bronchial airways of smokers with lung cancer and, importantly, was decreased in the airways of high-risk smokers whose dysplastic lesions regressed following treatment with the PI3K inhibitor myoinositol [96]. Microarray and gene expression profiling methodologies were also used to demonstrate the wide anatomical spread of the lung field cancerization. Common gene expression alterations were identified in bronchial, nasal and buccal epithelia of smokers [97] and in a separate study, the expression of 119 genes was demonstrated to be affected by smoking similarly in both bronchial and nasal epithelium [98]. Recently, Beane *et al.* applied next-generation RNA sequencing technology to analyze bronchial airway epithelial cell brushings from healthy never-smokers and smokers with and without lung cancer [99]. The study highlighted transcripts whose expression was either not interrogated or not found to be significantly altered when using microarrays, demonstrating that next-generation sequencing (NGS), as in established lung tumors, has the potential to provide new insights into the biology of the airway field cancerization associated with smoking and lung cancer [99].

Field cancerization compartmentalization

In light of the prevalence of mutations in the *EGFR* oncogene in adenocarcinomas and in particular those occurring in never-smokers, Tang and colleagues investigated the presence of *EGFR* mutations in normal bronchial and bronchiolar epithelium adjacent to *EGFR* mutant tumors. *EGFR* mutations were detected in histologically normal peripheral epithelia in 44% of lung adenocarcinoma patients with mutations but none in patients lacking mutations in the oncogene [28]. Moreover, the same study highlighted more frequent *EGFR* mutations in normal epithelium within the tumor (43%) than in adjacent sites (24%) suggesting a localized field effect phenomenon for this abnormality in the respiratory epithelium of the lung [28]. These findings suggest that adenocarcinomas may be associated with a field cancerization dissimilar from that linked to SCCs.

The low frequency of molecular abnormalities detected in the centrally located bronchial respiratory epithelium in patients with peripheral lung adenocarcinomas, compared with specimens from patients with SCCs [6], suggests the presence of two compartments in the lung with different degrees of smoking-related genetic damage. Thus, smokers who develop SCCs display more smoking-related genetic damage in the respiratory epithelium of the central airway, whereas patients who develop adenocarcinomas exhibit molecular and histological damage mainly in the peripheral airways. While some molecular changes (e.g., inflammation and signaling pathways activation) have been detected throughout the lung airway and include both compartments (central and peripheral airway), other aberrations have been more frequently altered in either central (e.g., LOH, genetic instability evidenced by microsatellite repeats) or peripheral (e.g., *EGFR* mutations as mentioned above) airways

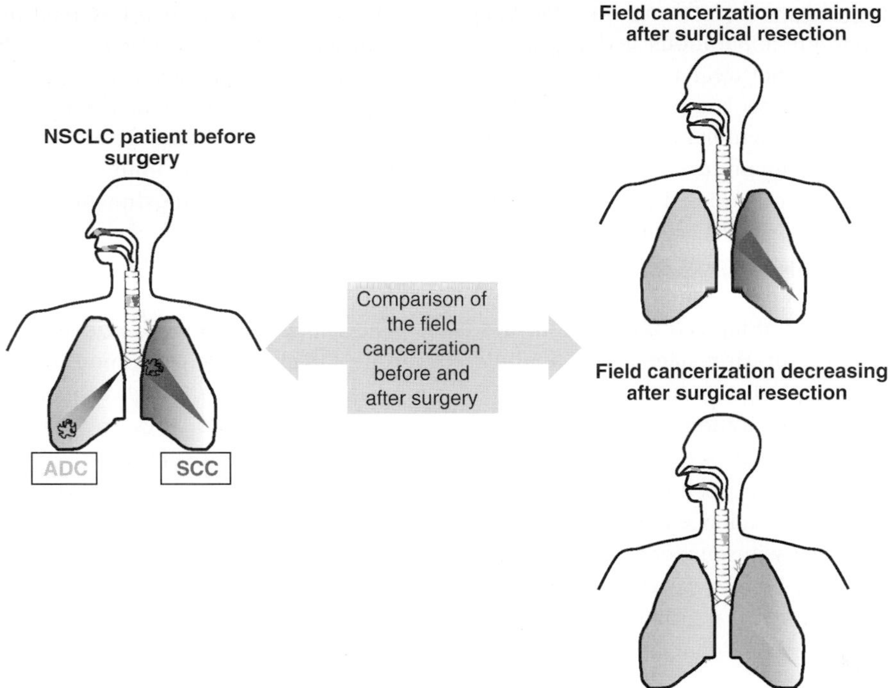

Figure 6.4 Field cancerization phenomenon in early-stage NSCLC patients. The relevance of the lung field cancerization to the development of a particular subtype of NSCLC, i.e., adenocarcinomas compared to SCCs, is still unknown yet possible. Analyzing local and distant field of cancerization by analysis of the transcriptome of airway brushings from multiple sites independently for lung adenocarcinoma (yellow spots) and SCC (red spots) cases, may shed light on events common or unique to the molecular pathogenesis of the two major subtypes of NSCLC (left panel). The potential important clinical relevance of the field cancerization to early-stage NSCLC can be investigated by studying the molecular cancerization before and after surgery to determine whether the cancerization effect persists (upper right) or decreases (bottom right) following surgical removal of the lung tumor. Such analysis may aid to determine whether the persistence of a molecular field cancerization effect in NSCLC patients after surgery is associated with disease relapse, and if so, whether the effect can be leveraged for development of novel prevention strategies. (For a color version, see the color plate section.)

[2, 9]. These interesting observations indicate a possible compartmentalization of the field cancerization and its dissimilarity between adenocarcinomas and SCCs which may well reflect the differential mechanisms of pathogenesis of both NSCLC subtypes (Figure 6.4, left) [2, 9].

We have recently studied the smoking-damaged field cancerization in early-stage NSCLC patients that were treated by definitive surgery and after which they were enrolled in a phase II surveillance trial (Department of Defense Vanguard cohort). Our recent study indicated significantly altered patterns of expression between airways adjacent to the primary resected tumors compared to airways contralateral to the tumor as well as alterations in the field of cancerization or injury with time up to 3 years from the baseline time point or enrollment into the study (within one year from respective surgery) [100]. In addition, immunohistochemical expression of phosphorylated ERK1/2 and AKT kinases exhibited statistically significantly different levels of expression in corresponding airway biopsies by distance from the primary tumor and by time the biopsy was sampled following inclusion of patients in the trial [100]. Our group's recent findings enrich the molecular definition of the airway field cancerization phenomenon [100, 101] and have important implications in lung cancer prevention. It is still not clear whether the differences in expression described in this study reflect an already present gradient field of injury that may have contributed to tumor development in light of the differential cancer-associated pathways identified or one that arises due to the molecular impact of the tumor on the adjacent field [9]. Future studies that will analyze in-depth the molecular spatial and temporal airway field of injury/cancerization prior to and after surgery in early stage patients would answer the above speculation and have favorable far-reaching clinical implications in lung cancer prevention in particular in the tertiary setting (Figure 6.4) [9]. It is intriguing to postulate that while the molecular field cancerization effect may decrease after definitive surgery in some early-stage NSCLC patients (Figure 6.4, bottom right), it may persist in other patients and be associated with higher risk of disease recurrence or relapse (Figure 6.4, top right).

Inflammation and lung cancer

The association between chronic inflammatory conditions of the lung and cancer has been studied extensively [102]. Several studies have found that smokers with chronic obstructive pulmonary disease (COPD) have an increased risk of lung cancer compared to smokers without COPD [102]. In COPD, at the level of the alveoli, inflammation leads to protease release and oxidative inactivation of antiproteases by inflammatory cells contributing to degradation of the extracellular matrix [103, 104]. At the level of the conducting airways, there is metaplasia of the airway epithelium to a mucus-secreting phenotype, thickening of the airway wall from the increased deposition of matrix molecules and the proliferation of mesenchymal cells, and narrowing from fibrosis [103, 104]. These changes are also present in the lungs of smokers without COPD but they are not as severe [105]. COPD patients with 40 or more pack-years of smoking history have demonstrated a high prevalence of premalignant dysplasia (24% severe and CIS) detectable through sputum cytology [106]. Compared with men, women smokers have a lower prevalence of high-grade preinvasive lesions in the observed airways (14% versus 31%), and women with preinvasive lesions had fewer such lesions. The prevalence of preinvasive lesions did not change substantially for more than 10 years after cessation of smoking. Lung function was associated with the prevalence of preinvasive lesions, but the association was weaker in women than in men [107].

A number of lines of evidence suggest that chronic inflammation contributes to the process of lung carcinogenesis through activation of a number of molecular pathways, including the nuclear factor kappa B (*NF-κB*) [102]. In NSCLC cell lines, it was shown that tobacco components stimulate NF-κB-dependent survival [108]. Moreover, NF-κB p65 protein nuclear overexpression was demonstrated to be an early and frequent phenomenon in the pathogenesis of lung cancer, being frequently detected in bronchial squamous dysplastic changes and peripheral lung AAH lesions in lung cancer patients [109], and in a limited number of squamous dysplasias obtained from smokers without cancer [110]. The eicosanoid pathway, specifically *COX-2*, has been also shown to be involved in the pathogenesis of lung cancer. *COX-2*, an intermediate early response gene induced by growth factors, oncogenes, carcinogens, and tumor-promoter phorbol esters [111], is overexpressed in lung adenocarcinoma and squamous cell carcinoma [112]. Both preclinical and clinical trials of the effect of celecoxib on lung cancer prevention have shown a marked reduction in PGE2 production [113]. COX-2 immunohistochemical expression has shown to be highly expressed in bronchial squamous dysplasias, especially those having high-grade histology (severe dysplasia and CIS) [114]. Recent findings suggest that the COX-2 inhibitor celecoxib may be capable of modulating the proliferation indices and apoptotic balance in bronchial tissue of active smokers [115–117].

Summary and perspectives

Lung cancer results from the accumulation of multiple genetic and epigenetic changes and different patterns of molecular alterations have been detected among the major lung cancer histology types. There are three main morphologic forms of preneoplastic lesions recognized in the lung: squamous dysplasias, AAH, and DIPENECH. However, these lesions account for the development of only a subset of lung cancers. For squamous cell carcinoma of the lung, the current working model indicates a stepwise sequence of molecular and histopathological changes, with the molecular abnormalities starting in histologically normal and mildly abnormal epithelia. AAH is considered a putative precursor of a subset of lung adenocarcinoma, and it exhibits similar molecular changes found in invasive tumors. At least, two different molecular pathways have been detected in lung adenocarcinoma pathogenesis: smoking-related pathways associated with *KRAS* mutations and nonsmoking-related pathways associated with *EGFR* mutations; the latter are detected in histologically normal respiratory epithelium. Molecular changes detected in lung tumors and associated preneoplastic lesions have been detected in smoking-damaged epithelium of smokers, including histologically normal bronchial epithelium. Molecular and histopathological changes in the respiratory epithelium are extensive and multifocal throughout the bronchial tree of smokers and lung cancer patients, indicating a field effect phenomenon. A number of lines of evidence suggest that chronic inflammation contributes to the process of lung carcinogenesis through activation of a number of molecular pathways.

NGS technology, through whole-genome, whole-exome and whole-transcriptome approaches, holds great promise for providing invaluable insights into lung cancer biology, diagnosis, prevention and therapy [118]. Recently, the genomic landscapes of lung adenocarcinoma, SCCs and SCLCs have been characterized by NGS including deep sequencing [81, 119–121]. Applying the same advanced high-throughput methodologies currently used in studying established tumors for the genetic analysis of lung cancer preneoplasia and intraepithelial lesions as well as histologically normal adjacent regions and airway epithelia is expected to expand our understanding of the biology of this prevalent disease.

Despite numerous efforts that have centered on increasing our understanding of the biology of lung cancer, this malignancy still comprises the biggest share of cancer-related deaths in the United States and worldwide. Compared to advances in targeted and personalized therapy of NSCLC, little progress has been made in the tailored prevention of this fatal malignancy. This may change with the recent encouraging and significant findings of the NLST [16]. Various molecular markers and expression classifiers previously described in the lung airways and in less invasive sites of the field cancerization can aid in selecting high-risk individuals best suited for CT screening. A comprehensive analysis of early molecular events in NSCLC pathogenesis will undoubtedly identify new and important biomarkers for lung cancer detection and prevention.

References

1 Minna JD, Roth JA, Gazdar AF (2002) Focus on lung cancer. *Cancer Cell*, 1: 49–52.
2 Wistuba, II, Gazdar AF (2006) Lung cancer preneoplasia. *Annu Rev Pathol*, 1: 331–48.
3 Colby TV, Wistuba, II, Gazdar A (1998) Precursors to pulmonary neoplasia. *Adv Anat Pathol*, 5: 205–15.
4 Kerr KM (2001) Pulmonary preinvasive neoplasia. *J Clin Pathol*, 54: 257–71.
5 Wistuba, II, Behrens C, Milchgrub S, Bryant D, Hung J, Minna JD, *et al.* (1999) Sequential molecular abnormalities are involved in the multistage development of squamous cell lung carcinoma. *Oncogene*, 18: 643–50.
6 Wistuba, II, Behrens C, Virmani AK, Mele G, Milchgrub S, Girard L, *et al.* (2000) High resolution chromosome 3p allelotyping of human lung cancer and preneoplastic/preinvasive bronchial epithelium reveals multiple, discontinuous sites of 3p allele loss and three regions of frequent breakpoints. *Cancer Res*, 60: 1949–60.
7 Wistuba, II, Berry J, Behrens C, Maitra A, Shivapurkar N, Milchgrub S, *et al.* (2000) Molecular changes in the bronchial epithelium of patients with small cell lung cancer. *Clin Cancer Res*, 6: 2604–10.
8 Wistuba, II, Mao L, Gazdar AF (2002) Smoking molecular damage in bronchial epithelium. *Oncogene*, 21: 7298–7306.

9 Kadara H, Wistuba, II (2012) Field cancerization in non-small cell lung cancer: implications in disease pathogenesis. *Proc Am Thorac Soc*, 9: 38–42.

10 Steiling K, Ryan J, Brody JS, Spira A (2008) The field of tissue injury in the lung and airway. *Cancer Prev Res (Phila Pa)*, 1: 396–403.

11 Wistuba, II, Lam S, Behrens C, Virmani AK, Fong KM, LeRiche J, *et al.* (1997) Molecular damage in the bronchial epithelium of current and former smokers. *J Natl Cancer Inst*, 89: 1366–73.

12 Mao L, Lee JS, Kurie JM, Fan YH, Lippman SM, Lee JJ, *et al.* (1997) Clonal genetic alterations in the lungs of current and former smokers. *J Natl Cancer Inst*, 89: 857–62.

13 Gold KA, Kim ES, Lee JJ, Wistuba, II, Farhangfar CJ, Hong WK (2011) The BATTLE to personalize lung cancer prevention through reverse migration. *Cancer Prev Res (Phila)*, 4: 962–72.

14 Herbst RS, Heymach JV, Lippman SM (2008) Lung cancer. *N Engl J Med*, 359: 1367–80.

15 Kadara H, Kabbout M, Wistuba, II (2012) Pulmonary adenocarcinoma: a renewed entity in 2011. *Respirology*, 17: 50–65.

16 Aberle DR, Adams AM, Berg CD, Black WC, Clapp JD, Fagerstrom RM, *et al.* (2011) Reduced lung-cancer mortality with low-dose computed tomographic screening. *N Engl J Med*, 365: 395–409.

17 Travis WD, Brambilla E, Noguchi M, Nicholson AG, Geisinger KR, Yatabe Y, *et al.* (2011) International Association for the Study of Lung Cancer/American Thoracic Society/European Respiratory Society International Multidisciplinary Classification of Lung Adenocarcinoma. *J Thorac Oncol*, 6: 244–85.

18 Westra WH (2000) Early glandular neoplasia of the lung. *Respir Res*, 1: 163–9.

19 Keith RL, Miller YE, Gemmill RM, Drabkin HA, Dempsey EC, Kennedy TC, *et al.* (2000) Angiogenic squamous dysplasia in bronchi of individuals at high risk for lung cancer. *Clin Cancer Res*, 6: 1616–25.

20 Hanahan D, Weinberg RA (2011) Hallmarks of cancer: the next generation. *Cell*, 144: 646–74.

21 Lam S, MacAulay C, leRiche JC, Palcic B (2000) Detection and localization of early lung cancer by fluorescence bronchoscopy. *Cancer*, 89: 2468–73.

22 Kitamura H, Kameda Y, Ito T, Hayashi H (1999) Atypical adenomatous hyperplasia of the lung. Implications for the pathogenesis of peripheral lung adenocarcinoma. *Am J Clin Pathol*, 111: 610–22.

23 Osanai M, Igarashi T, Yoshida Y (2001) Unique cellular features in atypical adenomatous hyperplasia of the lung: ultrastructural evidence of its cytodifferentiation. *Ultrastruct Pathol*, 25: 367–73.

24 Yatabe Y (2010) EGFR mutations and the terminal respiratory unit. *Cancer Metastasis Rev*, 29: 23–36.

25 Chapman AD, Kerr KM (2000) The association between atypical adenomatous hyperplasia and primary lung cancer. *Br J Cancer*, 83: 632–6.

26 Yatabe Y, Borczuk AC, Powell CA (2011) Do all lung adenocarcinomas follow a stepwise progression? *Lung Cancer*, 74: 7–11.

27 Yatabe Y, Mitsudomi T, Takahashi T (2002) TTF-1 expression in pulmonary adenocarcinomas. *Am J Surg Pathol*, 26: 767–73.

28 Tang X, Shigematsu H, Bekele BN, Roth JA, Minna JD, Hong WK, *et al.* (2005) EGFR tyrosine kinase domain mutations are detected in histologically normal respiratory epithelium in lung cancer patients. *Cancer Res*, 65: 7568–72.

29 Tang X, Varella-Garcia M, Xavier AC, Massarelli E, Ozburn N, Moran C, *et al.* (2008) Epidermal growth factor receptor abnormalities in the pathogenesis and progression of lung adenocarcinomas. *Cancer Prev Res (Phila Pa)*, 1: 192–200.

30 Armas OA, White DA, Erlandson RA, Rosai J (1995) Diffuse idiopathic pulmonary neuroendocrine cell proliferation presenting as interstitial lung disease. *Am J Surg Pathol*, 19: 963–70.

31 Gazdar AF, Thun MJ (2007) Lung cancer, smoke exposure, and sex. *J Clin Oncol*, 25: 469–71.

32 Le Calvez F, Mukeria A, Hunt JD, Kelm O, Hung RJ, Taniere P, *et al.* (2005) TP53 and KRAS mutation load and types in lung cancers in relation to tobacco smoke: distinct patterns in never, former, and current smokers. *Cancer Res*, 65: 5076–83.

33 Mounawar M, Mukeria A, Le Calvez F, Hung RJ, Renard H, Cortot A, *et al.* (2007) Patterns of EGFR, HER2, TP53, and KRAS mutations of p14arf expression in non-small cell lung cancers in relation to smoking history. *Cancer Res*, 67: 5667–72.

34 Ridanpaa M, Karjalainen A, Anttila S, Vainio H, Husgafvelpursiainen K (1994) Genetic alterations in p53 and k-ras in lung-cancer in relation to histopathology of the tumor and smoking history of the patient. *Int J Oncol*, 5: 1109–17.

35 Rodenhuis S, Slebos RJ, Boot AJ, Evers SG, Mooi WJ, Wagenaar SS, *et al.* (1988) Incidence and possible clinical significance of K-ras oncogene activation in adenocarcinoma of the human lung. *Cancer Res*, 48: 5738–41.

36 Shigematsu H, Lin L, Takahashi T, Nomura M, Suzuki M, Wistuba, II, *et al.* (2005) Clinical and

biological features associated with epidermal growth factor receptor gene mutations in lung cancers. *J Natl Cancer Inst*, 97: 339–46.

37 Tam IY, Chung LP, Suen WS, Wang E, Wong MC, Ho KK, *et al.* (2006) Distinct epidermal growth factor receptor and KRAS mutation patterns in non-small cell lung cancer patients with different tobacco exposure and clinicopathologic features. *Clin Cancer Res*, 12: 1647–53.

38 Shigematsu H, Takahashi T, Nomura M, Majmudar K, Suzuki M, Lee H, *et al.* (2005) Somatic mutations of the HER2 kinase domain in lung adenocarcinomas. *Cancer Res*, 65: 1642–6.

39 Wistuba, II, Behrens C, Virmani AK, Milchgrub S, Syed S, Lam S, *et al.* (1999) Allelic losses at chromosome 8p21–23 are early and frequent events in the pathogenesis of lung cancer. *Cancer Res*, 59: 1973–9.

40 Lerman MI, Minna JD (2000) The 630-kb lung cancer homozygous deletion region on human chromosome 3p21.3: identification and evaluation of the resident candidate tumor suppressor genes. The International Lung Cancer Chromosome 3p21.3 Tumor Suppressor Gene Consortium. *Cancer Res*, 60: 6116–33.

41 Zochbauer-Muller S, Fong KM, Maitra A, Lam S, Geradts J, Ashfaq R, *et al.* (2001) 5′ CpG island methylation of the FHIT gene is correlated with loss of gene expression in lung and breast cancer. *Cancer Res*, 61: 3581–5.

42 Miyazu YM, Miyazawa T, Hiyama K, Kurimoto N, Iwamoto Y, Matsuura H, *et al.* (2005) Telomerase expression in noncancerous bronchial epithelia is a possible marker of early development of lung cancer. *Cancer Res*, 65: 9623–7.

43 Yashima K, Milchgrub S, Gollahon LS, Maitra A, Saboorian MH, Shay JW, *et al.* (1998) Telomerase enzyme activity and RNA expression during the multistage pathogenesis of breast carcinoma. *Clin Cancer Res*, 4: 229–34.

44 Lantuejoul S, Soria JC, Morat L, Lorimier P, Moro-Sibilot D, Sabatier L, *et al.* (2005) Telomere shortening and telomerase reverse transcriptase expression in preinvasive bronchial lesions. *Clin Cancer Res*, 11: 2074–82.

45 Park IW, Wistuba, II, Maitra A, Milchgrub S, Virmani AK, Minna JD, *et al.* (1999) Multiple clonal abnormalities in the bronchial epithelium of patients with lung cancer. *J Natl Cancer Inst*, 91: 1863–8.

46 Belinsky SA, Nikula KJ, Palmisano WA, Michels R, Saccomanno G, Gabrielson E, *et al.* (1998) Aberrant methylation of p16(INK4a) is an early event in lung cancer and a potential biomarker for early diagnosis. *Proc Natl Acad Sci USA*, 95: 11891–6.

47 Belinsky SA, Liechty KC, Gentry FD, Wolf HJ, Rogers J, Vu K, *et al.* (2006) Promoter hypermethylation of multiple genes in sputum precedes lung cancer incidence in a high-risk cohort. *Cancer Res*, 66: 3338–44.

48 Hirsch FR, Prindiville SA, Miller YE, Franklin WA, Dempsey EC, Murphy JR, *et al.* (2001) Fluorescence versus white-light bronchoscopy for detection of preneoplastic lesions: a randomized study. *J Natl Cancer Inst*, 93: 1385–91.

49 Merrick DT, Haney J, Petrunich S, Sugita M, Miller YE, Keith RL, *et al.* (2005) Overexpression of vascular endothelial growth factor and its receptors in bronchial dypslasia demonstrated by quantitative RT-PCR analysis. *Lung Cancer*, 48: 31–45.

50 Hirsch FR, Lippman SM (2005) Advances in the biology of lung cancer chemoprevention. *J Clin Oncol*, 23: 3186–97.

51 Khuri FR, Cohen V (2004) Molecularly targeted approaches to the chemoprevention of lung cancer. *Clin Cancer Res*, 10: 4249s–53s.

52 Merrick DT, Kittelson J, Winterhalder R, Kotantoulas G, Ingeberg S, Keith RL, *et al.* (2006) Analysis of c-ErbB1/epidermal growth factor receptor and c-ErbB2/HER-2 expression in bronchial dysplasia: evaluation of potential targets for chemoprevention of lung cancer. *Clin Cancer Res*, 12: 2281–8.

53 Tsao AS, McDonnell T, Lam S, Putnam JB, Bekele N, Hong WK, *et al.* (2003) Increased phospho-AKT (Ser(473)) expression in bronchial dysplasia: implications for lung cancer prevention studies. *Cancer Epidemiol Biomarkers Prev*. 12: 660–4.

54 Lee HY, Moon H, Chun KH, Chang YS, Hassan K, Ji L, *et al.* (2004) Effects of insulin-like growth factor binding protein-3 and farnesyltransferase inhibitor SCH66336 on Akt expression and apoptosis in non-small-cell lung cancer cells. *J Natl Cancer Inst*, 96: 1536–48.

55 Wislez M, Spencer ML, Izzo JG, Juroske DM, Balhara K, Cody DD, *et al.* (2005) Inhibition of mammalian target of rapamycin reverses alveolar epithelial neoplasia induced by oncogenic K-ras. *Cancer Res*, 65: 3226–35.

56 Abbruzzese JL, Lippman SM (2004) The convergence of cancer prevention and therapy in early-phase clinical drug development. *Cancer Cell*, 6: 321–6.

57 Bass AJ, Watanabe H, Mermel CH, Yu S, Perner S, Verhaak RG, *et al.* (2009) SOX2 is an amplified lineage-survival oncogene in lung and esophageal squamous cell carcinomas. *Nat Genet*, 41: 1238–42.

58 Hussenet T, Dali S, Exinger J, Monga B, Jost B, Dembele D, *et al.* (2010) SOX2 is an oncogene activated by recurrent 3q26.3 amplifications in human lung squamous cell carcinomas. *PLoS One*, 5: e8960.

59 Yuan P, Kadara H, Behrens C, Tang X, Woods D, Solis LM, *et al.* (2010) Sex determining region Y-Box 2 (SOX2) is a potential cell-lineage gene highly expressed in the pathogenesis of squamous cell carcinomas of the lung. *PLoS One*, 5: e9112.

60 Lu Y, Futtner C, Rock JR, Xu X, Whitworth W, Hogan BL, *et al.* (2010) Evidence that SOX2 overexpression is oncogenic in the lung. *PLoS One*, 5: e11022.

61 Xiang R, Liao D, Cheng T, Zhou H, Shi Q, Chuang TS, *et al.* (2011) Downregulation of transcription factor SOX2 in cancer stem cells suppresses growth and metastasis of lung cancer. *Br J Cancer*, 104: 1410–17.

62 McCaughan F, Pole JC, Bankier AT, Konfortov BA, Carroll B, Falzon M, *et al.* (2010) Progressive 3q amplification consistently targets SOX2 in preinvasive squamous lung cancer. *Am J Respir Crit Care Med*, 182: 83–91.

63 Westra WH, Baas IO, Hruban RH, Askin FB, Wilson K, Offerhaus GJ, *et al.* (1996) K-ras oncogene activation in atypical alveolar hyperplasias of the human lung. *Cancer Res*, 56: 2224–8.

64 Chiosea S, Jelezcova E, Chandran U, Luo J, Mantha G, Sobol RW, *et al.* (2007) Overexpression of Dicer in precursor lesions of lung adenocarcinoma. *Cancer Res*, 67: 2345–50.

65 Selamat SA, Galler JS, Joshi AD, Fyfe MN, Campan M, Siegmund KD, *et al.* (2011) DNA methylation changes in atypical adenomatous hyperplasia, adenocarcinoma in situ, and lung adenocarcinoma. *PLoS One*, 6: e21443.

66 Rudin CM, Avila-Tang E, Harris CC, Herman JG, Hirsch FR, Pao W, *et al.* (2009) Lung cancer in never smokers: molecular profiles and therapeutic implications. *Clin Cancer Res*, 15: 5646–61.

67 Sun S, Schiller JH, Gazdar AF (2007) Lung cancer in never smokers – a different disease. *Nat Rev Cancer*, 7: 778–90.

68 Yatabe Y, Kosaka T, Takahashi T, Mitsudomi T (2005) EGFR mutation is specific for terminal respiratory unit type adenocarcinoma. *Am J Surg Pathol*, 29: 633–9.

69 Yoshida Y, Shibata T, Kokubu A, Tsuta K, Matsuno Y, Kanai Y, *et al.* (2005) Mutations of the epidermal growth factor receptor gene in atypical adenomatous hyperplasia and bronchioloalveolar carcinoma of the lung. *Lung Cancer*, 50: 1–8.

70 Minoo P, Su G, Drum H, Bringas P, Kimura S (1999) Defects in tracheoesophageal and lung morphogenesis in Nkx2.1(−/−) mouse embryos. *Dev Biol*, 209: 60–71.

71 Yuan B, Li C, Kimura S, Engelhardt RT, Smith BR, Minoo P (2000) Inhibition of distal lung morphogenesis in Nkx2.1(−/−) embryos. *Dev Dyn*, 217: 180–90.

72 Kimura S, Hara Y, Pineau T, Fernandez-Salguero P, Fox CH, Ward JM, *et al.* (1996) The T/ebp null mouse: thyroid-specific enhancer-binding protein is essential for the organogenesis of the thyroid, lung, ventral forebrain, and pituitary. *Genes Dev*, 10: 60–9.

73 Ikeda K, Clark JC, Shaw-White JR, Stahlman MT, Boutell CJ, Whitsett JA (1995) Gene structure and expression of human thyroid transcription factor-1 in respiratory epithelial cells. *J Biol Chem*, 270: 8108–14.

74 Kwei KA, Kim YH, Girard L, Kao J, Pacyna-Gengelbach M, Salari K, *et al.* (2008) Genomic profiling identifies TITF1 as a lineage-specific oncogene amplified in lung cancer. *Oncogene*, 27: 3635–40.

75 Weir BA, Woo MS, Getz G, Perner S, Ding L, Beroukhim R, *et al.* (2007) Characterizing the cancer genome in lung adenocarcinoma. *Nature*, 450: 893–8.

76 Tanaka H, Yanagisawa K, Shinjo K, Taguchi A, Maeno K, Tomida S, *et al.* (2007) Lineage-specific dependency of lung adenocarcinomas on the lung development regulator TTF-1. *Cancer Res*, 67: 6007–11.

77 Winslow MM, Dayton TL, Verhaak RG, Kim-Kiselak C, Snyder EL, Feldser DM, *et al.* (2011) Suppression of lung adenocarcinoma progression by Nkx2–1. *Nature*, 473: 101–4.

78 Meuwissen R, Linn SC, Linnoila RI, Zevenhoven J, Mooi WJ, Berns A (2003) Induction of small cell lung cancer by somatic inactivation of both Trp53 and Rb1 in a conditional mouse model. *Cancer Cell*, 4: 181–9.

79 Park KS, Martelotto LG, Peifer M, Sos ML, Karnezis AN, Mahjoub MR, *et al.* A crucial requirement for Hedgehog signaling in small cell lung cancer. *Nat Med*, 17: 1504–8.

80 Watkins DN, Berman DM, Burkholder SG, Wang B, Beachy PA, Baylin SB (2003) Hedgehog signalling within airway epithelial progenitors and in small-cell lung cancer. *Nature*, 422: 313–17.

81 Peifer M, Fernandez-Cuesta L, Sos ML, George J, Seidel D, Kasper LH, *et al.* (2012) Integrative genome analyses identify key somatic driver mutations of small-cell lung cancer. *Nat Genet*, 44: 1104–10.

82 Slaughter DP, Southwick HW, Smejkal W (1953) Field cancerization in oral stratified squamous

epithelium; clinical implications of multicentric origin. *Cancer*, 6: 963–8.

83 Auerbach O, Stout AP, Hammond EC, Garfinkel L (1961) Changes in bronchial epithelium in relation to cigarette smoking and in relation to lung cancer. *N Engl J Med*, 265: 253–67.

84 Nelson MA, Wymer J, Clements N, Jr (1996) Detection of K-ras gene mutations in non-neoplastic lung tissue and lung cancers. *Cancer Lett*, 103: 115–21.

85 Belinsky SA, Palmisano WA, Gilliland FD, Crooks LA, Divine KK, Winters SA, *et al.* (2002) Aberrant promoter methylation in bronchial epithelium and sputum from current and former smokers. *Cancer Res*, 62: 2370–7.

86 Powell CA, Klares S, O'Connor G, Brody JS (1999) Loss of heterozygosity in epithelial cells obtained by bronchial brushing: clinical utility in lung cancer. *Clin Cancer Res*, 5: 2025–34.

87 Franklin WA, Gazdar AF, Haney J, Wistuba, II, La Rosa FG, Kennedy T, *et al.* (1997) Widely dispersed p53 mutation in respiratory epithelium. A novel mechanism for field carcinogenesis. *J Clin Invest*, 100: 2133–7.

88 Zochbauer-Muller S, Lam S, Toyooka S, Virmani AK, Toyooka KO, Seidl S, *et al.* (2003) Aberrant methylation of multiple genes in the upper aerodigestive tract epithelium of heavy smokers. *Int J Cancer*, 107: 612–16.

89 Soria JC, Rodriguez M, Liu DD, Lee JJ, Hong WK, Mao L (2002) Aberrant promoter methylation of multiple genes in bronchial brush samples from former cigarette smokers. *Cancer Res*, 62: 351–5.

90 Heller G, Zielinski CC, Zochbauer-Muller S (2010) Lung cancer: from single-gene methylation to methylome profiling. *Cancer Metastasis Rev*, 29: 95–107.

91 Hackett NR, Heguy A, Harvey BG, O'Connor TP, Luettich K, Flieder DB, *et al.* (2003) Variability of antioxidant-related gene expression in the airway epithelium of cigarette smokers. *Am J Respir Cell Mol Biol*, 29: 331–43.

92 Spira A, Beane J, Shah V, Liu G, Schembri F, Yang X, *et al.* (2004) Effects of cigarette smoke on the human airway epithelial cell transcriptome. *Proc Natl Acad Sci USA*, 101: 10143–8.

93 Beane J, Sebastiani P, Liu G, Brody JS, Lenburg ME, Spira A (2007) Reversible and permanent effects of tobacco smoke exposure on airway epithelial gene expression. *Genome Biol*, 8: R201.

94 Schembri F, Sridhar S, Perdomo C, Gustafson AM, Zhang X, Ergun A, *et al.* (2009) MicroRNAs as modulators of smoking-induced gene expression changes in human airway epithelium. *Proc Natl Acad Sci USA*, 106: 2319–24.

95 Spira A, Beane JE, Shah V, Steiling K, Liu G, Schembri F, *et al.* (2007) Airway epithelial gene expression in the diagnostic evaluation of smokers with suspect lung cancer. *Nat Med*, 13: 361–6.

96 Gustafson AM, Soldi R, Anderlind C, Scholand MB, Qian J, Zhang X, *et al.* (2010) Airway PI3K pathway activation is an early and reversible event in lung cancer development. *Sci Transl Med*, 2: 26ra5.

97 Sridhar S, Schembri F, Zeskind J, Shah V, Gustafson AM, Steiling K, *et al.* (2008) Smoking-induced gene expression changes in the bronchial airway are reflected in nasal and buccal epithelium. *BMC Genomics*, 9: 259.

98 Zhang X, Sebastiani P, Liu G, Schembri F, Dumas YM, Langer EM, *et al.* (2010) Similarities and differences between smoking-related gene expression in nasal and bronchial epithelium. *Physiol Genomics*, 41: 1–8.

99 Beane J, Vick J, Schembri F, Anderlind C, Gower A, Campbell J, *et al.* (2011) Characterizing the impact of smoking and lung cancer on the airway transcriptome using RNA-Seq. *Cancer Prev Res (Phila)*, 4: 803–17.

100 Kadara H, Shen L, Fujimoto J, Saintigny P, Chow CW, Lang W, *et al.* (2013) Characterizing the molecular spatial and temporal field of injury in early-stage smoker non-small cell lung cancer patients after definitive surgery by expression profiling. *Cancer Prev Res (Phila)*, 6: 8–17.

101 Gomperts BN, Walser TC, Spira A, Dubinett SM (2013) Enriching the molecular definition of the airway "field of cancerization:" establishing new paradigms for the patient at risk for lung cancer. *Cancer Prev Res (Phila)*, 6: 4–7.

102 Anderson GP, Bozinovski S (2003) Acquired somatic mutations in the molecular pathogenesis of COPD. *Trends Pharmacol Sci*, 24: 71–6.

103 Barnes PJ (2000) Chronic obstructive pulmonary disease. *N Engl J Med*, 343: 269–80.

104 Hogg JC (2004) Pathophysiology of airflow limitation in chronic obstructive pulmonary disease. *Lancet*, 364: 709–21.

105 Hida T, Kozaki K, Muramatsu H, Masuda A, Shimizu S, Mitsudomi T, *et al.* (2000) Cyclooxygenase-2 inhibitor induces apoptosis and enhances cytotoxicity of various anticancer agents in non-small cell lung cancer cell lines. *Clin Cancer Res*, 6: 2006–11.

106 Kennedy TC, Proudfoot SP, Franklin WA, Merrick TA, Saccomanno G, Corkill ME, *et al.* (1996) Cytopathological analysis of sputum in patients with

airflow obstruction and significant smoking histories. *Cancer Res*, 56: 4673–8.

107 Lam S, leRiche JC, Zheng Y, Coldman A, MacAulay C, Hawk E, *et al.* (1999) Sex-related differences in bronchial epithelial changes associated with tobacco smoking. *J Natl Cancer Inst*, 91: 691–6.

108 Tsurutani J, Castillo SS, Brognard J, Granville CA, Zhang C, Gills JJ, *et al.* (2005) Tobacco components stimulate Akt-dependent proliferation and NFkappaB-dependent survival in lung cancer cells. *Carcinogenesis*, 26: 1182–95.

109 Tang X, Liu D, Shishodia S, Ozburn N, Behrens C, Lee JJ, *et al.* (2006) Nuclear factor-kappaB (NF-kappaB) is frequently expressed in lung cancer and preneoplastic lesions. *Cancer*, 107: 2637–46.

110 Tichelaar JW, Zhang Y, leRiche JC, Biddinger PW, Lam S, Anderson MW (2005) Increased staining for phospho-Akt, p65/RELA and cIAP-2 in preneoplastic human bronchial biopsies. *BMC Cancer*, 5: 155.

111 Dannenberg AJ, Altorki NK, Boyle JO, Dang C, Howe LR, Weksler BB, *et al.* (2001) Cyclo-oxygenase 2: a pharmacological target for the prevention of cancer. *Lancet Oncol*, 2: 544–51.

112 Hasturk S, Kemp B, Kalapurakal SK, Kurie JM, Hong WK, Lee JS (2002) Expression of cyclooxygenase-1 and cyclooxygenase-2 in bronchial epithelium and nonsmall cell lung carcinoma. *Cancer*, 94: 1023–31.

113 Mao JT, Cui X, Reckamp K, Liu M, Krysan K, Dalwadi H, *et al.* (2005) Chemoprevention strategies with cyclooxygenase-2 inhibitors for lung cancer. *Clin Lung Cancer*, 7: 30–9.

114 Mascaux C, Martin B, Verdebout JM, Ninane V, Sculier JP (2005) COX-2 expression during early lung squamous cell carcinoma oncogenesis. *Eur Respir J*, 26: 198–203.

115 Mao JT, Fishbein MC, Adams B, Roth MD, Goodglick L, Hong L, *et al.* (2006) Celecoxib decreases Ki-67 proliferative index in active smokers. *Clin Cancer Res*, 12: 314–20.

116 Kim ES, Hong WK, Lee JJ, Mao L, Morice RC, Liu DD, *et al.* (2010) Biological activity of celecoxib in the bronchial epithelium of current and former smokers. *Cancer Prev Res (Phila)*, 3: 148–59.

117 Mao JT, Roth MD, Fishbein MC, Aberle DR, Zhang ZF, Rao JY, *et al.* (2011) Lung cancer chemoprevention with celecoxib in former smokers. *Cancer Prev Res (Phila)*, 4: 984–93.

118 Meyerson M, Gabriel S, Getz G (2010) Advances in understanding cancer genomes through second-generation sequencing. *Nat Rev Genet*, 11: 685–96.

119 Govindan R, Ding L, Griffith M, Subramanian J, Dees ND, Kanchi KL, *et al.* (2012) Genomic landscape of non-small cell lung cancer in smokers and never-smokers. *Cell*, 150: 1121–34.

120 Hammerman PS, Hayes DN, Wilkerson MD, Schultz N, Bose R, Chu A, *et al.* (2012) Comprehensive genomic characterization of squamous cell lung cancers. *Nature*, 489: 519–25.

121 Imielinski M, Berger AH, Hammerman PS, Hernandez B, Pugh TJ, Hodis E, *et al.* (2012) Mapping the hallmarks of lung adenocarcinoma with massively parallel sequencing. *Cell*, 150: 1107–20.

CHAPTER 7

Detection and Treatment of Preneoplastic Lesions

Rachel Jen and Stephen Lam
Department of Medicine, University of British Columbia, Vancouver, British Columbia, Canada

Introduction

Currently, lung cancer survival is poor with only 15% of patients surviving 5 years or more after diagnosis [1]. While new systemic therapy agents and radiotherapy have improved survival and quality of life of patients, the overall impact in the last decade has been mainly on palliation rather than reduction in mortality. Lung cancer survival is strongly associated with stage. The Surveillance Epidemiology and End Results (SEER) data indicate that only 16% of lung cancer patients present with localized disease while the remaining presents with either regional or distant metastasis [2]. Improving cure rates would involve diagnosing patients at an earlier stage, when the cancer is still localized.

There are unique challenges to localize preneoplastic lesions in the lung. In contrast to other epithelial organs, the lung is an internal organ consisting of a complex branching system of conducting airways leading to peripheral gas exchange units with a surface area of the size of a tennis court. In addition, instead of a single cell type, lung cancer consists of several cell types and they are preferentially located in different parts of the airways and lung parenchyma. There is no single method that can scan the entire bronchial epithelium for preneoplastic lesions and allow tissue sampling for pathological diagnosis and molecular profiling. Several biophotonic imaging methods have been developed such as autofluorescence bronchoscopy (AFB) and optical coherence tomography (OCT) for localization of preneoplastic lesions in areas accessible by fiberoptic probes. Multidetector spiral CT is a sensitive tool to detect preneoplastic lesions in the peripheral lung. CT can serve as a virtual map to enable biopsy of peripheral lung lesions using navigational systems. In this chapter, current evidence supporting the use of these methods and direction for future research is discussed.

Detection of preneoplastic lesions in central airways

Principles of biophotonic imaging

When the bronchial surface is illuminated by light, the light can be absorbed, reflected, back scattered, or induce fluorescence [3]. These optical properties can be used for determining the structural features as well as the biochemical composition and functional changes in normal and abnormal bronchial tissues. White-light bronchoscopy (WLB) makes use of differences in specular reflection, back scattering, and absorption properties of broadband visible light to define the structural features of the bronchial surface to discriminate between normal and abnormal tissues. Although it is the simplest

Lung Cancer, Fourth Edition. Edited by Jack A. Roth, Waun Ki Hong and Ritsuko U. Komaki.

imaging technique, less than 40% of carcinoma in situ (CIS) is detectable by standard WLB [4]. AFB makes use of fluorescence and absorption properties to provide information about the biochemical composition and metabolic state of bronchial tissues. Collagen and elastin are the most important structural fluorophores. Fluorophores involve in cellular metabolism include nicotinamide adenine dinucleotide (NADH) and flavins. Other fluorophores include the aromatic amino adds (e.g., tryptophan, tyrosine, phenylalanine), various porphyrins, and lipopigments (e.g., ceroids, lipofuscin). The fluorescence properties of bronchial tissue is determined by the concentration and distribution of these fluorophores, their distinct excitation and emission spectra, metabolic state as well as the tissue architecture and the distribution of nonfluorescent chromophores such as hemoglobin [3]. Upon illumination by violet or blue light, normal bronchial tissues fluoresce strongly in the green. As the bronchial epithelium changes from normal to dysphasia, and then to CIS and invasive cancer, there is a progressive decrease in green autofluorescence but proportionately less decrease in red fluorescence intensity [5]. This change is due a decrease in strongly fluorescent extracellular matrix in the submucosa such as collagen and elastin, alteration of the light scattering process from an increase in nuclear size, cellular density and cell distribution as well as increase in the microvascular density [6, 7]. The presence of an increased concentration and distribution of hemoglobin results in increased absorption of the blue excitation light and reduced fluorescence. For example, angiogenic squamous dysplasia was found to have decreased autofluorescence [8]. In addition, there is a reduction in the amount of flavins and NADH in premalignant and malignant cells. Other factors such as pH and oxygenation may also alter the fluorescence quantum yield [9]. In bronchoscopy, the excitation wavelengths producing the highest tumor to normal tissue contrasts are between 400 and 480 nm with a peak at 405 nm [5, 10]. The spectral differences between 500 and 700 nm in normal, preneoplastic and neoplastic tissues serve as the basis for the design of several autofluorescence endoscopic imaging devices for localization of early lung cancer in the bronchial tree [5, 11, 12]. Recent versions of these devices usually use a combination of reflectance and fluorescence for imaging to make use of all the optical properties to optimize detection of subtle preneoplastic lesions [12–18].

Autofluorescence bronchoscopy (AFB)

AFB allows rapid scanning of large areas of the bronchial surface for subtle abnormalities that are difficult to detect by white-light examination (WLB). Current devices make use of CCD tipped videobronchoscopes with higher resolution than fiberoptic bronchoscopes. They allow rapid switching between white-light and fluorescence examination or simultaneous display of the white-light and fluorescence images [13, 18]. Small amounts of reflected light (blue, green, or near infrared) is used to enhance the chromatic contrast and to normalize the green autofluorescence image to correct for nonuniformity caused by optical and geometrical factors such as variable distances and angles between the endoscope tip to the bronchial surface. Depending on the type of reflected light used to combine with the fluorescence image for display, abnormal areas appear brownish red, red, purple or magenta while normal areas appear green or light blue [12–18].

In addition to multiple single center studies [19], there are two randomized trials [20, 21], and three large multicenter trials [11, 12, 22] comparing WLB and AFB. The studies showed an improvement in the detection rate of high-grade dysplasia, CIS and microinvasive cancer with AFB compared to WLB. In general, there is a twofold improvement in the relative sensitivity with AFB. However, the specificity of AFB is lower – ~60% versus ~90% for WLB. A recent meta-analysis reported a pooled sensitivity on a per-lesion basis to detect pre-invasive lesions of 85% for AFB. The relative sensitivity compared to WLB was 2.04 (95% CI: 1.56–11.55) [23]. However, the sensitivity AFB vs. WLB alone for invasive squamous cell carcinoma (SCC) was only marginally improved (95% vs. 89%, respectively; relative sensitivity 1.15, 95% CI: 1.05–1.26). The specificity of AFB (61%) was lower than WLB (80%) [23].

The lower specificity of AFB is due to false positive fluorescence with inflammation, mucous gland hyperplasia, suction trauma and interobserver variation. The specificity of AFB can be improved to 80% by quantifying the red to green fluorescence ratio (R/G) during the bronchoscopic procedure [24]. Combining the R/G ratios with the visual score improved the specificity further to 88%. A higher false-positive rate was also found in a multicenter trial where the R/G ratios were hidden from the bronchoscopists when making the visual classification of the bronchial mucosal changes [12]. Quantitative imaging decreases intra- and interobserver variation.

The presence of autofluorescence abnormalities in some cases may be an indicator of field cancerization and increased cancer risk. Lesions that are positive on AFB but only mild dysplasia or lower grade pathology in the biopsies were found to have more genetic alterations than similar lesions with normal fluorescence [25, 26]. They may have a higher potential for progression. The presence of multiple areas of abnormal autofluorescence, notwithstanding the histopathology grade, appears to be a risk factor for subsequent development of lung cancer. Pasic *et al.* reported that the risk of developing lung cancer over the next 4 years is 50% in those with two or more areas of abnormal autofluorescence compared to 8% in those with only one abnormal site [27].

Narrow band imaging (NBI)

Angiogenesis is a relatively early event during lung cancer pathogenesis and neovascularization correlates with tumor progression [28]. NBI, also known as image enhanced endoscopy, was developed to enhance the superficial microvasculature [29]. It is widely used in gastrointestinal endoscopy for classification of early neoplasia in Barrett's esophagus [30], but its place in routine bronchoscopic examination has not been established. NBI uses narrow band blue light centered at 415 nm (400 nm to 430 nm) and green light centered at 540 nm (530 nm to 550 nm) corresponding to the maximal hemoglobin absorption peaks. The blue light highlights the superficial capillaries while the green light can penetrate deeper to highlight the larger blood vessels in the submucosa. The narrow bandwidths reduce the scattering of light from other wavelengths that are present in a broad spectrum white-light and enable enhanced visualization of blood vessels [31]. NBI may improve the detection of pre-invasive lesions and differentiation of these lesions from invasive carcinoma. Dotted vessels, increased vessel growth and complex networks of tortuous vessels of various sizes are observed with angiogenic squamous dysplasia. With CIS, dotted vessels and small spiral or corkscrew type tumor vessels are observed. Prominent spiral or cork-screw type tumor vessels of various sizes and grades are visible in micro-invasive or invasive lung cancer [31]. A prospective study compares the accuracy of WLB followed by either AFB or NBI as determined by a randomized code to detect intraepithelial neoplasia [32]. The sensitivity of WLB to detect high-grade dysplasia or CIS was 0.18 and the specificity was 0.88. The relative sensitivity of WLB+AFB versus WLB alone was 3.7 compared to 3.0 with WLB+NBI but the difference was not statistically significant. The relative specificities of WLB+AFB and WLB+NBI were 0.5 and 1.0 respectively. WLB+NBI showed a significantly higher specificity compared to WLB+AFB ($p < 0.001$).

Currently it is not known as to how NBI compares to high-definition WLB that makes use of CCD with markedly higher pixel densities and high-definition images. With the shift in lung cancer cell types from the more centrally located squamous cell and small cell carcinomas to adenocarcinomas that are generally located in smaller airways and lung parenchyma, the prevalence of preneoplastic lesions found by AFB with a standard adult size bronchoscope (5.8 mm to 6 mm) has been decreasing steadily in the last decade as noted by experience in the British Columbia Cancer Agency (Figure 7.1). To make use of AFB or NBI, a reduction in the size of the bronchoscope to <4 mm outer diameter with a 2 mm biopsy channel is needed.

Optical coherence tomography (OCT)

OCT is an optical imaging method that can offer near histologic resolution for visualizing cellular and extracellular structures at and below the tissue surface [33–35]. OCT is similar to ultrasound,

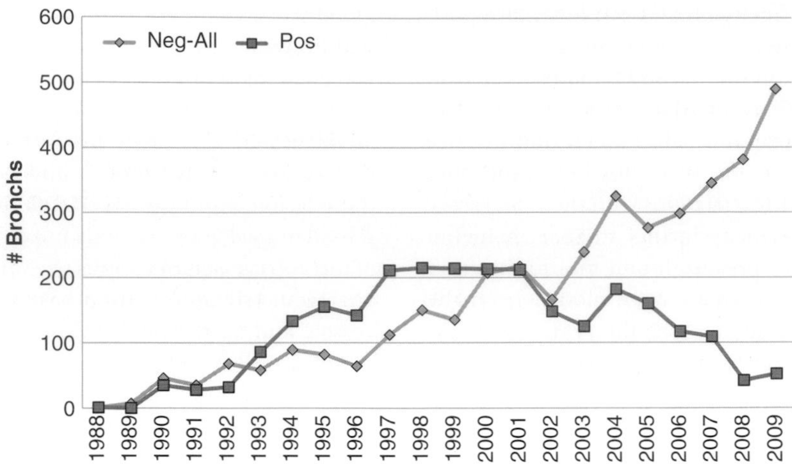

Figure 7.1 Proportion of heavy smokers participating in the BCCA Lung Health Study between 1998 and 2009 found to have one or more sites of bronchial dysplasia on autofluorescence bronchoscopy and biopsy using a 5.8 mm bronchoscope showing a steady decline in the prevalence of bronchial dysplasia since 2000.

but instead of sound, near infrared light is used. The light that is back scattered or reflected by the tissue is used to generate a one-dimensional tissue profile using optical interferometry. By scanning the light beam over the tissue, two-dimensional images or three-dimensional volumetric images can be displayed. The procedure is performed using fiberoptic probes that can be miniaturized to enable imaging of airways down to the terminal bronchioles. These probes can be inserted to airways of interest through the biopsy channel of a standard bronchoscope during the examination under conscious sedation. The axial and lateral resolutions of OCT range from approximately 5 μm to 30 μm depending on imaging conditions. The imaging depth is 2 to 3 millimeters [35]. This combination of resolution and imaging depth is ideal for examining preneoplastic changes originating in epithelial tissues or tumors involving smaller airways. Additionally, unlike ultrasound, light does not require a liquid coupling medium and thus is more compatible with airway imaging. There are no associated risks from the weak near-infrared light sources that are used for OCT.

OCT images of normal bronchus, primary tumors and alveoli from seven human lung cancer lobectomy specimens have been compared with the histopathology [33–36]. OCT imaging revealed a layered bronchial wall structure in normal bronchi that is lost in lung cancer. In peripheral lung, air-containing alveoli are imaged by OCT as a honeycomb structure beyond the bronchial wall. Lam *et al.* investigated the ability of OCT to discern invasive cancer versus CIS or dysplasia [34]. Normal or hyperplasia is characterized by one or two cell layers above a highly scattering basement membrane and upper submucosa. As the epithelium changes from normal/hyperplasia to metaplasia, various grades of dysplasia, and CIS, the thickness of the epithelial layer increases. Quantitative measurement of the epithelial thickness showed that invasive carcinoma is significantly thicker than carcinoma in situ ($p = 0.004$) and dysplasia is significantly thicker than metaplasia or hyperplasia ($p = 0.002$). The nuclei become more readily visible in high-grade dysplasia or CIS. The basement membrane is still intact in CIS but became discontinuous or no longer visible with invasive cancer [34, 35]. Squamous cell carcinoma (SCC) has different volumetric features than adenocarcinoma [36]. OCT may be useful for confirming the nature of the lesion before taking a biopsy.

Indications for autofluorescence bronchoscopy

Evaluation of patients with abnormal sputum cytology

There is no controversy that a finding of cells suspicious or diagnostic of malignancy on sputum cytology examination requires further investigation, usually bronchoscopy and CT scanning. Sato *et al.* reported a marked improvement in survival of patients with a sputum diagnosis of SCC and negative chest radiographs that were treated following bronchoscopic localization of the cancer compared to a group with the same diagnosis but declined treatment. The treated group had a 94.9% survival at 10 years versus 33.5% in the untreated group [37].

Severe atypia on sputum cytology examination has been reported in several studies to have an approximately 45% risk of developing lung cancer within 2 years [38, 39]. In the Johns Hopkins Early Lung Cancer Detection Project, moderate atypia was also found to have an increased risk of the subsequent development of lung cancer. Fourteen percent of the participants with moderate atypia developed lung cancer compared to 3% of participants without atypia [38]. In the Colorado SPORE cohort of high-risk smokers and ex-smokers with airflow obstruction, the relative risks of developing lung cancer, adjusted for age, gender, pack-years, and smoking status, was found to increase from 1.10 for mild atypia, 1.68 for moderate atypia, 3.18 for moderate atypia or worse, and 31.4 for severe atypia or worse [40]. Sputum cytology of severe atypia or worse clearly carries a risk of lung cancer that is high enough to warrant an aggressive diagnostic approach with WLB+AFB. A case may also be made for bronchoscopic examination of patients with moderate atypia although the evidence is not as strong as patients with severe atypia. In a series of 79 subjects with moderate sputum atypia with chest radiographs negative for cancer, lung cancer was found at bronchoscopy in 5 (6.3%; 95% CI, 0.7–11%) [41]. Two of the cancers were CIS lesions and three were invasive. This rate of discovery of cancer at bronchoscopy exceeds the rate of discovery of colon cancer when colonoscopy is performed for a positive fecal occult blood test.

Evaluation of patients with suspected, known or previously completely resected lung cancer

AFB can play a useful role in both the delineation of tumor margins and to assess the presence of synchronous lesions in patients with early lung cancer who are being assessed for curative surgical resection [27,41–43]. A careful clinical-pathological study by Ikeda *et al.* in 30 patients with NSCLC who had preoperative AFB examination and subsequently surgical resection showed more accurate delineation of the tumor extent as well as finding other sites of dysplasia with AFB compared to WLB [44]. Synchronous cancer can be found on AFB in up to 15% of patients with early lung cancer [43–45]. The discovery of synchronous lesions altered the therapeutic plan in these patients.

Following successful curative resection of NSCLC, a high rate (1–3% per year) of second primary (metachronous) tumors is reported [46]. In the subset of patients with prior early SCC, the reported rate of metachronous lesions appears to be even higher with nearly 30% develop a second central carcinoma within 4 years [47, 48]. Postoperative surveillance WLB and AFB was performed in patients with completely resected NSCLC [27, 48, 49]. In 25 patients, Weigel *et al.* found 12% of the patients subsequently developed three lesions of moderate/severe dysplasia and one micro-invasive cancer over an average of 20.5 months of follow-up [48]. Pasic *et al.*, found that 28% of patients with a previous lung cancer developed metachronous SCC within a median of 47 months [27]. The predominance of metachronous lesions in the central airways in patients with previous SCC versus those with peripheral adenocarcinoma is suggested by a study that showed 30% of the patients with a previously resected SCC had high-grade dysphasia or worse compared to only 4% with a previously resected adenocarcinoma [50]. Patients with a previous curative resection for lung cancer are at high risk of developing second primary lung cancers. Surveillance AFB may be useful in those with previous SCC who have good performance status and no significant comorbidities.

Assessment of patients with early central lung cancer prior to endobronchial therapy

When considering an early central carcinoma for curative endobronchial therapy, AFB plays an important role in determining the extent of the lesion. Complete response after endobronchial therapy such as photodynamic therapy is influenced by the surface area of the lesion and whether all margins can be visualized [51]. These factors cannot be accurately assessed with WLB alone. Sutedja *et al.* performed AFB on 23 patients referred for intraluminal therapy of NSCLC following WLB [52]. The lesions were determined to be too extensive for intraluminal therapy by CT scan and AFB examination in 4 (17%) and 19 (68%) patients, respectively.

Surveillance of bronchial intraepithelial neoplasia

Dysplasia and CIS have been considered as precursors of SCC of the lung. The risk and rate of progression of preneoplastic lesions to invasive SCC as well as the mechanism of progression or regression are incompletely understood due to small number of patients in longitudinal studies. A review of the published reports showed that on the average, 60% of severe dysplasia regressed spontaneously and 40% progressed or persisted [53]. The extent to which repeat biopsies of the same site actually removed the lesion cannot be estimated. The natural history of CIS is even more difficult to evaluate as all studies except one [54] intervened with treatment at the time of the diagnosis or when CIS persisted on repeat bronchoscopy and biopsy within 3 months. CIS is different than severe dysplasia at the molecular level and appears to have different clinical outcome. The spontaneous regression rate of CIS is ~13% versus >50% for high grade dysplasia [53]. In the single study in 16 patients with 36 high-grade lesions (7 severe dysplasia and 29 CIS) who were not treated initially, 11 cancers were diagnosed in 9 of 16 patients. Six high-grade lesions in 5 patients progressed to invasive cancers at intervals ranging from 4 to 17 months; 3 of these 5 patients had incurable disease despite treatment [54]. Thus, CIS, when allowed to progress to invasive cancer can become incurable by local therapy [53, 54]. While it may be appropriate to perform surveillance bronchoscopy in those with severe dysplasia, treatment is preferable for CIS lesions instead of observation with repeat bronchoscopies and biopsies. As discussed below, endobronchial therapy such as electrocautery treatment and cryotherapy is simple, low cost and safe [55, 56].

Genetic alterations such as loss of heterozygosity in chromosome 3p or chromosomal aneusomy as well as host factors such as the inflammatory load and levels of anti-inflammatory proteins in the lung influence the progression or regression of preneoplastic lesions [53, 57]. In a study at the BC Cancer Agency, a significantly higher progression rate was found to occur in those who developed SCC compared with those who developed adenocarcinoma [53]. The progression rate of mild dysplasia was 30.9% for those who developed SCC versus 3.3% in those who developed adenocarcinoma ($P = 0.041$). The underlying mechanism has not been identified yet. Some lesions appear to progress rapidly from hyperplasia/metaplasia to CIS/invasive cancer within 2 years [53, 58], which is much shorter than the traditional thinking of 10–20 years. The addition of nuclear morphometry or molecular analysis to histopathologic grading allows more accurate classification of preneoplastic lesions and better identification of lesions that are biologically more aggressive. A recent study by van Boerdonk *et al.* [26] compared the genetic alterations in squamous metaplasia lesions from 6 subjects that progressed to CIS or invasive carcinoma in the same site with squamous metaplasia lesions from 20 subjects that did not progress. p53, p63, and Ki-67 immunostaining were not predictive for a differential clinical outcome of the lesions. The mean copy number alterations (CNA) in baseline squamous metaplasia lesions of cases that progressed was significantly higher than the control subjects ($P < 0.01$). A model based on CNAs at 3p26.3–p11.1, 3q26.2–29, and 6p25.3–24.3 predicted cancer development with 97% accuracy. If these findings can be validated, it would provide the evidence to support the use of surveillance AFB or endobronchial therapy in patients with these apparently low grade lesions.

The presence of high-grade dysplasia or CIS is a risk marker for lung cancer both in the central airways and peripheral lung [53, 54]. Close follow-up with AFB and CT imaging should be considered in patients with these lesions.

Detection of preneoplastic lesions in peripheral lung

Atypical adenomatous hyperplasia (AAH) is considered to be the preinvasive lesion of adenocarcinoma [59, 60]. These lesions are usually less than 7 mm in diameter and are detectable on CT scan as small, "ground glass" densities [61, 62]. In resected lungs, the incidence of AAH was estimated to be 9–21% in patients with primary lung cancer and 4–10% in patients without lung cancer [59]. Laboratory investigations demonstrate that AAH cells have the ultrastructural features of Clara cells or Type II pneumocytes [63] and that many of the molecular changes present in lung adenocarcinomas are present in these lesions supporting the concept that AAH lesions are precursor lesions of peripheral adenocarcinoma. The finding of ground glass densities, small semi-solid or noncalcified nodules on a CT scan is not specific for AAH, adenocarcinoma in-situ, minimally invasive or invasive adenocarcinoma. The majority of these small lung densities are not preneoplastic or neoplastic [61, 62]. Diagnosis of subcentimeter lung nodules that grow or increase in density requires a biopsy.

CT guided transthoracic needle/core biopsy for lesions ≤15 mm has a sensitivity of 70–82% [64, 65]. Transthoracic needle biopsy has an average pneumothorax rate of 15%. Chest tube drainage is required in approximately 6.6% [66]. Several bronchoscopic biopsy methods show diagnostic yields approaching that of CT guided transthoracic lung biopsy with a significantly lower complication rate. With the advancement of thin slice CT and image reconstruction technology, virtual bronchoscopy navigation (VBN) uses a computer-generated 3D road map to locate the lung lesion. At each branching point, the bronchoscopist can match the actual videobronchoscopy image with the virtual image to steer the bronchoscope [67]. A randomized trial by Ishida *et al.* showed that the diagnostic yield was significantly higher with VBN compared to no VBN assistance (75.9% versus 59.3 mm for lesions < 20 mm) [68]. A further development is the ability to overlay the videobronchoscopy and virtual images to indicate which airway to follow in real time as well as displaying the location and distance of the lesion behind the bronchial wall if there is no airway leading to the lesion directly [69]. VBN significantly shortens the bronchoscopy time.

VBN can also be used with co-registration of a steerable catheter, a bronchoscope or biopsy forceps with a sensor at the tip that can be tracked by an external electromagnetic device similar in concept to a Global Positioning System. The procedure is known as Electromagnetic Navigation (EMN). Once the target lesion is reached on the virtual image, the location may be further confirmed by radial endoscopic ultrasound (R-EBUS) or fluoroscopy before taking a biopsy to minimize registration error [70]. R-EBUS can visualize lesions that are not well-defined on fluoroscopy [71]. A meta-analysis of EMN showed an average diagnostic yield of 67% (95% CI 62.6% to 71.4%) [72]. In the community setting, the diagnostic yield is lower. A recent multicenter experience with EMN showed a sensitivity of 50% for lesions ≤ 2 cm [73]. A combination of technologies can improve the diagnostic yield. Randomized trials showed improved sensitivity of 90% for lesions ≤ 20 mm with VBN+EMN+R-EBUS compares to 78% with R-EBUS alone and 75% for EMN alone [74]. A recent meta-analysis of guided bronchoscopy showed similar results [72].

Two small randomized trials comparing transthoracic needle biopsy and R-EBUS bronchoscopy show a similar overall diagnostic yield [75, 76]. The incidence of pneumothorax and other complications are significantly lower. The average incidence of pneumothorax is 1% (range 0–5%) with R-EBUS [72, 75, 76].

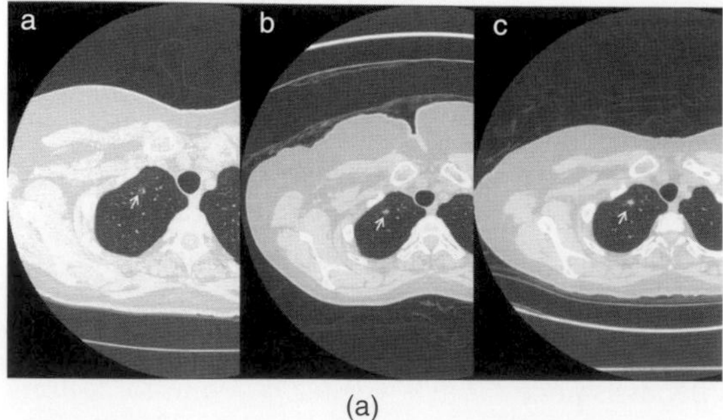

(a)

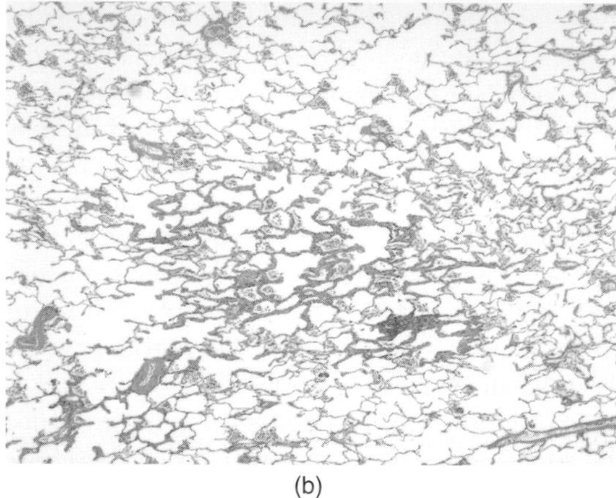

(b)

Figure 7.2 a: Progressive increase in size and density of the lung nodule in the right upper lobe [arrow] between two consecutive annual repeat low dose spiral CT scans [b, c]. b: Wedge resection showed atypical adenomatous hyperplasia.

Newer technologies such as OCT [35, 36], which allows visualization with micron resolution or SpyGlass [77] that allows direct visualization of the airways as small as 1 mm using a fiberoptic probe, has the potential to further improve the diagnostic yield and real time sampling. Coupling the navigation system with OCT may allow better localization and characterization of the growth behavior of small lung densities to separate preneoplastic lesions and early adenocarcinoma from benign lesions. As illustrated in Figure 7.2, calculation of volume doubling time of adenocarcinoma based on serial CT scans without a biopsy of the lung nodule detected on the first CT can be erroneous as the nodule may represent AAH before progression to invasive carcinoma.

Treatment of preinvasive bronchial lesions

Surgery remains the gold standard for the treatment of CIS and results in 80~90% 5-year survival rate [47, 78, 79]. However, a significant limitation is the need to remove a substantial amount of lung tissue for curative treatment. Up to 30% may require a bilobectomy or pneumonectomy to achieve cure, and the remaining 70% require a lobectomy [47, 78, 79]. Segmentectomy has only been used in small series of selected patients. Excellent 5-year survival rate of >90% was reported [79].

Some patients may not be candidates for surgical resection due to co-morbidities or limited pulmonary reserves. Up to 30% of patients with central SCC will develop metachronous cancer and approximately 15% will be found to have synchronous cancer [42, 43, 45, 47, 78–80]. Therefore, lung sparing local treatment modality should be considered with surgery reserved for patients who fail endobronchial therapy.

Prior to endobronchial therapy with curative intent, it is important to rule out peribronchial tumor extension, regional or systemic spread. Thoracic CT and PET imaging are useful techniques [81]. CT scan has been shown to alter clinical management in 22~35% of cases being considered for curative therapy [81]. Positive lymph nodes either on CT or PET imaging should be investigated to exclude metastases.

Endobronchial therapy is usually not curative for lesions that have invaded into the bronchial cartilage or beyond [81–83]. Konaka *et al.* suggested that flat lesions >10 mm in length and nodular or polypoid tumors are associated with a higher risk of cartilaginous invasion [84]. EBUS has been shown to be a helpful tool to evaluate cartilaginous involvement in the assessment of small central SCC with a sensitivity and specificity of 89% and 100% respectively [82, 85]. In addition, EBUS can be used for staging with lymph node sampling. EBUS resulted in a change in management in 36% of tumors thought to be curable by endobronchial therapy after WLB and thoracic CT [82].

In addition to determining the depth of tumor infiltration into the bronchial wall and rule out extrabronchial spread, the margins of the lesion must be visualized and accessible for endoscopic therapy. Lesions that do not fit these criteria should be referred for curative surgery if the patient is an operable candidate. AFB is the best modality to evaluate to accurately visualize all margins [44, 52].

Endobronchial therapies

Although there are no prospective, randomized studies comparing surgery to endobronchial therapy for CIS, outcomes of similar cases of early central lung cancer treated with endobronchial therapy or surgery appear to be comparable [47, 56]. In addition to the benefits of lung tissue conservation and low risks associated with the procedure, endobronchial therapy is cost-effective, with up to 70% cost saving compared to surgical resection [56].

Commonly used and well-described endobronchial techniques include photodynamic therapy (PDT), electrocautery, argon plasma coagulation (APC), cryotherapy, brachytherapy, and Nd-YAG laser therapy. All these techniques when used for CIS lesions are generally performed with flexible bronchoscopy under conscious sedation compared to bulkier obstructive lesions that may require rigid bronchoscopy. Among them, PDT has the most worldwide clinical experience, but cost and skin photosensitivity are the main disadvantages. Electrocautery/APC and cryotherapy are cheaper and simpler alternatives to PDT but there are less data for their efficacy. Nd-YAG laser therapy is not generally considered appropriate for curative therapy for superficial CIS due to the increased risk of perforation and hemorrhage [86].

Photodynamic therapy (PDT)

PDT refers to intravenous administration of a photosensitizer such as Photofrin that is preferentially retained in higher concentrations in the tumor than the surrounding tissue, and activation of the drug in 24–72 hours with light of a specific wavelength to produce a photochemical reaction to destroy the tumor [51, 87, 88]. Newer photosensitizer such as mono-L-aspartyl chlorine e6 (talaporfin sodium, NPe6), has much shorter skin photosensitivity, compared to Photofrin [89, 90].

Kato *et al.* reported complete responses (CR) were obtained in 85% of the 264 centrally located early-stage cancers [91]. With increasing size of the cancers, CR rates fall from 94% for tumors with a longitudinal length of <10 mm, 80% for those between 10–20 mm, and 44% for tumors >20 mm. Smaller studies from North America and Europe reported CR rates in 62% to 100% [92, 93]. Local recurrence occurred in approximately 12% [88, 91] and most occurred with 12 months [94]. These were thought to be due to inadequate visualization of the peripheral margin or depth leading to inadequate irradiation. To improve the efficacy of PDT, EBUS, OCT and AFB have been used in conjunction to better delineate the lesions [82, 91].

Electrocautery

Bronchoscopic electrocautery causes tissue destruction through direct contact of the probe to deliver heat energy generated by a high frequency alternating current. Through a wide variety of applicators such as forceps, cutting loops, and blunt heat probes, electrocautery achieves tissue destruction and coagulation through adjustment of the wattage, contact surface area, and duration of energy application. It is an inexpensive technique with low complication rates. One report by Van Boxem *et al.* showed a complete response rate of 80% in 13 patients with 15 small intraluminal lesions $\leq$10 mm^2 and normal CT scans. No residual disease was seen at a median follow-up of 22 months [95]. A subsequent report by the same group evaluated multiple curative endobronchial modalities including electrocautery of small intraluminal, microinvasive stage 1A disease (CIS excluded) in 32 inoperable patients. Seventy-five percent of these patients were treated with electrocautery and more than 95% achieved bronchoscopic eradication. Half the patients died in the mean follow-up of 5 years but only one death was attributable to the failure or complications of the bronchoscopic treatment [80].

Argon plasma coagulation (APC) is another relatively low cost noncontact thermal ablation technique [96]. Ionized argon gas that jets out of the probe conducts electrons between the active electrode of the probe and the tissue. These electrons encountering high resistance in human tissue generate heat that leads to superficial tissue damage. Data on the efficacy of APC in treatment of bronchial CIS [97] is scanty but in theory, the result should be similar to electrocautery.

Cryotherapy

Cryotherapy uses nitrous oxide or liquid nitrogen to achieve rapid freezing and thawing to cause tissue destruction. It is an inexpensive and safe technique. Bronchial cartilage and extracellular matrix are highly cold resistant making cryosurgery relatively safe from airway perforation or stricture formation [98]. In contrast to the denaturation of proteins seen with heat-based techniques, the preservation of the extracellular matrix engenders an environment that promotes ablation of an unwanted tissue without significant scarring [99, 100].

There are limited studies of cryotherapy as curative therapy for CIS or micro-invasive bronchial cancer. Deygas *et al.* [100] reported no severe adverse events and 91% CR in 35 patients with 41 CIS or micro-invasive disease at 12 months follow-up. Ten patients (28%) developed local recurrence within 12 months and the overall long-term cure rate was 80%. Cryotherapy with an endobronchial cryo-probe is not efficient and can be difficult to perform depending on the tumor location. Recently, spray cryotherapy (SCT) was developed to deliver liquid nitrogen at a much lower temperature than a cryo-probe through an endoscopic catheter. The noncontact approach facilitates more precise treatment in larger areas. Clinical experience with SCT has been mainly with large obstructive bronchial tumors [101, 102]. Applying shorter but more cycles of SCT and proper positioning of the catheter are important to avoid pneumothorax due to rapid gas expansion.

Brachytherapy

Endobronchial brachytherapy (EBBT) delivers local irradiation through the insertion of a polyurethane catheter to the tumor site in the airway by flexible bronchoscopy to serve as a conduit for the radioactive source (usually Iridium^{192}). This technique has been used effectively for palliative treatment of obstructive endobronchial tumors but there are limited reports on EBBT as a treatment of CIS and micro-invasive tumors. The unique advantage of EBBT is its ability to treat tumors that have invaded beyond the bronchial cartilage. One of the largest series was from Hennequin *et al.* on curative EBBT treatment of 106 patients with localized central airway tumors, not visible on CT and <10 mm in thickness [103]. The patients were not candidates for surgery or external beam radiotherapy due to medical contraindications. EBBT achieved complete histologic response in 59% of the patients. Shorter endobronchial tumor length and tumors that were not visible on CT scan showed significant better response to EBBT. Response rates of 83–85% were observed in two smaller studies [104, 105]. Potential complications of EBBT include hemoptysis and radiation-induced bronchitis/stenosis.

Follow-up after endobronchial treatment

Careful surveillance with repeat biopsies after the initial endobronchial therapy is required as 10–15% of patients may require a second treatment to achieve cure [80, 92, 100]. In addition, longer-term surveillance is recommended after curative therapy as up to 30% subjects will develop metachronous disease at other sites. Follow-up bronchoscopy and biopsy are generally performed at 4–6 weeks after the initial treatment, every 3~6 month for the first 1–2 years, and then yearly for up to 5 years. Although there is no published data of its utilities, surveillance CT scan may offer additional benefits given high risk of metachronous diseases in these patients.

References

1 Siegel R, Naishadham D, Jemal A (2012) Cancer statistics, 2012. *CA: a Cancer Journal for Clinicians*, Jan–Feb; 62(1): 10–29.

2 Surveillance, Epidemiology, and End Results (SEER) Program (www.seer.cancer.gov) SEER*Stat Database: Incidence—SEER 17 Regs Public-Use, Nov

2005 Sub (1973–2003 varying). released April 2006, based on the November 2005 submission.

3 Wagnieres G, McWilliams A, Lam S (2003) Lung cancer imaging with fluorescence endoscopy. In: Mycek M, Pogue B (eds), *Handbook of Biomedical Fluorescence*. New York: Marcel Dekker, pp. 361–96.

4 Woolner L (1983) Pathology of cancer detected cytologically. In: *Atlas of Early Lung Cancer*. Tokyo: Igaku-Shoin: National Institutes of Health, US Department of Health and Human Services, pp. 107–213.

5 Hung J, Lam S, LeRiche JC, Palcic B (1991) Autofluorescence of normal and malignant bronchial tissue. *Lasers in Surgery & Medicine*, 11(2): 99–105.

6 Qu J, MacAulay C, Lam S, Palcic B (1995) Laser-induced fluorescence spectroscopy at endoscopy: tissue optics, Monte Carlo modeling, and in vivo measurements. *Optical Engineering*, 34: 3334–43.

7 Qu J, Macaulay C, Lam S, Palcic B (1994) Optical properties of normal and carcinomatous bronchial tissue. *Appl Opt*, Nov 1; 33(31): 7397–7405.

8 Keith RL, Miller YE, Gemmill RM, Drabkin HA, Dempsey EC, Kennedy TC, *et al.* (2000) Angiogenic squamous dysplasia in bronchi of individuals at high risk for lung cancer. *Clinical Cancer Research*, May; 6(5): 1616–25.

9 Gardner CM, Jacques SL, Welch AJ (1996) Fluorescence spectroscopy of tissue: recovery of intrinsic fluorescence from measured fluorescence. *Appl Opt*, Apr 1; 35(10): 1780–92.

10 Zellweger M, Grosjean P, Goujon D, Monnier P, van den Bergh H, Wagnieres G (2001) In vivo autofluorescence spectroscopy of human bronchial tissue to optimize the detection and imaging of early cancers. *J Biomed Opt*, Jan; 6(1): 41–51.

11 Lam S, Kennedy T, Unger M, Miller YE, Gelmont D, Rusch V, *et al.* (1998) Localization of bronchial intraepithelial neoplastic lesions by fluorescence bronchoscopy. *Chest*, Mar; 113(3): 696–702.

12 Edell E, Lam S, Pass H, Miller YE, Sutedja T, Kennedy T, *et al.* (2009) Detection and localization of intraepithelial neoplasia and invasive carcinoma using fluorescence-reflectance bronchoscopy: an international, multicenter clinical trial. *Journal of Thoracic Oncology*, Jan; 4(1): 49–54.

13 Chiyo M, Shibuya K, Hoshino H, Yasufuku K, Sekine Y, Iizasa T, *et al.* (2005) Effective detection of bronchial preinvasive lesions by a new autofluorescence imaging bronchovideoscope system. *Lung Cancer*, Jun; 48(3): 307–13.

14 Ikeda N, Honda H, Hayashi A, Usuda J, Kato Y, Tsuboi M, *et al.* (2006) Early detection of bronchial lesions using newly developed videoendoscopy-based autofluorescence bronchoscopy. *Lung Cancer*, Apr; 52(1): 21–7.

15 Haussinger K, Stanzel F, Huber RM, Pichler J, Stepp H (1999) Autofluorescence detection of bronchial tumors with the D-Light/AF. *Diagnostic & Therapeutic Endoscopy*, 5(2): 105–12.

16 Goujon D, Zellweger M, Radu A, Grosjean P, Weber BC, van den Bergh H, *et al.* (2003) In vivo autofluorescence imaging of early cancers in the human tracheobronchial tree with a spectrally optimized system. *J Biomed Opt*, Jan; 8(1): 17–25.

17 Tercelj M, Zeng H, Petek M, Rott T, Palcic B (2005) Acquisition of fluorescence and reflectance spectra during routine bronchoscopy examinations using the ClearVu Elite device: pilot study. *Lung Cancer*, Oct; 50(1): 35–42.

18 Lee P, Brokx HA, Postmus PE, Sutedja TG (2007) Dual digital video-autofluorescence imaging for detection of pre-neoplastic lesions. *Lung Cancer*, Oct; 58(1): 44–9.

19 Lam S (2006) The role of autofluorescence bronchoscopy in diagnosis of early lung cancer. In: Hirsch F, Bunn PJ, Kato H, *et al.* (eds), *IASLC Textbook for Prevention and Detection of Early Lung Cancer*. London: Taylor & Francis; pp. 149–58.

20 Hirsch FR, Prindiville SA, Miller YE, Franklin WA, Dempsey EC, Murphy JR, *et al.* (2001) Fluorescence versus white-light bronchoscopy for detection of preneoplastic lesions: a randomized study. *J Natl Cancer Inst*, Sep 19; 93(18): 1385–91.

21 Haussinger K, Becker H, Stanzel F, Kreuzer A, Schmidt B, Strausz J, *et al.* (2005) Autofluorescence bronchoscopy with white light bronchoscopy compared with white light bronchoscopy alone for the detection of precancerous lesions: A European randomised controlled multicentre trial. *Thorax*, Jun; 60(6): 496–503.

22 Ernst A, Simoff M, Mathur P, Yung R, Beamis JJ (2005) D-light autofluorescence in the detection of premalignant airway changes: a multicenter trial. *Journal of Bronchology*, 12(3): 133–8.

23 Sun J, Garfield DH, Lam B, Yan J, Gu A, Shen J, *et al.* (2011) The value of autofluorescence bronchoscopy combined with white light bronchoscopy compared with white light alone in the diagnosis of intraepithelial neoplasia and invasive lung cancer: a meta-analysis. *Journal of Thoracic Oncology*, Aug; 6(8): 1336–44.

24 Lee P, van den Berg RM, Lam S, Gazdar AF, Grunberg K, McWilliams A, *et al.* (2009) Color fluorescence

ratio for detection of bronchial dysplasia and carcinoma in situ. *Clinical Cancer Research*, Jul 15; 15(14): 4700–5.

25 Helfritzsch H, Junker K, Bartel M, Scheele J (2002) Differentiation of positive autofluorescence bronchoscopy findings by comparative genomic hybridization. *Oncol Reports*, 9(4): 697–701.

26 van Boerdonk RA, Sutedja TG, Snijders PJ, Reinen E, Wilting SM, van de Wiel MA, *et al.* (2011) DNA copy number alterations in endobronchial squamous metaplastic lesions predict lung cancer. *American Journal of Respiratory & Critical Care Medicine*, Oct 15; 184(8): 948–56.

27 Pasic A, Vonk-Noordegraaf A, Risse EK, Postmus PE, Sutedja TG (2003) Multiple suspicious lesions detected by autofluorescence bronchoscopy predict malignant development in the bronchial mucosa in high risk patients. *Lung Cancer*, Sep; 41(3): 295–301.

28 Gazdar AF, Minna JD (2000) Angiogenesis and the multistage development of lung cancers. *Clinical Cancer Research*, May; 6(5): 1611–12.

29 Tajiri H, Niwa H (2008) Proposal for a consensus terminology in endoscopy: How should different endoscopic imaging techniques be grouped and defined? *Endoscopy*, Sep; 40(9): 775–8.

30 Curvers WL, Singh R, Song LM, Wolfsen HC, Ragunath K, Wang K, *et al.* (2008) Endoscopic tri-modal imaging for detection of early neoplasia in Barrett's oesophagus: a multi-centre feasibility study using high-resolution endoscopy, autofluorescence imaging and narrow band imaging incorporated in one endoscopy system. *Gut*, Feb; 57(2): 167–72.

31 Shibuya K, Nakajima T, Fujiwara T, Chiyo M, Hoshino H, Moriya Y, *et al.* (2010) Narrow band imaging with high-resolution bronchovideoscopy: a new approach for visualizing angiogenesis in squamous cell carcinoma of the lung. *Lung Cancer*, Aug; 69(2): 194–202.

32 Herth FJ, Eberhardt R, Anantham D, Gompelmann D, Zakaria MW, Ernst A (2009) Narrow-band imaging bronchoscopy increases the specificity of bronchoscopic early lung cancer detection. *Journal of Thoracic Oncology*, Sep; 4(9): 1060–5.

33 Tsuboi M, Hayashi A, Ikeda N, Honda H, Kato Y, Ichinose S, *et al.* (2005) Optical coherence tomography in the diagnosis of bronchial lesions. *Lung Cancer*, Sep; 49(3): 387–94.

34 Lam S, Standish B, Baldwin C, McWilliams A, leRiche J, Gazdar A, *et al.* (2008) In vivo optical coherence tomography imaging of preinvasive bronchial lesions. *Clinical Cancer Research*, Apr 1; 14(7): 2006–11.

35 Ohtani K, Lee A, Lam S (2012) Frontiers in bronchoscopic imaging. *Respirology*, 17(2): 261–9.

36 Hariri L, Applegate M, Mino-Kenudson M, Mark E, Medoff B, Luster A, *et al.* (2013) Volumetric optical frequency domain imaging of pulmonary pathology with precise correlation to histopathology. *Chest*, 143(1): 64–74.

37 Sato M, Sakurada A, Sagawa M, Minowa M, Takahashi H, Oyaizu T, *et al.* (2001) Diagnostic results before and after introduction of autofluorescence bronchoscopy in patients suspected of having lung cancer detected by sputum cytology in lung cancer mass screening. *Lung Cancer*, Jun; 32(3): 247–53.

38 Frost JK, Ball WC, Jr, Levin ML, Tockman MS, Erozan YS, Gupta PK, *et al.* (1986) Sputum cytopathology: use and potential in monitoring the workplace environment by screening for biological effects of exposure. *Journal of Occupational Medicine*, Aug; 28(8): 692–703.

39 Risse EK, Vooijs GP, van't Hof MA (1988) Diagnostic significance of "severe dysplasia" in sputum cytology. *Acta Cytol*, Sep–Oct; 32(5): 629–34.

40 Prindiville SA, Byers T, Hirsch FR, Franklin WA, Miller YE, Vu KO, *et al.* (2003) Sputum cytological atypia as a predictor of incident lung cancer in a cohort of heavy smokers with airflow obstruction. *Cancer Epidemiology, Biomarkers & Prevention*, Oct; 12(10): 987–93.

41 Kennedy TC, Franklin WA, Prindiville SA, Cook R, Dempsey EC, Keith RL, *et al.* (2005) High prevalence of occult endobronchial malignancy in high risk patients with moderate sputum atypia. *Lung Cancer*, Aug; 49(2): 187–91.

42 Pierard P, Faber J, Hutsebaut J, Martin B, Plat G, Sculier JP, *et al.* (2004) Synchronous lesions detected by autofluorescence bronchoscopy in patients with high-grade preinvasive lesions and occult invasive squamous cell carcinoma of the proximal airways. *Lung Cancer*, Dec; 46(3): 341–7.

43 van Rens MT, Schramel FM, Elbers JR, Lammers JW (2001) The clinical value of lung imaging fluorescence endoscopy for detecting synchronous lung cancer. *Lung Cancer*, Apr; 32(1): 13–18.

44 Ikeda N, Hiyoshi T, Kakihana M, Honda H, Kato Y, Okunaka T, *et al.* (2003) Histopathological evaluation of fluorescence bronchoscopy using resected lungs in cases of lung cancer. *Lung Cancer*, Sep; 41(3): 303–9.

45 Pierard P, Vermylen P, Bosschaerts T, Roufosse C, Berghmans T, Sculier JP, *et al.* (2000) Synchronous

roentgenographically occult lung carcinoma in patients with resectable primary lung cancer. *Chest*, Mar; 117(3): 779–85.

46 Johnson BE (1998) Second lung cancers in patients after treatment for an initial lung cancer. *J Natl Cancer Inst*, Sep 16; 90(18): 1335–45.

47 Nakamura H, Kawasaki N, Hagiwara M, Ogata A, Saito M, Konaka C, *et al.* (2001) Early hilar lung cancer-risk for multiple lung cancers and clinical outcome. *Lung Cancer*, Jul; 33(1): 51–7.

48 Weigel TL, Yousem S, Dacic S, Kosco PJ, Siegfried J, Luketich JD (2000) Fluorescence bronchoscopic surveillance after curative surgical resection for non-small-cell lung cancer. *Annals of Surgical Oncology*, Apr; 7(3): 176–80.

49 Weigel TL, Kosco PJ, Dacic S, Rusch VW, Ginsberg RJ, Luketich JD (2001) Postoperative fluorescence bronchoscopic surveillance in non-small cell lung cancer patients. *Ann Thorac Surg*, Mar; 71(3): 967–70.

50 Moro-Sibilot D, Fievet F, Jeanmart M, Lantuejoul S, Arbib F, Laverribre MH, *et al.* (2004) Clinical prognostic indicators of high-grade pre-invasive bronchial lesions. *European Respiratory Journal*, Jul; 24(1): 24–9.

51 Kato H, Okunaka T, Shimatani H (1996). Photodynamic therapy for early stage bronchogenic carcinoma. *J Clin Laser Med Surg*, Oct; 14(5): 235–8.

52 Sutedja TG, Codrington H, Risse EK, Breuer RH, van Mourik JC, Golding RP, *et al.* (2001) Autofluorescence bronchoscopy improves staging of radiographically occult lung cancer and has an impact on therapeutic strategy. *Chest*, Oct; 120(4): 1327–32.

53 Ishizumi T, McWilliams A, MacAulay C, Gazdar A, Lam S (2010) Natural history of bronchial preinvasive lesions. *Cancer & Metastasis Reviews*, Mar; 29(1): 5–14.

54 Jeremy George P, Banerjee AK, Read CA, O'Sullivan C, Falzon M, Pezzella F, *et al.* (2007) Surveillance for the detection of early lung cancer in patients with bronchial dysplasia. *Thorax*, Jan; 62(1): 43–50.

55 Sutedja G, Postmus PE (1994) Bronchoscopic treatment of lung tumors. *Lung Cancer*, Jul; 11(1–2): 1–17.

56 Pasic A, Brokx HA, Vonk Noordegraaf A, Paul RM, Postmus PE, Sutedja TG (2004) Cost-effectiveness of early intervention: Comparison between intraluminal bronchoscopic treatment and surgical resection for T1N0 lung cancer patients. *Respiration*, Jul–Aug; 71(4): 391–6.

57 Salaun M, Sesboue R, Moreno-Swirc S, Metayer J, Bota S, Bourguignon J, *et al.* (2008) Molecular predictive factors for progression of high-grade preinvasive bronchial lesions. *American Journal of Respiratory & Critical Care Medicine*, Apr 15; 177(8): 880–6.

58 Breuer RH, Pasic A, Smit EF, van Vliet E, Vonk Noordegraaf A, Risse EJ, *et al.* (2005) The natural course of preneoplastic lesions in bronchial epithelium. *Clinical Cancer Research*, Jan 15; 11(2 Pt 1): 537–43.

59 Miller RR (1990) Bronchioloalveolar cell adenomas. *Am J Surg Pathol*, Oct; 14(10): 904–12.

60 Travis WD, Brambilla E, Noguchi M, Nicholson AG, Geisinger KR, Yatabe Y, *et al.* (2011) International Association for the Study of Lung Cancer/American Thoracic Society/European Respiratory Society International Multidisciplinary Classification of Lung Adenocarcinoma. *Journal of Thoracic Oncology*, Feb; 6(2): 244–85.

61 Vazquez MF, Flieder DB (2000) Small peripheral glandular lesions detected by screening CT for lung cancer: A diagnostic dilemma for the pathologist. *Radiol Clin North Am*, May; 38(3): 579–89.

62 McWilliams AM, Mayo JR, Ahn MI, MacDonald SL, Lam SC (2006) Lung cancer screening using multi-slice thin-section computed tomography and autofluorescence bronchoscopy. *Journal of Thoracic Oncology*, Jan; 1(1): 61–8.

63 Mori M, Kaji M, Tezuka F, Takahashi T (1998) Comparative ultrastructural study of atypical adenomatous hyperplasia and adenocarcinoma of the human lung. *Ultrastruct Pathol*, Nov–Dec; 22(6): 459–66.

64 Kothary N, Lock L, Sze DY, Hofmann LV (2009) Computed tomography-guided percutaneous needle biopsy of pulmonary nodules: impact of nodule size on diagnostic accuracy. *Clinical Lung Cancer*, Sep; 10(5): 360–3.

65 Heyer CM, Reichelt S, Peters SA, Walther JW, Muller KM, Nicolas V (2008) Computed tomography-navigated transthoracic core biopsy of pulmonary lesions: which factors affect diagnostic yield and complication rates? *Acad Radiol*, Aug; 15(8): 1017–26.

66 Wiener RS, Schwartz LM, Woloshin S, Welch HG (2011) Population-based risk for complications after transthoracic needle lung biopsy of a pulmonary nodule: an analysis of discharge records. *Ann Intern Med*, Aug 2; 155(3): 137–44.

67 Asano F (2010) Virtual bronchoscopic navigation. *Clin Chest Med*, Mar; 31(1): 75–85.

68 Ishida T, Asano F, Yamazaki K, Shinagawa N, Oizumi S, Moriya H, *et al.* (2011) Virtual bronchoscopic navigation combined with endobronchial ultrasound to diagnose small peripheral pulmonary lesions: a randomised trial. *Thorax*, Dec; 66(12): 1072–7.

69 Eberhardt R, Kahn N, Gompelmann D, Schumann M, Heussel CP, Herth FJ (2010) LungPoint – a new approach to peripheral lesions. *Journal of Thoracic Oncology*, Oct; 5(10): 1559–63.

70 Becker HD, Herth F, Ernst A, Schwarz Y (2005) Bronchoscopic biopsy of peripheral lung lesions under electromagnetic guidance: A pilot study. *Journal of Bronchology & Interventional Pulmonology*, Jan; 12(1): 9–13.

71 Herth FJ, Eberhardt R, Becker HD, Ernst A (2006) Endobronchial ultrasound-guided transbronchial lung biopsy in fluoroscopically invisible solitary pulmonary nodules: a prospective trial. *Chest*, Jan; 129(1): 147–50.

72 Wang Memoli J, Nietert P, Silvestri G (2012) Meta-analysis of guided bronchoscopy for the evaluation of the pulmonary nodule. *Chest*, Aug; 142(2): 385–93.

73 Jensen KW, Hsia DW, Seijo LM, FellerKopman DJ, Lamb C, Berkowitz D, *et al.* (2012) Multicenter experience with electromagnetic navigation bronchoscopy for the diagnosis of pulmonary nodules. *Journal of Bronchology & Interventional Pulmonology*, Jul; 19(3): 195–9.

74 Eberhardt R, Anantham D, Ernst A, Feller-Kopman D, Herth F (2007) Multimodality bronchoscopic diagnosis of peripheral lung lesions: A randomized controlled trial. *American Journal of Respiratory & Critical Care Medicine*, Jul 1; 176(1): 36–41.

75 Steinfort DP, Vincent J, Heinze S, Antippa P, Irving LB (2011) Comparative effectiveness of radial probe endobronchial ultrasound versus CT-guided needle biopsy for evaluation of peripheral pulmonary lesions: a randomized pragmatic trial. *Respir Med*, Nov; 105(11): 1704–11.

76 Fielding DI, Chia C, Nguyen P, Bashirzadeh F, Hundloe J, Brown IG, *et al.* (2012) Prospective randomised trial of endobronchial ultrasound-guide sheath versus computed tomography-guided percutaneous core biopsies for peripheral lung lesions. *Intern Med J*, Aug; 42(8): 894–900.

77 Delage A, Godbout K, Martel S, Laviolette M, Simon M, Lampron N (2012) Evaluation of pulmonary nodules using the spyglass direct visualization system combined with radial endobronchial ultrasound: A feasibility study. *American Journal of Respiratory and Critical Care Medicine*, 05/01; 185(1): A1103.

78 Cortese DA, Pairolero PC, Bergstralh EJ, Woolner LB, Uhlenhopp MA, Piehler JM, *et al.* (1983) Roentgenographically occult lung cancer. A ten-year experience. *Journal of Thoracic & Cardiovascular Surgery*, Sep; 86(3): 373–80.

79 Fujimura S, Sakurada A, Sagawa M, Saito Y, Takahashi H, Tanita T, *et al.* (2000) A therapeutic approach to roentgenographically occult squamous cell carcinoma of the lung. *Cancer*, Dec 1; 89(11 Suppl): 2445–8.

80 Vonk-Noordegraaf A, Postmus PE, Sutedja TG (2003) Bronchoscopic treatment of patients with intraluminal microinvasive radiographically occult lung cancer not eligible for surgical resection: A follow-up study. *Lung Cancer*, Jan; 39(1): 49–53.

81 Sutedja G, Golding RP, Postmus, PE (1996) High resolution computed tomography in patients referred for intraluminal bronchoscopic therapy with curative intent. *European Respiratory Journal*, May; 9(5): 1020–3.

82 Miyazu Y, Miyazawa T, Kurimoto N, Iwamoto Y, Kanoh K, Kohno N (2002) Endobronchial ultrasonography in the assessment of centrally located early-stage lung cancer before photodynamic therapy. *American Journal of Respiratory and Critical Care Medicine*, 15 Mar, 165(6): 832–7.

83 Kurimoto N, Murayama M, Yoshioka S, Nishisaka T, Inai K, Dohi K (1999) Assessment of usefulness of endobronchial ultrasonography in determination of depth of tracheobronchial tumor invasion. *Chest*, 115(6): 1500–6.

84 Konaka C, Hirano T, Kato H, Furuse K, Takada M, Saito Y, *et al.* (1999) Comparison of endoscopic features of early-stage squamous cell lung cancer and histological findings. *Br J Cancer*, Jul; 80(9): 1435–9.

85 Herth F, Ernst A, Schulz M, Becker H (2003) Endobronchial ultrasound reliably differentiates between airway infiltration and compression by tumor. *Chest*, Feb; 123(2): 458–62.

86 Bolliger CT, Sutedja TG, Strausz J, Freitag L (2006) Therapeutic bronchoscopy with immediate effect: laser, electrocautery, argon plasma coagulation and stents. *European Respiratory Journal*, Jun; 27(6): 1258–71.

87 Lam S (1994) Photodynamic therapy of lung cancer. *Semin Oncol*, Dec; 21(6 Suppl 15): 15–19.

88 Furuse K, Fukuoka M, Kato H, Horai T, Kubota K, Kodama N, *et al.* (1993) A prospective phase II study on photodynamic therapy with photofrin II for centrally located early-stage lung cancer. The Japan Lung Cancer Photodynamic Therapy Study Group. *Journal of Clinical Oncology*, Oct; 11(10): 1852–7.

89 Ikeda N, Usuda J, Kato H, Ishizumi T, Ichinose S, Otani K, *et al.* (2011) New aspects of photodynamic therapy for central type early stage lung cancer. *Lasers in Surgery & Medicine*, Sep; 43(7): 749–54.

90 Kato H, Furukawa K, Sato M, Okunaka T, Kusunoki Y, Kawahara M, *et al.* (2003) Phase II clinical study of photodynamic therapy using mono-l-aspartyl chlorin e6 and diode laser for early superficial squamous cell carcinoma of the lung. *Lung Cancer*, 42(1): 103–11.

91 Kato H, Usuda J, Okunaka T, Furukawa K, Honda H, Sakaniwa N, *et al.* (2006) Basic and clinical research on photodynamic therapy at Tokyo Medical University Hospital. *Lasers in Surgery & Medicine*, Jun; 38(5): 371–5.

92 Cortese DA, Edell ES, Kinsey JH (1997) Photodynamic therapy for early stage squamous cell carcinoma of the lung. *Mayo Clin Proc*, Jul; 72(7): 595–602.

93 Moghissi K, Dixon K, Thorpe JA, Stringer M, Oxtoby C (2007) Photodynamic therapy (PDT) in early central lung cancer: a treatment option for patients ineligible for surgical resection. *Thorax*, May; 62(5): 391–5.

94 Furukawa K, Kato H, Konaka C, Okunaka T, Usuda J, Ebihara Y (2005) Locally recurrent central-type early stage lung cancer <1.0 cm in diameter after complete remission by photodynamic therapy. *Chest*, Nov; 128(5): 3269–75.

95 Van Boxem TJ, Venmans BJ, Schramel FM, Van Mourik JC, Golding RP, Postmus PE, *et al.* (1998) Radiographically occult lung cancer treated with fibreoptic bronchoscopic electrocautery: A pilot study of a simple and inexpensive technique. *European Respiratory Journal*, 11(1): 169–72.

96 Sutedja G, Bolliger C (2000) Endobronchial electrocautery and argon plasma coagulation. Interventional bronchoscopy. *Progress in Respiratory Research*, 30: 120–32.

97 Schuurman B, Postmus PE, Van Mourik JC, Risse EK, Sutedja TG (2004) Combined use of autofluorescence bronchoscopy and argon plasma coagulation enables less extensive resection of radiographically occult lung cancer. *Respiration* 71(4): 410–11.

98 Shepherd JP, Dawber RP (1984) Wound healing and scarring after cryosurgery. *Cryobiology*, Apr; 21(2): 157–69.

99 Vergnon JM, Huber RM, Moghissi K (2006) Place of cryotherapy, brachytherapy and photodynamic therapy in therapeutic bronchoscopy of lung cancers. *European Respiratory Journal*, Jul; 28(1): 200–18.

100 Deygas N, Froudarakis M, Ozenne G, Vergnon JM (2001) Cryotherapy in early superficial bronchogenic carcinoma. *Chest*, Jul; 120(1): 26–31.

101 Au JT, Carson J, Monette S, Finley DJ (2012) Spray cryotherapy is effective for bronchoscopic, endoscopic and open ablation of thoracic tissues. *Interactive Cardiovascular & Thoracic Surgery*, Oct; 15(4): 580–4.

102 Finley DJ, Dycoco J, Sarkar S, Krimsky WS, Sherwood JT, Dekeratry D, *et al.* (2012) Airway spray cryotherapy: Initial outcomes from a multiinstitutional registry. *Ann Thorac Surg*, Discussion 203–4; Jul; 94(1): 199–203.

103 Hennequin C, Bleichner O, Tredaniel J, Quero L, Sergent G, Zalcman G, *et al.* (2007) Long-term results of endobronchial brachytherapy: A curative treatment? *Int J Radiat Oncol Biol Phys*, Feb 1; 67(2): 425–30.

104 Marsiglia H, Baldeyrou P, Lartigau E, Briot E, Haie-Meder C, Le Chevalier T, *et al.* (2000) High-dose-rate brachytherapy as sole modality for early-stage endobronchial carcinoma. *International Journal of Radiation Oncology Biology Physics*, 47(3): 665–72.

105 Perol M, Caliandro R, Pommier P, Malet C, Montbarbon X, Carrie C, *et al.* (1997) Curative irradiation of limited endobronchial carcinomas with high-dose rate brachytherapy: Results of a pilot study. *Chest*, 111(5): 1417–23.

CHAPTER 8
Pathology of Adenocarcinoma

William D. Travis
Department of Pathology, Memorial Sloan-Kettering Cancer Center, New York, NY, USA

Introduction

Adenocarcinoma is the most common histologic subtype of lung cancer in most countries. In 2013 the American Cancer Society estimated there would be 228 190 new lung cancers in the United States (US) and 159 480 lung cancer deaths [1]. With 41% of lung cancers estimated to be adenocarcinomas according to the NCI SEER Cancer Statistics Review 1975–2010 [2], there would be over 93 000 lung adenocarcinomas expected in the US in 2013.

Lung adenocarcinoma is very heterogeneous from every perspective, including clinical, radiologic, pathologic, surgical and molecular aspects. Even within an individual tumor there is considerable histologic heterogeneity that has presented challenges to pathologists in developing a clinically meaningful classification that is prognostically relevant. In the past decade many advances have occurred that gave a need for an international multidisciplinary classification effort. This led to a new lung adenocarcinoma classification sponsored by the IASLC/ATS and ERS that has made major changes in how lung adenocarcinoma is diagnosed [3–5]. This classification addresses not only resection specimens (Table 8.1), but also small biopsies and cytology specimens (Table 8.2). This chapter will primarily address the classification in resection specimens with brief discussion of the small biopsy and cytology aspects.

The 2011 IASLC/ATS/ERS lung adenocarcinoma classification recommends multiple major changes (Table 8.1) [3–6]. First, it is recommended to no longer use the term bronchioloalveolar carcinoma (BAC) since the tumors formerly classified under this term are now classified into five different tumors. Second, there are new concepts of AIS and minimally invasive adenocarcinoma (MIA). Third, it is recommended to no longer use the term "mixed subtype," but rather to use comprehensive histologic subtyping to estimate the percentage of histologic patterns in 5% increments within a tumor with final classification according to the predominant subtype. Fourth, tumors with a predominant component formerly called nonmucinous BAC, should be classified as lepidic predominant adenocarcinoma. Fifth, micropapillary adenocarcinoma is recognized as a new subtype with a poor prognosis. Sixth, *invasive mucinous adenocarcinoma* is the term recommended for those tumors formerly classified as mucinous BAC (formerly mucinous BAC). Finally, specific terminology and diagnostic criteria are proposed for tumors in small biopsies and cytology specimens along with recommendations for strategic management of tissue and *EGFR* mutation testing in patients with advanced adenocarcinoma [3–6].

Lung Cancer, Fourth Edition. Edited by Jack A. Roth, Waun Ki Hong and Ritsuko U. Komaki.

Table 8.1 Histologic classification of lung adenocarcinoma in resection specimens*

Preinvasive lesions
Atypical adenomatous hyperplasia
Adenocarcinoma *in situ* (≤3 cm pure lepidic tumor without invasion)
Nonmucinous, mucinous or mixed nonmucinous/mucinous
Minimally invasive adenocarcinoma (≤3 cm lepidic predominant tumor with ≤5 mm invasion)
Nonmucinous, mucinous, mixed mucinous/nonmucinous
Invasive adenocarcinoma
Lepidic predominant (formerly nonmucinous BAC pattern, with >5 mm invasion)
Acinar predominant
Papillary predominant
Micropapillary predominant
Solid predominant with mucin
Variants of invasive adenocarcinoma
Invasive mucinous adenocarcinoma (formerly mucinous BAC)
Colloid
Fetal
Enteric

*Modified from the 2004 World Health Organization Classification [10] and the 2011 International Association for the Study of Lung Cancer/American Thoracic Society/European Respiratory Society Classification of Lung Adenocarcinoma [4]. This classification primarily addresses histology in resected specimens.

Adenocarcinoma classification in resected specimens

Preinvasive lesions

In the 2011 IASLC/ATS/ERS Classification of Lung Adenocarcinoma, adenocarcinoma in situ (AIS) was added as a new preinvasive lesion for adenocarcinoma (Table 8.1) [4]. Atypical adenomatous hyperplasia is comparable to squamous dysplasia and adenocarcinoma *in situ* the counterpart to squamous cell carcinoma *in situ*.

Atypical adenomatous hyperplasia

Atypical adenomatous hyperplasia (AAH) is an atypical pneumocyte proliferation that resembles but falls short of criteria for adenocarcinoma in situ [4, 7–12] AAH is typically an incidental histologic finding in the lung parenchyma surrounding a lung cancer in a resection specimen [13–15]. Most AAH lesions measure less than 5 mm in diameter and they are often multiple [15, 16]. Histologically AAH consists of a focal proliferation of slightly atypical cuboidal to low columnar pneumocytes spreading along the surface of alveolar walls. There may be slight thickening of alveolar septa.

The differential diagnosis for AAH includes nonmucinous AIS, minimally invasive adenocarcinoma (MIA) or lepidic predominant adenocarcinoma [17]. Separation between AAH and AIS can be challenging due to the potential overlap in the morphologic features between AAH and the lepidic pattern of adenocarcinoma [13, 14, 18, 19].

Adenocarcinoma *in situ*

AIS is defined in the new IASLC/ATS/ERS adenocarcinoma classification as a glandular proliferation measuring 3 centimeters or less that has a pure lepidic growth pattern lacking invasion (Figure 8.1) [4]. In most cases the tumor cells are nonmucinous, with a proliferation of type II pneumocytes or Clara cells. Rare cases of mucinous AIS occur consisting of tall columnar goblet cells having abundant apical mucin. With mucinous AIS one has to be very cautious to be sure the lesion is solitary and sharply circumscribed without miliary spread in the surrounding parenchyma. If lesions of AIS are completely resected, patients have been reported to have 100% 5-year disease free survival [20–27]. The typical CT appearance of nonmucinous AIS is a ground glass nodule if nonmucinous and for mucinous AIS a solid nodule of consolidation [4].

Most lesions that meet the historical strict definition of BAC according to the 1999 and 2004 WHO classification [10] criteria, these would correspond to the current definition of AIS. The concept of AIS was proposed based on multiple observational studies on solitary lung adenocarcinomas with pure lepidic growth, smaller than either 2 cm or 3 cm that documented 100% disease free survival when completely resected [20–26, 28]. While most of the published data focused on nonmucinous tumors, two of the 28 tumors reported in Noguchi's 1995 paper as type A and B were

Table 8.2 Proposed IASLC/ATS/ERS classification for small biopsies/cytology*

2004 WHO classification	SMALL BIOPSY/CYTOLOGY: IASLC/ATS/ERS
Adenocarcinoma Mixed subtype Acinar Papillary Solid	*Morphologic adenocarcinoma patterns clearly present:* Adenocarcinoma, describe identifiable patterns present (including micropapillary pattern not included in 2004 WHO classification) *If pure lepidic growth – mention an invasive component cannot be excluded in this small specimen*
Bronchioloalveolar carcinoma (nonmucinous)	Adenocarcinoma with lepidic pattern (if pure, add note: an invasive component cannot be excluded)
Bronchioloalveolar carcinoma (mucinous)	Mucinous adenocarcinoma (describe patterns present)
Fetal	Adenocarcinoma with fetal pattern
Mucinous (colloid)	Adenocarcinoma with colloid pattern
Signet ring	Adenocarcinoma with (describe patterns present) and signet ring features
Clear cell	Adenocarcinoma with (describe patterns present) and clear cell features
No 2004 WHO counterpart – most will be solid adenocarcinomas	*Morphologic adenocarcinoma patterns not present (supported by special stains):* Non-small cell carcinoma, favor adenocarcinoma
SQUAMOUS CELL CARCINOMA Papillary Clear cell Small cell Basaloid	*Morphologic squamous cell patterns clearly present:* Squamous cell carcinoma
No 2004 WHO counterpart	*Morphologic squamous cell patterns not present (supported by stains):* Non-small cell carcinoma, favor squamous cell carcinoma
SMALL CELL CARCINOMA	Small cell carcinoma
LARGE CELL CARCINOMA	Non-small cell carcinoma, not otherwise specified (NOS)
Large cell neuroendocrine carcinoma (LCNEC)	Non-small cell carcinoma with neuroendocrine (NE) morphology (positive NE markers), possible LCNEC
Large cell carcinoma with NE morphology (LCNEM)	Non-small cell carcinoma with NE morphology (negative NE markers) – see comment Comment: This is a non-small cell carcinoma where LCNEC is suspected, but stains failed to demonstrate NE differentiation
ADENOSQUAMOUS CARCINOMA	*Morphologic squamous cell and adenocarcinoma patterns present:* Non-small cell carcinoma, NOS, (comment that glandular and squamous components are present) Comment: this could represent adenosquamous carcinoma
No counterpart in 2004 WHO classification	*Morphologic squamous cell or adenocarcinoma patterns not present but immunostains favor separate favor glandular and adenocarcinoma component* Non-small cell carcinoma, NOS, (specify the results of the immunohistochemical stains and the interpretation) Comment: this could represent adenosquamous carcinoma
Sarcomatoid carcinoma	Poorly differentiated NSCLC with spindle and/or giant cell carcinoma (mention if adenocarcinoma or squamous carcinoma are present)

*From reference: [4]. Reproduced with permission of Lippincott Williams and Wilkins.

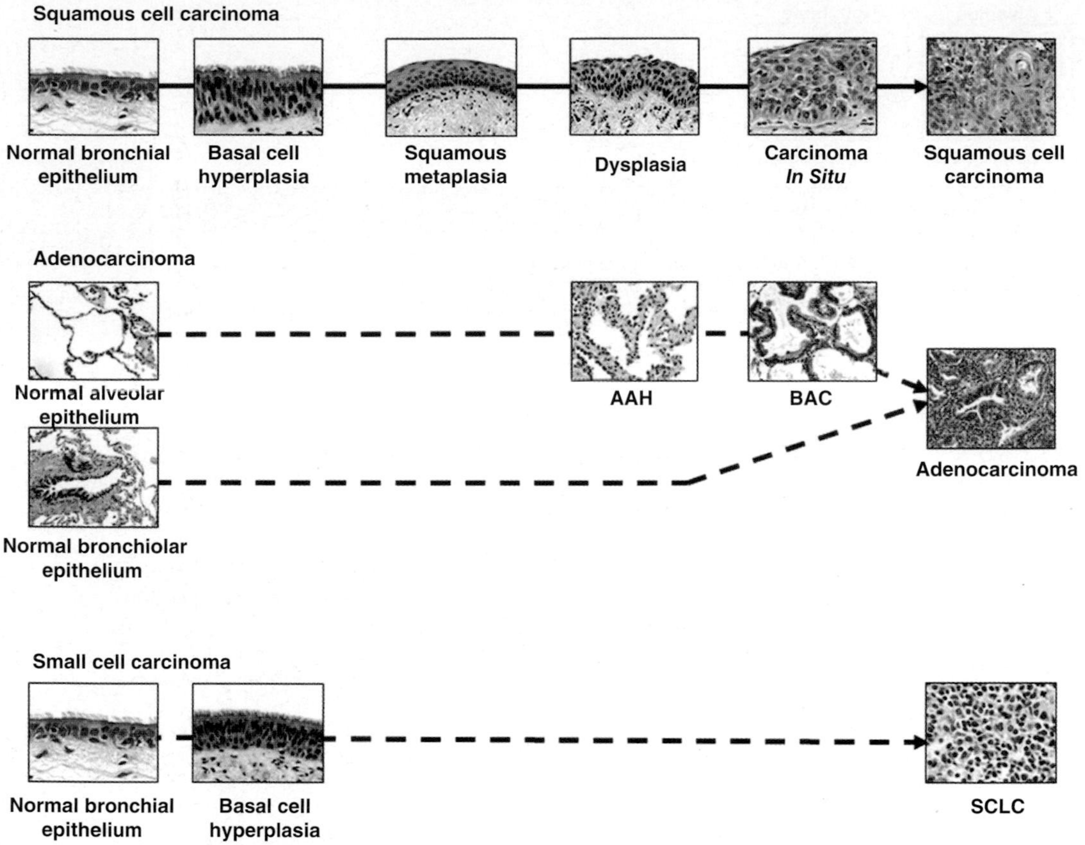

Squamous cell carcinoma

Normal bronchial epithelium — Basal cell hyperplasia — Squamous metaplasia — Dysplasia — Carcinoma *In Situ* — Squamous cell carcinoma

Adenocarcinoma

Normal alveolar epithelium — AAH — BAC — Adenocarcinoma

Normal bronchiolar epithelium — Adenocarcinoma

Small cell carcinoma

Normal bronchial epithelium — Basal cell hyperplasia — SCLC

Plate 6.1 Summary of histopatholologic changes involved in the pathogenesis of lung cancer. The sequence of preneoplastic lesions involved in the development of squamous cell carcinoma of the lung has been elucidated. For adenocarcinoma histology, the only known preneoplastic lesion is AAH (atypical adenomatous hyperplasia), which seems to be the precursor for a subset of lung adenocarcinomas. No preneoplastic lesion has been recognized for SCLC (microphotographs of histological tissue sections stained with hematoxylin and eosin).

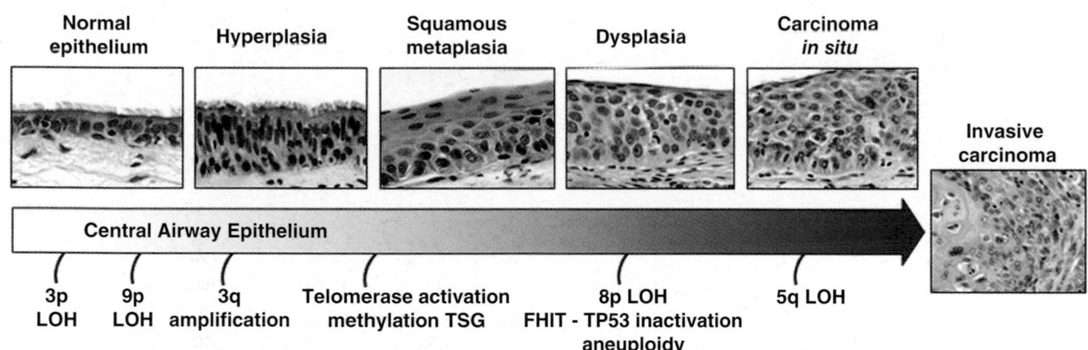

Plate 6.2 Molecular pathogenesis of squamous cell carcinoma of the lung. Several sequential molecular abnormalities have been recognized in the multistep pathogenesis of squamous cell carcinoma of the lung and have been detected in high-risk individuals.

Lung Cancer, Fourth Edition. Edited by Jack A. Roth, Waun Ki Hong and Ritsuko U. Komaki.

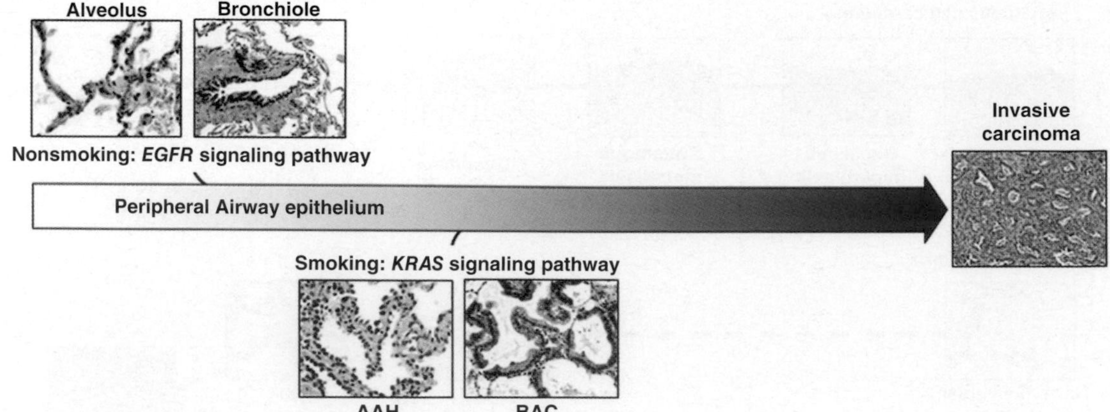

Plate 6.3 Molecular pathogenesis of adenocarcinoma of the lung. At least two molecular pathways have been identified in the development of lung adenocarcinoma, smoking and nonsmoking-related (AAH, atypical adenomatous hyperplasia; BAC, bronchioloalveolar carcinoma).

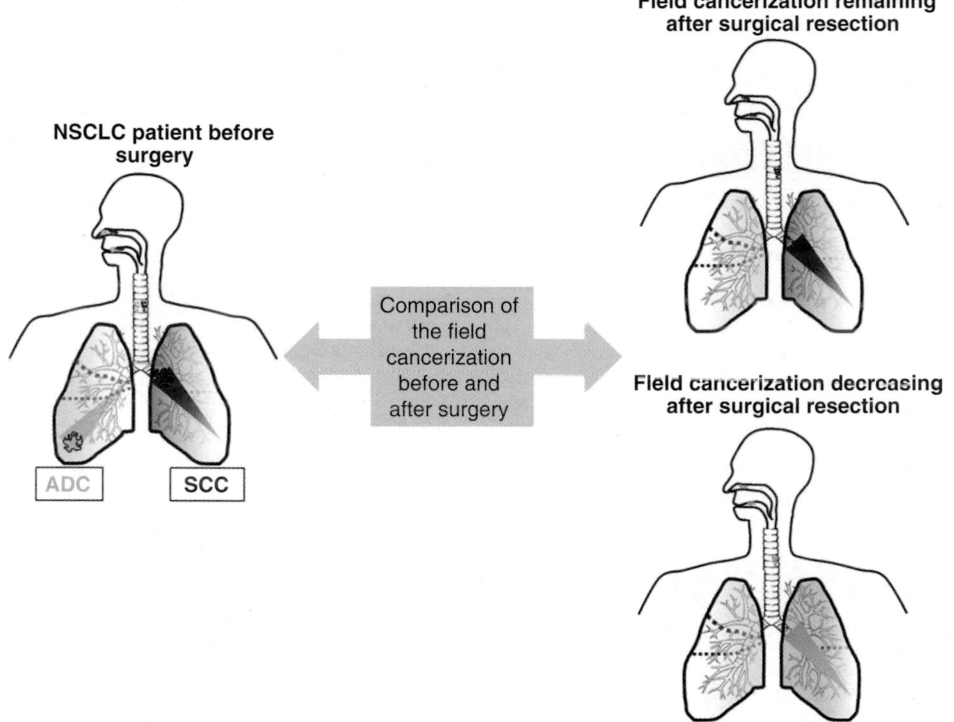

Plate 6.4 Field cancerization phenomenon in early-stage NSCLC patients. The relevance of the lung field cancerization to the development of a particular subtype of NSCLC, i.e., adenocarcinomas compared to SCCs, is still unknown yet possible. Analyzing local and distant field of cancerization by analysis of the transcriptome of airway brushings from multiple sites independently for lung adenocarcinoma (yellow spots) and SCC (red spots) cases, may shed light on events common or unique to the molecular pathogenesis of the two major subtypes of NSCLC (left panel). The potential important clinical relevance of the field cancerization to early-stage NSCLC can be investigated by studying the molecular cancerization before and after surgery to determine whether the cancerization effect persists (upper right) or decreases (bottom right) following surgical removal of the lung tumor. Such analysis may aid to determine whether the persistence of a molecular field cancerization effect in NSCLC patients after surgery is associated with disease relapse, and if so, whether the effect can be leveraged for development of novel prevention strategies.

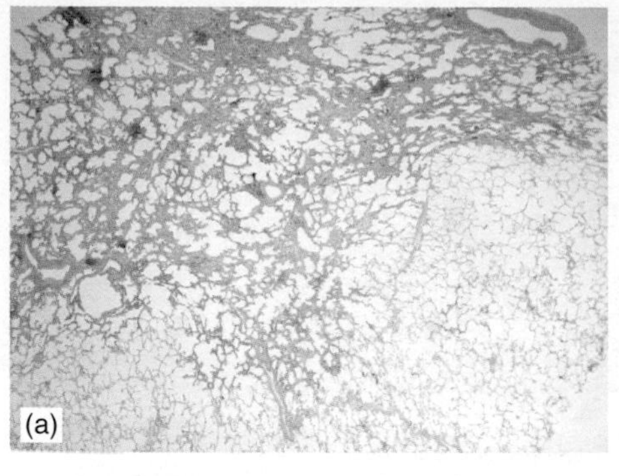

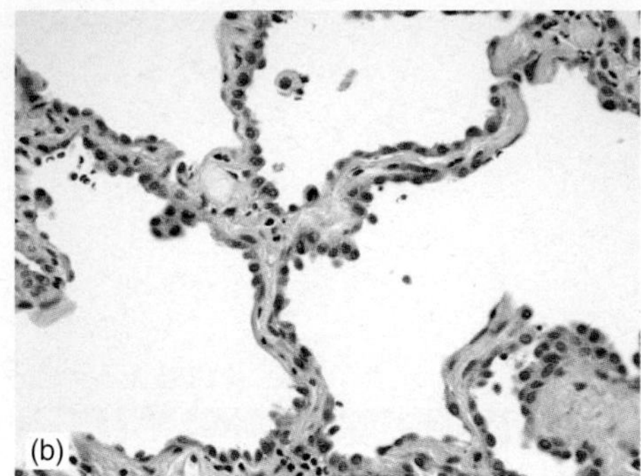

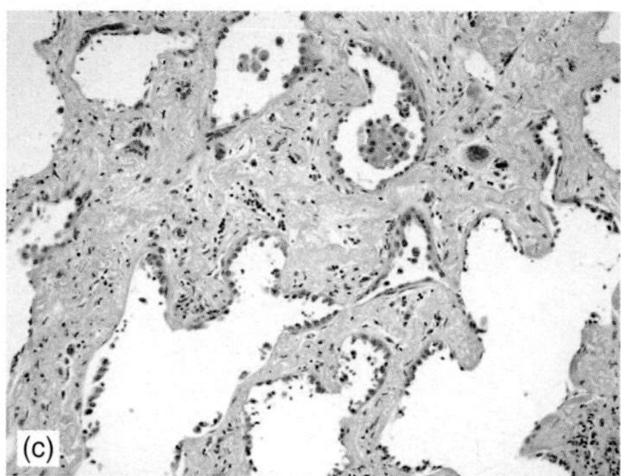

Plate 8.1 Nonmucinous adenocarcinoma *in situ*. a: This circumscribed nonmucinous tumor grows purely with a lepidic pattern. No foci of invasion or scarring are seen. Hematoxylin and eosin X 1.25. b: This area shows lepidic growth or atypical pneumocytes along thin alveolar walls. Hematoxylin and eosin X20. c: This area shows fibrotic thickening of the alveolar walls but no clear invasive growth, only a lepidic pattern. Hematoxylin and eosin X20.

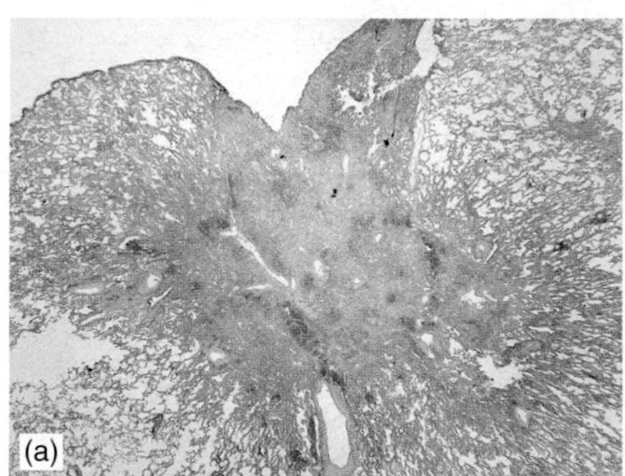

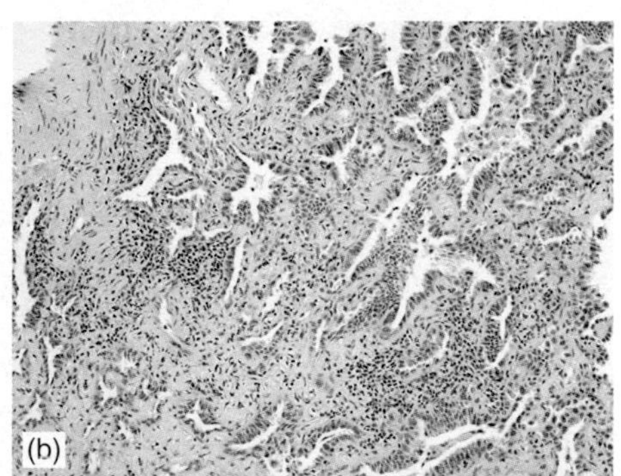

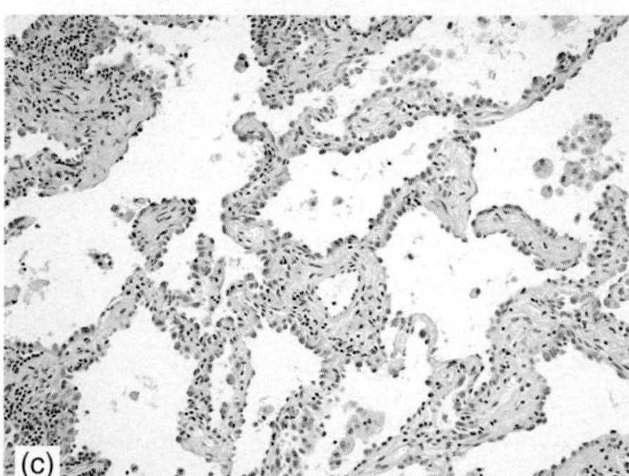

Plate 8.2 Nonmucinous minimally invasive adenocarcinoma. a: This adenocarcinoma tumor consists primarily of lepidic growth with a central scar which is mostly benign with small foci of invasion at the edges of the scar (<0.5 cm) area of invasion. Hematoxylin and eosin X 1.25. b: From the area of invasion, these acinar glands are invading in the fibrous stroma. Hematoxylin and eosin X 20. c: Other areas show a lepidic pattern with thin alveolar walls. Hematoxylin and eosin X20.

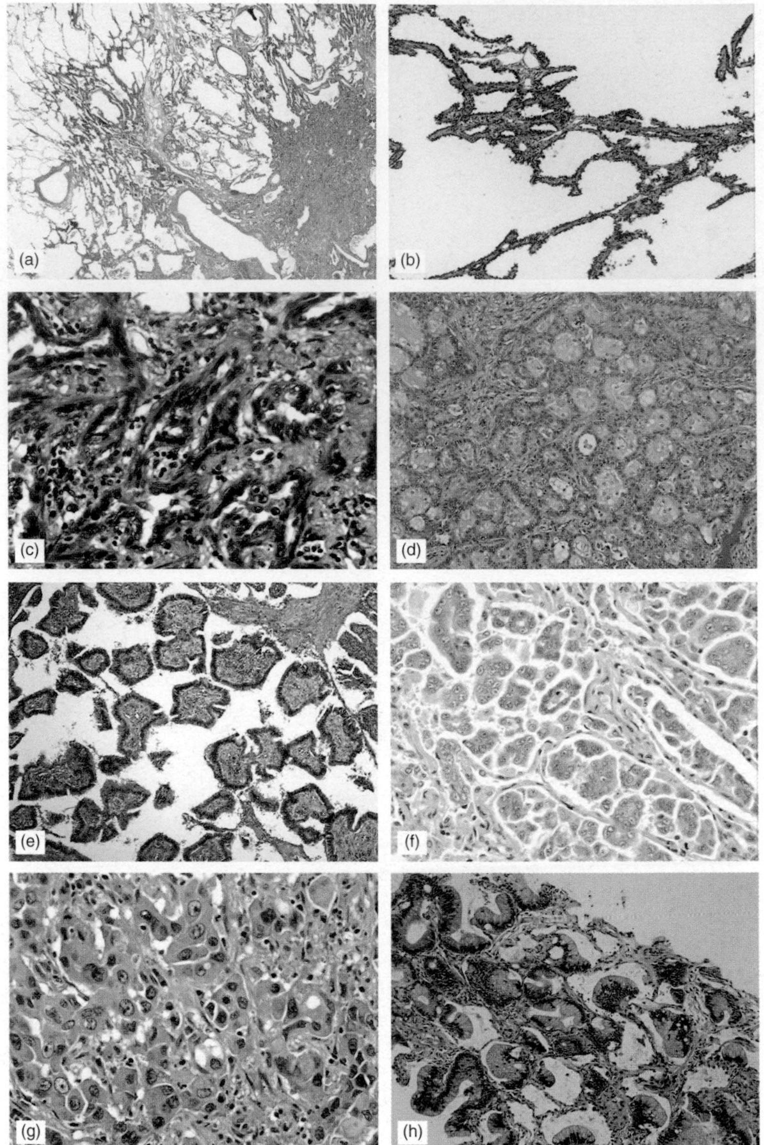

Plate 8.3 Major histologic patterns of invasive adenocarcinoma. a: Lepidic predominant pattern with mostly lepidic growth (left) and an area of invasive acinar adenocarcinoma (right). Hematoxylin and eosin X 100. b: Lepidic pattern consists of a proliferation type II pneumocytes and Clara cells along the surface alveolar walls. Hematoxylin and eosin X 200. c: Area of invasive acinar adenocarcinoma (same tumor as in 3A&B). Hematoxylin and eosin X 400. d: Acinar adenocarcinoma composed of round to oval shaped malignant glands invading a fibrous stroma. Hematoxylin and eosin X 200, e: Papillary adenocarcinoma consists of malignant cuboidal to columnar tumor cells growing on the surface of fibrovascular cores. Hematoxylin and eosin X 100, f: Micropapillary adenocarcinoma consists of small papillary clusters of glandular cells growing within this airspace, most of which do not show fibrovascular cores. Hematoxylin and eosin X 200. g: Solid adenocarcinoma with mucin consisting of sheets of tumor cells with abundant cytoplasm and mostly vesicular nuclei with several conspicuous nucleoli. No acinar, papillary or lepidic patterns are seen, but multiple cells have intracytoplasmic basophilic globules that suggest intracytoplasmic mucin. Hematoxylin and eosin X 400, h: Invasive mucinous adenocarcinoma demonstrates lepidic and acinar growth. The tumor consists of columnar cells filled with abundant mucin in the apical cytoplasm and shows small basal oriented nuclei. Hematoxylin and eosin X 200.

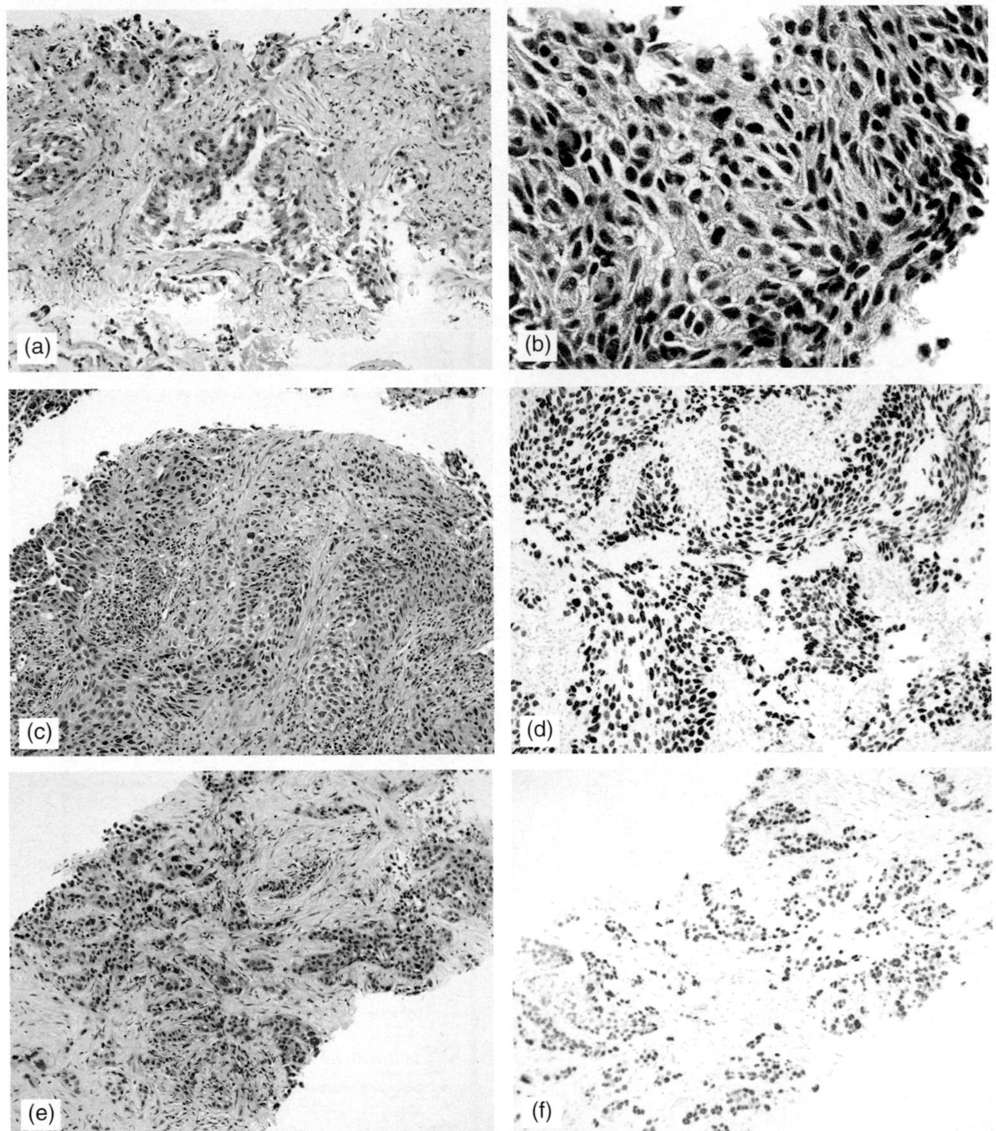

Plate 8.4 a: Adenocarcinoma: This tumor shows an acinar pattern of growth indicating adenocarcinoma. Hematoxylin and Eosin X20. b: Squamous cell carcinoma: This tumor shows keratinization indicating squamous cell carcinoma. c: Non-small cell carcinoma, favor adenocarcinoma. This carcinoma shows no clear squamous or glandular differentiation. Hematoxylin and eosin X 200. d: The diffuse positive TTF-1 staining, allows for the diagnosis of non-small cell carcinoma, favor adenocarcinoma. Hematoxylin and eosin X 200. e: Non-small cell carcinoma, favor squamous cell carcinoma. This carcinoma shows no clear squamous or glandular differentiation. Hematoxylin and eosin X 200 f: The diffuse positive p63 staining and negative TTF-1 staining (not shown), allows for the diagnosis of non-small cell carcinoma, favor squamous cell carcinoma. Immunohistochemistry for p63 × 200.

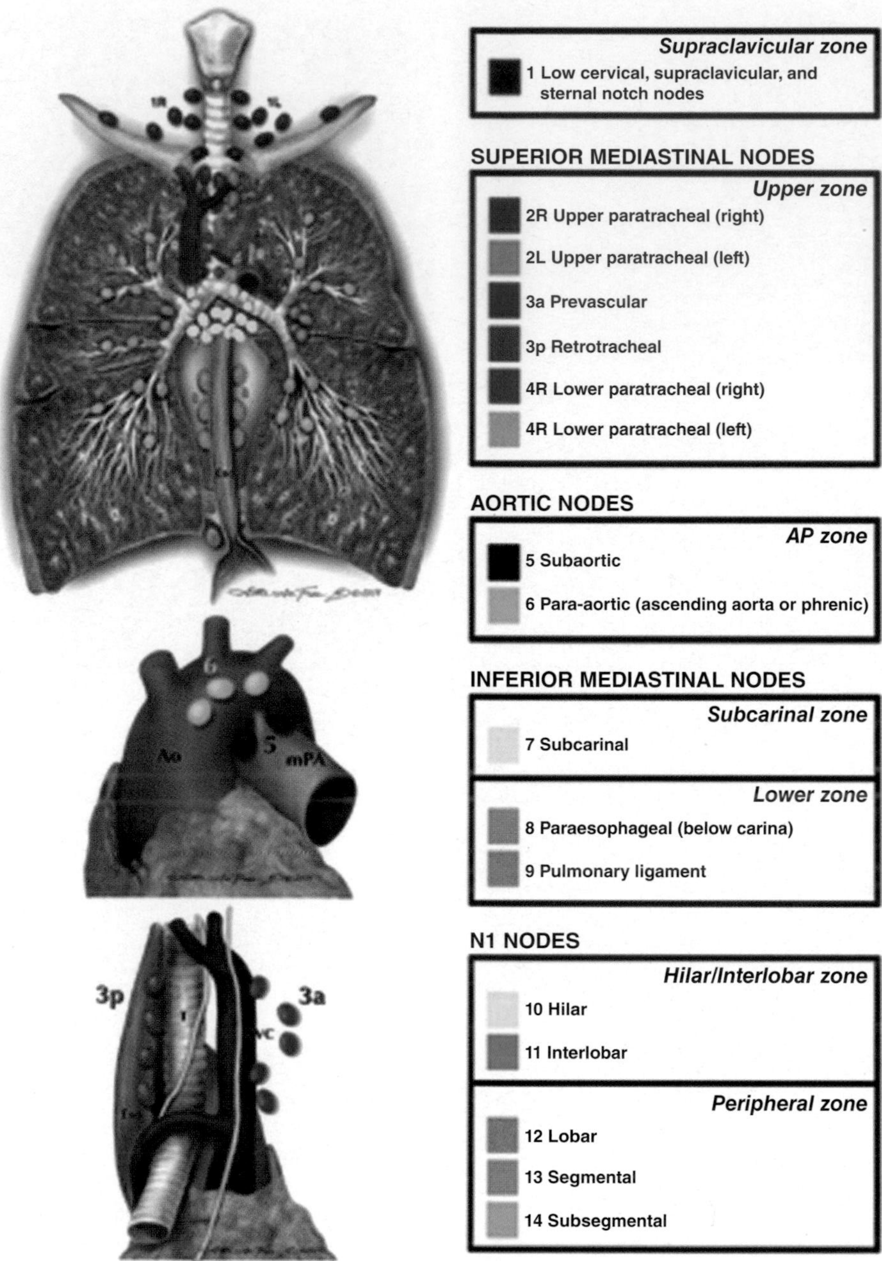

Plate 12.3 a–f: The International Association for the Study of Lung Cancer (IASLC) lymph node map as applied to clinical staging by computed tomography scan in axial (a–c), coronal (d), and sagittal (e, f) views. The border between the right and left paratracheal region is shown in a and b. Ao, aorta; AV, azygos vein; Br, bronchus; IA, innominate artery; IV, innominate vein; LA, ligamentum arteriosum; LIV, left innominate vein; LSA, left subclavian artery; PA, pulmonary artery; PV, pulmonary vein; RIV, right innominate vein; SVC, superior vena cava [55].
Source: Rusch, 2009 [55]. Reproduced with permission of Lippincott Williams and Wilkins.

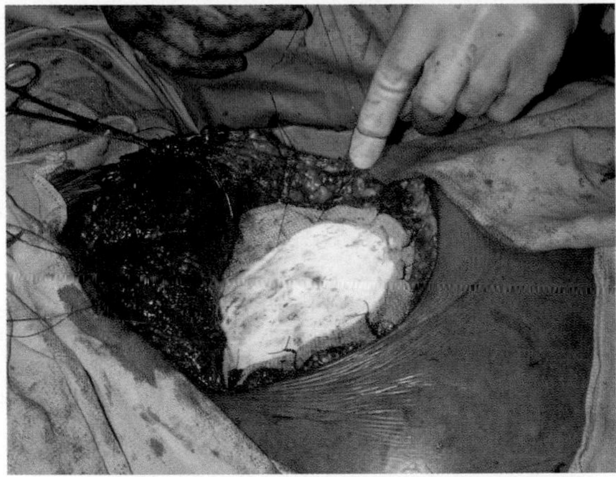

Plate 15.1 Polypropylene mesh reconstruction with methylmethacrylate.

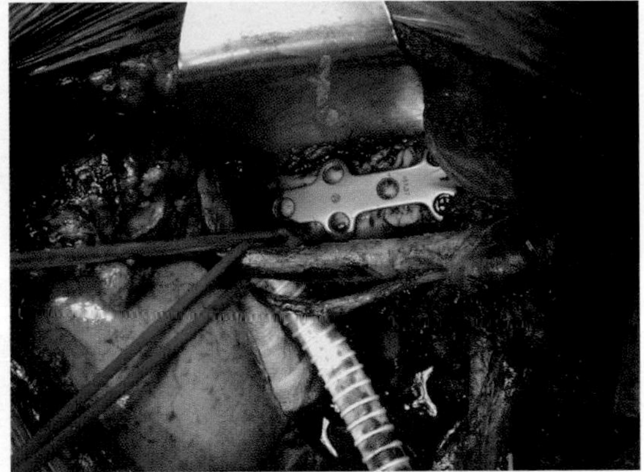

Plate 15.4 Resection of superior sulcus tumor in conjunction with spine (stabilization hardware shown) and subclavian vessel (replaced by ringed PTFE graft).

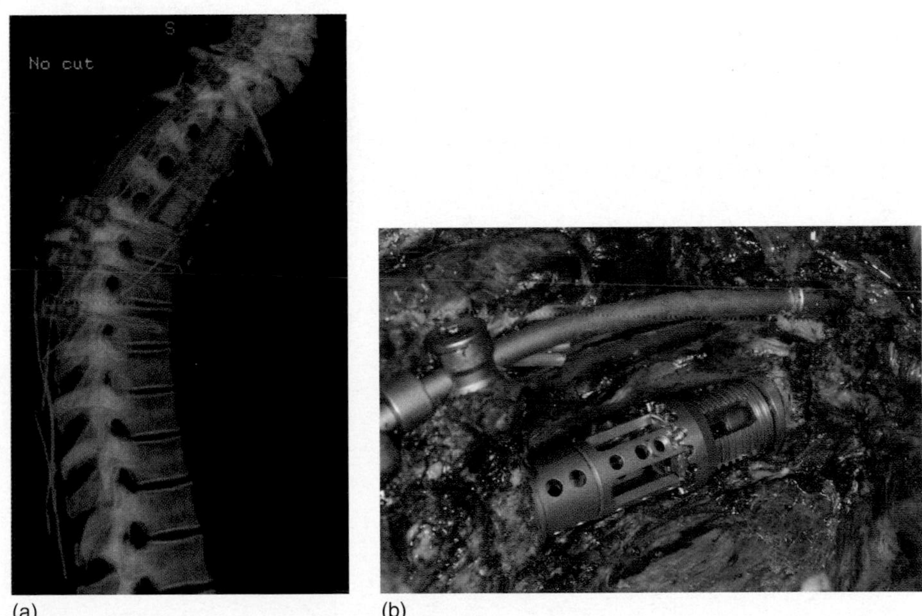

Plate 15.3 Extensive resection of the spine due to local invasion requires stabilization with hardware as demonstrated in postoperative imaging (a) and intraoperative photograph (b).

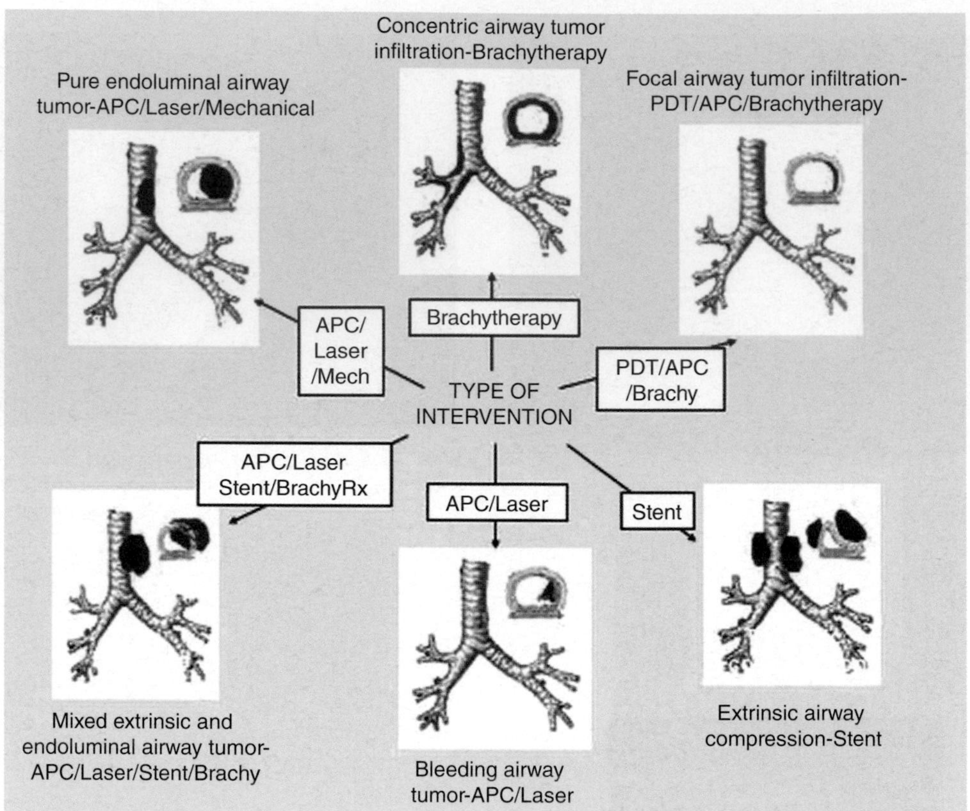

Plate 16.1 Selection of appropriate endobronchial therapeutic options based on location and type of lesion. *Source:* Reproduced with permission of Dr R. Morice.

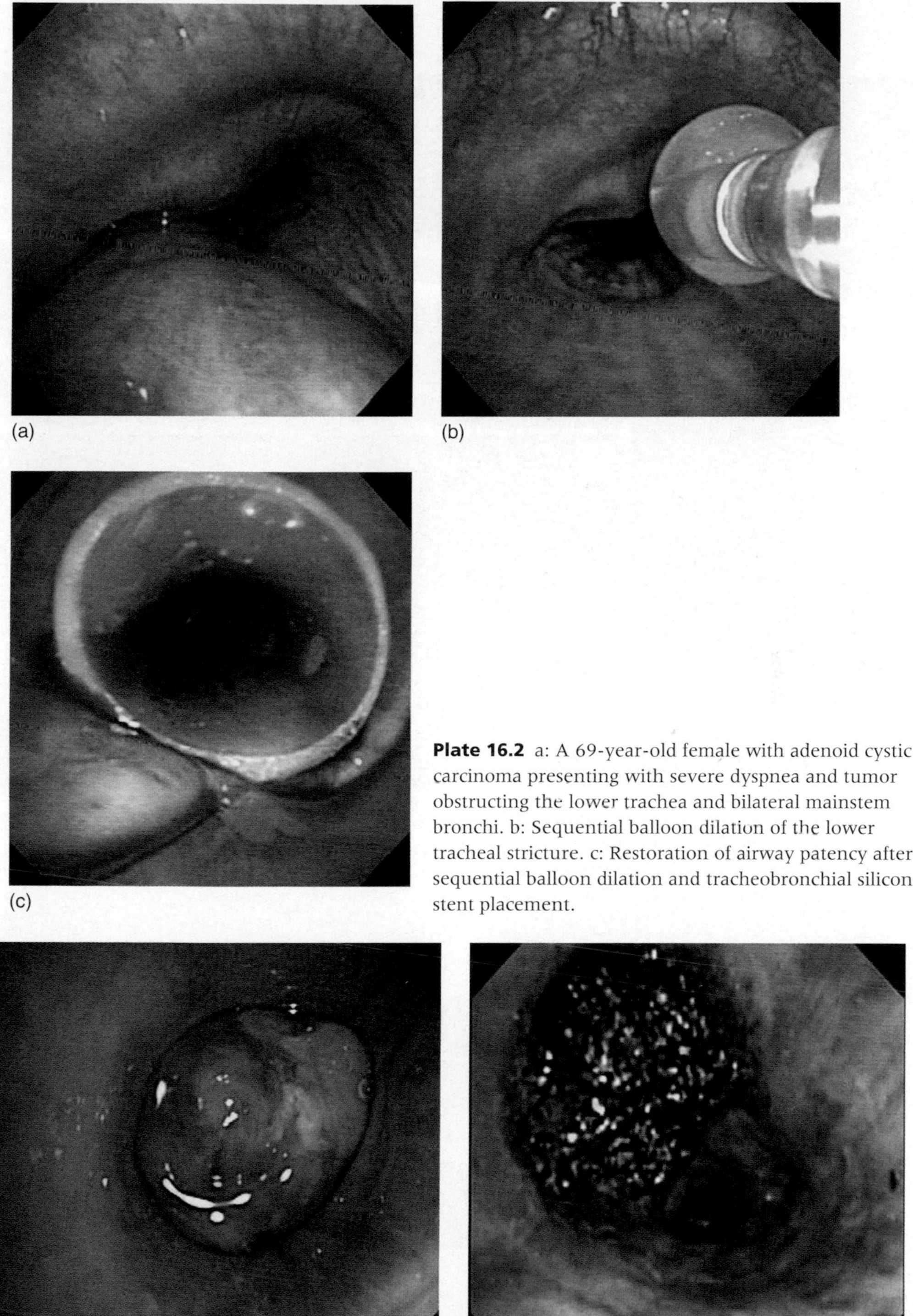

Plate 16.2 a: A 69-year-old female with adenoid cystic carcinoma presenting with severe dyspnea and tumor obstructing the lower trachea and bilateral mainstem bronchi. b: Sequential balloon dilation of the lower tracheal stricture. c: Restoration of airway patency after sequential balloon dilation and tracheobronchial silicone Y stent placement.

Plate 16.3 a: A 49-year-old female presenting with dyspnea and complete obstruction of the right bronchus intermedius from a right middle lobe adenocarcinoma. b: Complete recanalization of the right bronchus intermedius and right lower lobe following snare electrocautery and argon plasma coagulation of the endoluminal mass.

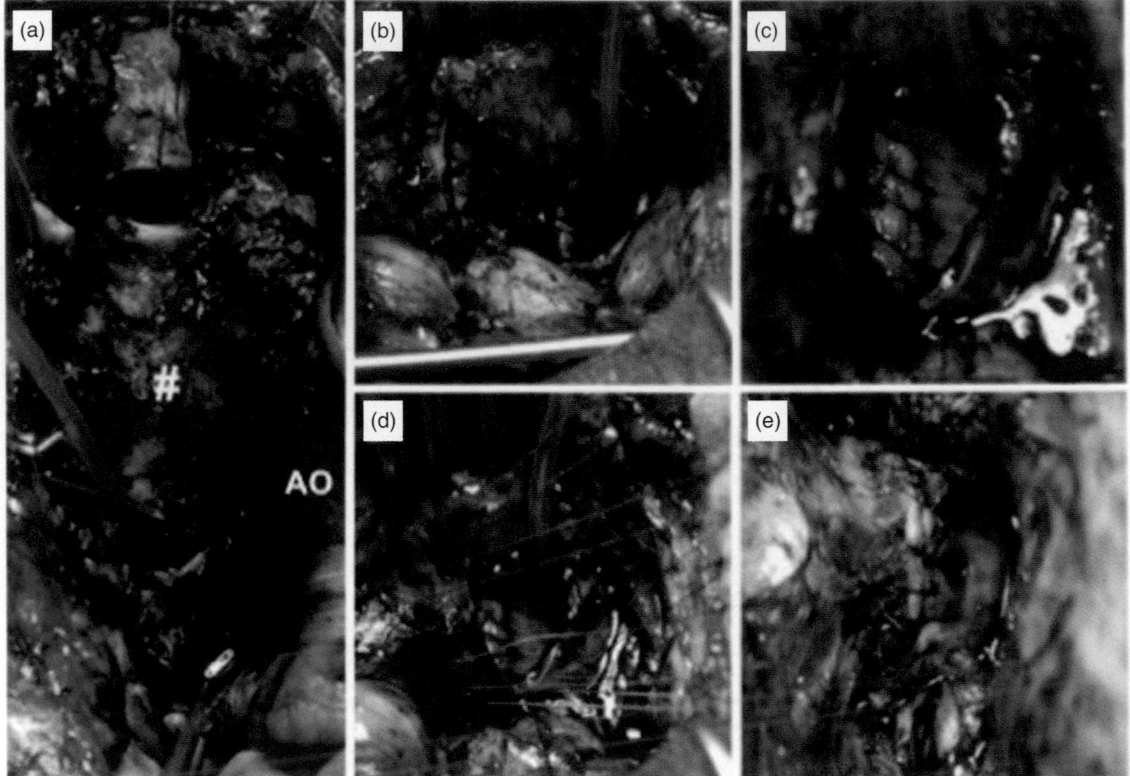

Plate 17.2 a: Anterior view on the middle and distal part of intrathoracic trachea after mobilizing ascending aorta (AO). # = part of trachea to be removed due to a tracheal tumor. b: Lateral intraoperative view of the dissected trachea and a placed running suture at the posterior wall. c: Tightened running suture. d: Single sutures (7x) at the anterior wall of the trachea. e: Tightened single sutures and closed anastomosis.

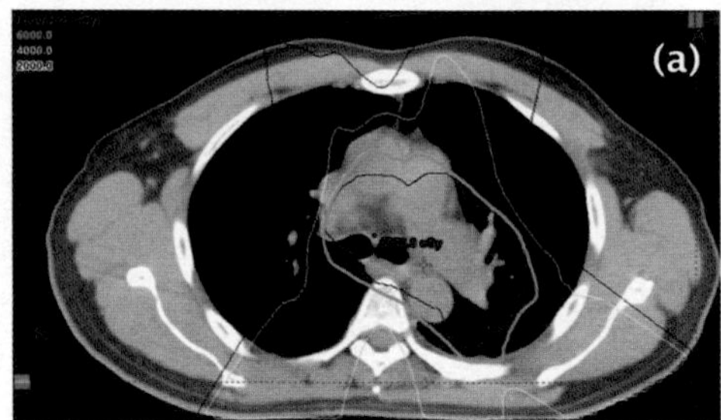

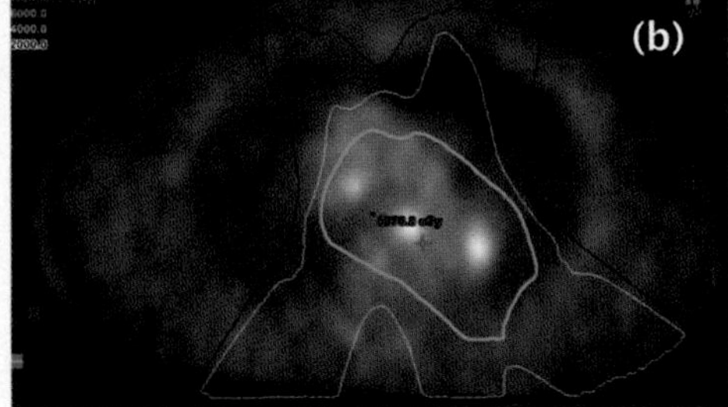

Plate 20.1 A 62-year-old male with inoperable Stage IIIB NSCLC. 60 Gy in 30 fractions was delivered to this site safely. Treatment planning was done using PET-CT registration. a: A CT scan slice from the treatment planning simulation with the planning target volume outlined in red. b: The FDG-PET image of the corresponding slice. The 6000 cGy, 4000 cGy and 2000 cGy isodose curves are shown in green, cyan and blue respectively.

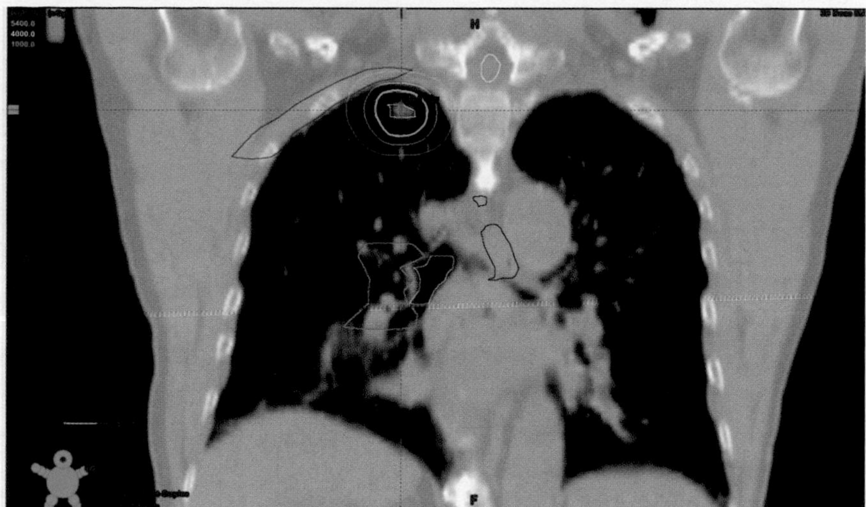

Plate 20.2 An 89-year-old male with medically inoperable early stage NSCLC. 54 Gy in three fractions was delivered to this site safely. The yellow contour represents the gross tumor volume. The green, white and blue isodose curves represent 1000 cGy, 4000 cGy and 5400 cGy respectively. The normal structures which need to have their radiation dose minimized include the chest wall (magenta), spinal cord (yellow), esophagus (blue), bronchial tree (orange and blue).

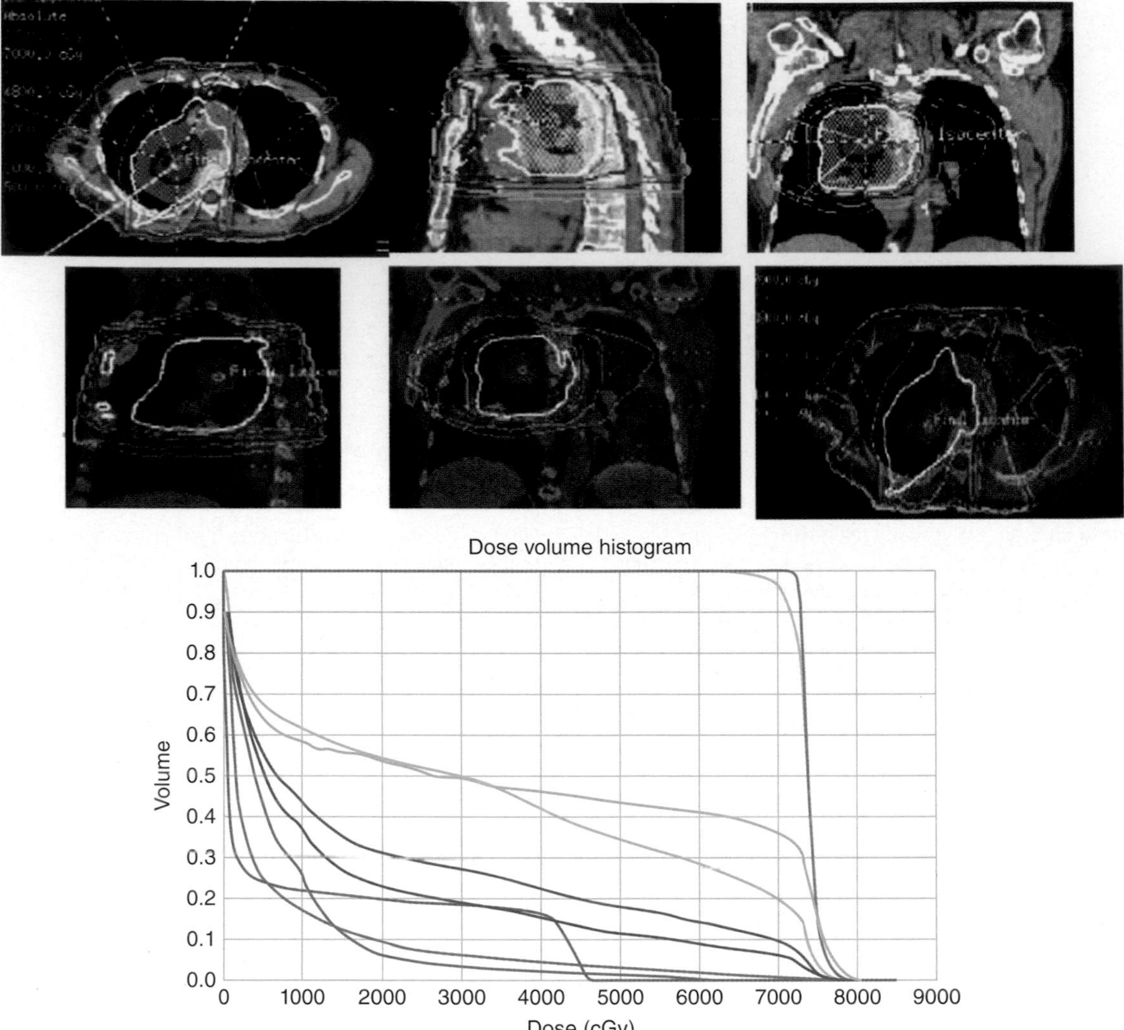

Plate 23.3 Typical dose-distribution images and dose-volume histograms for use in planning treatment of stage III non-small cell lung cancer (NSCLC). Upper panel, intensity-modulated radiation therapy (IMRT) plan based on CT images; middle panel, IMRT plan based on lung single positron emission computed tomography images; lower panel, a typical dose-volume histogram. Different colors in the histogram indicate different organ structures.

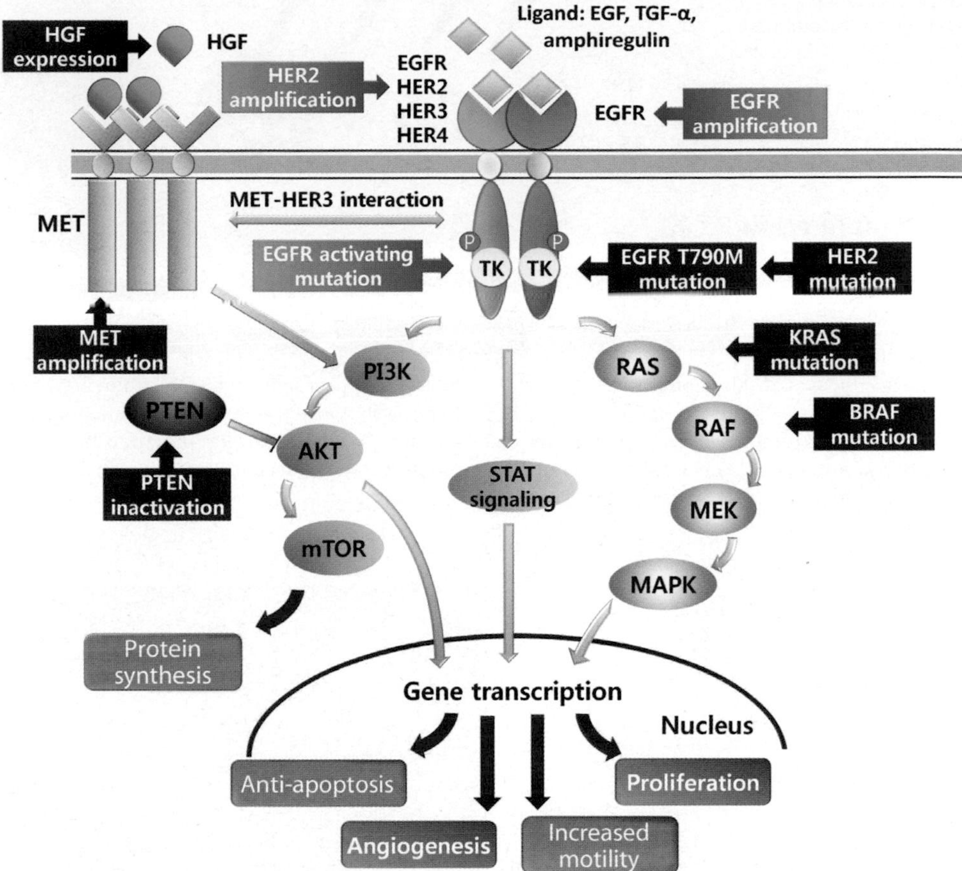

Plate 28.1 Signaling pathway of EGFR and related molecules. Binding of ligand to EGFR induce the receptors to form homodimers or heterodimers, which activate the intrinsic intracellular TK by autophosphorylation of tyrosine residues. The activation of EGFR drives signaling cascades involving downstream RAS, PI3K/AKT and STAT pathways and eventually results in cellular response such as proliferation, anti-apoptosis, increased cell motility and angiogenesis. *MET* amplification triggers HER3-dependent activation of PI3K/AKT pathway bypassing EGFR, which results in acquired resistance in *EGFR* mutant tumors. Genetic and epigenetic abnormalities targeting EGFR and downstream molecules which are associated with sensitivity (blue box) or resistance (red box) to EGR-TKIs are indicated.

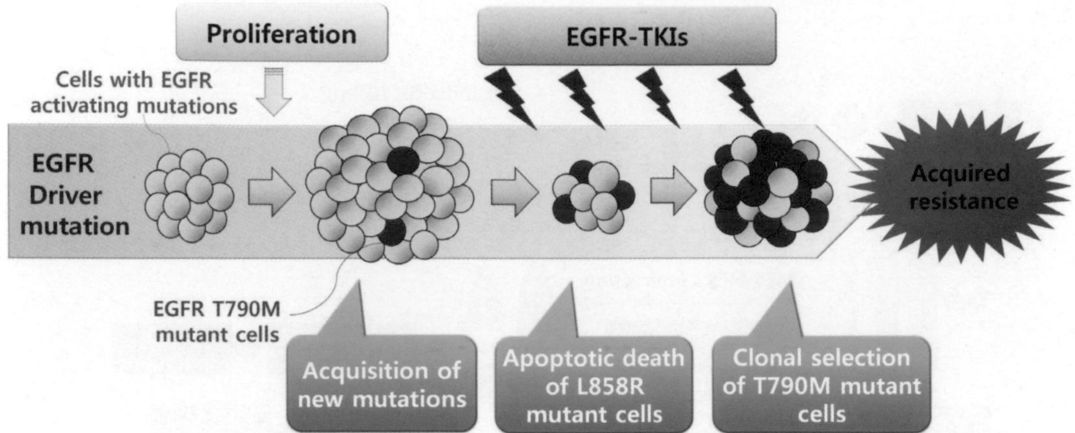

Plate 28.2 The overview of acquired resistance mechanism induced by *EGFR* T790M mutation. Proliferation of tumor cells induces emergence of mixed population of clones with diverse genetic abnormalities and a small number of tumor cells harboring T790M mutation appear in it. Under the influence of EGFR-TKIs, tumor cells with *EGFR* sensitizing mutations undergo apoptosis, while the T790M mutant cells continue to proliferate with selective pressure, which causes drug resistance.

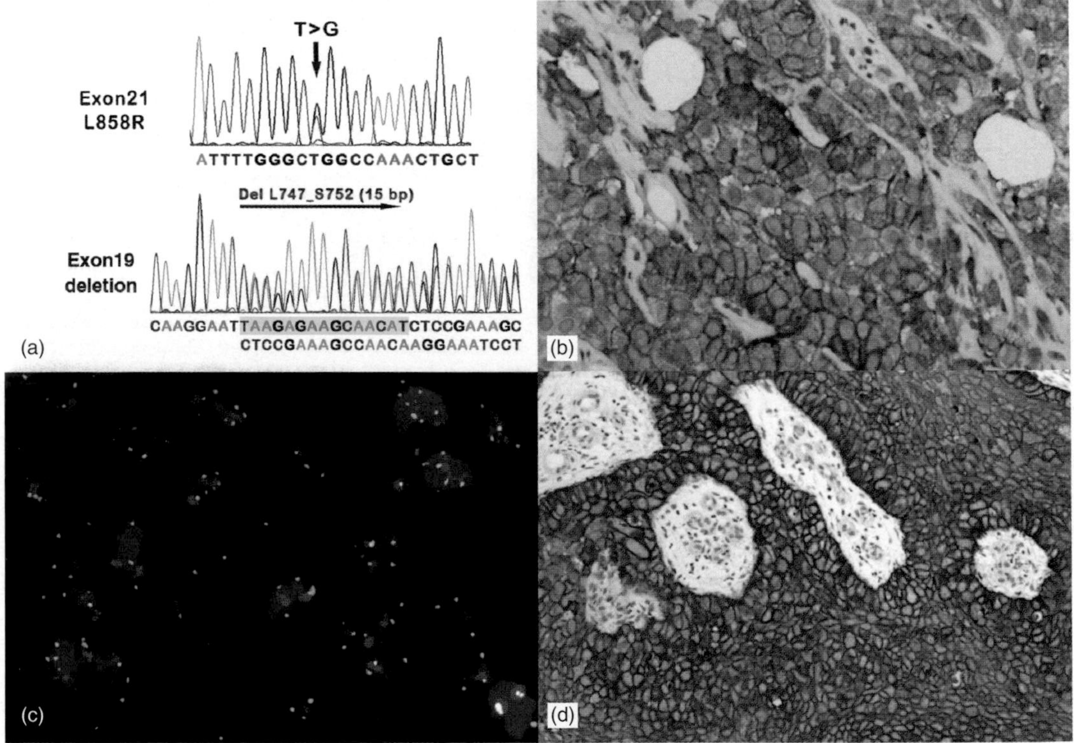

Plate 28.3 Common detection methods for *EGFR* mutation, gene copy number change, and protein expression. a: Direct sequencing results of *EGFR* L858R point mutation and Exon 19 deletion mutation. b: Immunohistochemistry with *EGFR* L858R mutation-specific antibody shows distinct membranous and cytoplasmic staining pattern in *EGFR* mutant tumor cells. c: *EGFR* amplification detected by fluorescence in situ hybridization. (Red signals, *EGFR* gene probe; green signals, chromosome 7 centromere probe.) d: EGFR protein expression assessed by immunohistochemistry shows distinct membranous staining pattern in the lung squamous cell carcinoma cells.

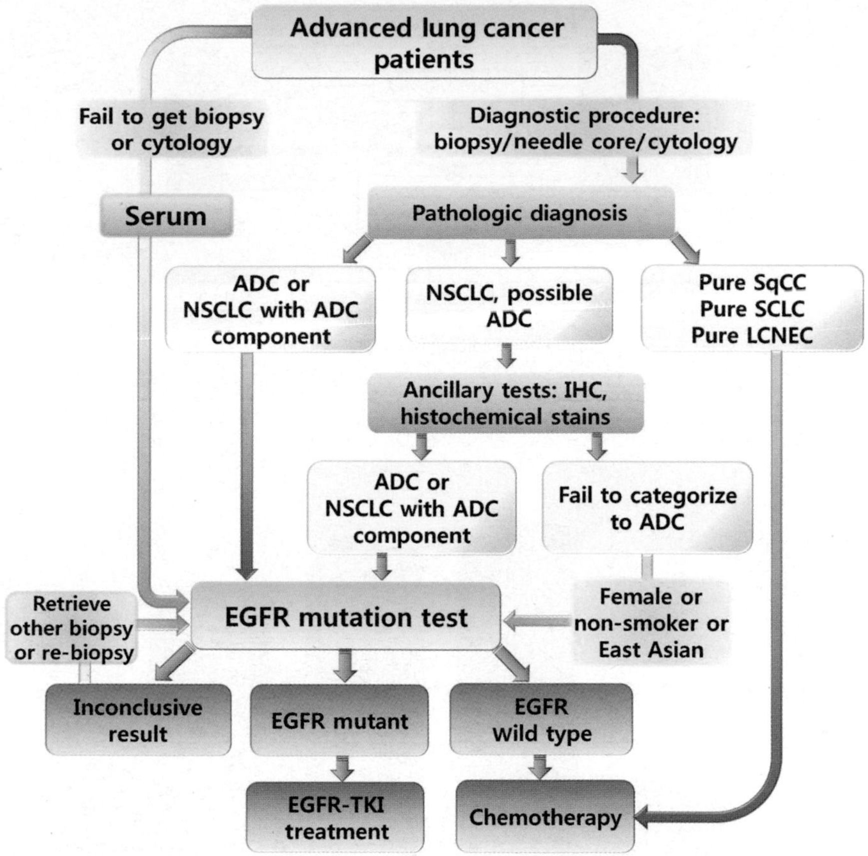

Plate 28.4 Decision-making algorithm for patients with newly diagnosed advanced NSCLC regarding *EGFR* mutation tests for directing first-line EGFR-TKI therapy.

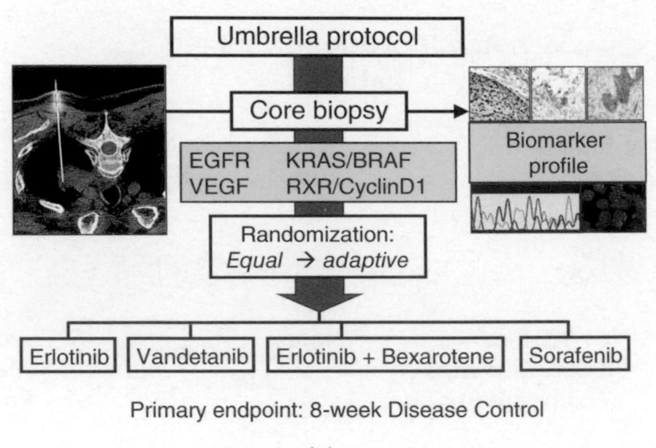

(a)

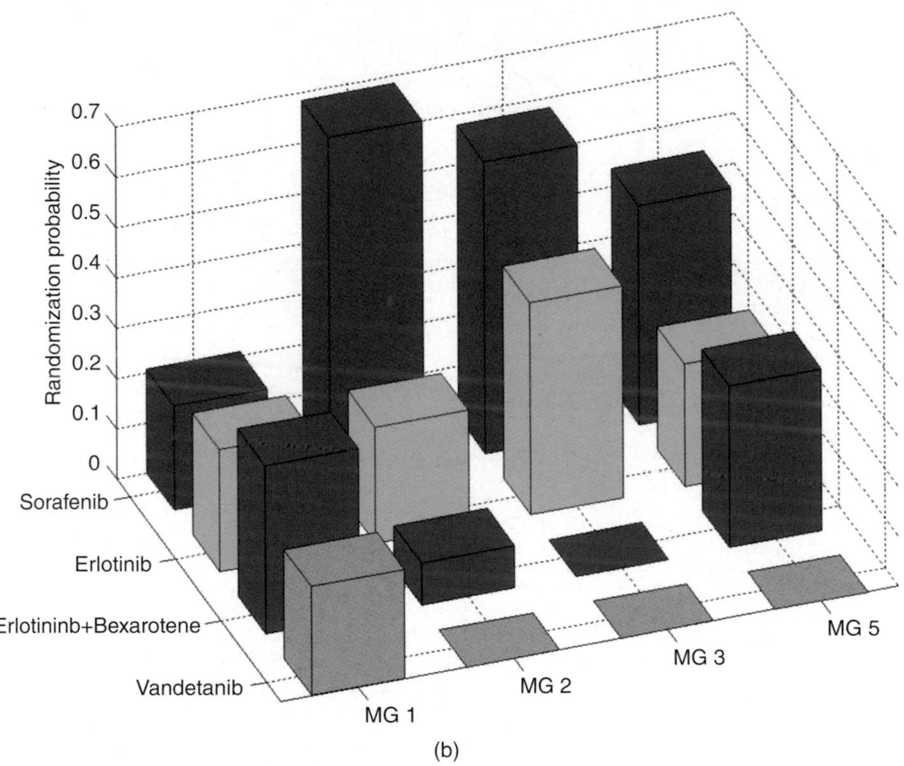

(b)

Plate 32.3 BATTLE trials. a: BATTLE trial design schema. b: Probability of adaptive randomization by treatment and marker group at the end of the BATTLE trial.

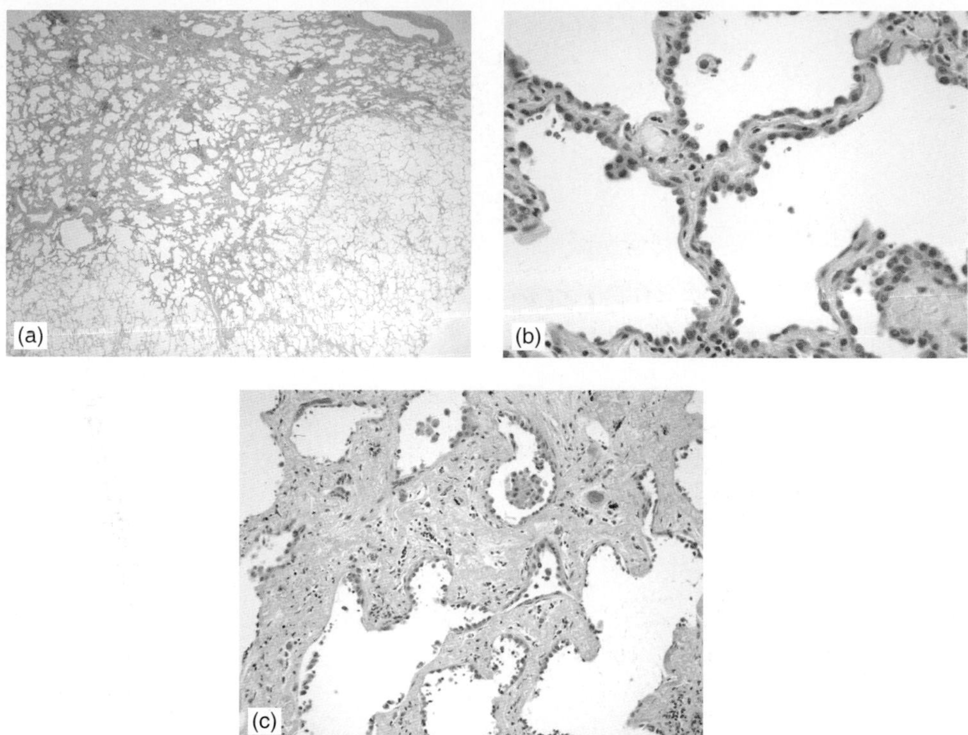

Figure 8.1 Nonmucinous adenocarcinoma *in situ*. a: This circumscribed nonmucinous tumor grows purely with a lepidic pattern. No foci of invasion or scarring are seen. Hematoxylin and eosin X 1.25. b: This area shows lepidic growth or atypical pneumocytes along thin alveolar walls. Hematoxylin and eosin X20. c: This area shows fibrotic thickening of the alveolar walls but no clear invasive growth, only a lepidic pattern. Hematoxylin and eosin X20. (For a color version, see the color plate section.)

mucinous [26]. In the new definition of AIS, small size (≤3 cm) and a discrete circumscribed border is important, to exclude cases with miliary spread into adjacent lung parenchyma and/or lobar consolidation, particularly for mucinous AIS. Most of the data that indicates 100% 5-year disease free survival in resected AIS is in series of tumors 2 cm or less with fewer studies including tumors up to 3 cm in diameter; however little data is published regarding mucinous AIS [20–26, 28].

Minimally invasive adenocarcinoma

Minimally invasive adenocarcinoma (MIA) is defined as a lepidic predominant adenocarcinoma measuring 3 cm or less that has an invasive component measuring 5 mm or less (Figure 8.2) [4]. Only a few studies were available at the time of the initial proposal of the IASLC/ATS/ERS classification to support that patients with MIA would have a near 100% 5-year disease free survival [4, 27, 29] and some did not use the exact same criteria [30, 31]. Similar to AIS, most of these are nonmucinous, but rarely mucinous cases may occur [4]. Nonmucinous MIA typically shows by CT a ground glass nodule (GGN) with a solid component measuring 5 mm or less; but mucinous MIA presents as a solid nodule on CT [4].

Invasion in MIA that needs to be measured is defined as follows: (1) invasive histological subtypes (i.e., acinar, papillary, micropapillary and/or solid) other than a lepidic pattern or (2) tumor cells invading myofibroblastic stroma. The diagnosis of MIA should not be made in the presence of (1) invasion of lymphatics, blood vessels, or pleura or (2)

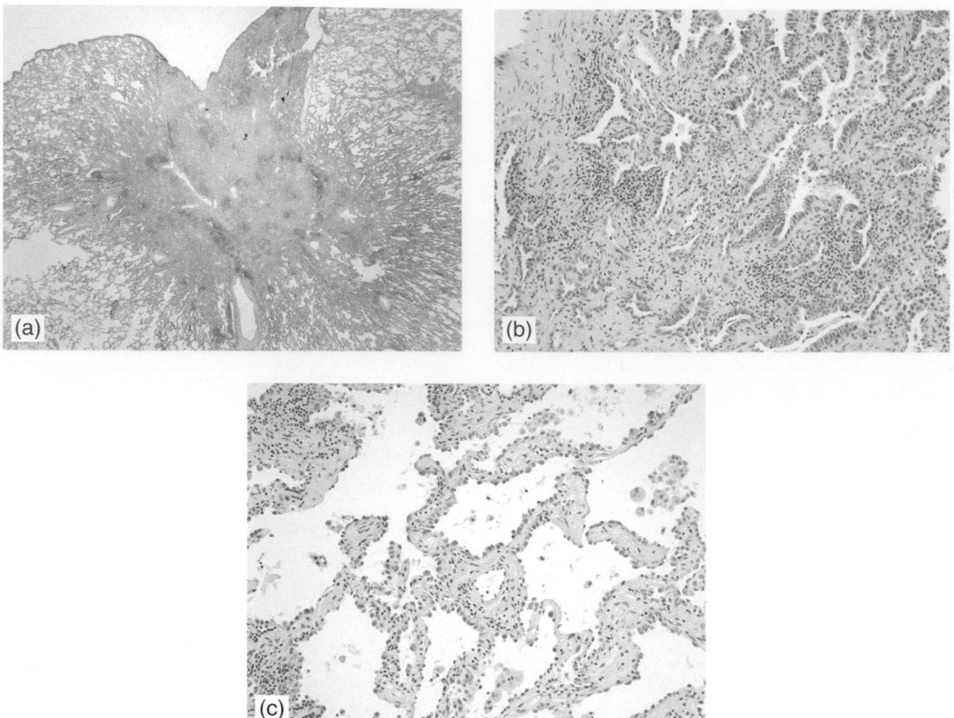

Figure 8.2 Nonmucinous minimally invasive adenocarcinoma. a: This adenocarcinoma tumor consists primarily of lepidic growth with a central scar which is mostly benign with small foci of invasion at the edges of the scar (<0.5 cm) area of invasion. Hematoxylin and eosin X 1.25. b: From the area of invasion, these acinar glands are invading in the fibrous stroma. Hematoxylin and eosin X 20. c: Other areas show a lepidic pattern with thin alveolar walls. Hematoxylin and eosin X20. (For a color version, see the color plate section.)

the presence of tumor necrosis. If there are multiple microinvasive foci in one tumor, the size of the largest invasive area should be measured in its greatest dimension and it should be $\leq$ 5 mm in size. Arbitrarily it was suggested that the size of invasion is not the summation of all such foci, if more than one occurs. This approach was arbitrarily adopted from the approach recommended by the Collage of American Pathologists for measurement of the invasive component of breast cancers that have multiple foci [32]. Another approach is to estimate the invasive size by multiplying the total percentage of the invasive (nonlepidic) components times the total tumor size.

Also, it remains to be determined if patients with MIA will still have a 100% disease free survival if the area of invasion shows a poorly differentiated component such as solid or micropapillary adenocarcinoma or if there is a giant and spindle cell component that does not meet criteria for pleomorphic carcinoma.

If there are multiple lung tumors the criteria for AIS as well as MIA can be applied only if the other tumors are regarded as synchronous primaries rather than intrapulmonary metastases.

Before making the diagnosis of AIS or MIA the entire tumor needs to be examined histologically, however, in a research setting, tissue procurement for frozen tissue banking is encouraged. In such cases, if there is a question regarding possible invasion, a frozen section could be performed to address this question.

Review of a CT scan may be helpful in tumors with a prominent lepidic component to assess tumor size and the extent of an invasive versus lepidic component because it is difficult to see these lesions grossly.

For tumors larger than 3.0 cm where the diagnoses of AIS or MIA are being considered, it is recommended to render the diagnosis of lepidic predominant adenocarcinoma. This is because most of the literature that was used to establish the criteria for AIS and MIA addressed tumors measuring 2.0 or 3.0 cm or less. Since the classification was an evidence-based effort, there was insufficient evidence to support that 100% disease free survival can occur in completely resected solitary tumors suspected to be AIS or MIA that are larger than 3.0 cm. The term "lepidic predominant adenocarcinoma" should be used for tumors where the diagnosis of AIS or MIA is being considered if they are larger than 3.0 cm or if they have not been completely sampled histologically, with a comment that an invasive component cannot be excluded.

Invasive adenocarcinoma

Overtly invasive adenocarcinomas are now classified according to the predominant subtype after using comprehensive histologic subtyping to estimate the percentages of the various histologic subtypes within a tumor in a semiquantitative fashion in 5–10% increments. Lepidic predominant adenocarcinoma (LPA) consists of tumors formerly classified as mixed subtype tumors containing a predominant lepidic growth pattern (formerly known as nonmucinous BAC) that have an invasive component greater than 5 mm or that measure greater than 3 cm (Figure 8.3a–c). The other major subtypes include acinar (Figure 8.3d), papillary (Figure 8.3e), micropapillary (Figure 8.3f) and solid with mucin predominant adenocarcinomas (Figure 8.3g). The micropapillary predominant subtype has been shown in multiple studies to be associated with poor prognosis in early stage adenocarcinomas (Figure 8.3f) [4, 29 33, 34]. Signet ring and clear cell carcinoma subtypes are now documented as cytologic features rather than as histologic subtypes and mentioned whenever present with a comment about the percentage identified. Although clear and signet ring cell cytologic changes are seen mostly in the solid subtype, they can also be seen in acinar or papillary patterns as well [35, 36].

There is a good correlation between amount of the ground glass vs solid component seen on CT and the lepidic vs invasive components seen on biopsy [29, 37].

Adenocarcinoma variants

The variants of lung adenocarcinoma consist of invasive mucinous adenocarcinoma (formerly mucinous BAC), colloid adenocarcinoma, fetal adenocarcinoma and enteric adenocarcinoma [4]. Invasive mucinous adenocarcinomas (formerly mucinous BAC) are separated from the nonmucinous invasive adenocarcinomas for several reasons. These tumors frequently associated with *KRAS* mutation, lack of TTF-1 and multicentric lung lesions. These tumors histologically show varying amounts of lepidic, acinar, papillary or micropapillary growth consisting of columnar cells with abundant apical mucin and small basally oriented nuclei (Figure 8.3h) [4]. By CT these tumors often show localized or multifocal consolidation with air bronchograms and lobar consolidation.

Prognosis of adenocarcinoma subtypes in resected specimens

Several studies have shown prognostic significance to this approach to histologic subtyping of resected lung adenocarcinomas with some variation in results [29, 38–41]. In a study of 514 Stage I adenocarcinomas reported by Yoshizawa A *et al.*, three groups of tumors were identified according to grades of clinical behavior: (1) low grade AIS and MIA with 100% 5-year disease free survival (DFS); (2) intermediate grade nonmucinous lepidic predominant, papillary predominant and acinar predominant with 90%, 83% and 84% 5-year DFS respectively; and (3) high grade: invasive mucinous adenocarcinoma, colloid predominant, solid predominant and micropapillary predominant with 75%, 71%, 70% and 67% 5-year DFS, respectively [29]. Similar results were found in two other datasets [40, 42]. In a Japanese cohort of 440 patients Yoshizawa found 5-year DFS was

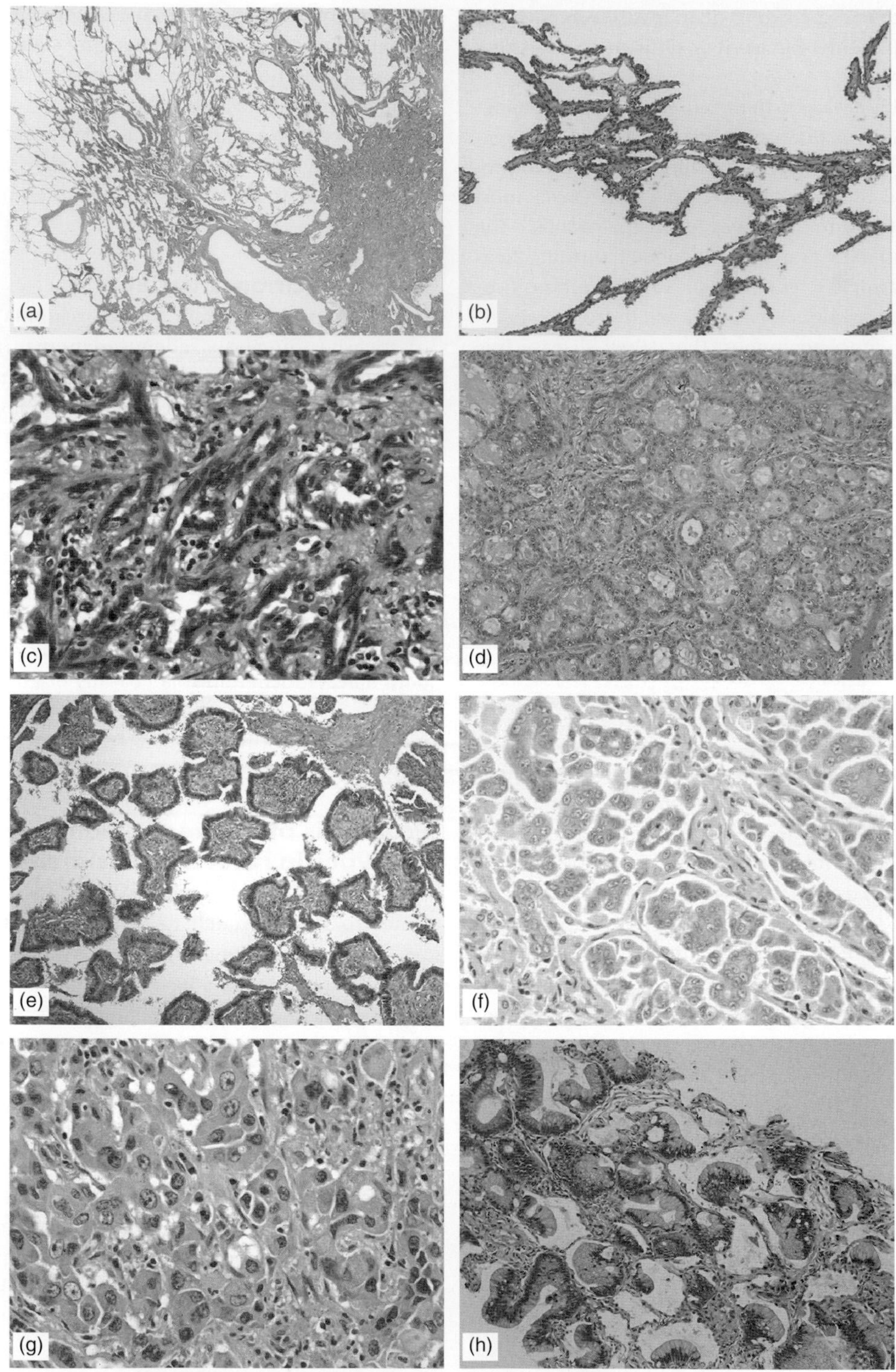

Figure 8.3

100% for AIS and MIA, 94% for LPD, 86.67% for papillary, 88.7% for acinar, 43.3% for solid predominant, and 0% for micropapillary (at 3 years) with 88.8% for invasive mucinous adenocarcinoma [40]. Kadota *et al.* found similar findings in a separate dataset of 540 Stage I lung adenocarcinomas where there was 100% DFS for AIS and MIA, 91% for LPD, 87% for acinar, 80% for papillary, 59% for micropapillary, and 69% for solid with a 62% 3-year DFS for invasive mucinous and colloid adenocarcinoma [42].

TNM staging: impact of 2011 adenocarcinoma classification

TNM staging of lung adenocarcinoma can be impacted in two major ways by the 2011 IASLC/ATS/ERS lung adenocarcinoma classification. First, morphologic assessment is a powerful tool for determining if two adenocarcinoma nodules represent metastatic disease or separate primaries. One tool is the use of comprehensive histologic subtyping to compare the percentage of histologic patterns. It is also useful to compare cytologic and stromal characteristics. These correlate well with molecular and clinical data in making this distinction [43–45]. The issue whether or not a second tumor is classified as a separate primary or an intrapulmonary metastasis has great importance for TNM staging and patient management, particularly for separate lobe or contralateral tumors.

In addition the 2012 UICC TNM Supplement states that "when size is a criterion for the T/pT category, it is a measurement of the invasive component" [46]. In lung cancer we have traditionally used total tumor size for determining T-factor size. Now it is possible that in invasive lung adenocarcinomas with a prominent lepidic component, that comprehensive histologic subtyping may help to determine the size of the invasive component. The invasive tumor size can be estimated by subtracting the percentage of the lepidic component from the total gross size. This approach has been used in breast cancer for many years. So the size T factor for early lung adenocarcinomas may be best determined by the size of the invasive component rather than the total tumor size and this may be more predictive of survival than total tumor size as suggested in several studies demonstrating that the invasive size is an independent prognostic factor [29, 30]. Several studies suggest that clinical stage by CT measurement is more predictive of prognosis according to invasive size rather than total size where the ground glass vs solid component by CT corresponds to lepidic vs invasive growth by histology. This also needs to be studied by CT to determine if prognosis is best predicted according to the size of the solid component rather than total tumor size including the ground glass component [4, 47, 48]. Hopefully these accumulating data will be sufficient to help include this issue in the next TNM revision.

Figure 8.3 Major histologic patterns of invasive adenocarcinoma. a: Lepidic predominant pattern with mostly lepidic growth (left) and an area of invasive acinar adenocarcinoma (right). Hematoxylin and eosin X 100. b: Lepidic pattern consists of a proliferation type II pneumocytes and Clara cells along the surface alveolar walls. Hematoxylin and eosin X 200. c: Area of invasive acinar adenocarcinoma (same tumor as in 3A&B). Hematoxylin and eosin X 400. d: Acinar adenocarcinoma composed of round to oval shaped malignant glands invading a fibrous stroma. Hematoxylin and eosin X 200, e: Papillary adenocarcinoma consists of malignant cuboidal to columnar tumor cells growing on the surface of fibrovascular cores. Hematoxylin and eosin X 100, f: Micropapillary adenocarcinoma consists of small papillary clusters of glandular cells growing within this airspace, most of which do not show fibrovascular cores. Hematoxylin and eosin X 200. g: Solid adenocarcinoma with mucin consisting of sheets of tumor cells with abundant cytoplasm and mostly vesicular nuclei with several conspicuous nucleoli. No acinar, papillary or lepidic patterns are seen, but multiple cells have intracytoplasmic basophilic globules that suggest intracytoplasmic mucin. Hematoxylin and eosin X 400, h: Invasive mucinous adenocarcinoma demonstrates lepidic and acinar growth. The tumor consists of columnar cells filled with abundant mucin in the apical cytoplasm and shows small basal oriented nuclei. Hematoxylin and eosin X 200. (For a color version, see the color plate section.)

Adenocarcinoma classification in small biopsies and cytology

A major new aspect of lung cancer classification has been focused on small biopsies and cytology since 70% of non-small cell lung carcinomas (NSCLC) present in advanced stages [4]. In recent years, there has been a major transformation in the approach to diagnosis of NSCLC, so now more attention is given to its precise classification in small biopsies and cytology [3–6]. The main reason for this new importance to classify NSCLC further is because the choice of therapies now is dependent on histology. For example, according to the new classification patients with adenocarcinoma, non-small cell carcinoma, favor adenocarcinoma and NSCLC-not otherwise specified (NSCLC-NOS) should be tested for EGFR mutation and if one is identified, these patients are eligible for *EGFR* tyrosine kinase inhibitors [49–53]. If no mutation is present they are also eligible for either pemetrexed [54–57] or bevacizumab based regimens [58]. In contrast, if the diagnosis is squamous cell carcinoma, tumors should not be tested for EGFR mutation and patients are not eligible for these therapies, but there is hope that newly recognized markers such as FRFR1 amplification and DDR2 mutation may represent potentially effective molecular targets [59–61]. The implications of these new therapeutic paradigms for lung cancer classification are profound.

Because of these therapeutic advances, in the 2011 IASLC/ATS/ERS lung adenocarcinoma classification, formal criteria for diagnosis of lung cancer in small biopsies and cytology were proposed (Table 8.2) [4]. Development of these new terms and criteria were driven by the need to separate adenocarcinoma from squamous cell carcinoma because of the therapeutic implications largely dependent on histology. Patients who have either *adenocarcinoma, NSCLC, favor adenocarcinoma* or *NSCLC-NOS* rather than squamous cell carcinoma are eligible at the moment for three therapeutic options. Patients with advanced stage lung adenocarcinoma that have one of these histologic diagnoses should be tested for *EGFR* mutation, and if the result is positive, EGFR tyrosine kinase inhibitor therapy has predictive benefit for response rate and progression free survival [49–52]. Patients who do not have EGFR mutation should also be tested for ALK rearrangement as this is a predictor or responsiveness to crizotinib [62, 63]. Further more it has been shown that in patients with adenocarcinoma or NSCLC-NOS, histology is a strong predictor of response to pemetrexed in advanced lung cancer patients [54–57].

The new classifications recommends to simply use the terms adenocarcinoma (Figure 8.4a) or squamous cell carcinoma (Figure 8.4b) if the tumors that show clear differentiation by morphology. However, if the tumor only shows a carcinoma with no clear squamous or adenocarcinoma features (NSCLC-NOS), a minimal immunohistochemical workup is recommended using a single adenocarcinoma marker and squamous marker, which should allow for classification of most tumors. At the moment the best markers for adenocarcinoma and squamous cell carcinoma are TTF-1 and p40, respectively [4, 64–66]. In a tumor that shows no clear squamous or adenocarcinoma morphology, but the staining results favor adenocarcinoma (i.e., TTF-1 positive, p63 negative), the tumor should be classified as *NSCLC, favor adenocarcinoma* (Figures 8.4c and 8.4d). Likewise, if the stains in such a tumor favor squamous cell carcinoma, the diagnosis would be *NSCLC, favor squamous cell carcinoma* (Figure 8.4e and 8.4f). Then for tumors where there is no clear differentiation by light microscopy or special stains, or if the results are conflicting, the diagnosis remains NSCLC-NOS. In addition to immunohistochemistry, cytology is another powerful tool in subclassifying poorly differentiated NSCLC. Cytology may be able to help classify some tumors better than can be done in the biopsy alone [3, 67]. It is recommended to avoid use of the term "non-squamous carcinoma" and state the specific diagnosis in precise terms as outlined above [4]. Also use of the term NSCLC should be minimized and instead the specific diagnosis (adenocarcinoma or squamous cell carcinoma) should be used whenever possible [4].

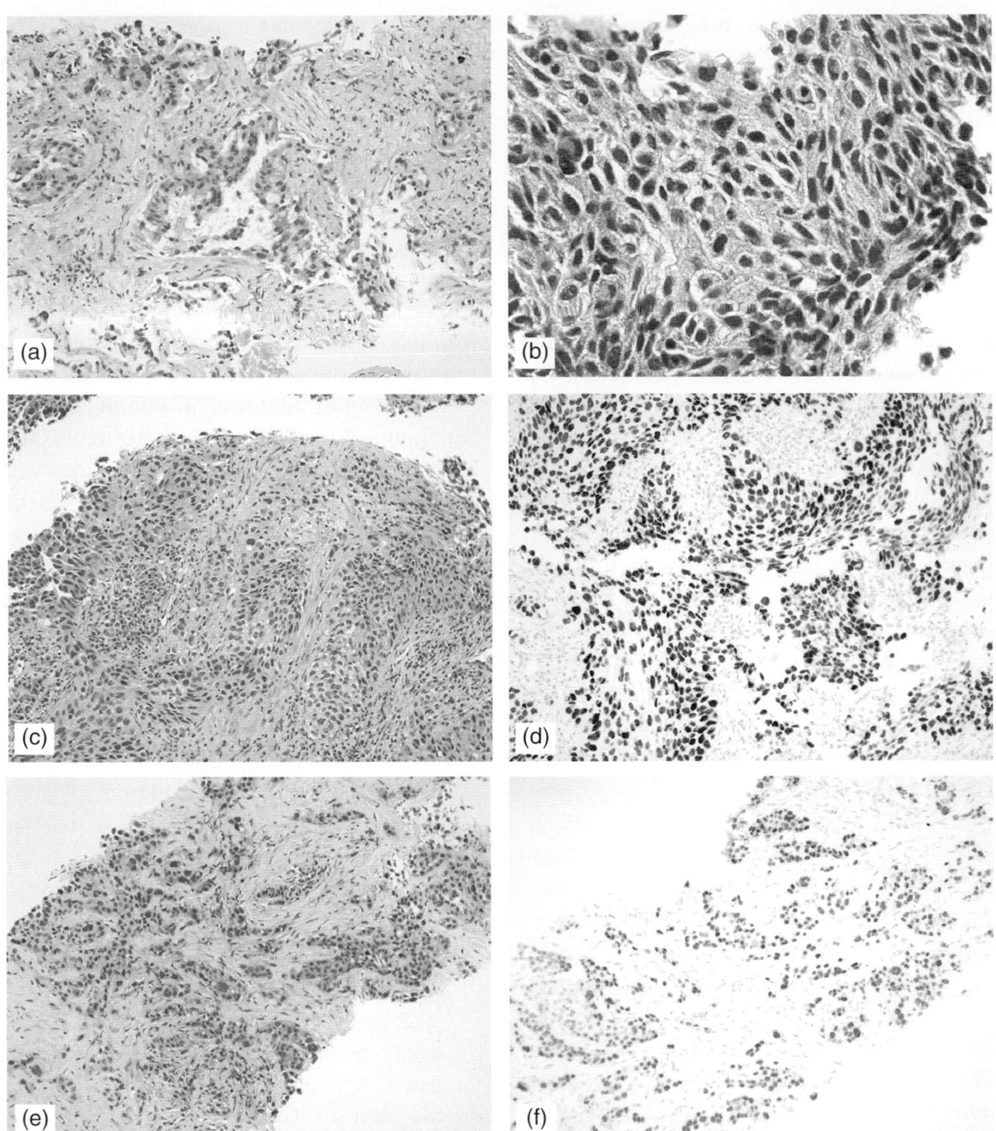

Figure 8.4 a: Adenocarcinoma: This tumor shows an acinar pattern of growth indicating adenocarcinoma. Hematoxylin and Eosin X20. b: Squamous cell carcinoma: This tumor shows keratinization indicating squamous cell carcinoma. c: Non-small cell carcinoma, favor adenocarcinoma. This carcinoma shows no clear squamous or glandular differentiation. Hematoxylin and eosin X 200. d: The diffuse positive TTF-1 staining, allows for the diagnosis of non-small cell carcinoma, favor adenocarcinoma. Hematoxylin and eosin X 200. e: Non-Small cell carcinoma, favor squamous cell carcinoma. This carcinoma shows no clear squamous or glandular differentiation. Hematoxylin and eosin X 200 f: The diffuse positive p63 staining and negative TTF-1 staining (not shown), allows for the diagnosis of non-small cell carcinoma, favor squamous cell carcinoma. Immunohistochemistry for p63 × 200. (For a color version, see the color plate section.)

Since not all tumors in the lung are adenocarcinoma or squamous carcinoma, pathologists must approach interpretation of small biopsies and cytology with consideration of diagnoses other than NSCLC, such as neuroendocrine tumors (carcinoid, small cell carcinoma or large cell neuroendocrine carcinoma) as well as metastatic tumors including metastatic breast cancer, malignant melanoma, or prostate cancer [3]. Therefore it the initial evaluation does not clearly point to adenocarcinoma or squamous cell carcinoma, some of these other diagnoses may need to be considered.

Using the new IASLC/ATS/ERS criteria and utilization of immunohistochemistry as well as cytology correlation, the percentage of NSCLC diagnosed as NSCLC-NOS, should be less than 5% of cases [3, 67]. This is a major change from the historical use of the diagnosis of NSCLC-NOS where in studies of advanced NSCLC, this diagnosis has been made in 20–40% of cases and some data suggest its use has been increasing [56, 68].

A multidisciplinary strategic plan is needed for each institution to manage these small biopsies and cytology specimens that addresses (1) obtaining the specimen, (2) processing it in the pathology laboratory, (3) providing material to the molecular diagnostic laboratory and (4) getting the results back into a pathology report and into the medical record [3, 4]. This process requires ongoing communication between experts involved with lung cancer patients and specimens to assure optimal management of tissues and efficient reporting of results. The specialists obtaining the biopsies such as the radiologists, pulmonologists or surgeons, need to obtain sufficient tissue not only for diagnosis, but also for molecular studies. Therefore the planned biopsy procedures should result either in a core biopsy or a cell block from tissue samples obtained for cytology [4, 69]. With voluminous pleural fluids that are positive by cytology for tumor, the fluid should be preserved rather than discarded to allow for generating cell blocks so immunostaining and molecular studies can be performed.

Another major change in clinical practice for pathologists is to minimize the amount of tissue used for making the diagnosis including use of as few special stains as possible in order to maximize tissue for molecular testing [3, 4]. It can be helpful to cut multiple unstained slides from the block after initial review in cases that are potential candidates for molecular testing, so valuable tissue is not lost by facing the block multiple times [3]. This would include tumors that are either clearly adenocarcinoma or those with NSCLC-NOS patterns on H&E that will require special stains. If adenocarcinoma is suspected, by performing only a TTF-1 stain, if the result is positive, it would confirm not only the adenocarcinoma diagnosis, but also a pulmonary origin. If by morphology the tumor could be either adenocarcinoma or squamous cell carcinoma, it may be best to perform one adenocarcinoma (i.e., TTF-1) and one squamous (i.e., p40) marker as recommended in the new classification [4, 64]. In the small percentage of cases where this limited panel does not allow for precise classification it is best to be conservative in using additional stains to further classify the tumor [3, 4].

References

1 Siegel R, Naishadham D, Jemal A (2013) Cancer statistics. *CA Cancer J Clin*, 63: 11–30.

2 Howlader N, Noone AM, Krapcho M, Garshell J, Neyman N, Altekruse SF, *et al.* (2013) Lung cancer. In: *SEER Cancer Statistics Review, 1975–2010*. National Cancer Institute, Bethesda, MD. 2013. Internet Communication.

3 Travis WD, Rekhtman N (2011) Pathological diagnosis and classification of lung cancer in small biopsies and cytology: strategic management of tissue for molecular testing. *Semin Respir Crit Care Med*, 32: 22–31.

4 Travis WD, Brambilla E, Noguchi M, Geisinger KR, Beer D, Powell CA, *et al.* (2011) The New IASLC/ATS/ERS international multidisciplinary lung adenocarcinoma classification. *J Thoracic Oncol*, 6: 244–85.

5 Travis WD, Brambilla E, Van SP, Scagliotti GV, Huber RM, Sculier JP, *et al.* (2011) Paradigm shifts in lung cancer as defined in the new IASLC/ATS/ERS lung adenocarcinoma classification. *Eur Respir J*, 38: 239–43.

6 Travis WD, Rekhtman N, Riley GJ, Geisinger KR, Asamura H, Brambilla E, *et al.* (2010) Pathologic diagnosis of advanced lung cancer based on small biopsies and cytology: a paradigm shift. *J Thorac Oncol*, 5: 411–14.

7 Noguchi M (2010) Stepwise progression of pulmonary adenocarcinoma – clinical and molecular implications. *Cancer Metastasis Rev*, 29: 15–21.

8 Yoo SB, Chung JH, Lee HJ, Lee CT, Jheon S, Sung SW (2010) Epidermal growth factor receptor mutation and p53 overexpression during the multistage progression of small adenocarcinoma of the lung. *J Thorac Oncol*, 5: 964–9.

9 Lantuejoul S, Salameire D, Salon C, Brambilla E (2009) Pulmonary preneoplasia – sequential molecular carcinogenetic events. *Histopathology*, 54: 43–54.

10 Travis WD, Brambilla E, Müller-Hermelink HK, Harris CC (2004) *Pathology and Genetics: Tumours of the Lung, Pleura, Thymus and Heart*. Lyon: IARC.

11 Travis WD, Brambilla E (2006) Pathology of lung preneoplasia. In: Hirsch FR, Bunn PA, Kato H, Mulshine JL (eds), *Textbook of Prevention and Detection of Early Lung Cancer*. International Association for the Study of Lung Cancer. 1 ed. London and New York: Taylor & Francis, pp. 75–89.

12 Ruffini E, Bongiovanni M, Cavallo A, Filosso PL, Giobbe R, Mancuso M, *et al.* (2004) The significance of associated pre-invasive lesions in patients resected for primary lung neoplasms. *Eur J Cardiothorac Surg*, 26: 165–72.

13 Travis WD, Colby TV, Corrin B, Shimosato Y, Brambilla E, in collaboration with L.H.Sobin and pathologists from 14 countries (1999) *Histological Typing of Lung and Pleural Tumors*, 3rd edn. Berlin: Springer.

14 Kitamura H, Kameda Y, Ito T, Hayashi H (1999) Atypical adenomatous hyperplasia of the lung: Implications for the pathogenesis of peripheral lung adenocarcinoma. *Am J Clin Pathol*, 111: 610–22.

15 Miller RR (1990) Bronchioloalveolar cell adenomas. *Am J Surg Pathol*, 14: 904–12.

16 Weng SY, Tsuchiya E, Kasuga T, Sugano H (1992) Incidence of atypical bronchioloalveolar cell hyperplasia of the lung: relation to histological subtypes of lung cancer. *Virchows Arch A Pathol Anat Histopathol*, 420: 463–71.

17 Mori M, Chiba R, Tezuka F, Kaji M, Kobubo T, Nukiwa T, *et al.* (1996) Papillary adenoma of type II pneumocytes might have malignant potential. *Virchows Arch*, 428: 195–200.

18 Mori M, Chiba R, Takahashi T (1993) Atypical adenomatous hyperplasia of the lung and its differentiation from adenocarcinoma: Characterization of atypical cells by morphometry and multivariate cluster analysis. *Cancer*, 72: 2331–40.

19 Ritter JH (1999) Pulmonary atypical adenomatous hyperplasia. A histologic lesion in search of usable criteria and clinical significance. *Am J Clin Pathol*, 111: 587–9.

20 Watanabe S, Watanabe T, Arai K, Kasai T, Haratake J, Urayama H (2002) Results of wedge resection for focal bronchioloalveolar carcinoma showing pure ground-glass attenuation on computed tomography. *Ann Thorac Surg*, 73: 1071–5.

21 Sakurai H, Dobashi Y, Mizutani E, Matsubara H, Suzuki S, Takano K, *et al.* (2004) Bronchioloalveolar carcinoma of the lung 3 centimeters or less in diameter: A prognostic assessment. *Ann Thorac Surg*, 78: 1728–33.

22 Vazquez M, Carter D, Brambilla E, Gazdar A, Noguchi M, Travis WD, *et al.* (2009) Solitary and multiple resected adenocarcinomas after CT screening for lung cancer: histopathologic features and their prognostic implications. *Lung Cancer*, 64: 148–54.

23 Yamato Y, Tsuchida M, Watanabe T, Aoki T, Koizumi N, Umezu H, *et al.* (2001) Early results of a prospective study of limited resection for bronchioloalveolar adenocarcinoma of the lung. *Ann Thorac Surg*, 71: 971–4.

24 Yoshida J, Nagai K, Yokose T, Nishimura M, Kakinuma R, Ohmatsu H, *et al.* (2005) Limited resection trial for pulmonary ground-glass opacity nodules: fifty-case experience. *J Thorac Cardiovasc Surg*, 129: 991–6.

25 Koike T, Togashi K, Shirato T, Sato S, Hirahara H, Sugawara M, *et al.* (2009) Limited resection for noninvasive bronchioloalveolar carcinoma diagnosed by intraoperative pathologic examination. *Ann Thorac Surg*, 88: 1106–11.

26 Noguchi M, Morikawa A, Kawasaki M, Matsuno Y, Yamada T, Hirohashi S, *et al.* (1995) Small adenocarcinoma of the lung. Histologic characteristics and prognosis. *Cancer*, 75: 2844–52.

27 Yim J, Zhu LC, Chiriboga L, Watson HN, Goldberg JD, Moreira AL (2007) Histologic features are important prognostic indicators in early stages lung adenocarcinomas. *Mod Pathol*, 20: 233–41.

28 Yamada S, Kohno T (2004) Video-assisted thoracic surgery for pure ground-glass opacities 2 cm or less in diameter. *Ann Thorac Surg*, 77: 1911–15.

29 Yoshizawa A, Motoi N, Riely GJ, Sima CS, Gerald WL, Kris MG, *et al.* (2011) Impact of proposed IASLC/ATS/ERS classification of lung adenocarcinoma: prognostic subgroups and implications for further revision of staging based on analysis of 514 stage I cases. *Mod Pathol*, 24: 653–64.

30 Borczuk AC, Qian F, Kazeros A, Eleazar J, Assaad A, Sonett JR, *et al.* (2009) Invasive size is an independent

predictor of survival in pulmonary adenocarcinoma. *Am J Surg Pathol*, 33: 462–9.

31 Suzuki K, Yokose T, Yoshida J, Nishimura M, Takahashi K, Nagai K, *et al.* (2000) Prognostic significance of the size of central fibrosis in peripheral adenocarcinoma of the lung. *Ann Thorac Surg*, 69: 893–7.

32 Lester SC, Bose S, Chen YY, Connolly JL, de Baca ME, Fitzgibbons PL, *et al.* (2009) Protocol for the examination of specimens from patients with invasive carcinoma of the breast. *Arch Pathol Lab Med*, 133: 1515–38.

33 Miyoshi T, Satoh Y, Okumura S, Nakagawa K, Shirakusa T, Tsuchiya E, *et al.* (2003) Early-stage lung adenocarcinomas with a micropapillary pattern, a distinct pathologic marker for a significantly poor prognosis. *Am J Surg Pathol*, 27: 101–9.

34 Tsutsumida H, Nomoto M, Goto M, Kitajima S, Kubota I, Hirotsu Y, *et al.* (2007) A micropapillary pattern is predictive of a poor prognosis in lung adenocarcinoma, and reduced surfactant apoprotein A expression in the micropapillary pattern is an excellent indicator of a poor prognosis. *Mod Pathol*, 20: 638–47.

35 Cohen PR, Yoshizawa A, Motoi N, Riely GJ, Kris M, Park BJ, *et al.* (2010) Signet ring cell features (SRCF) in lung adenocarcinoma: a cytologic feature or a histologic subtype? *Mod Pathol*, 23: 400A.

36 Deshpande CG, Yoshizawa A, Motoi N, Gerald WL, Kris M, Park B, *et al.* (2009) Clear cell change in lung adenocarcinoma: A cytologic change rather than a histologic variant. *Mod Pathol*, 22: 352A.

37 Naidich DP, Bankier AA, MacMahon H, Schaefer-Prokop CM, Pistolesi M, Goo JM, *et al.* (2013) Recommendations for the management of subsolid pulmonary nodules detected at CT: A statement from the Fleischner Society. *Radiology*, 266: 304–17.

38 Russell PA, Wainer Z, Wright GM, Daniels M, Conron M, Williams RA (2011) Does lung adenocarcinoma subtype predict patient survival?: A clinicopathologic study based on the new International Association for the Study of Lung Cancer/American Thoracic Society/European Respiratory Society international multidisciplinary lung adenocarcinoma classification. *J Thorac Oncol*, 6: 1496–1504.

39 Warth A, Muley T, Meister M, Stenzinger A, Thomas M, Schirmacher P, *et al.* (2012) The novel histologic IASLC/ATS/ERS classification system of invasive pulmonary adenocarcinoma is a stage-independent predictor of survival. *J Clin Oncol*, 30: 1438–46.

40 Yoshizawa A, Sumiyoshi S, Sonobe M, Kobayashi M, Fujimoto M, Kawakami F, *et al.* Validation of the IASLC/ATS/ERS lung adenocarcinoma classification for prognosis and association with EGFR and KRAS gene mutations: Analysis of 440 Japanese patients. *J Thorac Oncol*, 8: 52–61.

41 Xu L, Tavora F, Battafarano R, Burke A (2012) Adenocarcinomas with prominent lepidic spread: retrospective review applying new classification of the American Thoracic Society. *Am J Surg Pathol*, 36: 273–82.

42 Kadota K, Suzuki K, D'Angelo SP, Rekhtman N, Moreira AL, Sima CS, *et al.* (2011) Validation of the proposed IASLC/ American Thoracic Society (ATS)/ European Respiratory Society (ERS) international multidisciplinary classification of lung adenocarcinoma (ADC). *Journal of Thoracic Oncology*, 6: S286.

43 Girard N, Deshpande C, Azzoli CG, Rusch VW, Travis WD, Ladanyi M, *et al.* (2010) Use of epidermal growth factor receptor/Kirsten rat sarcoma 2 viral oncogene homolog mutation testing to define clonal relationships among multiple lung adenocarcinomas: comparison with clinical guidelines. *Chest*, 137: 46–52.

44 Girard N, Deshpande C, Lau C, Finley D, Rusch V, Pao W, *et al.* (2009) Comprehensive histologic assessment helps to differentiate multiple lung primary nonsmall cell carcinomas from metastases. *Am J Surg Pathol*, 33: 1752–64.

45 Girard N, Ostrovnaya I, Lau C, Park B, Ladanyi M, Finley D, *et al.* (2009) Genomic and mutational profiling to assess clonal relationships between multiple non-small cell lung cancers. *Clin Cancer Res*, 15: 5184–90.

46 Wittekind Ch, Compton CC, Brierley J, Sobin LH (2012) *UICC TNM Supplement, A Commentary on Uniform Use*, 4th edn. Oxford, UK: Wiley-Blackwell.

47 Tsutani Y, Miyata Y, Nakayama H, Okumura S, Adachi S, Yoshimura M, *et al.* (2012) Prognostic significance of using solid versus whole tumor size on high-resolution computed tomography for predicting pathologic malignant grade of tumors in clinical stage IA lung adenocarcinoma: a multicenter study. *J Thorac Cardiovasc Surg*, 143: 607–12.

48 Yanagawa N, Shiono S, Abiko M, Ogata SY, Sato T, Tamura G (2013) New IASLC/ATS/ERS classification and invasive tumor size are predictive of disease recurrence in Stage I lung adenocarcinoma. *J Thorac Oncol*, 8: 612–18.

49 Mok TS, Wu YL, Thongprasert S, Yang CH, Chu DT, Saijo N, *et al.* (2009) Gefitinib or carboplatin-paclitaxel in pulmonary adenocarcinoma. *N Engl J Med*, 361: 947–57.

50 Mitsudomi T, Morita S, Yatabe Y, Negoro S, Okamoto I, Tsurutani J, *et al.* (2010) Gefitinib versus cisplatin plus docetaxel in patients with non-small-cell lung cancer harbouring mutations of the epidermal growth

factor receptor (WJTOG3405): an open label, randomised phase 3 trial. *Lancet Oncol*, 11: 121–8.

51 Maemondo M, Inoue A, Kobayashi K, Sugawara S, Oizumi S, Isobe H, *et al.* (2010) Gefitinib or chemotherapy for non-small-cell lung cancer with mutated EGFR. *N Engl J Med*, 362: 2380–8.

52 Zhou C, Wu YL, Chen G, Feng J, Liu XQ, Wang C, *et al.* (2011) Erlotinib versus chemotherapy as first-line treatment for patients with advanced EGFR mutation-positive non-small-cell lung cancer (OPTIMAL, CTONG-0802): a multicentre, open-label, randomised, phase 3 study. *Lancet Oncol*, 12: 735–42.

53 Rosell R, Carcereny E, Gervais R, Vergnenegre A, Massuti B, Felip E, *et al.* (2012) Erlotinib versus standard chemotherapy as first-line treatment for European patients with advanced EGFR mutation-positive non-small-cell lung cancer (EURTAC): A multicentre, open-label, randomised phase 3 trial. *Lancet Oncol*, 13: 239–46.

54 Ciuleanu T, Brodowicz T, Zielinski C, Kim JH, Krzakowski M, Laack E, *et al.* (2009) Maintenance pemetrexed plus best supportive care versus placebo plus best supportive care for non-small-cell lung cancer: A randomised, double-blind, phase 3 study. *Lancet*, 374: 1432–40.

55 Scagliotti G, Hanna N, Fossella F, Sugarman K, Blatter J, Peterson P, *et al.* (2009) The differential efficacy of pemetrexed according to NSCLC histology: a review of two Phase III studies. *Oncologist*, 14: 253–63.

56 Scagliotti GV, Parikh P, von PJ, Biesma B, Vansteenkiste J, Manegold C, *et al.* (2008) Phase III study comparing cisplatin plus gemcitabine with cisplatin plus pemetrexed in chemotherapy-naive patients with advanced-stage non-small-cell lung cancer. *J Clin Oncol*, 26: 3543–51.

57 Scagliotti G, Brodowicz T, Shepherd FA, Zielinski C, Vansteenkiste J, Manegold C, *et al.* (2011) Treatment-by-histology interaction analyses in three phase III trials show superiority of pemetrexed in nonsquamous non-small cell lung cancer. *J Thorac Oncol*, 6: 64–70.

58 Johnson DH, Fehrenbacher L, Novotny WF, Herbst RS, Nemunaitis JJ, Jablons DM, *et al.* (2004) Randomized phase II trial comparing bevacizumab plus carboplatin and paclitaxel with carboplatin and paclitaxel alone in previously untreated locally advanced or metastatic non-small-cell lung cancer. *J Clin Oncol*, 22: 2184–91.

59 Hammerman PS, Hayes DN, Wilkerson MD, Schultz N, Bose R, Chu A, *et al.* (2012) Comprehensive genomic characterization of squamous cell lung cancers. *Nature*, 489: 519–25.

60 Dutt A, Ramos AH, Hammerman PS, Mermel C, Cho J, Sharifnia T, *et al.* (2011) Inhibitor-sensitive FGFR1 amplification in human non-small cell lung cancer. *PLoS One*, 6: e20351.

61 Hammerman PS, Sos ML, Ramos AH, Xu C, Dutt A, Zhou W, *et al.* (2011) Mutations in the DDR2 Kinase gene identify a novel therapeutic target in squamous cell lung cancer. *Cancer Discov*, 1: 78–89.

62 Sasaki T, Janne PA (2011) New strategies for treatment of ALK rearranged non-small cell lung cancers. *Clin Cancer Res*, 17: 7213–18.

63 Shaw AT, Yeap BY, Solomon BJ, Riely GJ, Gainor J, Engelman JA, *et al.* (2011) Effect of crizotinib on overall survival in patients with advanced non-small-cell lung cancer harbouring ALK gene rearrangement: a retrospective analysis. *Lancet Oncol*, 12: 1004–12.

64 Bishop JA, Teruya-Feldstein J, Westra WH, Pelosi G, Travis WD, Rekhtman N (2012) p40 (DeltaNp63) is superior to p63 for the diagnosis of pulmonary squamous cell carcinoma. *Mod Pathol*, 25: 405–15.

65 Rekhtman N, Ang DC, Sima CS, Travis WD, Moreira AL (2011) Immunohistochemical algorithm for differentiation of lung adenocarcinoma and squamous cell carcinoma based on large series of whole-tissue sections with validation in small specimens. *Mod Pathol*, 24: 1348–59.

66 Pelosi G, Fabbri A, Bianchi F, Maisonneuve P, Rossi G, Barbareschi M, *et al.* (2012) DeltaNp63 (p40) and thyroid transcription factor-1 immunoreactivity on small biopsies or cellblocks for typing non-small cell lung cancer: A novel two-hit, sparing-material approach. *J Thorac Oncol*, 7: 281–90.

67 Rekhtman N, Brandt SM, Sigel CS, Friedlander MA, Riely GJ, Travis WD, *et al.* (2011) Suitability of thoracic cytology for new therapeutic paradigms in non-small cell lung carcinoma: High accuracy of tumor subtyping and feasibility of EGFR and KRAS molecular testing. *J Thoracic Oncol*, 6: 451–8.

68 Ou SH, Zell JA (2009) Carcinoma NOS is a common histologic diagnosis and is increasing in proportion among non-small cell lung cancer histologies. *J Thorac Oncol*, 4: 1202–11.

69 Solomon SB, Zakowski MF, Pao W, Thornton RH, Ladanyi M, Kris MG, *et al.* (2010) Core needle lung biopsy specimens: adequacy for EGFR and KRAS mutational analysis. *AJR Am J Roentgenol*, 194: 266–9.

CHAPTER 9

Management of Multifocal Bronchioloalveolar Carcinoma (BAC)

Howard West
Swedish Cancer Institute, Seattle, WA, USA

Introduction

The management of advanced bronchioloalveolar carcinoma (BAC) must begin with the caveat that this clinical entity has been the subject of changing definitions and is no longer recognized as a discrete subtype of lung cancer by the new classification system for adenocarcinomas developed by the International Association for the Study of Lung Cancer (IASLC)/American Thoracic Society (ATS)/European Respiratory Society (ERS) [1]. While BAC had historically been defined histologically as an adenocarcinoma that does not invade the basement membrane or lung parenchyma, the new IASLC/ATS/ERS classification of adenocarcinomas classifies a noninvasive adenocarcinoma as *adenocarcinoma in situ* for a solitary lesion and *lepidic predominant adenocarcinoma* (LPA) for a multifocal process with the same histologic appearance if nonmucinous, or alternatively mucinous adenocarcinoma for what were previously termed nonmucinous and mucinous BAC, respectively.

Nevertheless, there has historically been a discordance between the recommendations of many leading pathologists and the use of terms like BAC in clinical practice [2], and it remains to be seen whether the new classification will be widely adopted by the clinical oncology community. As patients continue to be diagnosed by pathologists with BAC and clinicians routinely approach and publish about this group of patients as a distinct clinical entity, it remains relevant to discuss their clinical management within the functional definitions that persist in practice.

It is also necessary to offer several caveats in discussing management recommendations in this setting. The term BAC is applied to a broad range of patients who are heterogeneous in their histologic findings, natural history, molecular features, and responses to therapy [2], while trials dedicated to BAC are very infrequent, small in number, and may include such a variable population that definitive conclusions remain elusive. Moreover, even within the same individual patient, different lesions may demonstrate variable pace of progression, invasiveness, radiologic features, and molecular profiles, though these observations remain poorly characterized in publications. By necessity, therefore, as is true of the new proposed reclassification of lung adenocarcinomas, no recommendations made about multifocal BAC can be offered on the basis of level 1 evidence but rather can only be provided on the basis of significant clinical experience with this patient population, combined with extensive conversations with others who share a similarly extensive experience.

Lung Cancer, Fourth Edition. Edited by Jack A. Roth, Waun Ki Hong and Ritsuko U. Komaki.

Heterogeneity in the presentation with advanced BAC

Multifocal BAC, at least as it is recognized functionally in clinical practice, is an extremely heterogeneous disease setting. Radiographic findings may demonstrate a very indolent process that may include a few scattered subcentimeter ground glass opacities, a widespread miliary pattern, or diffuse parenchymal infiltrates that are extremely difficult to distinguish from bacterial pneumonia [3,4]. BAC may progress at a rate that can vary from barely perceptible growth over years to virulent progression over weeks. Pathologically, what is termed BAC often includes not only a strictly noninvasive component ("pure BAC"), but often also microscopic areas of invasive disease. It may be mucinous, nonmucinous, or a mix of both components. As with other lung adenocarcinomas, multifocal BAC may sometimes present with an *EGFR* mutation, *KRAS* mutation, *ALK* rearrangement, or sometimes other identifiable but rare molecular features that have significant implications for responsiveness to our available systemic therapies.

Even within the same patient, different areas of disease may demonstrate varying rates of progression, metabolic uptake on positron emission tomography (PET) scans, solid vs. nonsolid component on imaging, invasiveness vs. noninvasiveness on pathologic examination, and molecular marker profiles. In addition, areas of indolent disease may, over time, become invasive and more aggressive in rate of progression [5]. This wide array of clinicopathologic scenarios, despite all being loosely classified under the same category of multifocal BAC, is likely to be best managed through a corresponding diversity of management strategies. What is optimal management for a steadily progressing, widely multifocal miliary pattern of progression and an activating *EGFR* mutation is not likely to be the optimal treatment for a patient with 4–5 very small ground-glass opacities in different lung lobes that are growing imperceptibly over three years of follow-up scans.

Our staging system, published case series, and clinical trial eligibility do not make distinctions among the varied presentations and natural histories of what is defined as multifocal BAC (Figure 9.1). Nevertheless, proposed treatment considerations are discussed below based on a range of clinical presentations that merit individualized therapeutic strategies rather than a unified approach based on amalgamation of distinct patterns.

Because of the heterogeneity of the disease and its potential indolence, there is a significant potential for patients to be overtreated based on patient and/or physician anxiety and a compulsion to "treat the scan" or the stated diagnosis even when the objective findings indicate a natural history of the disease that on a trajectory of many years. In fact, this leads some patients with a more indolent process to experience significant limitations based on serial resections or prolonged systemic therapy for asymptomatic and even clinically irrelevant disease. Conversely, many clinicians remain nihilistic of the potential utility of chemotherapy for advanced BAC or reflexively dismiss the concept of local therapy for what may technically be multifocal but actually has only a single clinically significant focus that is growing at a far greater pace than any other background disease, and for which local therapy may be a very appropriate recommendation.

Evaluating Multifocal BAC

Though BAC is most commonly (50–85% of cases) diagnosed as a solitary nodule highly amenable to surgical resection, multifocal disease may present as satellites within a single lobe (60–65% of multifocal disease), multiple lobes of one lung (20–25%), or bilateral lung nodules (10–15%) [6–8].

In light of the variability of presentations, natural history, and heterogeneity of the disease process in an individual patient (potentially with one or a few areas of disease progressing at a fast rate against a relatively indolent disease process in the background), it becomes particularly helpful to characterize the features of multifocal BAC in an individual patient before developing and committing to therapeutic interventions. This initial characterization includes careful assessment of symptomatology, evaluation of the pace of the cancer and

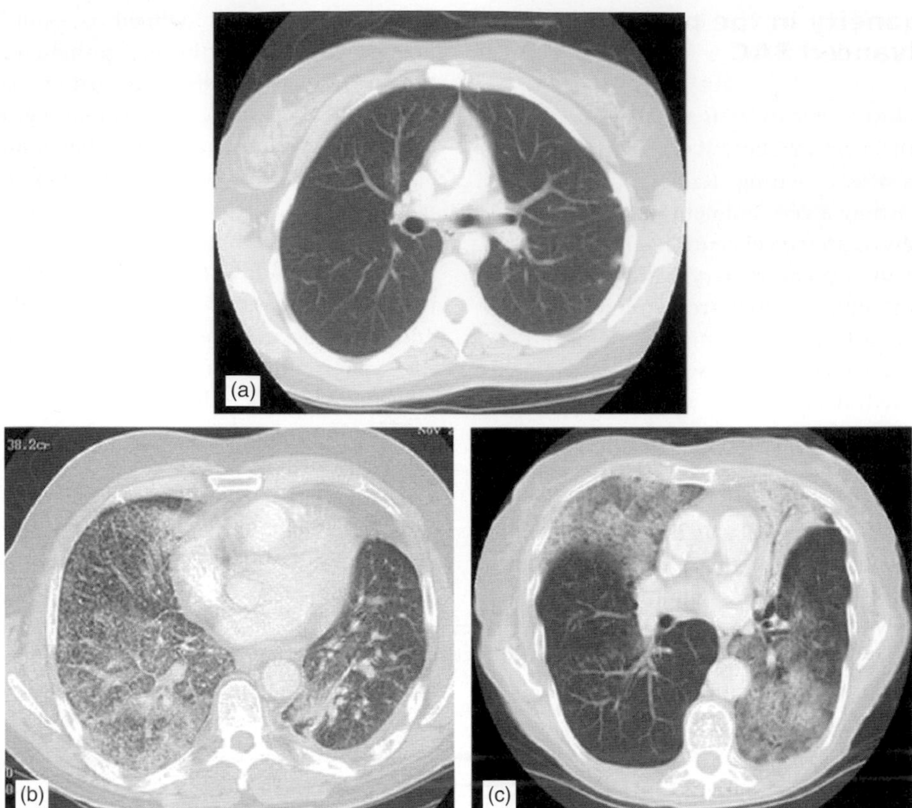

Figure 9.1 Range of case scenarios presenting with advanced BAC. a: Asymptomatic woman with minimal scattered ground-glass nodules (GGNs) (shown in left lower lobe). b: Miliary pattern of diffuse nonmucinous BAC in very symptomatic patient with dyspnea and nonproductive cough. c: Multilobal consolidation from mucinous BAC in patient with productive cough and dyspnea.

whether that is uniform or discordant across a patient's foci of disease, and, to the extent available, an assessment of the pathological findings that includes meticulous assessment of invasiveness and determination of a molecular profile that can shape recommendations for systemic therapy.

Symptomatology

BAC is commonly detected as an incidental finding in an asymptomatic patient who undergoes chest imaging for a routine pre-operative evaluation or nonspecific complaints. Up to two-thirds of patients with BAC (any stage) present with asymptomatic imaging findings, with symptomatic patients most commonly presenting with cough (30–50%), dyspnea (15%), weight loss (10–15%), hemoptysis (5–10%), or chest pain (5–10%) [9–11].

Bronchorrhea, a symptom of multifocal BAC characterized by copious production of thick, frothy sputum, is observed in approximately 5–10% of patients with BAC. In severe cases, patients may produce up to 1–2 liters of fluid per day, leading to significant electrolyte imbalances, as well as hypoxemia from intrapulmonary shunting [12–14]. Specific management considerations for bronchorrhea are discussed further below.

Natural history and imaging findings

Very commonly, the symptomatic and radiographic resemblance of advanced BAC to an infectious or inflammatory process leads to an initial trial of antibiotics and/or steroids, and sometimes multiple courses, for several weeks to months before it is concluded that the clinical and radiographic findings are not readily reversible with these treatments and a period of follow-up. The severity of initial symptoms and trajectory of progression, or lack thereof, are very relevant factors to be considered prior to initiating interventions with anticipated morbidity.

PET scans have become integrated in the workup of lung nodules, infiltrates of unknown etiology, as well as the routine staging of established lung cancers. It is common for pulmonary lesions to be discounted and a PET scan interpreted as inconsistent with malignancy if they do not demonstrate significant uptake. BAC lesions, however, are often characterized by an indolent natural history, very often with a volume doubling time of one to several years [15–17], which is typically associated with a metabolic rate too low to register as abnormally elevated on a PET scan [18]. Moreover, subcentimeter, nonsolid lesions will often not be of sufficient size and cellular density to reach the threshold of detection of a PET scan. In contrast, more significant hypermetabolism of known or presumed BAC lesions on PET scan is highly associated with invasive disease, greater malignant behavior, and inferior survival [19–21].

In this setting, a PET scan without appreciable hypermetabolism of lesions noted on chest CT may be considered as a false negative [22, 23]. Nevertheless, the lower uptake often seen on PET scans is consistent with the slower natural history and overall significantly more favorable prognosis of many patients with BAC, potentially with a survival of many years, including with multifocal disease [9, 10, 24]. This prolonged natural history is indicated by the terminology of the new classification of solitary lesions that reclassifies smaller unifocal lesions of nonmucinous, noninvasive adenocarcinomas from BAC to *adenocarcinoma in situ*, underscoring the very significant potential for overtreatment if therapeutic strategies intended for an invasive cancer process are applied. Though the practical implications for managing multifocal BAC/LPA are not specifically addressed in the new classification proposal [1], this designation is associated with a very favorable survival when reviewed specifically for differences in clinical outcomes when divided among lung adenocarcinoma subtypes under the new schema [25].

Another implication of the term of *adenocarcinoma in situ* is the implication from this terminology that the noninvasive *in situ* form of this disease, often referred to as BAC or pure BAC, represents a pre-malignant condition that evolves into invasive, malignant lung adenocarcinoma. Though this is presumed to be the case [26], it remains unclear whether the noninvasive adenocarcinomas are particularly prone to evolve into invasive lung adenocarcinoma, as more than half of a series of cases of both noninvasive lesions and synchronous invasive adenocarcinoma did not share the same K-ras mutation [27].

Interventions to manage multifocal BAC

There are several critical questions that should emerge early in the process of determining an optimal approach for managing what is functionally termed multifocal BAC (see proposed algorithm in Figure 9.2).

Is the multifocal disease encompassed within a single lobe or lung?

The most current revision of the NSCLC staging system (7th edition) reflects the potential utility of surgery for multifocal disease in one lobe or pneumonectomy if several lobes of the same lung involved in absence of disease in other areas [28–35].

Changes made in the most recent revision of the AJCC staging system for non-small cell lung cancer (NSCLC) consider satellite nodules within the same lobe as the primary tumor as T3 disease, and in the absence of nodal or distant metastatic involvement, this is now considered stage IIB, compared with stage IIIB in the 6th edition of AJCC staging [36]. Similarly, nodules in a separate lobe of the same lung as the primary tumor are now defined as T4 rather than M1 disease, defined as stage IIIA disease in the absence of nodal or distant metastatic disease, compared with stage IV NSCLC in the prior version of the NSCLC staging system [37].

These revisions reflect the more favorable prognosis of patients, who most commonly have AIS/BAC histology in these additional nodules,

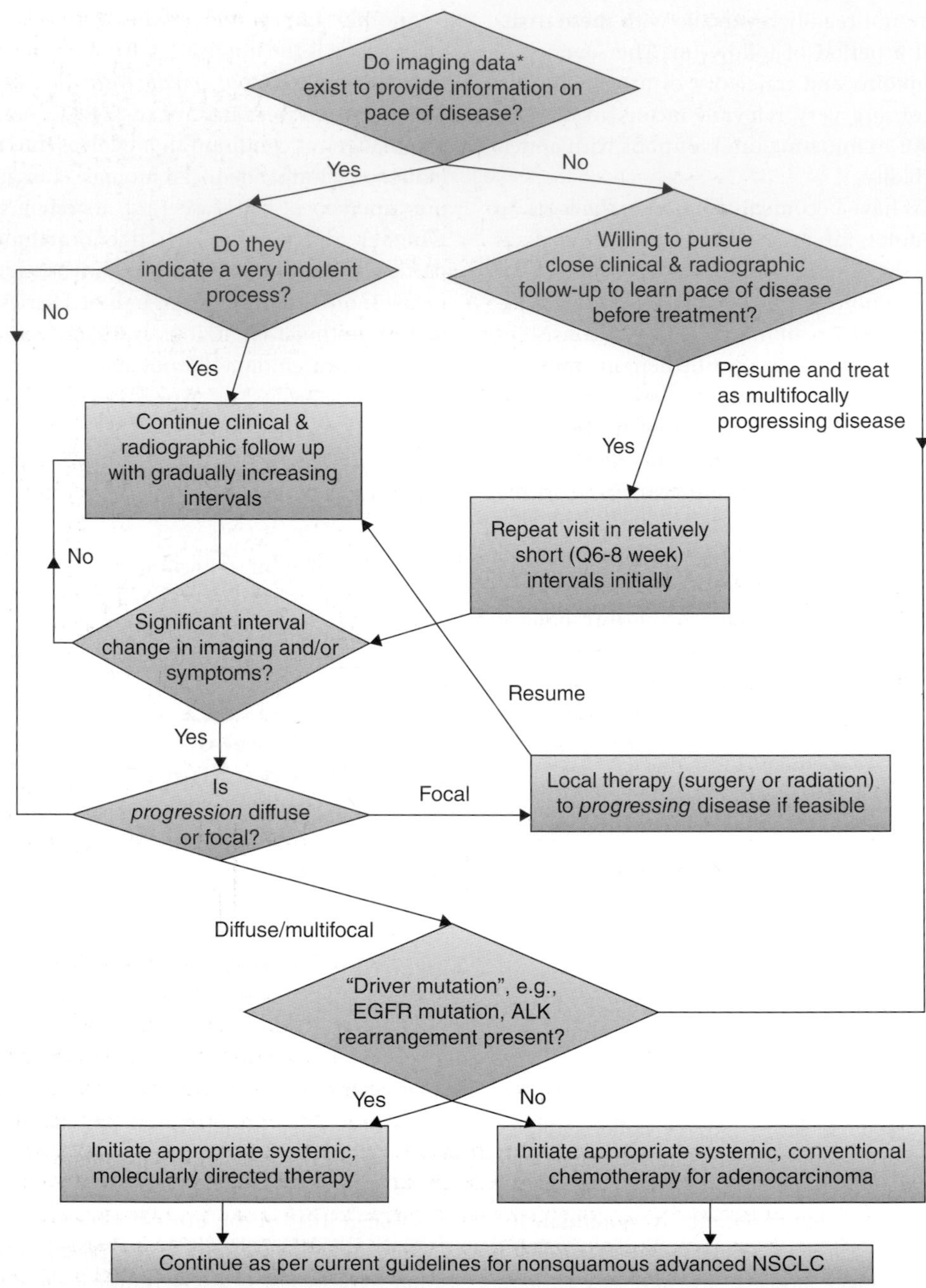

Figure 9.2 Proposed algorithm for management of asymptomatic multifocal BAC.

compared with patients who shared the same stage in the 6th edition of the AJCC staging system. However, it is important to note that the lower stage does not imply that the biology of the underlying disease clearly makes local therapy an optimal approach. Patients with AIS/BAC histology demonstrate a distinct natural history and pattern of progression compared with other NSCLC histologic subtypes that makes it appropriate to consider treatment strategies as distinct compared with the recommendations for other NSCLC subtypes, but the new staging system is not predicated on evidence that patients with satellite AIS/BAC nodules in the same lobe or other lobes of the same lung clearly benefit from surgery. The staging system is based on overall survival alone, whether this is improved by surgery or not.

Several studies have demonstrated that patients with satellite nodules in the same lobe can feasibly undergo resection and demonstrate no evidence of recurrence for many years [28, 38–42]. In the face of an indolent multifocal disease process, however, patients may potentially live as well and as long with no surgery. In the absence of comparative data to direct recommendations for or away from resection, it is certainly reasonable to defer to judgment of the treating physicians, along with patient preference and consideration of performance status, patient comorbidities, and the pattern of disease, to pursue primary surgery, favor systemic therapy, or pursue a strategy of initial attentive clinical and radiographic follow-up with consideration of treatment based on the pattern of change over time.

Is the patient symptomatic, or is there any progression at a clinically significant rate?

Because the natural history of *adenocarcinoma in situ*/multifocal BAC is often extremely indolent, it is important to first clarify whether treatment with a potentially morbid therapy is indicated. While advanced BAC may present as a symptomatic and sometimes even fulminant disease, patients may also be classified as having multifocal BAC on the basis of asymptomatic, scattered subcentimeter GGNs that demonstrate a doubling time of several years and may not change perceptibly over the course of one or more years. Even in patients with larger and/or more widespread lung nodules, these radiologic findings may remain asymptomatic and minimally changing on follow-up imaging for many years.

In patients with minimally progressing multifocal BAC, it is challenging to justify therapeutic interventions accompanied by treatment-related toxicities that can only worsen patient quality of life in the setting of an asymptomatic process that poses an exceptionally minimal threat to survival over a trajectory of many years. While it is always appropriate to review a range of treatment options with an individual patient, it is critical to recognize that this situation represents a fundamentally different situation than a highly PET-avid, metastatic invasive lung adenocarcinoma that clearly demonstrates progression between scans obtained over an interval of one or a few months during the initial workup.

In many cases, patients have had a PET scan that documents a very low SUV consistent with an indolent natural history, or serial imaging that has documented extremely indolent progression over many years prior to the pursuit of a tissue diagnosis. With the benefit of hindsight to illustrate the course over many years, the primary motivation for intervention is often based on patient and/or physician anxiety or is reflexive, based on a tissue diagnosis that mentions carcinoma, despite all signals suggesting that this may not be a clinically relevant threat in terms of either cancer-related symptoms or survival.

If there is evidence of progression at a clinically significant pace, is this a unifocal (or arguably "oligo-focal") or multifocal process?

In light of the heterogeneity of the disease, it is appropriate to ask whether, even in the setting of multifocal disease, the clinically relevant progression is unifocal or multifocal. Here again, as the revised lung adenocarcinoma classification attempts to highlight, it is valuable to distinguish between an indolent process (implied by the *in situ* moniker) that may progress in the background over many years to decades and a faster-progressing process that poses a more immediate threat in terms of cancer-related symptoms and survival.

The critical distinction between progression as a more focal versus diffuse process emerges because it may be very appropriate to favor a local therapy, most commonly surgery or radiation, in the setting of *unifocal* progression, even if this is against a background of multifocal disease (Figure 9.3). While a discordantly faster growth rate than other lesions may potentially be interpreted as sufficient evidence of unique biology in the progressing lesion, additional evidence may be available in terms of a transition from nonsolid to solid, greater metabolic uptake on PET, and/or evidence of invasive carcinoma based on a biopsy of the progressing lesion.

Functionally, unifocal progression may be interpreted as analogous to a solitary lesion. While the oncology community has historically defined multifocal BAC as clearly stage IV and therefore appropriately limited to systemic therapies, it is helpful to consider the implications of the revised classification. In the setting of a diffuse premalignant *in situ* process, the presence of a solitary focus of clinically significant progression against a background of minimal change should not preclude local treatment of the focus of progression. The central issue is whether a solitary area of progression is estimated to be the likely driver of a patient's prognosis, or alternatively, whether it is more likely that diffuse progression aside from the leading area of progression is likely to limit a patient's quality of life and/or survival. This is essentially a question of the differential growth rate between the leading area of progression and additional areas of disease: if the difference is very significant, it is quite appropriate to consider local therapy, even if there are additional lung lesions detectable.

Approach to unifocal progression in the setting of multifocal disease

The question of whether to pursue surgery, radiation, or an alternative local therapy such as radiofrequency ablation, cryotherapy, or another less established intervention may be approached in essentially the same way as someone who does not have background lesions consistent with multifocal disease, as long as the background lesions demonstrate a very indolent growth pattern. A recently published single center series [43] demonstrated that among 39 patients with suspected multifocal BAC but a single "dominant nodule", only 9 patients (23%) demonstrated radiographic progression of an unresected nodule over a mean duration of followup of over 30 months.

Given the significant risk of multifocal progression in the future f compared with patients who have no visible lesions, the potential to treat definitively with stereotactic body radiation therapy (SBRT) has emerged as an appealing option with minimal morbidity and a realistic potential for definitive treatment here. In a setting in which the value of local therapy remains poorly established, there may be a particular value to interventions that are associated with minimal risk. Analogous to the well described clinical setting of "precocious metastasis" that is sometimes associated with very prolonged survival following local therapy of the solitary metastatic focus [44, 45], this situation may be considered as "precocious progression" and approached similarly.

In an era of minimally invasive video-assisted thoracoscopic (VATS) surgery and greater availability of stereotactic radiosurgery (SRS), it is increasingly feasible and even tempting to pursue serial local therapies for multifocal disease that demonstrate metachronous multifocal progression over time. While this may be a very reasonable and even optimal approach if the interval between treatments is measured in years and treatments are limited to areas of demonstrated progression and not just identifiable, stable GGNs, there is a danger that may appear in clinical practice of multiple resections and/or radiation-directed treatments for what is, in essence, truly diffuse and multifocal progression if these lesions demonstrate changes over an interval of only several months.

It is necessary to acknowledge that there are no evidence-based guidelines to dictate a doubling time or interval for which it is appropriate to recommend serial local therapies. However, the value of serial local interventions is dubious if progression in multiple lesions is demonstrated over a course of less than a year. Moreover, there is a very real risk that the functional loss of significant amounts of functional lung parenchyma from serial surgeries or radiation treatments may lead to an overall harm of the patient if further progression within the lungs is very likely to lead to more loss of functional lung tissue. It is regrettable to have patients undergo resections of two lobes or a pneumonectomy for a process that should, on careful reflection, be recognized as highly likely to demonstrate multifocal progression.

Similarly, isolated small series have described the potential to pursue lung transplantation surgery for patients with pneumonic BAC or multifocal BAC [46–51]. Though they note encouraging short-term results, recurrence has been a very common outcome with prolonged follow up [47, 52]. Nevertheless, data from the United Network for Organ Sharing Registry notes a 5–7 year posttransplant survival of 57% among a total of 29 patients who underwent lung transplantation for multifocal BAC, compared with 50% for the entire population of lung transplant recipients. Overall, while the role for lung transplantation for patients with advanced BAC remains undefined, this is not a strategy amenable to widespread application.

As noted above, several groups have also reported on the feasibility of multiple resections, either synchronously or sequentially, for multifocal lung nodules [28, 38–42]. These series have not distinguished between lesions that are growing at a clinically significant rate and those that are visible but demonstrate little or no progression over prolonged follow-up. Notably, the surgical literature largely refers to such cases as separate primary tumors, often citing the circular argument that those patients who demonstrate favorable prognosis must by definition have had separate primary cancers, rather than considering that this is actually an indolent clonal but multifocal process. Unfortunately, recurrence of lung nodules is a common occurrence after surgery for multifocal disease [34, 53].

It is critical to recognize that BAC may often follow an indolent pattern of progression that would be associated with a favorable outcome in the short term whether *any* intervention is pursued or not. In addition, the patients offered such interventions may well be subject to selection bias and be uncharacteristically young and fit or have a disease indolent enough to be amenable to traveling for opinions at multiple centers. It therefore remains unknown whether more heroic interventions in the setting of multifocal BAC translate to clinical benefit or whether such patients are likely to do unusually well regardless of treatment, perhaps specifically enriched by selection bias for these more aggressive interventions.

In this setting, it is important to highlight the distinction between what *can be done* and what *should be done*. Though many patients and physicians may feel a bias toward pursuing the most aggressive strategy possible, overtreatment has a very real potential to cause harm if local therapies are truly futile because they are applied in a setting of multifocally progressing disease. Nevertheless, if we consider specifically the pattern of progression in an individual case, multifocal BAC arguably represents a setting in which a local therapy may be quite defensible and even optimal if considered judiciously for selected patients.

Palliative surgery

In rare cases, surgery may be a consideration as a palliative intervention even if more diffuse progression is seen. Particularly in the unique setting of "pneumonic BAC", a clinical picture in which a patient demonstrates an extensive infiltration that looks extremely consistent with pneumonia involving one or more lobes (Figure 9.1c), surgery may be considered as a palliative intervention to alleviate severe cough, bronchorrhea, or dyspnea caused by "shunting", where blood perfusing these extensively infiltrated areas of lung is not aerated. Though progression shortly after surgery is the pattern most typically seen in such cases [54], isolated reports have supported the concept of palliative surgery as a means of controlling severe symptoms in patients without other appealing treatment options [55, 56].

Systemic therapy for multifocal BAC

Because of the potential for AIS/BAC to demonstrate a very indolent natural history, an initial

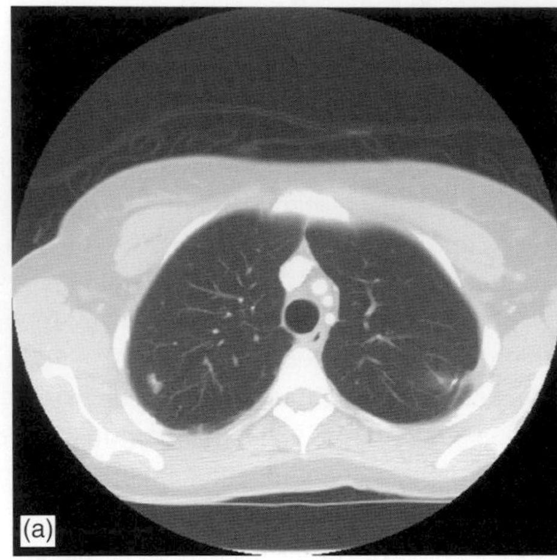

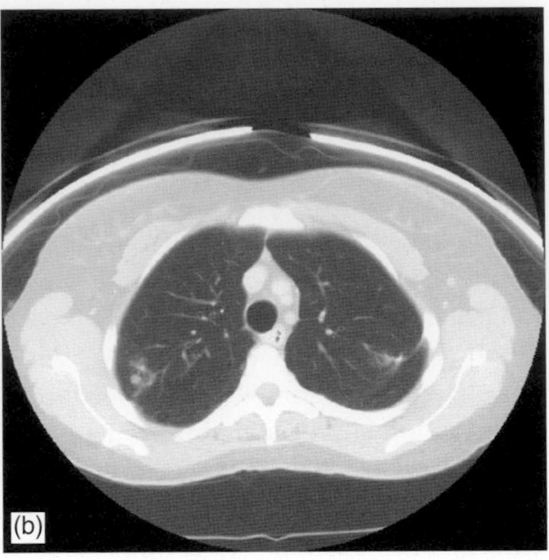

Figure 9.3 Progression over 17 months (from A to B) of a single focus of disease in the right upper lobe of a in a woman with multifocal BAC. All other lesions remained stable over this interval. She was treated with stereotactic body radiation therapy (SBRT) to the only lesion demonstrating appreciable interval progression.

question is whether immediate treatment with systemic therapy is clearly indicated, even with multifocal disease and a more diffuse pattern of progression. Whether imaging demonstrates a few limited foci of asymptomatic subcentimeter GGNs or a more extensive pattern of disease visible on CT imaging, it is appropriate to consider an interval of clinical and radiologic follow-up without immediate treatment in asymptomatic or minimally symptomatic patients. If a slow pace of interval change on scans obtained prior to diagnosis is available, this can often provide confidence that rapid radiologic change and clinical decline during initial observation with a repeat CT scan in 6–8 weeks is very unlikely. Though resistance from anxious patients (and physicians) may limit the application of this strategy, many patients can avoid treatment-related side effects for months or years, while the additional observation can provide valuable insight into the natural history for an individual patient's case. Particularly if patients are instructed to convey any significant change in symptoms, an initial period of attentive follow up is extremely unlikely to obviate the opportunity for the treatment options available.

Similarly, it is helpful to avoid discarding a generally effective therapy prematurely, based on the appearance of an equivocal small nodule or subtle progression of existing GGNs. If the natural history of multifocal BAC is likely to follow a trajectory of several years, whether due to effective therapy, the biology of the underlying disease, or both, it is easy to exhaust multiple appealing treatment options long before a patient has a decline in performance status or diminished motivation to receive further therapy. While it is appropriate to recognize clinically significant progression and not continue to administer clearly futile therapy, it is also optimal to be resistant to discontinuing a well-tolerated treatment that is associated with very modest, equivocal progression in an era in which the high resolution of our scans may document clinically irrelevant progression based on subtle appearance of new tiny lesions or minimal interval growth or PET-identified increased hypermetabolism in existing lung lesions.

Historically, multifocal BAC has not been consistently distinguished from other subtypes of NSCLC in trials of systemic therapy for advanced NSCLC. In most cases, patients with multifocal BAC have been eligible for trials for a broad range of NSCLC subtypes, despite demonstrating a more favorable prognosis for this stage compared with patients with metastatic invasive adenocarcinoma [57].

The more favorable prognosis of patients with multifocal BAC is also now reflected in the most recent revision of the AJCC staging system for NSCLC, which designates disease outside of a single lung but within the chest as M1a disease, which is associated with a more favorable prognosis than is seen in stage M1b, defined by metastatic spread outside of the chest. While this change reflecting superior survival in patients with cancer limited to the chest includes patients with pleural effusions and/or pleural implants, many of the patients with stage M1a NSCLC in the database that led to the staging revision [37] had what was considered to be multifocal BAC, associated with a relatively indolent pattern of disease and a comparably favorable survival compared with other NSCLC subtypes presenting with stage IV disease [57–59].

Importantly, the definition of BAC in both retrospective and prospective clinical trials of systemic therapy has generally not been subject to central histologic review, instead relying on the terminology used in pathology reports or physician assignment of histology. Studies that have subjected tumor tissue to central histologic review have clearly demonstrated that there is considerable variability in what is called BAC in practice, with a more loose use of this pathologic descriptor in broad clinical settings than is felt to be warranted by expert reviewers of lung pathology [2,60]. Studies directed at multifocal BAC have continued to generally pursue a practice of more lenient, local definition of BAC, but the work on central review of BAC pathology has underscored the heterogeneity of what is called BAC in trials of advanced NSCLC. Moreover, within the realm of advanced BAC, patients may have extremely variable natural histories and disease burdens yet still remain eligible for the same trials.

There has been a prevalent view of BAC as being unresponsive to conventional chemotherapy, or at least less responsive to chemotherapy than other NSCLC histologies. In part, this may be related to the association of greater chemo-responsiveness with fast cell turnover and disease natural history [61], but it is likely to be in part related to the difficulty in assessing response to therapy in patients whose cancer is less likely to appear as solid, discrete and measurable lesions than invasive NSCLC.

Despite the prevalent view in the oncology community that BAC is poorly responsive to chemotherapy, the limited data on the subject indicate that the response rate (RR) to conventional chemotherapy is actually comparable to that seen in other NSCLC histologic types. A retrospective review of patients treated at Mayo Clinic revealed a response rate of 32% for patients with BAC, versus 33% for patients with other NSCLC subtypes [62].

Limited prospective trial data on patients with advanced BAC also supports the view that conventional chemotherapy may have activity in BAC that is in the same range as what is expected in broader NSCLC populations. A study of single agent paclitaxel in 58 patients with advanced BAC who received by continuous infusion over 96 hours revealed a RR of 14% and stable disease (SD) in another 40%, and a median overall survival (OS) of 12 months [63]. A smaller trial of paclitaxel administered over 3 hours demonstrated a RR of 11%, with SD in another 50%, and a median OS of 8.6 months [64]. Finally, a report describes the results with a range of chemotherapy approaches given as second line therapy in 43 of 47 patients who had progressed on first line gefitinib in the French IFCT-0401 trial [65] described further below. The specific chemotherapy administered included platinum-based doublet chemotherapy in 38 (with a taxane in 29, gemcitabine in 9), five receiving single agent chemotherapy (gemcitabine in 3, pemetrexed in 2). The RR was 21% for the broad range of regimens administered, with a median PFS of 3 months. Although the small numbers preclude any conclusive thoughts on the comparison of different chemotherapeutic options, it is interesting that the RR with a platinum/taxane regimen was 28%, vs. 0% with the platinum/gemcitabine combination, and prolonged responses were seen in both patients receiving pemetrexed (PFS 10 and 32 months). Though limited to anecdotal reports, others have also noted particularly gratifying responses to pemetrexed in some patients with advanced BAC, including mucinous BAC with a pneumonic clinical picture [66,67].

Early work with oral epidermal growth factor receptor (EGFR) tyrosine kinase inhibitors (TKIs) such as gefitinib and erlotinib identified that BAC histology was among the clinico-pathologic features associated with a high probability of response to EGFR TKIs [68,69]. Combined with frequent anecdotal reports of dramatic and prolonged responses to EGFR TKIs in patients with BAC, this work led to the development of multiple trials of EGFR TKIs in advanced BAC, which all confirmed encouraging efficacy. A four-center phase II trial of erlotinib 150 orally per day in 101 patients with advanced BAC, most of whom previously untreated (N = 74), demonstrated a RR of 22% and median OS of 17 months [60]. A multicenter SWOG phase II trial of 136 patients with advanced BAC, 101 of whom were chemotherapy-naïve, administered gefitinib at 500 mg/day, yielding a RR of 17% in chemo-naïve patients and 9% among patients who had received prior chemotherapy [70]. Finally, a multicenter French study of 99 previously untreated patients with advanced BAC who received gefitinib 250 mg/day demonstrated a RR of 13%, with another 16% experiencing SD [71].

Over the last several years, however, clinical variables such as histology have largely been superseded by molecular marker results with regard to association of substantial clinical benefit from targeted therapies like EGFR TKIs. For instance, in the IPASS trial of Asian never-smokers or remote prior smokers with a lung adenocarcinoma, a very significant difference in outcome with gefitinib vs. standard chemotherapy was seen in patients with an activating mutation in the *EGFR* gene compared with those with *EGFR* wild type [72], a finding that definitively illustrated that the presence or absence of this molecular marker trumps clinical and pathologic variables in predicting clinical benefit with EGFR TKI therapy.

In terms of the potential utility of the anti-angiogenic agent bevacizumab, a SWOG follow-up phase II study to the S0126 trial of single agent gefitinib tested the combination of erlotinib and the anti-angiogenic agent bevacizumab in 78 patients with advanced BAC [73]. The results revealed a RR of 18%, with a median PFS of 5 months, and median OS of 17 months. Though not remarkably superior to the prior SWOG experience with gefitinib alone, the more recent trial included relatively few never-smokers, who were preferentially enrolled on a competing trial of the same regimen, so these results may be considered as encouraging. Nevertheless, in the absence of a prospective randomized trial, the incremental value of bevacizumab, whether added to chemotherapy or EGFR TKI-based therapy, in patients with advanced BAC otherwise remains undefined. Because such patients were eligible for the ECOG 4599 trial of carboplatin/paclitaxel with or without bevacizumab that demonstrated a survival benefit with the active drug it is certainly reasonable to include this agent in otherwise appropriate patients.

Though limited, data from studies of BAC have supported the concept that the association of BAC histology with benefit from EGFR TKIs is likely primarily due to the enrichment for patients with *EGFR* mutations among those with advanced BAC [74,75], and specifically the nonmucinous subtype of BAC [60,75–78]. *EGFR* mutations were detected in 26% of a series of 86 patients with BAC, all of whom had nonmucinous BAC (22/69 vs. 0/17) (71). Similar results were seen in smaller Italian series, in which *EGFR* mutations were seen in 30% of patients with nonmucinous and 0% of patients with mucinous BAC [54]. Finally, results from tissue from 44 of 59 Japanese patients with BAC or adenocarcinoma with BAC features revealed that *EGFR* mutations were present in 15% of patients with mucinous BAC vs. 58% with nonmucinous BAC, while *KRAS* mutations were present in 70% vs. 29%, respectively [79]. Nevertheless, recent reports have also documented the variability of molecular profiles of different lung nodules within the same patient [80–82].

These differences in molecular profiles have been associated with differences in responsiveness to EGFR TKI therapy in the trials that have evaluated this question. In the four-center study of single agent erlotinib described above [60], the RR among patients with an *EGFR* mutation was 87%, compared with 7% among those with *EGFR* wild type; the difference in median PFS was 13 vs. 2 months, respectively. Conversely, the presence of a *KRAS* mutation in this study was associated with a RR of 0%, compared with 32% in patients with *KRAS* wild type, consistent with the widely observed very low probability of objective response or significant clinical benefit from EGFR TKIs in advanced NSCLC [83–85].

A more recent French phase II trial, IFCT-0504, randomized patients with previously untreated advanced BAC to either erlotinib or standard chemotherapy carboplatin/paclitaxel, with all patients crossing over to the other therapy at progression and then receiving pemetrexed as third line therapy [86]. Among 130 eligible patients, 46% had nonmucinous BAC and 41% had mucinous BAC, with 13% undetermined subtype. This trial demonstrated a RR of 39% vs. 53%, median PFS of 3.2 vs. 6.1 months, and median OS of 20.2 vs. 16.4 months for erlotinib vs. chemotherapy, respectively. Subset analysis revealed that a significant interaction with nonmucinous vs. mucinous subtype: specifically, patients with nonmucinous BAC demonstrated a comparable PFS from the two approaches, while patients with mucinous BAC demonstrated a superior PFS with chemotherapy (HR 2.86). However, molecular marker studies were not reported, so it is very possible, if not probable, that differences in efficacy were fundamentally correlated with differences in the relative incidence of activating *EGFR* mutations in patients with nonmucinous vs. mucinous BAC.

Another recently identified driver mutation of lung cancer is a rearrangement of the *anaplastic lymphoma kinase* (*ALK*) gene. The oral ALK inhibitor crizotinib has recently been identified as an optimal systemic therapy approach for patients with an *ALK* rearrangement [87], for which this agent is now FDA approved [88]. Though only recently identified and still not well studied for individual and relatively uncommon lung cancer subtypes, several reports have highlighted that an *ALK* rearrangement is disproportionately seen in patients with adenocarcinoma with bronchiololalveolar features [89, 90].

In summary, though data of any systemic therapies specifically for patients with multifocal BAC remains limited, the association in advanced BAC of dramatic and prolonged responses to EGFR TKIs with the presence of an activating mutation in the *EGFR* gene and the absence of a *KRAS* mutation strongly suggests that such patients be approached in the same way as other patients with advanced NSCLC. Specifically, if it is determined that a patient with multifocal BAC has symptoms and/or progression that warrants initiation of systemic therapy, the optimal treatment is likely to be guided by the presence or absence of a "driver mutation," just as is the current standard of care for a stage IV invasive lung adenocarcinoma. Patients with an *EGFR* mutation or *ALK* rearrangement are most likely to demonstrate significant an objective response and significant clinical benefit from an oral EGFR or ALK inhibitor, respectively; while patients whose cancer demonstrates wild type with regard to *EGFR* or *ALK* are most appropriately directed to conventional chemotherapy as initial treatment. Importantly, clinical data available at this time do not support the view that either chemotherapy or EGFR TKI therapy is futile in patients with advanced BAC.

Bronchorrhea

As noted previously, bronchorrhea can be a severe symptom most commonly associated with the BAC subtype of lung cancer. Though consistently effective therapy has remained elusive, some of the treatment approaches that have demonstrated limited success, essentially in the form of case studies, have included corticosteroids [91, 92] and nonsteroidal anti-inflammatory drugs [93, 94]. Otherwise, the most effective intervention for managing bronchorrhea has been successful treatment of the underlying disease, primarily with systemic therapy such as an EGFR TKI [95–97]. Successful treatment of bronchorrhea with crizotinib in *ALK*-positive patients with mucinous BAC have also been seen in anecdotal cases from clinical practice.

In some cases, surgery has been pursued as a palliative intervention, with mixed success [13, 98].

Overall, bronchorrhea remains a difficult symptom to manage and one for which there is no recognized beneficial intervention aside from effective treatment of the underlying BAC process, when possible.

Conclusions

Though the latest reclassification of lung adenocarcinoma [1] favors no longer using the term bronchioloalveolar carcinoma, it almost exclusively discusses small and solitary lesions and provides very little discussion or insight about the multifocal disease process recognized clinically as advanced BAC. Though recognized in part for its significant variability in natural history and response to therapy, it is characterized as a distinct clinical entity by its significant potential to follow an indolent course, even when multifocal, and for its association with a relatively high incidence of *EGFR* mutations that are associated with often dramatic and prolonged responses to EGFR TKIs.

In light of the potentially indolent progression of multifocal disease, it is often extremely valuable to determine the pace of progression for the disease in an individual patient before initiating therapy, at least in someone what does not have a significant disease burden or symptoms clearly related to their cancer. If patient and physician anxiety can be allayed by the absence of clinically significant progression on interval scans leading up to or following diagnosis, many patients will demonstrate no clinically significant progression over a prolonged period of many months or even years, with some patients never demonstrating disease progression that causes symptoms or limits survival relative to other comordities or a normal lifespan.

Once the admittedly subjective threshold clinically significant and threatening progression is demonstrated, it can be useful to distinguish advanced BAC from most other NSCLC settings by questioning whether the progression is unifocal/limited or a more diffuse process. Many patients with multifocal BAC can have a single nodule progress at a pace that is uniquely faster than a background of nodules that continue to demonstrate relatively indolent or imperceptible change. Because very indolent nodules may well prove to be clinically insignificant, they can be discounted and a patient considered for local therapy if surgery or radiation would otherwise be appropriate for this treatment approach based on the location of the progressing disease, patient performance status, and competing comorbidities.

For patients who demonstrate diffuse, multifocal progression of disease that would be broadly defined as the clinical entity of advanced BAC, treatment recommendations are the same as those that would be recommended for patients with another form of advanced lung adenocarcinoma. The best evidence currently available suggests that the widely cited high probability of response of advanced BAC, and specifically nonmucinous BAC, to EGFR TKI therapy, is predicated upon the high incidence of activating mutations in the *EGFR* gene in such patients. Therefore, whether the diagnosis is clinically or pathologically defined as nonmucinous or mucinous BAC, decisions on systemic therapy are best directed by the presence or absence of molecular driver mutations such as an *EGFR* mutation or *ALK* rearrangement that should lead to a recommendation for an EGFR TKI or ALK inhibitor, respectively, if present, or conventional chemotherapy-based treatment with or without bevacizumab if a clinically relevant driver mutation is not identified.

Because the prevailing evidence suggests that patients with advanced BAC may respond to standard chemotherapy-based treatment comparably to other patients with advanced NSCLC, it is not recommended that patients be denied the opportunity to benefit from chemotherapy based on the widely held but not evidence-based perception that such patients do not respond to standard chemotherapy. This view may well be a product, in large part, of the difficulty in assessing response radiographically in many patients with multifocal BAC.

Overall, multifocal BAC represents a clinical setting in which there is a significant risk of overtreatment that may be detrimental to the patient if it is directed by anxiety or reflexive initiation of aggressive therapy, whether local or systemic. With an extremely variable clinical course that may potentially pose no threat to quality of life or survival over an extended period, pulmonary lesions that are asymptomatic and demonstrate little or no progression may be discounted, meaning that particular focus should be paid only to clearly progressing disease, which should otherwise be approached like other forms of NSCLC. The treatment strategy should include consideration of local therapy if the disease progression is very limited, while the optimal systemic therapy should be directed by the presence or absence of clinically relevant molecular markers if progression is diffuse.

References

1 Travis WD, Brambilla E, Noguchi M, *et al.* (2011) International Association for the Study of Lung Cancer/Americal Thoracic Society/Eruopean Respiratory Society international multidisciplinary classification of lung adenocarcinoma. *J Thorac Oncol*, 6(2): 244–85.

2 Travis WD, Garg K, Franklin WA, *et al.* (2006) Bronchiolalveolar carcinoma and lung adenocarcinoma: the clinical importance and research relevance of the 2004 World Health Organization Pathologic Criteria. *J Thorac Oncol*, 1(9): S13–S19.

3 Akira M, Atagi S, Kawahara M, *et al.* (1999) High-resolution CT findings of diffuse brinchioloalveolar carcinoma in 38 patients. *AJR Am J Roentgenol*, 173: 1623–9.

4 Thompson W (2004) Bronchioloalveolar carcinoma masquerading as pneumonia. *Respir Care*, 49: 1349–53.

5 Nakanishi K, Hiroi S, Kawai T, *et al.* (1998) Bronchogenic carcinoma and coexistent bronchioalveolar epithelial hyperplasia and adenocarcinoma of the lung. *Hum Pathol*, 29: 235–9.

6 Grover FL, Piantidosi S (1989) Lung Cancer Study Group. Recurrence and survival following resection of bronchioloalveolar carcinoma of the lung – the Lung Cancer Study Group experience. *Ann Surg*, 209: 779–90.

7 Akata S, Fukushima A, Kakizaki D, *et al.* (1995) CT scanning of bronchioloalveolar carcinoma: specific appearances. *Lung Cancer*, 12: 221–30.

8 Bonomo L, Storto ML, Ciccotosto C, *et al.* (1998) Bronchioloalveolar carcinoma of the lung. *Eur Radiol*, 8: 996–1001.

9 Greco RJ, Steiner RM, Goldman S, *et al.* (1986) Bronchoalveolar cell carcinoma of the lung. *Ann Thorac Surg*, 41: 615–2.

10 Dumont P, Gasser B, Rouge C, *et al.* (1998) Bronchioloalveolar carcinoma: histopathologic study of evolution in a series of 105 surgically treated patients. *Chest*, 113: 391–5.

11 Daly RC, Trastek VF, Pairolero PC, *et al.* (1991) Bronchioloalveolar carcinoma: factors affecting survival. *Ann Thorac Surg*, 51: 368–77.

12 Chetty K, Dick C, McGovern J, *et al.* (1997) Refractory hypoxemia due to intrapulmonary shunting associated with bronchiololaveolar carcinoma. *Chest*, 111(4): 1120–1.

13 Falcoz PE, Hoan NT, Le Pimpec-Barthes F, *et al.* (2009) Severe hypoxemia due to intrapulmonary shunting requires surgery for bronchioloalveolar carcinoma. *Ann Thorac Surg*, 88(1): 287–8.

14 Venkata C, Mireles JA, Venkateshiah SB (2009) Refractory hypoxemic respiratory failure due to adenocarcinoma of the lung with predominant bronchioloalveolar carcinoma component. *Respir Care*, 54(11): 1496–9.

15 Wilson DO, Ryan A, Furhman C, *et al.* (2012) Doubling times and CT screen-detected lung cancers in the Pittsburgh Lung Screening Study. *Am J Respir Crit Care Med*, 185(1): 85–9.

16 Oda S, Awai K, Murao K, *et al.* (2011) Volume-doubling time of pulmonary nodules with ground-glass opacity at multidetector CT: Assessment with computer-aided three-dimensional volumetry. *Acad Radiol*, 18(1): 63–9.

17 Lindell RM, Hartman TE, Swensen SJ, *et al.* (2007) Five-year lung cancer screening experience: CT appearance, growth rate, location, and histologic features of 61 lung cancers. *Radiology*, 242(2): 555–62.

18 Lee KS, Jeong YJ, Han J, *et al.* (2004) T1 non-small cell lung cancer: imaging and histopathologic findings and their prognostic implications. *Radiographics*, 24(6): 1632–6.

19 Okada M, Tauchi S, Iwanaga K, *et al.* (2007) Associations among bronchioloalveolar carcinoma components, positiron emission tomographic and computed tomorgraphic findings, and malignant behavior in small lung adenocarcinomas. *J Thorac Cardiovasc Surg*, 133(6): 1448–54.

20 Lee HY, Lee KS (2011) Ground-glass opacity nodules: histopathology, imaging evaluation, and clinical implications. *J Thorac Imaging*, 26(2): 106–18.

21 Sun JS, Park KJ, Sheen SS, *et al.* (2009) Clinical usefulness of fluorodeoxyglucose (FDG)-PET maximal standardized uptake value (SUV) in combination with CT features for the differentiation of adenocarcinoma with a bronchioloalveolar carcinoma from other subtypes of non-small cell lung cancer. *Lung Cancer*, 66(2): 205–10.

22 Aquino SL, Halpern EF, Kuester LB, *et al.* (2007) FDG-PET and CT features of non-small cell lung cancer based on tumor type. *Int J Mol Med*, 19(3): 495–9.
23 Huang TW, Lin LF, Hsieh CM, *et al.* (2012) Positron emission tomography in bronchioloalveolar carcinoma of the lung. *Eur J Surg Oncol*, 38(12): 1156–60.
24 Storey CF, Knudtson KP, Lawrence BJ (1953) Bronchiolar ("alveolar cell") carcinoma of the lung. *J Thorac Surg*, 26: 331–406.
25 Russell PA, Wainer Z, Wright G, *et al.* (2011) Does lung adenocarcinoma subtype predict survival? A clinicopathologic study based on the new International Association for the Study of Lung Cancer/American Thoracic Society/European Respiratory Society international multidisciplinary lung adenocarcinoma classification. *J Thorac Oncol*, 6: 1496–1504.
26 Wislez M, Beer DG, Wistuba I, *et al.* (2006) Molecular biology, genomics, and proteomics in bronchioloalveolar carcinoma. *J Thorac Oncol*, 1(9): S8–S12.
27 Westra WH, Baas IO, Hruban RH, *et al.* (1996) K-ras oncogene activation in atypical alveolar hyperplasias of the human lung. *Cancer Res*, 56(9): 2224–8.
28 Nakata M, Sawada S, Yamashita M, *et al.* (2004) Surgical treatments for multiple primary adenocarcinoma of the lung. *Ann Thorac Surg*, 78(4): 1194–9.
29 Osaki T, Sugio K, Hanagiri T, *et al.* (2003) Survival and prognostic factors of surgically resected T4 non-small cell lung cancer. *Ann Thorac Surg*, 75(6): 1745–51.
30 Rao J, Sayeed RA, Tomaszek S, Fischer S, *et al.* (2007) Prognostic factors in resected satellite-nodule T4 non-small cell lung cancer. *Ann Thorac Surg*, 84(3): 934–8.
31 Pennathur A, Lindeman B, Ferson P, *et al.* (2009) Surgical resection is justified in non-small cell lung cancer patients with node negative T4 satellite lesions. *Ann Thorac Surg*, 87(3): 893–9.
32 Volpino P, Cavallaro A, Cangemi R, *et al.* (2003) Comparative analysis of clinical features and prognostic factors in resected bronchioloalveolar carcinoma and adenocarcinoma of the lung. *Anticancer Res*, 23(6D): 4959–65.
33 Park JH, Lee KS, Kim JH, *et al.* (2009) Malignant pure pulmonary ground-glass opacity nodules; prognostic implications. *Korean J Radiol*, 10(1): 12–20.
34 Rusch VW, Tsuchiya R, Tsuboi M, *et al.* (2006) Surgery for bronchioloalveolar carcinoma and "very early" adenocarcinoma: an evolving standard of care? *J Thorac Oncol*, 1(9 Suppl): S27–31.
35 Lin ZC, Long H, Rong TH, *et al.* (2006) Surgical treatment efficacy of bronchioloalveolar carcinoma: a retrospective analysis of 130 patients. *Chinese J Cancer*, 25(9): 1123–6.
36 Goldstraw P, Crowley J, Chansky K, *et al.* (2007) The IASLC Lung Cancer Staging Project: proposals for the revision of the TNM stage groupings in the forthcoming (seventh) edition of the TNM classification of malignant tumours. *J Thorac Oncol*, 2(8): 706–14.
37 Rami-Porta R, Ball D, Crowley J, *et al.* (2007) The IASLC Lung Cancer Staging Project: proposals for the revision of the T descriptors in the forthcoming (seventh) edition of the TNM classification for lung cancer. *J Thorac Oncol*, 2(7): 593–602.
38 Roberts PF, Straznicka M, Lara PN, *et al.* (2003) Resection of multifocal non-small cell lung cancer when the bronchioloalveolar subtype is involved. *J Thorac Cardiovasc Surg*, 126(5): 1597–1602.
39 Mun M, Kohno T (2007) Single-stage surgical treatment of synchronous bilateral multiple lung cancer. *Ann Thorac Surg*, 83(3): 1146–51.
40 Mun M, Kohno T (2007) Efficacy of thoracoscopic resection for multifocal bronchioloalveolar carcinoma showing pure ground glass opacities of 20 mm or less in diameter. *J Thorac Cardiovasc Surg*, 134(4): 877–82.
41 Battafarano RJ, Meyers BF, Guthrie TJ, *et al.* (2002) Surgical resection of multifocal non-small cell lung cancer is associated with prolonged survival. *Ann Thorac Surg*, 74: 988–93.
42 Finley DJ, Yoshizawa A, Travis W, *et al.* (2010) Predictors of outcomes after surgical treatment of synchronous primary lung cancers. *J Thorac Oncol*, 5: 197–205.
43 Gu B, Burt BM, Merritt MD, *et al.* (2013) A dominant adenocarcioma with mutifocal ground glass lesions does not behave as advanced disease. *Ann Thorac Surg*. 96: 411–8.
44 Tanvetyanon T, Robinson LA, Schell MJ, *et al.* (2008) Outcomes of adrenalectomy for isolated syncrhonous vs. metachronous adrenal metastases in non-small cell lung cancer: a systematic review and pooled analysis. *J Clin Oncol*, 26(7): 1142–7.
45 Sofietti R, Ruda R, Mutani R (2002) Management of brain metastases. *J Neurol*, 249(10): 1357–69.
46 Zorn GL, McGifflin DC, Young KR, *et al.* (2003) Pulmonary transplantation for advanced bronchioloalveolar carcinoma. *J Thorac Cardiovasc Surg*, 125: 45–8.
47 Garver RI Jr., Zorn GL, Wu X, *et al.* (1999) Recurrence of bronchioloalveolar carcinoma in transplanted lungs. *N Engl J Med*, 340: 1071–4.
48 de Perrot M, Chernenko S, Waddell TK, *et al.* (2004) Role of lung transplantation in the treatment of bronchogenic carcinomas for patients with end-stage pulmonary disease. *J Clin Oncol*, 22: 4351–6.

49 Etienne B, Bertocchi M, Gamondes J-P, *et al.* (1997) Successful double-lung transplantation for bronchioloalveolar cell carcinoma. *Chest,* 112: 1423–4.

50 Geltner C, Jamnig H, Bucher B, *et al.* (2002) Lung transplantation from bronchiolo-alveolar lung carcinoma. *Lung Cancer,* 37 (Suppl 1): S27.

51 Paloyan EB, Swinnen LJ, Montoya A, *et al.* (2000) Lung transplantation for advanced bronchioloalveolar carcinoma confined to the lungs. *Transplantation,* 69: 2446–8.

52 Shin MS, Ho K-J (2004) Recurrent bronchioloalveolar carcinoma after lung transplantation: Radiographic and histologic features of the primary and recurrence. *J Thorac Imaging,* 19: 79–81.

53 Ebright MI, Zakowski MF, Martin J, *et al.* (2002) Clinical pattern and pathologic stage but not histologic features predict outcome for bronchioloalveolar carcinoma. *Ann Thorac Surg,* 74(5): 1640–6.

54 Casali C, Rossi G, Marchioni A, *et al.* (2010) A single institution-based retrospective study of surgically treated bronchioloalveolar adenocarcinoma of the lung: clinicopathologic analysis, molecular features, and possible pitfalls in routine practice. *J Thorac Oncol,* 5(6): 830–6.

55 Barlesi F, Doddoli C, Thomas P, *et al.* (2001) Bilateral bronchioloalveolar lung carcinoma: Is there a place for palliative pneumonectomy? *Eur J Cardiothorac Surg,* 20: 1113–16.

56 Takao M, Takagi T, Suzuki H, *et al.* (2010) Resection of mucinous lung adenocarcinoma presenting with intractable bronchorrhea. *J Thorac Oncol,* 5(4): 576–8.

57 Breathnach OS, Ishibe N, Williams J, *et al.* (1999) Clinical features of patients with stage IIIB and IV bronchioloalveolar carcinoma of the lung. *Cancer.* 86 (7): 1165–73.

58 Zell JA, Ou SHI, Ziogas A, *et al.* (2007) Validation of the proposed International Association for the Study of Lung Cancer non-small cell lung cancer staging system revisions for advanced bronchioloalveolar carcinoma using data from the California Cancer Registry. *J Thorac Oncol,* 2(12): 1078–85.

59 Chansky K, Sculier JP, Crowley JJ, *et al.* (2009) The International Association for the Study of Lung Cancer Staging Project: prognostic factors and pathologic TNM stage in surgically managed non-small cell lung cancer. *J Thorac Oncol,* 4(7): 792–801.

60 Miller VA, Riely GJ, Zakowski MF, *et al.* (2008) Molecular characteristics of bronchioloalveolar carcinoma and adenocarcinoma, bronchioloalveolar subtype, predict response to erlotinib. *J Clin Oncol,* 26(9): 1472–8.

61 Chu E, DeVita VT (2001) Principles of cancer management: Chemotherapy. In VT DeVita, Jr, S Helman, SA Ronsenberg (eds), *Cancer: Principals and Practice of Oncology,* 6th edn. Lippincott Williams & Wilkins, Philadelphia, pp. 289–306.

62 Feldman ER, Eagan RT, Schaid DJ (1992) Metastatic bronchiolalveolar carcinoma and metastatic adencoarcinoma of the lung: clinical manifestations, chemotherapeutic responses, and prognosis. *Mayo Clin Proc,* 67(1): 27–32.

63 West HL, Crowley JJ, Vance RB, et al. (2005) Advanced brocnhioloalveolar carcinoma: A phase II trial of paclitaxel by 96-hour infusion (SWOG 9714). *Annals of Oncology,* 16: 1076–80.

64 Scagliotti GV, Smit E, Bosque L, *et al.* (2005) A phase II study of paclitaxel in advanced bronchioloalveolar carcinoma (EORTC trial 08956). *Lung Cancer,* 50: 91–6.

65 Duruisseaux M, Baudrin L, Quoix E, *et al.* (2012) Chemotherapy effectiveness after first-line gefitinib treatment for advanced lepidic predominant adenocarcinoma (formerly advanced bronchioloalveolar carcinoma): exploratory analysis of the IFCT-0401 trial. *J Thorac Oncol,* 7(9): 1423–31.

66 Garfield D Franklin W (2011). Dramatic response to pemetrexed in a patient with pneumonic-type mucinous bronchioloalveolar carcinoma. *J Thorac Oncol,* 6(2): 397–8.

67 Okuda C, Kim YH, Takeuchi K, *et al.* (2011) Successful treatment with pemetrexed in a patient with mucinous bronchioloalveolar carcinoma: long-term response duration with mild toxicity. *J Thorac Oncol,* 6(3): 641–2.

68 Miller VA, Kris MG, Shah N, *et al.* (2004) Bronchioloalveolar pathologic subtype and smoking history predict sensitivity to gefitinib in advanced non-small-cell lung cancer. *J Clin Oncol,* 22(6): 1103–9.

69 Hsieh RK, Lim HK, Kuo HT, *et al.* (2005) Female sex and bronchioloalveolar subtype predict EGFR mutations in non-small cell lung cancer. *Chest,* 128(1): 317–21.

70 West HL, Franklin W, McCoy J, *et al.* (2006) Gefitinib therapy in advanced bronchioloalveolar carcinoma: Southwest Oncology Group Study S0126. *J Clin Oncol,* 24(12): 1807–13.

71 Cadranel J, Quoix E, Baudrin L, *et al.*, IFCT-0401 Trial Group. (2009) IFCT-0401 Trial: a phase II study of gefitinib administered as first-line treatment in advanced

adenocarcinoma with bronchioloalveolar carcinoma subtype. *J Thorac Oncol*, 4(4): 1126–35.

72 Mok TS, Wu Y-L, Thongprasert S, *et al.* (2009) Gefitinib or carboplatin-paclitaxel in pulmonary adenocarcinoma. *New Engl J Med*, 361: 947–57.

73 West H, Moon J, Hirsch FR, *et al.* (2012) SWOG 0635 and S0636: Phase II trials in advanced-stage NSCLC or erlotinib (OSI-774) and bevacizumab in bronchioloalveolar carcinoma (BAC) and adenocarcinoma with BAC features (adenoBAC), and in never-smokers with primary NSCLC adenocarcinoma. *J Clin Oncol*, 30(suppl): A#7517.

74 Marchetti A, Martella C, Felicioni L, *et al.* (2005) EGFR mutations in non-small-cell lung cancer: analysis of a large series of cases and development of a rapid and sensitive method for diagnostic screening with potential implications in pharmacologic treatment. *J Clin Oncol*, 23(4): 857–65.

75 Sun PL, Seol H, Lee HJ, *et al.* (2012) High incidence of EGFR mutations in Korean men smokers with no intratumoral heterogeneity of lung adenocarcinomas: correlation with histologic subtypes, EGFR/TTF-1 expressions, and clinical features. *J Thorac Oncol*, 7(2): 323–30.

76 Garfield DH, Cadranel J, West HL (2008) Bronchioloalveolar carcinoma: the case for two diseases. *Clin Lung Cancer*, 9(1): 24–9.

77 Matsumoto S, Iwakawa R, Kohno T, *et al.* (2006) Frequent EGFR mutations in noninvasive bronchioloalveolar carcinoma. *Int J Cancer*, 118(10): 2498–2504.

78 Sakuma Y, Matsukuma S, Yoshihara M, *et al.* (2007) Distinctive evaluation of nonmucinous and mucinous subtypes of bronchioloalveolar carcinomas in EGFR and K-ras gene-mutation analyses for Japanese lung adenocarcinomas: Confirmation of the correlations with histologic subtypes and gene mutations. *Am J Clin Pathol*, 128(1): 100–8.

79 Hata A, Katakami N, Fujita S, *et al.* (2010) Frequency of EGFR and KRAS mutations in Japanese patients with lung adenocarcinoma with features of the mucinous subtype of bronchioloalveolar carcinoma. *J Thorac Oncol*, 5(8): 1197–1200.

80 Chen Z-Y, Zhong W-Z, Chang X-C, *et al.* (2012) EGFR mutation heterogeneity and the mixed response to EGFR tyrosine kinase inhibitors of lung adenocarcinomas. *Oncologist*, 17: 978–85.

81 Nakano H, Soda H, Takasu M, *et al.* (2008) Heterogeneity of epidermal growth factor receptor mutations within a mixed adenocarcinoma lung nodule. *Lung Cancer*, 60(1): 136–40.

82 Ikeda K, Nomuri H, Ohba Y, *et al.* (2008) Epidermal growth factor receptor mutations in multicentric lung adenocarcinomas and atypical adenomatous hyperplasias. *J Thorac Oncol*, 3(5): 467–71.

83 Zhu CQ, da Cunha Santos G, *et al.* (2008) Role of KRAS and EGFR as biomarkers of response to erlotinib in National Cancer Institute of Cancer Clinical Trials Group Study BR.21. *J Clin Oncol*, 26: 4268–75.

84 Linardou H, Dahbreh IJ, Kanaloupiti D, *et al.* (2008) Assessment of k-RAS mutations as a mechanism associated with resistance to EGFR-targeted agents: A systematic review and meta-analysis of studies in advanced non-small-cell lung cancer and metastatic colorectal cancer. *Lancet Oncol*, 9: 962–72.

85 Brugger W, Triller N, Blasinka-Morawiec M, *et al.* (2011) Prospective molecular marker analysis of EGFR and KRAS from a randomized, placebo-controlled study of erlotinib maintenance therapy in advanced non-small cell lung cancer. *J Clin Oncol*, 29(31): 4113–20.

86 Cadranel J Gervais R, Wislez M, *et al.* (2011) IFCT-0504 trial: Mucinous (M) and nonmucinous (NM) cytologic subtypes interaction effect in first line treatment of advanced bronchioloalveolar carcinoma (BAC) by erlotinib (E) or carboplatin/paclitaxel (C/P). *J Clin Oncol*, 29(Suppl: abstr 7521): A#7521.

87 Kwak EL, Bang YJ, Camidge DR, *et al.* (2010) Anaplastic lymphoma kinase inhibition in non-small-cell lung cancer. *N Engl J Med*, 363: 1693–1703.

88 Pfizer I. (2011) Xalkori Prescribing Information. http://www.accessdata.fda.gov/drugsatfda_docs/label/2011/202570s000lbl.pdf (last accessed January 11, 2013).

89 Inamura K, Takeuchi K, Togashi Y, *et al.* (2008) EML4-ALK fusion is linked to histologic characteristics in a subset of lung cancers. *J Thorac Oncol*, 3(1): 13–17.

90 Sasaki T, Rodig SJ, Chirieac LR, Janne, PA (2010) The biology and treatment of EML4-ALK non-small cell lung cancer. *Eur J Cancer*, 46(10): 1773–80.

91 Marom ZM, Goswami SK (1991) Respiratory mucus hypersecretion (bronchorrhea): A case discussion – possible mechanisms(s) and treatment. *J Allergy Clin Immunol*, 87(6): 1050–5.

92 Nakajima T, Terashima T, Nishida J, *et al.* (2002) Treatment of bronchorrhea by corticosteroids in a case of bronchioloalveolar carcinoma producing CA19–9. *Intern Med*, 41(3): 225–8.

93 Homma S, Kawabata M, Kishi K, *et al.* (1999) Successful treatment of refractory bronchorrhea by inhaled

indomethacin in two patients with bronchioloalveolar carcinoma. *Chest*, 115(5): 1465–8.

94 Tamaoki J, Kohri K, Isono K, *et al.* (2000) Inhaled indomethacin in bronchorrhea in bronchioloalveolar carcinoma (letter). *Chest*, 117: 1213–14.

95 Kitazaki T, Fukuda M, Soda H, *et al.* (2005) Novel effects of gefitinib on mucin production in bronchioloalveolar carcinoma: two case reports. *Lung Cancer*, 49(1): 125–8.

96 Milton DT, Kris MG, Gomez JE, *et al.* (2005) Prompt control of bronchorrhea in patients with bronchioloalveolar carcinoma treated with gefitinib. *Support Care Cancer*, 13(1): 70–2.

97 Yano S, Kanematsu T, Miki T, *et al.* (2003) A report of two bronchioloalveolar carcinoma cases which were rapidly improved by treatment with the epidermal growth factor receptor tyrosine kinase inhibitor ZD1839 ("Iressa"). *Cancer Sci*, 94(5): 453–8.

98 Yokouchi H, Murata K, Murakami M, *et al.* (2012) A case of diffuse pneumonic type of mucinous adenocarcinoma treated with reduction surgery. *Gan To Kagaku Ryoho*, 39(12): 2396–8.

CHAPTER 10

Radiology and Lung Cancer Screening

Patricia de Groot[1] *and Reginald F. Munden*[2]

[1]Department of Diagnostic Radiology, The University of Texas MD Anderson Cancer Center, Houston, TX, USA
[2]Department of Radiology, The Houston Methodist Hospital, Houston, TX, USA

Introduction

Lung cancer is the leading cause of cancer mortality in the world, with more than 1.37 million deaths annually [1]. In the United States, it is responsible for just over one-quarter of all cancer deaths each year. Despite the declining incidence of lung cancer in American men since the 1980s, it is almost three times as deadly as prostate cancer, the second leading cause of male cancer deaths. In American women, lung cancer is nearly twice as lethal as breast cancer [2]. The disease burden in the US is seen disproportionately in minorities and less educated individuals [3]. In the European Union, the estimated annual toll from lung cancer in men is also approximately 25% of cancer deaths, but male lung cancer mortality has been decreasing over the last two decades. In contrast, lung cancer deaths in European women have increased 7% since 2009 and are projected to continue rising until 2020 [4]. Lung cancer 5-year survival rates within the 27 countries of the EU are quite variable, with the United Kingdom having one of the lowest in the developed world, approximately 8% survival at 5 years [5, 6]. Lung cancer incidence and mortality are also rising in China, Korea and some African nations as smoking has become more prevalent in these countries in recent decades [7].

Lung cancer is a heterogeneous disease morphologically, histologically, and with respect to behavior [8]. Multiple cell types are included within the designation, including small cell, squamous cell, large cell and adenocarcinoma of the lung. Current medical research is focused on the genomics and proteomics of tumors, and evidence shows that cell mutations in lung neoplasms have a marked effect on natural history, response to treatment and prognosis, even within the same histologic category of tumor [9].

Overall lung cancer survival is abysmally low, with an aggregate 5-year survival of 15% that has remained unchanged over decades, primarily because most lung carcinomas come to medical attention as advanced stage III or IV disease. However, treated Stage IA lung carcinoma has a considerable 5-year survival rate of over 70% [10], underscoring the need for a reliable method of identifying early stage disease.

Concept of screening

The fundamental aim of screening is to decrease disease-specific mortality by means of the screening test [11,12]. Until recently, all attempts to screen for lung cancer failed to demonstrate a statistically significant reduction in lung cancer deaths [8]. Acceptable screening tests must fulfill a number of well-established criteria to be justifiable, which had not occurred with lung cancer screening. For successful screening, the target disease must have considerable morbidity and mortality and must have a high

Lung Cancer, Fourth Edition. Edited by Jack A. Roth, Waun Ki Hong and Ritsuko U. Komaki.

prevalence in the population to be screened. It must have an established preclinical phase in which the disease is present but the patient is asymptomatic. It is also important that disease in the preclinical phase be able to be detected by the test before a critical point in the natural history, after which treatment is associated with a poorer prognosis. There must be an established effective treatment for the target disease when identified in earlier stages [11, 12].

Additionally, a screening test must be both sensitive and specific for the disease, to minimize false positive and false negative results [11, 12]. It must be accurate and reproducible. Finally, other psychosocial and economic features are required for effective screening. Procedures that are safe and painless are more likely to be acceptable to patients and clinicians, and the ease of performance and low cost are also necessary [12].

Bias

Trials to establish the validity of screening tests can be subject to several types of bias, leading to artificially inflated or possibly conflicting results. *Lead time bias* refers to diagnosis of the tested disease in the preclinical phase but the outcome is the same as if it had been diagnosed at the time clinical symptoms appeared. In other words, the time between diagnosis and death is longer, but there is no actual effect on survival. *Length time bias* is seen because of differing rates of disease progression, with indolent disease having a longer preclinical phase and increased detection rates during screening. This leads to overrepresentation of less aggressive forms of the disease, which may have better prognosis, in the screened population. Recurrent screening restricts length time bias by finding incident cancers that arise between test events.

The detection of disease that will have no effect on the life expectancy of the patient constitutes *overdiagnosis bias*. It is considered to be present when something other than the target disease is the actual cause of a patient's death [8, 11]. However, the concept of overdiagnosis is considered by some to be misleading in the context of lung cancer [13, 14]. Any lung cancer identified by screening has lethal potential based on both epidemiological and pathological evidence [15–17], even in the event that death is caused by another factor. The object screening population for lung carcinomas has competing comorbidities associated with tobacco consumption, including emphysema and cardiovascular disease. However, recent advances in understanding the natural history of adenocarcinoma, the most common type of lung cancer, suggest that length time and overdiagnosis bias may be significant in lung cancer. The mean volume doubling time of adenocarcinomas presenting as pure ground glass or subsolid lesions may be longer than 400 days in up to 27% of cases, particularly in women [18].

The accepted method to manage the effects of these limitations in a screening trial is a randomized, controlled clinical trial. Randomized controlled trials themselves are subject to drawbacks that include noncompliance by the participants and crossover, or contamination, from subjects obtaining relevant medical procedures outside the trial setting [8, 11].

Another form of bias may be inherent in voluntary screening trials: a type of *selection bias*, specifically self-selection by persons who choose to participate and undergo screening. It has also been called volunteer bias and participation bias. For instance, only 0.5% of those persons initially sent a letter of invitation finally took part in the US National Lung Screening Trial (NLST) [19]. While this may not affect comparison between the study arms of a randomized trial, it has implications for the generalizability of the study results to the population at large. A study of the Danish Lung Cancer Screening Trial (DLCST) suggests that there are significant sociodemographic and psychosocial factors that influence willingness to volunteer for screening [19].

Historical perspectives

The identification of a risk group for lung cancer occurred in 1950 when the landmark study by Doll and Hill incontrovertibly linked tobacco smoking with the development of lung carcinoma [20]. Current World Health Organization data estimates that tobacco use is responsible for 71% of global lung cancer deaths and 22% of all cancer deaths [1]. Attempts to validate effective screening measures in this high risk population began in the 1950s and continue today [21,22].

Radiographic screening

A large trial in the 1960s with 55 000 subjects in two arms differentiated by frequency of chest radiographic evaluation found that although more lung cancers and more resectable disease were identified in the group with more frequent radiographs, overall lung cancer mortality was not impacted, being very similar in both groups [22].

Four randomized clinical trials were initiated in the 1970s, three of them funded by the National Cancer Institute (NCI): the Johns Hopkins Lung Project, the Memorial Sloan Kettering Lung Project and the Mayo Lung Project [23–25]. The fourth took place in Czechoslovakia [26]. Of these, the Johns Hopkins and Memorial Sloan Kettering trials involved annual chest radiographs with and without sputum cytology (screening and control groups, respectively). The results failed to demonstrate any difference in the number of lung cancers detected, in the resectability of the disease, or in disease-specific mortality. The Mayo lung project evaluated frequency of chest radiography in conjunction with sputum analysis for screening purposes but was limited by noncompliance and crossover. Long term follow-up and analysis of the Mayo lung cohort has shown that, paradoxically, lung cancer mortality was actually slightly higher in the experimental (radiograph and sputum) arm. However, 5-year and 9-year survival in the screened group was improved. This dichotomy is attributed to a higher incidence of lung cancer in the experimental arm and possible unmeasured risk factors affecting randomization [27]. The Czech study was also based on chest radiographs together with sputum cytology performed at different intervals in the screened and nonscreened arms, and did not identify an improvement in overall lung cancer mortality based on screening [26].

Four government-funded population-based case-control studies of radiographic screening were performed in Japan in the 1990s, one each in the prefectures of Miyagi, Gunma, Niigata and Okayama [28]. Under the Japanese Health and Medical Service Law for the Elderly, annual chest screening for cancer has been available since 1987 to all persons over 40 years of age with miniature fluoro-photography (a procedure developed in 1935 similar to a frontal chest radiograph), and annual sputum cytology analysis is provided for smokers [29]. Even earlier, under the Tuberculosis Control Law of the 1950s, Japanese residents have undergone mass screening with a mini-chest X-ray annually [30]. However, despite these programs, there was insufficient evidence that the screening improved lung cancer-specific mortality, prompting initiation of the case-control projects [28]. Three of the four studies found that annual radiographic screening would reduce lung cancer deaths by statistically significant amounts. There has been hesitation, however, about applying this model to Western populations [28].

Computed tomography screening

The advent and especially the technological refinement of computed tomography (CT) of the chest has led to new efforts to establish effective screening measures. Chest CT is known to be much more sensitive than radiograph for the detection of small nodules less than 1 cm in diameter and also of nonsolid and part-solid nodules [31–33]. Low dose CT (LDCT) reduces the dose of ionizing radiation to the patient during the study, making it more feasible to employ the procedure in patients with risk factors but without known disease.

In the early to mid 1990s, three major lung cancer screening studies using low dose CT were performed in Japan [33–35], including an ambitious three-year population-based mass screening program with a mobile CT scanner undertaken in a rural Japanese prefecture [29, 33]. These studies integrated both chest fluoro-photography, performed under Japan's existing programs, and low-dose CT screening. All participants received the same screening protocol. There was no classification of high-risk populations, as smokers and nonsmokers alike were able to participate. In all of the studies, there was a large percentage of stage IA, resectable lung cancers among the identified lesions. They also showed evidence that low dose CT was more sensitive than chest radiograph for lung cancer detection. One of the more significant findings of the Japanese trials was the detection of lung cancers, primarily adenocarcinomas, in nonsmoking women. The results of these observational studies suggested an improvement in 10-year lung cancer survival rates [29].

At the same time, the Early Lung Cancer Action Project (ELCAP) was initiated in the United States. This study also incorporated conventional chest radiographs and low dose CT, and demonstrated the increased sensitivity of LDCT for lung cancer compared with radiographs, this time in a high-risk smoking population. It highlighted the value of LDCT in diagnosing early stage lung cancers, the majority of which (96%) were resectable. The study predicted that 5-year survival of the participants would be at least 80%; however, the sample size was small and the study had only a single arm [15, 36, 37]. The International-ELCAP promulgated this model and by 2005 had performed low dose CT screenings on approximately 25 000 individuals in eight countries in addition to the USA. Within this group, the majority of the lung cancers found were stage I and potentially curable [15].

The Mayo CT Screening study started in the late 1990s, using low-dose CT screening, annual sputum cytology, phlebotomy and spirometry in a high risk cohort for 5 consecutive years. Although a number of stage I lung cancers were identified during the course of the trial, the study concluded that no benefit in lung cancer mortality was observed [28]. Further, there was an exceptionally high rate of noncancerous, false-positive nodules identified during the course of the study, possibly due to endemic histoplasmosis in the geographical region of the trial [38]. A later study investigated and concluded that adherence to protocol would allow for successful CT screening in an area with endemic fungal disease, while minimizing benign biopsies [39].

None of the early trials using LDCT was able to demonstrate a benefit in disease-specific mortality or a decrease in the incidence of advanced lung cancer [40], because they were observational studies rather than randomized controlled studies.

The National Prostate, Lung, Colorectal and Ovarian (PLCO) Screening Trial was initiated in 1992 as a large randomized trial assessing screening modalities for four different malignancies. It enrolled 154 901 participants in the lung cancer screening portion of the study, which had an intervention arm offering either three or four chest radiograph screenings (for nonsmokers and ever-smokers, respectively) and a control arm with usual community care [41]. Of the trial participants, 50.5% were women. Approximately 45% were never-smokers, 42% were former smokers and 10% were active smokers. This is the only randomized controlled lung cancer screening trial and the only trial outside of Japan to include nonsmokers. The mean follow up of trial participants was 11.2 years [42]. In conjunction with the primary analysis comparing lung cancer mortality rates between the two randomized arms, there was additional evaluation of a subset of the participants who would have met eligibility criteria for the National Lung Screening Trial. The trial concluded that annual chest radiographic screening did not decrease lung cancer mortality [42].

The National Lung Screening Trial

The National Lung Screening Trial (NLST) was initiated specifically to answer the question of whether screening with low-dose CT could reduce lung cancer mortality. A randomized, controlled multicenter trial, it was launched in 2002 with collaboration between the National Cancer Institute Lung Screening Study (LSS) centers and the American College of Radiology Imaging Network (ACRIN) [43, 44]. With 53 454 participants randomized to two arms, it was sufficiently powered to detect a 20% reduction in disease-specific mortality [45].

The primary endpoint of the NLST was disease-specific mortality. Several secondary endpoints were also incorporated into the design, including lung cancer incidence and stage distribution, lung cancer survival and all-cause mortality. Additionally, the NLST-ACRIN centers are compiling data on the effects of screening and screening results on the smoking habits of trial subjects [44].

Trial design

Participants in the NLST were assigned randomly to one of two arms: annual screening with posteroanterior (PA) chest radiography or annual screening with low dose chest CT. There was a baseline examination and two additional annual screenings in each group [44]. Of the total number of participants, 26 732 received chest radiography and 26 722 received LDCT [46, 47]. Follow-up on the participants was conducted for a median duration of 6.5 years, through December 31, 2009 [47].

Chest radiographs used in the study were of several types, including screen-film, computed and digital radiographs, depending on the equipment available at each trial center. Multidetector CTs were used for all LDCT examinations, at first 4 channel scanners but over time 16 and 64 channel machines were also utilized. All radiographic and CT systems were certified by the NLST, met the trial protocol requirements and guidelines set out by the American College of Radiology (ACR) [44]. A rigorous quality assurance process was included in the trial protocol [43].

Radiologists interpreting the screening chest radiographs and LDCT examinations at each of the 33 trial centers were approved by the NLST [44]. The majority of them were specialists in thoracic radiology. They received specific training and quality assurance education in interpretation and reporting of the screening studies [48].

Participant cohort

Recruitment of volunteers was conducted via targeted mailings, public service television, radio and newspaper advertisements, internet advertising and community outreach [46]. Particular efforts were made to enroll minority participants based on regional demographics, through targeted mailings, advertisements and community ambassadors in order to have the trial population represent the general US population at high risk for lung cancer.

Study volunteers were eligible for trial participation if between 55 and 74 years of age, with a minimum of 30 pack-years of smoking. Former smokers meeting the 30 pack-year requirement could participate if they had quit within the previous 15 years [47]. Exclusion criteria included a previous diagnosis of lung cancer, history of any cancer other than nonmelanoma skin cancers and certain carcinomas *in situ* within the preceding 5 years, and prior lung surgery. Participation in another cancer screening trial, cancer prevention trial or having a chest CT within the previous 18 months was not allowed. Also excluded were those with home oxygen supplementation and metallic implants such as pacemakers. Symptoms of hemoptysis, an unexplained 15 pound weight loss, or a respiratory infection treated in the previous 12 weeks precluded enrollment [44].

Of the 55 456 participants, 31 533 (59%) were men. The majority, 39 234 (73%), were less than 65 years old. A total of 27 677 (52%) were former smokers; the rest were active smokers. Approximately 91% of participants were white, 4.4% were black and 1.7% were Hispanic or Latino [46]. Randomization between the two arms produced equivalent demographics. In comparison with the total high-risk population in the US, the trial participants tended to be younger in age. More of them were former rather than current smokers, and the level of education was higher, with 32% of the volunteers having at least a college degree.

Results

For each of the three screening rounds, there was a higher rate of positive findings in the LDCT group compared with the radiography group. The number of lung cancers found in the LDCT group was 1,060, compared with 941 in the radiography group. Of these, 367 carcinomas in the LDCT group and 525 in the CXR arm presented in patients after the screening ended or were missed during the screening and subsequently diagnosed in the years after the three screenings. The higher number of cancers found later in the radiograph group suggests that some cancers were missed by radiograph that would not have been missed on LDCT. The low dose CT group had more adenocarcinomas, particularly of the lepidic pattern. Fewer stage IV cancers were found in the LDCT group at the 2nd and 3rd screenings, leading to a better stage distribution vis-à-vis treatment options and prognosis [47].

Of all CT screenings, 24% had findings suggestive of lung cancer and were therefore classified as a positive screen. Of these cases, 96% were determined to be false positive screens. Additionally, in the CT arm, at least one positive CT was reported in 39% of the participants. These high rates have raised concern among some as to the effectiveness of screening in the general population. The cost effectiveness of lung cancer screening in the NLST is currently under review and may answer some of these concerns [47].

Of the cancers diagnosed by CT screening, 52% were Stage IA and 11.2% were Stage 1B compared to chest radiograph screening with 33% Stage 1A and 15% Stage 1B cancers. The complications from screening with CT were very low, 0.4%. In all, the NLST proved to meet the requirements for an effective screening test and programs are being implemented throughout the US [47].

The lower number of lung cancer deaths in the low-dose CT group represents a relative decrease in the lung cancer specific mortality rate of 20%. All-cause mortality was also improved in the low dose CT group, a 6.7% reduction compared with the radiography group. In light of these positive results, the trial was concluded in advance of the original plan [47].

Ongoing lung cancer screening trials and programs

There are a number of lung cancer screening trials using low-dose CT currently underway worldwide. The trial populations, inclusion and exclusion criteria, endpoints and amount of follow-up are varied. In Europe, randomized screening studies include the Nederlands-Leuvens Longkanker Screening Onderzoek (NELSON) trial in the Netherlands and Belgium; the Danish Lung Cancer Screening Trial (DLCST); Italian trials Italian Lung Cancer Computed Tomography (ITALUNG-Florence), Multicentric Italian Lung Detection (MILD), and DANTE-Milan; and the German Lung Cancer Screening Intervention (LUSI) study, a component of the European trial on the efficacy of multislice-CT for the early detection of lung cancer. These trials will publish final results in the next few years [10, 49]. A French randomized pilot trial of lung cancer screening with radiography and low dose CT, Dépiscan, published baseline results in 2007 that inform the larger trial Grandépiscan with 20 000 participants [49, 50]. The United Kingdom Lung Screen (UKLS) group is currently conducting a pilot study with 4200 subjects that will segue into a 10-year UKLS randomized controlled trial with 32 000 participants [51, 52]. The investigators in these trials have concluded that all trials will be continued, both to confirm the findings of the NLST, and to address numerous tangential questions relevant to ideal target populations for screening, optimal protocols and management of findings, and cost-effectiveness, among others [52, 53].

There is renewed interest in chest radiographic screening for lung cancer in China [54, 55]. There is better availability and lower cost associated with chest radiographs. Recent studies have attempted to better the accuracy of chest radiographic screening by using it in conjunction with a detailed self-assessment questionnaire about risk factors [54], or with computer-aided nodule detection systems [55]. In both cases, mature follow-up data is lacking.

Low dose CT lung cancer screening programs have been in place in Japan for over a decade, often administered by the government or employers. Employer sponsored programs may cover employees, retirees and their spouses aged 50 to 69 years, whereas other programs are available for community residents. A smoking history is not a prerequisite [56, 57].

Lung cancer screening recommendations in the US

In 2012 a number of groups for the first time issued guidelines recommending screening for lung cancer based on the positive results of the NLST. The National Comprehensive Cancer Network (NCCN) recommendations include annual LDCT screening for high risk patients aged 55–74 years who meet the NLST inclusion and exclusion criteria, and for adults 50 years and older with at least a 20 pack-year tobacco history in conjunction with one of the other known risk factors for lung cancer. Lung cancer survivors are not included in a screening group under the NCCN guidelines [58].

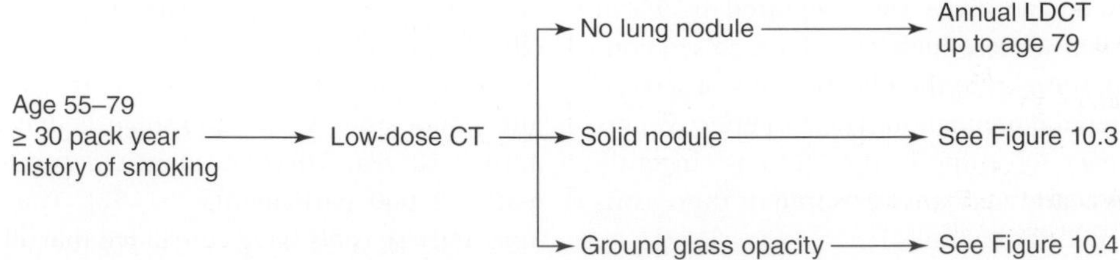

Figure 10.1 AATS lung cancer screening guidelines category 1 for highest risk. *CT*, Computed tomography; *LDCT*, low dose computed tomography.
Source: Reprinted from Jaklitsch MT *et al.* (2012) The American Association for Thoracic Surgery guidelines for lung cancer screening using low-dose computed tomography scans for lung cancer survivors and other high-risk groups, *J Thorac Cardiovasc Surg*, 144: 35, with permission from Elsevier.

Lung cancer screening with low-dose CT is not recommended by the NCCN for either moderate risk or low risk individuals, a category 2A recommendation. Patients over 50 years old with 20 pack-years of smoking or secondhand smoke exposure but without additional risk factors are considered to have moderate risk. The low risk category includes those under 50 years of age and/or a smoking history less than 20 pack-years [58].

The American Association for Thoracic Surgery (AATS) guidelines published in 2012 contain similar recommendations, but include lung cancer survivors as an at-risk population for screening purposes [59]. Tier 1 Guidelines for the highest risk population recommends annual lung cancer screening with low-dose CT beginning at age 55 and continuing to age 79 for current or former smokers with a 30 pack-year smoking history. This is considered to have level 1 evidence support [59] (see Figure 10.1).

The AATS Tier 2 Guidelines for lung cancer survivors recommends annual LDCT screening in patients who have already completed 4 years of radiologic surveillance following treatment for primary lung carcinoma without evidence of recurrence or metastatic disease. Tier 2 recommendations also apply to younger persons beginning at 50 years of age with at least a 20 pack-year smoking history and additional factors that increase the individual's risk of developing lung cancer within 5 years by at least 5%. Examples of risk factors include environmental or occupational exposures, COPD, prior radiation therapy or family history. Tier 2 recommendations are supported by level 2 evidence and have unanimous approval of the AATS Task Force [59] (see Figure 10.2).

Other organizations have also issued recommendations, including the American Cancer Society (ACS), the American Lung Association (ALA), and the American College of Chest Physicians (ACCP) and American Society of Clinical Oncology (ASCO) in a joint recommendation. They all follow the NLST guidelines and recommend annual LDCT screening only for high-risk individuals who meet the exact NLST inclusion and exclusion criteria. Further, most of these bodies recommend that screening candidates be referred only to centers that can provide the experienced, multidisciplinary care afforded to NLST participants [60].

Nodule detection and management

Low dose CT has greater sensitivity to detect pulmonary abnormalities than chest radiograph, both in terms of size and density [36]. Small nodules less than 1 cm are better seen on CT, as are nodules of ground glass or mixed ground glass and solid density. The malignant potential of nodules is related to both size and density.

Very small noncalcified solid nodules less than 5 mm have a smaller than 1% likelihood of being malignant. Nodules between 8 and 20 mm diameter have an 18% chance, and solid nodules greater than 20 mm have a 50% chance of malignancy [61]. Interval increase in size of a nodule at follow-up is a sign that favors malignant disease, although a very

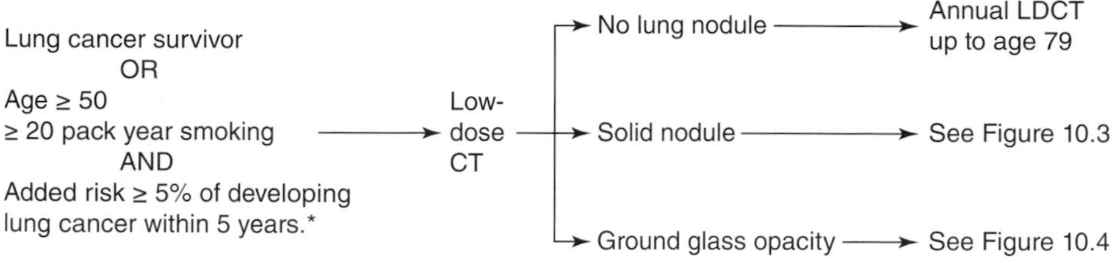

Figure 10.2 AATS lung cancer screening guidelines for combined risk or lung cancer survivor. *CT*, Computed tomography; *LDCT*, low-dose computed tomography; *COPD*, chronic obstructive pulmonary disease; *FEV_1*, forced expiratory volume in 1 second.
Source: Reprinted from Jaklitsch MT *et al.* (2012) The American Association for Thoracic Surgery guidelines for lung cancer screening using low-dose computed tomography scans for lung cancer survivors and other high-risk groups, *J Thorac Cardiovasc Surg*, 144: 35, with permission from Elsevier.

rapid increase may also indicate an infectious etiology. Protocols for follow-up of solid indeterminate nodules are well-established [61, 62]. The Fleischner Society recommends that high-risk patients having a history of smoking with small nodules less than or equal to 4 mm should receive a single follow-up at 12 months following the baseline examination; if unchanged, no further follow-up is needed. For nodules >4–6 mm, follow-up at 6–12 months and then at 18–24 months if unchanged. Nodules >6–8 mm should be followed at 3–6 months, 9–12 months and at 24 months to establish 2-year stability. Nodules greater than 8 mm should be reassessed at 3, 9 and 24 months with CT and/or with dynamic perfusion CT, PET/CT or biopsy [61] (see Figures 10.3 and 10.4 for AATS nodule management guidelines).

Overall, however, solid nodules have less malignant potential (7%) compared with ground glass nodules (18%). Part ground glass/part solid nodules have the highest malignancy rate of 63% [16].

An increasing number of adenocarcinomas of the lung present as ground glass and part-solid nodules on LDCT. There are three main categories. Pre-invasive lesions correspond with Noguchi type A and B tumors and include atypical adenomatous hyperplasia and adenocarcinoma *in situ* (AIS). The CT appearance ranges from pure ground glass opacities (GGO) to GGOs with small internal alveolar collapse. Many of these lesions have doubling times up to 2 years (see Figure 10.5). Minimally invasive adenocarcinoma with a predominantly lepidic pattern and an invasive component less than 5 mm is in the second category, and often appears as a GGO with a small solid focus. The last category is invasive adenocarcinoma of all subtypes (lepidic, acinar, papillary, micropapillary). These solid nodules may have lobulated or spiculated margins as well as air bronchograms, and correspond with some Noguchi type C tumors and Noguchi D through F categories [18, 63].

Pure GGO lesions greater than 10 mm in size that persist on follow up imaging are suspicious for AIS. PET/CT is often falsely negative in the evaluation of these lesions and needle biopsy is prone to sampling error. Any lesion with mixed solid and ground glass components is worrisome for malignancy with invasive potential and prompt work up is recommended [18, 64]. The Fleischner Society in 2013 issued the following recommendations based on size and density of the lesion. Pure GGOs of 5 mm or less do not require follow up. Solitary pure GGOs larger than 5 mm should have a repeat CT after 3 months, and if persistent and unchanged, should undergo annual surveillance for a minimum of 3 years. Single part-solid lesions

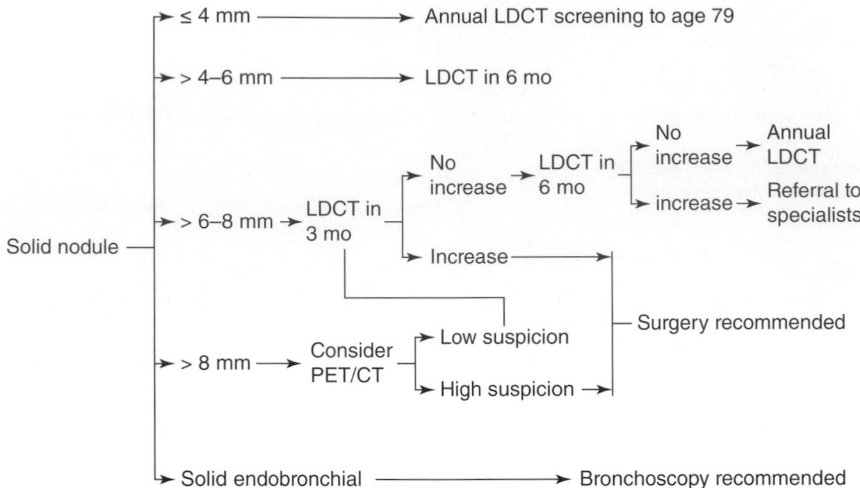

Figure 10.3 AATS lung cancer screening guidelines for solid nodules on low-dose computed tomography. *LDCT*, low-dose computed tomography; *PET/CT*, positron emission tomography/computed tomography. *Source*: Reprinted from Jaklitsch MT *et al.* (2012) The American Association for Thoracic Surgery guidelines for lung cancer screening using low-dose computed tomography scans for lung cancer survivors and other high-risk groups, *J Thorac Cardiovasc Surg*, 144: 36, with permission from Elsevier.

with a solid component greater than 5 mm should be considered malignant; a 3 month follow-up CT is advised if there is a question of infection and depending on the risk factors of the patient. When multiple ground glass lesions are present, an initial 3 month follow-up CT will confirm persistence. Management is then based on the characteristics of the dominant lesion [64] (see Figures 10.3 and 10.4 for AATS nodule management guidelines).

There has been an increase in the number of adenocarcinomas relative to squamous cell carcinomas over the last 30 years [65], and it is now the most common tumor histology in North America [66]. Although the lung cancer types most associated

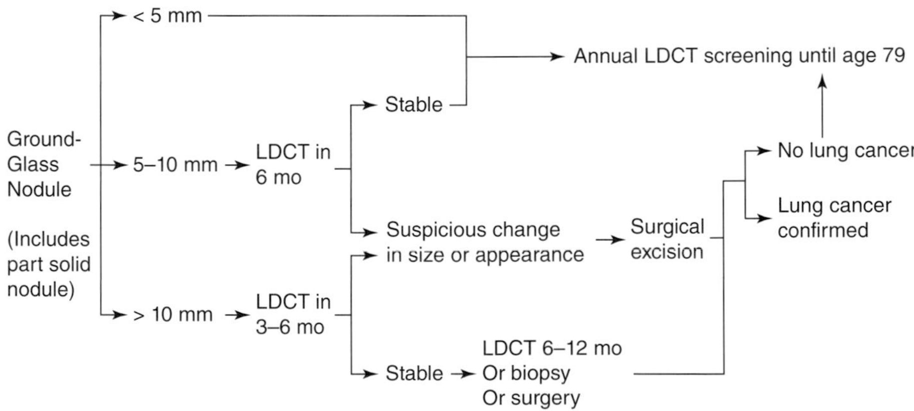

Figure 10.4 AATS lung cancer screening guidelines for ground-glass nodule. *LDCT*, Low-dose computed tomography. *Source*: Reprinted from Jaklitsch MT *et al.* (2012) The American Association for Thoracic Surgery guidelines for lung cancer screening using low-dose computed tomography scans for lung cancer survivors and other high-risk groups, *J Thorac Cardiovasc Surg*, 144: 36, with permission from Elsevier.

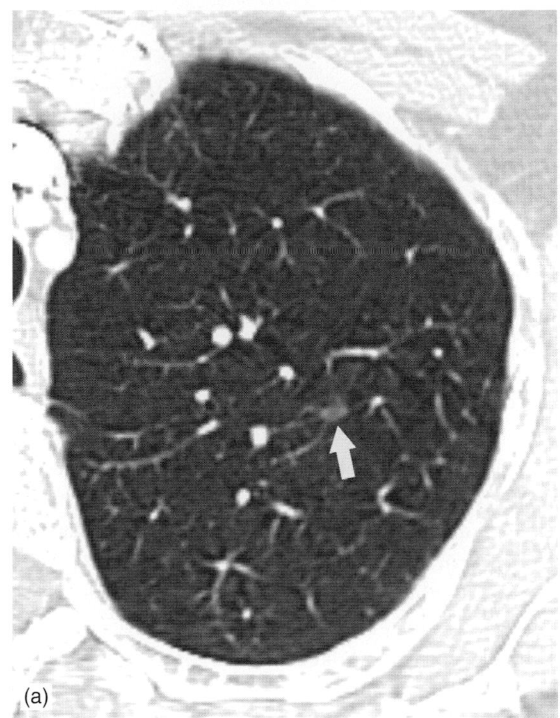

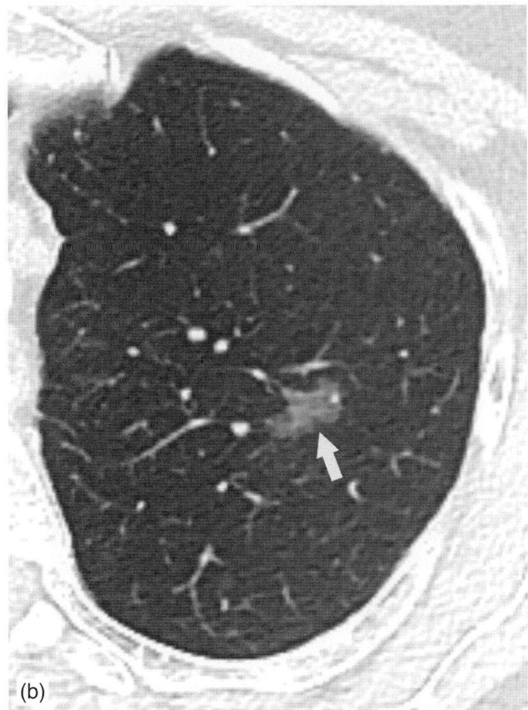

Figure 10.5 a: Low dose chest CT with lung windows demonstrates a small 6 mm left upper lobe ground glass nodule (white arrow). This nodule was not visible by conventional chest radiograph. b: Low dose chest CT with lung windows four years later shows the nodule (white arrow) with interval increase in size to 14 × 11 mm. The patient underwent left upper lobectomy, and pathology showed a moderately differentiated adenocarcinoma with predominantly acinar and lepidic subtypes.

with cigarette smoking have been squamous cell and small cell, adenocarcinomas are also strongly related to smoking [67].

Risks of LDCT screening

Risks of radiation

Low-dose CT screening is estimated to have an effective radiation dose to the patient of approximately 1.5 mSv (milliSieverts) per annual exam. This is lower than the average background radiation accumulated by every individual in the course of normal activity, which in the US is estimated to be 3.5 mSv annually. It can be compared with diagnostic chest CT, in which the effective dose is ~8 mSV, and PET/CT, which has an effective radiation dose of 14 mSv [48].

While the risk to the individual of radiation-induced cancer from a single CT examination is negligible, factors such as repeat examinations, age of the patient and synergistic effects of radiation and smoking may have an impact on relative risk [45, 68]. Models of increased risk of cancer from imaging-related radiation using the NLST exposure data predict one cancer death among 2500 screened [48]. Predictions of lung cancer risk from radiation by annual screening of high-risk populations show that radiation induced lung cancer would add to the number smoking-related lung cancers by 1.8% if screening started at 50 years of age, and by 0.8% if the screening started at age 60 [68]. Since radiation related carcinogenesis typically occurs 10–20 years after exposure, the risk–benefit ratio of screening for younger persons and low-risk populations may not be advantageous [48].

Psychological and procedural risks

Many of the abnormalities detected on low dose CT examinations are benign. Statistically, over 90% of pulmonary nodules are not cancerous [48]. Nevertheless, they may require follow up or diagnostic work-up for definitive characterization, and are thus classified as "positive" findings. In one study, half of screening participants reported dread and discomfort in waiting for the CT results [69]. The anxiety that may be provoked in the screening candidate by findings that are indeterminate or need further evaluation can be considerable.

Invasive diagnostic and therapeutic procedures carry a risk of morbidity and mortality. The complications during the NLST from screening with CT were very low, 0.4% [47]. Work up for findings in the NLST included 1.2% of patients who underwent needle biopsy or bronchoscopy and about 0.7% of persons who underwent thoracoscopy, thoracotomy or mediastinoscopy, and did not have lung cancer [48]. The risk of major complication or death following diagnostic interventions for nodules that turned out not to be cancer was 4.5 and 4.1 per 10 000 screened. The rate of major complications from surgery in patients with lung cancer found at screening was 14% [48].

Cost effectiveness of LDCT screening

The costs of a lung cancer screening program include not only the cost of the low-dose CT scanning, but also the costs of any follow-up imaging, diagnostic procedures and treatment that may ensue as well as the costs of tobacco cessation services. There are approximately 7 million high-risk ever-smokers in the US that would meet the NLST criteria, and a combined total of 94.9 million smokers and former smokers in the US alone. It is estimated that periodic annual LDCT screening of 25 million ever-smokers in the US would cost $115 billion dollars [70]. Some modeling studies based on monetized estimates of life-year and quality-adjusted life year (QALY) gained by screening have indicated that reduction in cancer mortality would have to exceed 40% in order for an LDCT screening program to be cost-effective [45]. Screening with CT can therefore be recommended only for high-risk cohorts [14]. Participation rates and compliance with screening will also affect the cost–benefit ratio.

Lung cancer screening and smoking cessation

The medical community agrees that smoking cessation programs and counseling should be a high priority in any lung cancer screening program [58–60]. There are 54.9 million active smokers in the US [71]. Worldwide, at least 1.3 billion people smoke tobacco [10]. Studies have found conflicting evidence about intention to quit on the part of potential and actual screening participants [72,73]. While many of them in theory are interested in smoking cessation services, some studies have found that up to a fifth of smokers would interpret a negative screening study as enabling them to continue smoking without concern [73,74]. Conversely, only 3% said they would continue to smoke if positive results were returned [73]. A study of NELSON trial participants noted that although smokers who received indeterminate screening results with request for follow up made more attempts to quit smoking than those who received negative results, there was no statistically significant difference in smoking cessation rates after two years of follow-up [75]. More intensive and integrative smoking cessation programs may be beneficial [73].

Translation from trial to practice

Recruitment

Improvement in lung cancer mortality and the cost-effectiveness of screening are dependent on successfully screening a sufficiently large high risk population. The experience of large-scale cancer screening programs for breast and colorectal carcinomas has revealed some prevalent obstacles to screening participation on the part of both patients and the health care system [74]. Lung cancer screening is unusual, however, in that the target disease is more strongly linked with a lifestyle habit, which may increase defensive attitudes in smokers.

Although the potential lung cancer screening populations in the US and other countries are sizeable, some qualitative studies have shown that active smokers may be less likely than anticipated to undergo screening [57, 74, 76]. In one report only 23% of interviewed smokers believed that they were at risk for lung cancer. Smokers also display fatalistic attitudes about lung cancer and are less likely to perceive that early detection and treatment can affect outcome. The accuracy of the screening test was less important to smokers than to nonsmokers in one survey, whereas the cost of the test was more important to them. Misconceptions about low-dose CT screening include anticipated pain and fear of radiation-induced cancer, which adversely affect intention to pursue screening. Mistrust of healthcare providers and anxiety and avoidance behaviors also play a part in decisions to decline screening [74, 76].

The majority of active smokers in one US study were nonwhite, male, poorly educated and the sole breadwinner of their family. Although they had employer-provided health insurance, they were much less likely than nonsmokers to have a designated healthcare provider. This demographic corresponds with the part of the population less likely to participate in screening of any sort [57]. In Britain, there is considerable interest in a subset of the smoking population, hard-core smokers. They tend to be white, male, older, poorly educated, have manual occupations and be single. They are less likely to believe that smoking affects their health, and more resistant to social pressures to quit [77]. A recent study evaluated a social marketing campaign in a poor English community focused on raising awareness of persistent cough as a symptom that should prompt a doctor's visit and a request for chest radiograph. Although the goal of the intervention was to promote earlier diagnosis of lung cancer and it was aimed at men over 50 who were ever-smokers, neither cancer nor smoking was specifically mentioned in the campaign materials [6].

Former smokers appear to be more willing to undergo screening [57], and former smokers slightly outnumbered active smokers among the NLST participants [46]. This high risk population is substantial in the US [71].

Academic center to community hospital

The NLST, like many of the previous lung cancer screening studies before it, was conducted primarily at large academic or university-based health centers [44]. Quality control and a nodule management algorithm were included in the trial design [48]. Studies were read by subspecialist trained radiologists, procedures were performed by highly experienced surgeons and interventionalists, and multidisciplinary teams collaborated on patient care. In particular, complication rates from surgical procedures within the trial setting are significantly lower than reported elsewhere [14, 48]. It may be difficult to develop a lung cancer screening program in settings without these advantages, and potential results may be affected. The ACS includes in its recommendations the caveat that whenever possible screening should be done at an institution with an organized lung cancer screening program having experience in LDCT interpretation and availability of multidisciplinary clinical expertise [60].

Conclusion

For the first time, there is evidence that screening with low-dose CT will reduce lung-cancer specific mortality. Although some questions remain to be answered, current guidelines recommend screening for certain high-risk populations. Concerted efforts to reach and educate eligible active smokers about the test and its benefits may be necessary to enroll substantial numbers in lung screening programs. Ultimately, smoking cessation and prevention should be emphasized.

References

1 Cancer Fact Sheet N 297. World Health Organization, 2013. (Accessed 02/15/2013, at http://www.who.int/mediacentre/factsheets/fs297/en/#.)

2 Siegel R, Naishadham D, Jemal A (2013) Cancer statistics, 2013. *CA: a Cancer Journal for Clinicians*, 63: 11–30.

3 Siegel R, Naishadham D, Jemal A (2012) Cancer statistics, 2012. *CA: a Cancer Journal for Clinicians*, 62: 10–29.

4 Malvezzi M, Bertuccio P, Levi F, La Vecchia C, Negri E (2013) European cancer mortality predictions for the year 2013. *Ann Oncol*, 24(3): 792–800, published online Feb. 12, 2013; doi:10.1093/annonc/mdt010.

5 Coleman MP, Forman D, Bryant H, *et al.* (2011) Cancer survival in Australia, Canada, Denmark, Norway, Sweden, and the UK, 1995–2007 (the International Cancer Benchmarking Partnership): An analysis of population-based cancer registry data. *Lancet*, 377: 127–38.

6 Athey VL, Suckling RJ, Tod AM, Walters SJ, Rogers TK (2012) Early diagnosis of lung cancer: Evaluation of a community-based social marketing intervention. *Thorax*, 67: 412–17.

7 Jemal A, Center MM, DeSantis C, Ward EM (2010) Global patterns of cancer incidence and mortality rates and trends. *Cancer Epidemiol Biomarkers Prev*, 19: 1893–1907.

8 Patz EF, Jr., Black WC, Goodman PC (2001) CT screening for lung cancer: not ready for routine practice. *Radiology*, 221: 587–91; discussion 98–9.

9 Herbst RS, Heymach JV, Lippman SM (2008) Lung cancer. *New England Journal of Medicine*, 359: 1367–80.

10 Jacobson FL, Jaklitsch MT (2012) Lung cancer screening trials: The United States and beyond. *Journal of Thoracic and Cardiovascular Surgery*, 144: S3–6.

11 Lee JM (2004) Screening issues for radiologists. *Academic Radiology*, 11: 162–8.

12 Hulka BS (1988) Cancer screening. Degrees of proof and practical application. *Cancer*, 62: 1776–80.

13 Stiles BM Altorki NK, Yankelevitz DF (2009) Screening for lung cancer: Challenges for thoracic surgery. In: Shields TW, LoCicero J, Reed CE, Feins RH (eds), *General Thoracic Surgery*. 7th edn. Philadelphia: Wolters Kluwer Health/Lippincott Williams & Wilkins, pp. 1299–1306.

14 Ganti AK, Mulshine JL (2006) Lung cancer screening. *Oncologist*, 11: 481–7.

15 Henschke CI, Sone S, Markowitz S (2004) International Early Lung Cancer Action Project (I-ELCAP): evaluation of low-dose CT screening. In: *Proceedings of the Annual Meeting of the Radiologic Society of North America; 2004, November 28–December 3, 2004*; Chicago, Illinois.

16 Henschke CI, Wisnivesky JP, Yankelevitz DF, Miettinen OS (2003) Small stage I cancers of the lung: Genuineness and curability. *Lung Cancer*, 39: 327–30.

17 Bianchi F, Hu J, Pelosi G, *et al.* (2004) Lung cancers detected by screening with spiral computed tomography have a malignant phenotype when analyzed by cDNA microarray. *Clinical Cancer Research*, 10: 6023–8.

18 Godoy MC, Naidich DP (2009) Subsolid pulmonary nodules and the spectrum of peripheral adenocarcinomas of the lung: Recommended interim guidelines for assessment and management. *Radiology*, 253: 606–22.

19 Hestbech MS, Siersma V, Dirksen A, Pedersen JH, Brodersen J (2011) Participation bias in a randomised trial of screening for lung cancer. *Lung Cancer*, 73: 325–31.

20 Doll R, Hill AB (1950) Smoking and carcinoma of the lung; preliminary report. *Br Med J*, 2: 739–48.

21 Boucot KR, Carnahan W, Cooper DA, Nealon T, Jr., Ottenberg DJ, Theodos PA (1955) Philadelphia pulmonary neoplasm research project; preliminary report. *J Am Med Assoc*, 157: 440–4.

22 Brett GZ (1968) The value of lung cancer detection by six-monthly chest radiographs. *Thorax*, 23: 414–20.

23 Frost JK, Ball WC, Jr., Levin ML, *et al.* (1984) Early lung cancer detection: Results of the initial (prevalence) radiologic and cytologic screening in the Johns Hopkins study. *American Review of Respiratory Disease*, 130: 549–54.

24 Melamed MR, Flehinger BJ, Zaman MB, Heelan RT, Perchick WA, Martini N (1984) Screening for early lung cancer. Results of the Memorial Sloan-Kettering study in New York. *Chest*, 86: 44–53.

25 Marcus PM, Bergstralh EJ, Fagerstrom RM, *et al.* (2000) Lung cancer mortality in the Mayo Lung Project: Impact of extended follow-up. *Journal of the National Cancer Institute*, 92: 1308–16.

26 Kubik A, Polak J (1986) Lung cancer detection: Results of a randomized prospective study in Czechoslovakia. *Cancer*, 57: 2427–37.

27 Strauss GM (2002) The Mayo Lung Cohort: A regression analysis focusing on lung cancer incidence and mortality. *Journal of Clinical Oncology*, 20: 1973–83.

28 Sagawa M, Nakayama T, Tsukada H, *et al.* (2003) The efficacy of lung cancer screening conducted in 1990s: Four case-control studies in Japan. *Lung Cancer*, 41: 29–36.

29 Sone S, Nakayama T, Honda T, *et al.* (2007) Long-term follow-up study of a population-based 1996–1998 mass screening programme for lung cancer using mobile low-dose spiral computed tomography. *Lung Cancer*, 58: 329–41.

30 Nakayama T, Baba T, Suzuki T, Sagawa M, Kaneko M (2002) An evaluation of chest X-ray screening for lung cancer in gunma prefecture, Japan: A population-based case-control study. *Eur J Cancer*, 38: 1380–7.
31 Quekel LG, Kessels AG, Goei R, van Engelshoven JM (1999) Miss rate of lung cancer on the chest radiograph in clinical practice. *Chest*, 115: 720–4.
32 Ko JP (2005) Lung nodule detection and characterization with multi-slice CT. *Journal of Thoracic Imaging*, 20: 196–209.
33 Sone S, Li F, Yang ZG, *et al.* (2001) Results of three-year mass screening programme for lung cancer using mobile low-dose spiral computed tomography scanner. *British Journal of Cancer*, 84: 25–32.
34 Kaneko M, Eguchi K, Ohmatsu H, *et al.* (1996) Peripheral lung cancer: Screening and detection with low-dose spiral CT versus radiography. *Radiology*, 201: 798–802.
35 Nawa T, Nakagawa T, Kusano S, Kawasaki Y, Sugawara Y, Nakata H (2002) Lung cancer screening using low-dose spiral CT: results of baseline and 1-year follow-up studies. *Chest*, 122: 15–20.
36 Henschke CI (2000) Early lung cancer action project: Overall design and findings from baseline screening. *Cancer*, 89: 2474–82.
37 Henschke CI, Naidich DP, Yankelevitz DF, *et al.* (2001) Early lung cancer action project: initial findings on repeat screenings. *Cancer*, 92: 153–9.
38 Swensen SJ, Jett JR, Hartman TE, *et al.* (2005) CT screening for lung cancer: five-year prospective experience. *Radiology*, 235: 259–65.
39 Starnes SL, Reed MF, Meyer CA, *et al.* (2011) Can lung cancer screening by computed tomography be effective in areas with endemic histoplasmosis? *Journal of Thoracic and Cardiovascular Surgery*, 141: 688–93.
40 Bach PB, Jett JR, Pastorino U, Tockman MS, Swensen SJ, Begg CB (2007) Computed tomography screening and lung cancer outcomes. *JAMA: The Journal of the American Medical Association*, 297: 953–61.
41 Prorok PC, Andriole GL, Bresalier RS, *et al.* (2000) Design of the Prostate, Lung, Colorectal and Ovarian (PLCO) cancer screening trial. *Controlled Clinical Trials*, 21: 273S–309S.
42 Oken MM, Hocking WG, Kvale PA, *et al.* (2011) Screening by chest radiograph and lung cancer mortality: The Prostate, Lung, Colorectal, and Ovarian (PLCO) randomized trial. *JAMA*, 306: 1865–73.
43 Gierada DS, Garg K, Nath H, Strollo DC, Fagerstrom RM, Ford MB (2009) CT quality assurance in the lung screening study component of the National Lung Screening Trial: Implications for multicenter imaging trials. *American Journal of Roentgenology*, 193: 419–24.
44 Aberle DR, Berg CD, Black WC, *et al.* (2011) The National Lung Screening Trial: overview and study design. *Radiology*, 258: 243–53.
45 Chiles C (2011) Lung cancer screening: achieving a reduction in mortality. *Seminars in Roentgenology*, 46: 230–40.
46 Aberle DR, Adams AM, Berg CD, *et al.* (2010) Baseline characteristics of participants in the randomized national lung screening trial. *Journal of the National Cancer Institute*, 102: 1771–9.
47 Aberle DR, Adams AM, Berg CD, *et al.* (2011) Reduced lung-cancer mortality with low-dose computed tomographic screening. *New England Journal of Medicine*, 365: 395–409.
48 Bach PB, Mirkin JN, Oliver TK, *et al.* (2012) Benefits and harms of CT screening for lung cancer: A systematic review. *JAMA*, 307: 2418–29.
49 Nair A, Hansell DM (2011) European and North American lung cancer screening experience and implications for pulmonary nodule management. *European Radiology*, 21: 2445–54.
50 Blanchon T, Brechot JM, Grenier PA, *et al.* (2007) Baseline results of the Depiscan study: A French randomized pilot trial of lung cancer screening comparing low dose CT scan (LDCT) and chest X-ray (CXR). *Lung Cancer*, 58: 50–8.
51 Baldwin DR, Duffy SW, Wald NJ, Page R, Hansell DM, Field JK (2011) UK Lung Screen (UKLS) nodule management protocol: modelling of a single screen randomised controlled trial of low-dose CT screening for lung cancer. *Thorax*, 66: 308–13.
52 Field JK, Baldwin D, Brain K, *et al.* (2011) CT screening for lung cancer in the UK: position statement by UKLS investigators following the NLST report. *Thorax*, 66: 736–7.
53 The European Lung Cancer Trials (2011) The PISA Position Statement. In: *State of the Art in Europe after Early Conclusion of the US National Lung Screening Trial: The European Lung Cancer Trials; March 4, 2011.* Pisa, Italy.
54 Chen B, Wang Y, Cao H, *et al.* (2013) Early lung cancer detection using the self-evaluation scoring questionnaire and chest digital radiography: A 3-year follow-up study in China. *Journal of Digital Imaging*, 26: 72–81.
55 Xu Y, Ma D, He W (2012) Assessing the use of digital radiography and a real-time interactive pulmonary nodule analysis system for large population lung cancer screening. *European Journal of Radiology*, 81: e451–6.

56 Nawa T, Nakagawa T, Mizoue T, *et al.* (2012) Long-term prognosis of patients with lung cancer detected on low-dose chest computed tomography screening. *Lung Cancer*, 75: 197–202.
57 Silvestri GA, Nietert PJ, Zoller J, Carter C, Bradford D (2007) Attitudes towards screening for lung cancer among smokers and their non-smoking counterparts. *Thorax*, 62: 126–30.
58 Wood DE, Eapen GA, Ettinger DS, *et al.* (2012) Lung cancer screening. *Journal of the National Comprehensive Cancer Network*, 10: 240–65.
59 Jaklitsch MT, Jacobson FL, Austin JH, *et al.* (2012) The American Association for Thoracic Surgery guidelines for lung cancer screening using low-dose computed tomography scans for lung cancer survivors and other high-risk groups. *The Journal of Thoracic and Cardiovascular Surgery*, 144: 33–8.
60 Wender R, Fontham ET, Barrera E, Jr., *et al.* (2013) American Cancer Society lung cancer screening guidelines. *CA: a Cancer Journal for Clinicians*, 63: 106–17.
61 MacMahon H, Austin JH, Gamsu G, *et al.* (2005) Guidelines for management of small pulmonary nodules detected on CT scans: a statement from the Fleischner Society. *Radiology*, 237: 395–400.
62 Stiles BM, Altorki NK (2011) Screening for lung cancer: challenges for the thoracic surgeon. *Surgical Oncology Clinics of North America*, 20: 619–35.
63 Travis WD, Brambilla E, Noguchi M, *et al.* (2011) International Association for the Study of Lung Cancer/American Thoracic Society/European Respiratory Society international multidisciplinary classification of lung adenocarcinoma. *Journal of Thoracic Oncology*, 6: 244–85.
64 Naidich DP, Bankier AA, MacMahon H, *et al.* (2013) Recommendations for the management of subsolid pulmonary nodules detected at CT: A statement from the Fleischner Society. *Radiology*, 266: 304–17.
65 Hoffmann D, Djordjevic MV, Hoffmann I (1997) The changing cigarette. *Preventive Medicine*, 26: 427–34.
66 Li YJ, Tsai YC, Chen YC, Christiani DC (2009) Human papilloma virus and female lung adenocarcinoma. *Seminars in Oncology*, 36: 542–52.
67 Yang P, Cerhan JR, Vierkant RA, *et al.* (2002) Adenocarcinoma of the lung is strongly associated with cigarette smoking: Further evidence from a prospective study of women. *American Journal of Epidemiology*, 156: 1114–22.
68 Brenner DJ (2004) Radiation risks potentially associated with low-dose CT screening of adult smokers for lung cancer. *Radiology*, 231: 440–5.
69 van den Bergh KA, Essink-Bot ML, Bunge EM, *et al.* (2008) Impact of computed tomography screening for lung cancer on participants in a randomized controlled trial (NELSON trial). *Cancer*, 113: 396–404.
70 Mahadevia PJ, Fleisher LA, Frick KD, Eng J, Goodman SN, Powe NR (2003) Lung cancer screening with helical computed tomography in older adult smokers: A decision and cost-effectiveness analysis. *JAMA*, 289: 313–22.
71 Patel JD (2005) Lung cancer in women. *Journal of Clinical Oncology*, 23: 3212–8.
72 Schnoll RA, Bradley P, Miller SM, Unger M, Babb J, Cornfeld M (2003) Psychological issues related to the use of spiral CT for lung cancer early detection. *Lung Cancer*, 39: 315–25.
73 Schnoll RA, Miller SM, Unger M, McAleer C, Halbherr T, Bradley P (2002) Characteristics of female smokers attending a lung cancer screening program: A pilot study with implications for program development. *Lung Cancer*, 37: 257–65.
74 Jonnalagadda S, Bergamo C, Lin JJ, *et al.* (2012) Beliefs and attitudes about lung cancer screening among smokers. *Lung Cancer*, 77: 526–31.
75 van der Aalst CM, van den Bergh KA, Willemsen MC, de Koning HJ, van Klaveren RJ (2010) Lung cancer screening and smoking abstinence: 2 year follow-up data from the Dutch-Belgian randomised controlled lung cancer screening trial. *Thorax*, 65: 600–5.
76 Patel D, Akporobaro A, Chinyanganya N, *et al.* (2012) Attitudes to participation in a lung cancer screening trial: a qualitative study. *Thorax*, 67: 418–25.
77 Jarvis MJ, Wardle J, Waller J, Owen L (2003) Prevalence of hardcore smoking in England, and associated attitudes and beliefs: cross sectional study. *BMJ*, 326: 1061.

CHAPTER 11
Imaging Lung Cancer

Sonia L. Betancourt Cuellar, Edith M. Marom, and Jeremy J. Erasmus
Department of Diagnostic Radiology, The University of Texas MD Anderson Cancer Center, Houston, TX, USA

Introduction

Imaging is important in the detection, diagnosis, and staging of non-small cell lung (NSCLC) as well as in assessing response to therapy and monitoring for tumor recurrence after therapy. In the management of patients with NSCLC at initial presentation, comprehensive evaluation, including imaging, is performed to define disease extent. In this regard, patients are staged clinically according to the 7th edition of the American Joint Committee on Cancer (AJCC) tumor-node-metastasis (TNM) staging system [1–3]. This chapter reviews the use of computed tomography (CT), magnetic resonance (MR) and 18F-2-deoxy-D-glucose (FDG) positron emission tomography (PET) in the initial evaluation of patients with NSCLC.

Imaging of the primary tumor (T)

The primary tumor is described according to its size, location and extent of local invasion (Table 1). Although chest radiographs can be useful in the evaluation of the primary tumor and in the detection of intrathoracic metastases, computed tomography (CT) is more reliable in the detection of locoregional invasion of the chest wall, mediastinum and diaphragm as well as nodal and lung metastases. Furthermore, there is an emphasis on accurate determination of primary tumor size in the current 7th AJCC staging system i.e., T1a (≤2 cm), T1b (>2 cm to ≤3 cm), T2a (>3 cm to ≤5 cm, T2b (>5 cm to ≤7 cm), T3 >7 cm and CT is the optimal modality in this assessment. In this regard, the relatively poor spatial resolution of MR and PET limit their utility in the evaluation of the primary tumor. Additionally, CT is almost universally used to evaluate patients with NSCLC because it is widely available and often used to direct invasive sampling (mediastinoscopy, endobronchial ultrasound-guided biopsy) and assist in surgical management decisions.

Although CT is useful in defining the T descriptors of the primary tumor, in many patients this assessment has limitations. In this regard, CT and MR are both useful in confirming gross chest wall (T3) or mediastinal invasion (T4) but are inaccurate in differentiating between anatomic contiguity and microscopic invasion (Figures 11.1 and 11.2). It is important to be aware that although a T4 descriptor generally precludes resection, patients with cardiac, tracheal and vertebral body invasion are potentially resectable when regional nodal metastases are absent or confined to the ipsilateral hilar nodes. In those patients being considered for surgical resection, MR can be an important adjunct to CT in showing the extent of vertebral body invasion, as

Lung Cancer, Fourth Edition. Edited by Jack A. Roth, Waun Ki Hong and Ritsuko U. Komaki.

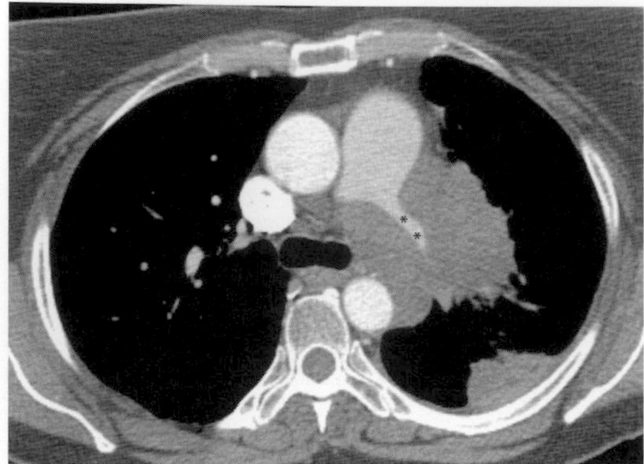

Figure 11.1 54-year-old woman with non-small cell lung cancer and extensive mediastinal invasion. Contrast-enhanced CT shows large, poorly marginated mass surrounding and narrowing the left main pulmonary artery (*). Mediastinal invasion is T4 and is nonresectable. Note opacity abutting pleural is due to post-obstructive consolidation.

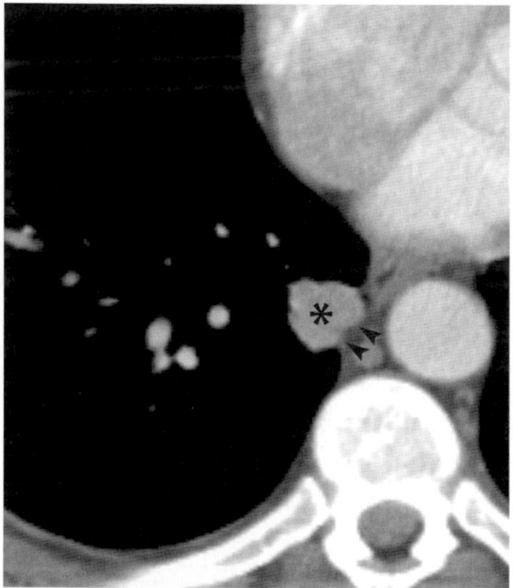

Figure 11.2 54-year-old man with primary non-small cell lung cancer presenting with a history of chronic cough. Contrast-enhanced CT (cropped to right lung) shows a right lower lobe nodule (*) abutting the pleura. Note poor margination of the interface of the nodule and pleura (arrowheads) raising the possibility of limited loco-regional invasion. At surgical resection there was no invasion of the pleura.

well as great vessel, pericardial or cardiac involvement. Additionally, because of its superior soft-tissue contrast resolution and multiplanar imaging ability, MR is particularly useful in the evaluation of patients with superior sulcus tumors [4–6]. MR is used to determine the degree of involvement of the brachial plexus, subclavian vessels and vertebral bodies in patients with superior sulcus tumors (Figure 11.3) [4, 5]. Importantly, absolute contraindications to surgery (invasion of the brachial plexus roots or trunks above the level of T1, invasion of greater than 50% of a vertebral body and invasion of the esophagus or trachea) are often accurately assessed by MR [7, 8].

Besides evaluation of the primary tumor, the T descriptor is also used to differentiate those patients with a solitary tumor from those with an additional lung nodule/s. Because of the recent changes incorporated in the 7th AJCC staging system, the presence and location of additional lung nodule/s can significantly change the T descriptor. Specifically, additional nodule/s are classified as T3 when in the primary tumor lobe, T4 when in the ipsilateral lung (different lobe) and M1a when in the contralateral lung. The higher spatial resolution of CT compared to MR and PET allows optimal evaluation of the lungs and the detection of lung metastases, particularly when they are small. Although CT detection of nodules is important, unfortunately the 7th AJCC staging system assigns a M1a descriptor for both single and multiple contralateral nodules. Furthermore, a solitary tumor and an additional nodule can be synchronous primary tumors or a primary tumor and a pulmonary metastasis (Figure 11.4). In this regard, patients with a single M1a nodule (which presumptively could be a synchronous primary rather than a metastasis) and no nodal metastasis have similar survival to those with satellite nodules in the primary (T3) and nonprimary (T4) lobes after resection [9].

Imaging of regional lymph nodes (N)

The presence and location of nodal metastases are important in determining management in patients

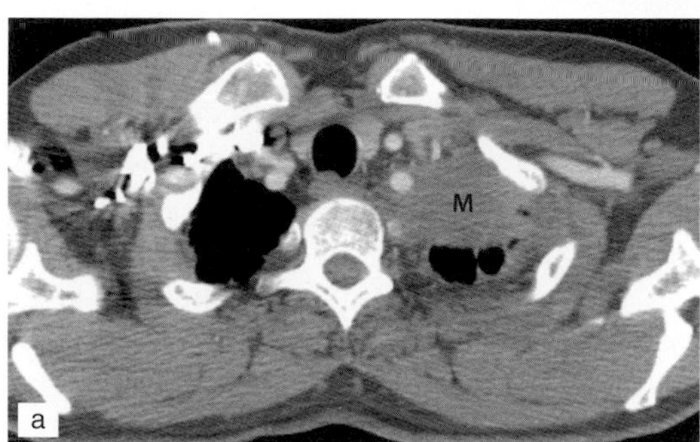

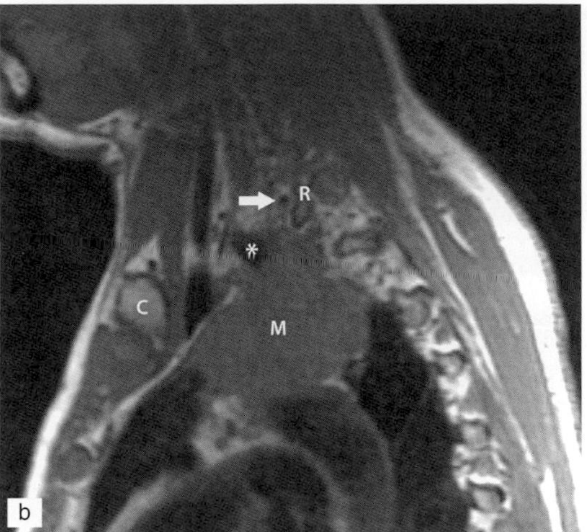

Figure 11.3 47-year-old man with a superior sulcus non-small cell lung cancer presenting with shoulder pain. a: Contrast-enhanced CT shows a mass (M) in the left lung apex. There are no findings of rib or vertebral body invasion. b: Sagittal T1-weighted MR shows the superior sulcus tumor (M) abutting the subclavian artery (∗) but clear of the C8 nerve root (arrow). MR allows optimal assessment of the brachial plexus and because there is no invasion of the C8 nerve root, the patient underwent surgical resection. C = clavicle, R = first rib.

with NSCLC (Table 11.1) [2]. In the imaging evaluation of nodal metastasis, nodes greater than 1 cm in short-axis diameter on a chest radiograph, CT or MR are considered abnormal. Chest radiographs are not sensitive or specific in evaluating nodal metastasis. Although CT and MR are better in detecting nodal metastasis, there is no definite correlation between lymph node size and metastatic involvement, i.e., enlarged nodes can be hyperplastic and small nodes can contain metastases. In this regard, Prenzel *et al.* reported that in 2891 resected hilar and mediastinal nodes obtained from 256 patients with NSCLC, 77% of the 139 patients with no nodal metastases had at least one node greater than 1 cm in diameter and 12% of the 127 patients with nodal metastases had no nodes greater than 1 cm [10]. The limitations of CT in the evaluation of mediastinal nodal metastasis in patients with NSCLC are shown in a meta-analysis by Toloza and colleagues [11]. Of the 3438 patients evaluated there was a pooled sensitivity of 57%, specificity of 82%, positive predictive value of 56% and negative predictive value of 83%.

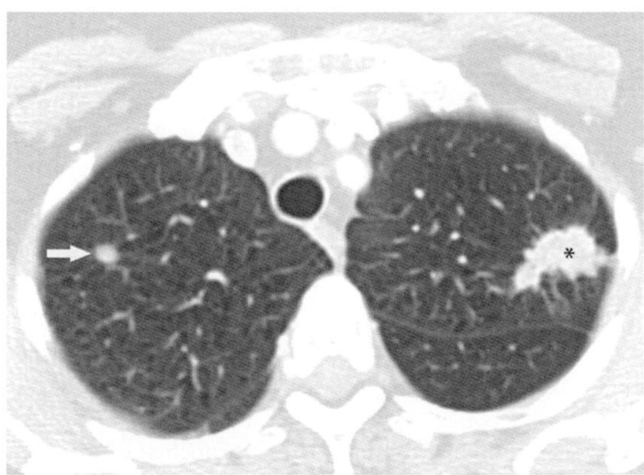

Figure 11.4 66-year-old asymptomatic woman with bilateral squamous cell lung cancers. Contrast-enhanced CT shows nodules in the left upper lobe (∗) and right upper lobe (arrow). Although classification is M1a (nonresectable) left upper lobectomy was performed and right lung malignancy was treated with stereotatic radiation. Note M1a designation may imply a worse prognosis than is warranted.

FDG-PET is being increasingly used to evaluate patients with NSCLC and improves the detection of nodal metastases (Figure 11.5). In a meta-analysis comparing PET and CT in nodal staging in patients with NSCLC, the sensitivity and specificity of FDG-PET for detecting mediastinal lymph node metastases ranged from 66% to 100% (overall 83%) and 81% to 100% (overall 92%), respectively

Table 11.1 TNM descriptors

T – Primary tumor	
TX	Primary tumor cannot be assessed, *or* tumor proven by the presence of malignant cells in sputum or bronchial washings but not visualized by imaging or bronchoscopy
T0	No evidence of primary tumor
Tis	Carcinoma in situ
T1	Tumor 3 cm or less in greatest dimension, surrounded by lung or visceral pleura, without bronchoscopic evidence of invasion more proximal than the lobar bronchus (i.e., not in the main bronchus) T1a tumor 2 cm or less in greatest dimension[1] T1b tumor more than 2 cm but not more than 3 cm in greatest dimension
T2	Tumor more than 3 cm but not more than 7 cm; or tumor with *any* of the following features[2]: • Involves main bronchus, 2 cm or more distal to the carina • Invades visceral pleura • Associated with atelectasis or obstructive pneumonitis that extends to the hilar region but does not involve the entire lung T2a Tumor more than 3 cm but not more than 5 cm in greatest dimension T2b Tumor more than 5 cm but not more than 7 cm in greatest dimension
T3	Tumor more than 7 cm or one that directly invades any of the following: chest wall (including superior sulcus tumors), diaphragm, phrenic nerve, mediastinal pleura, parietal pericardium; *or* tumor in the main bronchus less than 2 cm distal to the carina[1] but without involvement of the carina; *or* associated atelectasis or obstructive pneumonitis of the entire lung or separate tumor nodule(s) in the same lobe as the primary.
T4	Tumor of any size that invades any of the following: mediastinum, heart, great vessels, trachea, recurrent laryngeal nerve, esophagus, vertebral body, carina; separate tumor nodule(s) in a different ipsilateral lobe to that of the primary.
N – Regional lymph nodes	
NX	Regional lymph nodes cannot be assessed
N0	No regional lymph node metastasis
N1	Metastasis in ipsilateral peribronchial and/or ipsilateral hilar lymph nodes and intrapulmonary nodes, including involvement by direct extension
N2	Metastasis in ipsilateral mediastinal and/or subcarinal lymph node(s)
N3	Metastasis in contralateral mediastinal, contralateral hilar, ipsilateral or contralateral scalene, or supraclavicular lymph node(s)
M – Distant metastasis	
M0	No distant metastasis
M1	Distant metastasis M1a Separate tumor nodule(s) in a contralateral lobe; tumor with pleural nodules or malignant pleural or pericardial effusion[3] M1b Distant metastasis

Source: Reprinted with permission of the International Association for the Study of Lung Cancer. © Copyright 2009 IASLC.

Notes:

[1]The uncommon superficial spreading tumor of any size with its invasive component limited to the bronchial wall, which may extend proximal to the main bronchus, is also classified as T1a.

[2]T2 tumors with these features are classified T2a if 5 cm or less or if size cannot be determined, and T2b if greater than 5 cm but not larger than 7 cm.

[3]Most pleural (pericardial) effusions with lung cancer are due to tumor. In a few patients, however, multiple microscopical examinations of pleural (pericardial) fluid are negative for tumor, and the fluid is non-bloody and is not an exudate. Where these elements and clinical judgment dictate that the effusion is not related to the tumor, the effusion should be excluded as a staging element and the patient should be classified as M0.

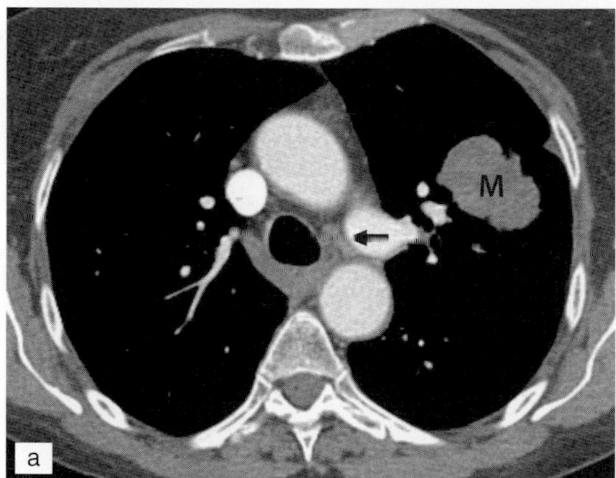

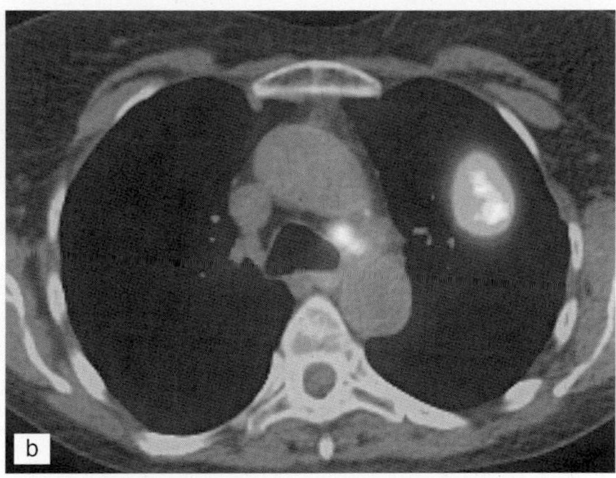

Figure 11.5 58-year-old woman with a left upper lobe non-small cell lung cancer being evaluated for surgical resection. a: CT shows a left upper lobe mass (M) and small (short axis diameter < cm) nodes in the ipsilateral mediastinum (arrow). b: Axial PET-CT shows increased [18F]-2-deoxy-D-glucose (FDG) uptake in the mass and in the left lower paratracheal lymph nodes. Biopsy was positive for nodal metastatic disease and the patient underwent induction chemotherapy followed by surgical resection.

compared to sensitivity and specificity of CT of 20% to 81% (overall 59%) and 44% to 100% (overall 78%), respectively [12]. Because surgical resection and potential use of adjuvant therapy are dependent on the N descriptor in patients with NSCLC, the performance of FDG-PET-CT should be considered in all patients without CT findings of distant metastasis [12, 13].

Currently, the performance of FDG-PET imaging is usually integrated with CT (rather than CT and PET performed separately). Integrated PET-CT allows precise anatomic localization of regions of focal increased FDG-uptake and is useful in confirming that FDG uptake correlates to nodal disease in the hila, mediastinum and supraclavicular regions [14]. However, a commonly encountered dilemma in the evaluation of nodes with PET-CT occurs when nodal imaging is discordant, i.e., enlarged nodes on CT that are not FDG avid on PET or small nodes on CT that are FDG avid on PET. Information that is potentially useful in understanding the likelihood of nodal metastasis when discordant nodal imaging findings are encountered was reported in a study by de Langen and colleagues regarding the size of mediastinal lymph nodes, FDG avidity and pathologic correlation [15]. In patients with NSCLC and small nodes on CT and a positive PET, the predicted post-test probability of N2 malignancy is 62% and when the nodes are ≥16 mm and the PET is negative, the posttest probability of N2 malignancy is 21% (Figure 11.6). Additionally, with concordant findings of enlarged nodes and positive PET, the posttest probability of N2 malignancy is only 90%. Accordingly, while the exact role of FDG-PET in nodal evaluation is not explicitly defined, FDG-PET should be used to direct invasive sampling rather than as an alternative to invasive nodal staging.

Imaging of distant metastasis (M)

Additional nodule/s in the contralateral lung, pleural nodules, malignant pleural or pericardial effusion and extrathoracic metastasis are common in patients with NSCLC at presentation. However, imaging performed in the detection of these metastases is not precisely defined. There is general agreement that CT of the thorax is the primary modality used in the detection of intra- and extrathoracic metastasis and that this imaging should routinely include the adrenals. In the evaluation of intrathoracic metastasis (M1a), malignant pleural effusions

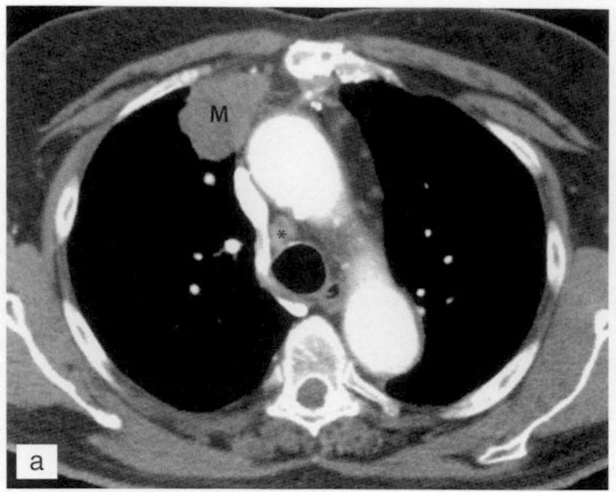

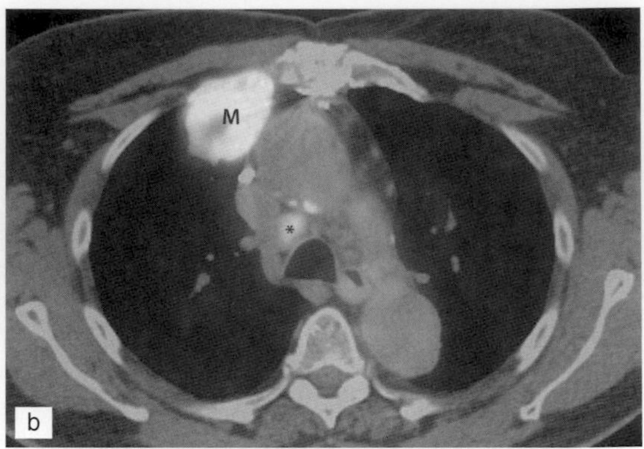

Figure 11.6 78-year-old man with a right upper lobe non-small cell lung cancer (NSCLC) being evaluated for surgical resection. a: CT shows a right upper lobe mass (M) and small (short axis diameter 1 cm) node in the ipsilateral mediastinum (*). b: Axial PET-CT shows increased [18F]-2-deoxy-D-glucose (FDG) uptake in the mass (M) and in the right lower paratracheal lymph node (*). Biopsy was negative for nodal metastatic disease and the patient underwent surgical resection. Note in patients with NSCLC and small nodes on CT and a positive PET, the predicted posttest probability of N2 malignancy is 62%.

are common and pleural thickening or nodularity on CT is suggestive of metastasis. However, the absence of pleural thickening or nodularity does not exclude pleural metastasis. Accordingly, it can be difficult, on the basis of CT findings, alone to diagnose pleural metastasis. FDG-PET has been reported in small series to be useful in the evaluation of pleural effusions in patients with NSCLC [16–18]. However, it is important to emphasize that FDG-PET is performed as part of the staging algorithm and not specifically to evaluate pleural effusions in patients with NSCLC.

Adrenal lesions have typically been characterized by CT and/or MR. Adrenal nodules or masses of low density (10 Hounsfield units or less) on non-contrast-enhanced CT are diagnosed as lipid-rich adenomas while those of higher attenuation are considered indeterminate in etiology (Figure 11.7) [19]. Indeterminate adrenal nodules or masses have typically been further evaluated with MR (chemical shift analysis, dynamic gadolinium-enhancement) or contrast-enhanced CT (adrenal enhancement and washout) [20, 21]. However, in a recent meta-analysis, FDG-PET was highly sensitive and specific for differentiating malignant from benign adrenal lesions and no further imaging evaluation was necessary in characterization [22]. In fact, if an adrenal mass in a patient with potentially resectable NSCLC has normal FDG uptake on PET, curative resection should be considered without further evaluation. If an adrenal mass has increased FDG uptake, biopsy should be performed to confirm metastatic disease.

The imaging performed to detect occult metastases to other organs such as the liver, brain, and bones is more variable than adrenal evaluation. Metastases to the liver typically occur when there is locally advanced, inoperable intrathoracic disease and/or metastases to other organs [23]. A meta-analysis that evaluated the utility of imaging in asymptomatic patients with NSCLC showed a pooled yield of only 3% in detecting hepatic metastases and routine imaging of the liver is generally not performed [24]. In addition, although FDG-PET has high specificity in detecting hepatic metastasis, the sensitivity is low and accordingly FDG-PET is not recommended.

Imaging to detect occult brain metastases is controversial. In patients with NSCLC without neurologic symptoms, a normal neurologic examination has high negative predictive value (79–100%) and CT or MR of the brain in these patients detects metastasis in only 0–10% [25]. However, occult brain metastasis in neurologically asymptomatic patients with NSCLC may be more common than

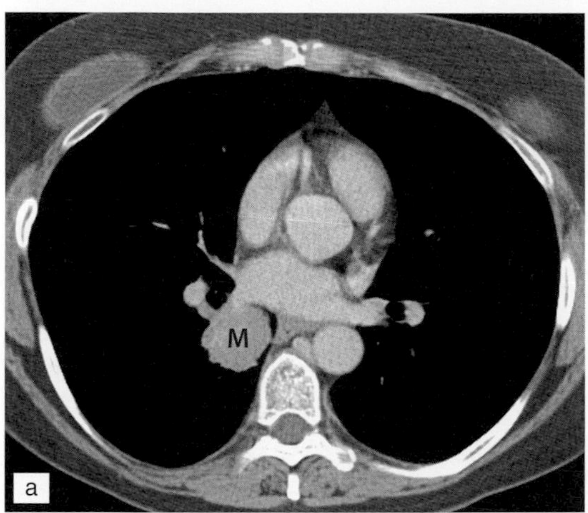

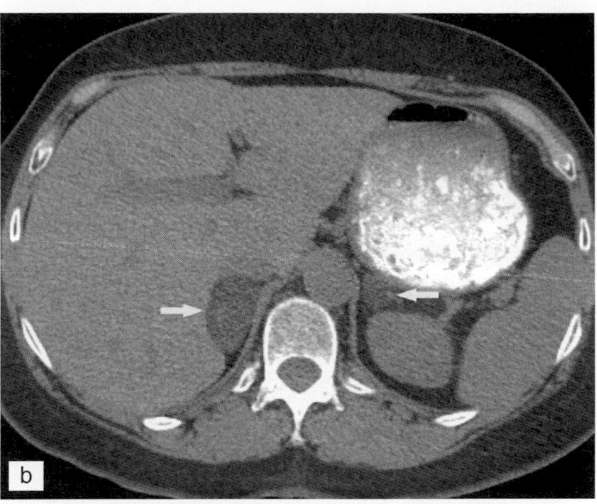

Figure 11.7 60-year-old woman with non-small cell cancer of the right lower lobe and adrenal adenomas. a: Contrast-enhanced CT shows a right lower lobe mass (M). b: Axial, unenhanced CT shows well-circumscribed, lipid-rich adrenal adenomas (arrows) with homogeneous low attenuation of approximately 2 Hounsfield units (HU). The unenhanced CT attenuation of less than 10 HU permits benign diagnostic characterization.

previously thought, especially in patients with adenocarcinoma [26]. In addition, because the brain is often the only site of distant disease and approximately one-third of these patients will have limited, potentially resectable disease, it has been suggested that routine imaging should be performed in the initial staging evaluation of patients with NSCLC [27]. The discrepancy in opinion regarding the importance of imaging in detecting occult brain metastasis may account for the lack of consensus in practice guidelines. In this regard, the American Thoracic and European Respiratory Societies advocate no routine screening in asymptomatic patients while American Society of Clinical Oncology recommends that asymptomatic patients with stage III NSCLC being considered for local therapy should have CT or MR imaging performed [28]. Although FDG-PET can occasionally detect brain metastases, the high background activity of FDG in normal brain tissue contributes to the low sensitivity and precludes routine use.

Occult metastases to the bones are rarely detected by radiographs, technetium (Tc)-99m labeled methylene diphosphonate (MDP) bone scintigraphy or MR and these imaging modalities should not be performed routinely in asymptomatic patients. In a recent study comparing whole-body FDG-PET/CT and Tc-99m MDP in patients with newly diagnosed NSCLC, the two studies had similar sensitivities (93.3% and 93.5%, respectively) but PET-CT had higher specificity (94.1% and 44.1%, respectively) and accuracy (93.4% and 52.2%, respectively) [29]. Once the mainstay for detection of bone metastasis, Tc-99m MDP now has no additional utility in NSCLC patients if FDG-PET is performed as part of the staging algorithm. In fact, discordant findings of skeletal metastasis between Tc-99m MDP scintigraphy and FDG-PET-CT are reported to occur in 20% of the patients with NSCLC. [30] This discordance is in large part due to the ability of FDG-PET to detect early bone metastasis and the failure of Tc-99m MDP scintigraphy to detect early neoplastic infiltration of bone marrow. However, it is important to emphasize that in patients with bone lesions detected on FGD-PET and potentially resectable disease, histologic confirmation or corroboration by additional imaging studies (radiographs, CT and/or MR) is required.

Whole-body FDG-PET has a higher sensitivity and specificity than CT in detecting metastases to the adrenals, bones and extrathoracic lymph nodes (Figure 11.8). Consequently, FDG-PET is

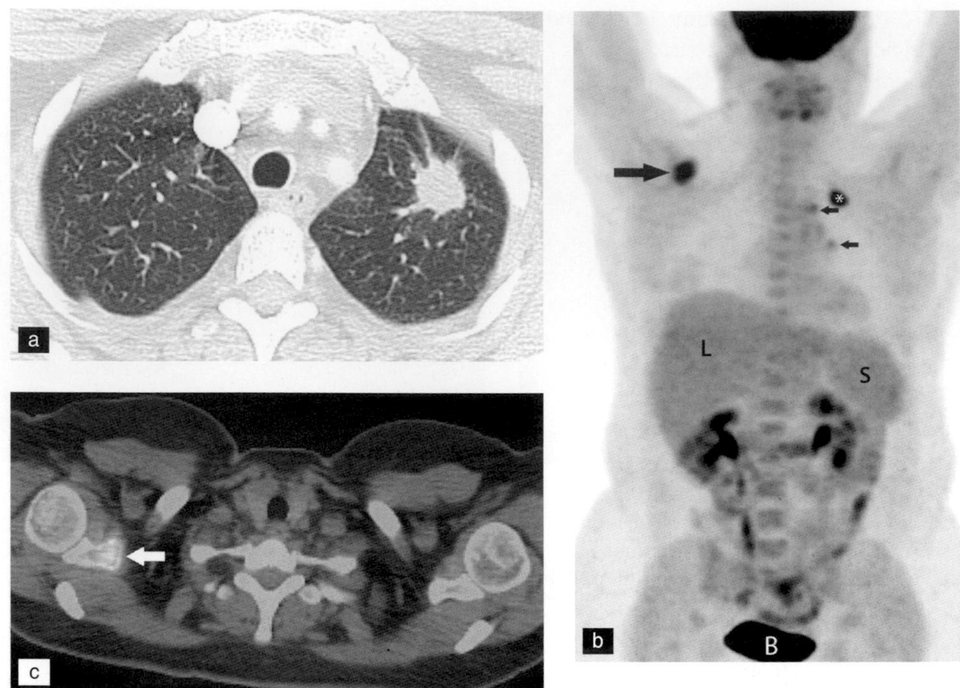

Figure 11.8 45-year-old woman with left upper lobe non-small cell lung cancer and solitary bone metastasis presenting with neck and shoulder pain. a: Contrast-enhanced CT shows a spiculated left upper lobe nodule. b: Whole-body PET maximum intensity projection image shows increased [18F]-2-deoxy-D-glucose (FDG) uptake in the left lung nodule (*), hilar and mediastinal nodes (short arrows) and in the right shoulder region (long arrow). B, accumulation of FDG in the bladder; L = liver, S = spleen. C. Axial PET-CT shows increased uptake of FDG in the corocoid process of the scapula (arrow) suspicious for a metastasis (arrow). Biopsy confirmed metastatic disease and the patient was treated palliatively.

increasingly being used to detect metastases and is usually performed in patients without metastases on CT and other imaging modalities. The American College of Surgeons Oncology Trial reports PET sensitivity, specificity, positive predictive value and negative predictive values of 83%, 90%, 36% and 99%, respectively for M1 disease [31]. Importantly, whole-body PET imaging is useful in the detection of occult extrathoracic metastases in patients considered resectable by standard imaging and clinical evaluation and is reported to prevent inappropriate resection in 20% of these patients [31, 32]. However, because the incidence of detection of occult metastases increases as the staging T and N descriptors increase, the utility of FDG-PET in patients with early stage disease has been questioned [33, 34]. In this regard, distant metastases were rarely detected (< 5%) in a randomized controlled trial of the role of PET in early stage lung cancer and management in the remaining patients was not substantially changed [34]. However, the subsequent use of neoadjuvant chemotherapy in stage IIIA N2 disease at the participating hospitals in the study would have resulted in a change in management in up to 20% of these patients.

Although whole-body FDG-PET imaging improves the accuracy of staging, focal increased uptake of FDG in extrathoracic lesions unrelated to the primary NSCLC can mimic distant metastasis. Accordingly, all extrathoracic FDG-avid lesions that potentially would alter patient management should be further imaged or biopsied to confirm the diagnosis of distant metastasis. The rationale for this management approach is supported by the results of a prospective study performed to assess the incidence and diagnosis of a single site of extrapulmonary accumulation of FDG in patients with newly diagnosed NSCLC [35]. In the 350 patients in the study group, 72 patients had solitary FDG-avid lesions. Sixty-nine of these lesions were biopsied and 37 (54%) had a solitary metastasis while 32 (46%) had lesions unrelated to the NSCLC (benign tumor or inflammatory lesion (n = 26), clinically unsuspected second malignancy or recurrence of a previously diagnosed carcinoma (n = 6)).

Conclusion

Imaging is an integral component of TNM staging and is important in the determination of therapeutic management in patients with NSCLC. However, there is substantial variability in the imaging performed to evaluate the primary tumor and to detect nodal and extrathoracic metastases. Chest CT is almost universally used to stage patients with NSCLC and is typically performed to assess the primary tumor, direct invasive sampling and detect intra- and extrathoracic metastases. Magnetic resonance (MR) imaging is particularly useful in the evaluation of superior sulcus tumors. Otherwise, MR imaging is generally used as an adjunct to CT in evaluating patients with equivocal CT findings. FDG-PET has limited utility in the evaluation of the primary tumor. However, whole-body FDG-PET imaging is better than CT and MR in the detection of nodal and extrathoracic metastasis and improves the accuracy of staging and the determination of the optimal therapeutic strategy.

References

1 Rami-Porta R, Ball D, Crowley J, Giroux DJ, Jett J, Travis WD, *et al.* (2007) The IASLC Lung Cancer Staging Project: Proposals for the revision of the T descriptors in the forthcoming (seventh) edition of the TNM classification for lung cancer. *J Thorac Oncol*, Jul; 2(7): 593–602.

2 Rusch VW, Crowley J, Giroux DJ, Goldstraw P, Im JG, Tsuboi M, *et al.* (2007) The IASLC Lung Cancer Staging Project: Proposals for the revision of the N descriptors in the forthcoming seventh edition of the TNM classification for lung cancer. *J Thorac Oncol*, Jul; 2(7): 603–12.

3 Postmus PE, Brambilla E, Chansky K, Crowley J, Goldstraw P, Patz EF, Jr., *et al.* (2007) The IASLC Lung Cancer Staging Project: proposals for revision of the M descriptors in the forthcoming (seventh) edition of the TNM classification of lung cancer. *J Thorac Oncol*, Aug; 2(8): 686–93.

4 Bruzzi JF, Komaki R, Walsh GL, Truong MT, Gladish GW, Munden RF, *et al.* (2008) Imaging of non-small cell lung cancer of the superior sulcus: Part 2: initial staging and assessment of resectability and therapeutic response. *RadioGraphics*, Mar–Apr; 28(2): 561–72.

5 Bruzzi JF, Komaki R, Walsh GL, Truong MT, Gladish GW, Munden RF, *et al.* (2008) Imaging of non-small cell lung cancer of the superior sulcus: Part 1: anatomy, clinical manifestations, and management. *RadioGraphics*, Mar–Apr; 28(2): 551–60; quiz 620.

6 Bolton WD, Rice DC, Goodyear A, Correa AM, Erasmus J, Hofstetter W, *et al.* (2009) Superior sulcus tumors with vertebral body involvement: A multimodality approach. *J Thorac Cardiovasc Surg*, Jun; 137(6): 1379–87.

7 Bilsky MH, Vitaz TW, Boland PJ, Bains MS, Rajaraman V, Rusch VW (2002) Surgical treatment of superior sulcus tumors with spinal and brachial plexus involvement. *J Neurosurg*, Oct; 97(3 Suppl): 301–9.

8 Dartevelle P, Macchiarini P (1999) Surgical management of superior sulcus tumors. *Oncologist*, 4(5): 398–407.

9 Finley DJ, Yoshizawa A, Travis W, Zhou Q, Seshan VE, Bains MS, *et al.* (2010) Predictors of outcomes after surgical treatment of synchronous primary lung cancers. *J Thorac Oncol*, Feb; 5(2): 197–205.

10 Prenzel KL, Monig SP, Sinning JM, Baldus SE, Brochhagen HG, Schneider PM, *et al.* (2003) Lymph node size and metastatic infiltration in non-small cell lung cancer. *Chest*, Feb; 123(2): 463–7.

11 Toloza EM, Harpole L, Detterbeck F, McCrory DC (2003) Invasive staging of non-small cell lung cancer: a review of the current evidence. *Chest*, Jan; 123 (1 Suppl): 157S–66S.

12 Birim O, Kappetein AP, Stijnen T, Bogers AJ (2005) Meta-analysis of positron emission tomographic and computed tomographic imaging in detecting mediastinal lymph node metastases in nonsmall cell lung cancer. *Ann Thorac Surg*, Jan; 79(1): 375–82.

13 Gould MK, Kuschner WG, Rydzak CE, Maclean CC, Demas AN, Shigemitsu H, *et al.* (2003) Test performance of positron emission tomography and computed tomography for mediastinal staging in patients with non-small-cell lung cancer: A meta-analysis. *Ann Intern Med*, Dec 2; 139(11): 879–92.

14 Perigaud C, Bridji B, Roussel JC, Sagan C, Mugniot A, Duveau D, *et al.* (2009) Prospective preoperative mediastinal lymph node staging by integrated positron emission tomography-computerised tomography in patients with non-small-cell lung cancer. *Eur J Cardiothorac Surg*, Oct; 36(4): 731–6.

15 de Langen AJ, Raijmakers P, Riphagen I, Paul MA, Hoekstra OS (2006) The size of mediastinal lymph nodes and its relation with metastatic involvement: A meta-analysis. *Eur J Cardiothorac Surg*, Jan; 29(1): 26–9.

16 Erasmus JJ, Goodman PC, Patz EF, Jr (2000) Management of malignant pleural effusions and pneumothorax. *Radiol Clin North Am*, Mar; 38(2): 375–83.

17 Gupta NC, Rogers JS, Graeber GM, Gregory JL, Waheed U, Mullet D, *et al.* (2002) Clinical role of F-18 fluorodeoxyglucose positron emission tomography imaging in patients with lung cancer and suspected malignant pleural effusion. *Chest*, Dec; 122(6): 1918–24.

18 Kim BS, Kim IJ, Kim SJ, Pak K, Kim K (2011) Predictive value of F-18 FDG PET/CT for malignant pleural effusion in non-small cell lung cancer patients. *Onkologie*, 34(6): 298–303.

19 Low G, Sahi K. Clinical and imaging overview of functional adrenal neoplasms. *Int J Urol*, Aug; 19(8): 697–708.

20 Remer EM, Obuchowski N, Ellis JD, Rice TW, Adelstein DJ, Baker ME (2000) Adrenal mass evaluation in patients with lung carcinoma: a cost-effectiveness analysis. *AJR Am J Roentgenol*, Apr; 174(4): 1033–9.

21 Low G, Dhliwayo H, Lomas DJ. Adrenal neoplasms. *Clin Radiol*, Oct; 67(10): 988–1000.

22 Boland GW, Dwamena BA, Jagtiani Sangwaiya M, Goehler AG, Blake MA, Hahn PF, *et al.* (2011) Characterization of adrenal masses by using FDG PET: A systematic review and meta-analysis of diagnostic test performance. *Radiology*, Apr; 259(1): 117–26.

23 Quint LE, Tummala S, Brisson LJ, Francis IR, Krupnick AS, Kazerooni EA, *et al.* (1996) Distribution of distant metastases from newly diagnosed non-small cell lung cancer. *Annals of Thoracic Surgery*, 62: 246–50.

24 Hillers TK, Sauve MD, Guyatt GH (1994) Analysis of published studies on the detection of extrathoracic metastases in patients presumed to have operable non-small cell lung cancer. *Thorax*, Jan; 49(1): 14–19.

25 Silvestri GA, Gould MK, Margolis ML, Tanoue LT, McCrory D, Toloza E, *et al.* (2007) Noninvasive staging of non-small cell lung cancer: ACCP evidenced-based clinical practice guidelines (2nd edn). *Chest*, Sep; 132(3 Suppl): 178S–201S.

26 Sanchez de Cos J, Sojo Gonzalez MA, Montero MV, Perez Calvo MC, Vicente MJ, Valle MH (2009) Non-small cell lung cancer and silent brain metastasis: Survival and prognostic factors. *Lung Cancer*, Jan; 63(1): 140–5.

27 Yokoi K, Kamiya N, Matsuguma H, Machida S, Hirose T, Mori K, *et al.* (1999) Detection of brain metastasis in potentially operable non-small cell lung cancer. A comparison of CT and MRI. *Chest*, 115: 714–19.

28 Pfister DG, Johnson DH, Azzoli CG, Sause W, Smith TJ, Baker S, Jr., *et al.* (2003) American Society of Clinical Oncology treatment of unresectable non-small-cell lung cancer guideline: update 2003. *J Clin Oncol*, Jan 15; 22(2): 330–53.

29 Min JW, Um SW, Yim JJ, Yoo CG, Han SK, Shim YS, *et al.* (2009) The role of whole-body FDG PET/CT, Tc 99m MDP bone scintigraphy, and serum alkaline phosphatase in detecting bone metastasis in patients with newly diagnosed lung cancer. *J Korean Med Sci*, Apr; 24(2): 275–80.

30 Ak I, Sivrikoz MC, Entok E, Vardareli E (2010) Discordant findings in patients with non-small-cell lung cancer: absolutely normal bone scans versus disseminated bone metastases on positron-emission tomography/computed tomography. *Eur J Cardiothorac Surg*, Apr; 37(4): 792–6.

31 Reed CE, Harpole DH, Posther KE, Woolson SL, Downey RJ, Meyers BF, *et al.* (2003) Results of the American College of Surgeons Oncology Group Z0050 trial: The utility of positron emission tomography in staging potentially operable non-small cell lung cancer. *J Thorac Cardiovasc Surg*, Dec; 126(6): 1943–51.

32 van Tinteren H, Hoekstra OS, Smit EF, van den Bergh JH, Schreurs AJ, Stallaert RA, *et al.* (2002) Effectiveness of positron emission tomography in the preoperative assessment of patients with suspected non-small-cell lung cancer: The PLUS multicentre randomised trial. *Lancet*, 359(9315): 1388–93.

33 MacManus MP, Hicks RJ, Matthews JP, Hogg A, McKenzie AF, Wirth A, *et al.* (2001) High rate of detection of unsuspected distant metastases by PET in apparent stage III non-small-cell lung cancer: Implications for radical radiation therapy. *Int J Radiat Oncol Biol Phys*, Jun 1; 50(2): 287–93.

34 Viney RC, Boyer MJ, King MT, Kenny PM, Pollicino CA, McLean JM, *et al.* (2004) Randomized controlled trial of the role of positron emission tomography in the management of stage I and II non-small-cell lung cancer. *J Clin Oncol*, Jun 15; 22(12): 2357–62.

35 Lardinois D, Weder W, Roudas M, von Schulthess GK, Tutic M, Moch H, *et al.* (2005) Etiology of solitary extrapulmonary positron emission tomography and computed tomography findings in patients with lung cancer. *J Clin Oncol*, Oct 1; 23(28): 6846–53.

CHAPTER 12
Staging of the Mediastinum

Mauricio Pipkin and Shaf Keshavjee
University of Toronto, Toronto, ON, Canada

Introduction

Lung cancer is the leading cause of cancer death among both men and women. Each year, more people die of lung cancer than from colon, breast, and prostate cancers combined [1]. The treatment of lung cancer is directed by the TNM staging system [2]. Clinical and pathological staging concordance is low and hence patients usually are clinically understaged [3]. Mediastinal lymph nodal status indicates the potential for curative treatment if there are no distant metastases. Patients with no mediastinal involvement are candidates for curative treatment with surgery alone. Patients with lymph node involvement are generally associated with a poorer prognosis, and accurate staging of the nodes will determine the treatment plan for the patient with respect for the potential for combined modality therapies, such as neoadjuvant chemoradiation.

Imaging

A CT scan of the chest is a basic examination that should be performed on all patients with suspected lung cancer. Accurate evaluation of lymph node disease usually requires a contrast-enhanced scan. A generally accepted parameter to describe a lymph node suspicious for metastases is a short axis diameter greater than 1 cm on a transverse CT scan. However, not all lymph nodes greater than one centimeter are malignant. About 40% of all lymph nodes considered to be malignant on CT are actually benign. On the other hand, about 20% of all lymph considered to be "benign" are malignant [4]. Considering central tumors or a tumor with enlarged N1 nodes, but a normal mediastinum makes the chance of N2–N3 nodal involvement in a range of 20% to 25% [57]. A recent review of pooled data reported a sensitivity of 57%, a specificity of 82%, a positive predictive value of 56% and a negative predictive value (NPV) of 83%, with marked heterogeneity across individual studies [5]. The subgroup of patients with peripheral tumors less than 3 cm in size and lymph nodes less than 1 cm may have mediastinal metastasis in 9% of cases [6].

The addition of PET represents an overall advance over CT alone. This modality is more sensitive and specific in detecting metastatic lymph nodes. A meta-analysis showed that FDG-PET was more accurate than CT, reporting sensitivity values of 79% and 60% and specificity 91% and 77% for PET vs. CT, respectively [7]. It should be noted that PET alone is not as helpful as a combined PET-CT.

Integrated PET-CT provides the ability to identify and anatomically localize metastatic lymph nodes. The anatomical location of a metastatic lymph node is delineated in an image where the FDG uptake is fused with the CT image. An appropriately targeted biopsy can be performed to confirm the diagnosis [8, 9]. A prospective study showed that integrated PET-CT improved specificity compared with

Lung Cancer, Fourth Edition. Edited by Jack A. Roth, Waun Ki Hong and Ritsuko U. Komaki.

CT alone, 85% vs. 61% respectively [10]. Integrated PET-CT compared with PET alone showed increased sensitivity, however a decrease in specificity [11]. This underscores the need for tissue confirmation (invasive staging) in order to confirm mediastinal node metastasis. Cerfolio *et al.* compared PET-CT and PET alone specifically for N2 lymph node, and demonstrated a higher accuracy for PET-CT being 96% vs 93% [12]. Darling *et al.* reported that PET-CT has a false-positive rate of 50%, 20% and 29% for cN0, cN1 and cN2 patients, respectively [13]. In patients with stage I tumors with normal lymph node size and hence a low risk of mediastinal metastasis, a negative PET scan presents a false negative rate of 5% [14]. This has been corroborated by others reporting that a negative result in the mediastinum is generally reliable for the cN0 patient with a false negative rate of 3% [13]. The ACCP recommendation thus for these patients with stage I tumors, with a negative CT scan and a negative mediastinal PET where the tumor is PET positive, is that mediastinoscopy is not needed. In the current (7th) edition of the TNM staging system, patients with T2aN0 are stage IB but are excluded from this recommendation [15].

Endoscopic evaluation

Endobronchial ultrasound with trans-bronchial fine needle aspiration (EBUS-TBNA or EBUS-FNA) is an alternative technique that provides ultrasound visualization of mediastinal and peri-bronchial lymph nodes with the possibility of needle aspiration biopsy performed trans-bronchoscopically [16]. The procedure is performed under sedation or general anesthesia. The bronchoscope is introduced orally, through a laryngeal mask or through an endotracheal tube. An ultrasound-imaged inspection is performed to localize and characterize lymph nodes at N3, N2 and N1 stations. A special ultrasound-visible needle is introduced through the bronchoscope (Figure 12.1). Once a lymph node is identified, a needle aspiration biopsy is performed. The material can be evaluated ideally by an on-site cytopathologist to confirm that the material is adequate (contains lymphocytes at least) and to confirm a diagnosis of cancer if present.

EBUS-TBNA was first reported in 2004 to be a novel minimally invasive staging modality with a high diagnostic yield for the evaluation of mediastinal and hilar lymph nodes [17]. Its minimally invasive nature, real-time targeting of lymph nodes and safety are significant benefits. Interestingly, EBUS can also access hilar, interlobar and lobar lymph nodes in this minimally invasive fashion – a capability not available before this technology came along [18]. A meta-analysis showed that EBUS-TBNA has a pooled sensitivity of 93% and specificity of 100%. This sensitivity increased to 94% if patient selection is based on positive CT or PET. In the subgroup without any selection, sensitivity reported was 76% [19]. Adams *et al.* published a systematic review and meta-analysis comparing EBUS-TBNA yield versus CT and PET. A total of 10 studies (n = 817) were reviewed showing that EBUS-TBNA had an excellent pooled specificity of 1.00 (95% CI 0.92 to 1.00) and a good pooled sensitivity of 0.88 (95% CI 0.79 to 0.94) [20]. In 2011 a study showed excellent agreement between EBUS-TBNA and mediastinoscopy for mediastinal staging. The sensitivity, negative predictive value, and diagnostic accuracy for mediastinal lymph node staging for EBUS-TBNA and mediastinoscopy were 81%, 91%, 93%, and 79%, 90%, 93%, respectively. Specificity and positive predictive value for both techniques, when metastatic cancer was identified, were 100 % [21]. The authors concluded that both techniques have similar results and that EBUS-TBNA could replace cervical mediastinoscopy in mediastinal staging for lung cancer. However, in high-risk patients, EBUS-TBNA negative aspirations should be confirmed by mediastinoscopy. Andrade *et al.*, commented that EBUS-TBNA should be done by a physician involved in a multidisciplinary lung cancer team [22].

Endoscopic esophageal ultrasound-guided fine needle aspiration (EUS-FNA) is a diagnostic procedure that provides an alternate route to biopsies of lymph node stations 2R, 2L, 3p, 4R, 4L. In addition however, one can access the lower part of station 5, station 7 – particularly the posterior part, as well as paraesophageal stations 8 and 9

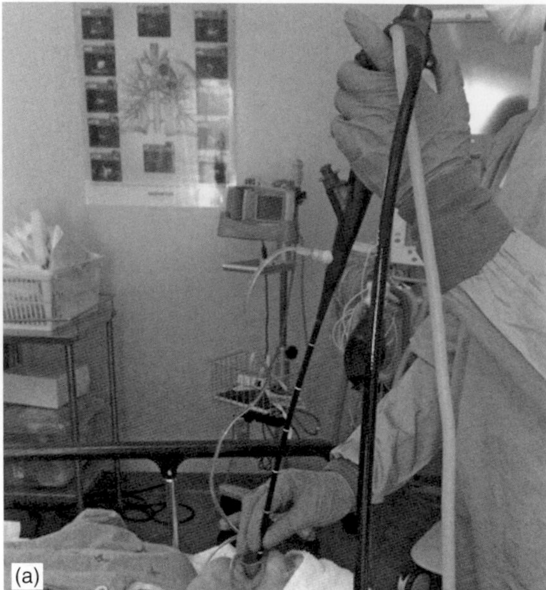

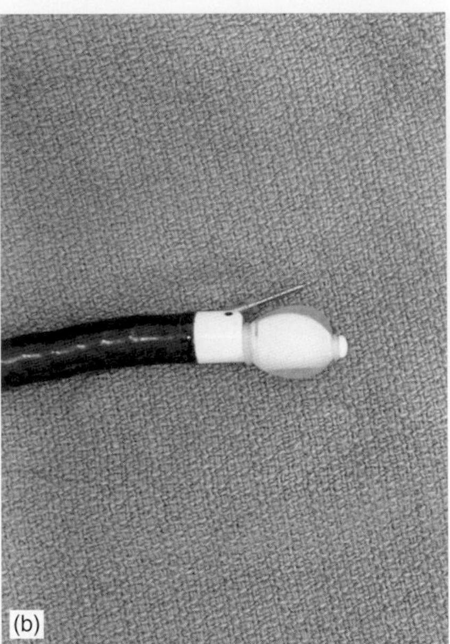

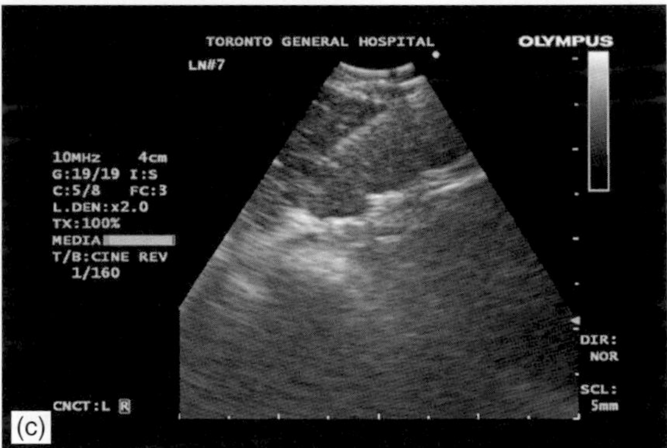

Figure 12.1 a: EBUS-TBNA scope during a procedure. b: Needle aspect on the scope. c: Ultrasound image of a lymph nodal biopsy.

[23, 24]. A meta-analysis including 18 studies and 1201 patients showed a sensitivity of 83% and a specificity of 97% [25]. Considering unenlarged lymph nodes the sensitivity was 58% [25]. When integrating EBUS-TBNA and EUS-FNA it is possible to biopsy additional lymph nodes that are not accessible by mediastinoscopy like station 3p, 8 and 9. Szlubowski showed that in a normal mediastinum the sensitivity was 68%, specificity 98%, accuracy 91%, PPV 91%, NPV 91% [26]. Herth *et al.* performed mediastinal staging in 139 patients diagnosed with NSCLC. In his study the sensitivity was 89% for EUS-FNA and 92% for EBUS-TBNA. With the combined approach, sensitivity rose to 96% with a NPV of 95% [27]. A combined approach therefore is feasible [23, 28–31]; however, there is no specific recommendation for using the combination routinely. It is useful to be aware of the capabilities and limitations of each in the event that a specific nodal area is identified on CT and PET. Essentially, EBUS and EUS provide the surgeon with a route for minimally invasive biopsy of tissue for confirmation and staging of every lymph node station in the mediastinum.

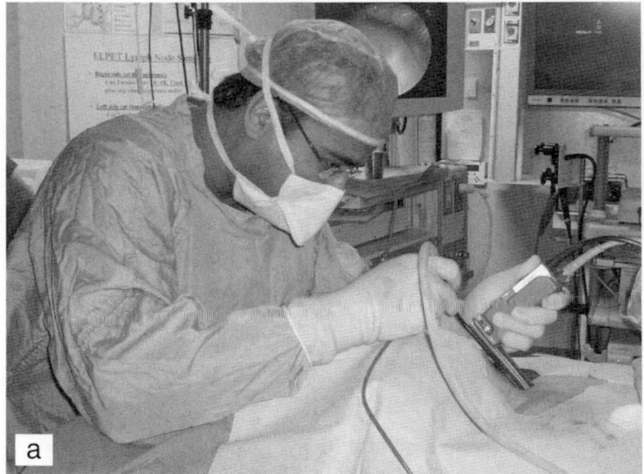

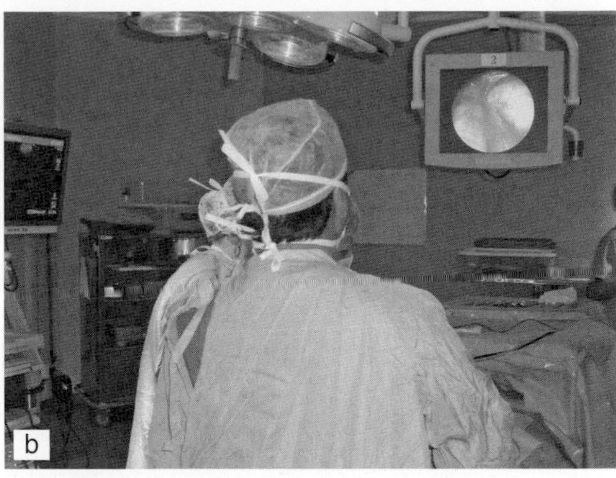

Figure 12.2 Videomediastinoscopy: visualization can be done directly through the scope (a) or on the HD monitor (b) [37].

Source: Yasufuku, 2010 [37]. Reproduced with permission of Lippincott Williams and Wilkins.

In a study done by Filho *et al.*, mediastinal staging was performed using mediastinoscopy and video-assisted thoracoscopy to access the posterior lymph node areas, particularly in the posterior subcarinal area. In 11 patients out of 62, mediastinoscopy showed no involvement of the subcarinal nodes, which were identified by VATS approach, presenting a positive predictive value of 89%, negative predictive value of 94%, prevalence of 18%, sensitivity of 73% and specificity of 99%. This approach could be used in institutions where EBUS-TBNA and/or EUS-FNA are not available [32].

Mediastinoscopy

Mediastinoscopy is an outpatient procedure performed under general anesthesia. A skin incision about 3 cm is made in the suprasternal notch. Dissection is carried down to the pre-tracheal fascia, which is incised to expose the trachea. Blunt finger dissection is used to open this paratracheal plane down to the carina. Digital palpation for abnormal lymph nodes or masses is performed. A video mediastinoscope is then inserted into the mediastinum to biopsy lymph nodes under direct vision. A video mediastinoscope is preferred due to the superior visualization, although a surgeon may look down directly through the mediastinoscope in the traditional fashion if desired (Figure 12.2). A systematic evaluation and dissection of the mediastinum is performed using a mediastinoscopy dissector (a tubular suction instrument which is insulated and has an exposed metal tip that is used to dissect the tissues and cauterize as needed). The lymph nodes in each station are systematically identified for biopsy. Stations 2R and 4R, 7, 2L and 4L can be assessed by mediastinoscopy. Stations 1 and 10 can be also assessed and biopsied by mediastinoscopy as required. Station 3, 5, 6, 8, and 9 cannot be assessed by mediastinoscopy. Ideally, 5 lymph node stations (2R, 4R, 7, 4L and 2L) should be sampled during a mediastinoscopy [15] (Figure 12.3).

Advances in imaging technology have led to the development of cervical video-mediastinoscopy. Conceptually, this is a conventional mediastinoscope with a high definition video camera that can transmit images to a screen. The surgeon and team in the operating suite can clearly visualize the dissection on a video monitor as well as under direct vision [33]. The clarity of visualization improves the precision and safety of the procedure. This also facilitates teaching as the surgeon can clearly see and direct the learner who is performing the procedure. More than one person can watch the procedure simultaneously. Video-mediastinoscopy permits rapid learning and

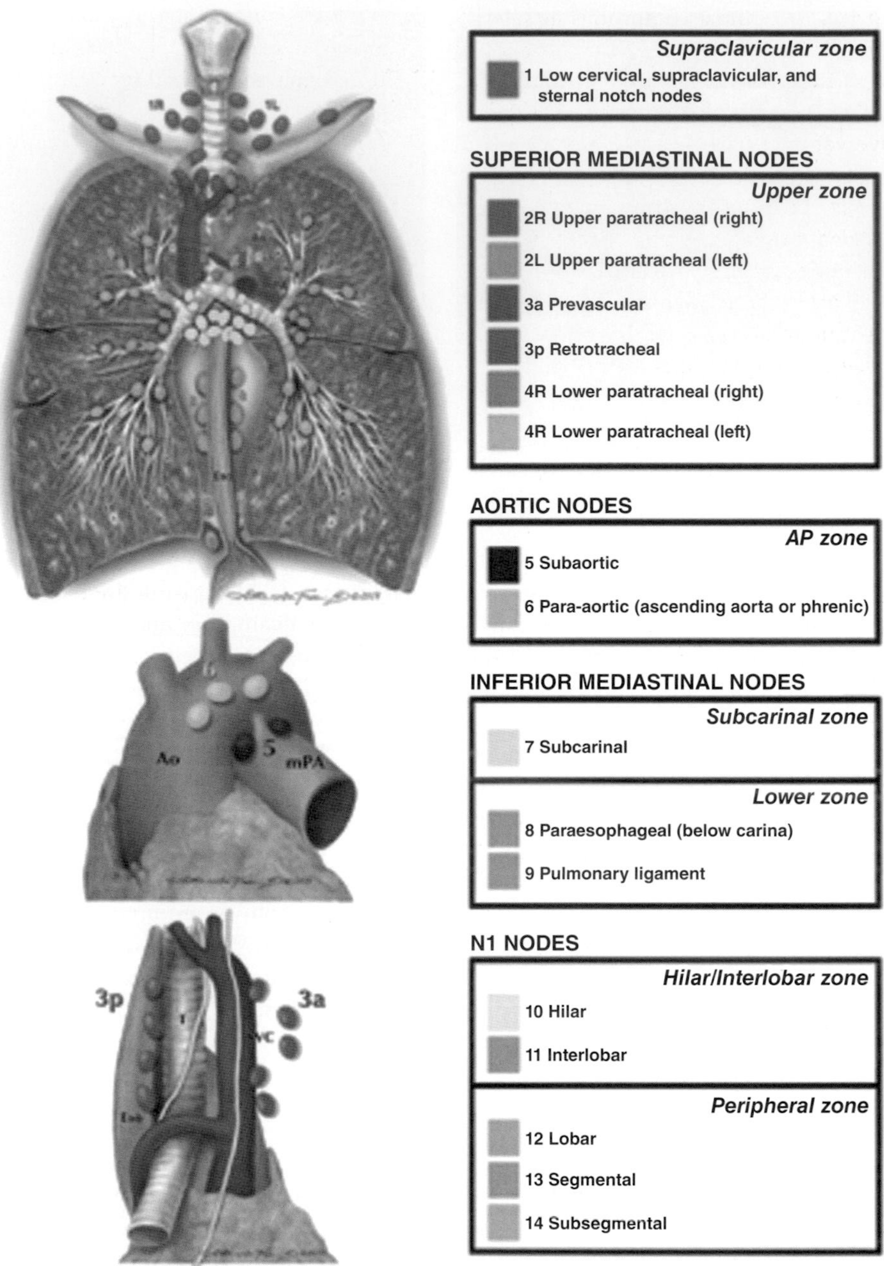

Figure 12.3 a–f: The International Association for the Study of Lung Cancer (IASLC) lymph node map as applied to clinical staging by computed tomography scan in axial (a–c), coronal (d), and sagittal (e, f) views. The border between the right and left paratracheal region is shown in a and b. Ao, aorta; AV, azygos vein; Br, bronchus; IA, innominate artery; IV, innominate vein; LA, ligamentum arteriosum; LIV, left innominate vein; LSA, left subclavian artery; PA, pulmonary artery; PV, pulmonary vein; RIV, right innominate vein; SVC, superior vena cava [55]. (For a color version, see the color plate section.)

Source: Rusch, 2009 [55]. Reproduced with permission of Lippincott Williams and Wilkins.

adequate supervision without compromising safety, operative time or completeness of the procedure [34]. A comparison between regular mediastinoscopy and video-mediastinoscopy showed a negative predictive value of 0.81 and 0.83 respectively. Accuracy was 83.8% and 87.9% [35].

Complications of mediastinoscopy are extremely low if performed by experienced surgeons [36]. Morbidity and mortality are 1.5% and 0.4% respectively [37]. Complications include left recurrent nerve injury, pneumothorax, and wound infection. More serious complications include tracheal-bronchial injury, esophageal trauma and bleeding from injury of the great vessels or azygous vein. The major complications are potentially life threatening and often require median sternotomy or right thoracotomy for repair [38].

Cervical mediastinoscopy is considered the gold standard method for staging the mediastinum. A review revealed that the sensitivity of cervical mediastinoscopy varied between 72% to 89%, with an average of 81% with a NPV of 91% [39]. The specificity of mediastinoscopy is reported as 100%. One explanation for the false-negatives cases related to metastatic lymph nodes that are not accessed by mediastinoscopy – usually stations 5 and 6 and sometimes posterior station 7 nodes. It can also be explained by incomplete nodal sampling, as this method is skill-dependent. On the other hand, the high negative predictive value makes this procedure reliable in excluding mediastinal metastases [37].

Anterior mediastinotomy, extended cervical mediastinoscopy, thoracoscopy and re-do mediatinoscopy

The parasternal anterior mediastinotomy approach was first described in 1966 by McNeil and Chamberlain [40]. A small incision in the left anterior chest wall in the second intercostal space giving access to the stations 5 and 6 (aorto-pulmonary window and para-aortic lymph nodes). Some surgeons remove the costal cartilage. A mediastinoscope is inserted to proceed with dissection and biopsies. This procedure is effective and safe, with a low morbidity and mortality. Sometimes video-thoracoscopy (VATS) can be used to evaluate lymph node stations 5 and 6. An added value of this modality is the ability to also evaluate and biopsy stations 8, 9, posterior station 7 and the pleural space if pleural disease is suspected.

Extended cervical mediastinoscopy is a procedure described by Robert Ginsberg, which accesses stations 5 and 6 through a conventional cervical mediastinoscopy incision. A blunt dissection is performed creating a space posterior to the innominate vein and anterior to the aorta between the left carotid and innominate arteries. This is a challenging procedure to carry out and with the advent of other techniques this procedure is rarely indicated.

Re-do mediastinoscopy is a procedure that may be considered in a patient after neoadjuvant treatment or sometimes for staging a patient with a second primary lung cancer. Both of these situations call for restaging of a previously staged mediastinum. This procedure can be challenging secondary to the scarring from the previous dissection of the mediastinal tissue planes. Adhesions involving the innominate artery and vein, azygous vein and the pulmonary artery are all areas of concern. Technically, the dissection is generally initiated going down the left side into the mediastinum and carefully extendeding over to the right side. Even though re-do mediastinoscopy is technically more challenging, studies have shown a sensitivity of 73%, a specificity of 100%, an accuracy of 85%, and positive and negative predictive values of 100 and 75%, respectively. [41] Mateu-Navarro et al. reported on 24 patients who underwent re-mediastinoscopy after neoadjuvant therapy for N2 lung cancer. Fifty percent were positive. Sensitivity was 70%, specificity 100% and accuracy 80%. [42] An additional report by DeWaele et al reported that re-do mediastinoscopy was positive in 40 patients and negative in 64. There were 17 false-negative re-do mediastinoscopies. Sensitivity of re-do mediastinoscopy was 71%, specificity 100% and accuracy 84%. [43] In the current era, we prefer to use PET plus EBUS-TBNA for the first staging of the mediastinum and plan to do the video mediastinoscopy post induction therapy to be able to perform a thorough and safe staging of the mediastinum in these higher oncologic-risk patients.

Video Assisted Mediastinal Lymphadenectomy (VAMLA) – a staging procedure?

Video Assisted Mediastinoscopic Lymphadenectomy (VAMLA) and Transcervical Extended Mediastinal Lymphadenectomy (TEMLA) are relatively recently described techniques proposed for mediastinal staging [44]. The proponents advocate complete removal not only of mediastinal lymph nodes, but also of the surrounding adipose tissue, claiming an improvement in accuracy [45]. In the VAMLA technique, the lymph nodes dissected are the same as in conventional mediastinoscopy, but essentially an en-bloc excisional biopsy is done [46]. In the TEMLA procedure an extensive lymph node dissection is performed: lymph node stations 1, 2R, 4R, 2L, 4L, 7, 8, 3A, 3P, 5, 6, 7, 8 through a combination of an open and mediastinoscope assisted technique. A study done by Zielinski with 256 patients reported an accuracy of 98% in a patient population with a disease prevalence of N2-N3 involvement of 31.3% [47]. VAMLA has a reported specificity of 93.75% and a sensitivity of 100% [48]. Both methods involve a "minimally invasive" or "hybrid" procedure, although TEMLA uses a bigger incision and sternal retraction in contrast to the other techniques. The mediastinal dissection in both TEMLA and VAMLA are extensive and, as suggested in the literature, the morbidity is high compared with other methods of staging the mediastinum. Laryngeal nerve injury is the most common complication with a rate of 3% and 5% for TEMLA and VAMLA, respectively [49]. The added value of these procedures to justify the added morbidity is not clear at this time.

Discussion

Staging of the mediastinum is a prerequisite in treatment decision making for a lung cancer patient. Patients with a tissue diagnosis and extensive inoperable infiltration of the mediastinum evident on CT scan, even with no distant metastases, don't need extensive invasive staging [14]. If the mediastinal lymph nodes are enlarged, some form of invasive staging is required. As discussed before, even if a PET/CT shows lymph node involvement, the false positive rate is high and a tissue diagnose should be obtained to confirm this before assuming the patient has advanced disease. This can be performed by several methods. Mediastinoscopy is still the gold standard approach for mediastinal staging; however EBUS-TBNA analyzed in a prospective study, compared favorably to mediastinoscopy in diagnostic accuracy [21]. It should be noted that this endoscopic approach was performed in an experienced center using a rapid on-site cytological evaluation of the specimen. A combined approach using EBUS-TBNA and EUS-FNA showed increased sensitivity and specificity as well. EBUS-TBNA and EUS-FNA are still very much operator skill-dependent procedures. As such, there is no consensus yet that mediastinoscopy can be substituted in a generalizable fashion by one or a combination of those methods.

In cases where mediastinal lymph nodes are normal in size on CT scan and PET negative, but associated with a central tumor or suspicious for N1 nodes, invasive mediastinal staging should be performed. Furthermore, in this setting if the EBUS-TBNA is nondiagnostic or negative and suspicion is high, then a mediastinoscopy should be performed to confirm or rule out N2 and particularly N3 disease.

Patients with a peripheral T1 tumor with normal sized mediastinal lymph nodes that are PET positive should have a tissue confirmation of the PET positivity to rule out a false positive PET (EBUS-TBNA or mediastinoscopy – recognizing that EBUS-TBNA is more challenging to do with normal/small sized mediastinal nodes). However, if the primary tumor is PET positive (hot) and mediastinum is PET negative, invasive staging can be omitted.

An additional concept to consider is that the endoscopic approach with EBUS-TBNA now gives us relatively easy access to sample N1 nodes – hilar and intrapulmonary nodes – in a minimally invasive way. This is a capability that was not available before this technology became a reality. This presents the possibility to identify N1 disease preoperatively and hopefully future trials will determine if this added information will be helpful in prognostication or treatment planning for lung cancer patients. Certainly, as we increasingly consider sublobar resections for T1 tumors, the ability to confirm the absence of N1 node positivity would be helpful in operative planning and even in planning of non-resecting techniques such as SBRT. Furthermore, it is conceivable that identification of and neoadjuvant treatment of patients with N1 disease might prove to be more beneficial than adjuvant therapy, although this remains to be studied.

Sampling of N1 nodes could also be used to obtain tissue for biomarker studies to predict response to targeted therapies. Our experience in lung cancer patients with N2 or N3 disease proven by EBUS-TBNA has shown that molecular diagnosis for targeted therapy, prognostic information by immunohistochemistry, as well as the assessment of chemosensitivity-related aberrant methylation is possible from the tissue samples obtained through EBUS-TBNA [37, 50].

A systematic review was done comparing different methods of restaging the mediastinum after neoadjuvant therapy for stage III NSCLC. It showed that a complete response presents with a false negative rate of 50% and 30% for CT and PET, respectively [53]. Mediastinal lymph node involvement carries a false negative rate of 33% and 25% for CT and PET respectively and false positive rates of 33% and 33% respectively. For invasive staging the results appeared to be better. Re-do mediastinoscopy showed a false negative rate of 22%, EUS-FNA 14% and primary mediastinoscopy 9% [53]. Furthermore, evaluation of down-staging should not be based on the assumption that imaging tests can accurately predict the status of the mediastinal nodes [53]. Even though systematic preoperative staging is done, there are still incidences wherein false negative mediastinal lymph node involvement is confirmed by surgical resection [54] (Figure 12.4).

EBUS-TBNA for post induction staging is also an option. In a review by Herth *et al.*, 124 NSCLC patients with N2 disease were restaged after induction chemotherapy. EBUS-TBNA detected 72% of patients with persistent nodal disease. In this group, of 35 patients with negative EBUS-TBNA mediastinal staging, 28 were found to have residual N2 disease at thoracotomy. Overall sensitivity, specificity, positive predictive value, negative predictive value, and diagnostic accuracy of EBUS-TBNA for mediastinal restaging after induction chemotherapy were 76%, 100%, 100%, 20%, and 77%, respectively [51]. Given this, the authors concluded that if presented with negative findings on EBUS-TBNA, because of the low NPV, mediastinoscopy should be performed before thoracotomy. Szlubowski *et al.* performed a prospective study in 61 patients that were restaged by EBUS-TBNA. Mediastinal involvement was detected in 18 patients (30%). In 43 patients with negative or uncertain mediastinal involvement, TEMLA was performed showing metastatic disease in 9 patients (15%) of which 7 patients (12%) were positive in the EBUS-TBNA accessible stations [52]. It should be noted that the false-negative results of biopsies were found only in small nodes. Also, all positive N2 nodes diagnosed by TEMLA contained only micrometastatic deposits. A diagnostic sensitivity, specificity, accuracy, positive predictive value (PPV) and negative predictive value (NPV) of the restaging EBUS-TBNA was 67%, 86%, 80%, 91% and 78%, respectively. In summary, EBUS-TBNA appears to be an effective technique for restaging of the mediastinum. With increasing experience with this technique, the performance may further improve.

Patients with stage IIIA N2 disease should be restaged after completing neoadjuvant treatment. It is well known that patients with a complete or near complete pathological response to induction chemoradiation have the best long-term prognosis for cure. Restaging of the mediastinum is particularly important to rule out the presence of N3 disease for which the benefit of surgical resection has not yet been demonstrated. Again, persistence of mediastinal lymph node positivity may lead to abandoning the plan for extensive resection in some high-risk patients or to consideration of further induction therapy in others. We prefer in these patients to stage the mediastinum pre-induction with CT, PET and EBUS–FNA, and post induction with CT, PET and mediastinoscopy. This avoids the need for re-do mediastinoscopy which as described above is technically more challenging and associated with a lower sensitivity and diagnostic accuracy [24, 28].

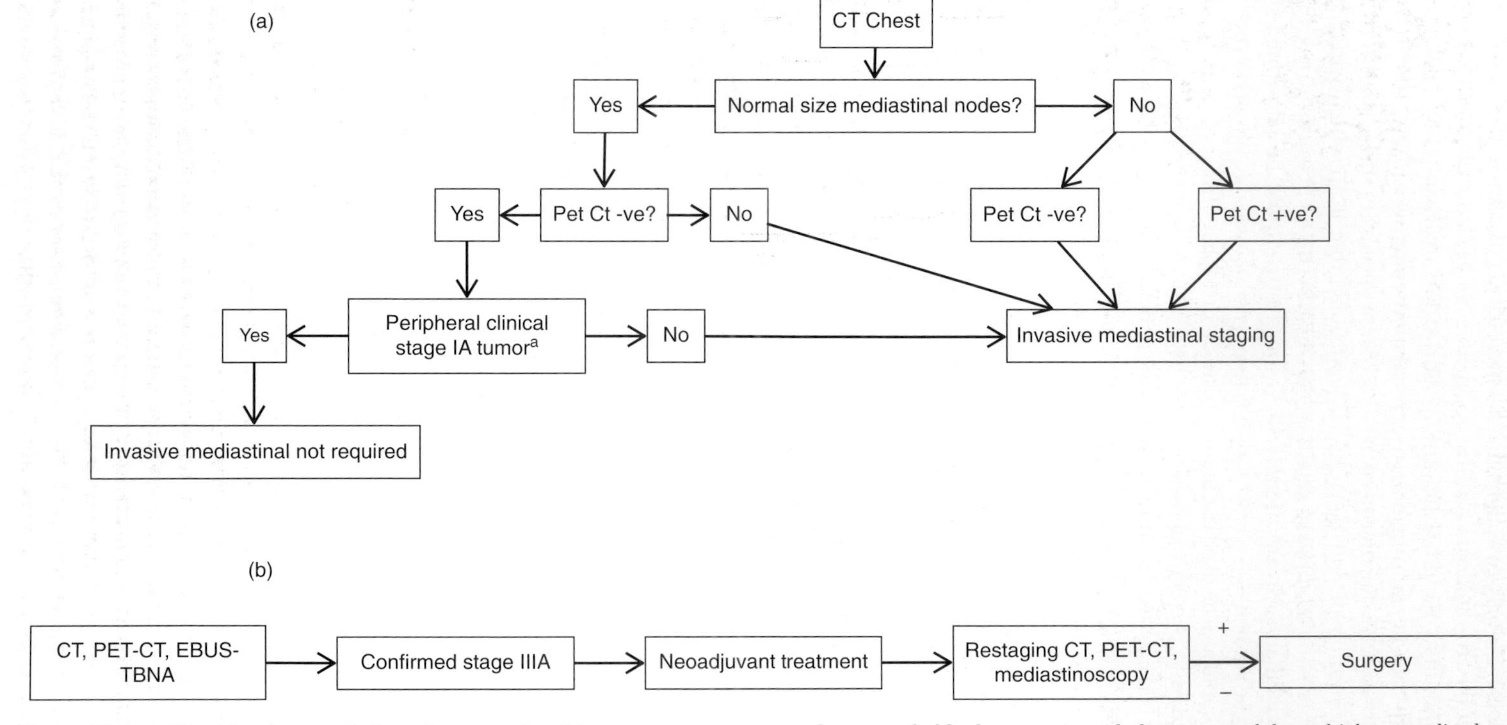

Figure 12.4 a: Algorithm for population of non-small-cell lung cancer clinically staged T1–4, N0–3, with no distant metastases, potentially surgically resectable patients. [a]T1: primary tumour diameter 3 cm or smaller and surrounded by lung or visceral pleura, or endobronchial tumor distal to the lobar bronchus. Modified from Darling *et al.* [14]. b: A mediastinal staging approach for patients with stage IIIA N2 disease.

References

1 Siegel R, Naishadham D, Jemal A (2012) Cancer statistics, 2012. *CA Cancer J Clin*, Jan 1; 62(1): 10–29.

2 Sobin LH, Gospodarowicz MK, Wittekind C (2009) *UICC TNM Classification of Malignant Tumours*, 7th edn. New York: Wiley-Liss.

3 Santos PARD, Rocha RSD, Pipkin M, Silveira MLD, Cypel M, Rios JO, *et al.* Concordance between clinical and pathological staging in patients with stages I or II non small cell lung cancer subjected to surgical treatment. *J Bras Pneumol*, Dec; 33(6): 647–54.

4 Silvestri GA, Gould MK, Margolis ML, Tanoue LT, McCrory D, Toloza E, *et al.* (2007) Noninvasive staging of non-small cell lung cancer: ACCP evidenced-based clinical practice guidelines (2nd edn). *Chest*, 178S–201S.

5 De Leyn P, Lardinois D, Van Schil PE, Rami-Porta R, Passlick B, Zielinski M, *et al.* (2007) ESTS guidelines for preoperative lymph node staging for non-small cell lung cancer. *European Journal of Cardio-Thoracic Surgery*, Jul; 32(1): 1–8.

6 Tournoy KG, Keller SM, Annema JT (2012) Mediastinal staging of lung cancer: novel concepts. *Lancet Oncol*, May; 13(5): e221–9.

7 Dwamena BAB, Sonnad SSS, Angobaldo JOJ, Wahl RLR (1999) Metastases from non-small cell lung cancer: mediastinal staging in the 1990s-meta-analytic comparison of PET and CT. *Radiology*, Nov 1; 213(2): 530–6.

8 Freudenberg LS, Rosenbaum SJ, Beyer T, Bockisch A, Antoch G (2010) PET versus PET/CT dual-modality imaging in evaluation of lung cancer. *Thorac Surg Clin*, Feb; 20(1): 25–30.

9 Broderick SR, Meyers BF (2012) PET Staging of mediastinal lymph nodes in thoracic oncology. *Thorac Surg Clin*, May; 22(2): 161–6.

10 Whitson BA, Groth SS, Maddaus MA (2008) Recommendations for optimal use of imaging studies to clinically stage mediastinal lymph nodes in non-small-cell lung cancer patients. *Lung Cancer*, Aug 1; 61(2): 9.

11 Lee BE, Haag von D, Lown T, Lau D, Calhoun R, Follette D (2007) Advances in positron emission tomography technology have increased the need for surgical staging in non-small cell lung cancer. *J Thorac Cardiovasc Surg*, Mar 1; 133(3): 746–52.

12 Cerfolio RJ, Ojha B, Bryant AS, Raghuveer V, Mountz JM, Bartolucci AA (2004) The accuracy of integrated PET-CT compared with dedicated pet alone for the staging of patients with nonsmall cell lung cancer. *Annals of Thoracic Surgery*, Sep; 78(3): 1017–23.

13 Darling GEG, Maziak DED, Inculet RIR, Gulenchyn KYK, Driedger AAA, Ung YCY, *et al.* (2011) Positron emission tomography-computed tomography compared with invasive mediastinal staging in non-small cell lung cancer: Results of mediastinal staging in the early lung positron emission tomography trial. *J Thorac Oncol*, Aug 1; 6(8): 1367–72.

14 Detterbeck FC, Jantz MA, Wallace M, Vansteenkiste J, Silvestri GA (2007) Invasive mediastinal staging of lung cancer: ACCP evidence-based clinical practice guidelines (2nd edn). *Chest*, Sep 1; 132(3_suppl): 202S–220S.

15 Darling GE, Dickie AJ, Malthaner RA, Kennedy EB, Tey R (2011) Invasive mediastinal staging of non-small-cell lung cancer: A clinical practice guideline. *Curr Oncol*, Dec; 18(6): e304–10.

16 Nakajima T, Yasufuku K (2011) The techniques of endobronchial ultrasound-guided transbronchial needle aspiration. *Innovations (Phila)*, Jan; 6(1): 57–64.

17 Yasufuku K, Chiyo M, Sekine Y, Chhajed PN, Shibuya K, Iizasa T, *et al.* (2004) Real-time endobronchial ultrasound-guided transbronchial needle aspiration of mediastinal and hilar lymph nodes. *Chest*, Jul; 126(1): 122–8.

18 Ernst A, Eberhardt R, Krasnik M, Herth FJF (2009) Efficacy of endobronchial ultrasound-guided transbronchial needle aspiration of hilar lymph nodes for diagnosing and staging cancer. *J Thorac Oncol*, Aug; 4(8): 947–50.

19 Gu P, Zhao Y-Z, Jiang L-Y, Zhang W, Xin Y, Han B-H (2009) Endobronchial ultrasound-guided transbronchial needle aspiration for staging of lung cancer: A systematic review and meta-analysis. *Eur. J. Cancer*, May; 45(8): 1389–96.

20 Adams K, Shah PL, Edmonds L, Lim E (2009) Test performance of endobronchial ultrasound and transbronchial needle aspiration biopsy for mediastinal staging in patients with lung cancer: Systematic review and meta-analysis. *Thorax*, Sep; 64(9): 757–62.

21 Yasufuku K, Pierre A, Darling G, de Perrot M, Waddell T, Johnston M, *et al.* (2011) A prospective controlled trial of endobronchial ultrasound-guided transbronchial needle aspiration compared with mediastinoscopy for mediastinal lymph node staging of lung cancer. *Journal of Thoracic and Cardiovascular Surgery*, Dec; 142(6): 1393–400.e1.

22 Andrade RS, Odell DD, D'Cunha J, Maddaus MA (2012) Endobronchial ultrasonography (EBUS) – its role in staging of non-small cell lung cancer and who should do it? *Journal of Thoracic and Cardiovascular Surgery*, Sep; 144(3): S9–13.

23 Kuźdżał J, Szlubowski A (2012) Ultrasound-guided transbronchial and transesophageal needle biopsy in the mediastinal staging of lung cancer. *Thorac Surg Clin*, May; 22(2): 191–203.
24 Groth SS, Andrade RS (2010) Endobronchial and endoscopic ultrasound-guided fine-needle aspiration: A must for thoracic surgeons. *Annals of Thoracic Surgery*, Jun; 89(6): S2079–83.
25 Micames CG (2007) Endoscopic ultrasound-guided fine-needle aspiration for non-small cell lung cancer staging – a systematic review and metaanalysis. *Chest*, Feb 1; 131(2): 539.
26 Szlubowski AA, Zieliński MM, Soja JJ, Annema JTJ, Sośnicki WW, Jakubiak MM, *et al.* (2010) A combined approach of endobronchial and endoscopic ultrasound-guided needle aspiration in the radiologically normal mediastinum in non-small-cell lung cancer staging – a prospective trial. *Eur J Cardiothorac Surg*, May 1; 37(5): 5.
27 Herth FJF (2010) Combined endoscopic-endobronchial ultrasound-guided fine-needle aspiration of mediastinal lymph nodes through a single bronchoscope in 150 patients with suspected lung cancer. *Chest*, Oct 1; 38(4): 90.
28 Herth FJF (2011) Nonsurgical staging of the mediastinum: EBUS and EUS. *Semin Respir Crit Care Med*, Feb; 32(1): 62–8.
29 Ohnishi R, Yasuda I, Kato T, Tanaka T, Kaneko Y, Suzuki T, *et al.* (2011) Combined endobronchial and endoscopic ultrasound-guided fine needle aspiration for mediastinal nodal staging of lung cancer. *Endoscopy*, © Georg Thieme Verlag KG; Oct 4; 43(12): 1082–9.
30 Hwangbo B (2010) Transbronchial and transesophageal fine-needle aspiration using an ultrasound bronchoscope in mediastinal staging of potentially operable lung cancer. *Chest*, Oct 1; 138(4): 795.
31 Cerfolio RJ, Bryant AS, Eloubeidi MA, Frederick PA, Minnich DJ, Harbour KC, *et al.* (2010) The true false negative rates of esophageal and endobronchial ultrasound in the staging of mediastinal lymph nodes in patients with non-small cell lung cancer. *Annals of Thoracic Surgery*, Aug; 90(2): 427–34.
32 Filho DRDP, Avino AJGA, Brandão SLBS, Spiandorello WPW (2009) Joint use of cervical mediastinoscopy and video-assisted thoracoscopy for the evaluation of mediastinal lymph nodes in patients with non-small cell lung cancer. *J Bras Pneumol*, Nov 1; 35(11): 1068–74.
33 Lerut T, De Leyn P, Coosemans W, Decaluwé H, Decker G, Nafteux P, *et al.* (2010) Cervical videomediastinoscopy. *Thorac Surg Clin*, May; 20(2): 195–206.
34 Martin-Ucar AE, Chetty GK, Vaughan R, Waller DA (2004) A prospective audit evaluating the role of video-assisted cervical mediastinoscopy (VAM) as a training tool. *Eur J Cardiothorac Surg*, Aug; 26(2): 393–5.
35 Leschber G, Sperling D, Klemm W, Merk J (2008) Does video-mediastinoscopy improve the results of conventional mediastinoscopy? *Eur J Cardiothorac Surg*, Feb; 33(2): 289–93.
36 Rami-Porta R, Call S (2012) Invasive staging of mediastinal lymph nodes: Mediastinoscopy and remediastinoscopy. *Thorac Surg Clin*, May; 22(2): 177–89.
37 Yasufuku K, Keshavjee S (2010) Staging non-small cell lung cancer. *Clinical Pulmonary Medicine*, Sep; 17(5): 223–31.
38 Lemaire A, Nikolic I, Petersen T, Haney JC, Toloza EM, Harpole DH, *et al.* (2006) Nine-year single center experience with cervical mediastinoscopy: complications and false negative rate. *Annals of Thoracic Surgery*, Oct; 82(4): 1185–9, discussion 1189–90.
39 Toloza EME, Harpole LL, Detterbeck FF, McCrory DCD (2003) Invasive staging of non-small cell lung cancer: A review of the current evidence. *Chest*, Jan 1; 123(1 Suppl): 157S–166S.
40 McNeill TM, Chamberlain JM (1966) Diagnostic anterior mediastinotomy. *Annals of Thoracic Surgery. Soc Thorac Surgeons*, Jul 1; 2(4): 532.
41 Van Schil P, van der Schoot J, Poniewierski J, Pauwels M, Carp L, Germonpré P, *et al.* (2002) Remediastinoscopy after neoadjuvant therapy for non-small cell lung cancer. *Lung Cancer*, Sep; 37(3): 281–5.
42 Mateu-Navarro M, Rami-Porta R, Bastus-Piulats R, Cirera-Nogueras L, González-Pont G (2000) Remediastinoscopy after induction chemotherapy in non-small cell lung cancer. *ATS*, Aug; 70(2): 391–5.
43 De Waele M, Serra-Mitjans M, Hendriks J, Lauwers P, Belda-Sanchis J, Van Schil P, *et al.* (2008) Accuracy and survival of repeat mediastinoscopy after induction therapy for non-small cell lung cancer in a combined series of 104 patients. *Eur J Cardiothorac Surg*, May; 33(5): 824–8.
44 Rami-Porta R (2007) Supermediastinoscopies: A step forward in lung cancer staging. *J Thorac Oncol*, Apr 1; 2(4): 355–6.
45 Zielinski M (2012) Video-assisted mediastinoscopic lymphadenectomy and transcervical extended mediastinal lymphadenectomy. *Thorac Surg Clin*, May; 22(2): 219–25.
46 Yoo DG, Kim Y-H, Kim DK, Kim HR, Park S-I (2011) Clinical feasibility and surgical benefits of

video-assisted mediastinoscopic lymphadenectomy in the treatment of resectable lung cancer. *Eur J Cardio-thorac Surg*, Dec 1; 40(6): 4.

47 Zielinski M (2007) Transcervical extended mediastinal lymphadenectomy: Results of staging in two hundred fifty-six patients with non-small cell lung cancer. *J Thorac Oncol*, Apr; 2(4): 370–2.

48 Witte BB, Wolf MM, Huertgen MM, Toomes HH (2006) Video-assisted mediastinoscopic surgery: Clinical feasibility and accuracy of mediastinal lymph node staging. *ATS*, Nov 1; 82(5): 7.

49 Yendamuri S, Demmy TL (2012) Is VAMLA/TEMLA the new standard of preresection staging of non-small cell lung cancer? *Journal of Thoracic and Cardiovascular Surgery*, Sep; 144(3): S14–17.

50 Mohamed S, Yasufuku K, Nakajima T, Hiroshima K, Kubo R, Iyoda A, *et al.* (2008) Analysis of cell cycle-related proteins in mediastinal lymph nodes of patients with N2-NSCLC obtained by EBUS-TBNA: Relevance to chemotherapy response. *Thorax*, Jul 1; 63(7): 642–7.

51 Herth FJF, Annema JT, Eberhardt R, Yasufuku K, Ernst A, Krasnik M, *et al.* (2008) Endobronchial ultrasound with transbronchial needle aspiration for restaging the mediastinum in lung cancer. *J Clin Oncol*, Jul 10; 26(20): 3346–50.

52 Szlubowski A, Herth FJF, Soja J, Kołodziej M, Figura J, Ćmiel A, *et al.* (2010) Endobronchial ultrasound-guided needle aspiration in non-small-cell lung cancer restaging verified by the transcervical bilateral extended mediastinal lymphadenectomy – a prospective study. *European Journal of Cardio-thoracic Surgery*, 37: 1180–4.

53 de Cabanyes Candela S, Detterbeck FC (2010) A systematic review of restaging after induction therapy for stage IIIa lung cancer: prediction of pathologic stage. *J Thorac Oncol*, Mar; 5(3): 389–98.

54 Kirmani BH, Rintoul RC, Win T, Magee C, Magee L, Choong C, *et al.* (2013) Stage migration: results of lymph node dissection in the era of modern imaging and invasive staging for lung cancer. *European Journal of Cardio-Thoracic Surgery*, Jan; 43(1): 104–10.

55 Rusch VW, Asamura H, Watanabe H, Giroux DJ, Rami-Porta R, Goldstraw P, *et al.* (2009) The IASLC lung cancer staging project: A proposal for a new international lymph node map in the forthcoming 7th edition of the TNM classification for lung cancer. *J Thorac Oncol*, May; 4(5): 568–77.

56 Darling G, Dickie A, Malthaner R, Kennedy E, Tey R, Invasive Mediastinal Staging Expert Panel (2010) *Invasive Mediastinal Staging of Non-small-cell Lung Cancer: A Clinical Practice Guideline*. Toronto (ON): Cancer Care Ontario; 2010 Oct 18. Program in Evidence-based Care Evidence-based Series No. 17–6.

57 Silvestri GA, Gonzalez AV, Jantz MA, Margolis ML, Gould MK, Tanoue LT, *et al.* (2013) Methods for staging non-small cell lung cancer: diagnosis and management of lung cancer, 3rd ed: American College of Chest Physicians evidence-based clinical practice guidelines. *Chest*, May; 143(5 Suppl): e211S–50S.

CHAPTER 13

Management of the Solitary Pulmonary Nodule

Min P. Kim

Department of Surgery, Division of Thoracic Surgery, Houston Methodist Hospital, Houston, TX, USA

Introduction

A solitary pulmonary nodule is defined as a single opacity on a chest radiograph that is smaller than or equal to 3 cm, and surrounded by aerated lung [1–3]. A lesion larger than 3 cm is called a lung mass. Successful management of solitary pulmonary nodules is based on accurate assessment of the risk of a solitary pulmonary nodule being a malignant lesion and based on the risk assessment providing appropriate tests and interventions. The ultimate goal is to provide early diagnosis and treatment for patients with malignant tumors and reduce morbidity for patients with benign nodules. It is a fine balance of considering all of the available information about the patient and setting a management plan that provides the best outcome.

A solitary pulmonary nodule could be a benign lesion such as hamartoma, chondroma, granuloma, pneumonia, abscess, rheumatoid arthritis, Wegener granulomatosis, arteriovenous malformation, vascular infarction, hematoma, congenital bronchial atresia, or sequestration. It also could be a malignant lesion such as lung cancer or solitary metastatic cancer to the lung from other organs [4]. The clinical and radiographic features can provide information on the probability that the nodule is malignant.

Prevalence of lung nodules

The National Lung Cancer Screening trial has shown that individuals with a high risk of lung cancer benefit from low-dose computed tomography (CT) screening [5]. The study showed that there was a 20% relative decrease in mortality in the individuals who underwent low-dose CT screening for lung cancer. This trial enrolled more than 50 000 patients between 55 and 74 years of age with at least 30-pack-year of smoking history who had smoked within the previous 15 years. The trial excluded patients who had a previous diagnosis of lung cancer, a chest CT in the previous 18 months, recent hemoptysis, or a 15-lb weight loss in the past year. They were randomized to either three annual screening low-dose CT scans or a single chest radiographic screening. In the low-dose CT group, 39% of the patients had at least one positive screening result. In the patients with a positive result, 96% had a benign lesion. The screening eventually resulted in finding tumors in 649 patients (2.4%). However, it missed cancer in 44 patients (0.2%); 367 patients (1.4%) developed cancer after the trial-screening phase. This trial did not develop an algorithm to manage lung nodules. The radiologist reported the results to the participant and his or her health care provider, but there was no specific

Lung Cancer, Fourth Edition. Edited by Jack A. Roth, Waun Ki Hong and Ritsuko U. Komaki.

evaluation approach. The most common approach was additional imaging, with few patients undergoing invasive procedures [5].

This study, along with other large screening studies [6–9], showed that the nodules that are identified in a screening trial tend to be smaller with a lower prevalence of malignancy. A review of eight other large screening trials showed that the prevalence of solitary pulmonary nodules in the screened population varied from 8% to 51%, with 1.1% to 12% of the nodules identified as malignant [10]. However, when solitary lung nodules that have an intermediate or high probability of being malignant are resected, the probability of the nodule being malignant can be as high as 55% [11].

Since the National Lung Screening Trial showed that low-dose CT screening for high-risk patients reduces mortality, more individuals will be diagnosed with a solitary pulmonary nodule. There are no set rules in terms of how to manage a solitary pulmonary nodule. However, there are some guidelines to help balance between performing excessive diagnostic procedures and delaying cancer diagnosis and treatment. These guidelines are based on the data of clinical features and diagnostic imaging features that help provide an assessment of risk of the nodule being malignant.

Risk of malignancy

For an individual with a solitary lung nodule, the clinician should take account of both clinical and radiologic features to assess the probability of the nodule being malignant. The management of the solitary lung nodule should be based on this assessment.

Clinical features

Several clinical features increase the risk of the nodule being a malignancy, including age of the individual, smoking status, occupational exposure, medical history of chronic obstructive pulmonary disease (COPD), and history of extrathoracic malignancy. On the other hand, individuals with a recent history of pneumonia or history of fungal infections will show decreased risk of malignant nodules.

Smoking is the single greatest risk factor for lung cancer. Thus, a patient with a solitary pulmonary nodule with a long history of smoking multiple packs per day has a very high risk of the nodule being malignant. Current high-rate smokers (> 1 pack per day) have the highest risk of a solitary lung nodule being malignant compared to current smokers who smoke less then a pack per day and patients who were never-smokers [1]. The individual who quit smoking less then 7 years ago has a higher risk of a nodule being malignant compared to patients who quit more then 7 years ago [1]. Thus, former smokers are at a much lower risk for malignancy than the current smoker.

In addition to smoking status, the age of the individual contributes to the probability of the solitary lung nodule malignancy. The lung cancer rates are very high for patients between 65 and 70 years old, while it is rarely diagnosed before the age of 40 [12]. Thus, a 30-year-old individual with a solitary lung nodule is less likely to have primary lung cancer than a 65-year-old with a solitary lung nodule.

An individual's medical history also contributes to the probability of the patient having a malignant solitary pulmonary nodule. An individual with COPD is more likely to have a malignant nodule than one without COPD [1]. An individual with a history of asbestos exposure has a higher risk of developing a cancer than patients who never had asbestos exposure [1]. Finally, an individual with a history of extrathoracic cancer with a solitary pulmonary nodule on a CT scan has an increased probability of a malignant nodule [13]. Thus, a patient who had a colon cancer resected with a pulmonary nodule that has increased over serial CT scans will most likely have a metastatic colon cancer. However, individuals with a recent history of bacterial or fungal pneumonia are less likely to have a malignancy. Further imaging should be obtained and, if the nodule decreases in size or disappears, it is most likely related to patient's pneumonia.

Radiographic features

The radiographic feature of a solitary lung nodule is best assessed using CT. An individual who is diagnosed with a solitary pulmonary nodule on a chest

X-ray should have a CT of the chest to further evaluate the probability of the nodule being malignant. In addition, any previous imaging of the chest should be obtained to estimate the growth rate of the nodule [14]. The size of the tumor, nodule characteristics, and growth rate help determine the probability of a malignant solitary nodule.

The probability of the nodule being a tumor increases with its size. In eight large clinical lung cancer screening studies, it was shown that nodules < 5 mm had a prevalence of malignancy 0–1% of the time, 5–10 mm nodules had a prevalence of 6–28%, 11–20 mm nodules had a prevalence of 33–64%, and those greater than 20 mm had a prevalence of 64–82% [10, 15]. Thus, the larger the lesion, the greater the likelihood that the solitary lung nodule is malignant.

The features of the nodule also provide information on the probability of a malignant nodule. A review of six lung cancer screening studies showed that a nodule with a smooth edge had a 20–30% probability of malignancy, while a nodule with irregular, lobulated, or spiculated borders had a 33–100% chance of malignancy [10]. Malignant tumor with smooth edge tends to be metastatic cancer to the lung from other organs. Certain patterns of calcification of the solitary pulmonary nodule denote that the nodule is benign. Individuals with nodules with a diffuse, centrally laminated and popcorn pattern of calcification are likely to have a benign nodule while patients with nodules with stippled and eccentric patterns of calcification are less likely to have a benign nodule [14].

The growth rate of the solitary nodule will provide information about its probability of malignancy. Most malignant solitary pulmonary nodules will double in size between 40 and 400 days. When a nodule grows more rapidly, it is usually infectious; if it grows more slowly, it is usually benign [16–19]. A pulmonary nodule's stability for more than two years or 730 days is a reliable indicator for being benign [16, 20]. However, this is not absolute: this indication is accurate only 65% of the time [17]. This may be due to the fact that the doubling time for smaller solitary lung nodules is difficult to assess. For example, a 5 mm solitary nodule will double in volume and will then measure 6 mm. However, the CT scan might not be able to detect the difference between these two sizes and, thus, it may appear stable on the CT scan. Thus, smaller nodules may require longer follow-up to establish the nodule's benign nature, based on imaging criteria alone [17].

Management

Patient preference and shared decision-making

After assessing the probability of a malignant nodule, the clinician should discuss the risks and benefits of each of the management plans. Some patients may be uncomfortable with a plan of watchful waiting with any probability that that nodule is malignant, while some patients would be similarly risk adverse about undergoing surgery unless there is confirmation that the nodule is a tumor. Thus, each of the management plans outlined below should also take into account the patient's preference [14].

Management plan

Based on the patient's clinical history and radiographic studies, the risk of a solitary pulmonary nodule being a malignancy should be determined and an individualized management plan should be offered. Individuals with a very low probability of having a malignancy should be managed with serial imaging. Individuals with an intermediate probability of having a malignancy should be managed with an additional non-invasive test of FDG-PET; if it is still indeterminate, then a sampling of the nodule should be obtained. Finally, individuals with a very high probability of having a malignancy should be managed based on the surgical candidacy of the patient and the location of the lesion.

Low probability

After an assessment of the risk of a malignant solitary pulmonary nodule, if an individual has a high probability of having a benign lung lesion, the patient should undergo serial CT scans. The rationale for this strategy is based on the fact that the malignant nodules tend to double in size between 40 and 400 days. Thus, if a nodule doubles in size during serial CT scans, then the probability that the nodule is indeed a malignancy increases and the person should undergo the management strategy that is outlined in a high-risk probability group. The only downside of this strategy of watchful waiting is that there are hazards with delaying a diagnosis of malignancy [15]. There is a possibility that a patient with a lung nodule that is surgically curable at the time of initial detection may develop a metastatic lesion during the interval CT scan. This makes an individual's curative lung cancer become noncurable, significantly decreasing the likelihood of overall survival for that individual. With this in mind, the individual should be imaged at a set interval.

There are no standard set time interval recommendations for imaging patients, but there are general guidelines and societal recommendations. A strategy for a patient with a smaller nodule (< 8 mm) is described by the Fleischner Society [21]. In patients with clinical risk for malignancy such as smoking, the patients with < 4 mm nodule should have a follow-up CT scan in 12 months and no additional follow-up if the nodule is stable. For a > 4–6 mm lesion, the patients should have a follow-up scan at 6–12 months, with another follow-up at 18–24 months. For a > 6–8 mm lesion, the patients should have a follow-up scan at 3–6 months, 9–12 months, and 24 months, if stable. Four years since the recommendation came out, about 80% of the radiologists who were surveyed were aware of the recommendation and 50% of them have incorporated it into their practice [22]. For small nodules (< 8 mm), the Fleischner Society recommendation is a reasonable approach, with a caveat that there can still be malignant nodules that can be missed with this approach. If there is any question about the stability of the nodule, then an additional scan at a longer interval may be needed to confirm that the nodule is nonmalignant [17]. For larger nodules, more frequent intervals should be adopted to follow the growth of the nodule; stability in two years is a reasonable metric for a nonmalignant solitary pulmonary nodule. For an individual with a solitary pulmonary nodule that measures 8–10 mm, serial CT scans at least 3, 6, 12, and 24 months is a reasonable strategy [14]. Patients with > 1 cm nodules tend to have shorter initial intervals for imaging, but there is no set recommendation for how to image this group of patients. Typically a CT of the chest is obtained in 2–3 month intervals for this group of patients with larger nodules. Such a nodule increasing its size over subsequent imaging increases the risk of it being malignant. Thus, the individual should be managed based on an intermediate or high-probability algorithm as outlined below.

Intermediate probability

Individuals with clinical and radiographic evidence of a nodule's intermediate probability of malignancy should undergo further studies to help determine whether the lesion is a malignancy. The additional tests would include a FDG-PET with or without sampling of a tissue. This strategy will either increase or decrease the probability of malignant solitary pulmonary nodule.

FDG-PET

The FDG-PET is a nuclear medicine scan in which ^{18}F-fluorodeoxyglucose (FDG), a glucose analog, is injected in the patient and the amount of the FDG uptake on the scan suggests the possibility of the nodule being malignant. The FDG-PET has very high sensitivity between 80% and 100% for detecting a malignancy with specificity between 40% and 100%, depending on the series [10, 23]. The lower specificity in some series is due to the fact that glucose uptake also takes place in inflammation and infection; thus, a patient with pneumonia can have false-positive FDG-PET results. The maximum standardized uptake (maxSUV) can also provide information on the probability of the nodule being malignant. In one series, a nodule with maxSUV between 0 and 2.5 had a 24% probability of the nodule being malignant; if it was between 2.6 and 4.0, it had an 80% chance of being malignant; and if it was greater than 4.1, it had a 96% chance of being malignant [24]. Another study showed that the highest diagnostic accuracy for malignancy was found for solitary pulmonary nodules with SUV > 4 [25].

A negative FDG-PET can significantly decrease the probability that the nodule is malignant; thus patients with a negative FDG-PET scan may be monitored with serial imaging. In one series, the 85% of the patients with negative FDG-PET scans were managed by watchful waiting. Five percent of the individuals in the study had a false negative scan, but the survival in this group did not differ significantly from the patients with a true-positive FDG-PET scan [26]. The FDG-PET scan often misses the small malignant tumors (< 8 mm), certain types of metastatic tumor, and certain types of lung cancer, such as carcinoid and bronchoalveolar carcinomas [24].

If the nodule is malignant, the FDG-PET is an effective test for providing staging information for patients with primary lung cancer. One series showed that including the FDG-PET can provide improved diagnostic accuracy in detecting mediastinal lymph node metastasis in patients with lung cancer [27], thus providing better staging information for patients with lung cancer before operating for therapeutic resection. Cost-effectiveness of using FDG-PET in staging and management of solitary pulmonary nodules have shown that overall the PET imaging is cost effective in context of proper medical indication [28].

Sampling of a tissue

Information obtained on the FDG-PET scan can significantly increase the probability that the nodule is malignant, which may change the algorithm from the intermediate-probability to the high-probability algorithm. However, after the FDG-PET, if the probability of a malignant nodule is still intermediate, the individual should obtain a tissue sampling. The modality to sample the tissue can be separated, based on the location of the lesion.

Central

Individuals with a central pulmonary lung nodule should obtain a biopsy either through bronchoscopy or radial endobronchial ultrasound (EBUS)-guided biopsy. The bronchoscopy will help obtain a diagnosis of a solitary pulmonary nodule with endobronchial component, while the radial EBUS will help in obtaining a diagnosis with a pulmonary nodule that is located near the trachea and the main bronchus.

Bronchoscopy and bronchial washing with or without a transbronchial needle biopsy has diagnostic yield of up to 74% for patients with an endobronchial component [29]. However, for patients with a solitary pulmonary nodule without an endobronchial component, the diagnostic yield is about 30–40% [29, 30]. The advantage of this method of obtaining a tissue is that it can be performed in an awake patient with conscious sedation, with very low morbidity.

The radial EBUS combines the direct visualization of the airway along with the ability to perform an ultrasound of the structures next to the airway. Thus, it offers the ability to perform ultrasound-guided visualization of a solitary pulmonary nodule and subsequent biopsy of the nodule. However, this is limited to the solitary pulmonary nodules located near the major airway. Overall, EBUS has a very low complication rate and very good diagnostic yield. In addition, if the nodule is indeed malignant, the patient can undergo staging of the mediastinal lymph nodes at the same setting to complete the lung cancer staging. The EBUS allows examination of the mediastinal lymph nodes and some hilar lymph nodes.

Mid to peripheral

There are two major modalities that can be used to obtain a diagnosis for a mid to peripheral nodule: the CT-guided transthoracic biopsy and the guided transbronchial biopsy. Currently, the transthoracic biopsy has higher diagnostic yield than the guided transbronchial biopsy, but it carries a significantly higher pneumothorax rate.

Transthoracic biopsy

Transthoracic needle biopsy using CT provides a diagnostic yield 36–86% of the time, depending on the series [10, 14], with an accepted diagnostic yield of about 80%. It is performed in an awake patient with light sedation and local anesthetic. In spite of a high diagnostic yield, transthoracic needle biopsy has a pneumothorax rate of about 30–50% [31, 32]. Another downside of the CT-guided needle biopsy is the difficulty in obtaining a biopsy in certain locations such as central lesions and lesions located between the fissure. This risk of pneumothorax increases, depending on the size of the lesion, amount of emphysema, distance of the nodule from the pleura, and number of passes [33]. In one study, a diagnostic specimen was obtained in patients with nodules greater then 1.5 cm in 73% of the time compared to the patient with 51% of the time for nodules less then 1.5 cm. The overall diagnostic yield in that study was 68%, with 35% of the patients getting a pneumothorax and 5% of patients requiring a thoracostomy tube [32].

Guided transbronchial biopsy

There are three types of guided transbronchial biopsy. The technology allows the placement of a sheath to the nodule and allowing the biopsy of the nodule using a needle, forcep and brush. Meta-analysis of electromagnetic navigation bronchoscopy (ENB) (SuperDimension, Minneapolis, MN), virtual bronchoscopy navigation (VBN) using LungPoint (Broncus Technologies, Mountain View, CA), and radial endobronchial ultrasound (Olympus Medical, Tokyo, Japan) shows significant improvement of diagnostic yield compared to bronchoscopy alone. The diagnostic yield ranged from 46% to 80%, with pooled diagnostic yield of 70%, but the overall incidence of pneumothorax was 1.5% [34].

ENB allows guided placement of a sheath to the nodule and, then, different tools can be placed to take a biopsy. The procedure involves taking a thin-slice CT of the chest and converting it to a three-dimensional rendering of the lung. Next, the patient is placed in an electromagnetic field, which allows merging the real bronchoscopy image to the virtual computer-generated image. This allows for guiding the sheath with turn by turn directions into the lung nodule beyond the area that can be visualized on simple bronchoscopy [35]. There are several factors that can enhance the diagnostic yield of this procedure. Two major factors are size of the nodule and the presence of a CT scan image that shows an airway going to the nodule [36]. This technology also allows for placement of a fiducial marker for individuals who are diagnosed with lung cancer who are not operative candidates. This technology can be used with conscious sedation; however, it is much easier to perform the procedure with general anesthesia. Overall, it has very good diagnostic yield with very low pneumothorax rate.

VBN, on the other hand, does not use real-time positioning information provided by the ENB but simply uses a CT scan alone to make a map of the bronchial tree. LungPoint software (Broncus Technologies), takes a thin-slice CT image and creates a map of the bronchial tree [37]. The virtual image is superimposed over the live bronchoscopic view and the ultrathin bronchoscope is guided to the nodule [38]. Depending on the location of the lesion, standard bronchoscope or ultrathin bronchoscope can be used to get to the nodule, and the nodule is biopsied under X-ray fluoroscopy [37]. In one series, the overall diagnostic yield was 63%, with no pneumothorax rate [37].

The radial endobronchial ultrasound-guided sheath (Olympus Medical) and biopsy allows biopsy of the lesion under conscious sedation. An individual undergoing a standard bronchoscopy will have a plastic sheath with mini radial EBUS placed through the bronchoscope and the sheath guided to the lesion. Then, the EBUS is removed and disposable biopsy forceps and cytology brushes are used to obtain the biopsy. A fluoroscopy is used to ensure that the ultrasound miniprobe has not reached the visceral pleura and that the forceps is working during the biopsy. Diagnostic sensitivity was 64%, with a 1% pneumonthorax rate for one series using this technology [39]. Radial endobronchial ultrasound can be combined with ENB or VBN. In one study, combining the VBN and radial EBUS led to 80% diagnostic yield, with faster time to localization than radial EBUS alone [38].

High probability

Individuals with a high probability of having a malignant solitary pulmonary nodule should be managed based on whether the individual can tolerate surgical resection. The individual should undergo the standard pulmonary and cardiac workup to see whether he or she is a surgical candidate if the solitary pulmonary nodule is indeed primary lung cancer. If the FDG-PET was not used to make the determination of a high probability of having a malignant nodule, a FDG-PET should be performed for staging of possible lung cancer. If the FDG-PET shows a widely metastatic disease to other sites, then the individual should have a biopsy of the most accessible place and be subsequently treated for metastatic lung cancer. If the FDG-PET shows uptake only at the solitary pulmonary nodule, the individual should be managed based on the ability of the individual to tolerate the surgical resection of the lesion.

Nonsurgical patients

If the patient is determined to not be a surgical candidate, every effort should be made to obtain a diagnosis of the solitary pulmonary nodule. There are several different methods of obtaining a diagnosis, which are outlined above. Depending of the location of the lesion, the individual should have bronchoscopy, radial EBUS, or CT-guided transthoracic or guided transbronchial biopsy of the pulmonary nodule. An advantage of guided bronchoscopy for a nonsurgical patient with a solitary pulmonary nodule is that the individual can get a fiducial marker to receive radiation therapy if the patient has an early-stage lung cancer. Guided bronchoscopy, such as electromagnetic navigation bronchoscopy, has been used with a very high success rate of placement of the fiducial marker without migration [28]. Once the diagnosis of the solitary pulmonary nodule is made in the nonsurgical patient with a high probability of a malignant solitary pulmonary nodule, the patient should undergo staging and appropriate treatment of the nodule.

Surgical patients

After evaluation of the cardiopulmonary status, if the individual is a surgical candidate, the management of the solitary pulmonary nodule should be based on the location of the lesion.

Peripheral nodules

An individual with a high probability of having a malignant solitary pulmonary nodule in the periphery of the lung after FDG-PET who can tolerate a surgical resection should undergo VATS (video assisted thoracic surgery) wedge resection and subsequent VATS completion lobectomy and mediastinal lymph node dissection, if the lesion is a primary lung cancer. For example, a 65-year-old man with a 40-pack-a-year smoking history with a 2 cm spiculated, noncalcified peripheral nodule, which has grown in size over 3 months on serial CT scans with maxSUV of 8 on FDG-PET, without any signs of metastasis, and who can tolerate a lobectomy, may benefit from going directly to the operating room for both diagnostic and surgical treatment for the early-stage lung cancer.

The individual should undergo VATS wedge resection, which can be performed with low morbidity for a peripheral lesion, and undergo intra-op freezing of the nodule. The introduction of VATS wedge resection has increased the overall success rate of resection of a benign lesion [40], but when performed, it results in decreased morbidity and mortality compared to open thoracotomy and lung resection [41]. If the nodule is a primary lung cancer, the patient should undergo completion lobectomy and mediastinal lymph node dissection for definitive treatment of early-stage lung cancer, since that is the standard of care for a patient with a < 3 cm tumor without evidence of mediastinal lymph node spread [42]. This will provide both definitive diagnosis and treatment of the cancer. If the VATS wedge resection shows a metastasis from extrathoracic malignancy, the procedure provides both diagnosis and treatment of the solitary lung nodule. If the VATS wedge resection shows a benign nodule, the individual has a definitive diagnosis of the solitary lung nodule and the individual does not have to undergo additional CT scans.

This method avoids obtaining a transthoracic or transbronchial needle biopsy of the nodule in this select group of patients with high risk of malignancy. The argument for this strategy is that, if the needle biopsy shows nondiagnostic tissue then the patient will be scheduled for VATS wedge resection. If the needle biopsy shows a benign lesion, there is still a possibility that the needle biopsy missed the malignant cells. Thus the results may be due to an error in the biopsy technique or misinterpretation of the cytology, and the individual will be scheduled for VATS wedge resection. If the needle biopsy shows diagnostic tissue that is consistent with malignancy, the patient will undergo an operation. Regardless of the results of the needle biopsy, the patient will undergo surgery. Thus, needle biopsy result of a nodule that is at high risk of being malignant may not alter the management of the individual. Most likely the individual will take on all of the risks of the needle biopsy with minimal benefit from the biopsy. However, certain individuals would be risk-averse to any type of surgical intervention without proof of presence of malignancy. In this group, patients should get a needle biopsy to confirm the presence of malignancy.

Mid to central nodules

An individual with a high risk of having a malignant nodule located in the mid to central lung who is a surgical candidate and requires either segmentectomy or lobectomy to obtain a diagnosis should undergo transbronchial or transthoracic biopsy of the nodule to confirm the diagnosis. Since VATS segmentectomy and lobectomy carries significantly higher morbidity and mortality than VATS wedge resection, the individual should undergo a needle biopsy of the lesion to confirm the presence of malignancy. If the biopsy shows that the individual has early-stage lung cancer, the individual should undergo VATS or open lobectomy and mediastinal lymph node dissection.

Conclusion

As more institutions adopt screening for lung cancer, there will be an increase in the diagnosis of solitary pulmonary nodule. Management of this group of individuals should be based on accurate assessment of clinical risk factors such as age, smoking status, occupational exposure, history of extrathoracic malignancy or COPD, and assessment of nodule size, characteristics, and growth rate on a CT scan of the chest. If the clinical and radiographic assessment shows a low probability of a malignant nodule, the individual should undergo serial CT scans or a watchful waiting strategy. If the individual has an intermediate probability of a malignant nodule, the individual should get a FDG-PET with or without sampling of the nodule. If the individual has a high probability of having a malignant nodule, the nonsurgical patients should undergo every attempt possible to get a sampling of the tissue, while the surgical patients should undergo either VATS wedge for a peripheral nodule or transthoracic or transbronchial sampling of the tissue for a mid to central nodule. After the diagnosis is obtained, the patient will receive the appropriate therapy for the nodule as per the diagnosis. This strategy will provide diagnosis and treatment of patients with early-stage lung cancer while providing low morbidity for the individual with a benign lesion.

References

1 Ost DE, Gould MK (2012) Decision making in patients with pulmonary nodules. *Am J Respir Crit Care Med*, 185(4): 363–72. PMCID: 3361350.

2 Ost D, Fein AM, Feinsilver SH (2003) Clinical practice. The solitary pulmonary nodule. *New England Journal of Medicine*, 348(25): 2535–42.

3 Gould MK, Fletcher J, Iannettoni MD, Lynch WR, Midthun DE, Naidich DP, *et al.* (2007) Evaluation of patients with pulmonary nodules: when is it lung cancer?: ACCP evidence-based clinical practice guidelines (2nd edn). *Chest*, 132(3 Suppl): 108S–30S.

4 Erasmus JJ, Connolly JE, McAdams HP, Roggli VL (2000) Solitary pulmonary nodules: Part I. Morphologic evaluation for differentiation of benign and malignant lesions. *Radiographics*, 20(1): 43–58.

5 Aberle DR, Adams AM, Berg CD, Black WC, Clapp JD, Fagerstrom RM, *et al.* (2011) Reduced lung-cancer mortality with low-dose computed tomographic screening. *New England Journal of Medicine*, 365(5): 395–409.

6 Henschke CI, Yankelevitz DF, Naidich DP, McCauley DI, McGuinness G, Libby DM, *et al.* (2004) CT screening for lung cancer: Suspiciousness of nodules according to size on baseline scans. *Radiology*, 231(1): 164–8.

7 Gohagan J, Marcus P, Fagerstrom R, Pinsky P, Kramer B, Prorok P (2004) Baseline findings of a randomized feasibility trial of lung cancer screening with spiral CT scan vs chest radiograph: The Lung Screening Study of the National Cancer Institute. *Chest*, 126(1): 114–21.

8 Sone S, Li F, Yang ZG, Honda T, Maruyama Y, Takashima S, *et al.* (2001) Results of three-year mass screening programme for lung cancer using mobile low-dose spiral computed tomography scanner. *Br J Cancer*, 84(1): 25–32. PMCID: 2363609.

9 Swensen SJ, Jett JR, Hartman TE, Midthun DE, Sloan JA, Sykes AM, *et al.* (2003) Lung cancer screening with CT: Mayo Clinic experience. *Radiology*, 226(3): 756–61.

10 Wahidi MM, Govert JA, Goudar RK, Gould MK, McCrory DC (2007) Evidence for the treatment of patients with pulmonary nodules: when is it lung cancer?: ACCP evidence-based clinical practice guidelines (2nd edn). *Chest*, 132(3 Suppl): 94S–107S.

11 Varoli F, Vergani C, Caminiti R, Francese M, Gerosa C, Bongini M, *et al.* (2008) Management of solitary pulmonary nodule. *Eur J Cardiothorac Surg*, 33(3): 461–5.

12 Parkin DM, Muir CS (1992) Cancer Incidence in Five Continents. Comparability and quality of data. *IARC Sci Publ*, 120: 45–173.

13 Swensen SJ, Silverstein MD, Ilstrup DM, Schleck CD, Edell ES (1997) The probability of malignancy in solitary pulmonary nodules. Application to small radiologically indeterminate nodules. *Arch Intern Med*, 157(8): 849–55.

14 Gould MK, Fletcher J, Iannettoni MD, Lynch WR, Midthun DE, Naidich DP, *et al.* (2007) Evaluation of patients with pulmonary nodules: when is it lung cancer?: ACCP evidence-based clinical practice guidelines (2nd edn). *Chest*, 132(3 Suppl): 108S–30S.

15 Ost DE, Gould MK (2012) Decision making in patients with pulmonary nodules. *Am J Respir Crit Care Med*, 185(4): 363–72. PMCID: 3361350.

16 Erasmus JJ, McAdams HP, Connolly JE (2000) Solitary pulmonary nodules: Part II. Evaluation of the indeterminate nodule. *Radiographics*, 20(1): 59–66.

17 Yankelevitz DF, Henschke CI (1997) Does 2-year stability imply that pulmonary nodules are benign? *AJR Am J Roentgenol*, 168(2): 325–8.

18 Howard TA, Woodring JH (1992) Clinical and imaging evaluation of the solitary pulmonary nodule. *Am Fam Physician*, 46(6): 1753–9.

19 Caskey CI, Templeton PA, Zerhouni EA (1990) Current evaluation of the solitary pulmonary nodule. *Radiol Clin North Am*, 28(3): 511–20.

20 Good CA, Wilson TW (1958) The solitary circumscribed pulmonary nodule; study of seven hundred five cases encountered roentgenologically in a period of three and one-half years. *J Am Med Assoc*, 166(3): 210–15.

21 MacMahon H, Austin JHM, Gamsu G, Herold CJ, Jett JR, Naidich DP, *et al.* (2005) Guidelines for management of small pulmonary nodules detected on CT scans: a statement from the Fleischner Society. *Radiology*, 237(2): 395–400.

22 Eisenberg RL, Bankier AA, Boiselle PM (2010) Compliance with Fleischner Society guidelines for management of small lung nodules: a survey of 834 radiologists. *Radiology*, 255(1): 218–24.

23 Kubota K, Murakami K, Inoue T, Saga T, Shiomi S (2011) Additional effects of FDG-PET to thin-section CT for the differential diagnosis of lung nodules: a Japanese multicenter clinical study. *Ann Nucl Med*, 25(10): 787–95.

24 Bryant AS, Cerfolio RJ (2006) The maximum standardized uptake values on integrated FDG-PET/CT is useful in differentiating benign from malignant pulmonary nodules. *Ann Thorac Surg*, 82(3): 1016–20.

25 Grgic A, Yuksel Y, Groschel A, Schafers HJ, Sybrecht GW, Kirsch CM, *et al.* (2010) Risk stratification of solitary pulmonary nodules by means of PET using (18)F-fluorodeoxyglucose and SUV quantification. *Eur J Nucl Med Mol Imaging*, 37(6): 1087–94.

26 Barnett PG, Ananth L, Gould MK (2010) Veterans affairs positron emission tomography imaging in the management of patients with solitary pulmonary nodules cooperative study G. Cost and outcomes of patients with solitary pulmonary nodules managed with PET scans. *Chest*, 137(1): 53–9.

27 Kubota K, Murakami K, Inoue T, Itoh H, Saga T, Shiomi S, *et al.* (2011) Additional value of FDG-PET to contrast enhanced-computed tomography (CT) for the diagnosis of mediastinal lymph node metastasis in non-small cell lung cancer: a Japanese multicenter clinical study. *Ann Nucl Med*, 25(10): 777–86.

28 Schwarz Y (2010) Electromagnetic navigation. *Clin Chest Med*, 31(1): 65–73.

29 van der Drift MA, van der Wilt GJ, Thunnissen FB, Janssen JP (2005) A prospective study of the timing and cost-effectiveness of bronchial washing during bronchoscopy for pulmonary malignant tumors. *Chest*, 128(1): 394–400.

30 Chechani V (1996) Bronchoscopic diagnosis of solitary pulmonary nodules and lung masses in the absence of endobronchial abnormality. *Chest*, 109(3): 620–5.

31 Edell E, Krier-Morrow D (2010) Navigational bronchoscopy: overview of technology and practical considerations – new Current Procedural Terminology codes effective 2010. *Chest*, 137(2): 450–4.

32 Kothary N, Lock L, Sze DY, Hofmann LV (2009) Computed tomography-guided percutaneous needle biopsy of pulmonary nodules: impact of nodule size on diagnostic accuracy. *Clin Lung Cancer*, 10(5): 360–3.

33 Cox JE, Chiles C, McManus CM, Aquino SL, Choplin RH (1999) Transthoracic needle aspiration biopsy: variables that affect risk of pneumothorax. *Radiology*, 212(1): 165–8.

34 Wang Memoli JS, Nietert PJ, Silvestri GA (2012) Meta-analysis of guided bronchoscopy for the evaluation of the pulmonary nodule. *Chest*, 142(2): 385–93.

35 Pearlstein DP, Quinn CC, Burtis CC, Ahn KW, Katch AJ (2012) Electromagnetic navigation bronchoscopy performed by thoracic surgeons: one center's early success. *Annals of Thoracic Surgery*, 93(3): 944–9; discussion 9–50.

36 Seijo LM, de Torres JP, Lozano MD, Bastarrika G, Alcaide AB, Lacunza MM, *et al.* (2010) Diagnostic yield of electromagnetic navigation bronchoscopy is highly dependent on the presence of a Bronchus sign on CT imaging: Results from a prospective study. *Chest*, 138(6): 1316–21.

37 Tachihara M, Ishida T, Kanazawa K, Sugawara A, Watanabe K, Uekita K, *et al.* (2007) A virtual bronchoscopic navigation system under X-ray fluoroscopy for transbronchial diagnosis of small peripheral pulmonary lesions. *Lung Cancer*, 57(3): 322–7.

38 Ishida T, Asano F, Yamazaki K, Shinagawa N, Oizumi S, Moriya H, *et al.* (2011) Virtual bronchoscopic navigation combined with endobronchial ultrasound to diagnose small peripheral pulmonary lesions: A randomised trial. *Thorax*, 66(12): 1072–7. PMCID: 3221323.

39 Fielding DI, Robinson PJ, Kurimoto N (2008) Biopsy site selection for endobronchial ultrasound guide-sheath transbronchial biopsy of peripheral lung lesions. *Intern Med J*, 38(2): 77–84.

40 Kuo E, Bharat A, Bontumasi N, Sanchez C, Zoole JB, Patterson GA, *et al.* (2012) Impact of video-assisted thoracoscopic surgery on benign resections for solitary pulmonary nodules. *Annals of Thoracic Surgery*, 93(1): 266–72; discussion 72–3.

41 Sedrakyan A, van der Meulen J, Lewsey J, Treasure T (2004) Video assisted thoracic surgery for treatment of pneumothorax and lung resections: Systematic review of randomised clinical trials. *BMJ*, 329(7473): 1008. PMCID: 524550.

42 Ginsberg RJ, Rubinstein LV (1995) Randomized trial of lobectomy versus limited resection for T1 N0 non-small cell lung cancer. Lung Cancer Study Group. *Annals of Thoracic Surgery*, 60(3): 615–22; discussion 22–3.

CHAPTER 14

Minimally Invasive Resections for Lung Cancer

Shanda H. Blackmon
Houston Methodist Hospital, Weill Cornell Medical College of Cornell University, Houston, TX, USA
The University of Texas MD Anderson Cancer Center, Houston, TX, USA

Introduction

Primary lung cancer remains the most lethal of all malignancies, predicted to accounting for nearly 160 000 deaths and 226 000 new diagnoses in 2012 [1]. The cornerstone of therapy for early-stage lung cancer is anatomic individual vessel ligation and division by surgical lobectomy with concomitant removal of the draining nodal basin. Thoracoscopic lobectomy is defined as individual vessel ligation with no rib spreading and complete visualization with a camera inside the chest for visualization. There are generally two approaches to thoracoscopic lobectomy; the multiple incision approach with three or more incisions and a utility port (which is larger than the others and averages 3–4 cm in length) or the two-incision technique (which includes a utility incision and a camera incision) (Figures 14.1a and b). The double-action instrumentation and slightly curved instruments as well as articulating stapler now make approaching the hilum much easier and the location of the ports more forgiving.

The steps to perform a thoracoscopic right upper lobectomy (Figures 14.2a–d) include positioning the patient in the lateral decubitus position tilted posteriorly, using an arm board, and securing the hip to prevent rotation. After creating the necessary ports (when operating on the left side of the patient, these are positioned more posteriorly to correct for the pericardium), the hilum is dissected posteriorly to reveal the branch of the right upper lobe from the bronchus intermedius. Instead of standing on the posterior side of the patient, the surgeon stands on the anterior side of the patient during the dissection. The nodal dissection can also be done at this time. After releasing the pleura, the rest of the surgery can be approached from the front of the patient's hilum proceeding towards the back. This is the hallmark difference between thoracoscopic lobectomy and open lobectomy. The first structure to be identified is the superior pulmonary vein. It is important to make sure there is no common vein, and then to make sure the branches to the right middle lobe are spared. A vascular load stapler is ideal for dividing the veins and artery. The truncus anterior branch of the right pulmonary artery is then dissected and divided, followed by additional nodal dissection. Each time a node is removed, a branch point of the vessels is revealed. Finally, either the right upper lobe bronchus is taken or the posterior ascending pulmonary artery; this depends on the position of the structures, the size of the artery, and the stapler angle. Once the lobe has been removed, it is placed into a bag to prevent port site recurrence. All nodes are labeled according to station and sent

Lung Cancer, Fourth Edition. Edited by Jack A. Roth, Waun Ki Hong and Ritsuko U. Komaki.

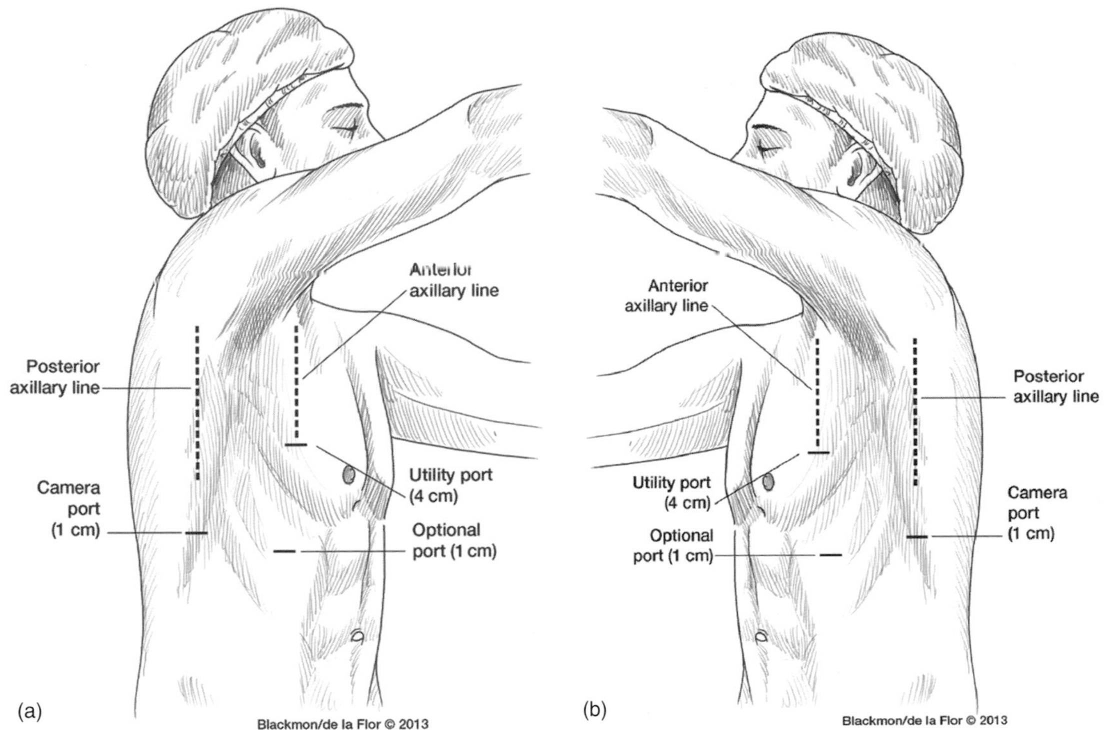

Figure 14.1 a: Thoracoscopic lobectomy port placement options for right-sided surgery. b: Thoracoscopic lobectomy port placement options for left-sided surgery. *Source*: Blackmon/de la Flor © 2013.

as separate specimens. When resecting other lobes of the lung, the hilar structures are removed in a similar manner proceeding from the front of the patient to the back. The steps for removing the remaining lobes of the lung are illustrated in Figures 14.3, 14.4, 14.5 and 14.6.

Surgeons have successfully performed thoracoscopic lobectomy for more than a decade, with such technology disseminating throughout the thoracic surgical community establishing it as a standard for the management of early-stage non-small cell lung cancer (NSCLC) [2, 3]. Thoracoscopic lobectomy is now clearly supported by evidence-based treatment guidelines [4], as three of the four published randomized clinical trials of thoracoscopic lobectomy versus open lobectomy demonstrated an advantage in the VATS (Video Assisted Thoracoscopic Surgery) group [5–8]. Some of the advantages of thoracoscopic lobectomy compared to thoracotomy include less postoperative pain [9–11], less blood loss [5, 8, 10, 12], improved inflammatory response [13], shorter chest tube duration [9, 10, 13–15], improved postoperative independence [14], better pulmonary function [16–19], comparable operative times [9, 13, 14, 20], shorter hospitalization [2,3, 5, 13–15, 21–24], more cost-effective [16], and improved delivery of adjuvant chemotherapy to eligible patients [15, 17]. A recent assessment of morbidity and mortality after thoracoscopic lobectomy demonstrated improved results for many additional outcomes [18, 20, 25–30]. Despite the milieu of published advantages, thoracoscopic lobectomy is underutilized. Analyzing the board-certified thoracic surgeons participating in the General Thoracic Surgery component of the Society of Thoracic Surgeons database from 1999 to 2006, only 20% of all lobectomies for NSCLC were thoracoscopically performed [31]. Because of these many advantages, thoracoscopic lobectomy is now considered a gold standard for patients with NSCLC [32].

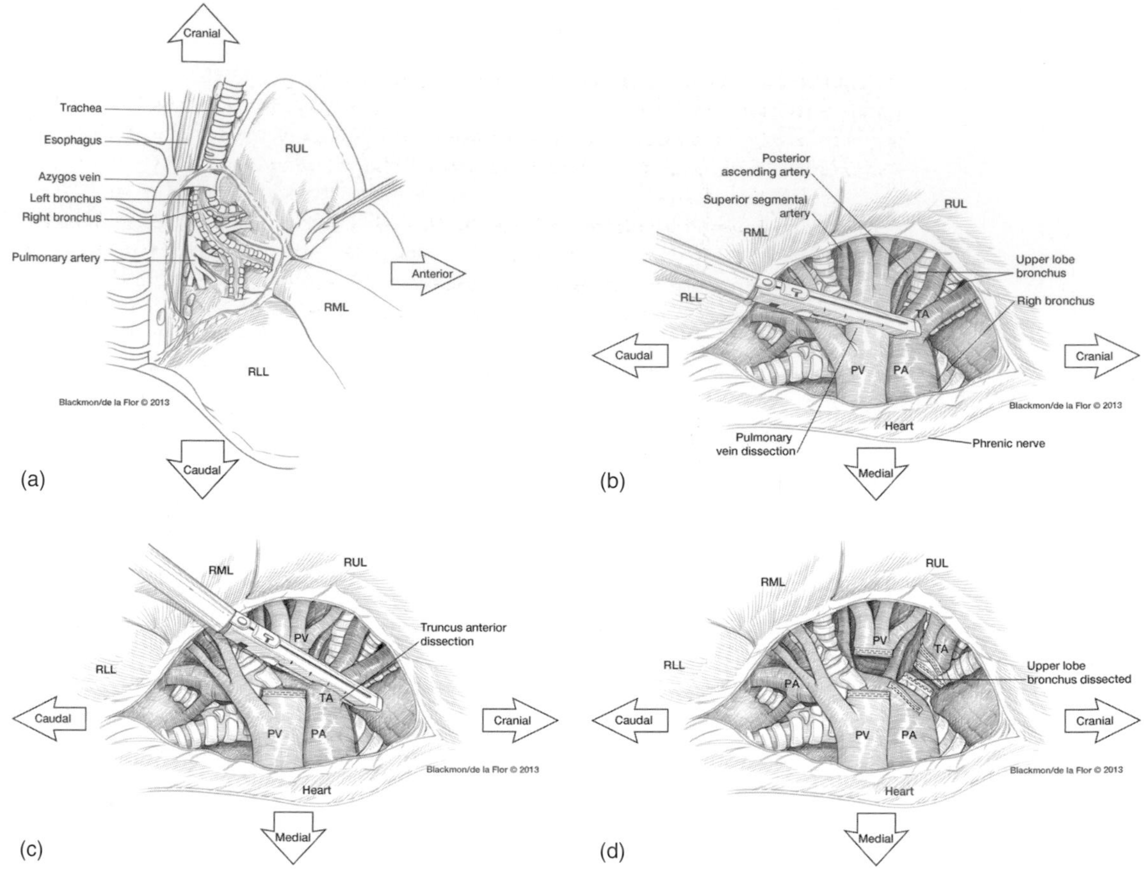

Figure 14.2 a: Steps for thoracoscopic right upper lobectomy; posterior pleural dissection. b: Steps for thoracoscopic right upper lobectomy; right upper lobe pulmonary vein dissection. c: Steps for thoracoscopic right upper lobectomy; right upper lobe truncus arteriosus pulmonary artery dissection. d: Steps for thoracoscopic right upper lobectomy; posterior ascending pulmonary artery branch and right upper lobe bronchus dissection. *Abbreviations*: PA, pulmonary artery; PV, pulmonary vein; RLL, right lower lobe; RML, right middle lobe; RUL, right upper lobe; TA, truncus anterior. *Source*: Blackmon/de la Flor © 2013.

Postoperative pain

Demmy and colleagues [9] reported their results in a series of patients who underwent either thoracoscopic lobectomy or conventional thoracotomy. Using similar pain control treatment, the percentage of patients reporting severe pain was 6% after thoracoscopic lobectomy and 65% after thoracotomy. Moreover, the percentage of patients reporting minimal or no pain was 63% after thoracoscopic lobectomy and 6% after thoracotomy. Other studies analyzing acute pain have concluded that video-assisted thoracoscopic surgery either causes less pain or lower analgesia requirement in the early postoperative period [11, 17, 18]. There is evidence this improved pain control extends beyond one year [10].

Estimated blood loss and chest tube duration

Tajiri and colleagues found less blood loss in a VATS group (168) compared to a thoracotomy group (61)

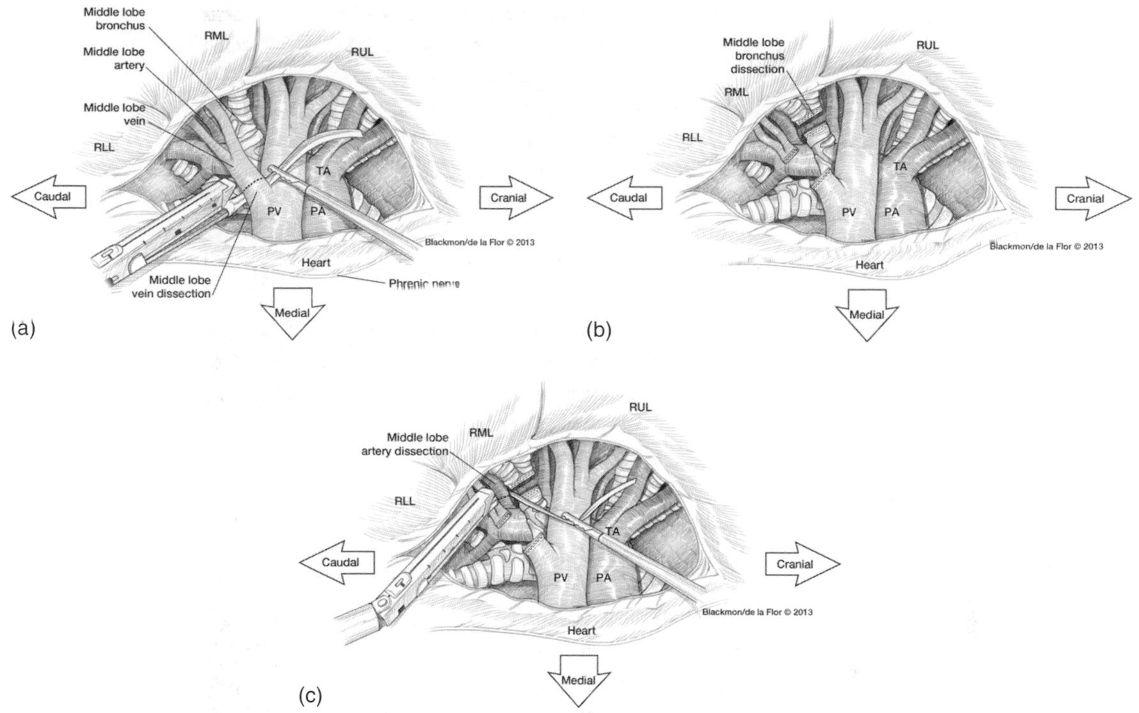

Figure 14.3 Steps for thoracoscopic right middle lobectomy. *Abbreviations*: PA, pulmonary artery; PV, pulmonary vein; RLL, right lower lobe; RML, right middle lobe; RUL, right upper lobe; TA, truncus anterior. *Source*: Blackmon/de la Flor © 2013.

[10]. Other studies have shown either less blood loss or no significant difference between the two groups [5, 8, 10, 11]. With regard to chest tube duration, many studies have shown equivalent outcomes relating to chest tube duration and some with statistically significant improved chest tube output at the end of three days [3, 10, 13–15].

Postoperative independence and return to pre-operative function

Improved postoperative independence is seen in a study published by Demmy and colleagues, which analyzed the number of patients requiring postoperative discharge with home health care or transfer to a separate care facility [9]. Additional studies show improved return to pre-operative function [14].

Pulmonary function

Because thoracoscopic lobectomy may be easier to tolerate, the traditional accepted pulmonary function minimum values may no longer apply, as more patients are able to tolerate a less invasive resection. Less pain and smaller incisions logically lead to better postoperative respiratory mechanics for patients undergoing minimally invasive lung resections. This is demonstrated by testing performed immediately after the operation as well as up to 3 months postoperatively. In 1996, Tschernko and colleagues compared patients from their prospective series of 47 patients assigned to VATS or axillary thoracotomy and showed that the thoracoscopic lobectomy group demonstrated superior oxygen saturation at all time points up to 72 hours after lung resection [17]. Furthermore, forced expiratory volumes in 1 second have been

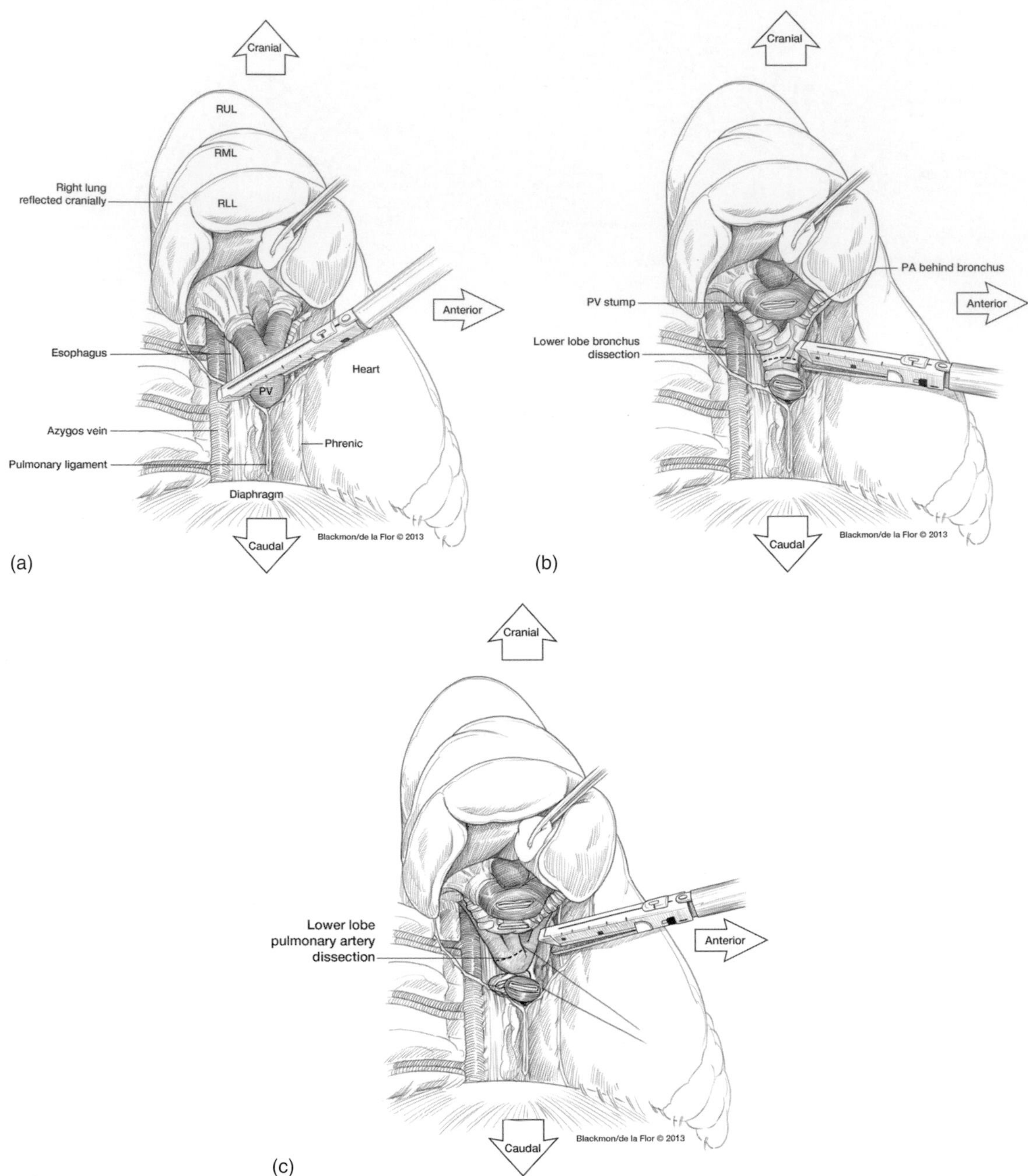

Figure 14.4 Steps for thoracoscopic right lower lobectomy. *Abbreviations*: PA, pulmonary artery; PV, pulmonary vein; RLL, right lower lobe; RML, right middle lobe; RUL, right upper lobe. *Source*: Blackmon/de la Flor © 2013.

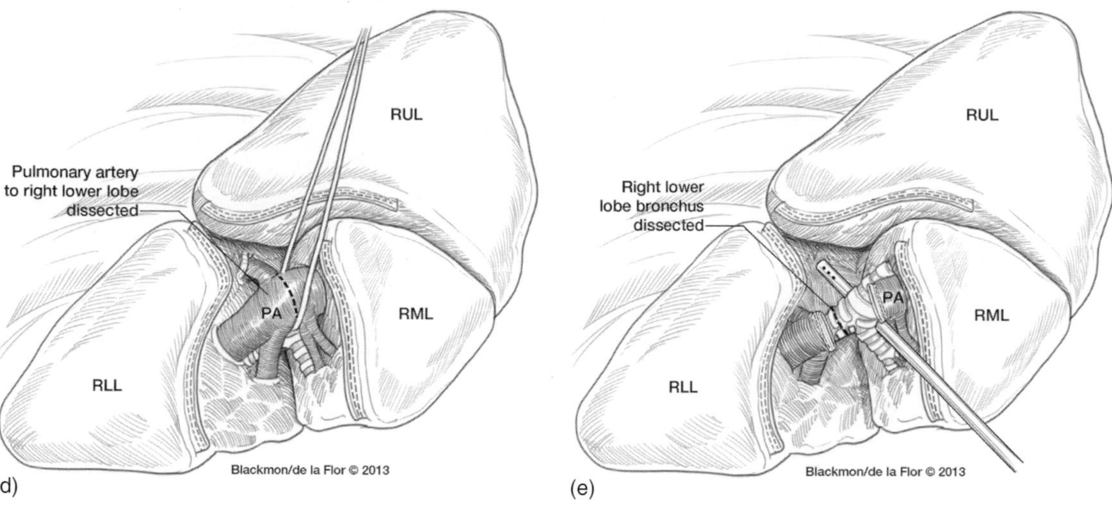

Figure 14.4 *(Continued)*

studied and compared. Nagahiro and colleagues showed that at 14 days postoperatively, the VATS patients recovered 95% of their preoperative forced expiratory volume in 1 second compared with 80% for those undergoing thoracotomy [11]. Findings from another Japanese group support the improved recovery of forced expiratory volume in 1 second in those undergoing thoracoscopic lobectomies out to 3 months after the operation [18]. Improved 1 year pulmonary function was reported by Kaseda and colleagues [18]. Poor pulmonary function predicts respiratory complications regardless of approach. Respiratory complications increase at a significantly greater rate in lobectomy patients with poor pulmonary function after thoracotomy compared with VATS. Planned surgical approach should be considered while determining whether a high-risk patient is an appropriate resection candidate [33].

Operative time and length of stay

Operative times are overall not expected to be different given a surgeon has advanced along the learning curve and is proficient with the technique and has a trained team [5, 9, 13, 14]. The Cancer and Leukemia Group B reported the results of a multi-institutional series of 97 patients who underwent thoracoscopic lobectomy [8]. Mortality was 2%, the operative time was 130 minutes, and the median length of stay was 3 days. The three-day length of stay is commensurate with many other published series [2, 3, 5, 13–15, 23, 24]. Onaitis and colleagues reported the results of thoracoscopic lobectomy in 500 consecutive patients [3]. The 30-day mortality was 1%, with no intraoperative deaths. The conversion rate was less than 2%, and none was emergent. The median chest tube duration was 2 days, and median length of stay was 3 days. Overall, most studies are presenting a shorter expected length of stay with thoracoscopic lobectomy [14, 15].

Cost-effectiveness

Burfeind and colleagues performed a retrospective analysis of cost associated with thoracoscopic lobectomy and open lobectomy in 113 patients having surgery between 2002 and 2004 [16]. In this study, cost and cost-utility analysis was performed by using prospectively acquired quality of life measurements and calculating a quality-adjusted life-year for each patient. Total costs were significantly

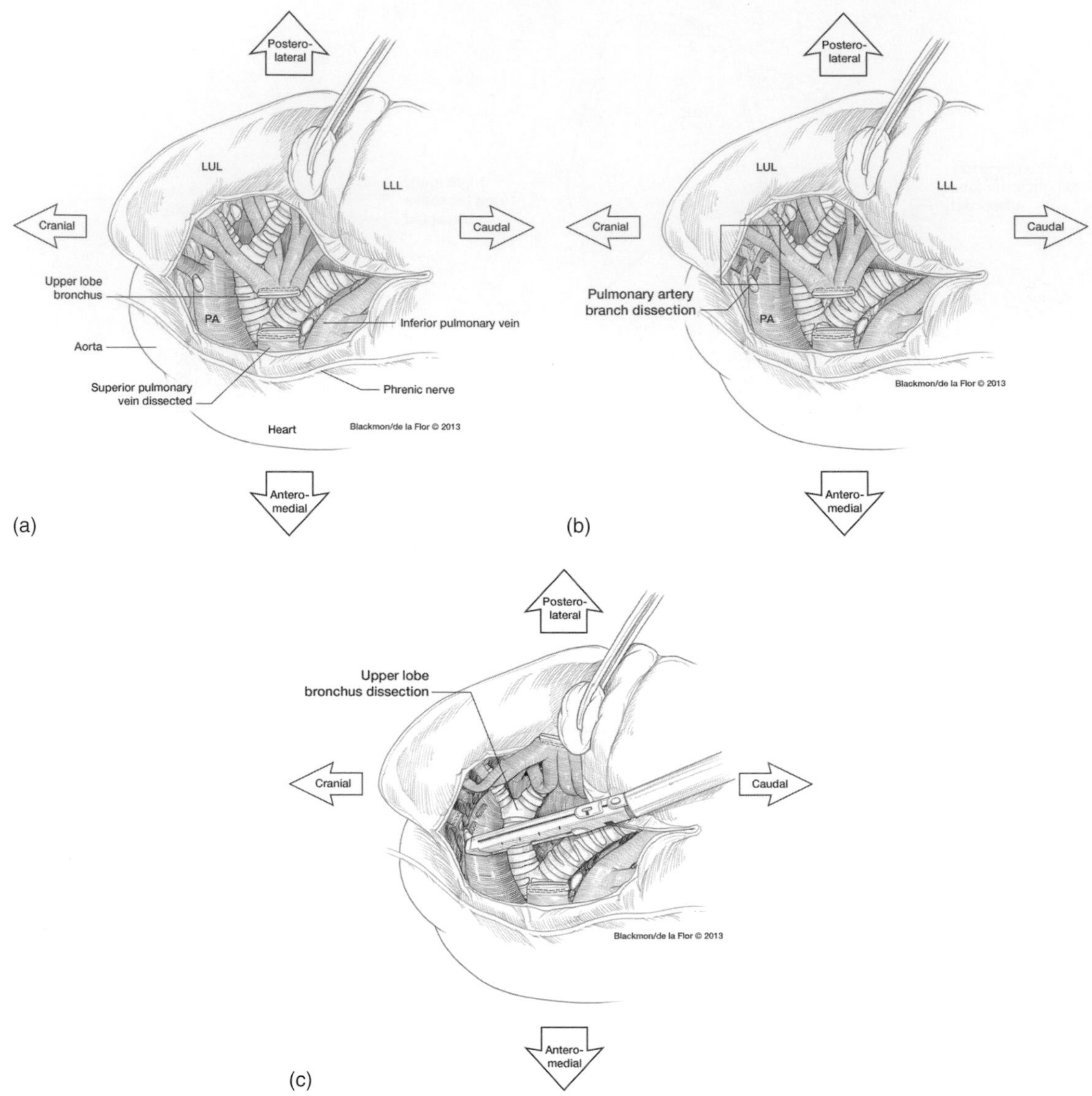

Figure 14.5 Steps for thoracoscopic left upper lobectomy. *Abbreviations*: LLL: left lower lobe; LUL, left upper lobe; PA, pulmonary artery; PV, pulmonary vein. *Source*: Blackmon/de la Flor © 2013.

greater for thoracotomy (US $12 119) vs thoracoscopy (US $10 084; $p = 0.0012$). The use of minimally invasive techniques for the 50 000 lobectomies performed in the United States each year was estimated to represent a savings of approximately $100 million.

Administration of adjuvant chemotherapy

Improved compliance with adjuvant chemotherapy appears to be one of the most promising advantages associated with thoracoscopic

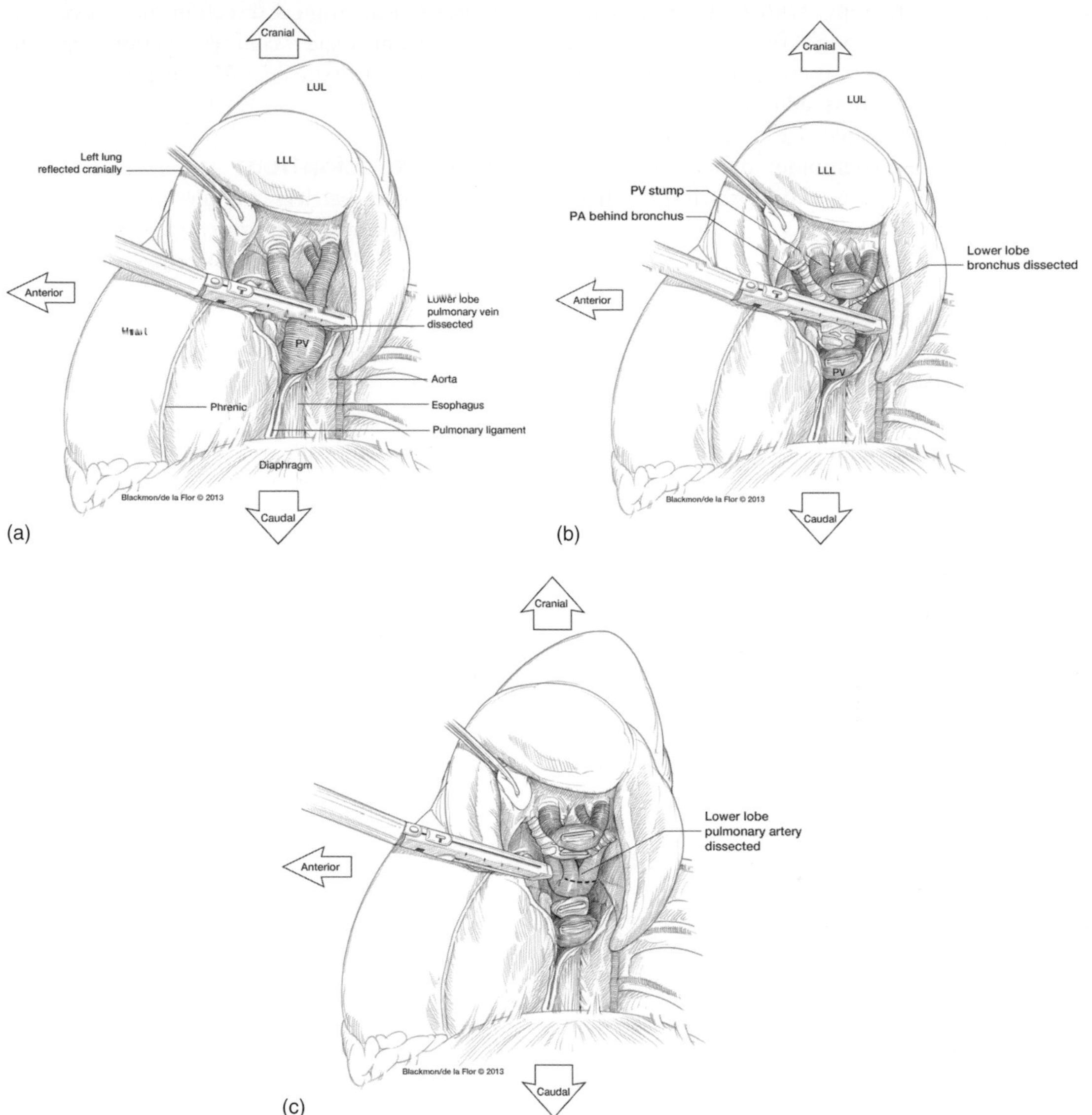

Figure 14.6 Steps for thoracoscopic left lower lobectomy. *Abbreviations*: LLL: left lower lobe; LUL, left upper lobe; PA, pulmonary artery; PV, pulmonary vein. *Source*: Blackmon/de la Flor © 2013.

lobectomy [15]. Petersen's study compared the ability to deliver adjuvant chemotherapy in 100 patients who underwent complete resection for NSCLC by thoracotomy(43) or thoracoscopy(57) [15]. Those undergoing thoracoscopic lobectomy had significantly fewer delayed (18% vs 58%; $p = 0.001$) and reduced (26% vs 49%; $p = 0.02$) chemotherapy doses. A higher percentage of patients undergoing thoracoscopic resection received 75% or more of their planned adjuvant regimen without delayed or reduced doses (61% vs 40%; $p = 0.03$). A separate group also looked at adjuvant chemotherapy received after VATS and noted that 85% of patients received all cycles of planned chemotherapy, with or without some delay [17]. Although long-term survival was not an end point of either of these studies, similar differences in chemotherapy administered for other tumor types are associated with improved survival [34, 36]. Also, these chemotherapy administration rates compare favorably with historical controls in which only 55–70% of patients received full regimens of chemotherapy after thoracotomy [37, 38].

Complications

Several studies ranging from case-matched to analyzing the large prospective STS database have recently demonstrated that the incidence of postoperative complications is lower after thoracoscopic lobectomy than after thoracotomy [18, 20, 25–30]. A recent meta-analysis of morbidity and mortality after thoracoscopic lobectomy combined the results of reported incidence of morbidity and mortality from 21 eligible comparative studies (2 randomized and 19 nonrandomized) [35]. In this meta-analysis, thoracoscopic lobectomy was not associated with a difference in locoregional recurrence ($p = 0.24$) compared with the open lobectomy arm, but the data suggested a reduced systemic recurrence rate ($p = 0.03$) and an improved 5-year mortality rate for the thoracoscopic approach ($p = 0.04$) [35].

Intraoperative events of significant consequence occur in less than 1% of cases [39]. Although catastrophic intraoperative complications of VATS lobectomy are uncommon, awareness of the possibility of such injuries is critical to avoid them. Specific techniques designed to lessen such complications include a solid knowledge of anatomic relationships, careful dissection, awareness of certain potential complications, and judicious conversion to thoracotomy.

Special circumstances

Reoperation

Another advantage of thoracoscopic resections is during the development of a second primary that requires repeat surgical resection. It is possible the decreased scar tissue facilitates a better reoperation due to less scar tissue against the chest wall and in the hilum as well.

Barriers to adoption

There remain barriers to adoption of thoracoscopic lobectomy. The misconception that pulmonary artery bleeding is uncontrollable thoracoscopically is an obstacle that is likely to dissuade surgeons from considering learning thoracoscopic lobectomy. Most practicing thoracic surgeons in the United States completed their training before the advent of thoracoscopic lobectomy, and postgraduate training along with credentialing is an extensive process. Although it is probable that most training programs in thoracic surgery in the United States provide exposure to thoracoscopic lobectomy, it is unknown what the actual operative experience is for residents. The American Board of Thoracic Surgery has recently included thoracoscopic lobectomy as a required index case. Advanced training pathways and credentialing guidelines are needed to guide hospitals and programs as they seek to train their older generation of surgeons.

Thoracoscopic segmentectomy

A study by Yang and colleagues analyzed outcomes of published studies including segmentectomy patients and found, when compared with open segmentectomy, thoracoscopic segmentectomy was found to have equivalent oncologic results, with shorter hospital length of stay, reduced rates of morbidity, and lower cost [40]. When compared with thoracoscopic lobectomy, thoracoscopic segmentectomy had equivalent rates of morbidity, recurrence, and survival. Preliminarily, thoracoscopic segmentectomy was found to result in greater preservation of lung function and exercise capacity than the thoracoscopic lobectomy. What remains to be determined is the overall oncologic outcome, evidenced by equivalent recurrence-free survival, associated with a segmentectomy compared to a lobectomy. CALGB 140503 and JCOG0802/WJOG4607L are two well-designed studies that aim to determine the benefit of VATS segmentectomy that have yet to publish results.

Thoracoscopic pneumonectomy

Nwogu and colleagues retrospectively analyzed 70 patients over a six-year period at a single institution according to the type of resection, and found those patients having a thoracoscopic pneumonectomy had a shorter length of stay and less blood loss with equivalent complications when compared to the open pneumonectomy group [41]. Pneumonectomy performed either by means of thoracoscopy or thoracotomy resulted in equivalent survival.

Thoracoscopic bronchoplasty

Although there are single case studies and videos discussing technique and methods to perform bronchoplastic resections using a minimally invasive technique [42], nothing beyond feasibility has been discussed in the literature. This may be one of the key areas in minimally invasive surgery where robotic suturing or advanced articulating devices may play a role.

Thoracoscopic chest wall resections

Although the more basic operations like thoracoscopic lobectomy and segmentectomy have clearly shown improved outcomes compared to open procedures, the advantage of minimally invasive surgery for more complex chest wall resections or extended resections is not as clearly defined. Advanced thoracoscopic instrumentation is more essential for chest wall resections than lobectomy or segmentectomy. Minimally invasive bone manipulation instrumentation commonly available in scoliosis surgery is helpful when performing thoracoscopic chest wall resections. Such necessary equipment includes either an endoscopic rib cutter (now made by Medtronic), a long rotating burr that can divide ribs, an orthopedic Kerrison No.5, or a gigli saw. When reconstructing the chest wall with mesh, trans-thoracic fixation sutures, tacking devices, and laparoscopic suturing devices may facilitate placement and fixation [43, 44].

Thoracoscopic lymphadenectomy

Boffa and colleagues determined the frequency of nodal metastases identified in 11 531 clinically node-negative tumors by thoracotomy (7137) and thoracoscopic approaches (4394) to approximate the completeness of surgical nodal dissections over a nine-year period using the Society of Thoracic Surgeons (STS) database [45]. During lobectomy or segmentectomy for clinical N0 lung cancer, mediastinal nodal evaluation by VATS and thoracotomy resulted in equivalent upstaging. In contrast, lower rates of N1 upstaging in the VATS group possibly indicated variability in the completeness of the peribronchial and hilar lymph node evaluation. Because of these results, concern about the completeness of nodal dissection has been raised as more surgeons adopt the VATS approach. To compensate for a less thorough nodal dissection performed by some surgeons who do not feel comfortable performing an extensive lymphadenectomy, the robotic approach offers an alternative yet still minimally invasive technique.

Robotic-assisted lobectomy

Robotic-assisted lobectomy (RATS) is an alternative to VATS, with a similar technique of video-guided resection, but has improved three-dimension viewing, instrumentation with seven degrees of freedom, high definition imaging, and a master slave surgical cart. Using a 3–4 arm totally robotic approach, a 325 multi-institutional international series of patients reported an 8% conversion rate, 3.7% (12/325) major complication rate, and one in-hospital death [46]. Although some centers have reported excessive cost associated with this new technology, RATS can be performed with low morbidity and mortality. Long-term stage-specific survival is acceptable and consistent with prior results for VATS and thoracotomy.

Conclusions

Minimally invasive lung resections have demonstrated safety, efficacy, and less cost of care for patients with early stage NSCLC. Thoracoscopic lobectomy is designed to achieve the same oncologic result as conventional lobectomy: complete hilar dissection and individual vessel control. The recognized advantages of thoracoscopic anatomic resection include less short-term postoperative pain, shorter hospital stay, faster return to full activity, preserved pulmonary function, and fewer postoperative complications. In addition, thoracoscopic lobectomy has demonstrated improved compliance with adjuvant therapy. A randomized clinical trial is needed, but unlikely to be performed. Thoracoscopic lobectomy is considered an acceptable standard for patients with early stage lung cancer.

References

1 Siegel R, Naishadham D, Jemal A (2012) Cancer statistics, 2012. *CA Cancer J Clin*, Jan–Feb; 62(1): 10–29. doi: 10.3322/caac.20138. Epub 2012 Jan 4.

2 McKenna RJ, Houck W, Fuller CB (2006) Video-assisted thoracic surgery lobectomy: Experience with 1,100 cases. *Ann Thorac Surg*, 81: 421–6.

3 Onaitis MW, Petersen PR, Balderson SS, *et al.* (2006) Thoracoscopic lobectomy is a safe and versatile procedure: Experience with 500 consecutive patients. *Ann Surg*, 244: 420–5.

4 Ettinger DS, Akerly W, Bepler G, *et al.* (2008) National Comprehensive Cancer Network (NCCN). Non-small cell lung cancer clinical practice guidelines in oncology. *J Natl Compr Canc Netw*, 6: 228–69.

5 Kirby TJ, Mack MJ, Landreneau RJ, Rice TW (1995) Lobectomy – video-assisted thoracic surgery versus muscle-sparing thoracotomy: A randomized trial. *J Thorac Cardiovasc Surg*, 109: 997–1001

6 Sugi K, Kaneda Y, Esato K (2000) Video-assisted thoracoscopic lobectomy achieves a satisfactory long-term prognosis in patients with clinical stage IA lung cancer. *World J Surg*, 24: 27–31.

7 Craig SR, Leaver HA, Yap PL, *et al.* (2001) Acute phase responses following minimal access and conventional thoracic surgery. *Eur J Cardiothorac Surg*, 20: 455–63.

8 Shigemura N, Akashi A, Nakagiri T, *et al.* (2004) Complete vs. assisted thoracoscopic approach: a prospective randomized trial comparing a variety of video-assisted thoracoscopic lobectomy techniques. *Surg Endosc* 18: 1492–7.

9 Demmy TL, Curtis JJ (1999) Minimally invasive lobectomy directed toward frail and high-risk patients: A case control study. *Ann Thorac Surg*, 68: 194–200.

10 Tajiri M, *et al.* (2007) Decreased invasiveness via two methods of thoracoscopic lobectomy for lung cancer, compared with open thoracotomy. *Respirology*, 12: 207–11.

11 Nagahiro I, Andou A, Aoe M, *et al.* (2001) Pulmonary function, postoperative pain, and serum cytokine level after lobectomy: A comparison of VATS and conventional procedure. *Ann Thorac Surg*, 72: 362–5.

12 Nomori H, Horio H, Naruke T, Suemasu K. (2001) What is the advantage of a thoracoscopic lobectomy over a limited thoracotomy procedure for lung cancer surgery? *Ann Thorac Surg*, 72(3): 879–84.

13 Yim APC, *et al.* (2000) VATS lobectomy reduces cytokine responses compared with conventional surgery. *Ann Thorac Surg*, 70: 243–7.

14 Demmy TJ, *et al.* (2004) Discharge independence with minimally invasive lobectomy. *Am J Surg*. 188: 689–702.

15 Petersen RP, Pham D, Burfeind WR, *et al.* (2007) Thoracoscopic lobectomy facilitates the delivery of chemotherapy after resection for lung cancer. *Ann Thorac Surg*, 83: 1245–9.

16 Burfeind W, Jaik N, Villamizar N, Toloza E, Harpole D, D'Amico TA (2010) A cost-minimization analysis of lobectomy: Thoracoscopic vs. posterolateral thoracotomy. *Eur J Cardiothorac Surg* (E-pub; doi: 10.1016/j.ejcts.2009.10.017).

17 Tschernko E, Hofer S, Beiglmayer C, Wisser W, Haider W (1996) Video-assisted wedge resection/lobectomy versus conventional axillary thoracotomy. *Chest*, 109: 1636–42.

18 Kaseda S, Aoki T, Hangai N, Shimizu K (2000) Better pulmonary function and prognosis with video-assisted thoracic surgery than with thoracotomy. *Ann Thorac Surg*, 70: 1644–6.

19 Nakata M, *et al.* (2000) Pulmonary function after lobectomy: Video-assisted thoracic surgery versus thoracotomy. *Ann Thorac Surg*, 70: 938–41.

20 Cattaneo SM, Park BJ, Wilton AS, *et al.* (2008) Use of video-assisted thoracic surgery for lobectomy in the elderly results in fewer complications. *Ann Thorac Surg*, 85: 231–6.

21 Park BJ, Zhang H, Rusch VW, Amar D (2007) Video-assisted thoracic surgery does not reduce the incidence of postoperative atrial fibrillation after pulmonary lobectomy. *J Thorac Cardiovasc Surg*, 133: 775–9.

22 Nicastri DG, Wisnivesky JP, Litle VR, *et al.* (2008) Thoracoscopic lobectomy: report on safety, discharge independence, pain, and chemotherapy tolerance. *J Thorac Cardiovasc Surg*, 135: 642–7.

23 Swanson SJ, Herndon JE, D'Amico TA, *et al.* (2007) Video-assisted thoracic surgery (VATS) lobectomy – report of CALGB 39802: a prospective, multi-institutional feasibility study. *J Clin Oncol*, 25: 4993–7.

24 Cajipe MD, Chu D, Bakaeen FG, Casal RF, LeMaire SA, Coselli JS, Cornwell LD (2012) Video-assisted thoracoscopic lobectomy is associated with better perioperative outcomes than open lobectomy in a veteran population. *Am J Surg*, Nov; 204(5): 607–12.

25 Villamizar NR, Darrabie MD, Burfeind WR, *et al.* (2009) Thoracoscopic lobectomy is associated with lower morbidity compared to thoracotomy. *J Thorac Cardiovasc Surg*, 138: 419–14.

26 Paul S, Altorki NK, Sheng S, *et al.* (2010) Thoracoscopic lobectomy is associated with lower morbidity than open lobectomy: A propensity-matched analysis from the STS Database. *J Thorac Cardiovasc Surg*, 139: 366–78.

27 Berry MF, Hanna J, Tong BC, *et al.* (2009) Risk factors for morbidity after lobectomy for lung cancer in elderly patients. *Ann Thorac Surg*, 88: 1093–9.

28 Muraoka M, Oka T, Akamine S, *et al.* (2006) Video-assisted thoracic surgery lobectomy reduces the morbidity after surgery for stage I non-small cell lung cancer. *Jpn J Thorac Cardiovasc Surg*, 54: 49–55.

29 Whitson BA, Andrade RS, Boettcher A, *et al.* (2007) Video-assisted thoracoscopic surgery is more favorable than thoracotomy for resection of clinical stage I non-small cell lung cancer. *Ann Thorac Surg*, 83: 1965–70.

30 D'Amico TA (2008) Long-term outcomes after thoracoscopic lobectomy. *Thorac Surg Clin*, 18: 259–62.

31 Boffa DJ, Allen MS, Grab JD, *et al.* (2008) Data from the Society of Thoracic Surgeons General Thoracic Surgery database: the surgical management of primary lung tumors. *J Thorac Cardiovasc Surg*, 135: 247–54.

32 Hartwig MG, D'Amico TA (2010) Thoracoscopic lobectomy: The gold standard for early-stage lung cancer? *Ann Thorac Surg*, Jun; 89(6): S2098–S2101.

33 Ceppa DP, Kosinski AS, Berry MF, Tong BC, Harpole DH, Mitchell JD, D'Amico TA, Onaitis MW (2012) Thoracoscopic lobectomy has increasing benefit in patients with poor pulmonary function: a Society of Thoracic Surgeons Database analysis. *Ann Surg*, Sep; 256(3): 487–93.

34 Bonadonna G, Valagussa P, Moliterni A, *et al.* Adjuvant cyclophosphamide, methotrexate, and fluorouracil in nodepositive breast cancer: the results of 20 years of follow-up. *N Engl J Med*, 332: 901–26.

35 Yan TD, Black D, Bannon PG, McCaughan BC (2009) Systematic review and meta-analysis on safety and efficacy of VATS lobectomy for NSCLC. *J Clin Oncol*, 27: 2553–62.

36 Lohrisch, C, Paltiel, C, Gelmon, K, *et al.* (2006) Impact on survival of time from definitive surgery to initiation of adjuvant chemotherapy for early-stage breast cancer. *J Clin Oncol*, 24: 4888–94.

37 Strauss GM, Herndon J, Maddaus MA, *et al.* (2004) Randomized clinical trial of adjuvant chemotherapy with paclitaxel and carboplatin following resection in stage 1B non-small cell lung cancer (NSCLC): Report of Cancer and Leukemia Group B (CALGB) Protocol 9633. *J Clin Oncol*, 22(suppl 14): 621s [abstract].

38 Scagliotti GV, Fossati R, Torri V, *et al.* (2003) Randomized study of adjuvant chemotherapy for completely resected stage I, II, or IIIA non-small-cell lung cancer. *J Natl Cancer Inst*, 95: 1453–61.

39 Flores RM, Ihekweazu U, Dycoco J, *et al.* (2011) Video-assisted thoracoscopic surgery (VATS) lobectomy: catastrophic intraoperative complications. *J Thorac Cardiovasc Surg*, 142: 1412–17.

40 Yang CF, D'Amico TA (2012) Thoracoscopic segmentectomy for lung cancer. *Ann Thorac Surg*, Aug; 94(2): 668–81.

41 Nwogu CE, Yendamuri S, Demmy TL (2010) Does thoracoscopic pneumonectomy for lung cancer affect survival? *Ann Thorac Surg*, Jun; 89(6): S2102–6.

42 Kamiyoshihara M, Ibe T, Takeyoshi I (2008) Video-assisted thoracoscopic lobectomy with bronchoplasty for lung cancer; tip regarding bronchial anastomosis. *Gen Thorac Cardiovasc Surg*, Sep; 56(9): 476–8.

43 Demmy, TL, Nwogu CE, Yendamuri S (2010) Thoracoscopic chest wall resection: What is its role? *Annals of Thoracic Surgery*, 89(6): S2142–5.

44 Cerfolio RJ, Bryant AS, Minnich DJ (2012) Minimally invasive chest wall resection: Sparing the overlying, uninvolved musculature of the chest. *Ann Thorac Surg*, Nov; 94(5): 1744–7.

45 Boffa DJ, Kosinski AS, Paul S, Mitchell JD, Onaitis M (2012) Lymph node evaluation by open or video-assisted approaches in 11,500 anatomic lung cancer resections. *Ann Thorac Surg*, Aug; 94(2): 347–53; discussion 353.

46 Park BJ, Melfi F, Mussi A, *et al.* (2012) Robotic lobectomy for non-small cell lung cancer (NSCLC): Long-term oncologic results. *J Thorac Cardiovasc Surg*, Feb; 143(2): 383–9.

CHAPTER 15
Extended Resections for Lung Cancer

Matthew A. Steliga[1] *and David C. Rice*[2]
[1]Division of Thoracic Surgery, University of Arkansas, Little Rock, AR, USA
[2]Department of Thoracic and Cardiovascular Surgery, The University of Texas MD Anderson Cancer Center, Houston, TX, USA

Introduction

Lung cancer is a leading cause of cancer mortality with over 160 000 deaths annually in the United States and over 1.3 million deaths worldwide [1,2]. With the recent benefit of screening demonstrated in high-risk individuals, the future of lung cancer treatment may involve an increasing proportion of small, localized early stage cancers. However, screening is not widely performed, and lung cancer can certainly develop in individuals not eligible for screening programs. Therefore, despite screening efforts, many cases of lung cancer may continue to present as locally advanced disease. While most individuals with advanced lung cancer may not benefit from surgical resection, particularly those with advanced mediastinal nodal disease or distant metastases, some presenting with locally advanced lung cancer may be candidates for curative surgical resection. Since survival of locally advanced lung cancer without resection is not common, it is critical for all clinicians who treat lung cancer to appreciate the potential ability of locally advanced tumors to be resected in order to provide the best opportunity for cure.

This chapter focuses on extended resection for lung cancer, specifically anatomic resection of the tumor and lung, with resection and reconstruction of adjacent structures as needed. Overall, practice guidelines such as the NCCN guidelines for non-small cell lung cancer [3] are excellent sources to provide consistent care, but even within the context of guidelines, care must be individualized based upon performance status, local expertise, and patient wishes. Patient selection is a challenging decision-making process. One must balance risks and benefits which must be weighed for each individual patient in order to extend survival options to those who may benefit, while judiciously refraining from surgical resection which may be harmful. Using the AJCC 7th Edition Cancer Staging Manual [4] criteria as a framework, we will discuss strategies to evaluate and treat several types of locally invasive T3 and T4 non-small cell lung cancer (see Table 15.1).

General principles for all extended resections

Standard lobectomy carries approximately a 2% mortality rate and 32% morbidity rate as reported in a retrospective review of the Society of Thoracic Surgeons Database [5]. Locally advanced lung cancers are by definition higher stage and have a greater chance of subsequent development of metastatic disease and local recurrence. Extended resection of lung cancer, whether it involves chest wall, great vessels, airway, or other structures, can be done but often carries higher perioperative

Lung Cancer, Fourth Edition. Edited by Jack A. Roth, Waun Ki Hong and Ritsuko U. Komaki.

Table 15.1 Staging of locally advanced NSCLC per AJCC 7th edition. [4]

	T3	T4
Involvement of:	Chest wall	Mediastinum
	Diaphragm	Heart
	Phrenic nerve	Great vessels
	Mediastinal pleura	Trachea
	Parietal pericardium	Recurrent laryngeal nerve
	Main bronchus <2 cm from carina	Esophagus
	Obstructive collapse entire lung	Vertebral body
	Separate tumor nodule: same lobe	Carina
		Separate tumor nodule: ipsilateral different lobe

Source: Staging of locally advanced NSCLC per AJCC 7th Edition [4].

risk than standard lobectomy. The combination of higher risk, more complex surgery with a greater propensity for nodal and/or metastatic disease in locally advanced cancers mandates a thorough and efficient preoperative assessment.

In general, any patient being evaluated for extended resection of any type should undergo dedicated chest computed tomography (CT) with intravenous contrast to best define the tumor in relationship to its surrounding anatomy and integrated positron emission tomography / CT (PET/CT) to evaluate the patient for nodal and distant metastatic disease. Any mediastinal nodes greater than 1 centimeter on short axis, or with elevated standard uptake value (SUV) on PET are suspect and warrant histologic confirmation. In the setting of clinical T4 tumors, surgical outcomes for known positive N2 or N3 disease are poor, and typically resection is not offered if discovered preoperatively. Even in the face of negative imaging, mediastinal node biopsy is critical in patients considered for extended resection. Staging procedures have low morbidity, and if positive, thoracotomy may be avoided with sooner initiation of chemotherapy and radiotherapy. Mediastinoscopy has been the standard for mediastinal nodal staging for many years and in certain cases, can be useful preoperatively to directly assess invasion of the trachea and mediastinal tissues. Increasingly, endobronchial ultrasound (EBUS) and esophageal ultrasound (EUS) are used in place of mediastinoscopy with similar sensitivity and specificity to mediastinoscopy while being less invasive. Radial endobronchial ultrasound has greater sensitivity than CT for assessing tracheal invasion. More detail regarding sensitivity and specificity of mediastinal staging is discussed in Chapter 12.

Due to the poor sensitivity of PET for detecting intracranial metastases, preoperative imaging of the brain, preferably by magnetic resonance imaging (MRI), should be routinely performed in any patient presenting for extended resection. It is not routine to obtain MRI of the chest for all patients, but rather this modality is used selectively to determine tissue invasion and relationship of the tumor to the spine, and central vasculature.

Patients with locally advanced tumors that are node-negative, but found to have distant metastatic spread are not considered for curative surgery except in very rare circumstances. A contralateral lung nodule may not be a metastasis, but instead a synchronous primary tumor, and, if fulfilling the accepted criteria established by Martini and Melamed [6], can be treated as such, with staged resection or possibly a combination of resection and stereotactic radiation. Those with a negative mediastinum and an isolated brain metastasis that is resected, or completely treated with gamma knife radiation, could be considered for extended resection, but these are truly rare circumstances and require a judicial evaluation of the anticipated benefit versus the potential morbidity of resection of the lung lesion in a multi-disciplinary thoracic tumor board conference.

Selection of patients for surgery requires a rigorous oncologic and physiologic evaluation. The traditional criteria for lung resection include a predicted postoperative forced expiratory volume in 1 second (FEV1) and diffusion capacity in the lungs for carbon monoxide (DLCO) of greater than 40% predicted, however, this value should not be used as an absolute contraindication for resection in all cases. This is particularly relevant for locally advanced tumors leading to obstructive atelectasis of the lung parenchyma to be resected. Calculation of postoperative predicted pulmonary function is familiar to practicing thoracic surgeons and the details of this are beyond the scope of this chapter; however, when discussing preoperative evaluation, a quantitative ventilation/perfusion (V/Q) scan can be critical to determine if a patient would tolerate resection. Often, the locally advanced tumor has impeded either the ventilation or the blood flow to the anatomic portion of the lung to be resected. Typically V/Q scans are not necessary for routine lobectomy, but are often used to help surgeons best determine resectability for more advanced tumors, particularly those requiring pneumonectomy.

Once deemed a candidate for curative surgery, certain principles guide surgical resection. Regardless of the structure invaded, anatomic resection the tumor involving dissection and division of pulmonary artery, pulmonary vein and airway at the hilum, with microscopically negative margins is the goal. Even in the face of negative preoperative mediastinal staging with imaging and biopsy, mediastinal lymphadenectomy is an integral part of any oncologically sound lung cancer resection, and particularly for extended resections. Osarogiagbon and colleagues recently reported a retrospective database review of lung cancer resection in the United States. The subgroup of patients who had undergone resection which "extended to chest wall, carina, or further" comprised 5% of their overall study population and had a disappointing rate of 54% (n = 316/582) of cases in which no mediastinal nodes were examined from surgery [7]. Adequate surgical mediastinal staging at the time of resection is critical to determine prognosis and for making evidence-based decisions regarding the appropriateness and extent of adjuvant therapy. Despite thorough preoperative staging with imaging and mediastinal node biopsy, some clinically node negative patients are found to harbor unexpected microscopic positive N2 nodes at the time of surgery. The combination of increased risk from extended resection, and the poorer survival of T3N2 and T4N2 lung cancer would lead many to abandon resection.

Chest wall invasion

Direct extension to the chest wall by primary pulmonary malignancy is the most commonly resectable scenario of locally advanced lung cancer that presents to the thoracic surgeon. Historically, this seemingly incurable situation was initially challenged by Coleman in 1947 who reported extended resection in seven patients, five of which underwent combined lung and chest wall resection [8]. Currently, lung and en-bloc chest wall resection is commonly performed and is considered the standard of care for T3N0 and T3N1 tumors with direct extension to the chest wall. Approximately 5% of patients presenting for lung resection have tumors of T3 status due to involvement of the chest wall [9], which is defined as invasion into the parietal pleura, and deeper.

Direct extension is obvious in some cases with evidence of bony destruction on the CT imaging, but can be subtle in cases where the tumor appears to abut the visceral pleural surface. While obvious bony destruction clearly indicates involvement, many patients have more subtle radiographic findings. The most sensitive CT finding is felt to be obliteration of the extrapleural fat plane (sensitivity of 85% versus rib invasion which had a sensitivity of 16%) [10]. The peripheral location of tumors invading the chest wall make symptoms such as cough, hemoptysis and postobstructive pneumonia rare, whereas focal chest wall pain is the most common symptom of chest wall invasion. Pain radiating along intercostal dermatomes or brachial plexus distribution can be seen with invasion as well. Since the parietal pleura and chest wall are richly innervated with sensory fibers, a patient's symptom of focal pain localized to the area may be more reliable to determine chest wall invasion than CT imaging. Focal chest wall pain has been shown to be a reliable indicator of chest wall involvement independent of CT imaging [11]. While PET is obtained on all patients with chest wall invasion to evaluate for distant metastatic disease, it is not sensitive for determining local invasion. Magnetic resonance imaging can provide information about local invasion, but is most useful for evaluating superior sulcus tumors to determine involvement of the brachial plexus, and subclavian vessels. It is not routinely used for preoperative evaluation of tumors with lower chest wall invasion. Most tumors with chest wall invasion should be biopsied percutaneously, rather than by bronchoscope due to their peripheral location. In occasional cases with questionable chest wall invasion, reviewing the CT images obtained during biopsy can demonstrate separation of the lung from the chest wall if a pneumothorax has occurred. Ultrasonography (US) can determine chest wall invasion by visualizing the pleural plane and lung movement during respiration. This dynamic examination in the hands of experienced clinicians is felt to have better sensitivity and similar specificity to the use of CT scan (US: 89% sensitivity, 95% specificity versus CT, 42% sensitivity, 100% specificity) [12], and this may be more useful for tumors lower in the chest which may move in real time imaging with diaphragmatic excursion during breathing. The apices of the lungs do not move during respiration and utility of this test may be more limited for those tumors. Routine ultrasonography for preoperative imaging is not necessary, since chest wall invasion is not a contraindication for curative surgery, and the decision about resection can often be made intraoperatively.

For the patient whose predicted postoperative pulmonary FEV1 (ppoFEV1) or DLCO is borderline after a prospective lung resection, it is important to recognize that typical calculations and guidelines relate to lung resection alone, and this does not take into account the physiologic insult of chest wall resection [13]. A single rib resection likely has minimal negative impact on breathing physiology, but resection of several ribs can lead to a physiologic scenario similar to flail chest from trauma, with paradoxical breathing motion, unless reconstructed. For the borderline patient, chest wall resection can greatly increase chances of respiratory failure and need for mechanical ventilation. Rigid stabilization with mesh and cement can decrease paradoxical movement to a large degree. It is still crucial for the clinician to appreciate that respiratory physiology will be more impaired postoperatively after a large chest wall resection combined with lung resection than simply lung resection alone. Martin-Ucar and colleagues found that low body mass index, age greater than 75 years, and preoperative FEV1 less than 70% predicted were independently associated with increased risk for postoperative mortality most often secondary to respiratory complications [13]. In rare cases which may have truly borderline pulmonary function and may not tolerate concomitant chest wall resection, additional preoperative imaging beyond CT alone such as MRI or US may determine eligibility for surgery.

In some cases, benign adhesions may tether the lung to the chest wall without tumor invasion. In cases of questionable invasion, the surgeon will have to decide whether to proceed with full thickness chest wall resection versus dissection in an extrapleural plane. In the absence of chest wall pain and firm fixation of the mass to the chest wall, combined with no clear radiographic evidence of invasion or violation of extrapleural fat planes, it may be acceptable to initiate dissection in an extrapleural plane, converting to a full thickness resection if there is later evidence of deeper invasion on frozen section. This may avoid unnecessary chest wall resection. If there is indeed invasion, the tumor plane has been breached, or there is microscopic deeper invasion, intrapleural resection could lead to a higher risk of local recurrence [11, 14, 15]. Frozen section histology can be useful in this situation to confirm completeness of resection.

The goal of surgery with chest wall invasion is complete en-bloc resection of the tumor with negative margins (R0 resection). Anatomic resection with lobectomy is standard, and can be accomplished several ways. Either a traditional open thoracotomy or a thoracoscopic approach for division of structures at the hilum and lymphadenectomy, with a more limited open incision for resection of the chest wall. Pleural disease is rare and precludes curative resection. Discovery of this thoracoscopically may allow quicker recovery than nontherapeutic thoracotomy. Entry into the chest is in a remote location from the tumor and thoracoscopic visualization can also guide margins of the chest wall resection rather than palpation. It can also confirm absence of pleural metastases [16]. For resection with an open thoracotomy, careful preoperative planning and review of imaging is crucial in order to enter the pleural space in a location remote from the tumor to avoid breaching tumor planes. After entering the pleural space, palpation of the chest wall and tumor typically guides resection. Typical margins are one grossly negative rib space above and below the affected area of chest wall invasion, and at least 3–4 cm anteriorly and posteriorly [16, 17], although some advocate 1 cm gross negative margins [15]. One of the many challenges with resection of the chest wall and anatomic lung resection can be exposure of the hilum with a bulky mass fixed to the chest wall. In select cases, the chest wall resection is carried out first, then the lung is divided in a nonanatomic (wedge) resection to separate the tumor and contiguous chest wall from the remaining lung tissue at the hilum. This can greatly improve visualization of the hilum to remove the remaining amount of the lobe in an anatomic fashion and facilitate mediastinal lymphadenectomy.

Reconstruction with prosthetic mesh is generally not required for resection of a single rib. Defects of 5 cm or greater, which typically result from resecting multiple ribs, may benefit from reconstruction in certain locations. Some authors do not routinely reconstruct the chest wall with mesh and reporting minimal morbidity [17]. Typically, defects at the apex and those posterior defects covered by the scapula and paraspinous musculature may not need reconstruction even if more than one rib is resected. Anterior, lateral and inferior defects may benefit from reconstruction due to deformity and greater paradoxical breathing motion. Reconstruction may be indicated in some posterior defects at or just above the level of the scapular tip to prevent scapular entrapment from occurring. Alternatively, the tip of the scapula may be resected to mitigate against this. Some surgeons prefer to perform chest wall reconstructions with polytetrafluoroethylene (PTFE). It is available as solid sheets, impervious to fluid, has minimal ingrowth, and minimal incorporation into surrounding tissues. However, the prosthesis most frequently used is polypropylene mesh, a less expensive material than PTFE that has excellent tissue incorporation and resists infection well. As the tissue heals, there is ingrowth of tissue into the interstices of this mesh, which can add to the rigidity of the reconstruction. The open lattice of the mesh provides a framework for methylmethacrylate cement (sandwich technique) stiffening the reconstruction prosthesis of the chest wall (see Figure 15.1).

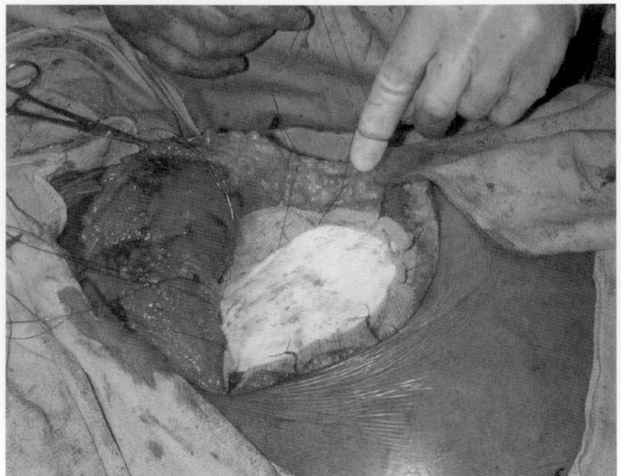

Figure 15.1 Polypropylene mesh reconstruction with methylmethacrylate. (For a color version, see the color plate section.)

Weyant *et al.* discussed chest wall resection in 262 patients and found a low incidence of respiratory failure (3.1%) following chest wall resection, which they attributed to selective use of mesh reconstruction, with and without methylmethacrylate. Although this was a heterogenous group containing patients with a variety of tumor types, their use of chest wall reconstruction was felt to improve respiratory mechanics and decrease postoperative pulmonary complications. [19]. While this cement can provide contour for anterior and lateral defects, and stiffen the mesh for less paradoxical movement,

Table 15.2 Outcomes of lung resection for direct invasion of the chest wall

Author	Year	Number	Mortality (%)	Overall survival (%)	N0	N1	N2
Chapelier [18]	2000	100	2	18	22	9	0
Facciolo [17]	2001	104	0	61.4	67	100	17
Magdeleniat [22]	2001	201	7	21	25	21	20
Elia [23]	2001	110	0	35	47	0	
Burkhart [24]	2002	94	6.3	38.7	44.0	26*	26*
Riquet [15]	2002	125	7	22.5	30.7	0	11.5
Rovario [25]	2003	146	0.7	NS	78.5	7.2*	7.2*
Matsuoka [26]	2004	97	NS	34.2	44.2	40.0	6.2
Doddoli [27]	2005	309	8	30.7	40	23.8	8.4
Volotini [28]	2006	68	4	37	42	17*	17*
Lin [29]	2006	42	NS	28.4	39	17.1	
Lee [30]	2012	107	5	26.3	37.4	21.1	4.6

NS: not stated.
*Study reported node negative versus node positive, N1 and N2 not specified.

it is not perfect. The rigidity of the cement plate can be painful if placed in direct contact with the ribs, which move during respiration and body movement. Typically, if cement is to be used, it is contoured so that the edges of the methylmethacrylate do not abut or overlap the rib edges. A more anatomic reconstruction involves use of polypropylene mesh and injection of methylmethacrylate into silicone tubes to act as molds, which are formed to the desired contour of the chest wall and allowed to harden. The silicone tubes then are interposed between the cut ends of the ribs and sutured into place to create new rib-shaped prostheses [20]. Newer options for chest wall reconstruction include acellular collagen sheets which have been used after vertebral and chest wall resection for a primary chest wall neoplasm [21]. The biologic materials, such as the acellular collagen products, may be more resistant to infection than the synthetic prosthetic materials; however, due to increased costs, variable long term strength and limited availability, its routine use for chest wall reconstruction is not preferred over a traditional polypropylene mesh. If possible, a preserved muscle layer between the mesh and skin closure may improve healing and decrease the possibility for wound and mesh infection. The latissimus dorsi, serratus anterior, and pectoralis major muscles all have reliable blood supply and can be rotated to cover the mesh prosthesis. In the event of a superficial cutaneous and subcutaneous wound disruption, the mesh is not exposed. The need to preserve chest wall musculature is best considered from the outset of the operation in order to mobilize and spare the muscle when performing thoracotomy. Omental flaps and rectus abdominus muscle flaps may also be useful to cover mesh, but this also requires appropriate planning of the operative site. The placement of chest drainage tubes is a seemingly small detail, but important to keep the tube insertion site remote from the chest wall mesh site to minimize possibility of contamination. Finally, frozen section margins are obtained on soft tissue, but bone will take days to de-calcify.

Outcomes of lung resection for T3 tumors due to chest wall invasion are summarized in Table 15.2. Not all of the listed studies are directly comparable, since some studies included extrapleural dissection for what was deemed to be pleural invasion only, whereas other studies only included full thickness chest wall resection. Several studies report N status individually, whereas others report N1 and N2 combined [24, 25, 28]. The reported mortality from surgical resection ranges from 0 to 8%, with a five year survival of 22–61% for all patients. Not surprisingly, survival was best for node negative (N0) patients, with five-year survival of 78%, while it is worse for patients with N2 metastases (0–20%). [15, 17, 18, 22–30]. The overall poor survival of this group of patients reinforces the importance of careful preoperative mediastinal staging.

Superior sulcus tumor resection

Superior sulcus tumors were first described by Henry Pancoast, a radiologist who noted a pattern of apical chest masses associated with significant pain. He did not attribute the masses to invasive lung cancer and initially felt they may be tumors of embryonal epithelial rests of the last branchial cleft [31]. Apical lung masses which invade adjacent structures have historically been called Pancoast tumors or superior sulcus tumors. Recently, however, there has been further discussion that a more accurate name would be apical chest tumors since there is no clear anatomic or radiographic correlation to a "superior sulcus" [32]. Despite different perspectives on terminology, most literature published regarding these tumors has used the phrase "superior sulcus tumors" which we will use for continuity. The strategy of radiation followed by surgical resection for these painful apical tumors was first discussed by Shaw, Paulson, and Kee in 1961 [33]. This extended posterior thoracotomy remained the most common surgical approach for this type of tumor for several decades. The Shaw Paulson approach is still used in many centers today.

While most would agree that these advanced locally aggressive tumors should be treated with trimodality therapy (involving surgery, radiation therapy and chemotherapy), there are different approaches and opinions regarding the order of the treatment components. The prospective, phase II Southwest Oncology Group trial (SWOG 9416), treated patients with cT3-4N0-1 superior sulcus tumors with concurrent cisplatin, etoposide and radiation to 45 Gy. Perioperative mortality was 1.8% and 5-year survival was 44% [34]. A European study included 31 patients with superior sulcus tumors, which included some N2 and N3 patients (cT3-4N0-3), incorporated three cycles of chemotherapy followed by chemoradiation to 45 Gy followed by resection after restaging. Complete resection was noted in 94% and 5-year survival was 46% [35]. The multidisciplinary approach from Toronto included induction chemoradiation according to the same protocol as SWOG 9416 and reported 5% operative mortality and 59% 5-year survival [36]. Lastly, a phase II Japanese trial of induction chemoradiation with platinum-based chemotherapy administered concurrently with 45 Gy of radiation showed similar outcomes to SWOG 9416 and had a 3.5% operative mortality rate with a 5-year survival of 56%. For bulky apical tumors that may be questionably resectable based upon imaging studies, there is theoretical appeal to delivering preoperative chemoradiation with the hope of tumor shrinkage, thus increasing the complete resection rate. Response to therapy can also inform the clinician regarding the efficacy of that particular treatment regimen on the individual tumor. Finally, there may be some patients who, despite upfront therapy with chemoradiation, may show signs of distant progression while on treatment. These patients may already have had undetectable subclinical distant disease, would have progressed after surgery and thus were spared a futile thoracotomy and its associated pain and complications. Despite these potential benefits of induction treatment, other centers hold the perspective that initial surgery allows upfront resection without the challenges and complications of operating in a radiated field. Post-radiation changes are not infrequently difficult to distinguish from tumor and tissue planes may be obliterated, making resection more difficult. Microscopic or macroscopic tumor left after surgery is impossible to treat effectively with radiation following preoperative radiation treatment. Proponents of postoperative radiation maintain that saving radiation until after surgery allows delivery of higher doses of radiotherapy than can be delivered in a preoperative setting. In addition, these patients frequently have severe unrelenting pain, and initial surgery may offer quicker and more durable palliation [37]. Finally, there are more supportive data for delivery of adjuvant therapy compared to preoperative delivery of therapy for non-small cell lung cancer in general. A recent prospective phase II study was conducted by a multidisciplinary group at the M.D. Anderson Cancer Center. Initial surgery for superior sulcus tumors was followed by radiation therapy (RT) of 60 to 64.8 Gray (Gy) with two cycles of etoposide and cisplatin administered concurrently with RT and 3 additional cycles after completion of RT. The results demonstrated 2-year, 5 year, and 10-year rates of locoregional control of 84%, 76%, and 76%; with overall survival of 72%, 50%, and 45%, respectively. This approach of trimodality therapy allows delivery of higher doses of RT than the strategies in which pre-operative radiation is used limiting the radiation dose to 45 Gy [38].

Involvement of the subclavian artery or vein, once felt to be a contraindication to curative resection is routinely resected in some centers. The anterior cervical incision extending along the sternocleidomastoid muscle, over the clavicle, and across the anterior chest wall as described by Dartevelle and colleagues provides excellent exposure to the apex of the chest. It provides proximal and distal control of the vasculature as well. A modification to this anterior approach presented by Grunenwald *et al.* [39] involving division of the manubrium (but preservation of the clavicle and sternoclavicular joint) and rotation of the entire clavicle and musculature, which is known as a "trap door" approach. The rotation of this ostemuscular flap provides excellent exposure, with the benefit of easier stabilization with wires to reapproximate the cut manubrium. An additional benefit of the cervicothoracic approach is the ability to dissect and submit scalene nodes through this approach. Some centers use the cervicothoracic approach for most superior sulcus tumors and usually perform the apical dissection and hilar dissection from that single incision. Some use combined cervicothoracic approach for vascular dissection and separate thoracotomy for hilar dissection, even A hybrid approach combining a transmanubrial cervicothoracic incision with the addition of thoracoscopic dissection of the hilum is another option [40, 41]. It has been proposed by de Perrot and colleagues that the thoracic inlet can be divided into different zones, with more anterior involvement being better approached via an anterior cervicothoracic incision with preservation of the clavicle, central involvement which is most challenging is best exposed with transclavicular exposure, and posterior involvement along the spine and nerve roots being better exposed posteriorly [42]. Despite the variety of perspectives, local expertise and familiarity with the different approaches certainly can play a role in the choice of surgical approach. Resection and reconstruction of the artery and vein are routinely done in centers with significant expertise. Simple ligation of the vein can be done, if necessary, and may be tolerated due to significant collateral venous flow around the shoulder girdle. Due to a risk of postoperative upper extremity edema, most would reconstruct the subclavian vein.

Vertebral body involvement

Invasion of the chest wall alone constitutes T3 status whereas vertebral body invasion is considered T4 (see Figure 15.2). There is a spectrum of vertebral invasion ranging from focal invasion of the transverse process or vertebral body to near replacement of the entire vertebra by tumor. In some cases, extension of the tumor into the spinal

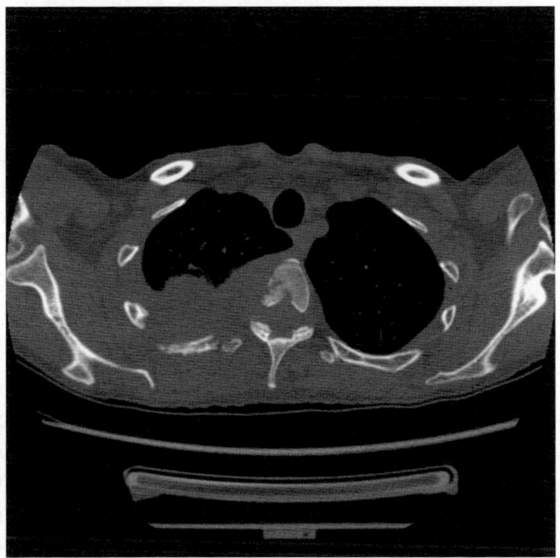

Figure 15.2 Axial imaging CT demonstrates bony involvement of both rib and vertebra.

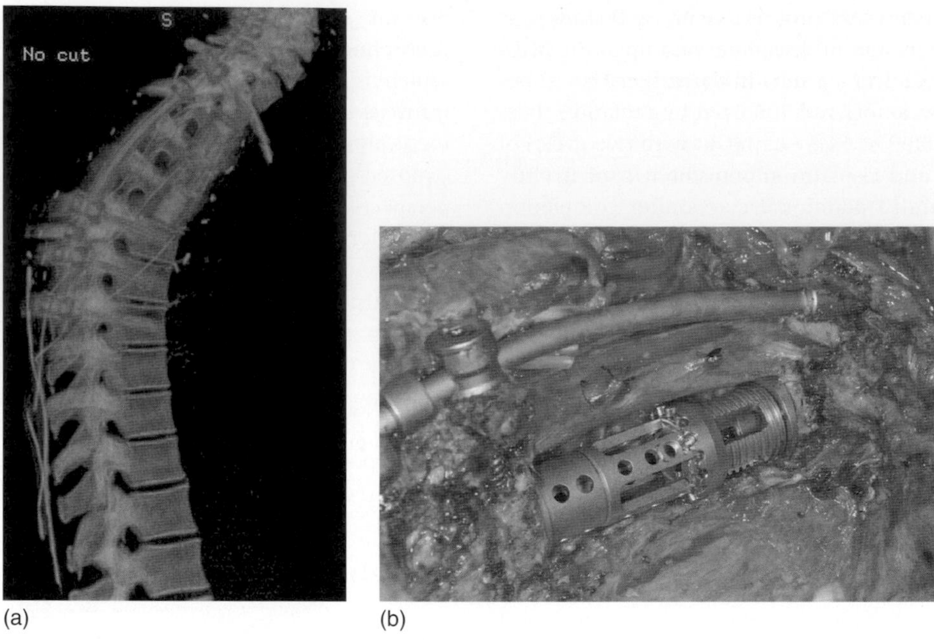

(a) (b)

Figure 15.3 Extensive resection of the spine due to local invasion requires stabilization with hardware as demonstrated in postoperative imaging (a) and intraoperative photograph (b). (For a color version, see the color plate section.)

canal with impending cord compromise is seen. Invasion into the vertebral body is not a contraindication for curative resection, but does require careful planning for safe complete resection. This should be performed in an experienced center and in collaboration with spine surgeons. In a few select centers, tumors with invasion into the vertebral body have been successfully treated by either partial vertebrectomy or total vertebrectomy with prosthetic reconstruction hardware to stabilize the spine (see Figure 15.3). [37, 43–45]. Resection is typically only done for curative intent. Palliative surgery for pain control or to limit spinal cord compromise is reported in 10% (4/39) of those undergoing vertebrectomy in one series [37]. A retrospective review of 39 cases of superior sulcus tumors with vertebral invasion was reported by Bolton and colleagues from the M.D. Anderson Cancer Center. Surgery was performed with adjuvant radiation and chemotherapy administered following resection, R0 resection was achieved in 22 of 39 cases (56%). Median survival was 18 months and 5-year survival of 27% was highly dependent on the presence or absence of nodal metastases. Patients who underwent resection, who had negative nodes had a 5-year survival of 41%, whereas there were no long-term survivors in patients who had positive mediastinal or hilar nodes [37].

The complications of chest wall and spine resection in conjunction with anatomic lung resection include all of the common complications of lung resection (such as arrhythmia, pneumonia, atelectasis, or air leak) however, certain complications are unique to chest wall and vertebral resection or reconstruction. Infection of the mesh prosthesis can be challenging. Prosthetic material such as polytetraflouroethylene (PTFE) has poor tissue ingrowth and almost always requires complete removal. Polypropylene mesh, if infected, may require removal. If the mesh is partially incorporated, it can often be treated with surgical irrigation or a negative pressure wound therapy system (VAC- Kinetic Concepts Inc., San Antonio, Texas, USA) can be used to promote granulation tissue through the mesh and healing with the mesh in place. The rigidity of methylmethacrylate can be painful if placed in close proximity to ribs or sternum. The painful clicking or popping can occasionally necessitate a second operation. This is best avoided by keeping the rigid material away from bony structures. Due to the location of the thoracic duct and its junction with the left subclavian-jugular vein confluence, dissection of apical structures on the left side must be done with care. The surgeon should be vigilant for any pooling of lymphatic fluid and ligate any lymphatic leaks during the operation with permanent suture. Postoperative low volume chyle leaks from minor ducts can be treated nonoperatively with minimizing oral intake, parenteral nutrition, and octreotide. However, if the leak is high output and does not respond to these initial measures, it may be due to an injury of the main duct. Reoperation and ligation of the duct (usually through the right chest) is often required and can readily be performed thoracoscopically.

Dissection of posterior chest wall tumors can require disarticulation of the rib heads from the costotransverse and costovertebral joints. Care should be taken to identify and ligate the nerve roots and intercostal vessels. Cerebrospinal fluid (CSF) leaks have occurred following transection of nerve roots. The accompanying dural sheath encasing the nerve root can be damaged by proximal division of the nerve and lead to a CSF leak if it is not ligated first. The clinical scenario of high output from the chest tubes and severe postural headache worsening in the upright position should raise suspicion. The combination of positive pressure of the CSF and negative intrathoracic pressure leads to a challenging situation unlikely to resolve without some form of intervention. Placement of a lumbar CSF drain and/or autologous blood patch may used to treat some dura leaks, but if it does not respond to these measures, reoperation may be required. A case report of neurologic dysfunction due to pneumocephalus following superior sulcus tumor resection [46] included a literature review and cited 17 other cases of pneumocephalus following thoracotomy for superior sulcus tumors due to dura leak. Some cases with minimal symptoms demonstrated spontaneous resolution, but cases with more serious neurologic dysfunction required reoperation. If a dural tear is encountered during vertebrectomy this is best treated with immediate repair and coverage with a pedicled soft tissue rotational flap such as intercostal or serratus muscle.

Diaphragm Involvement

Few reports are available regarding lung resection for tumors with direct extension into the diaphragm. While this is not common for lung cancer, this is a common scenario in patients with malignant pleural mesothelioma and imaging tumors with CT or MR does not always demonstrate diaphragmatic invasion. Diaphragmatic invasion by lung cancer may not be suspected initially, and is primarily encountered intraoperatively. Diaphragm invasion is a rare situation, presenting in less than 0.2% of all lung cancer resections at a single institution (n = 8/4668) reviewed retrospectively by Weksler *et al.* [47]. Portions of the diaphragm can easily be resected, and small defects can be repaired primarily with nonabsorbable suture using horizontal mattress sutures of nonabsorbable material such as braided polyester. If a defect is larger than can be repaired primarily, mesh can be used, but a smooth solid mesh prosthesis such as PTFE is preferable over coarser polypropylene mesh due to potential contact with abdominal viscera. Long-term survival is reported to range from 20 to 39% at five years following en-bloc resection of lung cancer with the diaphragm [48, 49]. Poorer survival of patients with diaphragmatic invasion compared to other sites of T3 invasion may be related to the lymphatic drainage of the diaphragm itself, which drains not only to the mediastinal nodes, but also the internal mammary chain and the infradiaphragmatic para-aortic nodes [50]. Finally, depending upon the location of the diaphragm resection and potential denervation of remaining diaphragm muscle, resection may impair breathing physiology. This should be considered in more marginal patients.

Phrenic nerve involvement

Lung tumors abutting the mediastinum with concomitant ipsilateral elevated hemidiaphragm signify phrenic nerve invasion. A quantitative V/Q scan may demonstrate that the affected lung may contribute less to their breathing physiology than the contralateral side. Alternatively, a "sniff" test may be performed using fluoroscopy to document paradoxical movement of the ipsilateral hemidiaphragm upon inspiration. In these patients, resection of the tumor en-bloc with the nerve is done to offer a curative resection if the patient meets other oncologic and physiologic criteria for surgery. No attempt is made to dissect and spare the nerve if it is nonfunctional.

Unexpected phrenic nerve involvement (the diaphragm is in a normal position preoperatively) can be encountered, and, if possible, careful dissection and neurolysis is sometimes possible if the tumor does not directly invade the nerve. There is risk of short-term and even long-term paresis because of devascularization of the nerve. However, if invasion is present, the nerve can be sacrificed safely in most patients unless their pulmonary reserve is borderline. Plication of the affected diaphragm after unilateral nerve resection was reported in 6/13 patients undergoing resection of lung and mediastinal tumors by Tokunaga *et al.* They noted a need for mechanical ventilation longer than 7 days in 2/13 (15%) of their patients overall but in 2/6 (33%) of those who had undergone lung resection with phrenic nerve sacrifice [51].

Recurrent laryngeal nerve involvement

The right recurrent laryngeal nerve (RLN) descends as fibers of the vagus nerve. After coursing around the right subclavian artery, it ascends in the tracheoseophageal groove to innervate the larynx. The left RLN descends along with the left vagus anterior to the aortic arch before wrapping around the inferior arch and ascending again in the left tracheo-esophageal groove. Preoperative hoarseness is an ominous sign, for it signifies not just invasion of the nerve, but often invasion of associated mediastinal structures (subclavian artery, aorta, esophagus or trachea). Invasion of only the nerve usually does not preclude surgery, but the limitation to resectability may be the direct extension into associated vascular structures, viscera or the presence of nodal and distant disease. Intraoperative discovery of tumor abutting a preoperatively functioning nerve can happen, and if a tissue plane exists, neurolysis can spare the nerve. However, if the RLN is sacrificed the risk of aspiration in the postoperative period is high. These patients should remain fasting and nutritionally maintained using either enteral feeding or total parenteral nutrition until a speech therapist has been able to document their aspiration risk. Frequently, a contrast fluoroscopic modified barium swallow examination is required. If patients aspirate, then temporary medialization of the affected vocal cord can be performed using Teflon or fat injection. Definitive vocal cord medialization may be required but is best performed after 2–3 months have passed so that the degree of lateralization of the affected cord stablizes allowing the otolaryngologist to perform an optimized medialization procedure. Early vocal cord injection can improve voice quality, decrease aspiration, and improve the ability to cough and clear secretions in the postoperative period.

Pericardium

Direct extension of tumor onto the pericardium is considered stage T3 and is amenable to resection. However, presence of pericardial fluid on imaging may represent a malignant pericardial effusion. If confirmed, this is considered M1a and is not surgically curable. Unfortunately, the diagnosis of transmural pericardial invasion with epicardial involvement can be difficult to diagnose accurately in the preoperative setting. While pericardial resection due to direct invasion is not commonly described in the literature, surgical principles such as resection to a negative margin are followed. Often this will require resection of the phrenic nerve as well. Lung resection combined with resection of a portion of the pericardium can result in a pericardial defect, and if left untreated could be a risk for cardiac herniation, which is of particular concern on the right side following pneumonectomy where herniation may lead to torsion of the heart on the caval axis resulting in rapid hemodynamic collapse and death. Most surgeons choose to repair the pericardial defects with smooth PTFE mesh or softer absorbable material such as polyglycolic acid or polyglactin mesh. If a solid material such as PTFE is used, it is prudent to create multiple small fenestrations to evacuate postoperative fluid. This avoids tamponade from accumulated intrapericardial fluid. Bulky tumors at the hilum can be more easily resected if the pericardium is opened. Intrapericardial dissection of the pulmonary artery and veins is performed as well. Closure of the pericardial defect is a simple but important step to avoid cardiac herniation, which is often lethal. On the left side, even if pneumonectomy is performed, pericardial reconstruction is not required, however, the defect should be widely opened to prevent partial herniation of the heart. On the right, if sufficient pulmonary parenchyma remains, the defect does not generally require repair. Repair is advised if a lower and middle lobe bilobectomy is performed and is mandatory in conjuncton with a pneumonectomy.

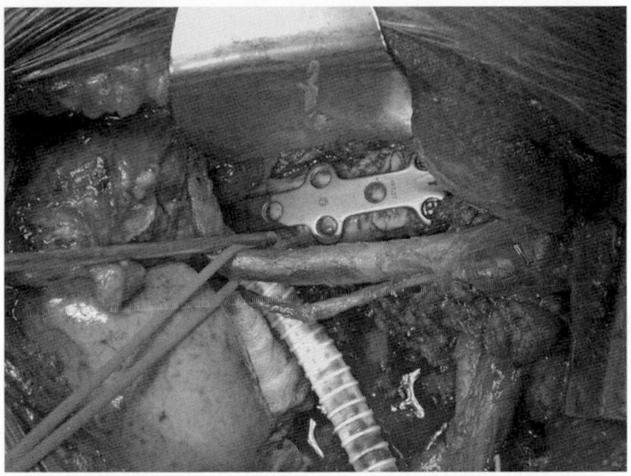

Figure 15.4 Resection of superior sulcus tumor in conjunction with spine (stabilization hardware shown) and subclavian vessel (replaced by ringed PTFE graft). (For a color version, see the color plate section.)

Heart and great vessels

Invasion of the vena cava, aorta, or subclavian artery have been deemed incurable clinical scenarios at one time or another. Currently, tumors with great vessel invasion are often not amenable to surgical cure due to bulky nodal or distant disease. For select T4N0 or T4N1 patients without metastatic disease and adequate respiratory reserve, resection to negative margins for curative intent (see Figure 15.4) has been done in specialized thoracic centers with acceptable morbidity and long-term survival.

Direct ingrowth of the tumor into the superior vena cava (SVC) does not preclude curative resection. Preoperative planning is critical. Obtaining large bore intravenous access in the lower body allows intravenous fluids and pharmacologic agents to be infused during SVC clamping. Depending on tumor location and size, either sternotomy, or an anterior thoracosternotomy, also known as hemiclamshell incision can be used to provide better access to the upper mediastinum and hilum than a traditional thoracotomy. Limited involvement can be addressed by resection to negative margins with primary repair. Larger defects may require patch repair with either prosthetic material or autologous tissue such as pericardium, saphenous vein as a spiral graft, or azygous vein. Complete segmental resection and reconstruction is possible with good results using dacron grafts, PTFE, or bovine pericardium, however, clamping the SVC can lead to a rapid drop in preload and subsequent hypotension. Generally, this will require resection of the right phrenic nerve as well. The combination of arterial hypotension and acute venous congestion can lead to cerebral edema. Protective strategies such as intravenous steroids, heparin, and use of vasoconstrictors may decrease this risk [52]. Furthermore, it is essential that infra-diaphramatic venous access be established in cases where SVC resection is anticipated. Series reporting SVC resection for lung cancer have reported an operative mortality ranging from 7.7 to 14% and a 5-year survival from 24–31% [53–56]. For complex cases entailing SVC reconstruction as well as carina resection, care must be taken to minimize contamination from the airway to decrease risk of graft infection, which could be a truly disastrous complication. Tumors invading the SVC may present with SVC syndrome, which is swelling and congestion of the face and upper extremities, though the absence of these symptoms do not imply lack of SVC invasion. Development of collateral supply over a the slow course of tumor progression may prevent such facial swelling. Rarely, SVC syndrome presents with negative mediastinal nodes, no distant metastases and is compatible with resection of localized disease. In cases not surgically resectable, symptomatic patients are referred for palliative SVC angioplasty and stenting to relieve the symptoms due to venous congestion. Surgical bypass of the SVC may also be performed.

Aortic invasion was previously felt to be a contraindication for curative resection, yet select cases of NSCLC invading the aorta have been resected with acceptable long term survival. Aortic invasion is suspected in patients with an absent fat plane between the aorta and tumor on imaging, flattening of the concave wall of the aorta when filled with contrast, intraluminal irregularity, and interscapular back pain. The imaging characteristics for aortic invasion on CT and MRI have low sensitivity. Intravascular ultrasound has improved sensitivity, but this may not be widely available at all centers. Often, the only way one can definitively establish the presence or absence of invasion is intraoperative examination by an experienced thoracic surgeon. Most often, lung cancers abut but do not invade the aorta. Encountering focal adhesions between the tumor and descending aorta can be readily addressed with careful dissection along the vessel, and a clear plane may exist beneath the adventitia, however, deeper invasion into the media may require with full thickness excision and repair with a prosthetic graft. Simply cross-clamping the aorta puts significant afterload on the left ventricle while the lower half of the body is ischemic. Either passive arterial shunting or bypass from atrium to descending aorta should be considered to avoid deleterious hemodynamic effects of clamping, and perfuse the lower body. Misthos and colleagues reported resection of T4 lung cancer with aortic invasion in 13 patients with 0% complication rate and 100% survival at 5 years for the subgroup of T4N0 and 30.7% five year survival overall [57]. Ohta and colleagues also reported their series of 16 resections of T4 with aortic invasion (n = 16). In their series, they report a 12.5% mortality rate and 31% complication rate. Despite significant perioperative morbidity and mortality, five year survival for pT4N0 (n = 10) was 70%. The other 6 patients were staged as pT4N2-3 with only one surviving five years (17% survival) [58]. Preoperative endovascular stent grafting has been reported in a case of the descending aorta to facilitate resection of a left lower lobe tumor with invasion of the aorta and avoid the hemodynamic challenges of cross-clamping the aorta, while avoiding complications associated with bypass. A redo thoracotomy and completion left pneumonectomy permitted an R0 resection of a T4N1 without the need for bypass and the patient was reported alive and well, disease free at 23 months [59].

Cardiopulmonary bypass (CPB) has been employed to allow some tumors to be resected. A recent literature review yielded 20 articles discussing CPB with resection of non-small cell lung cancer [60]. Overall five-year survival was 37% with a significant difference between planned and unplanned use of CPB (54% vs 11%). Overall 90-day perioperative mortality was 1%, indicating that even with CPB short-term and long-term survival is acceptable, and for select patients with potential for cure, CPB can be a valuable operative strategy [60]. Despite the appeal of CPB to facilitate complex resections, systemic heparinization and resultant inflammatory response from the perfusion pump is associated with its own risks and challenges, including pulmonary edema which is poorly tolerated following pneumonectomy. A report by de Perrot and colleagues of seven cases involving CPB and lung resection involved two cases where CPB was used for carinal resection; both of these patients developed respiratory complications and had a prolonged postoperative course, but did survive [61]. A series of 19 patients with advanced thoracic malignancies underwent resection with CPB. These cases were predominantly sarcomas, but one case in the series was a primary lung cancer invading the descending thoracic aorta. The patient underwent resection for curative intent and was alive at 25 months

[62]. Cardiopulmonary bypass can be utilized in cases of lung cancer invading the heart, pulmonary veins or main pulmonary artery or in scenarios as a strategy to maintain oxygenation while resecting and reconstructing the airway. While this is a seemingly aggressive approach, long term survival is clearly demonstrated in some patients. Proper patient selection, combined with surgical expertise, may allow these patients a curative option

Infiltration of tumor along the pulmonary veins and direct extension into the left atrium is another scenario of limited T4 invasion amenable to local resection. Stella and colleagues report 31 patients with invasion along the intrapericardial pulmonary vein or left atrium. Transesophageal echocardiography was used intraoperatively, and R0 resection was noted in 94% (29/31). Cardiopulmonary bypass was not required. Their three deaths were all right side intrapericardial pneumonectomies. Despite negative margins and a low rate of N2 disease (26% 8/31), the three-year survival rate was only 30% [63]. A similar cohort requiring left atrial resection (n = 46) was reported by Wu and colleagues. In their series they noted 0% operative mortality and 38% three-year survival and 22% five-year survival[64].

Trachea

Tracheal and carinal resection is certainly a technically challenging situation but the combination of proper patient selection and treatment in a high volume center with expertise in these approaches can lead to resection with negative margins and long term disease free survival. The details of tracheal and carinal surgery are covered in detail in Chapter 18.

Surgical perspectives for synchronous tumors

Clinical scenarios presenting two localized tumors in separate lobes (or separate lungs) have interesting diagnostic and therapeutic challenges and may be surgically curable. These warrant referral to a thoracic surgeon for evaluation. While these scenarios are not technically demanding in the manner that T4 tumors with visceral invasion are, they do present their own unique challenges. Certainly, preoperative staging is critical and aforementioned principles of staging the mediastinum with CT and PET and tissue sampling with EBUS, EUS or cervical mediastinoscopy are necessary for accurate patient selection. Different histologic cell types certainly indicate separate primary tumors, whereas the same cell type may represent solitary metastasis or synchronous primary tumors. Molecular testing may be of use to determine if two same histology nodules are likely separate primary tumors or a solitary metastasis; however, this clinical picture can still be approached with curative intent in the absence of mediastinal or other distant disease. The most recent changes to the AJCC staging system have addressed the status of separate nodules. Same lobe satellite nodules, previously considered T4 have been changed to T3 status to reflect overall better prognosis, and can routinely be treated with lobectomy after thorough preoperative staging. Nodules in the same lung, but different lobe, are categorized as T4, and contralateral disease is considered M1a but may be surgically resected for cure.

Lesions in different lobes of the same lung may be addressed with lobectomy for the larger or more central lesion and sublobar resection for the smaller or more peripheral lesion. If two separate primary lesions are found in different lungs, most surgeons would address this as staged procedures rather than trying to resect both sides in the same setting, due to pain and respiratory compromise from bilateral thoracotomies. A midline sternotomy can be performed with access to both pleural spaces, and this approach has routinely been done for wedge resections of bilateral pulmonary metastases from extrathoracic tumors. While bilateral wedge resections can be performed this way, access to the hila of the lungs and ability to do anatomic resection with thorough mediastinal lymphadenectomy is limited and most thoracic surgeons would not approach bilateral lung cancers in this fashion for these reasons. Depending upon the size and location of the tumors, a patient with two separate sites of NSCLC may be treated with surgical resection of both tumors as discussed. If a sublobar resection is performed, segmentectomy may be oncologically preferable to nonanatomic wedge resection, if possible. A combination of resection and other localized nonsurgical ablative techniques such as stereotactic radiation or percutaneous radiofrequency ablation may also be appropriate. While these situations are rare, it may be favorable to perform anatomic resection of the larger or more central tumor whereas, a smaller more peripheral tumor may be amenable to ablation as a staged procedure.

A single center retrospective review of 116 patients with synchronous primary lung cancers in different ipsilateral lobes (T4) or contralateral lung (M1a) demonstrated better survival than would otherwise be predicted by the AJCC staging of these tumors with mean overall survival of 65 months [65]. A systematic review pooled data from six separate studies to determine prognostic factors for survival in patients undergoing resection for synchronous primary lung cancer. Male gender, increased age, and node positivity were all associated with poorer prognosis. Bilateral location of the tumors was associated with decreased mortality: HR 0.69 (95% CI 0.50–0.94) and the median overall survival was 52 months for all patients [66]. The data suggests that while these patients are considered stage IIIB or IVa, their long term survival after curative resection is much more favorable than others with IIIB or IVa, and they should routinely be evaluated for surgical resection if possible.

Summary

Invasion of lung cancer into adjacent organs signifies a locally aggressive tumor. The greatest determinant of survival is not always the degree of local invasion, but instead the lymphatic and hematogenous spread of tumor. This principle is demonstrated by presenting effective curative strategies for locally aggressive and destructive tumors. After thorough preoperative staging has excluded mediastinal nodal or distant disease, complete en bloc resection of the tumor with adjacent structures is the best possible strategy to provide long-term cure. Advances in surgical technique, perioperative care, collaboration with other experts, and appropriate delivery of multimodality therapy has allowed the thoracic surgeon to expand boundaries of resection and offer curative resection or longer survival to many with locally advanced lung cancer.

References

1 Siegel R, Naishadham D, Jemal A (2012) Cancer statistics, 2012. *CA Cancer J Clin*, 62: 10–29.

2 Jemal A, Bray F, Center MM, Ferlay J, Ward E, Forman D (2011) Global cancer statistics. *CA Cancer J Clin*, 61: 69–90.

3 NCCN Clinical Practice Guidelines in Oncology. Non-Small Cell Lung Cancer Version 1.2013. National Comprehensive Cancer Network; 2013. Available from: http://www.nccn.org/professionals/physician_gls/pdf/nscl.pdf (accessed Dec 15, 2012).

4 Edge SB, Byrd DR, Compton CC, Fritz AG, Greene FL, Trotti A (eds) (2010) *AJCC Cancer Staging Manual* (7th ed). New York, NY: Springer.

5 Boffa DJ, Allen MS, Grab JD, *et al.* (2008) Data from the Society of Thoracic Surgeons General Thoracic Surgery Database: The surgical management of primary lung tumors. *J Thorac Cardiovasc Surg*, 135: 247–54.

6 Martini N, Melamed MR (1975) Multiple primary lung cancers. *J Thorac Cardiovasc Surg*, 70: 606–12.

7 Osariogiagbon RU, Yu X (2012) Mediastinal lymph node examination and survival in resected early stage non-small cell lung cancer in the Surveillance, Epidemiology, and End Results database. *J Thorac Oncol*, 7(12): 1978–1806.

8 Coleman FP (1947) Primary carcinoma of the lung with invasion of the ribs: Pneumonecotmy and simultaneous block resection of the chest wall. *Ann Surg*, 126(2): 156–68.

9 Stoelben E, Ludwig C (2009) Chest wall resection for lung cancer: Indications and techniques. *Eur J Cardiothorac Surg*, 35(3): 450–6.

10 Ratto GB, Piacenza G, Frola C, *et al.* (1991) Chest wall involvement by lung cancer: Computed tomography detection and results of operation. *Ann Thorac Surg*, 51: 182–8.

11 Kawaguchi K, Mori S, Usami N, Fukui T, Mitsudomi T, Yokoi K (2009) Preoperative evaluation of the depth of chest wall invasion and the extent of combined resections in lung cancer patients. 64(1): 41–4.

12 Bandi V, Lunn W, Ernst A, *et al.* (2008) Ultrasound vs CT in detecting chest wall invasion by tumor. *Chest*, 133: 881–6.

13 Martin-Ucar AE, Nicum R, Oey I, Edwards JG, Waller DA (2003) En-bloc chest wall and lung resection for non-small cell lung cancer. Predictors of 60-day non-cancer related mortality. *Eur J Cardiothorac Surg,* 23: 859–64.

14 D'Andrilli A, Venuta F, Menna C, Rendina EA (2011) Extensive resections: Pancoast tumors, chest wall resections, en bloc vascular resections. *Surg Onc Clin N Am,* 20: 733–56.

15 Riquet M, Arame A, Barthes FLP (2010) Non-small cell lung cancer invading the chest wall. *Thorac Surg Clin,* 20: 519–27.

16 Berry MF, Onaitis MW, Tong BC, Balderson SS, Harpole DH, D'Amico TA (2012) Feasibility of hybrid thoracoscopic lobectomy and en-bloc chest wall resection. *Eur J Cardiothorac Surg,* 41(4): 888–92.

17 Facciolo F, Cardillo G, Lopergolo M, *et al.* (2001) Chest wall invasion in non-small cell lung carcinoma: A rationale for en bloc resection. *J Thorac Cardiovasc Surg,* 121: 649–56.

18 Chapelier A, Fadel E, Macchiarini P, *et al.* (2000) Factors affecting long-term survival after en bloc resection of lung cancer invading the chest wall. *Eur J Cardiothorac Surg,* 18: 513–18.

19 Weyant MJ, Bains MS, Venkatraman E, *et al.* (2006) Results of chest wall resection and reconstruction with and without rigid prosthesis. *Ann Thorac Surg,* 81: 279–85.

20 Dartevelle PG, Bedrettin Y, Mussot S (2008) Extended resections for lung cancer. In: Roth JA, Cox J, Hong WK (eds), *Lung Cancer,* 3rd edn. London: Blackwell Science, p. 195.

21 Rocco G, Serra L, Fazioli F (2011) The use of Veritas collagen matrix to reconstruct the posterior chest wall after costovertebrectomy. *Ann Thorac Surg,* 92: e17–18.

22 Magdeleniat P, Ailfano M, Benbrahem C, *et al.* (2001) Surgical treatment of lung cancer invading the chest wall: Results and prognostic factors. *Ann Thorac Surg,* 71: 1094–9.

23 Elia S, Griffo S, Gentile M, Costabile R, Ferrante G (2001) Surgical treatment of lung cancer invading the chest wall: A retrospective analysis of 110 patients. *Eur J Cardiothorac Surg,* 20: 356–60.

24 Burkhart HM, Allen MS, Nichols FC, *et al.* (2002) Results of en bloc resection for bronchogenic carcinoma with chest wall invasion. *J Thorac Cardiovasc Surg,* 123: 670–5.

25 Roviaro G, Varoli F, Grignani F, *et al.* (2003) Non-small cell lung cancer with chest wall invasion: evolution of surgical treatment and prognosis in the last 3 decades. *Chest,* 123: 1341–7.

26 Matsuoka H, Nishio W, Okada M, *et al.* (2004) Resection of chest wall invasion in patients with non-small cell lung cancer. *Eur J Cardiothorac Surg,* 26(6): 1200–4.

27 Doddoli C, D'Journo B, Le Pimpec-Barthes F, *et al.* (2005) Lung cancer invading the chest wall: A plea for en-bloc resection but the need for new treatment strategies. *Ann Thorac Surg,* 80: 2032–40.

28 Volotini L, Rapicetta C, Luzzi L, *et al.* (2006) Lung cancer with chest wall involvement: Predictive factors of long term survival after surgical resection. *Lung Cancer,* 52: 359–64.

29 Lin YT, Hsu PK, Hsu HS, *et al.* (2006) En bloc resection for lung cancer with chest wall invasion. *J Chin Med Assoc,* 69(4): 157–62.

30 Lee CY, Byun CS, Lee JG, *et al.* (2012) The prognostic factors of resected non-small cell lung cancer with chest wall invasion. *World J Surg Oncol,* 10: 9.

31 Pancoast HK (1932) Superior pulmonary sulcus tumor. *JAMA,* 99: 1391.

32 Van Schil PE, Sigal-Cinqualbre A, Dartevelle P, Pac-Ferrer JJ (2012) Superior sulcus tumors: Do they really exist? *J Thorac Oncol,* 7(5): 777.

33 Shaw RR, Paulson DL, Kee JL (1961) Treatment of the superior sulcus tumor by irradiation followed by resection. *Ann Surg,* 154(1): 29–40.

34 Rusch VW, Giroux DJ, Kraut MJ, *et al.* (2007) Induction chemoradiation and surgical resection for superior sulcus non-small cell lung carcinomas: Long term results of the Southwest Oncology Group Trial 9416 (Intergroup Trial 0160). *J Clin Oncol,* 25(3): 313–18.

35 Marra A, Eberhardt W, Pottgen C, *et al.* (2007) Induction chemotherapy, concurrent chemoradiation and surgery for Pancoast tumor. *Eur Respir J,* 29: 117–27.

36 Fischer S, Darling G, Pierre AF, *et al.* (2008) Induction chemoradiation therapy followed by surgical resection for non-small cell lung cancer (NSCLC) invading the thoracic inlet. *Eur J Cardiothorac Surg,* 33: 1129–34.

37 Bolton WD, Rice DC, Goodyear A, *et al.* (2009) Superior sulcus tumors with vertebral body involvement: A multimodality approach. *J Thorac and Cardiovasc Surg,* 137(6): 1379–87.

38 Gomez DR, Cox JD, Roth JA, *et al.* (2012) A prospective phase 2 study of surgery followed by chemotherapy and radiation for superior sulcus tumors. *Cancer,* 118: 444–51.

39 Grunenwald MD, Spaggiari, MD (1997) Transmanubrial osteomuscular sparing approach for apical chest tumors. *Ann Thorac Surg,* 63(2): 563–6.

40 Shikuma K, Miyahara R, Osako T (2012) Transmanubrial approach combined with video-assisted approach for superior sulcus tumors. *Ann Thorac Surg,* 94(1): e29–30.

41 Truin W, Siebenga J, Belgers E, Bollen EC (2010) The role of video-assisted thoracic surgery in the surgical treatment of superior sulcus tumors. *Interact Cardiovasc Thorac Surg*, 11(4): 512–14.

42 dePerrot M, Rampersaud R (2012) Surgical approaches to apical thoracic malignancies. *J Thorac Cardiovasc Surg*, 144: 72–80.

43 Fadel E, Missenard G, Chapelier A, *et al.* (2002) En-Bloc resection of non-small cell lung cancer invading the thoracic inlet and intervetrebal foramina. *J Thorac Cardiovasc Surg*, 123: 676–85.

44 Grunenwald DH, Mazel C, Girard P, *et al.* (2002) Radical en bloc resection for lung cancer invading the spine. *J Thorac Cardiovasc Surg*, 123: 271–9.

45 Bilsky MH, Vitaz TW, Boland PJ, Bains MS, Rajaraman V, Rusch VW (2002) Surgical treatment of superior sulcus tumors with spinal and brachial plexus involvement. *J Neurosurg*, 97: 301–9.

46 Navarro BO, Atance PL, Trueba AA (2004) Pneumocephalus and cerebrospinal fluid fistula following removal of a superior sulcus tumor(Pancoast tumor). *Arch Bronconeumol*, 40(9): 422–5.

47 Weksler B, Bains M, Burt M, *et al.* (1997) Resection of lung cancer invading the diaphragm. *J Thorac Cardiovasc Surg*, 114: 500–1.

48 Rocco G, Rendina EA, Meroni A. *et al.* (1999) Prognostic factors after surgical treatment of lung cancer invading the diaphragm. *Ann Thorac Surg*, 68: 2065–8.

49 Riquet M, Porte H, Chapelier A (2000) Resection of lung cancer invading the diaphragm. *J Thorac Cardiovasc Surg*, 120(2): 417–18.

50 Brotons ML, Bolca C, Frechette E, Deslauriers J (2012) Anatomy and physiology of the thoracic lymphatic system. *Thorac Surg Clin*, 22: 155–60.

51 Tokunaga T, Sawabata N, Kadota Y, *et al.* (2010) Efficacy of intra-operative unilateral diaphragm plication for patients undergoing unilateral phrenicotomy during extended surgery. *Eur J Cardiothorac Surg*, 38: 600–3.

52 D'Andrilli A, Venuta F, Menna C, Rendina EA (2011) Extensive resections: Pancoast tumors, chest wall resections, en bloc vascular resections. *Surg Onc Clin N Am*, 20: 733–56.

53 Shargall Y, de Perrot M, Keshavjee S, *et al.* (2004) 15 years single center experience with surgical resection of the superior vena cava for non-small cell lung cancer. *Lung Cancer*, 45: 357–63.

54 Suzuki K, Asamura H, Watanabe S, *et al.* (2004) Combined resection of superior vena cava for lung carcinoma: Prognostic significance of patterns of superior vena cava invasion. *Ann Thorac Surg*, 78: 1184–9.

55 Spaggiari L, Thomas P, Magdeleinat P, *et al.* (2002) Superior vena cava resection with prosthetic replacement for non–small cell lung cancer: long-term results of a multicentric study. *Eur J Cardiothorac Surg*, 21: 1080–6.

56 Yıldızeli B, Dartevelle PG, Fadel E, Mussot S (2008) Results of primary surgery with T4 non–small cell lung cancer during a 25-year period in a single center: The benefit is worth the risk. *Ann Thorac Surg*, 86: 1065–75.

57 Misthos P, Papagiannakis G, Kokotsakis J, Lazopoulos G, Skouteli E, Lioulias A (2007) Surgical management of lung cancer invading the aorta or the superior vena cava. *Lung Cancer*, 56(2): 223–7.

58 Ohta M, Hirabayasi H, Shiono H, *et al.* (2005) Surgical resection for lung cancer with infiltration of the thoracic aorta. *J Thorac Cardiovasc Surg*, 129(4): 804–8.

59 Berna P, Bagan P, De Dominicis F, Dayden C, Douadi Y, Riquet M (2011) Aortic endostent followed by extended pneumonectomy for T4 lung cancer. *Ann Thorac Surg*, 91(2): 591–3.

60 Muralidaran A, Detterbeck FC, Boffa DJ, Wang Z, Kim AW (2011) Long-term survival after lung resection for non-small cell lung cancer with circulatory bypass: A systematic review. *J Thorac Cardiovasc Surg*, 142: 1137–42

61 de Perrot M, Fadel E, Mussot S, de Palma A, Chapelier A, Dartevelle P (2005) Resection of locally advanced (T4) non-small cell lung cancer with cardiopulmonary bypass. *Ann Thorac Surg*, 79(5): 1691–6.

62 Vaporciyan AA, Rice DC, Correa AM, *et al.* (2002) Resection of advancer thoracic malignancies requiring cardiopulmonary bypass. *Eur J Cardio-Thorac Surg*, 22: 47–52.

63 Stella F, Dell'Amore A, Caroli G, *et al.* (2012) Surgical results and long-term follow-up of T4-non-small cell lung cancer invading the left atrium or the intrapericardial base of the pulmonary veins. *Interactive Cardiovascular and Thoracic Surgery*, 14: 415–19.

64 Wu L, Xu Z, Zhao X, *et al.* (2009) Surgical treatment of lung cancer invading the left atrium or base of the pulmonary vein. *World J Surg*, 33: 492–6.

65 Tanvetyanon T, Robinson L, Sommers KE, *et al.* (2010) Relationship between tumor size and survival among patients with resection of multiple synchronous lung cancers. *J Thorac Oncol*, 5: 1018–24.

66 Tanvetyanon T, Finley DJ, Fabian T, *et al.* (2012) Prognostic factors for survival after complete resections of synchronous lung cancers in multiple lobes: pooled analysis based on individual patient data. *Ann Oncol.* epub Nov 7: 1–6.

CHAPTER 16

Bronchoscopic Interventions for Lung Cancer

Donald R. Lazarus and George A. Eapen
Department of Pulmonary Medicine, The University of Texas MD Anderson Cancer Center, Houston, TX, USA

Introduction

Lung cancer is the leading cause of cancer mortality in the United States, with more than 150 000 people dying from lung cancer annually [1]. As many as 60% of patients with non-small cell lung cancer (NSCLC) have symptoms related to locoregional involvement at the time of diagnosis [2]. Among the complications of lung cancer that may be amenable to palliation with therapeutic bronchoscopy are central airway obstruction, hemoptysis, and bronchial fistulas [3–5]. Bronchoscopic techniques may also be used to treat central early stage central lung cancers, although the use of such treatment is only recommended for those patients who cannot tolerate standard treatment with surgery or definitive external radiation [6, 7]. The only such lesions amenable to bronchoscopic treatment are those within reach of the rigid or flexible bronchoscope – primarily the trachea, main bronchi, bronchus intermedius, and occasionally the proximal lobar bronchi [3, 8, 9]. In this chapter we will briefly review the types of central airway lesions that are amenable to bronchoscopic intervention (listed in Table 16.1). We will then discuss in more detail the bronchoscopic techniques used for the palliation and treatment of central airway disease in lung cancer. Other causes of central airway disease are beyond the scope of this chapter.

Central airway disease in lung cancer amenable to bronchoscopic treatment

The most common indication for therapeutic bronchoscopy in patients with lung cancer is for palliation of symptoms related to tumor involvement of the central airways. Selection of the bronchoscopic method depends on type of symptoms present, the nature and location of the lesion causing the symptoms, and the locally available equipment and expertise (Figure 16.1) Central airway obstruction (CAO) involving the trachea or mainstem bronchi may cause complications in as many as 20–30% of patients with lung cancer [8]. These complications include dyspnea, atelectasis, and postobstructive pneumonia. Patients often do not develop symptoms until the narrowing is severe [8]. The type of central airway obstruction determines the most effective and appropriate therapy. Bolliger *et al.* describe three types of airway stenosis: those with primarily intraluminal tumor growth, those with primarily extraluminal compression, and those with elements of both [3]. Those lesions with primarily intraluminal involvement are best treated by utilizing mechanical and ablative methods to debulk and destroy the tumor, thereby restoring luminal patency. Lesions characterized primarily by extraluminal compression

Lung Cancer, Fourth Edition. Edited by Jack A. Roth, Waun Ki Hong and Ritsuko U. Komaki.

Table 16.1 Bronchoscopic interventions used in lung cancer

Mechanical interventions
Rigid bronchoscopy
Balloon bronchoplasty
Airway stenting
Microdebrider bronchoscopy
Thermal interventions
Laser bronchoscopy
Endobronchial electrocautery
Argon plasma coagulation
Endobronchial cryotherapy
Nonmechanical, nonthermal interventions
Photodynamic therapy
Endobronchial brachytherapy

of the airway require dilation to restore airway patency followed by stenting if significant residual stenosis remains. Combined modality treatment is usually required for patients with lesions characterized by both intraluminal tumor and extraluminal compression of the airway. Hemoptysis is also a common locoregional complication of lung cancer. Although more commonly seen in esophageal cancer, tracheo-esophageal and broncho-esophageal fistulas may occur in patients with lung cancer [10]. These most often develop after treatment with chemoradiotherapy and may have devastating consequences related to continuous contamination of the respiratory tract [5, 10]. Endobronchial therapy with stenting can be used to palliate these lesions and improve the quality of life for patients with such fistulas [11, 12].

While massive hemoptysis is relatively rare, submassive hemoptysis occurs in as many as 20% of patients with lung cancer at some time during

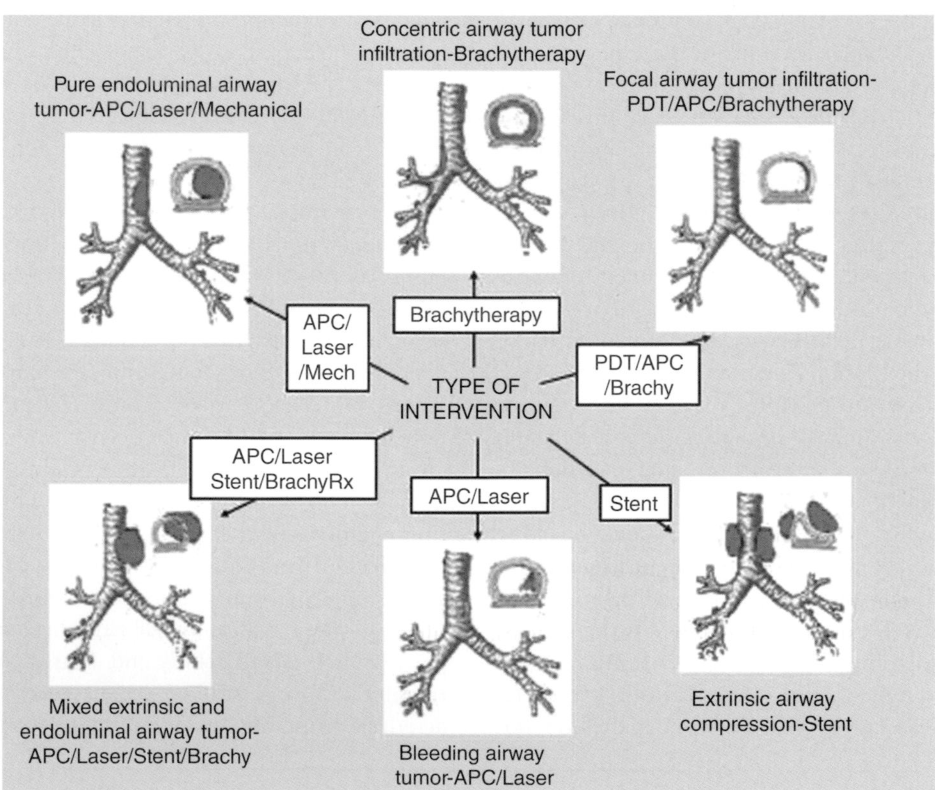

Figure 16.1 Selection of appropriate endobronchial therapeutic options based on location and type of lesion. (For a color version, see the color plate section.) *Source:* Reproduced with permission of Dr R. Morice.

their disease [13]. The precise definition of massive hemoptysis is controversial, with various authors advocating from 100 to 1000 ml of expectorated blood in a 24-hour period or a bleeding rate greater than 100 ml/hr. From a clinical perspective, massive hemoptysis is better defined as hemoptysis associated with respiratory insufficiency or hemodynamic instability [14]. Hemoptysis originating from discrete lesions in the visible central airways may be amenable to bronchoscopic palliation. Localizing the source of bleeding to a central airway lesion requires rapid clinical evaluation including imaging studies and flexible or rigid bronchoscopy. Imaging and bronchoscopy should be considered complementary techniques, and clinicians are more effective at localizing the bleeding source when both are used [4, 15]. Bronchoscopy is most helpful in localizing the site of bleeding if the rate of bleeding is 200 mL/day or more [16]. Once the site has been localized, efforts should initially focus on isolating the bleeding side and protecting the good lung. Useful techniques can include placing the bleeding side down, selectively intubating the nonbleeding mainstem bronchus, or deploying an endobronchial blocker on the bleeding side to tamponade the hemorrhage. Once the patient has been stabilized, sources of bleeding in the central airways can be managed using a variety of bronchoscopic techniques, including thermal therapies, mechanical resection of bleeding tumors, photodynamic therapy, and brachytherapy. More distal sources of bleeding are better managed with bronchial artery embolization or surgery.

Endobronchial treatment with brachytherapy or photodynamic therapy is also indicated for patients who present with early stage lung cancer confined to the central airways and who are not candidates for standard surgical or radiation treatment due to the location of the tumor, poor lung function, or otherwise poor performance status. The intent of treatment in this situation is curative [9]. The types of lesions that respond best to endobronchial treatment with curative intent are less than 1 cm in diameter, do not invade beyond the cartilaginous layer of the bronchial wall, and have not metastasized to regional lymph nodes [17]. Brachytherapy and photodynamic therapy can also be used to augment the effect of traditional external beam radiotherapy for tumors involving the central airways or to treat postsurgical endobronchial recurrence [9].

Mechanical bronchoscopic interventions in lung cancer

Mechanical bronchoscopic techniques can be used to debulk endobronchial tumors and dilate and reinforce narrowed or compromised airways in patients with lung cancer and airway obstruction. These techniques include rigid bronchoscopy, airway stents, and microdebrider bronchoscopy.

Rigid bronchoscopy is among the most important tools available for treating symptomatic central airway lesions of all three types. Rigid bronchoscopes are hollow metal tubes with side ports used for ventilation and the introduction of suction and other tools into the airway. They also permit the establishment of a safe airway and ventilation strategy prior to resection of obstructing tracheal tumors. Jet ventilation rather than volume cycled ventilation can be used with an open circuit to facilitate the passage of instruments through the working channel. They are typically used with a lighted telescope to enable good visualization of the airway distant to the tip of the bronchoscope. Rigid bronchoscopes come in varying sizes ranging from 2 mm external diameter to 14 mm external diameter. The flexible bronchoscope can also be passed through the rigid scope in order to facilitate examination of the more distal bronchi. The relatively large caliber of the interior channel of the rigid bronchoscope is of particular importance and allows it to serve as a conduit for other therapeutic instruments. Interventional bronchoscopists will often use more than one tool at a time through the lumen of the rigid scope, and some interventions, most notably silicone stents, can only be placed via the rigid bronchoscope. The rigid bronchoscope allows the bronchoscopist to secure the airway and facilitates oxygenation and ventilation while interventions are performed. In addition to its function as a conduit for other therapeutic instruments, the rigid bronchoscope itself can be used to treat central airway obstruction from lung cancer by "coring-out" the tumor. Most commercially available rigid bronchoscopes have a beveled tip. The operator can use the rigid bronchoscope to resect endoluminal tumor by placing the beveled edge of the tip against the portion of the endoluminal tumor. A corkscrew motion of the scope is then used to shave off portions of the tumor which are then removed using forceps or suction via the interior channel of the rigid bronchoscope [18, 19]. It is important to maintain proper orientation of the rigid bronchoscope during endobronchial tumor resection. If the bronchoscope is not held parallel to the airway wall there is a risk of airway perforation. The pressure of the barrel of the bronchoscope on the airway wall also helps to tamponade the lesion and reduce bleeding after resection [8]. The rigid bronchoscope can also be used to dilate narrowed portions of the airway without resecting endoluminal tumor. Rigid bronchoscopes of sequentially larger size may be passed through a stenotic portion of airway, producing progressive mechanical dilation. The disadvantage of this technique is that it does not allow for visualization of the mucosa during dilation and may cause more mucosal damage than sequential dilation with balloon catheters [8, 18, 19].

Balloon bronchoplasty is another technique used to treat bronchial obstruction due to extrinsic compression by tumor. In this technique, a flexible inflatable balloon catheter is introduced via either the flexible or rigid bronchoscope and inflated in order to dilate a narrowed segment of the airway. The tip of the balloon catheter should reach beyond the stenosis, and the catheter should be inflated to a diameter greater than that of the stenotic airway in order to achieve dilation. While balloon dilation alone is often enough to achieve an acceptable degree of improvement in airway stenosis due to external compression, many patients with compression due to malignancy also require stents to maintain airway patency after balloon dilation [20] (Figure 16.2a–c)

Airway stents have become an increasingly popular technique for palliating airway stenosis from malignant disease. The most popular types of stents currently in use are silicone stents and self-expanding metal stents (SEMS). Bronchoscopically placed silicone stents were first developed by Dumon and reported in 1990 [21]. Once they are deployed using a rigid bronchoscope, they are relatively easy to remove or adjust. In addition to the traditional straight cylinder, silicone stents can also be configured in a Y-shape to accommodate the trachea and bilateral mainstem bronchi [22]. Most types of silicone stent have studs lining the external wall in order to reduce the chance of migration [21]. Silicone stents can also be customized on-site to optimize their conformation to the patient's airways and allow successful treatment of more complex airway stenosis [23]. Disadvantages of silicone stents are that they may be difficult to deploy at times, are prone to migration, and do not conform well to tortuous airways [22]. Self-expandable metal stents are usually made from alloys such as nitinol (nickel and titanium) which are more elastic than steel while still providing sufficient radial force to resist extrinsic compression from tumor. Some SEMS are uncovered metal, and others are partially or completely coated with polyurethane. They are easier to deploy than silicone stents and can be placed during flexible bronchoscopy. SEMS are also less prone to migration than silicone stents. They cannot be customized on-site, however, and the woven metal design of uncovered SEMS can allow some tumors to grow through the stent wall and into the lumen. They are also more difficult to remove or adjust than silicone stents and more likely to erode through the airway wall [22]. Indications for airway stenting in patients with lung cancer are primarily to relieve airway obstruction and to seal airway fistulas. Stents are not effective for relieving obstruction due primarily to intraluminal tumor. They are best used for bronchial obstruction caused by extrinsic compression of the airway, with or without an associated intraluminal component. It also must be noted that stenting is ineffective in patients who do not have patent airway and viable normal lung distal to the bronchial stenosis. An area of lung that has been collapsed for a prolonged period of time may not recover even if stenting is performed [22]. Stenting can also be a successful palliative measure for patients with lung cancer who form fistulas from the tracheobronchial tree to the esophagus. Esophageal stents

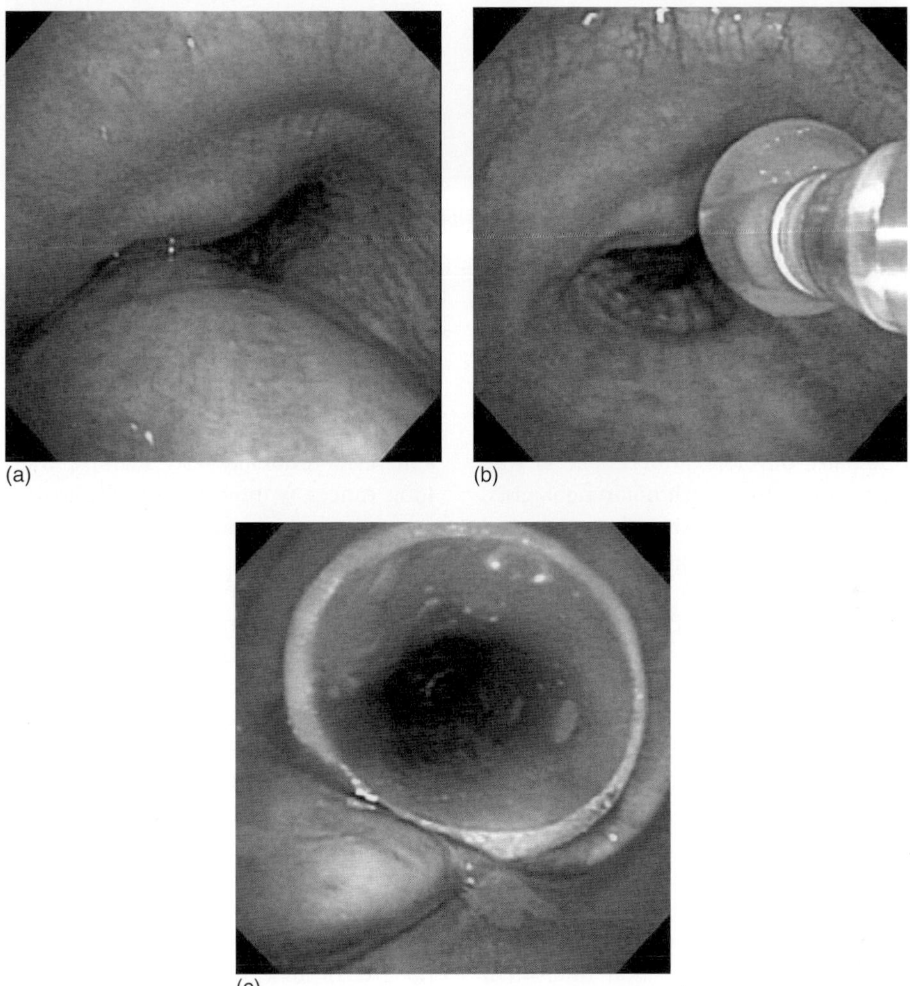

Figure 16.2 a: A 69-year-old female with adenoid cystic carcinoma presenting with severe dyspnea and tumor obstructing the lower trachea and bilateral mainstem bronchi. b: Sequential balloon dilation of the lower tracheal stricture. c: Restoration of airway patency after sequential balloon dilation and tracheobronchial silicone Y stent placement. (For a color version, see the color plate section.)

are more commonly used than airway stents for palliation of airway-esophageal fistulas, but they may erode into the bronchi (reopening the fistula) or compress the airway (resulting in dyspnea from obstruction) [24]. Double stenting with both airway and esophageal stents or initial treatments with an airway stent prior to placing an esophageal stent have been used in attempting to avoid these complications. Both silicone stents and SEMS have been used successfully for this purpose. It should be emphasized that stenting of bronchial fistulas is at best a palliative procedure for patients who cannot tolerate surgery, which remains the only potentially curative therapy [11, 12, 24, 25]. Once an airway stent has been placed follow up care is not standardized and based largely on local experience. Pulmonary toilet is of utmost importance, since airway stents impair natural mucociliary clearance. No single approach to this has been proven superior. Nebulized bronchodilators, nebulized hypertonic saline, and nebulized acetylcystine have all been reported [22]. Close scheduled clinical follow up is required for as long as the stent is in place, with bronchoscopy generally reserved for patients who have an increase in airway symptoms.

Microdebrider bronchoscopy is the newest mechanical method used for palliation of symptoms due to endobronchial lung cancer. It is a device consisting of a rotary blade enclosed in a hollow metal tube with integrated suction. The blade cuts at between 1000 and 5000 rpm and is controlled by a console and foot pedal. There is a single-side window allowing the blade access to the bronchial wall, and this can be rotated 360 degrees. Although originally developed for upper airway problems and used by otorhinolaryngologists, the newer microdebrider has since been adapted for use in the bronchi by lengthening the tube, allowing it to access the trachea and main bronchi through the rigid bronchoscope [26]. The blade can reach lesions in the trachea, mainstem bronchi, and bronchus intermedius. It is capable of very precise tissue debridement. The integrated suction removes blood and debris rapidly, allowing for an optimal field of view [27]. It is best used for resecting the intraluminal portion of tumors within the proximal airways, and samples obtained can be used for tissue diagnosis without the charring artifacts seen with thermal therapy. Its disadvantages are primarily its inability to reach distal lesions and the possibility of accidental resection of normal tissue [26]. It must also be used with caution in proximity to airway stents, which can be damaged by the cutting blade.

Thermal bronchoscopic interventions in lung cancer

Thermal bronchoscopic techniques are primarily used to palliate obstruction due to intraluminal central airway tumors and to treat hemoptysis arising from bleeding lesions in the central airways. Thermal therapies include laser, electrocautery, argon plasma coagulation, and cryotherapy.

Laser is an acronym for Light Amplified by Stimulated Emission of Radiation [8]. Atoms are stimulated to release photons in phase. The released light travels in the same plane and at the same wavelength. This may be converted into thermal energy, and this is the mechanism by which endobronchial laser therapy has its effect. This may result in cutting, coagulation, or vaporization of the targeted tissue [3]. Laser has long been used for endobronchial lesions causing obstruction or hemoptysis [28]. The neodynium:yttrium aluminum garnet (Nd:YAG) laser is most commonly used in bronchoscopy because it has sufficient power to vaporize tissue while retaining an excellent coagulation effect. Its wavelength is 1064 nanometers, and rigid and flexible probes are available. Endobronchial laser therapy in patients with lung cancer is indicated for the treatment of airway obstruction or hemoptysis arising from proximal lesions which have a significant intraluminal component [3]. The best results with endobronchial laser therapy are likely for exophytic lesions within the trachea or mainstem bronchi with a visible distal lumen in patients who are hemodynamically stable [19, 29]. Laser is less useful for lesions characterized by extrinsic compression within the upper lobe or segmental bronchi or who have a completely obstructed lumen [8, 28]. The optical fiber transmitting laser light is extended beyond the tip of the bronchoscope and a visible aiming laser is used to target the desired lesion. The fraction of inhaled oxygen (FiO2) must be kept at 0.4 or less to reduce the risk of airway fire. Aim should be parallel to the airway, and coagulation is typically followed by mechanical debridement [3]. Many small case studies have demonstrated the effectiveness of laser therapy for palliation of central airway obstruction in lung cancer, although a clear survival benefit has not been established [8, 29, 30]. Potential complications of laser therapy include bleeding, hypoxemia, perforation, airway fire, eye injury (for patients or medical staff who are required to wear protective eyewear during the procedure), and gas embolism [3, 18, 19, 28, 31].

Endobronchial electrocautery uses high frequency electrical current to generate heat. This enables a cautery probe to cut or coagulate tissue at the point of contact [32]. The tissue effect is affected by the voltage, the duration of contact, the area of contact, and the tissue density [32, 33]. Temperatures above 40 degrees centigrade lead to irreversible tissue injury, with coagulation coming between 70 and 100 degrees centigrade and carbonization and vaporization beginning at temperatures above 200 degrees centigrade [32]. Multiple electrocautery tools are available, including a blunt probe, a flat knife, cautery forceps, and a snare [34]. Endobronchial electrocautery is useful in debulking intraluminal tumors, snaring polypoid tumors, and treating hemoptysis [3, 32, 35]. It does require direct contact between the instrument and the tissue to be cauterized, and its use is limited to those airways that can be reached with the flexible bronchoscope. Endobronchial electrocautery is comparable to Nd:YAG laser in effectiveness for treating airway obstruction from endoluminal tumors at a somewhat reduced cost [34, 35]. The risks of electrocautery include bleeding, perforation, hypoxemia, pacemaker malfunction, and airway fire [3]. As with endobronchial laser therapy, the FiO2 should be kept at or below 0.4 to reduce the risk of airway fire. The patient must be grounded, and the use of monopolar electrocautery is not recommended for patients who have pacemakers or automated implanted cardioverter-defibrillators [32].

Argon plasma coagulation (APC) is a noncontact form of electrocautery which has become very popular for endobronchial use in recent years. Argon is ionized by an electric field, resulting in a homogenous monopolar current traveling from the probe to the tissue [32]. The current travels to the point of nearest contact, which may or may not be directly ahead of the probe. Side firing is possible with APC [3, 36]. The current is transformed into heat upon contact with the tissue, leading to superficial coagulation and fulguration to a depth of 5 millimeters or less [32, 36]. Once a certain depth of coagulation is achieved the current demonstrates a preference for superficial spreading rather than continued deeper penetration because the coagulated tissue has greater resistance. This characteristic reduces the risk of perforation during APC [36]. APC is used via a flexible probe introduced via the working channel of the bronchoscope. The patient must be grounded, and the FiO2 should be maintained at 0.4 or less to reduce the risk of airway fire. The probe is extended until the tip is around 1 centimeter from the end of the bronchoscope and held approximately 3–4 millimeters from the target. The tip of the probe should be closer to the target than to any other tissue, since the current will flow to the nearest point of contact. The application time is for 3–4 seconds. Applying continuous suction during coagulation will help clear airway smoke, reduce the risk of airway fire, and improve visualization of the airway [32,36]. APC has found its greatest use in treating hemoptysis from proximal endobronchial lesions. It is also used to coagulate and debulk intraluminal tumors, with or without adjunct mechanical debulking [32, 36]. Potential complications of APC include airway fire, perforation, bleeding, and gas embolism [37,38]. Complications are rare, however, and occur in fewer than 3% of all APC procedures [36, 37] (Figures 16.3a and b).

Cryotherapy is another endobronchial thermal technique that uses cold to destroy tissues via repeated cycles of freezing and thawing [9]. Rapid freezing followed by slow thawing results in the formation of both intracellular and extracellular ice crystals, leading to cellular damage and dehydration. This process also leads to local vascular damage, including vasoconstriction and increased capillary permeability. Delayed local thrombosis later leads to infarction of the treated tissues, resulting in nonhemorrhagic necrosis in 7–14 days [39]. The success of the resulting freeze injury is increased by rapid cooling, slow thawing, achieving a low tissue temperature of less than -40 degrees centigrade, and repeated freezing [39–41]. The effect of cryotherapy also depends on the type of tissue exposed. Tissues with higher water content tend to be more cryosensitive, and these include skin, mucosa, tumor, and granulation tissue. Conversely, tissues such as fat, cartilage, and connective tissue have lower water content and are relatively cryoresistant [39, 40]. Endobronchial cryotherapy is delivered via a flexible contact probe connected by a transfer line to a console containing a gas cylinder. The gas cools rapidly when it moves from high to low pressure – at the tip of the cryoprobe. Nitrous oxide is the most commonly used cooling agent in bronchoscopy [9, 41]. The safety of spray

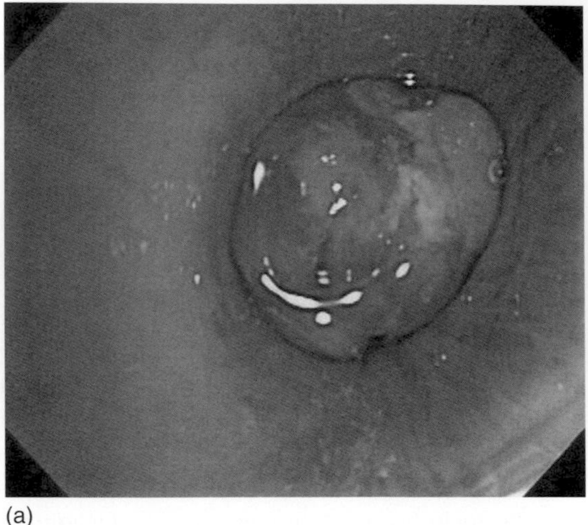

(a)

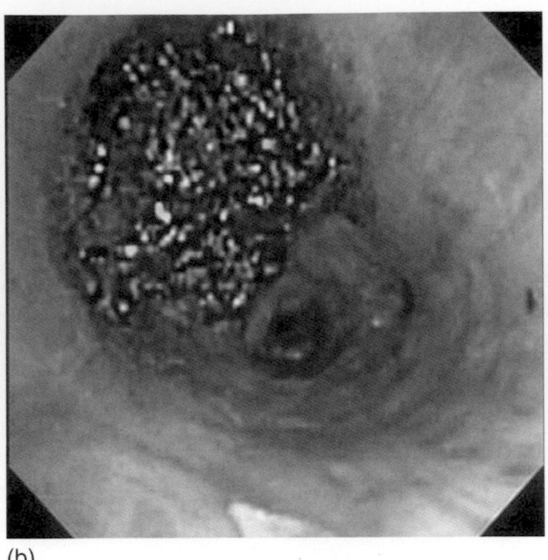

(b)

Figure 16.3 a: A 49-year-old female presenting with dyspnea and complete obstruction of the right bronchus intermedius from a right middle lobe adenocarcinoma. b: Complete recanalization of the right bronchus intermedius and right lower lobe following snare electrocautery and argon plasma coagulation of the endoluminal mass. (For a color version, see the color plate section.)

cryotherapy in the airways using liquid nitrogen has not been established and so its use cannot be recommended, and concerns about rapid expansion of the gas causing pneumothorax and cardiovascular complications have been raised. Once the lesion of interest is located bronchoscopically, the cryoprobe is advanced through the working channel of the bronchoscope until the tip is a safe distance beyond the end of the scope. The tip of the probe is then placed in contact with the target lesion and the coolant is activated. Approximately 30 seconds of freezing is followed by passive thawing. Until thawing is completed the probe will be frozen to the targeted tissue. Between 1 and 3 freeze-thaw cycles are completed under direct vision, and the operator then moves the probe to the next site, overlapping with the initial treated area so as to ensure the entire surface of the tumor is treated. Cryotherapy may be repeated if needed [9]. Endobronchial cryotherapy is used primarily to treat airway obstruction from intraluminal tumor. Although its necrotic effect is delayed, it can also be used to accomplish immediate "cryorecanalization" by freezing a portion of the obstructing lesion and then removing the probe before thawing can occur. The attached frozen portion of the treated tumor is removed along with the probe, resulting in rapid recanalization. This technique may result in bleeding, so the operator should be prepared to intervene if necessary [42]. Cryotherapy in lung cancer is primarily indicated for treating tumor obstruction of the tracheobronchial tree, either through its delayed effect or via "cryorecanalization" [9,42–45]. It has also demonstrated effectiveness as an adjunct to more established therapies for lung cancer with endobronchial involvement, particularly in conjunction with radiation therapy [45, 46]. One very small study of cryotherapy as monotherapy for early superficial proximal lung cancer demonstrated good local control at one year, but its use for this indication must still be regarded as experimental [47]. Cryotherapy is generally considered to be safer and less expensive than most other ablative endobronchial techniques, partly because there is no risk of airway fire (the patient may remain on 100% oxygen if necessary during the procedure) and partly because many of the normal surrounding tissues are relatively cryoresistant and unlikely to be damaged inadvertently. Complications are primarily limited to bleeding, reactive edema or sloughing of necrotic tissue, and very rare fistulas [42,46].

Nonthermal, nonmechanical bronchoscopic interventions in lung cancer

Photodynamic therapy and brachytherapy use nonmechanical and nonthermal mechanisms to treat and palliate lung cancer involving the airways. Both of these modalities are delivered bronchoscopically, and have shown effectiveness for both palliation and treatment in selected cases [9]. Both of these techniques have a delayed effect, and so should not be used for patients who need immediate palliation of central airway obstruction.

Photodynamic therapy (PDT) is based on damage to tissue arising from interactions between individually innocuous components. These include a photosensitizer, a light source, and oxygen [9, 48]. Light in a specific wavelength excites a photosensitive chemical found in tumor cells from its ground state to an excited state. The excited photosensitizer then interacts with tissue oxygen to form free radicals and singlet oxygen resulting in toxicity. Local effects include direct cellular damage to membranes and mitochondria, induction of apoptosis, local vascular injury, and a tumor-sensitized immune and inflammatory response [9, 48, 49]. An ideal photosensitizer should be selective for tumors, have a light absorption spectrum within a clinically useful range, and have a high yield of singlet oxygen [49]. Most commercially available photosensitizers are derived from hematoporphyrins. Porfimer sodium (Photofrin™, Axcan Pharma, Birmingham, AL) is the most commonly used photosensitizer in the United States. It is given as a slow injection of 2 milligrams/kilogram. Porfimer sodium is cleared from most normal tissues within 72 hours of administration, but it is retained in tumor cells, vascular endothelium, and skin for much longer. After a 48-hour latent period, the tumor is exposed to light at a wavelength of 630 nanometers, activating the compound. This produces tumor destruction to a depth of around 5–10 millimeters [9, 48, 49]. Photoactivation is accomplished by a nonthermal light source, most often a laser. Commonly used lasers for PDT are an argon pumped dye laser, a potassium-titanyl-phosphate (KTP) laser, and a diode laser. Light is delivered to the tumor by a fiber system advanced through the working channel of the bronchoscope. A diffuser at the tip of the fiber disseminates the light [9]. The approved light dose is 200 Joules/centimeter. This is typically reached with 8 to 12 minutes of light per fiber placement [9, 50]. PDT is indicated for palliation of advanced central lung cancer with existing or impending symptoms. It should only be used for treatment of tumors that have a predominantly intraluminal component because of its minimal depth of penetration. PDT is also indicated for the treatment of early stage central lung cancer for curative intent in patients who are not candidates for surgery or definitive radiotherapy and have sufficiently superficial tumor for PDT to treat them effectively [9, 50]. It is difficult to precisely assess the depth of tumor invasion using standard bronchoscopy or computed tomography alone. Radial probe endobronchial ultrasound (RP-EBUS) has been demonstrated to be very accurate for assessing the depth of invasion of endobronchial tumors [51]. Miyazu *et al.* evaluated the use of RP-EBUS as part of the pre-treatment evaluation of 18 patients who were thought to be good candidates for PDT. Half of the cohort were found to have invasion beyond the cartilaginous layer by RP-EBUS and therefore determined to be poor candidates for PDT, despite CT and standard bronchoscopy consistent with only superficial invasion [52]. It is therefore prudent to formally assess the depth of invasion of superficial endobronchial tumors with endobronchial ultrasound before beginning PDT to confirm their indication for this treatment. PDT should not be used for patients with impending life-threatening central airway obstruction because of its delayed effect. Treatment of tumors which are invading adjacent vascular structures or hypersensitivity to porphyrins are other contraindications to PDT [50]. Once an appropriate central superficial lesion is identified, the photosensitizer is injected. After the latent period, a bronchoscopy is performed and the lesion to be treated is visualized. The light fiber is advanced into the airway via the working channel and the diffuser at the tip of the fiber is embedded in the tumor. Light is applied for 8–12 minutes, and the catheter is removed. A repeat bronchoscopy is recommended in 24–48 hours in order to remove necrotic debris. Repeat illumination may also be performed at that time if viable residual tumor is seen [9, 50]. Most of the evidence assessing the effectiveness of PDT for palliation of central airway obstruction in lung cancer is in the form of observational case series. In these limited studies PDT is effective at reducing the observed degree of endoluminal obstruction while also reducing symptoms of dyspnea [9, 50, 53–55]. When used for curative intent in patients with early stage central lung cancer who were not candidates for surgery PDT has shown rates of complete local control ranging from 44% to 100% in mostly small studies [52, 56–60]. The most common complication of PDT is photosensitivity. Others include cough, delayed bleeding from the treated tumor, chest discomfort, and airway compromise from edema and necrotic secretions [50].

Endobronchial brachytherapy uses a radiation source placed very close to the targeted tumor to provide local radiation treatment with less toxicity to surrounding tissues. The radiation source is placed within the bronchus, and gamma rays are the primary type of radiation used to damage the tumor cells. The inverse square law states that the dose rate of radiation decreases as a function of the inverse square of the distance to the center of the source: this allows a high radiation dose near the center of the source with a rapid decrease in dose further away. The radiation emitted during brachytherapy does not directly kill the cancer cells. Rather, it damages their DNA leading to apoptosis and decreased cellular proliferation. The effect is delayed, and reaches its maximum at 3 to 4 weeks after treatment. One of the advantages endobronchial brachytherapy offers over PDT is its longer effect and deeper penetration – brachytherapy can destroy tissue beyond cartilage [9]. Early attempts at brachytherapy were limited by the effects of radiation exposure on the medical personnel handling the radiation source. Introduction of automated remote afterloaders increased the safety of endobronchial brachytherapy for medical personnel and have led to increases in its use [61, 62]. Endobronchial brachytherapy is typically given at a high dose rate, meaning greater than 12 Gy/hour but more often greater than 100 Gy/hour. The source used is most often iridium-192. Using high dose rate brachytherapy allows for a short treatment time, enabling outpatient therapy. Treatment is usually divided into between 2 and 4 fractions of 5 to 15 Gy each [9,62,63]. Brachytherapy is indicated for the palliation of symptoms related to malignant endobronchial lesions (including airway obstruction, hemoptysis, and cough) in patients who are not candidates for external beam radiation and as an adjunct to surgery or external beam radiation for both cure and palliation. Brachytherapy is also used as a potentially curative therapy for patients with early stage lung cancer in the central airways within reach of the bronchoscope who are not candidates for surgery or external beam radiation [9]. Before brachytherapy can be administered the endobronchial afterloading catheter must be positioned bronchoscopically. Once the operator has localized the tumor, the afterloading catheter is placed within the airway with the distal tip at least 3 centimeters beyond the tumor and then secured to the nose with tape. Dummy wires are introduced in order to confirm the location with fluoroscopy, and the desired irradiation length may also be marked using external tags secured to the skin. Then the patient is transported to the radiation therapy suite, where a dummy seed is inserted into the afterloading catheter and correct placement is confirmed by X-ray. After the dummy seed is removed, the applicator is connected to the radiation source and advanced to the proper position under computer control. It remains in each position long enough to apply the prescribed dose and is then withdrawn at 5 millimeter intervals. Catheters are then removed after treatment [9]. Brachytherapy is effective at palliating symptoms in patients with predominantly endoluminal central airway obstruction. Several studies have shown symptomatic improvement in 65–85% of patients with predominantly endoluminal disease, and one study demonstrated successful palliation requiring no further treatment in 67% of a large 324 patient cohort [63–66]. Brachytherapy may also augment the effect of external beam radiation when used in patients with obstructing tumors in the main bronchi [67]. When used for curative intent the results are less promising, with 2-year survival ranging from 58% to 78% [6,68,69]. Complications of brachytherapy are common and include hemoptysis, bronchial stenosis, bronchomalacia, and fistula formation. Hemoptysis is the most feared complication of brachytherapy, with incidence of between 10% and 50%. Fatal massive hemoptysis is reported in 0–8% of patients treated with brachytherapy [9, 66, 70]. Because brachytherapy is often used to palliate hemoptysis it is difficult to determine how much is due to the treatment and how much to the underlying malignancy. Clinicians should remain vigilant for hemoptysis in patients who have received brachytherapy.

Conclusion

Bronchoscopic interventions are important adjuncts for the palliation of symptoms due to central airway involvement in patients with lung cancer. They are most effective for proximal central airway obstruction and hemoptysis. The choice of which intervention is most appropriate is based on the nature and location of the lesion, the type of symptoms encountered, and the locally available equipment and expertise. Photodynamic therapy and endobronchial brachytherapy are also indicated for treatment with curative intent for early stage superficial lung cancers of the central airways, but only in patients who are unable to tolerate standard treatment. It should be emphasized that all of these techniques augment but do not replace standard treatments such as surgery, chemotherapy, and radiation therapy.

References

1 Siegel R, Naishadham D, Jemal A (2013) Cancer statistics, 2013. *CA Cancer J Clin*, Jan; 63(1): 11–30.

2 Numico G, Russi E, Merlano M (2001) Best supportive care in non-small cell lung cancer: Is there a role for radiotherapy and chemotherapy? *Lung Cancer*, Jun; 32(3): 213–26.

3 Bolliger CT, Sutedja TG, Strausz J, Freitag L (2006) Therapeutic bronchoscopy with immediate effect: Laser, electrocautery, argon plasma coagulation and stents. *Eur Respir J*, Jun; 27(6): 1258–71.

4 Hirshberg B, Biran I, Glazer M, Kramer MR (1997) Hemoptysis: etiology, evaluation, and outcome in a tertiary referral hospital. *Chest*, Aug; 112(2): 440–4.

5 Schreiber J, Waldburg N (2012) Bronchoesophageal fistula and fatal hemoptysis after bevacizumab-containing chemotherapy without radiation in lung cancer. *J Clin Oncol*, Nov 10; 30(32): e324.

6 Perol M, Caliandro R, Pommier P, Malet C, Montbarbon X, Carrie C, *et al.* (1997) Curative irradiation of limited endobronchial carcinomas with high-dose rate brachytherapy. Results of a pilot study. *Chest*, May; 111(5): 1417–23.

7 Simone CB, 2nd, Friedberg JS, Glatstein E, Stevenson JP, Sterman DH, Hahn SM, *et al.* (2012) Photodynamic therapy for the treatment of non-small cell lung cancer. *J Thorac Dis*, Feb; 4(1): 63–75.

8 Ernst A, Feller-Kopman D, Becker HD, Mehta AC (2004) Central airway obstruction. *Am J Respir Crit Care Med*, Jun 15; 169(12): 1278–97.

9 Vergnon JM, Huber RM, Moghissi K (2006) Place of cryotherapy, brachytherapy and photodynamic therapy in therapeutic bronchoscopy of lung cancers. *Eur Respir J*, Jul; 28(1): 200–18.

10 Burt M, Diehl W, Martini N, Bains MS, Ginsberg RJ, McCormack PM, *et al.* (1991) Malignant esophagorespiratory fistula: management options and survival. *Ann Thorac Surg*, Dec; 52(6): 1222–8; discussion 8–9.

11 Freitag L, Tekolf E, Steveling H, Donovan TJ, Stamatis G (1996) Management of malignant esophagotracheal fistulas with airway stenting and double stenting. *Chest*, Nov; 110(5): 1155–60.

12 Herth FJ, Peter S, Baty F, Eberhardt R, Leuppi JD, Chhajed PN (2010) Combined airway and oesophageal stenting in malignant airway-oesophageal fistulas: a prospective study. *Eur Respir J*, Dec; 36(6): 1370–4.

13 Cahill BC, Ingbar DH (1994) Massive hemoptysis. Assessment and management. *Clin Chest Med, Mar*; 15(1): 147–67.

14 Ibrahim WH (2008) Massive haemoptysis: the definition should be revised. *Eur Respir J*, Oct; 32(4): 1131–2.

15 Set PAK, Flower CDR, Smith IE, Cahn AP, Twentyman OP, Shneerson JM (1993) Hemoptysis – comparative-study of the role of Ct and fiberoptic bronchoscopy. *Radiology*, Dec; 189(3): 677–80.

16 Poe RH, Israel RH, Marin MG, Ortiz CR, Dale RC, Wahl GW, *et al.* (1988) Utility of fiberoptic bronchoscopy in patients with hemoptysis and a nonlocalizing chest roentgenogram. *Chest*, Jan; 93(1): 70–5.

17 McWilliams A, Lam B, Sutedja T (2009) Early proximal lung cancer diagnosis and treatment. *Eur Respir J*, Mar; 33(3): 656–65.

18 Bolliger CT, Mathur PN, Beamis JF, Becker HD, Cavaliere S, Colt H, *et al.* (2002) ERS/ATS statement on interventional pulmonology. European Respiratory Society/American Thoracic Society. *Eur Respir J*, Feb; 19(2): 356–73.

19 Ernst A, Silvestri GA, Johnstone D (2003) Interventional pulmonary procedures: Guidelines from the American College of Chest Physicians. *Chest*, May; 123(5): 1693–1717.

20 Hautmann H, Gamarra F, Pfeifer KJ, Huber RM (2001) Fiberoptic bronchoscopic balloon dilatation in malignant tracheobronchial disease: indications and results. *Chest*, Jul; 120(1): 43–9.

21 Dumon JF (1990) A dedicated tracheobronchial stent. *Chest*, Feb; 97(2): 328–32.

22 Casal RF (2010) Update in airway stents. *Current Opinion in Pulmonary Medicine*, July; 16: 321–8.

23 Breen DP, Dutau H (2009) On-site customization of silicone stents: Towards optimal palliation of complex airway conditions. *Respiration*, 77(4): 447–53.

24 Oida T, Mimatsu K, Kano H, Kawasaki A, Kuboi Y, Fukino N, *et al.* (2011) Double stents: airway stenting after esophageal-stent implantation for esophageal cancer. *Hepatogastroenterology*, Nov–Dec; 58(112): 1985–8.

25 Kim KR, Shin JH, Song HY, Ko GY, Kim JH, Yoon HK, *et al.* (2009) Palliative treatment of malignant esophagopulmonary fistulas with covered expandable metallic stents. *AJR Am J Roentgenol*, Oct; 193(4): W278–82.

26 Lunn W, Garland R, Ashiku S, Thurer RL, Feller-Kopman D, Ernst A (2005) Microdebrider bronchoscopy: A new tool for the interventional bronchoscopist. *Ann Thorac Surg*, Oct; 80(4): 1485–8.

27 Melendez J, Cornwell L, Green L, Casal RF (2012) Treatment of large subglottic tracheal schwannoma with microdebrider bronchoscopy. *J Thorac Cardiovasc Surg*, Aug; 144(2): 510–12.

28 Dumon JF, Shapshay S, Bourcereau J, Cavaliere S, Meric B, Garbi N, *et al.* (1984) Principles for safety in application of neodymium – YAG laser in bronchology. *Chest*, Aug; 86(2): 163–8.

29 Desai SJ, Mehta AC, VanderBrug Medendorp S, Golish JA, Ahmad M (1988) Survival experience following Nd:YAG laser photoresection for primary bronchogenic carcinoma. *Chest*, Nov; 94(5): 939–44.

30 Ross DJ, Mohsenifar Z, Koerner SK (1990) Survival characteristics after neodymium: YAG laser photoresection in advanced stage lung cancer. *Chest*, Sep; 98(3): 581–5.

31 Tellides G, Ugurlu BS, Kim RW, Hammond GL (1998) Pathogenesis of systemic air embolism during bronchoscopic Nd:YAG laser operations. *Ann Thorac Surg*, Apr; 65(4): 930–4.

32 Sheski FD, Mathur PN (2004) Endobronchial electrosurgery: Argon plasma coagulation and electrocautery. *Semin Respir Crit Care Med*, Aug; 25(4): 367–74.

33 van Boxem TJ, Venmans BJ, Schramel FM, van Mourik JC, Golding RP, Postmus PE, *et al.* (1998) Radiographically occult lung cancer treated with fibreoptic bronchoscopic electrocautery: A pilot study of a simple and inexpensive technique. *Eur Respir J*, Jan; 11(1): 169–72.

34 Coulter TD, Mehta AC (2000) The heat is on: Impact of endobronchial electrosurgery on the need for Nd-YAG laser photoresection. *Chest*, Aug; 118(2): 516–21.

35 Boxem T, Muller M, Venmans B, Postmus P, Sutedja T. Nd-YAG laser vs bronchoscopic electrocautery for palliation of symptomatic airway obstruction: A cost-effectiveness study. *Chest*, Oct; 116(4): 1108–12.

36 Morice RC, Ece T, Ece F, Keus L (2001) Endobronchial argon plasma coagulation for treatment of hemoptysis and neoplastic airway obstruction. *Chest*, Mar; 119(3): 781–7.

37 Reichle G, Freitag L, Kullmann HJ, Prenzel R, Macha HN, Farin G. (2000) Argon plasma coagulation in bronchology: a new method-alternative or complementary? *Pneumologie*, Nov; 54(11): 508–16.

38 Reddy C, Majid A, Michaud G, Feller-Kopman D, Eberhardt R, Herth F, *et al.* (2008) Gas embolism following bronchoscopic argon plasma coagulation: A case series. *Chest*, Nov; 134(5): 1066–9.

39 Theodorescu D (2004) Cancer cryotherapy: Evolution and biology. *Rev Urol*, 6(Suppl 4): S9–S19.

40 Gage AA, Baust J (1998) Mechanisms of tissue injury in cryosurgery. *Cryobiology*, Nov; 37(3): 171–86.

41 Gage AA, Guest K, Montes M, Caruana JA, Whalen DA, Jr (1985) Effect of varying freezing and thawing rates in experimental cryosurgery. *Cryobiology*, Apr; 22(2): 175–82.

42 Hetzel M, Hetzel J, Schumann C, Marx N, Babiak A (2004) Cryorecanalization: A new approach for the immediate management of acute airway obstruction. *J Thorac Cardiovasc Surg*, May; 127(5): 1427–31.

43 Walsh DA, Maiwand MO, Nath AR, Lockwood P, Lloyd MH, Saab M (1990) Bronchoscopic cryotherapy for advanced bronchial carcinoma. *Thorax*, Jul; 45(7): 509–13.

44 Mathur PN, Wolf KM, Busk MF, Briete WM, Datzman M (1996) Fiberoptic bronchoscopic cryotherapy

in the management of tracheobronchial obstruction. *Chest*, Sep; 110(3): 718–23.

45 Asimakopoulos G, Beeson J, Evans J, Maiwand MO (2005) Cryosurgery for malignant endobronchial tumors: analysis of outcome. *Chest*, Jun; 127(6): 2007–14.

46 Vergnon JM, Schmitt T, Alamartine E, Barthelemy JC, Fournel P, Emonot A (1992) Initial combined cryotherapy and irradiation for unresectable non-small cell lung cancer. Preliminary results. *Chest*, Nov; 102(5): 1436–40.

47 Deygas N, Froudarakis M, Ozenne G, Vergnon JM (2001) Cryotherapy in early superficial bronchogenic carcinoma. *Chest*, Jul; 120(1): 26–31.

48 Dolmans DE, Fukumura D, Jain RK (2003) Photodynamic therapy for cancer. *Nat Rev Cancer*, May; 3(5): 380–7.

49 Pass HI (1993) Photodynamic therapy in oncology: Mechanisms and clinical use. *J Natl Cancer Inst*, Mar 17; 85(6): 443–56.

50 Loewen GM, Pandey R, Bellnier D, Henderson B, Dougherty T (2006) Endobronchial photodynamic therapy for lung cancer. *Lasers Surg Med*, Jun; 38(5): 364–70.

51 Kurimoto N, Murayama M, Yoshioka S, Nishisaka T, Inai K, Dohi K (1999) Assessment of usefulness of endobronchial ultrasonography in determination of depth of tracheobronchial tumor invasion. *Chest*, Jun; 115(6): 1500–6.

52 Miyazu Y, Miyazawa T, Kurimoto N, Iwamoto Y, Kanoh K, Kohno N (2002) Endobronchial ultrasonography in the assessment of centrally located early-stage lung cancer before photodynamic therapy. *Am J Respir Crit Care Med*, Mar 15; 165(6): 832–7.

53 Furukawa K, Okunaka T, Yamamoto H, Tsuchida T, Usuda J, Kumasaka H, *et al.* (1999) Effectiveness of photodynamic therapy and Nd-YAG laser treatment for obstructed tracheobronchial malignancies. *Diagn Ther Endosc*, 5(3): 161–6.

54 Moghissi K, Dixon K, Stringer M, Freeman T, Thorpe A, Brown S (1999) The place of bronchoscopic photodynamic therapy in advanced unresectable lung cancer: experience of 100 cases. *Eur J Cardiothorac Surg*, Jan; 15(1): 1–6.

55 Minnich DJ, Bryant AS, Dooley A, Cerfolio RJ (2010) Photodynamic laser therapy for lesions in the airway. *Ann Thorac Surg*, Jun; 89(6): 1744–8; discussion 8–9.

56 Furuse K, Fukuoka M, Kato H, Horai T, Kubota K, Kodama N, *et al.* (1993) A prospective phase II study on photodynamic therapy with photofrin II for centrally located early-stage lung cancer. The Japan Lung Cancer Photodynamic Therapy Study Group. *J Clin Oncol*, Oct; 11(10): 1852–7.

57 Kato H (1998) Photodynamic therapy for lung cancer-a review of 19 years' experience. *J Photochem Photobiol B*, Feb; 42(2): 96–9.

58 Cortese DA, Edell ES, Kinsey JH (1997) Photodynamic therapy for early stage squamous cell carcinoma of the lung. *Mayo Clin Proc*, Jul; 72(7): 595–602.

59 Hayata Y, Kato H, Furuse K, Kusunoki Y, Suzuki M, Mimura S (1996) Photodynamic therapy of 168 early stage cancers of the lung and oesophagus: A Japanese multi-centre study. *Lasers in Medical Science*, 11: 255–9.

60 McCaughan JS, Jr., Williams TE (1997) Photodynamic therapy for endobronchial malignant disease: A prospective fourteen-year study. *J Thorac Cardiovasc Surg*, Dec; 114(6): 940–6; discussion 6–7.

61 Henschke UK, Hilaris BS, Mahan GD (1964) Remote afterloading with intracavitary applicators. *Radiology*, Aug; 83: 344–5.

62 Ung YC, Yu E, Falkson C, Haynes AE, Stys-Norman D, Evans WK (2006) The role of high-dose-rate brachytherapy in the palliation of symptoms in patients with non-small-cell lung cancer: A systematic review. *Brachytherapy*, Jul–Sep; 5(3): 189–202.

63 Kelly JF, Delclos ME, Morice RC, Huaringa A, Allen PK, Komaki R (2000) High-dose-rate endobronchial brachytherapy effectively palliates symptoms due to airway tumors: The 10-year M. D. Anderson cancer center experience. *Int J Radiat Oncol Biol Phys*, Oct 1; 48(3): 697–702.

64 Escobar-Sacristan JA, Granda-Orive JI, Gutierrez Jimenez T, Delgado JM, Rodero Banos A, Saez Valls R (2004) Endobronchial brachytherapy in the treatment of malignant lung tumours. *Eur Respir J*, Sep; 24(3): 348–52.

65 Paradelo JC, Waxman MJ, Throne BJ, Beller TA, Kopecky WJ (1992) Endobronchial irradiation with 192Ir in the treatment of malignant endobronchial obstruction. *Chest*, Oct; 102(4): 1072–4.

66 Gollins SW, Burt PA, Barber PV, Stout R (1994) High dose rate intraluminal radiotherapy for carcinoma of the bronchus: Outcome of treatment of 406 patients. *Radiother Oncol*, Oct; 33(1): 31–40.

67 Langendijk H, de Jong J, Tjwa M, Muller M, ten Velde G, Aaronson N, *et al.* (2001) External irradiation versus external irradiation plus endobronchial brachytherapy in inoperable non-small cell lung cancer: A prospective randomized study. *Radiother Oncol*, Mar; 58(3): 257–68.

68 Aumont-le Guilcher M, Prevost B, Sunyach MP, Peiffert D, Maingon P, Thomas L, *et al.* (2011) High-dose-rate brachytherapy for non-small-cell lung carcinoma: A retrospective study of 226 patients. *Int J Radiat Oncol Biol Phys*, Mar 15; 79(4): 1112–6.
69 Marsiglia H, Baldeyrou P, Lartigau E, Briot E, Haie-Meder C, Le Chevalier T, *et al.* (2000) High-dose-rate brachytherapy as sole modality for early-stage endobronchial carcinoma. *Int J Radiat Oncol Biol Phys*, Jun 1; 47(3): 665–72.
70 Speiser BL (1999) Brachytherapy in the treatment of thoracic tumors. Lung and esophageal. *Hematol Oncol Clin North Am*, Jun; 13(3): 609–34.

CHAPTER 17
Primary Tracheal Tumors

Francesco Sammartino[1] *and Paolo Macchiarini*[2]
[1]Department of General and Mininvasive Surgery, San Giovanni di Dio Hospital, Orbetello, Italy
[2]Division Ear, Nose and Throat (CLINTEC), Karolinska University Hospital, Stockholm, Sweden

Epidemiology

Due to their rare incidence, few epidemiological studies have reported on primary tracheal tumors. Primary tracheal tumors represent about 2% of upper airway tumors and 0.1–0.4% of all malignant diseases. Tracheal tumors occur at a rate of 2.7 new cases per 1 000 000 people per year and 8% of these cases represent tumors in children [1, 2]. In adults, 90% of primary tracheal tumors are malignant in contrast to 30% in children [3, 4].

Anatomy and physiology

To appreciate the difficulties associated with tracheal surgery, it is mandatory to understand the anatomy and physiology of the upper respiratory tract. The trachea in adults measures approximately 11–12 cm from the cricoid cartilage to the superior edge of the carina. The distal two-thirds are positioned within the thorax, whereas the proximal third is found in the extrathoracic region of the neck. Its full length is composed of 18–22 C-shaped cartilage rings, with almost two rings per cm [5]. The trachea measures about 1.5–2.5 cm in diameter, which allows air to pass without turbulence or associated noise. The posterior wall of the trachea consists of a membranous portion with the embedded trachealis muscle, which connects both ends of the cartilage rings and the intercartilagenous spaces via a longitudinal and transverse layer of smooth muscle. The internal lumen of the trachea is covered by specialized tracheal mucosa composed of ciliated pseudo-stratified columnar epithelium. Underlying the respiratory epithelium, a network of longitudinal elastic fibers, blood vessels, lymphoid tissue, nerves and mucous glands is found.

At a glance, the trachea seems to be a simple conduit for passing air, but a closer look reveals it has many functions. Due to its position in the neck, its lateral rigidity and longitudinal flexibility permit movement and esophageal distention during swallowing. It is flexible enough to allow movement, but strong enough to avoid collapse during positive and negative pressure cycles of respiration. Its exposure to ambient air containing dust particles and harmful organisms require the trachea to perform a clearing function and possess immunocompetence. This is accomplished by mucous glands in the trachea and bronchi which produce a viscous mucous to trap bacteria and foreign particles. They are then transported toward the pharynx via the ciliary apparatus and by coughing (*clearance*).

Vascularization of the trachea is supplied by a delicate network of fine vessels, which is more pronounced (mostly right) in children than in adults [6]. Branches of the inferior thyroid artery supply the majority upper half of the tracheal lateral longitudinal vessels, whereas bronchial arteries from the aorta supply the lower part of the trachea and carina.

Lung Cancer, Fourth Edition. Edited by Jack A. Roth, Waun Ki Hong and Ritsuko U. Komaki.

Structures surrounding the trachea require special attention during surgical interventions. Bilateral recurrent laryngeal nerves, which innervate the inner muscles of the larynx, course down each side of the trachea. Along the posterior wall, the esophagus is directly connected and provides a fine vascular network to the trachea. The upper anterior portion is covered by the thyroid gland and has a close proximity to bilateral carotid arteries. The lower portion of the trachea is initially intersected by the brachiocephalic artery (synonym: innominate artery) and then by the left brachiocephalic vein. The aortic arch, superior vena cava and pulmonary artery cross anteriorly over the distal third of the trachea [3].

Lymph nodes are found pretracheal, paratracheal and subcarinal. Pathways of lymph drainage of nodes are similar to those found for bronchial carcinomas, which usually drain to the nodes nearest to the tumor [7].

Table 17.1 Signs and symptoms

– Wheezing
– Stridor
– Dyspnea
– Hoarseness
– Change in voice
– Hemoptysis
– Dysphagia
– Pneumonia

Symptoms

Most patients with primary malignant tracheal tumors present with advanced or inoperable disease, due to the difficulty in its diagnosis. Benign and malignant tracheal tumors often cause the same signs and symptoms initially – a dry cough and irritation of the throat are common. As the lesion grows within the tracheal lumen, wheezing or stridor may arise, which is often mistaken for asthma. Signs and symptoms vary with the type, but not with the site of the tumor [9, 10]. Squamous cell carcinoma can cause startling hemoptysis which usually leads to an early diagnosis [11]. Less than 25% of patients with adenoid-cystic carcinoma have hemoptysis during their clinical course [2, 8]. Dysphagia, hoarseness and change in voice are signs of advanced disease but do not preclude resectability. The nonspecificity of these symptoms leads to a prolonged period between symptom onset and eventual diagnosis (up to 18 months), at which time most patients are already in a late stage of disease. By contrast, squamous cell carcinoma has a mean duration of symptoms before diagnosis of only 4 months. Adenoid cystic carcinoma is detected by symptoms of wheezing or stridor, but dyspnea is a more prominent symptom. Dysphagia, hoarseness and change in voice may occur due to direct invasion and involvement of the esophagus and recurrent laryngeal nerve.

A delay in diagnosis can also be attributed to the functional reserve of the tracheal lumen, as a tumor does not cause symptoms until it occludes around 50–70% of the luminal diameter. Wheezing often erroneous diagnoses of asthma, leads to chronic obstructive pulmonary disease or bronchitis first.

Recurrent unilateral or bilateral pneumonitis may occur in patients who initially respond to antibiotic treatment. A summary of symptoms for primary tracheal cancers are summarized in Table 17.1.

Diagnosis and staging

Bronchoscopy is the most important and commonly used diagnostic tool. It is a fast and simple way to obtain crucial information such as trachea and tumor dimension and location for surgical resection planning as well as a means to obtain biopsies for tumor identification (Figure 17.1). *Fluorescence bronchoscopy* is an evaluation which differentiates normal (fluorescent green) and abnormal (brown and red in color) mucosal areas. The absence of auto-fluorescence occurs in dysplasia, carcinoma *in situ* and invasive carcinoma, and may enable earlier detection of endobronchial tumors.

Endotracheal ultrasonography (EU) involves either a radial probe covered in a water-filled balloon which

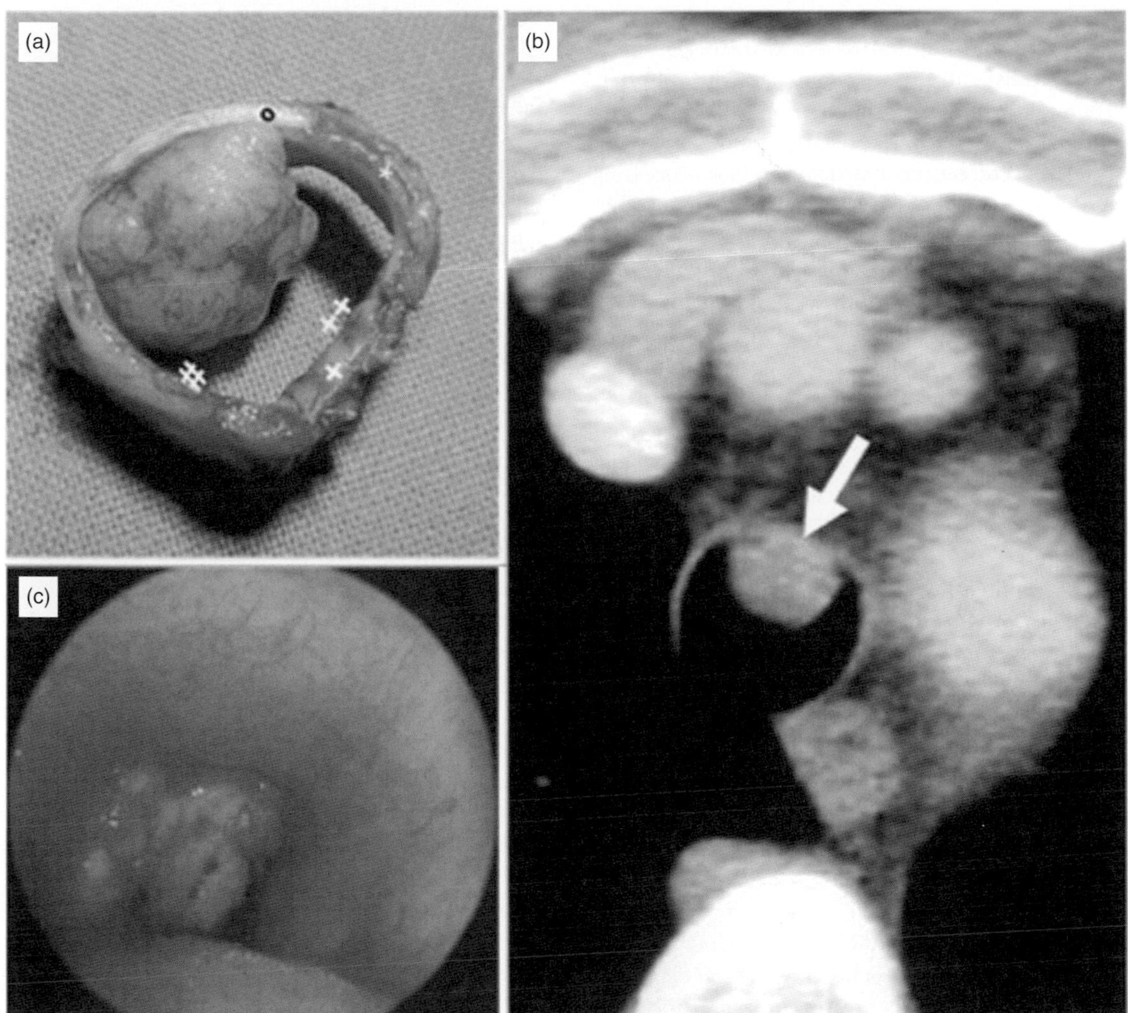

Figure 17.1 a: Cross section of a tracheal tumor. * = submucosa, # = mucosa, ∘ = c-shaped cartilage ring, + = membranosus part, ++ = trachealis muscle. b: CT-scan showing a well-defined tracheal tumor at the anterior wall of the trachea. white arrow indicating tracheal tumor. c: Bronchoscopic view on an intraluminal tracheal tumor with high grade luminal occlusion.

provides a 360° view of the structures beyond the tracheal and bronchial wall or a linear probe which provides a longitudinal view of structures within the wall and outside the trachea for a distance up to 4–5 cm. EU reveals the laminar structure of the tracheal wall and accurately predicts carcinoma invasion. A systematic mediastinal evaluation is also imperative in patients with tracheal tumors and EU provides valuable information about mediastinal and hilar node involvement. Each lymph node is sampled 1–3 times if cytology is positive for malignancy and 3 times if cytology is benign or nondiagnostic. Sampling more than 3 times usually does not ensure a reliable pathologic diagnosis [12]. *New integrated bronchoscopes*, with a linear-array ultrasound probe, allow excellent evaluation of mediastinal nodes down to 5 mm in size, and enable needle aspiration under image guidance.

Computertomographic (CT)-scan (spiral or helical) is the most useful method to assess tracheal tumors radiologically, since it can rapidly acquire volumetric data of the entire thorax in a single breath-hold, minimizing respiratory and cardiac motion artifact. These data can be reconstructed by postprocessing techniques allowing the trachea to be visualized in the axial plane. Axial images allow assessment of the size and shape of the trachea and measurement of the tracheal wall thickness. Adjacent tracheal structures and the presence of extrinsic compression are clearly delineated, especially following intravenous contrast enhancement.

Coronal and sagittal oblique multiplanar reformats (MPRs) can accurately determine the location (distance from vocal cords and carina) and length of a tracheal lesion, its relation to anatomic landmarks, the degree of luminal narrowing, and the extraluminal component of abnormal tissue growth. It can also detect multifocal lesions and prevent unnecessary surgery in one-third of patients at the time of diagnosis. The surgical planning of tracheal tumors and post therapeutic assessment is improved with two- and three- dimensional techniques, which allow creation of an external ("CT bronchography") and internal ("Virtual bronchoscopy") rendered CT-scan [13, 14]. Development of new aerosolized contrast agents or spectroscopic techniques, which can discriminate between benign and malignant mucosal tissues, might enhance the sensitivity and specificity of virtual bronchoscopy for the detection of preinvasive cancers within the respiratory tract. *Dynamic CT* imaging can be performed during inspiration and expiration to detect changes in tracheal diameter in patients with tracheomalacia [15, 16].

Magnetic resonance imaging (MRI) is used in the assessment of pediatric patients who often have vascular anomalies that cause tracheal narrowing and in whom radiation dose is a concern [17]. *Integrated F-FDG PET/CT imaging* allows evaluation of both the metabolic activity of a tumor, its anatomic extent and possible recurrence after treatment, but has not been extensively studied with tracheal tumors [18]. *Conventional chest radiograph* delays the definitive diagnosis of disease because it is often normal and tumors can be easily missed, making radiographs less helpful when following tracheal tumors.

Tumor pathology and classification

Primary tracheal tumors in adult and in children are malignant in 90% and 30% of cases, respectively [3, 4, 19], and originate either from the respiratory epithelium (epithelial origin), salivary glands (adenoid origin) or mesenchymal structures (mesenchymal origin). Squamous cell carcinoma and adenoid cystic carcinoma compose about two-thirds of adult primary tracheal tumors and occur in the same proportion. The remaining third is made up of a wide variety of tumors of other histology, most often benign, or of low-grade malignancy such as hemangiomas, leiomyomas and others. A complete list of all primary tracheal tumors can be found in Table 17.2.

Metastatic spread to the trachea rarely occurs through hematogenous spread from melanoma, renal cell carcinoma, breast and colon cancer. Hematogenous spread from tracheal tumors to other sites is also a rare event due to its unique vascular supply, but is mostly found in squamous cell carcinoma.

Squamous cell carcinoma has a behavior, etiology, curability, and associated aerodigestive carcinoma, similar to squamous lung cancer. It affects more men than women (3 male: 1 female ratio), mainly in their sixth and seventh decades, and is mostly associated with habitual cigarette smoking. It can be either exophitic or ulcerative, and multiple and scattered over a considerable length of trachea. The progression is rapid and about a third of patients have either mediastinal or pulmonary metastases at diagnosis. On CT-scan it typically appears as a polyploidy, focal sessile lesion, a mass causing eccentric narrowing of the lumen, or circumferential wall thickening.

In contrast, *adenoid cystic carcinoma* has the same incidence in men and women and it is most common in patients between 20 and 69 years old with a slight peak in the fifth decade. Its progress is very slow and the clinical symptoms have prolonged courses, sometimes for years. It may extend over a long distance by perineural and submucosal planes and only 10% of patients develop regional lymph node or remote metastases. The prolonged course

Table 17.2 List of primary tracheal tumors

Epithelial origin	benign	Papilloma Papillomatosis
	malignant	Squamous carcinoma in situ Squamous-cell carcinoma Adenocarcinoma Large-cell undifferentiated carcinoma *Neuroendocrine tumors:* Typical and atypical carcinoids Large-cell neuroendocrine tumor Small cell carcinoma
Adenoid origin	benign	Pleiomorphic adenoma Mucous-gland adenoma Myoepithelioma Oncocytoma Other
	malignant	Mucoepidermoid carcinoma Adenoid cystic carcinoma Carcinoma ex pleiomorphic adenoma
Mesenchymal origin	benign	Fibroma Fibromatosis Benign fibrous histiocytoma Hemangioma Hemangioperycitoma Paraganglioma (chemodectoma) Glomus tumor Lipoma Leiomyoma Granular-cell tumor Schwann-cell tumors Chondroma Chondroblastoma
	malignant	Soft-tissue type sarcomas Chondrosarcoma Malignant lymphomas Other

Source: Macchiarini 2006 [20]. Reproduced with permission of Elsevier.

of adenoid cystic carcinoma clearly requires prolonged observation for complete clinical definition. Usually it is detected on CT as an intraluminal mass or as circumferential wall thickening with a smooth contour. The length of the lesion can be accurately assessed on coronal 2D MPRs and 3D external rendering before resection. F-FDG PET uptake is variable and depends on the grade of differentiation.

In children, tracheal tumors develop between the neonatal period and 14 years of age, predominantly at the posterior wall of the cervical trachea [4]. The trachea may also be involved by a variety of secondary tumors, such as laryngeal, thyroid, lung and esophageal carcinomas, for which palliation therapies are recommended.

To date there have been only two recommendations for TNM- and Staging-classifications because of the rarity of tracheal tumors. A more simple approach of TNM-classification was established by Bhattacharyya N in 2004 [2], followed by a second,

Table 17.3a TNM classification

Tumor stage		
Tx	Cannot be assessed	
Tis	Any tumor without invasion	
T1a	< 3 cm limited to mucosa	
T1b	< 3 cm limited to mucosa	
T2*	Any tumor that invades cartilage or adventitia	
T3	Any tumor that invades trachea or larynx	
T4a	Any tumor that invades carina or main bronchus	
T4b	Any tumor that invades neighbouring structures	
Nodal stage		
Nx	Regional lymph nodes cannot be assessed	
N0	No evidence of node metastasis	
N1	Local nodes positive (N1a < 3 cm; N1b < 3 cm)	
	Upper third	Highest mediastinal nodes; upper paratracheal nodes, prevascular and retrotracheal
	Middle third	Upper paratracheal nodes; prevascular and retrotracheal; lower paratracheal nodes; paraaortic nodes (ascending aorta or phrenic)
	Lower third	Upper paratracheal nodes; prevascular and retrotracheal; subaortic nodes (aorto-pulmonalis window)
N1A	1–3 positive nodes in upper third	
N1B	< 3 positive nodes in upper third	
N2	Regional nodes positive	
	Upper third	Lower paratracheal nodes; subaortic nodes (aortopulmonalis window)
	Middle third	Highest mediastinal nodes; subaortic nodes (aortopulmonalis window)
	Lower third	Upper paratracheal nodes; pulmonary ligament
Metastasis		
Mx	Distant metastasis cannot be assessed	
M0	No distant metastasis	
M1	Metastasis to nodes other than N1 and N2	
M2	Distant metastasis (e.g., lung)	

*Tumor involvement of pars membranacea always classified at least as T2, irrespective of infiltration depth.
Source: Macchiarini [20]. Reproduced with permission of Elsevier.

more extensive, realization of TNM- and Staging-classification, developed by Macchiarini, P. in 2006 [20]. The impact on prognosis and survival of these classifications has to be determined clinically. In Table 17.3a and 17.3b the TNM- and Staging-classifications are shown.

Management

Because of the rarity of this disease, there are no clear criteria for the selection and treatment of patients. Standard surgical treatment with tracheal resection with primary reconstruction, should be considered in cases of benign tumors and localized malignant tumors. Often patients with resectable tumors are treated with palliative procedures, such as endotracheal stenting, debridement or brachytherapy [21], which leads to shortened life expectancy. The challenge of treating tracheal tumors provides an the initial purpose for tracheal resection, but its limited incidence provides little incentive to face this problem systematically. Experimental and clinical tracheal therapy started back in the late nineteenth century and different approaches have been attempted. Primary benign

Table 17.3b Staging system

Stage	T	N	M
0	Tis	N0	M0
Ia	T1a	N0	M0
Ib	T1b–2	N0	M0
IIa	T1b–2	N1	M0
IIb	T1b–2	N2	M0
IIIa	T3	N0	M0
IIIb	T3	N1-2	M0
IVa	Any	N1-2	M1
IVb	Any	N1-2	M2

N: nodal stage; M: metastasis stage: T: tumour stage.
Source: Macchiarini [20]. Reproduced with permission of Elsevier.

and malignant tumors can be treated by open or endoscopic resection and radiotherapy. However, surgical resection is safer and more effective for all benign and low grade malignant tumors, and therefore should be considered as the gold standard for these disorders. It allows for permanent relief of the airway obstruction to achieve long-term survival and provides pathological confirmation of complete tumor removal [22, 23] and staging.

Improved survival in patients who undergo tracheal resection suggests that surgery is the only therapeutic option. Co-morbidities, age, general health, previous treatment, histology and tumor extension are factors that may limit eligibility for resection and candidates should be carefully considered. In select patients where meticulous surgical care is provided, the operative mortality is 5%. A sufficient residual native trachea and adequate vascularization of the anastomosis must be ensured for a safe and successful primary reconstruction [3].

Several surgical techniques have been described for the treatment of the upper trachea, resection of the larynx and trachea, trachea, carina, or carina

Table 17.4 Contraindications for surgical resection

- More than 1/2 of trachea involved in adults
- More than 1/3rd of trachea involved in children
- Presence of positive mediastinal lymph nodes or systemic metastasis
- Mediastinal invasion of unresectable organs
- Mediastinum received more than 60 Gy of radiation
- Distant metastases in squamous cell carcinoma

and lung. An absolute contraindication to tracheal resection is the presence of positive lymph nodes, mediastinal invasion of unresectable organs, a mediastinum that has received the maximum radiation dose of more than 60 Gy or has been operated on, and distant metastases of squamous-cell carcinoma [3, 8, 23]. For those patients, laser resection plus stenting can delay the progression of the tumor, but only as a palliative measure. A summary of contraindications for tracheal resection is summarized in Table 17.4.

In order to stage and evaluate the extent of a tracheal tumor, a complete lymphadenectomy should be done, paying attention to avoid impairment of vascularization to the surrounding trachea.

Brachytherapy can be performed as an adjuvant therapy after incomplete removal of a tumor, for unresectable disease, for recurrent disease and to palliate severe symptoms. Endotracheal debridement and stenting can be used to treat and alleviate inoperable tumors to keep the airway patent until further therapy.

When an acute intervention is necessary to maintain air passage in a severely obstructed airway, a salvage endoscopic debulking is indicated. Any procedure that prohibits further surgical resection should be avoided (such as stenting and tracheostomy).

If spread to the esophagus is suspected, an esophagoscopy and endoesophageal ultrasound is indicated. If symptoms indicate bone or brain involvement from metastatic spread, bone scintigraphy or cerebral MRI respectively, should be performed.

Regarding secondary tracheal tumors, the rationale for resection and reconstruction is adherence to oncologic principles. The surgery is not high risk or radical in competent hands.

For many years, palliative surgery has been the most common surgical procedure used to treat patients with thyroid carcinoma invading the trachea. Given the proclivity of papillary tumors to become more aggressive in time, the shaving-off procedure is inadequate. Complete removal, including airway and esophagus if necessary, seems the only radical therapeutic treatment for invasive thyroid carcinoma. Surgeons without extensive experience in tracheal reconstruction still recommend "shave" procedures, in the case of superficial invasion, and "window" resection, in the case of deep invasion. However, tracheal resection with primary repair is now the treatment of choice for such patients showing improved survival in the long term.

Surgical techniques

General anesthesia is required for all tracheal resections. Airway control is critical and intubation should not be taken for granted. Maintaining endotracheal intubation beyond the stenosis can avoid sudden respiratory arrest.

Ventilation can be achieved via an endotracheal tube passed into the operative field and placed past the stenosis after the tracheal transection. JET ventilation or hyperventilation with periods of apnea are additional options for endotracheal ventilation. Lung assist devices (iLA) might also be an alternative in this context to provide CO2-removal during surgery. Rarely, extracorporeal membrane oxygenation (ECMO with cardiopulmonary bypass) needs to be established prior to or during intubation, although recent developments like the venous-venous ECMO may be considered in patients with borderline lung function. The longitudinal extension of the tumor up to one-half of the trachea in adults and one-third in infants and children is a contraindication to surgery as resection renders the residual length of the native airway inadequate for a primary reconstruction. However, resectability should be considered before starting any local or systemic treatment. A very recent novel approach of tissue engineered tracheal replacement provides evidence for a potential clinical alternative for patients with long-segment tracheal disorders, including cancer [24, 25].

Technique: A neck-collar incision usually with a mini-sternotomy, or full sternotomy are performed for tumors of the cervical and uppermost portion of the intrathoracic trachea. The innominate artery, superior vena cava, innominate vein, and pulmonary artery are retracted for exposure of the distal trachea. Dissection must be performed directly on the trachea, confined to the area of stenosis, and no more than 1–2 cm of normal trachea above and below the lesion, to preserve the lateral segmental blood supply. The cervical trachea can be approached through a low collar incision or a collar incision combined with an upper partial sternotomy. If a stoma is present, then it is usually incorporated into the collar incision or closed separately. The thyroid isthmus is divided and reflected laterally. The trachea is first divided below the stenosis in an area of normal trachea, and dissection is carried proximally to separate the esophagus posterior to the trachea. Throughout the entire airway procedure, gentle dissection paying attention to both recurrent laryngeal nerves is mandatory. Furthermore, blood should not be allowed to enter the distal opening, and the airway should be cleaned immediately if spillage occurs. The trachea is then divided proximally, and, after the tumorous stenotic segment is removed, cross-field ventilation via the operative field is placed into the distal trachea. Cervical neck flexion and anterior mobilization to the carina will allow, in most cases, a tension-free anastomosis of the cervical trachea. If additional length is required, a suprahyoid laryngeal release can be performed by the Montgomery technique and neck flexion performed for approximately one week postoperatively. To maintain consistent neck flexion after surgery, a reminder suture or collar brace may ensure the patient does not accidentally flex the neck. For tumors of the lower portion of the trachea, a median sternotomy or high right posterolateral thoracotomy is performed. The initial dissection is commenced by division of the azygous vein to expose the carina. The distal trachea and right and left mainstem bronchi are isolated. A flexible bronchoscope through the oral endotracheal tube can guide the incision into the distal

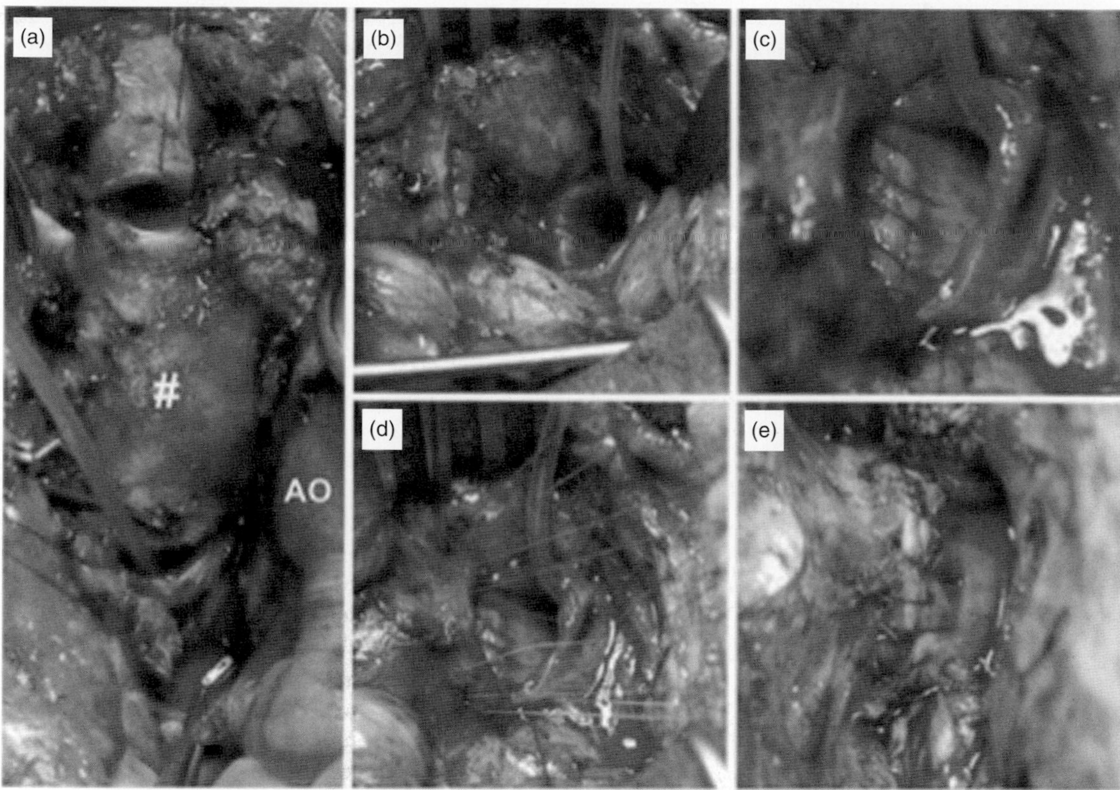

Figure 17.2 a: Anterior view on the middle and distal part of intrathoracic trachea after mobilizing ascending aorta (AO). # = part of trachea to be removed due to a tracheal tumor. b: Lateral intraoperative view of the dissected trachea and a placed running suture at the posterior wall. c: Tightened running suture. d: Single sutures (7x) at the anterior wall of the trachea. e: Tightened single sutures and closed anastomosis. (For a color version, see the color plate section.)

trachea. The technique for reconstructing the airway is the same regardless of the level. If excess anastomotic tension is thought to exist, release maneuvers may help reduce tension on the anastomosis. Division of the pulmonary ligament and hilar release accomplished by dividing the pericardium circumferentially around the hilum provide an additional centimeter or two of mobility to the distal airway. Suprahyoid release may also be used to add additional length for carinal resection procedures. Once determination has been made that the airway can be reapproximated, individual circumferential anastomotic sutures for the anterior nonmembranous part and a continuous suture for the posterior membranous part are placed (4-0 Vicryl in adults and 5-0 Vicryl in children) (Figure 17.2). All sutures are made to allow the knots to be on the outside of the anastomosis. Once the continuous suture of the back row is tied, the table neck is flexed, the operative field endotracheal tube is removed, and the oral endotracheal tube is advanced onto the left mainstem bronchus beyond the anastomosis. The front row sutures should then be tied and the endotracheal tube withdrawn to the trachea proximal to the anastomosis. When all of the sutures have been tied, the anastomosis should be checked to see if it is hermetically sealed. The anesthesiologist ventilates the patient to 20, 30, and 40 cm of pressure. The operative field is submersed in saline to allow identification of any leaks. Any leaks should be repaired even to the point of taking the entire anastomosis apart and starting all over if the leak can't be repaired. Once the anastomosis has been secured, soft tissue coverage of the anastomosis is achieved by a pedicled flap of pericardial fat, pleura, or intercostal muscle. Inspection of the anastomosis with bronchoscopy is performed prior to extubation. Frozen section to confirm complete resection for tracheal tumors is also generally indicated prior to completing the anastomosis. A radical lymphadenectomy is always recommended. Several postoperative complications may occur after tracheal resection, such as anastomotic separation, anastomotic granulation tissue formation, aspiration during swallowing and subsequent pneumonia, recurrent nerve paralysis, tracheo-innominate fistula, ventilatory support >48 hours, and the potential need for tracheostomy. In addition to pulmonary insufficiency, general complications such as wound infection or bleeding are possible.

Prognosis

Squamous cell carcinoma of the trachea has a subsequent reported 5-year survival rate of about 5%. Five-year survival rates for adenoid cystic carcinoma are improved by surgery combined with radiotherapy, but are associated with a continued decrease in survival at 10 years and thereafter, because of local recurrence and the appearance of metastases.

Conclusion

Tracheal primary tumors are rare and usually diagnosed at a late stage due to their unspecific clinical symptoms. However, for carefully selected patients, surgical resection with a subsequent re-anastomosis, combined with a adjuvant or neo-adjuvant therapeutic strategy (due to the type of tumor) is currently available and has the potential to cure the patient. For patients with advanced tracheal tumors, the therapeutic options are still poor but recent advances give hope. The treatment of patients suffering from a tracheal tumor must be determined by a multidisciplinary process, including diagnostic tools, staging, specific follow-up strategies and detailed therapeutic planning.

References

1 Manninen MP, Antila PJ, Pukander JS, *et al.* (1991) Occurrence of tracheal carcinoma in Finland. *Acta Otolaryngol,* 111: 1162–9.

2 Bhattacharyya N (2004) Contemporary staging and prognosis for primary tracheal malignancies: A population-based analysis. *Otolaryngol Head Neck Surg,* 131: 639–42.

3 Grillo HC (2004) Surgery of the trachea and bronchi. In: Grillo HC (ed.), *Surgery of the Trachea and Bronchi.* London: Hamilton, pp. 208–47.

4 Desai DP, Holinger LD, Gonzalez-Crussi F (1998) Tracheal neoplasms in children. *Ann Otol Rhinol Laryngol* 107: 790–6.

5 Grillo HC, Dignan EF, Miura T (1964) Extensive resection and reconstruction of mediastinal trachea without prosthesis or graft: an antomical study in man. *J Thorac Cardiovasc Surg,* 48: 741–9.

6 Gelder CM, Hetzel MR (1993) Primary tracheal tumours: A national survey. *Thorax,* 48: 688–92.

7 Salassa JR, Pearson BW, Payne WS (1977) Gross and microscopical blood supply of the trachea. *Annals of Thoracic Surgery,* Aug; 24: 100–7.

8 Gaissert HA, Grillo HC, Shadmehr MB, *et al.* (2004) Long-term survival after resection of primary adenoid cystic and squamous cell carcinoma of the trachea and carina. *Ann Thorac Surg,* 78: 1889–96.

9 Hollingsworth HM (1987) Wheezing and stridor. *Clin Chest Med,* 8: 231–40.

10 Geffin B, Grillo HC, Cooper JD, *et al.* (1971) Stenosis following tracheostomy for respiratory care. *JAMA,* 216: 1984–8.

11 Gaissert HA (2003) Primary tracheal tumors. *Chest Surg Clin N Am,* 13: 247–56.

12 Andrade RS (2010) Relevance of endobronchial ultrasonography to thoracic surgeons. *Semin Thorac Cardiovasc Surg,* 22: 150–4.

13 LoCicero J, Costello P, Campos CT, *et al.* (1996) Spiral CT with multiplanar and three-dimensional reconstructions accurately predicts tracheobronchial pathology. *Ann Thorac Surg,* 62: 818–22.

14 Remy-Jardin M, Remy J, Artaud D, *et al.* (1998) Volume rendering of the tracheobronchial tree: clinical evaluation of bronchographic images. *Radiology,* 208: 761–70.

15 Gilkeson RC, Ciancibello LM, Hejal RB, *et al.* (2001) Tracheobronchomalacia: Dynamic airway evaluation with multidetector CT. *AJR Am J Roentgenol*, 176: 205–10.
16 Zhang J, Hasegawa I, Hatabu H, *et al.* (2004) Frequency and severity of air trapping at dynamic expiratory CT in patients with tracheobronchomalacia. *AJR Am J Roentgenol*, 182: 81–5.
17 Yedururi S, Guillerman RP, Chung T, *et al.* (2008) Multimodality imaging of tracheobronchial disorders in children. *Radiographics*, 28: e29.
18 Lee EY, Litmanovich D, Boiselle PM (2009) Multidetector CT evaluation of tracheobronchomalacia. *Radiol Clin North Am*, 47: 261–9.
19 Gilbert JG, Kaufman B, Mazzarella LA (1949) Tracheal tumors in infants and children. *J Pediatr*, 35: 63–9.
20 Macchiarini P (2006) Primary tracheal tumours. *Lancet Oncol*, 7: 83–91.
21 Grillo HC (1993) Primary tracheal tumours. *Thorax*, 48: 681–2.
22 Grillo HC (2002) Tracheal replacement: A critical review. *Ann Thorac Surg*, 73: 1995–2004.
23 Mathisen DJ (1996) Tracheal tumors. *Chest Surg Clin N Am*, 6: 875–98.
24 Macchiarini P, Jungebluth P, Go T, *et al.* (2008) Clinical transplantation of a tissue-engineered airway. *Lancet*, 372: 2023–30.
25 Jungebluth P, Alici E, Baiguera S, *et al.* (2011) Tracheobronchial transplantation with a stem-cell-seeded bioartificial nanocomposite: A proof-of-concept study. *Lancet*, 378: 1997–2004.

CHAPTER 18

Adjuvant Chemotherapy Following Surgery for Lung Cancer

Kathryn A. Gold

Department of Thoracic/Head and Neck Medical Oncology, The University of Texas MD Anderson Cancer Center, Houston, TX, USA

Introduction

Surgical resection is the standard treatment for early stage non-small cell lung cancer (NSCLC). Unfortunately, 5-year survival following complete resection has been disappointing, ranging from 63% in patients with stage IA tumors to 19% in patients with stage IIIA [1]. Following surgery, 10–15% of patients will experience a local relapse, while a distant recurrence will occur in 15–60% of the cases, generally leading to death. Efforts at improving local and distant control as well as survival for patients with operable NSCLC have examined the addition of chemotherapy and/or radiation in the postoperative (adjuvant) setting.

Outcomes with postoperative radiation therapy have been disappointing, with some studies showing an improvement in local control [2] but a large meta-analysis suggesting a detrimental effect on survival [3]. Postoperative radiation may be indicated for some patients at a high risk of local relapse, including patients with mediastinal nodal involvement or positive surgical margins, but should not routinely be offered to patients with N0 or N1 disease.

The high rate of distant recurrence is thought to be due to unrecognized micro-metastatic disease present at the time of surgery. Following surgical resection, adjuvant chemotherapy can potentially reduce the risk of developing recurrent and metastatic disease, theoretically by treating micro-metastatic disease before it becomes clinical evident. Adjuvant chemotherapy following surgical resection is the standard of care for a number of malignancies, including breast cancer and colon cancer [4, 5], and it has been extensively studied for non-small cell lung cancer.

Clinical trials of adjuvant chemotherapy

Early clinical trials of postoperative adjuvant chemotherapy in NSCLC showed a detrimental effect on survival with the use of alkylating agents like cyclophosphamide or nitrosurea [6]. Subsequent randomized trials of postoperative cisplatin-based chemotherapy failed to demonstrate clear benefits in any single study. These studies were pooled in an individual patient data-based meta-analysis reported in 1995 [6]. Eight trials used cisplatin in a range of doses (50–240 mg/m^2 total dose) and in various combinations with doxorubicin, cyclophosphamide, and vindesine. The overall hazard ratio (HR) was 0.87 ($p = 0.08$) in favor of chemotherapy and corresponded to a 13%

Lung Cancer, Fourth Edition. Edited by Jack A. Roth, Waun Ki Hong and Ritsuko U. Komaki.

Table 18.1 Overview of recent randomized, platinum-based adjuvant chemotherapy trials

Trial	N	Stage	Regimen	Radiation therapy	Hazard ratio for death (95% CI)	p-value
ALPI (8)	1209	I-IIIA	MVP	Optional	0.96 (0.81, 1.13)	0.589
IALT (9)	1867	I-IIIA	Cisplatin-based*	Optional	0.89 (0.76, 0.98)	0.03
Big lung trial (11)	381	I-IIIA	Cisplatin-based*	Optional	1.02 (0.77, 1.35)	0.90
JBR.10 (12)	482	IB-II	Cisplatin-vinorelbine	None	0.69 (0.52-0.91)	0.04
ANITA (14)	840	IB-IIIA	Cisplatin-vinorelbine	Optional	0.80 (0.66-0.96)	0.017
CALGB (15)	344	IB	Carboplatin-paclitaxel	None	0.83 (0.64-1.08)	0.12

*Investigator's choice between several regimens; MVP, mitomycin C, vindesine, cisplatin.

reduction in the risk of death. This study suggested an absolute benefit for chemotherapy of 3% at 2 years (95% CI, 0.5% detriment to 7% benefit) and 5% at 5 years (95% CI, 1% detriment to 10% benefit). Although these results were not statistically significant, they prompted many groups to launch adjuvant platinum-based chemotherapy trials in completely resected NSCLC. See Tables 18.1 and 18.2 for a summary of these trials.

Japanese Clinical Oncology Group Trial 9304

Japan Clinical Oncology Group (JCOG) Trial 9304 aimed to determine whether adjuvant chemotherapy with three courses of cisplatin and vindesine was superior to observation only in patients with completely resected NSCLC patients with ipsilateral mediastinal lymph node involvement [7]. Three courses of chemotherapy (cisplatin 80 mg/m^2 day 1, vindesine 3 mg/m^2 days 1 and 8, administered

Table 18.2 Regimens used in adjuvant chemotherapy trials

Trial	Chemotherapy regimen: Cisplatin	Chemotherapy regimen: Other	# of cycles	Compliance
ALPI (8)	100 mg/m^2 d1	Mitomycin 8 mg/m^2 d1 and Vindesine 3 mg/m^2 d1, d8	3 21-day cycles	69% received all 3 cycles
IALT (9)	80–120 mg/m^2 d1	Vindesine 3 mg/m^2 wkly* OR Vinblastine 4 mg/m^2 wkly* OR Vinorelbine 30 mg/m^2 wkly OR Etoposide 100 mg/m^2 d1, d2,d3	4 21-day cycles OR 3 28-day cycles OR 4 28-day cycles	74% received ≥ 240 mg/m^2 of cisplatin
Big lung trial (11)	50–80 mg/m^2 d1	Mitomycin 6 mg/m^2, Ifosfamide 3 g/m^2 d1 OR Mitomycin 6 mg/m^2,Vinblastine 6 mg/m^2 d1 OR Vindesine 3 mg/m^2 d1, d8 OR Vinorelbine 30 mg/m^2 d1, d8	3 21-day cycles	64% received all 3 cycles
JBR.10 (12)	50 mg/m^2 d1, d8	Vinorelbine 25 mg/m^2 weekly	4 28-day cycles	58% received at least 3 cycles
ANITA (14)	100 mg/m^2 d1	Vinorelbine 30 mg/m^2 weekly	4 28-day cycles	50% received all 4 cycles
CALGB (15)	None	Carboplatin AUC 6 and paclitaxel 200 mg/m^2	4 21-day cycles	86% received all 4 cycles

*modified weekly schedule: weekly x 4 weeks, then every 2 weeks.

every four weeks) were administered in the experimental arm. Chemotherapy started within 6 weeks after surgery. Postoperative radiotherapy was not delivered. Eligible patients were under 75 years of age, had a performance status of 0 or 1, and had received no prior chemotherapy or radiotherapy. Patients were stratified by treatment center, and the two groups were well balanced. The trial closed before reaching the planned sample size because of slow accrual. From January 1994 to July 1998, 119 patients were randomized (59 in the chemotherapy arm and 60 in the surgery alone arm). The intended dose of chemotherapy was administered to 58% of patients. There were no statistically significant differences in overall and disease-free survival between the arms. Median survival was 36 months in both groups and 5-year survival was 28% in the chemotherapy arm and 36% in the control arm ($p = 0.89$). Median disease-free survival was 18 months in the chemotherapy arm and 16 months in the control arm ($p = 0.66$).

Adjuvant Lung Project Italy

Investigators from the Adjuvant Lung Project Italy (ALPI) and the European Organization for Research and Treatment of Cancer (EORTC) randomly assigned patients with completely resected stage I, II, or IIIA NSCLC to either MVP (mitomycin at 8 mg/m^2 on day 1, vindesine at 3 mg/m^2 on days 1 and 8, and cisplatin at 100 mg/m^2 on day 1) every 3 weeks for three cycles or observation [8]. Treatment had to begin within 42 days after surgical resection. Patients were stratified by center, tumor size, lymph node involvement, and the intention to perform radiotherapy. Patients received radiotherapy according to the policy of the individual participating center, which was decided prior to the enrollment of the first patient. For the patients in the MVP arm, radiotherapy was initiated 3–5 weeks after the last chemotherapy, and for patients in the control arm, radiotherapy was initiated 4 to 6 weeks after surgery. The primary endpoint was overall survival. Secondary endpoints were progression-free survival and toxicity associated with adjuvant treatment. The trial was designed to have 80% power to detect a 20% relative reduction in mortality (increasing 5-year survival from 50–57%) corresponding to a hazard rate of 0.8, with a two-sided alpha of 0.05.

From January 1994 to January 1999, 1209 patients were enrolled, 606 to the MVP arm, and 603 to the control arm. Patients were well balanced between the two arms of the study: 39% had stage I disease, 33% had stage II disease, and 28% had stage IIIA disease. Median age was 61 years. Sixty-nine percent of the MVP patients completed the three planned cycles of chemotherapy, though many required dose reductions. Sixty-five percent of patients received radiotherapy in the MVP arm, and 82% in the control arm. MVP chemotherapy was associated with grade 3 or 4 neutropenia in 16 and 12% of patients, respectively. There were 10 treatment-related deaths in the study; three in the chemotherapy arm and seven in the control arm. After a median follow-up of 64.5 months, no significant difference in overall survival was seen between the arms, with an HR of 0.96 (95% CI, 0.81–1.13; $p = 0.589$). Progression-free survival was also not significantly different between the arms ($HR = 0.89$, 95% CI, 0.76–1.03; $p = 0.128$). Median overall survival was 55 months in the MVP arm and 48 months in the control arm. Disease stage and sex were associated with survival in the multivariable analysis. Kras mutation status, p53 staining, and Ki-67 status were investigated as potential predictive or prognostic markers, but no significant associations were seen between these biomarkers and overall or disease-free survival.

International Adjuvant Lung Cancer Trial

The International Adjuvant Lung Cancer Trial (IALT) Collaborative Group evaluated the effect of cisplatin-based adjuvant chemotherapy on survival in completely resected NSCLC [9]. 1867 patients with completely resected stage I, II, or III NSCLC were randomly assigned to either 3 or 4 cycles of cisplatin-based chemotherapy or to observation. Chemotherapy was one of four different regimens combining cisplatin (80–120 mg/m^2, every 3–4 weeks) with either a vinca alkaloid or etoposide (vindesine 3 mg/m^2 weekly for 5 weeks then every 2 weeks, vinblastine 4 mg/m^2 weekly for 5 weeks then every 2 weeks, vinorelbine 30 mg/m^2 weekly, or etoposide 100 mg/m^2 days 1–3 per cycle). Because of uncertainty regarding optimal postoperative treatment and to facilitate accrual, each participating center could determine the pathologic stage of disease to include, the dose of cisplatin given per cycle, the drug that was combined with cisplatin, and the postoperative radiotherapy policy. Eligible patients had completely resected stage I, II, or III NSCLC, and were between 18 and 75 years of age. Patients were randomly assigned within 60 days of surgery and were stratified by treatment center, type of surgery, and pathological stage. Chemotherapy was to begin within 60 days of surgery. Postoperative radiotherapy, if indicated, consisted of 60 Gy or less, delivered to the mediastinal lymph nodes. The primary endpoint was overall survival. Secondary endpoints were disease-free survival, second primary cancers, and adverse effects. The trial was designed to demonstrate an absolute improvement in overall survival of 5%, from 50 to 55% at 5 years.

Enrollment began in February 1995 and the steering committee decided to discontinue recruitment on December 31, 2000, citing slow accrual. A total of 1867 patients had been randomly assigned, recruited by 148 centers in 33 countries. Patients were well balanced between the two arms of the study. Ten percent of patients had stage IA disease, 27% stage 1B, 24% stage II, and 39% stage III. Median age was 59 years, 20% were women, 40% had adenocarcinoma. A regimen combining 100 mg/m^2 cisplatin for three or four cycles with etoposide was the most commonly used regimen, selected for 49.3% of the patients. Of the patients assigned to the chemotherapy arm, 74% received at least 240 mg/m^2 of cisplatin. Twenty-seven percent of patients received postoperative radiotherapy. In the chemotherapy arm, 23% of patients experienced grade 3 or 4 toxicity, and 7 patients (0.8%) died of chemotherapy-related toxicity. In the chemotherapy group, 7.8% did not receive chemotherapy. The median duration of follow-up was 56 months. Patients assigned to chemotherapy had a significantly higher overall survival rate than patients assigned to observation (44.5% versus 40.4% at 5 yr, respectively; HR 0.86 [0.76–0.98], $p < 0.03$). Disease-free survival was also significantly improved with chemotherapy (HR = 0.83[0.74–0.94], $p < 0.003$). Median survival was 50.8 months in the chemotherapy arm and 44.4 months in the control arm, while median disease-free survival was 40.2 months and 30.5 months, respectively. Five-year disease-free survival rates were 39.4% and 34.3% in the chemotherapy group and in the control group, respectively.

An updated analysis published in 2009 with a median follow-up of 90 months showed that that benefits of chemotherapy on overall survival persisted, but were no longer statistically significant (HR 0.91, 95% CI 0.81–1.02, $p = 0.1$) [10]. There was a trend, however, towards increased risk of nonlung cancer related death in the chemotherapy arm (HR 1.34, 95% CI 0.99–1.81, $p = 0.06$).

Big Lung Trial

The British Big Lung Trial randomized patients with surgically resectable lung cancer to surgery with or without cisplatin-based chemotherapy [11]. Chemotherapy could be administered either prior to surgery (neoadjuvant chemotherapy) or postoperatively, at the treating physician's discretion. Clinicians could select between four chemotherapy regimens: MIC (cisplatin 50 mg/m^2, mitomycin 6 mg/m^2, and ifosfamide 3 g/m^2), MVP (cisplatin 50 mg/m^2, mitomycin 6 mg/m^2, and vinblastine 6 mg/m^2), CV (cisplatin 80 mg/m^2, vindesine 3 mg/m^2 on days 1 and 8), or NP (cisplatin 80 mg/m^2, vinorelbine 30 mg/m^2 on days 1 and 8), all of which were given every 3 weeks for 3 cycles.

The primary endpoint of this study was overall survival. This was an underpowered study – with about a 20% power to detect a 5% difference in survival – and the aim was to contribute to an updated meta-analysis. A total of 381 patients were randomized. Median age was 61 years, 69% of patients were male, 48% had squamous cell carcinoma and 37% had adenocarcinoma. Twenty-seven percent of patients had stage I disease, 38% stage II, and 34% stage III. A macroscopic complete resection was achieved in approximately 95% of patients, and an incomplete microscopic resection was reported in 15% of cases. Nearly two-thirds of patients in the chemotherapy group received all three planned cycles of chemotherapy with 40% of these patients requiring a dose reduction. A large majority of those assigned to chemotherapy received adjuvant therapy (97%), rather than neoadjuvant chemotherapy; only a small portion (14%) received postoperative radiation. With a median follow-up of 34.6 months, there was no significant benefit in overall survival to the chemotherapy group (HR: 1.02; p = 0.90). Median overall survival was 33.9 months for the chemotherapy group and 32.6 months for the surgery alone arm, and median progression free survival was 27 months for the surgery with chemotherapy group, and 24.7 months for the surgery alone arm.

JBR.10 Trial

In this North American intergroup trial, patients with completed resected T2N0, T1N1 or T2N1 NSCLC were randomized to adjuvant chemotherapy versus observation [12]. This trial was initially opened by the National Cancer Institute of Canada Clinical Trials Group (NCIC CTG) in 1994; United States cooperative groups (Cancer and Leukemia Group B [CALGB], Southwest Oncology Group [SWOG], and Eastern Cooperative Oncology Group [ECOG]) joined in 1998. Patients randomized to the chemotherapy arm received vinorelbine 25 mg/m^2 weekly and cisplatin 50 mg/m^2 on days 1 and 8, every 4 weeks for four cycles, to start within 6 weeks of surgery. Patients were stratified by nodal status (N0 versus N1) and *RAS* mutation (present versus absent versus unknown). The primary study endpoint was overall survival; secondary endpoints included recurrence-free survival, quality of life, and toxicity.

Between 1994 and 2001, 482 patients underwent randomization to chemotherapy (242 patients) or observation alone (240 patients). The two groups were well balanced and the median age was 61 years. Forty-five percent of the patients had T2N0 disease, 15% had T1N1, and 40% had T2N1 disease. Fifty-three percent had adenocarcinoma and *RAS* mutations (in codons 12, 13, and 61 of *NRAS*, *KRAS*, or *HRAS*) were present in 24% of the samples. Only 45% of patients were able to complete all four planned cycles of chemotherapy. Febrile neutropenia occurred in 7% of patients receiving chemotherapy and treatment-related death was rare (2 patients, 0.8%). With median follow-up over 5 years, significantly increased median overall survival was seen in the chemotherapy group (94 months versus 73 months; HR = 0.69; p = 0.011). There was also a significant improvement in recurrence free survival with chemotherapy (not reached versus 47 months; HR = 0.6; p = 0.0003). The 5-year survival rates were 69 and 54% in the chemotherapy and control group, respectively (p = 0.03). On subgroup analysis, there was no significant improvement in overall survival in patients with stage IB disease (p = 0.79) while patients with stage II disease had a significant improvement in median overall survival with chemotherapy (80 months vs 41 months, p = 0.004). On an updated survival analysis performed after a median follow-up of 9.3 years, adjuvant chemotherapy continued to show a survival benefit (HR 0.78, p = 0.04), though this benefit appeared to be confined to patients with node-positive disease [13].

Adjuvant Navelbine International Trialist's Association Study

In the Adjuvant Navelbine International Trialist's Association (ANITA) trial, investigators randomized patients with completely resected stage IB, II, or IIIA NSCLC to either adjuvant chemotherapy or observation [14]. Patients were enrolled from 101 centers in 14 countries. Patients assigned to the chemotherapy group received vinorelbine 30 mg/m^2 weekly and cisplatin 100 mg/m2 every four weeks for 16 weeks. Postoperative radiotherapy was undertaken according to each center's policy and was recommended for patients with node-positive disease. Patients were stratified by center, stage, and histology. The primary endpoint was overall survival, and secondary endpoints were disease-free survival and safety. The trial was designed to have a 90% power to detect an absolute improvement of 10% indicating a benefit for adjuvant chemotherapy, with a two-sided alpha of 0.05. The planned sample size for the study was 400 patients per treatment group. From December 1994 to December 2000, 840 patients were enrolled: 407 to the chemotherapy arm and 433 to the observation group. Patients were well balanced between the two arms of the study, with 36% having stage IB disease, 24% stage II disease, and 39% stage IIIA disease. Sixty-one percent of patients completed at least 3 of the planned four cycles. Chemotherapy was associated with grade 3 or 4 neutropenia in 85% of patients, and febrile neutropenia in 9% of patients. Two percent of patients died from toxic effects of chemotherapy.

At the time of analysis, median follow-up was over 6 years in both groups. Median survival was 65.7 months for patients in the chemotherapy group and 43.7 months for patients assigned to observation (HR = 0.80 [0.66–0.96], p = 0.017). The absolute overall survival benefit with chemotherapy at five years was 8.6%. There was also as statistically significant benefit in disease-free survival between the groups (p = 0.002). On subgroup analysis, patients with stage IB disease did not appear to benefit from adjuvant chemotherapy, while patients with stage II and IIIA disease had a statistically significant benefit in overall survival.

Cancer and Leukemia Group B-9633

The Cancer and Leukemia Group B (CALGB) trial 9633 randomly assigned patients with completely resected stage IB (T2N0) lung cancer to observation alone or chemotherapy with four cycles of paclitaxel (200 mg/m^2) and carboplatin (AUC = 6) [15]. This trial was initially presented at the ASCO Annual Meeting in 2004 as positive after a follow-up of 34 months [16], though final survival analysis was negative. Chemotherapy was started within 8 weeks of surgery and there was no planned thoracic radiotherapy. The trial started in September 1996 and planned accrual was 500 patients over 3.5 years. Because of slow accrual and reported results from other trials, the trial was closed following accrual of 344 patients in November 2003.

Patient characteristics were well balanced between the two arms of the study with regard to age, sex, race, weight loss, ethnicity, histology, tumor differentiation, and type of surgery. Adjuvant chemotherapy was well tolerated, and there were no chemotherapy-related deaths. Grade 3 or 4 neutropenia occurred in 35% of patients. With a median follow-up of 74 months, overall survival and disease free survival were not significantly different between the chemotherapy and observation groups. Median overall survival was 95 months for the chemotherapy group and 78 months in the observation group (HR 0.83, p = 0.124), and median disease free survival was 89 months with chemotherapy and 56 months with observation (HR 0.80, p = 0.065).

In an unplanned subgroup analysis, the CALGB investigators found significant benefits in overall and disease free survival for patients with tumors larger than 4 cm, and a trend towards inferior outcomes for those with tumors less than 4 cm. In contrast to other studies, this trial utilized carboplatin-paclitaxel rather than a cisplatin-based regimen.

Pooled analyses of adjuvant chemotherapy trials

Of the trials described above, several (ALPI, Big Lung Trial, and CALGB-9633) showed no clear benefit for adjuvant chemotherapy, while others (IALT, JBR.10, ANITA) showed significant improvement in survival with adjuvant chemotherapy. Some trials, like ALPI, used older, more toxic chemotherapy regimens. Others, like the Big Lung Trial and CALGB-9633, were underpowered to detect small differences in survival. A number of meta-analyses have pooled individual data from randomized trials to try to draw broad conclusions.

In the Lung Adjuvant Cisplatin Evaluation (LACE) analysis, individual data from five randomized cisplatin-based chemotherapy trials (ALPI, IALT, ANITA, Big Lung Trial, and JBR.10) were pooled [17]. These trials were all performed after the 1995 meta-analysis [6]. These trials included 4584 patients. Pathology stages between IA and III were represented (IA: 8%, IB: 29%, II: 35%, III: 28%). Adjuvant chemotherapy was associated with an 11% reduction in the risk of death and absolute overall survival benefit of 5.4% at 5 years. This survival benefit was statistically significant (HR = 0.89, p = 0.005). Patients receiving chemotherapy had an increased risk of death in the first 6 months (74 deaths in chemotherapy arm vs 29 in control arm), mostly due to chemotherapy toxicity and increased cardiovascular/pulmonary deaths. There was a trend in favor of use of higher dose cisplatin (planned dose greater than 300 mg/m^2) which did not meet statistical significance (p = 0.1). There was significant interaction between chemotherapy effect and stage. Though the numbers were small, patients with stage IA disease did not appear to benefit from chemotherapy (HR 1.40, 95% CI 0.95–2.06). Patients with stage IB disease had an insignificant trend towards benefit from chemotherapy (HR 0.93; 95% CI 0.78–1.10) and patients with stage II and III disease had statistically significant improvements in survival with adjuvant chemotherapy (HR 0.83, 95% CI 0.70–0.91 and HR 0.83, 95% CI 0.72–0.94, respectively). Patients with good performance status tended to benefit from chemotherapy, whereas the utility of chemotherapy in patients with borderline performance status (PS = 2) was unclear.

Another large meta-analysis by the NSCLC Meta-analyses Collaborative Group included 34 trials randomizing patients between surgery followed by adjuvant chemotherapy versus surgery alone as well as 13 trials randomizing patients to surgery plus radiotherapy and chemotherapy versus surgery plus radiotherapy [18]. A total of 11 107 patients were included in this meta-analysis. This trial found that chemotherapy was associated with a 4% absolute benefit in overall survival at 5 years. In contrast to the LACE meta-analysis, there was no significant interaction between benefit from chemotherapy and tumor stage or performance status.

Selection of patients to receive adjuvant chemotherapy

Stage II and III disease

Clinical trials and meta-analyses suggest a benefit in terms of both overall survival and disease free survival with adjuvant chemotherapy in patients with resected stage II or III non-small cell lung cancer. The magnitude of absolute survival benefit is around 5% at five years [17, 18]. For patients with good performance status and no contraindications, adjuvant chemotherapy is the standard of care.

Stage IA disease

The Big Lung Trial, ALPI, and IALT were the only cisplatin-based adjuvant chemotherapy trials to include stage IA disease [8, 9, 11]. This group accounted for 347 patients in total between these trials. Individual data have been analyzed in the LACE pooled analysis [17]. This meta-analysis suggested a detrimental effect in that subgroup, taking into account that some of the patients were treated with more toxic, older regimens. Nevertheless, there is no clear evidence of a benefit for adjuvant chemotherapy in resected stage IA non-small cell lung cancer.

Stage IB disease

CALGB-9633 is the only large platinum-based adjuvant trial focusing on patients with stage IB disease [15]. Though initial results were promising, final analysis did not show a benefit of adjuvant carboplatin and paclitaxel. Many hypotheses have been advanced to explain the negative results of this study, including the lower activity of the paclitaxel/carboplatin doublet in comparison with cisplatin-based doublets and the lack of power due to the early discontinuation of accrual. In a subgroup analysis of JBR.10 and ANITA trials, no benefit was observed for patients with stage IB disease, though statistical tests for interactions showed no clear relationship between stage and benefit from chemotherapy [12, 14]. In the LACE pooled analysis, a trend toward a benefit for adjuvant chemotherapy was reported but it was not statistically significant [17].

In an unplanned, post-hoc analysis of data from the CALGB-9633 study, tumor size greater than 4 centimeters was found to predict for benefit from chemotherapy [15]. A similar relationship was found between tumor size and benefit from chemotherapy in JBR.10. Patients with tumors larger than 4 centimeters tended to benefit from chemotherapy, while patients with small tumors did not, though these subset analyses did not reach statistical significance [13]. At our institution, decisions regarding adjuvant chemotherapy for stage IB disease are made on an individual basis, with chemotherapy considered for patients with high risk features such as large (greater than 4 cm) or poorly differentiated tumors, visceral pleural invasion, or vascular invasion.

Elderly patients

The median age at presentation for patients with lung cancer is 70 years old [19] but elderly patients are underrepresented in clinical trials. Older patients tend to have more comorbidities and may have difficulty tolerating chemotherapy. In a subgroup analysis of the JBR.10 trial, patients over the age of 65 were found to have a similar benefit from adjuvant chemotherapy (HR 0.61, 95% CI 0.38 to 098, p = 0.04) as younger patients, though they received fewer doses of chemotherapy on average [20]. On this trial, there were only 23 evaluable patients over the age of 75, and these patients had a trend towards decreased survival with chemotherapy (HR 2.35, 95% CI 0.84 to 6.58, p = 0.09). In the LACE meta-analysis, 414 of a total of 4,584 patients were age 70 or older [21]. There was no statistically significant interaction between age and benefit from chemotherapy, and these elderly patients had a trend towards improvement in overall survival (HR 0.87, 95% CI 0.68 to 1.11). Elderly patients received a lower total cisplatin dose, though adverse events were similar in younger and older patients.

In a large observational cohort study, 3324 patients aged more than 65 years with resected stage II or IIIA lung cancer were identified from the SEER database [22]. Only 21% of these patients received platinum-based adjuvant therapy. Chemotherapy was associated with an improved survival (HR 0.80, 95% CI, 0.72–0.89), similar to the benefit seen in clinical trials, though there was a higher rate of hospitalization for serious adverse events.

Based on these results, adjuvant chemotherapy should not be withheld from patients on the basis of age alone, though comorbidities should be considered, both when deciding whether to use adjuvant chemotherapy and in choosing a regimen.

Patients with poor performance status

The benefit of adjuvant chemotherapy is unclear in patients with WHO performance status (PS) of 2 or higher. JBR.10 and CALGB 9633 only allowed patients with PS 0 or 1 [12, 15] and other trials accrued only small numbers of patients with poor PS. In the LACE meta-analysis, only 183 out of 4584 patients had a PS of 2. These patients had a trend towards worsened outcomes with adjuvant chemotherapy [17].

Selection of adjuvant chemotherapy regimen

Cisplatin versus carboplatin

For patients with metastatic lung cancer, most studies suggest similar progression free and overall survival with the use of cisplatin versus carboplatin based doublets [23,24], though a meta-analysis suggested higher response rates with cisplatin-based therapy [25]. In the adjuvant setting, however, cisplatin based regimens have been used in most large clinical trials, including all the trials incorporated into the LACE meta-analysis [17]. The only large trial to use a carboplatin-based regimen was CALBG-9633, and this trial was not able to demonstrate a significant survival benefit with adjuvant chemotherapy [15]. Cisplatin is considered the preferred agent for adjuvant treatment, though carboplatin-based regimens can be considered for patients unable to tolerate cisplatin.

Choice of a second agent

The most studied adjuvant chemotherapy regimen is cisplatin and vinorelbine, which was used in all patients in the ANITA and JBR.10 trial, and in some patients in IALT and the Big Lung Trial [9, 11, 12, 14]. In the metastatic setting, cisplatin in combination with newer agents such as docetaxel, gemcitabine, or pemetrexed has similar or improved response rates and survival compared to cisplatin with vinorelbine [23, 26, 27]. These newer regimens are often better tolerated. Though these newer agents have not been studied in randomized trials in the adjuvant setting, they are often used in clinical practice. Acceptable options for adjuvant treatment include cisplatin with gemcitabine, cisplatin with docetaxel, and cisplatin with pemetrexed (for non-squamous tumors only). If patients are not able to tolerate cisplatin, carboplatin and paclitaxel, as used in CALGB-9633, is an acceptable regimen [15].

Unanswered questions

Predictive and prognostic biomarkers

There are at present no validated biomarkers to identify subgroups of patients who will derive particular benefit from adjuvant treatment. A treatment decision-making process based on the analysis of biomarkers of response and resistance to cytotoxic drugs would be quite valuable, ensuring that patients likely to benefit from adjuvant chemotherapy receive appropriate therapy and sparing toxicity for those unlikely to benefit. A number of studies have attempted to identify predictive or prognostic biomarkers. Common molecular changes such as *p53* mutations, p53 protein expression, or *KRAS* mutations have not proven to have a consistent prognostic or a predictive value in published adjuvant trials [8, 28–30].

The excision repair cross-complementation group 1 (ERCC1) enzyme, which plays a critical role in the nucleotide excision repair pathway, has been extensively studied as a marker of chemoresistance. In an analysis of ERCC1 protein expression in 761 tumors from IALT, cisplatin-based chemotherapy significantly prolonged survival among patients with ERCC1-negative tumors (56% of the cases, HR = 0.65 [0.50–0.86], p = 0.002) while in patients with ERCC1-positive tumors, adjuvant chemotherapy had no effect (HR = 1.14 [0.84–1.55], p = 0.40) [31]. Measurement of ERCC1 is technically difficult, however, and other studies have shown inconsistent results [32].

A number of groups have used gene expression data to create risk prediction models; however, results are inconsistent between the studies and none have been prospectively validated [33–36]. Currently, the use of biomarkers for selection of adjuvant chemotherapy should be considered experimental and is best done within a clinical trial.

Use of targeted therapies with adjuvant chemotherapy

Targeted therapies are increasingly used in the treatment of metastatic non-small cell lung cancer. Epidermal growth factor receptor (EGFR) inhibitors erlotinib and gefitinib are active in NSCLC, especially in patients with activating *EGFR* mutations [37–39]. Several trials using these agents as adjuvant therapy were initiated. In the Canadian BR.19 study, 503 patients with resected stage IB to IIIA lung cancer were randomized to either gefitinib 250 mg PO daily or placebo. Patients could receive adjuvant radiation or chemotherapy at the discretion of the treating clinician. This study has been presented only in abstract form, but the preliminary results were not promising – there was a trend towards shorter disease free and overall survival with gefitinib treatment [40]. This trend towards shorter overall survival was also seen in the small subgroup of patients with *EGFR* mutations. The RADIANT trial is a phase III trial randomizing patients with stage IB to IIIA resected NSCLC to either erlotinib 150 mg PO daily or placebo. Eligible patients must have EGFR-positive tumors, either by immunohistochemistry or FISH. Accrual to this study has been completed, though results have not yet been published. The SELECT trial is a single arm phase II study which is currently enrolling patients with *EGFR* mutant NSCLC. All patients will receive erlotinib 150 mg PO daily. Expected accrual is 100 patients.

Bevacizumab is an antivascular endothelial growth factor (VEGF) antibody. It has been approved for use in the front-line treatment of nonsquamous NSCLC, in combination with carboplatin and paclitaxel [41]. An ongoing Intergroup trial, E1505, is enrolling patients with resected stage IB to IIIA NSCLC of any histologic subtype. Patients will be randomized to either chemotherapy for four cycles or chemotherapy with bevacizumab for four cycles, followed by maintenance bevacizumab for one year. Planned accrual is 1500 patients.

Currently, there is no standard role for targeted therapies in the adjuvant treatment of lung cancer. These therapies should only be used in the context of a clinical trial.

Summary of recommendations

- Adjuvant chemotherapy with four cycles of a cisplatin-based regimen is the standard of care following surgical resection of stage II or IIIA non-small cell lung cancer in patients with good performance status.

- Adjuvant chemotherapy is not routinely recommended for patients with stage IA lung cancer.
- Patients with stage IB lung cancer with adverse features may benefit from adjuvant chemotherapy.
- The most studied adjuvant chemotherapy regimen is cisplatin with vinorelbine; however, cisplatin in combination with docetaxel, pemetrexed, or gemcitabine is also acceptable.
- Cisplatin-based regimens are preferred to carboplatin-based regimens, in the absence of contraindications.
- There are no proven biomarkers to predict for benefit from adjuvant chemotherapy.
- The role of targeted therapies in adjuvant treatment is under active investigation; however, these drugs are not the standard of care and should be used in the context of a clinical trial.

References

1 van Rens MT, de la Riviere AB, Elbers HR, van Den Bosch JM (2000) Prognostic assessment of 2,361 patients who underwent pulmonary resection for non-small cell lung cancer, stage I, II, and IIIA. *Chest*, Feb; 117(2): 374–9.

2 The Lung Cancer Study Group (1986) Effects of postoperative mediastinal radiation on completely resected stage II and stage III epidermoid cancer of the lung. The Lung Cancer Study Group. *N Engl J Med*, Nov 27; 315(22): 1377–81.

3 PORT Meta-analysis Trialists Group (1998) Postoperative radiotherapy in non-small-cell lung cancer: systematic review and meta-analysis of individual patient data from nine randomised controlled trials. PORT Meta-analysis Trialists Group. *Lancet*, Jul 25; 352(9124): 257–63.

4 International Multicentre Pooled Analysis of Colon Cancer Trial (IMPACT) Investigators (1995) Efficacy of adjuvant fluorouracil and folinic acid in colon cancer. International Multicentre Pooled Analysis of Colon Cancer Trials (IMPACT) investigators. *Lancet*, Apr 15; 345(8955): 939–44.

5 Early Breast Cancer Trialist's Collaborative Group (1992) Systemic treatment of early breast cancer by hormonal, cytotoxic, or immune therapy. 133 randomised trials involving 31,000 recurrences and 24,000 deaths among 75,000 women. Early Breast Cancer Trialists' Collaborative Group. *Lancet*, Jan 11; 339(8785): 71–85.

6 Non-small Cell Lung Cancer Collaborative Group (1995) Chemotherapy in non-small cell lung cancer: a meta-analysis using updated data on individual patients from 52 randomised clinical trials. *BMJ*, Oct 7; 311(7010): 899–909.

7 Tada H, Tsuchiya R, Ichinose Y, Koike T, Nishizawa N, Nagai K, *et al.* (2004) A randomized trial comparing adjuvant chemotherapy versus surgery alone for completely resected pN2 non-small cell lung cancer (JCOG9304). *Lung Cancer*, Feb; 43(2): 167–73.

8 Scagliotti GV, Fossati R, Torri V, Crino L, Giaccone G, Silvano G, *et al.* (2003) Randomized study of adjuvant chemotherapy for completely resected stage I, II, or IIIA non-small-cell Lung cancer. *J Natl Cancer Inst*, Oct 1; 95(19): 1453–61.

9 The International Adjuvant Lung Cancer Trial Collaborative Group (2004) Cisplatin-based adjuvant chemotherapy in patients with completely resected non-small-cell lung cancer. *N Engl J Med*, 350(4): 351–60.

10 Arriagada R, Dunant A, Pignon JP, Bergman B, Chabowski M, Grunenwald D, *et al.* (2010) Long-term results of the international adjuvant lung cancer trial evaluating adjuvant Cisplatin-based chemotherapy in resected lung cancer. *J Clin Oncol*, Jan 1; 28(1): 35–42.

11 Waller D, Peake MD, Stephens RJ, Gower NH, Milroy R, Parmar MK, *et al.* (2004) Chemotherapy for patients with non-small cell lung cancer: the surgical setting of the Big Lung Trial. *Eur J Cardiothorac Surg*, Jul; 26(1): 173–82.

12 Winton T, Livingston R, Johnson D, Rigas J, Johnston M, Butts C, *et al.* (2005) Vinorelbine plus cisplatin vs. observation in resected non-small-cell lung cancer. *N Engl J Med*, Jun 23; 352(25): 2589–97.

13 Butts CA, Ding K, Seymour L, Twumasi-Ankrah P, Graham B, Gandara D, *et al.* (2010) Randomized phase III trial of vinorelbine plus cisplatin compared with observation in completely resected stage IB and II non-small-cell lung cancer: updated survival analysis of JBR-10. *J Clin Oncol*, Jan 1; 28(1): 29–34.

14 Douillard JY, Rosell R, De Lena M, Carpagnano F, Ramlau R, Gonzales-Larriba JL, *et al.* (2006) Adjuvant vinorelbine plus cisplatin versus observation in patients with completely resected stage IB-IIIA non-small-cell lung cancer (Adjuvant Navelbine International Trialist Association [ANITA]): a randomised controlled trial. *Lancet Oncol*, Sep; 7(9): 719–27.

15 Strauss GM, Herndon JE, 2nd, Maddaus MA, Johnstone DW, Johnson EA, Harpole DH, *et al.* (2008) Adjuvant paclitaxel plus carboplatin compared with observation in stage IB non-small-cell lung cancer:

CALGB 9633 with the Cancer and Leukemia Group B, Radiation Therapy Oncology Group, and North Central Cancer Treatment Group Study Groups. *J Clin Oncol*, Nov 1; 26(31): 5043–51.

16 Strauss GM, Herndon JE, Maddaus MA, Johnstone DW, Johnson EA, Watson DM, *et al.* (2004) Randomized clinical trial of adjuvant chemotherapy with paclitaxel and carboplatin following resection in stage IB non-small cell lung cancer: report of Cancer and Leukemia Group B (CALGB) protocol 9633. *J Clin Oncol*, ASCO Annual Meeting Proceedings, 2004; 22(14S): 7019.

17 Pignon JP, Tribodet H, Scagliotti GV, Douillard JY, Shepherd FA, Stephens RJ, *et al.* (2008) Lung adjuvant cisplatin evaluation: A pooled analysis by the LACE Collaborative Group. *J Clin Oncol*, Jul 20; 26(21): 3552–9.

18 Arriagada R, Auperin A, Burdett S, Higgins JP, Johnson DH, Le Chevalier T, *et al.* (2010) Adjuvant chemotherapy, with or without postoperative radiotherapy, in operable non-small-cell lung cancer: two meta-analyses of individual patient data. *Lancet*, Apr 10; 375(9722): 1267–77.

19 Siegel R, DeSantis C, Virgo K, Stein K, Mariotto A, Smith T, *et al.* (2012) Cancer treatment and survivorship statistics, 2012. *CA Cancer J Clin*, Jul–Aug; 62(4): 220–41.

20 Pepe C, Hasan B, Winton TL, Seymour L, Graham B, Livingston RB, *et al.* Adjuvant vinorelbine and cisplatin in elderly patients: National Cancer Institute of Canada and Intergroup Study JBR.10. *J Clin Oncol*, Apr 20; 25(12): 1553–61.

21 Fruh M, Rolland E, Pignon JP, Seymour L, Ding K, Tribodet H, *et al.* (2008) Pooled analysis of the effect of age on adjuvant cisplatin-based chemotherapy for completely resected non-small-cell lung cancer. *J Clin Oncol*, Jul 20; 26(21): 3573–81.

22 Wisnivesky JP, Smith CB, Packer S, Strauss GM, Lurslurchachai L, Federman A, *et al.* (2011) Survival and risk of adverse events in older patients receiving postoperative adjuvant chemotherapy for resected stages II-IIIA lung cancer: observational cohort study. *BMJ*, 343: d4013.

23 Schiller JH, Harrington D, Belani CP, Langer C, Sandler A, Krook J, *et al.* (2002) Comparison of four chemotherapy regimens for advanced non-small-cell lung cancer. *N Engl J Med*, 346(2): 92–8.

24 Ohe Y, Ohashi Y, Kubota K, Tamura T, Nakagawa K, Negoro S, *et al.* (2007) Randomized phase III study of cisplatin plus irinotecan versus carboplatin plus paclitaxel, cisplatin plus gemcitabine, and cisplatin plus vinorelbine for advanced non-small-cell lung cancer: Four-Arm Cooperative Study in Japan. *Ann Oncol*, Feb; 18(2): 317–23.

25 Ardizzoni A, Boni L, Tiseo M, Fossella FV, Schiller JH, Paesmans M, *et al.* (2007) Cisplatin- versus carboplatin-based chemotherapy in first-line treatment of advanced non-small-cell lung cancer: an individual patient data meta-analysis. *J Natl Cancer Inst*, Jun 6; 99(11): 847–57.

26 Fossella F, Pereira JR, von Pawel J, Pluzanska A, Gorbounova V, Kaukel E, *et al.* (2003) Randomized, multinational, phase III study of docetaxel plus platinum combinations versus vinorelbine plus cisplatin for advanced non-small-cell lung cancer: The TAX 326 study group. *J Clin Oncol*, Aug 15; 21(16): 3016–24.

27 Scagliotti GV, Parikh P, Von Pawel J, Biesma B, Vansteenkiste J, Manegold C, *et al.* (2008) Phase III study comparing cisplatin plus gemcitabine with cisplatin plus pemetrexed in chemotherapy-naive patients with advanced-stage non-small-cell lung cancer. *J Clin Oncol*, 26(21): 3543–51.

28 Schiller JH, Adak S, Feins RH, Keller SM, Fry WA, Livingston RB, *et al.* (2001) Lack of prognostic significance of p53 and K-ras mutations in primary resected non-small-cell lung cancer on E4592: A laboratory ancillary study on an eastern cooperative oncology group prospective randomized trial of postoperative adjuvant therapy. *J Clin Oncol*, Jan 15; 19(2): 448–57.

29 Tsao MS, Aviel-Ronen S, Ding K, Lau D, Liu N, Sakurada A, *et al.* (2007) Prognostic and predictive importance of p53 and RAS for adjuvant chemotherapy in non small-cell lung cancer. *J Clin Oncol*, Nov 20; 25(33): 5240–7.

30 Cuffe S, Bourredjem A, Graziano S, Pignon JP, Domerg C, Ezzalfani M, *et al.* (2012) A pooled exploratory analysis of the effect of tumor size and KRAS mutations on survival benefit from adjuvant platinum-based chemotherapy in node-negative non-small cell lung cancer. *J Thorac Oncol*, Jun; 7(6): 963–72.

31 Olaussen KA, Dunant A, Fouret P, Brambilla E, Andre F, Haddad V, *et al.* (2006) DNA repair by ERCC1 in non-small-cell lung cancer and cisplatin-based adjuvant chemotherapy. *N Engl J Med*, Sep 7; 355(10): 983–91.

32 Hubner RA, Riley RD, Billingham LJ, Popat S (2011) Excision repair cross-complementation group 1 (ERCC1) status and lung cancer outcomes: a meta-analysis of published studies and recommendations. *PLoS One*, 6(10): e25164.

33 Shedden K, Taylor JMG, Enkemann SA, Tsao M-S, Yeatman TJ, Gerald WL, *et al.* (2008) Gene expression-based survival prediction in lung adenocarcinoma: a multi-site, blinded validation study. *Nature Medicine,* 14(8): 822–7.

34 Gold KA, Lee JJ, Ping Y, Behrens C, Liu D, Lee HY, *et al.* (2011) Biologic risk model for recurrence in resected early-stage non-small cell lung cancer. *J Clin Oncol,* ASCO Annual Meeting Proceedings, 2011. 29(15s): 7053.

35 Zhu CQ, Ding K, Strumpf D, Weir BA, Meyerson M, Pennell N, *et al.* (2010) Prognostic and predictive gene signature for adjuvant chemotherapy in resected non-small-cell lung cancer. *J Clin Oncol,* Oct 10; 28(29): 4417–24.

36 Kratz JR, He J, Van Den Eeden SK, Zhu ZH, Gao W, Pham PT, *et al.* (2012) A practical molecular assay to predict survival in resected non-squamous, non-small-cell lung cancer: Development and international validation studies. *Lancet,* Mar 3; 379(9818): 823–32.

37 Shepherd FA, Pereira JR, Ciuleanu T, Tan EH, Hirsch V, Thongprasert S, *et al.* (2005) Erlotinib in previously treated non-small-cell lung cancer. *N Engl J Med,* 353(2): 123–32.

38 Lynch TJ, Bell DW, Sordella R, Gurubhagavatula S, Okimoto RA, Brannigan BW, *et al.* (2004) Activating mutations in the epidermal growth factor receptor underlying responsiveness of non-small-cell lung cancer to gefitinib. *N Engl J Med,* 350(21): 2129–39.

39 Mok TS, Wu Y-L, Thongprasert S, Yang CH, Chu D-T, Saijo N, *et al.* (2009) Gefitinib or carboplatin-paclitaxel in pulmonary adenocarcinoma. *N Engl J Med,* 361(10): 947–57.

40 Goss GD, Lorimer I, Tsao MS, O'Callaghan CJ, Ding K, Masters GA, *et al.* (2010) A phase III, randomized, double-blind, placebo-controlled trial of the epidermal growth factor receptor inhibitor gefitinib in completely resected stage IB-IIIA non-small cell lung cancer. *J Clin Oncol,* ASCO Annual Meeting Proceedings. 28(18s): LBA7005.

41 Sandler A, Gray R, Perry MC, Brahmer JR, Schiller JH, Dowlati A, *et al.* (2006) Paclitaxel-carboplatin alone or with bevacizumab for non-small-cell lung cancer. *N Engl J Med,* 355(24): 2542–50.

CHAPTER 19

Neoadjuvant Chemotherapy for Resectable Non-Small Cell Lung Cancer

Christopher G. Azzoli[1] *and Katherine M.W. Pisters*[2]

[1]Department of Medicine, Harvard Medical School, Massachusetts General Hospital, Boston, MA, USA

[2]Department of Thoracic/Head and Neck Medical Oncology, The University of Texas MD Anderson Cancer Center, Houston, TX, USA

Introduction

In 2012, approximately 226 160 new cases of lung cancer were diagnosed in the United States; and 160 340 patients died of lung cancer [1]. Lung cancer is the leading cause of cancer-related death in both men and women. Non-small cell lung cancer (NSCLC) accounts for nearly 90% of these cases [2]. Recently, screening heavy smokers with low-dose CT scan has been shown to reduce the risk of death from lung cancer by detecting lung cancers at an earlier stage [3]. However, widespread lung cancer screening has yet to be implemented, and the majority of patients with lung cancer continue to be diagnosed with advanced, incurable disease [4].

For patients with early-stage NSCLC, surgery offers the best hope for cure. However, despite successful surgery, rates of cancer recurrence and death at 5 years are as high as 27% for pathologic stage IA, 42% for pIB, 54% for pIIA, 64% for pIIB, 76% for pIIIA, and 91% for pIIIB [5]. Clinical, or pre-operative staging often underestimates the extent of disease, particularly if fluorodeoxyglucose positron emission tomography (FDG-PET) and mediastinoscopy are not used. The estimated survival rates for a given clinical stage are worse than the corresponding surgical/pathological stage (Table 19.1) [5]. Given the poor survival rates seen with surgery alone, investigators have studied adjuvant therapies, such as chemotherapy and thoracic irradiation, in an attempt to improve survival.

For many years, postoperative adjuvant chemotherapy was studied, and the majority of trials did not find a survival benefit. A meta-analysis examining the role of chemotherapy in the treatment of NSCLC was published in 1995 [6]. Part of this meta-analysis examined the role of postoperative chemotherapy compared to surgery alone. For regimens containing cisplatin, the pattern of results was consistent with most trials favoring chemotherapy. In meta-analysis, the overall hazard ratio (HR) was 0.87 with an absolute benefit from cisplatin-based chemotherapy of 5% at 5 years, however the results did not achieve statistical significance ($p = 0.08$). This prompted a number of large, randomized studies of postoperative adjuvant chemotherapy using cisplatin-based combination chemotherapy. By 2003, the first and largest of these trials was reported showing the benefit of postoperative chemotherapy in patients with

Lung Cancer, Fourth Edition. Edited by Jack A. Roth, Waun Ki Hong and Ritsuko U. Komaki.

Table 19.1 Five-year survival based on clinical and pathological staging for resected NSCLC [5]

Stage	TNM	Estimated 5-yr survival proportion (%)	
		Pathological staging	Clinical staging
IA	T1N0M0	73%	50%
IB	T2N0M0	58%	43%
IIA	T1N1M0	46%	36%
IIB	T2N1M0, T3N0M0	36%	25%
IIIA	T3N1M0, T1-3N2M0	24%	19%

Source: Goldstraw 2007 [5]. Reproduced with permission of Elsevier.

completely-resected NSCLC [7–10]. Postoperative chemotherapy has since become a standard of care for stage II-III NSCLC. Postoperative adjuvant chemotherapy is reviewed in detail in Chapter 18 (this volume).

The focus of this chapter will be the use of neoadjuvant, also known as pre-operative, or induction chemotherapy for patients with resectable NSCLC. For over 30 years, pre-operative approaches have been explored, inspired by the poor survival following surgical resection and, before 2003, a lack of evidence to support postoperative chemotherapy. Interest in neoadjuvant therapy was bolstered by data in the early 1990s showing that patients with locally advanced, unresectable NSCLC treated with chemotherapy prior to chest radiation had improved survival compared to patients treated with radiation alone [11, 12]. In addition, there are several theoretical advantages to giving chemotherapy prior to surgery. Administration of chemotherapy prior to surgery allows assessment of radiographic and pathologic tumor response to chemotherapy, earlier treatment of clinically undetectable micrometastatic disease, and improved drug delivery compared to post-operative adjuvant therapy [13, 14].

Despite early, intense interest, neoadjuvant chemotherapy remains investigational, except in patients with stage IIIA/N2 disease. This is due, primarily, to the historical timing of the phase III clinical trials of neoadjuvant chemotherapy. Postoperative/adjuvant therapy trials had a head start on large, randomized trials comparing neoadjuvant chemotherapy followed by surgery, versus surgery alone, in patients with earlier stages of NSCLC. As a result, most of the large neoadjuvant chemotherapy trials were closed early when the benefit of adjuvant chemotherapy was discovered [15–17]. In addition, there has yet to be a large enough trial to allow a meaningful comparison between postoperative, and pre-operative chemotherapy [14].

It took eight years (1995–2003) for prospective randomized trials to prove the hypothesis that postoperative cisplatin improves survival in patients with resected NSCLC. With advances in new drug development now occurring from year to year, resources to conduct clinical trials must focus on which drugs to give to which patients, with less concern for the peri-operative timing of that treatment. Over the same eight years, phase III clinical trials of pre-operative chemotherapy have demonstrated the neoadjuvant approach to be safe, and beneficial to patients.

This chapter will review these data, and make a case for the advantages of a neoadjuvant approach to more immediately treat micro-metastatic disease, improve drug delivery, and perhaps most importantly, provide surrogate efficacy endpoints, such as radiographic response, pathologic response, and downstaging, to provide a platform for more immediate integration of new chemotherapy drugs into the treatment of patients with resectable NSCLC.

Phase II trials in resectable stage III disease

Initial phase II trials evaluating pre-operative chemotherapy in stage III NSCLC were launched in the 1980s following reports from Memorial Sloan-Kettering Cancer Center (MSKCC) of the poor outcome of surgery alone in this patient subset [18]. Martini *et al.* demonstrated that patients with ipsilateral mediastinal lymph node involvement could have 5-year survival rates as high as 24% following complete resection, but that a subgroup of patients with bulky ipsilateral nodal involvement (mediastinal lymphadenopathy so large as to be apparent on chest X-ray, or causing splaying of the carina at bronchoscopy) had only an 8% survival at 3 years [18]. Based on these observations, a pre-operative regimen of mitomycin, vinca alkaloid (vindesine or vinblastine) and high-dose cisplatin (MVP) was administered to this poor risk, bulky N2 patient population. In a large phase II trial of 136 patients, the investigators at MSKCC found a radiographic major response rate of 77%, with 65% of patients undergoing complete surgical resection [19]. Pathologically, 14% achieved a complete response with no evidence of viable tumor in the resected surgical specimen. Median survival for the 136 patients was 19 months. Three-year survival was 41% in patients who were completely resected; an improvement over the historical experience of 8% for surgery alone.

A confirmatory phase II trial was conducted by investigators in Canada [20]. The Toronto group enrolled 65 mediastinoscopy-proven stage IIIA NSCLC patients and treated them with two cycles of preoperative mitomycin, vindesine and cisplatin, followed by thoracotomy and two further cycles of postoperative chemotherapy. The radiographic response rate to induction chemotherapy was 68%, and 54% had complete surgical resection. The median survival of the entire patient group was 18.6 months, with a 5-year survival of 29%, and 10-year survival of 22%.

A number of other phase II trials have been completed assessing the role of neoadjuvant chemotherapy, with or without radiation therapy, followed by surgery for stage III disease [21–24]. These trials have demonstrated that radiographic response rates from chemotherapy are significantly higher than observed in patients with stage IV NSCLC, that surgical resection is feasible following neoadjuvant therapy, and pathologic complete responses and downstaging are seen. In trials utilizing neoadjuvant chemotherapy alone, the pathologic complete response rate has been reported as high as 18%, while those using chemotherapy and radiation have been as high as 26% [20, 24]. Patients who have been found to have pathologic complete responses have been noteworthy for significantly prolonged survival. Another important finding of these trials was that radiographic response did not always correlate with pathological response, with both more, and less extensive disease found at surgery than would have been predicted radiographically. Finally, survival does not appear to be substantially different in studies using combined radiation and chemotherapy, as compared with those using neoadjuvant chemotherapy alone. Integration of radiation therapy before, and after surgical resection is reviewed in greater detail elsewhere in this book.

The United States cooperative groups attempted to conduct a randomized study to compare induction chemoradiation, with induction chemotherapy alone, in patients with resectable stage IIIA/N2 NSCLC (Radiation Therapy Oncology Group (RTOG) 0412/Southwest Oncology Group S0332). The study was open from 2005 to 2006, but was closed due to poor accrual. The investigators learned that physician and patient preferences were so strong in selecting an approach to this stage of disease that neither physicians, nor patients, were comfortable with random assignment. The use of pre-operative radiation therapy in multimodality approaches to resectable stage III NSCLC is discussed in detail elsewhere in this textbook.

More recent phase II investigations have examined newer chemotherapy agents in the neoadjuvant setting. Some of these trials have employed a two-drug regimen, while others have examined three-drug combinations. Some trials have focused only on stage IIIA/N2 patients, while others have allowed selected entry of stage IIIB patients. Although comparison of these phase II trials is hampered by differences in patient selection, and subsequent use of either surgery or thoracic radiation, there have been no striking differences between the two- and three-drug regimens, and old versus newer chemotherapy agents, to merit a randomized trial.

A summary of phase II trials focusing on patients with stage III NSCLC is presented in Table 19.2. Betticher and colleagues from Switzerland have studied docetaxel and cisplatin in stage IIIA/N2 NSCLC [23]. In this trial, 90 patients with potentially operable IIIA/N2 NSCLC were treated with

Table 19.2 Prospective phase II neoadjuvant trials for resectable stage III NSCLC

Study	Stage	Regimen	N	ORR (%)	R0 (%)	MST (mo)	1-YS (%)	Path CR (%)
Betticher *et al.* [23]	IIIA- N2	DP	90	66	48	33	65	19% /75 resected
Van Zandwijk *et al.* [25]	IIIA- N2	GP	47	70	NR	19	69	NR
Migliorino *et al.* [26]	IIIA-N2/IIIB	GP	70	57	41	15	67	3%
Garrido *et al.* [27]	IIIA/B	DGP	136	72	50	16	NR	NR
Esteban *et al.* [28]	IIIA/B	GPVn	62	65	NR	NR	NR	25%
		GP	66	61	NR	NR	NR	18%
Lorent *et al.* [29]	IIIA-N2	VdIP	131	54	47	24	(21% 5 yr)	5%
Cappuzzo *et al.* [30]	IIIA-N2/IIIB	GPacP	42	71	38	22	92	7%
De Marinis *et al.* [31]	IIIA-N2	GPacP	49	74	55	23	85	16%

DP, docetaxel, cisplatin; GP, gemcitabine, cisplatin; DGP, docetaxel, gemcitabine, cisplatin; GPVn, gemcitabine, cisplatin, vinorelbine; GPacP, gemcitabine, paclitaxel, cisplatin; NR, not reported; VdIP, vindesine, ifosfamide, cisplatin.

three cycles of cisplatin with docetaxel. Chemotherapy was well tolerated with 96% of patients completing all three cycles. The radiographic response rate was 66%, and 48% underwent complete resection. With mature follow-up, those patients who were completely resected had a median survival of 5.2 years (range 0.3–6.3 years). Multivariate analysis found that mediastinal lymph node downstaging and complete resection were independent predictors for long-term survival.

Van Zandwijk and colleagues have evaluated cisplatin and gemcitabine as a pre-operative therapy in stage IIIA/N2 NSCLC (EORTC 08955) [25]. Patients received induction chemotherapy (three cycles) before re-evaluation and randomization to surgery or radiotherapy as part of the randomized EORTC 08941 trial. The results of the EORTC 08941 trial are discussed elsewhere in this textbook in chapters which address the role of surgery and radiation therapy for stage III NSCLC. In EORTC 08955, radiographic responses were seen in 70% of the 47 eligible patients. Thirty-three (70%; 95% confidence interval, 55% to 83%) had objective responses. Mediastinal nodes were tumor-free after induction therapy in 53% of cases. Resections were considered complete in 71% of the patients who underwent thoracotomy after induction therapy.

Cisplatin plus gemcitabine induction in stage IIIA/N2 and selected IIIB NSCLC has also been evaluated by investigators from Italy [26]. In a phase II trial of 70 patients, radiographic response was seen in 57% of patients. Twenty-eight patients were able to undergo complete resection (41%), with pathologic complete response seen in two patients. With a median follow-up of 16 months, the median survival was 15 months.

A three-drug regimen of docetaxel, cisplatin, and gemcitabine has been evaluated by investigators in Spain [27]. Mediastinoscopy-proven N2 (IIIA) or T4N0–1 (IIIB) disease was required. Among 129 patients assessable for response, the radiologic response rate was 56%. The overall complete resection rate was 69% of patients eligible for surgery (72% of stage IIIA patients and 66% of stage IIIB patients) and 48% of all assessable patients. Eight (12.9%) of 62 completely resected patients had a pathologic complete response. The median overall survival time was 16 months, 3-year survival rate was 37%, and 5-year survival rate was 21%, with no significant differences in survival between stage IIIA and stage IIIB patients. Median survival time was 48 months for 62 completely resected patients, 13 months for 13 incompletely resected patients, and 17 months for 15 nonresected patients ($P = 0.005$). Five-year survival rates were 41% for completely resected patients, 11% for incompletely resected patients, and 0% for nonresected patients. In the multivariate analysis, complete resection (hazard ratio [HR] = 0.35; $P < 0.0001$), clinical response (HR = 0.32; $P < 0.0001$), and age younger than 60 years (HR = 0.64; $P = 0.027$) were the most powerful prognostic factors.

Another group in Spain has studied cisplatin plus gemcitabine, with or without vinorelbine, as induction therapy in stage III NSCLC [28]. In this study of 154 patients, there was no difference in radiographic response between the two- and three-drug regimens (65% versus 61%, respectively). Hematologic toxicity and fatigue were slightly more frequent with the three-drug regimen, but this difference was not statistically significant. Most patients in both groups received radiotherapy as part of their local treatment. Of those resected, pathological complete response was confirmed by surgery in 18% in the two-drug, and 25% in the three-drug group. Median progression-free survival was 368 days in the two-drug, and 322 days in the three-drug group indicating similar efficacy.

Three cycles of pre-operative vindesine, ifosfamide, and cisplatin were given to 131 patients with stage IIIA/N2 NSCLC by investigators in Belgium [29]. Radiographic response occurred in 54% and the median and 5-year survival rates for the entire patient group were 24 months and 21%, respectively. Seventy-five patients underwent surgery, with complete resection in 47%. Although survival in the entire cohort appeared to correlate with response following chemotherapy, this effect was not seen in patients who underwent complete resection. Resection rates were lower in the subgroup of patients with stable disease; however, the authors emphasized that long-term survival following complete resection was seen in some patients who did not have major radiographic response.

Gemcitabine, paclitaxel, and cisplatin have also been studied as an induction regimen. In one study, this three-drug regimen was given to 42 patients with stage IIIA/N2 and IIIB NSCLC [30]. Major radiographic response was seen in 71%, and 21 patients underwent thoracotomy with 16 complete resections (38%). Pathologic complete responses were seen in 7%. With short median follow-up (14 mo), the median survival was 22 months. This same regimen was studied as an induction treatment in 49 patients with stage IIIA/N2 disease [31]. In this cohort of 49 patients, 74% achieved radiographic response, and 55% were completely resected. In this small study, 8/49 (16%) had pathologic complete response at surgery. With a median follow-up of 15.6 months, the median overall survival was 23 months.

Phase II trials in earlier stage disease

After the use of induction chemotherapy appeared promising in stage III NSCLC, clinical trials were designed and conducted which examined this approach in earlier stages of NSCLC. These trials are summarized in Table 19.3. The first such study was the Bimodality Lung Oncology Team trial (BLOT) [13]. This phase II trial enrolled two sequential cohorts of patients with clinical stage IB, II, and IIIA disease. Clinical staging was defined by CT imaging and all patients were required to undergo mediastinoscopy. PET imaging was not routinely performed in this study. Patients with mediastinoscopy-proven N2 disease or superior sulcus tumors were excluded from this trial. Patients were treated with carboplatin plus paclitaxel before

Table 19.3 Prospective phase II neoadjuvant trials in patients with earlier stages of resectable NSCLC

Study	Stage	Regimen	N	ORR (%)	R0 (%)	OS (%) Year	Path CR (%)
Pisters *et al.* [13]	IB-IIIA	PacCb	134	51	86	(42) 5	5
Kunitoh *et al.* [32]	IB-II	DP	40	45	95	NR	5
		D	39	15	85	NR	0
Abratt *et al.* [33]	IB-IIIA	PacGCb	44	75	82	NR	11
Ramnath *et al.* [34]	IB-III	GVn	62	34	77	(65) 2	3

DP, docetaxel, cisplatin; D, docetaxel; GVn, gemcitabine, vinorelbine; NR, not reported; PacCb, paclitaxel, carboplatin; PacGCb, paclitaxel, gemcitabine, carboplatin.

and after surgery (number of cycles in cohort I: 2 pre and 3 post; cohort II: 3 pre and 4 post). For the two cohorts combined, the radiographic response rate was 51%, complete resection rate was 86%, and pathologic complete response rate was 5%. Three- and five-year survival rates were 61 and 42%, respectively. There were no significant differences in patient characteristics or outcome between the two cohorts. Based on this encouraging data, a randomized phase III trial was initiated (S9900) with results discussed below.

Induction docetaxel and cisplatin has been compared to docetaxel alone in a randomized phase II trial from the Japan Clinical Oncology Group [32]. This study of 80 clinical stage IB and II NSCLC patients found improved results with the doublet. Pathologic complete response was observed in two patients treated with docetaxel-cisplatin, and radiologic response was superior to docetaxel (45 vs 15%). Disease-free survival at 1, 2, and 4 years were 78%, 65%, and 57% with two drugs, and 62%, 44%, and 36% with single-agent therapy.

A three-drug regimen, gemcitabine/carboplatin/paclitaxel was tested in patients with operable stage IB, II, or IIIA [33]. Each 21-day cycle consisted of gemcitabine 1000 mg/m^2 on days 1 and 8, carboplatin AUC 5 on day 1, and paclitaxel 175 mg/m^2 on day 1. Forty-four patients were enrolled with a radiologic response rate of 76%. Thirty-six patients had a complete tumor resection, five of whom had a complete pathological response with no viable tumor cells in the resected tumor on histological examination. The 1-year survival rate was 86%. The authors concluded that a cytotoxic triplet was both safe and effective as neoadjuvant chemotherapy in patients with operable NSCLC.

A nonplatinum regimen of gemcitabine and vinorelbine for two preoperative cycles was given to clinical stage IB-III NSCLC [34]. This study enrolled 62 patients. Although the radiographic response rate was low at 34%, 77% underwent complete resection, and 3% had pathologic complete response. The 1-year and 2-year overall survival rates were 80% and 65%, and the median overall survival was 38 months. These results using a nonplatinum regimen showed similar survival rates comparable to those obtained with platinum-containing doublets, but lower rates of radiographic and pathologic response rates compared with platinum-containing chemotherapy doublets.

Randomized phase II and phase III trials

Following the initial encouraging phase II reports of neoadjuvant chemotherapy, randomized trials were undertaken comparing neoadjuvant chemotherapy and surgery, to surgery alone. These trials are summarized in Table 19.4. These neoadjuvant chemotherapy trials were designed and launched before 2003, when the first positive results from individual studies of post-operative adjuvant chemotherapy were reported. After 2003, it was no longer reasonable to randomize patients with stage II-III NSCLC to surgery alone, and many of the larger studies which included stage I–III patients closed early with too small of a sample size to provide significant statistical comparisons.

Nevertheless, the earliest trials which were designed exclusively for patient with stage III NSCLC were able to demonstrate the benefit of neoadjuvant chemotherapy with surprisingly small sample sizes. Roth and colleagues conducted a phase III randomized trial of peri-operative chemotherapy with cyclophosphamide, etoposide, and cisplatin followed by surgery compared to a control arm of surgery alone in potentially resectable clinical stage IIIA NSCLC [35]. Patients randomized to chemotherapy were to receive three cycles of chemotherapy before surgery; and an additional three cycles were given after surgery to patients with pre-operative radiographic response. Following an interim analysis, the trial was closed after 60 patients had been accrued because of a clinically meaningful survival benefit in favor of the neoadjuvant chemotherapy arm. Long-term follow-up of this trial after a median time from randomization of 82 months confirmed the beneficial effect of neoadjuvant chemotherapy. Median and 5-year survival rates were 21 months and 36% versus 14 months and 15% for surgery alone.

Table 19.4 Randomized trials of neoadjuvant chemotherapy in operable NSCLC

Study	Stage	Regimen	N	ORR (%)	R0 (%)	MST (mo)	1YS (%)	Path CR (%)
Roth [35]	IIIA	CEP	28	35	39	21	36	0
		Control	32		31	14	15	
Rosell [36]	IIIA	MIP	30	60	77	22	17	3
		Control	30		90	10	0	
Pass [37]	IIIA/N2	EP	13	62	85	29	46 (2 yr)	8
		Control	14		86	16	21 (2 yr)	
Zhou [38]	III	Varied	414	73	94	NR	34	15
		Control	310		92	NR	24	
Nagai [39]	IIIA/N2	VdP	31	28	65	17	10	NR
		Surgery	31		77	16	22	
DePierre [41]	IB, II, IIIA	MIP	179	64	92	37	41	11
		Surgery	176		86	26	32	
Sorensen [43]	IB, II, IIIA	PacCb	44	46	79	34	36	NR
		Surgery	46		70	23	24	
Pisters [15]	IB, II, IIIA	PacCb	168	41	94	47	69 (2 yr)	NR
		Surgery	167		89	40	63 (2 yr)	
Gilligan [16]	IA – IIIB	P/Cb-based	258	49	82	54	75	4
		Surgery	261		80	55	75	1*
Scagliotti [17]	IB, II, IIIA	GP	129	35	88	94	68 (3 yr)	5
		Surgery	141		84	58	60 (3 yr)	1*
Felip [14]	IA(>2 cm),	PacCb pre	201	53	87	NR	47 (5 yr)	10.5
	IB, II,	PacCb post	211		90	NR	46 (5 yr)	
	IIIA(T3N1)	Surgery	212		90	NR	44 (5 yr)	

CEP, cyclophosphamide, etoposide, cisplatin; DP, docetaxel, cisplatin; EP, etoposide, cisplatin; GP, gemcitabine, cisplatin; MIP, mitomycin, ifosfamide, cisplatin; NR, not reported; PacCb, paclitaxel, carboplatin; P/Cb-based, cisplatin/carboplatin based; VdP, vindesine, cisplatin.

*2 trials reported 1 patient each with pathologic stage T0N0 in the surgery alone arm.

A similar phase III trial was conducted by Rosell and colleagues from Barcelona [36]. In this study, clinical stage IIIA NSCLC patients were randomized to immediate surgery or surgery preceded by three cycles of mitomycin, ifosfamide, and cisplatin chemotherapy. Both treatment groups received postoperative mediastinal radiation therapy to 50 Gy. Interim analysis after 24 months follow-up with 60 eligible patients showed a significant difference in survival favoring induction chemotherapy, and enrollment was stopped. Reassessment with 7-year follow-up found median and 5-year survival rates of 22 months and 17% in the chemotherapy arm, compared to 10 months and 0% in the surgery alone arm.

Another phase III randomized study of induction chemotherapy was conducted at the National Cancer Institute [37]. This trial randomized stage IIIA/N2 patients to receive two cycles of cisplatin plus etoposide chemotherapy prior to surgery (and four postoperative cycles if evidence of radiographic response) or surgery followed by 54–60 Gy of mediastinal radiation. After 4 years of accrual only 27 patients had agreed to participate. An interim analysis published in 1992 found a trend toward improved survival in the chemotherapy arm of the study, with median survivals of 29 versus 16 months, $p = 0.095$.

A large randomized trial of neoadjuvant chemotherapy in stage III NSCLC from China has been reported in abstract [38]. This study randomized 724 patients over a 12-year period to preoperative chemotherapy or a control group of surgery alone. Of the 414 patients assigned to two cycles of chemotherapy, 21 had bronchial artery interventional chemotherapy (details not reported).

The other 393 patients were given intravenous chemotherapy (130 patients cisplatin plus gemcitabine, 68 mitomycin, vinca alkaloid, cisplatin, 67 cisplatin and etoposide, 36 cyclophosphamide, doxorubicin, cisplatin, 32 vindesine, cisplatin, 30 paclitaxel, vinorelbine, and 30 paclitaxel, cisplatin). Response to induction chemotherapy was reported for 73% of patients with pathologic complete responses seen in 15%. Complete resection rates were 94% in the chemotherapy arm and 92% in the surgery group. No significant differences in operative complications or mortality were reported. Five- and ten-year survival rates were 34% and 29% versus 24% and 22%, $p < 0.01$. The response, resection, survival, and pathologic complete response rates are higher than what has been reported in other trials, and there was marked variation in induction regimen.

Nagai and colleagues from the Lung Cancer Surgical Study Group of the Japan Clinical Oncology Group have published their experience of a phase III randomized trial in stage IIIA/N2 NSCLC [39]. The trial was designed to accrue 200 patients over a 3-year period. However, the trial was closed secondary to slow accrual after only 62 patients had entered in 5 years. The authors cited lack of rewarding compensation to the patients, prolonged hospitalization in the induction chemotherapy group, and wide reports in the domestic media of the ineffectiveness of chemotherapy for NSCLC as the major reasons for poor accrual. With a median follow-up of 6.2 years, there was no difference in survival between the two arms in terms of median or 5-year survival rates (17 mo and 10% versus 16 mo and 22% in the surgery alone arm).

As for earlier stages of NSCLC (i.e., without mediastinal lymph node involvement), the first report of a randomized neoadjuvant chemotherapy trial came from the Royal Brompton Hospital in London, England [40]. This feasibility study was performed in 22 patients with early stage (IB, II, and IIIA) resectable NSCLC. Patients were randomized to either three cycles of mitomycin, vinblastine, and cisplatin chemotherapy followed by surgery ($n = 11$), or to surgery alone ($n = 11$). Of 40 patients who were potentially eligible for the study, 22 agreed to participate. Patients assigned to chemotherapy tolerated treatment well and did not have increased operative morbidity or mortality. Based on this limited experience, the authors recommended a large, multicenter phase III trial in all patients with operable NSCLC and supported accrual to the Medical Research Council Lung Group trial the UK Big Lung Trial.

In 2002, the results of a phase III randomized trial of induction mitomycin, ifosfamide, and cisplatin chemotherapy in resectable stage IB, II and IIIA were reported [41]; 355 eligible patients were randomized to surgery alone or combined modality therapy with two cycles of chemotherapy followed by surgery. Responding patients (radiographically or pathologically) received two additional cycles of chemotherapy postoperatively. The arms were well balanced for patient characteristics with the exception that fewer clinical N2 patients were assigned to the surgery-only arm (28% versus 40%, $p = 0.65$). A nonsignificant excess of postoperative morbidity in the chemotherapy arm was seen (24/167 versus 22/171). Postoperative mortality was 6.7% in the chemotherapy arm and 4.5% in the surgery arm ($p = 0.38$). Median survival was improved by 11 months (37 versus 26 months) and at 4 years, there was an 8.6% increase in survival in the chemotherapy arm, but this did not achieve statistical significance. In a subset analysis, the benefit of chemotherapy was confined to patients with N0 to N1 disease with a relative risk of death of 0.68, $p = 0.027$. After a nonsignificant excess of deaths in the combined modality arm during the treatment period, the effect of induction chemotherapy was favorable on survival. No difference was seen in local recurrence rates. A significant decrease in distant metastases was observed favoring the chemotherapy arm with a relative risk of 0.54, $p = 0.01$. Follow-up data on this trial was presented in 2003, when minimal follow-up exceeded 60 months [42]. The 3- to 5-year survival differences were stable around 10% ($p = 0.04$ at 3 years and $p = 0.06$ at 5 years). Statistically significant benefits in the N0–1 subgroup were confirmed with 5-year survival rates of 49% compared to 34% ($p = 0.02$).

The Scandinavians have reported their randomized trial of neoadjuvant carboplatin plus paclitaxel chemotherapy in clinical stage IB, II, and IIIA (excluding N2 patients) [43]. The study was closed prematurely secondary to slow accrual (90 patients in 6 years). Of the 44 patients randomized to chemotherapy, major radiographic responses were seen in 46%, and 79% had complete resection. In the 46 patients treated with surgery alone, complete resection was achieved in 70%. Median and 5-year survival rates were 34 months and 36% compared to 23 months and 24% in the control arm, a difference which was not statistically significant.

The Southwest Oncology Group trial, S9900, was a phase III randomized study comparing induction carboplatin and paclitaxel for three cycles followed by surgery to surgery alone in clinical stage IB, II, and IIIA NSCLC (excluding superior sulcus and N2 disease) [15]. The study called for 600 patients to detect a 33% increase in median survival or 10% increase in 5-year survival. Accrual to this trial was suspended after data from randomized adjuvant chemotherapy trials in completely-resected NSCLC revealed a survival benefit. Total accrual reached only 354 patients. Patient characteristics were well balanced between the two groups. Of the patients randomized to chemotherapy, 41% had radiographic response, 94% had complete resection, and no unexpected toxicity was observed. The median OS was 41 months in the surgery-only arm and 62 months in the pre-operative chemotherapy arm (HR = 0.79; 95% CI, 0.60 to 1.06; p = 0.11). The median PFS was 20 months for surgery alone and 33 months for pre-operative chemotherapy (HR = 0.80; 95% CI, 0.61 to 1.04; p = 0.10).

A multicenter randomized trial in Europe sponsored by the United Kingdom Medical Research Council, and the European Organization for Research and Treatment of Cancer (LU22/NVALT 2/EORTC 08012) randomized 519 patients with resectable stage I–III NSCLC to receive either surgery alone, or three cycles of platinum-based chemotherapy followed by surgery [16]. Before randomization, clinicians chose the chemotherapy that would be given from a list of six standard regimens, four of which contained cisplatin, and two carboplatin (with either paclitaxel or docetaxel). Most patients (61%) were clinical stage I, including 17% stage IA, and only 7% stage III. Most patients assigned to chemotherapy (75%) received all three cycles, with a response rate of 49%, and down-staging in 31%. Clinicians favored cisplatin regimens over carboplatin regimens (78% cisplatin, 12% carboplatin). Rates of successful surgery were identical between the two arms (lobectomy: 56%/60%, complete resection: 80%/82%, for surgery alone/chemotherapy). Postoperative complications were not increased in the chemotherapy group, and no impairment of quality of life was observed. In the final analysis, there was no evidence of a benefit in terms of PFS (HR = 0.96, 95% CI 0.77–1.21, p = 0.74), or OS (HR = 1.02, 95% CI 0.80–1.31, p = 0.86).

In contrast to the lack of efficacy observed in LU22/NVALT 2/EORTC 08012, an independent European trial completed in parallel was more promising. The Ch.E.S.T. (Chemotherapy in Early Stages in NSCLC Trial) was a phase III randomized trial which compared three cycles of neoadjuvant cisplatin plus gemcitabine followed by surgery, to surgery alone [17]. The primary endpoint of this study was progression-free survival, and the original study design required 700 randomized patients. Similar to the S9900 study, the Ch.E.S.T. trial was closed to patient accrual at 270 patients following the results of the positive adjuvant trials. In contrast to LU22, Ch.E.S.T. enrolled only patients stage IB-IIIA, and only 47% of patients had stage IB. Slightly more patients in the surgery alone arm had disease stage IB/IIA (55% v 49%). The chemotherapy response rate was 35%. The hazard ratios for PFS and OS were 0.70 (95% CI, 0.50 to 0.97; p = 0.003) and 0.63 (95% CI, 0.43 to 0.92; p = 0.02), respectively, both in favor of chemotherapy plus surgery. The greatest benefit was observed in the stage IIB/IIIA subgroup (3-year PFS rate: 36.1% v 55.4%; p = 0.002). There were no unexpected toxicities observed.

The NATCH trial (Neoadjuvant vs. Adjuvant Carbo Taxol Hope) was a three-arm trial which directly compared pre-operative chemotherapy plus surgery, postoperative chemotherapy plus surgery, and surgery alone in patients with earlier stages of resectable NSCLC [14]. Six hundred and twenty-four patients with stage IA (tumor size > 2 cm), IB, II, or T3N1 were randomly assigned to surgery alone, three cycles of pre-operative carboplatin and paclitaxel followed by surgery, or surgery followed by three cycles of postoperative carboplatin and paclitaxel. The primary endpoint was disease-free survival (DFS). In the pre-operative arm, 97% of patients started the planned chemotherapy, and radiologic response rate was 53%. In the adjuvant arm, 66% started the planned chemotherapy. Ninety four percent of patients underwent surgery; surgical procedures and postoperative mortality were similar across the three arms. Patients in the pre-operative arm had a nonsignificant trend toward longer disease-free survival than those assigned to surgery alone (5-year disease-free survival 38% v 34%; HR = 0.92; p = 0.176). Five-year disease-free survival rates were 37% in the adjuvant arm versus 34% in the surgery arm (HR = 0.96; p = 0.74). Although the NATCH study found no statistically significant differences in disease-free survival with these approaches, trends favored the neoadjuvant approach, and more patients were able to receive pre-operative than adjuvant treatment.

Meta-analyses of neoadjuvant chemotherapy

Given there are both negative, and positive individual studies testing neoadjuvant chemotherapy plus surgery versus surgery alone, and the preponderance of studies which closed early or were underpowered to detect the benefit of neoadjuvant chemotherapy, meta-analyses regarding this approach are of special importance. To date, there have been four meta-analyses examining the efficacy of induction chemotherapy in resectable NSCLC, all of them generated from summary statistics, and not from individual patient data [16, 44–46]. The results of these meta-analyses are summarized in Table 19.5.

The first meta-analysis by Berghmans *et al.* looked at both induction and adjuvant randomized studies reported between 1965 and June 2004 [44]. They found an HR of 0.66 (95% CI, 0.48–0.93) for the addition of induction chemotherapy and an HR of 0.84 (95% CI, 0.78–0.89) for the addition of adjuvant (postoperative chemotherapy). The randomized neoadjuvant trials included in this meta-analysis are a subset of those reviewed above, and included six trials enrolling 590 patients. When examining the effect of induction chemotherapy in the subgroup of patients with clinical stage III NSCLC, the HR became 0.65 (95% CI, 0.41–1.04) and although strongly trended in favor of the use of chemotherapy in stage III disease, did not achieve statistical significance.

A second meta-analysis was conducted by Burdett *et al.* and was also based on data extracted from abstracts and manuscripts from randomized trials [45]. Literature searches identified 12 eligible

Table 19.5 Meta-analyses of randomized trials of neoadjuvant chemotherapy in operable NSCLC

	Berghmans [44]	Burdett [45]	Gilligan [16]	Song [46]
Number of trials	**6**	**7**	**8**	**13**
Number of patients	**590**	**988**	**1507**	**3224**
Hazard ratio	**0.66 (0.48–0.93)**	**0.82 (0.69–0.97)**	**0.88 (0.76–1.01)**	**0.84 (0.77–0.92)**
Trials included	Dautzenberg [73]	Dautzenberg [73]	Dautzenberg [73]	Dautzenberg [73]
	Rosell [36]	Rosell [36]	Rosell [36]	Rosell [36]
	Roth [35]	Roth [35]	Roth [35]	Roth [35]
	Depierre [41]	Depierre [41]	Depierre [41]	Depierre [41]
	Nagai [39]	Nagai [39]	Nagai [39]	Nagai [39]
	Pass [37]	Sorensen [43]	Sorensen [43]	Sorensen [43]
		Pisters [13]	Pisters [13]	Pisters [13]
			Gilligan [16]	Gilligan [16]
				Zhou [38]
				Liao [74]
				Li [75]
				Yao [76]
				Scagliotti [17]

randomized controlled trials. Five of these trials were excluded as insufficient data could be extracted from the published results. The remaining seven trials on which the meta-analysis is based included 988 patients. The authors found that pre-operative chemotherapy improved survival with an HR of 0.82 (0.69–0.97, p = 0.02). This is equivalent to an absolute benefit of 6% at 5 years. An analysis grouping trials according to the type of chemotherapy administered was also performed. All patients received a platinum-based chemotherapy – either cisplatin or carboplatin – that was combined with other agents. These other agents were split into the three groups: vinca alkaloid/etoposide, taxane, or other. There was no clear evidence of a difference of treatment effect shown by chemotherapy group. The authors concluded that the meta-analysis suggests a significant survival benefit for patients with NSCLC who receive pre-operative chemotherapy compared to those who do not.

Given the negative result of the LU22/NVALT 2/ EORTC 08012 study, the authors of this study updated the meta-analysis by Burdett *et al.* and added their trial and re-estimated the HR using summary statistics. When the results of their trial were added to the Burdett meta-analysis, there was still a significant overall benefit observed for neoadjuvant chemotherapy (p = 0.07) with a hazard ratio of 0.88 (0.76–1.01), N = 1507.

The most recent meta-analysis is larger, but like the first three is not an individual patient data meta-analysis [46]. This study incorporated all of the studies that were considered by Burdett *et al.*, and added 6 new ones. The overall survival of NSCLC patients in the neoadjuvant chemotherapy arm was significantly better than in the surgery-alone arm (combined HR = 0.84; 95% confidence interval, 0.77–0.92; p = 0.0001), N = 3224. When only patients with stage III NSCLC were considered, the result was similar (combined HR = 0.84; 95% confidence interval, 0.75–0.95; p = 0.005).

Impact on surgical morbidity and mortality

A consistent, and reassuring finding in every randomized trial studying neoadjuvant chemotherapy, versus surgery alone, is that none of the studies discovered that pre-operative chemotherapy significantly affected the surgical plan of care, or increased surgical risk. As detailed above, several studies report identical rates of type of surgery (lobectomy versus pneumonectomy), complete resection, and similar rates of surgical morbidity and mortality, whether or not patients received pre-operative chemotherapy [14–17].

Independent retrospective studies have also addressed this issue. Siegenthaler *et al.* from M.D. Anderson Cancer Center (MDACC) reported on a series of 380 consecutive patients undergoing lobectomy or greater resection for NSCLC [47]. Following exclusion of 45 patients (history of prior lung cancer, prior radiation or chemoradiation to the chest, prior malignancy etc.), a population of 335 patients (259 surgery alone, 76 chemotherapy followed by surgery) was studied from the MDACC Thoracic Surgery database. The use of pre-operative chemotherapy did not significantly affect morbidity or mortality overall, based on clinical stage, postoperative stage, or extent of resection. No significant differences in overall or subset mortality or morbidity including pneumonia, acute respiratory distress syndrome, reintubation, tracheostomy, wound complication, or length of hospitalization were seen.

All patients undergoing thoracotomy after induction chemotherapy from 1993 through 1999 at MSKCC were the subject of a review [48]. Four hundred and seventy patients treated with induction chemotherapy and surgery were reviewed. Univariate and multivariate methods for logistic regression model were used to identify predictors of adverse events. Overall, the MSKCC group found a surgical mortality rate of 3.8%, which compared favorably to other primary surgery studies. Total morbidity and major complication rates were 38% and 27%; similar to previous primary surgery studies. The authors concluded that overall morbidity rates were not significantly affected by the use of induction therapy. Of note, they reported a high operative mortality rate of 24% for patients undergoing right pneumonectomy following induction therapy. This number was higher than previous mortality rates seen in trials where patients did not have induction therapy. The authors recommended that right pneumonectomy after induction therapy be performed very selectively, and only when no alternative resection is possible.

A third series from investigators in France reviewed 114 patients who underwent thoracotomy following induction chemotherapy [49]. In this series, there was only 1 death following pneumonectomy in 55 patients. Overall morbidity rate was 29%, similar to other surgical series. The authors concluded that preoperative chemotherapy did not increase postoperative morbidity and mortality.

Surrogate efficacy endpoints in neoadjuvant trials

One of the advantages of a neoadjuvant approach to chemotherapy is that it provides an experimental platform for testing new drugs, otherwise available only to patients with stage IV disease, in the care of patients with earlier stages of NSCLC. When patients receive chemotherapy prior to surgery, efficacy may be measured using a variety of surrogate efficacy endpoints, including radiographic response, pathologic response, and downstaging. These measures are immediately available to the clinician, and may predict future outcomes such as disease-free survival, and overall survival, which would otherwise take years to measure. In addition, observations made during neoadjuvant chemotherapy may, theoretically, be used to select patients for additional, or alternative postoperative therapies.

The question is not whether surrogate efficacy endpoints may be used in neoadjuvant clinical trials, but rather how best to use them. This is complicated by a lack of universal definitions of clinically meaningful radiographic response, FDG-PET response, or pathological response, in the neoadjuvant setting, or even in patients with stage IV disease [50–52]. In patients with stage IV NSCLC, radiographic response remains the most reliable, time-tested, and intuitive indicator that a new drug is effective, and therefore remains a popular measurement in neoadjuvant drug studies using standardized radiographic response criteria, like RECIST (Response Evaluation Criteria In Solid Tumors) [53, 54]. In contrast, methods or metrics for measuring pathologic response have not been standardized across clinical trials, although there have been attempts [55]. At the extreme, a complete pathologic response (path CR) means there is no viable cancer discovered at the time of surgery. Path CR is a fairly well-validated endpoint. A retrospective study of 492 patients treated with neoadjuvant chemotherapy in two consecutive neoadjuvant trials of platinum-based chemotherapy in France found a path CR rate of 8%, which reduced the risk of death by over 60% (RR = 0.34, 95% CI 0.18–0.64) [56]. However, rates of path CR in neoadjuvant drug trials are low (3–17%), and relying on this endpoint may miss efficacy indicated by a partial pathologic response [55].

In the NATCH study, which compared surgery alone vs. preoperative carboplatin and paclitaxel, vs. postoperative carboplatin and paclitaxel, the 5-year disease-free survival rates were 34% in the surgery alone arm, 38% in the pre-operative chemotherapy arm, and 37% in the postoperative chemotherapy arm [14]. Within the preoperative arm, the 5-year disease-free survival rate for the 106 patients achieving radiologic response was 51%, and the 5-year disease-free survival rate for the 19 patients with pathologic complete response was 59%. Statistical comparisons of these trends were not provided. Other phase III trials of neoadjuvant chemotherapy also did not report whether radiographic response by serial CT scan predicted survival among patients who received neoadjuvant therapy [15–17].

For patients with esophago-gastric carcinoma, serial FDG-PET scans are routinely used to assess the efficacy of neoadjuvant therapy [57]. Whether serial FDG-PET scans are useful during neoadjuvant therapy for resectable NSCLC is an area of active study. The major problem with FDG-PET is the lack of consistency in scanning protocols, standardized uptake value (SUV) measurement, and consensus regarding the best cutoff values for PET response. A recent review of the literature found 9 prospective studies, with wide ranges in sensitivity, specificity, positive predictive value, and negative predictive value, for PET to document clinical response or survival [58]. Pooling data for N2 restaging after neoadjuvant response, the overall sensitivity was 64% (95% CI, 53–74%) and overall specificity was 85% (95% CI, 80–89%). The authors concluded that FDG-PET is superior to CT for restaging after neoadjuvant therapy; however, unacceptably high rates of false-positive and false-negative results preclude the routine use of FDG-PET as the only reassessment tool for response to therapy [58]. CT scan, endoscopic ultrasound-guided aspiration biopsy or redo-mediastinoscopy should also be employed to verify response and down-staging, especially if the results would impact the surgical plan of care. In addition to FDG-PET, other new technologies, including serial diffusion-weighted MRI, and circulating tumor cells or other serially-measured blood biomarkers, may enhance the ability to measure the efficacy of novel therapies in the neoadjuvant setting [59, 60].

Whatever the biomarker, surrogate efficacy measures have never been as reliable as clinical stage, and/or pathologic stage, in predicting disease-free, and overall survival in patients with resectable NSCLC. When considering outcomes from clinical trials of novel agents used in the neoadjuvant setting, the stage admixture of patients enrolled is by far the most important factor to put the measured survival of the study population into context. Given the observed dramatic difference in outcomes between clinically staged, and pathologically staged patients (see Table 19.1), a major concern in neoadjuvant drug trials is ambiguous or inaccurate clinical stage at enrollment. Meticulous pre-operative staging, including FDG-PET, endobronchial ultrasound biopsy (to rule-in lymph node metastases), and mediastinoscopy (to rule-out lymph node metastases), are essential to avoid staging ambiguity in clinical research protocols, as well as routine clinical practice.

Despite these potential pitfalls, surrogate efficacy endpoints have been shown to predict overall survival in prospective studies of neoadjuvant therapy. Such observations are especially meaningful in stage-matched cohorts. For example, the phase II study by Betticher *et al.*, delivered neoadjuvant docetaxel and cisplatin exclusively to patients with resectable IIIA/N2 NSCLC confirmed by mediastinoscopy [61]. Among 75 patients who underwent successful surgery after chemotherapy, several factors were found to strongly correlate (i.e., predict) both overall survival, and disease-free survival, including complete (R0) resection, radiographic response, pathologic response, and mediastinal downstaging. These surrogate efficacy endpoints remain useful in ongoing neoadjuvant research protocols.

Window of opportunity trials

To date, the most important discovery in drug therapy for lung cancer is that oral inhibitors of the epidermal growth factor receptor (EGFR) tyrosine kinase are more effective than traditional chemotherapy for patients with stage IV NSCLC with activating/sensitizing *EGFR* mutations.[62] This topic is covered extensively in other chapters of this textbook. Patients with stage IV NSCLC who are never, or former light smokers, females, of Asian ethnicity, or adenocarcinoma histology, are more likely to have an activating/sensitizing *EGFR* mutation.

Soon after this discovery, a phase II study was initiated at MSKCC to determine if the efficacy of the EGFR TKI, gefitinib, could be detected in patients with early-stage NSCLC [63]. Patients with resectable stage I and II NSCLC with ≤ 15 pack-year cigarette smoking history received preoperative gefitinib for 21 days. Radiographic response during gefitinib was measured, and tumor specimens were analyzed for molecular markers. Fifty patients with stage I/II NSCLC were treated. After 21 days of preoperative gefitinib a response of 25% or more was observed in 21 of 50 (42%) patients. Seventeen of 21 patients with a response had an *EGFR* mutation and 4 of 21 patients with a response did not (P = 0.0001). Half of patients had either radiologic response to gefitinib, or had a detectable *EGFR* mutation, and went on to receive postoperative gefitinib. With a median follow-up of 44.1 months, the median disease free and overall survivals has not been reached, and 2-year disease free survival is not statistically different between clinically relevant subgroups (i.e., EGFR mutant/nonmutant, and adjuvant gefitinib subgroups). The authors concluded that neoadjuvant therapy provides a platform which may be used to evaluate the activity of new agents in the care of patients with early-stage NSCLC.

A separate phase II trial, performed in four hospitals in the Netherlands, enrolled 60 patients with early-stage, operable NSCLC to receive preoperative erlotinib for 3 weeks [64]. Response to treatment was evaluated using both fluorodeoxyglucose positron emission tomography (PET), computed tomography (CT) scans, and histologic examination of the resection specimen. PET evaluation revealed metabolic response (> 25% standardized uptake value decrease) in 16 patients (27%); CT evaluation showed CT response in three patients (5%), and pathologic examination showed more than 50% necrosis in 14 patients (23%), of whom three (5%) had more than 95% tumor necrosis. Evidence of clinical benefit based on radiographic or pathologic response was observed both in patients with, and without *EGFR* activating/sensitizing mutations. The authors concluded that the neoadjuvant platform was important for developing medical therapies in early-stage patients, especially when the therapy has apparent efficacy and low toxicity.

Another advance in the medical care of patients with stage IV NSCLC has been the development of bevacizumab, a mononclonal antibody directed against the angiogenic protein vascular endothelial growth factor (VEGF). Bevacizumab has been shown to improve overall survival in patients with stage IV, nonsquamous NSCLC when added to traditional chemotherapy [65]. The same group at MSKCC which studied gefitinib in the neoadjuvant setting tested the safety and efficacy of bevacizumab in early-stage patients by adding it to cisplatin/docetaxel neoadjvuant chemotherapy, and then offering it also after surgery to selected patients [66]. Another novel aspect of the study was to give single-agent bevacizumab with cycle 1, and assess radiologic response to bevacizumab alone. Due to concerns that an anti-angiogenic drug would impair wound healing, patients did not receive bevacizumab with their final cycle of neoadjuvant therapy to allow time for drug clearance prior to surgery. The primary endpoint of the study was the rate of pathological downstaging (decrease from pretreatment clinical stage to posttreatment pathological stage). Fifty patients were enrolled. Thirty-four (68%) were clinical stage IIIA. The primary endpoint, the rate of downstaging, was 38% (95% CI 23–53%). This did not meet the prespecified increase to 50% [66] (N.A. Rizvi, personal communicaton). Secondary endpoints, including radiologic response rate to chemotherapy (45%), and peri-operative complications (12%), were comparable to historical data. No partial responses were observed to single-agent bevacizumab but 18% developed new intratumoral cavitation with a trend toward improved pathologic response (57% vs. 21%, p = 0.07). A major pathologic response (≥90% treatment effect) was associated with survival at 3 years (100% vs. 49%, p = 0.01). No patients with KRAS-mutant NSCLC (0/10) had a pathologic response as compared with 11/31 with wild-type KRAS. The authors concluded that neoadjuvant chemotherapy with chemotherapy plus bevacizumab was not warranted in unselected patient populations.

Jones *et al.*, completed a phase 1 trial of neoadjuvant vorinostat (histone deacetylase inhibitor), plus bortezomib (proteasome inhibitor) followed by surgery in patients with resectable NSCLC [67]. Twenty-one patients were treated on study, and 20 underwent surgery on study. The maximum tolerated dose was bortezomib 1.3 mg/m^2 and vorinostat 300 mg twice daily. Thirty percent of patients (6 of 20) had more than 60% histologic necrosis of their tumor after treatment, with two having 90% or more tumor necrosis. Correlative laboratory studies included measurements of tumor metabolism, 20S proteasome activity, specific protein expression, and comparison of gene-expression arrays pre- and posttherapy. The authors concluded that pre-operative therapy with these targeted drugs was feasible, and may serve as a platform of discovery for the effect of these drugs on cell-signaling pathways.

Altorki *et al.* treated 29 patients with stages IB to IIIA NSCLC with two pre-operative cycles of paclitaxel and carboplatin, as well as daily celecoxib, followed by surgical resection [68]. The overall clinical response rate was 65% (48% with partial response; 17% with complete response). Grade 3 or 4 neutropenia was observed in 18 patients (62%). Twenty-eight patients were explored and underwent complete resection of their tumors. The addition of celecoxib to a regimen of paclitaxel and carboplatin abrogated the marked increase in levels of PGE2 detected in primary tumors after treatment with paclitaxel and carboplatin alone. The authors concluded that future combinations of chemotherapy and COX2 inhibitors was warranted, however a lack of activity of celecoxib in phase 3 trials in patients with stage IV NSCLC has dampened enthusiasm for simple inhibition of this pathway [69,70].

Another study by Altorki *et al.*, treated patients with early-stage, resectable NSCLC with the oral angiogenesis inhibitor, pazopanib [71]. Patients scheduled for resection received oral pazopanib 800 mg daily dose for 2 to 6 weeks preoperatively. Of 35 patients enrolled, 33 (94%) had clinical stage I NSCLC and two (6%) had clinical stage II NSCLC. Median treatment duration was 16 days (range, 3–29 days). Thirty patients (86%) achieved tumor-volume reduction on serial CT scan after pazopanib treatment. Two patients achieved tumor-volume reduction > or = 50%, and three patients had partial response according to Response Evaluation Criteria in Solid Tumors. Pazopanib was generally well tolerated with expected rates of hypertension, diarrhea, and fatigue. One patient developed pulmonary embolism 11 days after surgery. Several pazopanib target genes and other angiogenic factors were dysregulated posttreatment. Serial plasma cytokine analysis discovered that posttreatment changes in plasma sVEGFR2 and interleukin (IL)-4 significantly correlated with tumor shrinkage [72]. Baseline levels of IL-12, and several other cytokines, significantly correlated with tumor shrinkage. Using multivariate classification, a baseline signature consisting of hepatocyte growth factor and IL-12 was associated with tumor response to pazopanib and identified responding patients with 81% accuracy. The authors promised further clinical evaluation of pazopanib using a similar platform was warranted.

Conclusions

Pre-operative, neoadjuvant chemotherapy for patients with resectable NSCLC has been studied since the 1980s with numerous phase II and phase III trials published. No individual trial has demonstrated a statistically significant survival benefit for patients with resectable stage I-II NSCLC. The conduct of many of the phase III, randomized studies of neoadjuvant chemotherapy was cut short by the discovery of the survival benefit of postoperative adjuvant chemotherapy in 2003. Nevertheless, several basic facts have been established.

All prospective phase III trials have shown that neoadjuvant chemotherapy does not interfere with surgery, with the same rates of R0 resection, surgical morbidity and mortality observed in both arms of the study [14–17]. Single-modality, preoperative chemotherapy followed by surgery is a standard of care for patients with mediastinoscopy-proven resectable stage IIIA/N2 NSCLC [35, 36]. Whether patients with N2 disease should also receive pre-operative radiation therapy remains a matter of debate, and is the subject of other chapters in this textbook. With attention to the meta-analyses, the benefit of pre-operative chemotherapy appears to be similar to that observed with postoperative chemotherapy [46]. Similar to the data for postoperative therapy, the benefit of chemotherapy is more apparent in patients with stage II-III NSCLC. In the one, relatively small study which directly compared the pre-operative with the postoperative approach, efficacy trends favored neoadjuvant therapy and drug delivery was substantially better using a pre-operative approach.

Randomized trials comparing preoperative to postoperative chemotherapy are warranted. However, these protocols are difficult to accomplish. It has proven difficult for physicians and patients with strong opinions to subject themselves to random assignment of such disparate approaches to therapy. Some surgeons and patients want the lung cancer resected as soon as possible, with no delay in potentially curative treatment. Other clinicians are concerned enough about the high risk of lung cancer recurrence after surgery to refer their patients for pre-operative chemotherapy – especially in patients with larger tumors, or N1 disease proven by pre-operative endo-bronchial ultrasound (EBUS), where postoperative chemotherapy will most certainly be recommended.

Finally, and perhaps most importantly, neoadjuvant window-of-opportunity trials will serve as the best platform to test new drugs in patients with resectable NSCLC, using surrogate efficacy endpoints such as radiologic response, pathologic response, and downstaging. It took over 8 years and 4500 patients randomized to prove that postoperative cisplatin improves overall survival for patients with resected stage II-III NSCLC. With rapid advances in new drug development for patients with stage IV NSCLC now being observed from year to year, the unacceptably high rates of recurrence and death in patients with resectable NSCLC, and the anticipated increase in the number of patients with resectable NSCLC due to the advent of lung cancer screening, it is increasingly clear that oncologists must employ neoadjuvant platforms, along with biomarker development and flexible treatment strategies, to promote new drug development for patients with resectable NSCLC. It would be impossible to test all of the new, more effective drugs being discovered in head-to-head adjuvant trials. Fortunately, the evidence supports the neoadjuvant approach as a reasonable standard of care such that it may be boldly employed in this discovery effort.

References

1 Siegel R, Naishadham D, Jemal A (2012) Cancer statistics, 2012. *CA Cancer J Clin*, 62: 10–29.

2 Govindan R, Page N, Morgensztern D, *et al.* (2006) Changing epidemiology of small-cell lung cancer in the United States over the last 30 years: analysis of the surveillance, epidemiologic, and end results database. *J Clin Oncol*, 24: 4539–44.

3 Aberle DR, Adams AM, Berg CD, *et al.* (2011) Reduced lung-cancer mortality with low-dose computed tomographic screening. *N Engl J Med*, 365: 395–409.

4 Bach PB, Mirkin JN, Oliver TK, *et al.* (2012) Benefits and harms of CT screening for lung cancer: a systematic review. Jama 307: 2418–2429.

5 Goldstraw P, Crowley J, Chansky K, *et al.* (2007) The IASLC Lung Cancer Staging Project: Proposals for the revision of the TNM stage groupings in the forthcoming (seventh) edition of the TNM Classification of malignant tumours. *J Thorac Oncol*, 2: 706–14.

6 Chemotherapy in non-small cell lung cancer: A meta-analysis using updated data on individual patients from 52 randomised clinical trials. Non-small Cell Lung Cancer Collaborative Group. *BMJ*, 311: 899–909.

7 Arriagada R, Dunant A, Pignon JP, *et al.* (2010) Long-term results of the international adjuvant lung cancer trial evaluating adjuvant Cisplatin-based chemotherapy in resected lung cancer. *J Clin Oncol*, 28: 35–42.

8 Winton T, Livingston R, Johnson D, *et al.* (2005) Vinorelbine plus cisplatin vs. observation in resected non-small-cell lung cancer. *N Engl J Med*, 352: 2589–97.

9 Douillard JY, Rosell R, De Lena M, *et al.* (2006) Adjuvant vinorelbine plus cisplatin versus observation in patients with completely resected stage IB-IIIA non-small-cell lung cancer (Adjuvant Navelbine International Trialist Association [ANITA]): A randomised controlled trial. *Lancet Oncol*, 7: 719–27.

10 Pignon JP, Tribodet H, Scagliotti GV, *et al.* (2008) Lung adjuvant cisplatin evaluation: A pooled analysis by the LACE Collaborative Group. *J Clin Oncol*, 26: 3552–9.

11 Dillman RO, Herndon J, Seagren SL, *et al.* (1996) Improved survival in stage III non-small-cell lung cancer: seven-year follow-up of cancer and leukemia group B (CALGB) 8433 trial. *J Natl Cancer Inst*, 88: 1210–15.

12 Sause WT, Scott C, Taylor S, *et al.* (1995) Radiation Therapy Oncology Group (RTOG) 88–08 and Eastern Cooperative Oncology Group (ECOG) 4588: Preliminary results of a phase III trial in regionally advanced, unresectable non-small-cell lung cancer. *J Natl Cancer Inst*, 87: 198–205.

13 Pisters KM, Ginsberg RJ, Giroux DJ, *et al.* (2000) Induction chemotherapy before surgery for early-stage lung cancer: A novel approach. Bimodality Lung Oncology Team. *J Thorac Cardiovasc Surg*, 119: 429–39.

14 Felip E, Rosell R, Maestre JA, *et al.* (2010) Preoperative chemotherapy plus surgery versus surgery plus adjuvant chemotherapy versus surgery alone in early-stage non-small-cell lung cancer. *J Clin Oncol*, 28: 3138–45.

15 Pisters KM, Vallieres E, Crowley JJ, *et al.* (2010) Surgery with or without preoperative paclitaxel and carboplatin in early-stage non-small-cell lung cancer: Southwest Oncology Group Trial S9900, an intergroup, randomized, phase III trial. *J Clin Oncol*, 28: 1843–9.

16 Gilligan D, Nicolson M, Smith I, *et al.* (2007) Preoperative chemotherapy in patients with resectable non-small cell lung cancer: Results of the MRC LU22/NVALT 2/EORTC 08012 multicentre randomised trial and update of systematic review. *Lancet*, 369: 1929–37.

17 Scagliotti GV, Pastorino U, Vansteenkiste JF, *et al.* (2012) Randomized phase III study of surgery alone or surgery plus preoperative cisplatin and gemcitabine in stages IB to IIIA non-small-cell lung cancer. *J Clin Oncol*, 30: 172–8.

18 Martini N, Flehinger BJ, Zaman MB, Beattie EJ, Jr (1980) Prospective study of 445 lung carcinomas with mediastinal lymph node metastases. *J Thorac Cardiovasc Surg*, 80: 390–9.

19 Martini N, Kris MG, Flehinger BJ, *et al.* (1993) Preoperative chemotherapy for stage IIIa (N2) lung cancer: The Sloan-Kettering experience with 136 patients. *Ann Thorac Surg*, 55: 1365–73; discussion 1373–4.

20 Burkes RL, Shepherd FA, Blackstein ME, *et al.* (2005) Induction chemotherapy with mitomycin, vindesine, and cisplatin for stage IIIA (T1–3, N2) unresectable non-small-cell lung cancer: final results of the Toronto phase II trial. *Lung Cancer*, 47: 103–9.

21 Albain KS, Rusch VW, Crowley JJ, *et al.* (1995) Concurrent cisplatin/etoposide plus chest radiotherapy followed by surgery for stages IIIA (N2) and IIIB non-small-cell lung cancer: mature results of Southwest Oncology Group phase II study 8805. *J Clin Oncol*, 13: 1880–92.

22 Elias AD, Skarin AT, Leong T, *et al.* (1997) Neoadjuvant therapy for surgically staged IIIA N2 non-small cell lung cancer (NSCLC). *Lung Cancer*, 17: 147–61.

23 Betticher DC, Hsu Schmitz SF, Totsch M, *et al.* (2003) Mediastinal lymph node clearance after docetaxel-cisplatin neoadjuvant chemotherapy is prognostic of survival in patients with stage IIIA pN2 non-small-cell lung cancer: A multicenter phase II trial. *J Clin Oncol*, 21: 1752–9.

24 Eberhardt W, Wilke H, Stamatis G, *et al.* (1998) Preoperative chemotherapy followed by concurrent chemoradiation therapy based on hyperfractionated accelerated radiotherapy and definitive surgery in locally advanced non-small-cell lung cancer: mature results of a phase II trial. *J Clin Oncol*, 16: 622–34.

25 Van Zandwijk N, Smit EF, Kramer GW, *et al.* (2000) Gemcitabine and cisplatin as induction regimen for patients with biopsy-proven stage IIIA N2 non-small-cell lung cancer: a phase II study of the European Organization for Research and Treatment of Cancer Lung Cancer Cooperative Group (EORTC 08955). *J Clin Oncol*, 18: 2658–64.

26 Migliorino MR, De Marinis F, Nelli F, *et al.* (2002) A 3-week schedule of gemcitabine plus cisplatin as induction chemotherapy for Stage III non-small cell lung cancer. *Lung Cancer*, 35: 319–27.

27 Garrido P, Gonzalez-Larriba JL, Insa A, *et al.* (2007) Long-term survival associated with complete resection after induction chemotherapy in stage IIIA (N2) and IIIB (T4N0–1) non small-cell lung cancer patients: the Spanish Lung Cancer Group Trial 9901. *J Clin Oncol*, 25: 4736–42.

28 Esteban E, de Sande JL, Villanueva N, *et al.* (2007) Cisplatin plus gemcitabine with or without vinorelbine as induction chemotherapy prior to radical locoregional treatment for patients with stage III non-small-cell lung cancer (NSCLC): Results of a prospective randomized study. *Lung Cancer*, 55: 173–80.

29 Lorent N, De Leyn P, Lievens Y, *et al.* (2004) Long-term survival of surgically staged IIIA-N2 non-small-cell lung cancer treated with surgical combined modality approach: analysis of a 7-year prospective experience. *Ann Oncol*, 15: 1645–53.

30 Cappuzzo F, De Marinis F, Nelli F, *et al.* (2003) Phase II study of gemcitabine-cisplatin-paclitaxel triplet as induction chemotherapy in inoperable, locally-advanced non-small cell lung cancer. *Lung Cancer*, 42: 355–61.

31 De Marinis F, Nelli F, Migliorino MR, *et al.* (2003) Gemcitabine, paclitaxel, and cisplatin as induction chemotherapy for patients with biopsy-proven Stage IIIA(N2) nonsmall cell lung carcinoma: A Phase II multicenter study. *Cancer*, 98: 1707–15.

32 Kunitoh H, Kato H, Tsuboi M, *et al.* (2008) A randomised phase II trial of preoperative chemotherapy of cisplatin-docetaxel or docetaxel alone for clinical stage IB/II non-small-cell lung cancer results of a Japan Clinical Oncology Group trial (JCOG 0204). *Br J Cancer*, 99: 852–7.

33 Abratt RP, Lee JS, Han JY, *et al.* (2006) Phase II trial of gemcitabine-carboplatin-paclitaxel as neoadjuvant chemotherapy for operable non-small cell lung cancer. *J Thorac Oncol*, 1: 135–40.

34 Ramnath N, Sommers E, Robinson L, *et al.* (2005) Phase II study of neoadjuvant chemotherapy with gemcitabine and vinorelbine in resectable non-small cell lung cancer. *Chest*, 128: 3467–74.

35 Roth JA, Atkinson EN, Fossella F, *et al.* (1998) Long-term follow-up of patients enrolled in a randomized trial comparing perioperative chemotherapy and surgery with surgery alone in resectable stage IIIA non-small-cell lung cancer. *Lung Cancer*, 21: 1–6.

36 Rosell R, Gomez-Codina J, Camps C, *et al.* (1999) Preresectional chemotherapy in stage IIIA non-small-cell lung cancer: A 7-year assessment of a randomized controlled trial. *Lung Cancer*, 26: 7–14.

37 Pass HI, Pogrebniak HW, Steinberg SM, *et al.* (1992) Randomized trial of neoadjuvant therapy for lung cancer: interim analysis. *Ann Thorac Surg*, 53: 992–8.
38 Zhou Q, Liu L, Li L, *et al.* (2003) A randomized clinical trial of preoperative neoadjuvant chemotherapy followed by surgery in the treatment of stage III non-small cell lung cancer. *Lung Cancer*, 41: S45–S46.
39 Nagai K, Tsuchiya R, Mori T, *et al.* (2003) A random ized trial comparing induction chemotherapy followed by surgery with surgery alone for patients with stage IIIA N2 non-small cell lung cancer (JCOG 9209). *J Thorac Cardiovasc Surg*, 125: 254–60.
40 de Boer RH, Smith IE, Pastorino U, *et al.* (1999) Preoperative chemotherapy in early stage resectable non-small-cell lung cancer: a randomized feasibility study justifying a multicentre phase III trial. *Br J Cancer*, 79: 1514–18.
41 Depierre A, Milleron B, Moro-Sibilot D, *et al.* (2002) Preoperative chemotherapy followed by surgery compared with primary surgery in resectable stage I (except T1N0), II, and IIIa non-small-cell lung cancer. *J Clin Oncol*, 20: 247–53.
42 Depierre A, Westeel V, Milleron B, *et al.* (2003) 5-year results of the French randomized study comparing preoperative chemotherapy followed by surgery and primary surgery in resectable stage I (except T1N0), II and IIIA non-small cell lung cancer. *Lung Cancer*, 41: S62.
43 Sorensen J, Riska H, Ravn J, *et al.* (2005) Scandinavian phase III trial of neoadjuvant chemotherapy in NSCLC stages IB-IIIA/T3. *J Clin Oncol*, 23.
44 Berghmans T, Paesmans M, Meert AP, *et al.* (2005) Survival improvement in resectable non-small cell lung cancer with (neo)adjuvant chemotherapy: results of a meta-analysis of the literature. *Lung Cancer*, 49: 13–23.
45 Burdett S, Stewart LA, Rydzewska L (2006) A systematic review and meta-analysis of the literature: Chemotherapy and surgery versus surgery alone in non-small cell lung cancer. *J Thorac Oncol*, 1: 611–21.
46 Song WA, Zhou NK, Wang W, *et al.* (2010) Survival benefit of neoadjuvant chemotherapy in non-small cell lung cancer: an updated meta-analysis of 13 randomized control trials. *J Thorac Oncol*, 5: 510–16.
47 Siegenthaler MP, Pisters KM, Merriman KW, *et al.* (2001) Preoperative chemotherapy for lung cancer does not increase surgical morbidity. *Ann Thorac Surg*, 71: 1105–11; discussion 1111–2.
48 Martin J, Ginsberg RJ, Abolhoda A, *et al.* (2001) Morbidity and mortality after neoadjuvant therapy for lung cancer: the risks of right pneumonectomy. *Ann Thorac Surg*, 72: 1149–54.
49 Perrot E, Guibert B, Mulsant P, *et al.* (2005) Preoperative chemotherapy does not increase complications after nonsmall cell lung cancer resection. *Ann Thorac Surg*, 80: 423–7.
50 Mandrekar SJ, Qi Y, Hillman SL, *et al.* (2010) End-points in phase II trials for advanced non-small cell lung cancer. *J Thorac Oncol*, 5: 3–9.
51 Soria JC, Massard C, Le Chevalier T (2010) Should progression-free survival be the primary measure of efficacy for advanced NSCLC therapy? *Ann Oncol*, 21: 2324–32.
52 Lara PN, Jr., Redman MW, Kelly K, *et al.* (2008) Disease control rate at 8 weeks predicts clinical benefit in advanced non-small-cell lung cancer: Results from Southwest Oncology Group randomized trials. *J Clin Oncol*, 26: 463–7.
53 Oxnard GR, Morris MJ, Hodi FS, *et al.* (2012) When progressive disease does not mean treatment failure: reconsidering the criteria for progression. *J Natl Cancer Inst*, 104: 1534–41.
54 Eisenhauer EA, Therasse P, Bogaerts J, *et al.* (2009) New response evaluation criteria in solid tumours: revised RECIST guideline (version 1.1). *Eur J Cancer*, 45: 228–47.
55 Pataer A, Kalhor N, Correa AM, *et al.* (2012) Histopathologic response criteria predict survival of patients with resected lung cancer after neoadjuvant chemotherapy. *J Thorac Oncol*, 7: 825–32.
56 Mouillet G, Monnet E, Milleron B, *et al.* (2012) Pathologic complete response to preoperative chemotherapy predicts cure in early-stage non-small-cell lung cancer: combined analysis of two IFCT randomized trials. *J Thorac Oncol*, 7: 841–9.
57 Lordick F, Ott K, Krause BJ, *et al.* (2007) PET to assess early metabolic response and to guide treatment of adenocarcinoma of the oesophagogastric junction: The MUNICON phase II trial. *Lancet Oncol*, 8: 797–805.
58 Rebollo-Aguirre AC, Ramos-Font C, Villegas Portero R, *et al.* (2010) Is FDG-PET suitable for evaluating neoadjuvant therapy in non-small cell lung cancer? Evidence with systematic review of the literature. *J Surg Oncol* 101: 486–94.
59 Ohno Y, Koyama H, Yoshikawa T, *et al.* (2012) Diffusion-weighted MRI versus 18F-FDG PET/CT: performance as predictors of tumor treatment response and patient survival in patients with non-small cell lung cancer receiving chemoradiotherapy. *AJR Am J Roentgenol*, 198: 75–82.

60 Punnoose EA, Atwal S, Liu W, *et al.* (2012) Evaluation of circulating tumor cells and circulating tumor DNA in non-small cell lung cancer: association with clinical endpoints in a phase II clinical trial of pertuzumab and erlotinib. *Clin Cancer Res,* 18: 2391–2401.

61 Betticher DC, Hsu Schmitz SF, Totsch M, *et al.* (2006) Prognostic factors affecting long-term outcomes in patients with resected stage IIIA pN2 non-small-cell lung cancer: 5-year follow-up of a phase II study. *Br J Cancer,* 94: 1099–1106.

62 Mok TS, Wu YL, Thongprasert S, *et al.* (2009) Gefitinib or carboplatin-paclitaxel in pulmonary adenocarcinoma. *N Engl J Med,* 361: 947–57.

63 Rizvi NA, Rusch V, Pao W, *et al.* (2011) Molecular characteristics predict clinical outcomes: prospective trial correlating response to the EGFR tyrosine kinase inhibitor gefitinib with the presence of sensitizing mutations in the tyrosine binding domain of the EGFR gene. *Clin Cancer Res,* 17: 3500–6.

64 Schaake EE, Kappers I, Codrington HE, *et al.* (2012) Tumor response and toxicity of neoadjuvant erlotinib in patients with early-stage non-small-cell lung cancer. *J Clin Oncol,* 30: 2731–8.

65 Sandler A, Gray R, Perry MC, *et al.* (2006) Paclitaxel-carboplatin alone or with bevacizumab for non-small-cell lung cancer. *N Engl J Med,* 355: 2542–50.

66 Price K, Kris MG, Rusch V, *et al.* (2009) Phase II study of induction and adjuvant bevacizumab in patients with stage IB-IIIA non-small cell lung cancer (NSCLC) receiving induction docetaxel and cisplatin. *J Clin Oncol,* (abstract 7531); 27.

67 Jones DR, Moskaluk CA, Gillenwater HH, *et al.* (2012) Phase I trial of induction histone deacetylase and proteasome inhibition followed by surgery in non-small-cell lung cancer. *J Thorac Oncol,* 7: 1683–90.

68 Altorki NK, Keresztes RS, Port JL, *et al.* (2003) Celecoxib, a selective cyclo-oxygenase-2 inhibitor, enhances the response to preoperative paclitaxel and carboplatin in early-stage non-small-cell lung cancer. *J Clin Oncol,* 21: 2645–50.

69 Groen HJ, Sietsma H, Vincent A, *et al.* (2011) Randomized, placebo-controlled phase III study of docetaxel plus carboplatin with celecoxib and cyclooxygenase-2 expression as a biomarker for patients with advanced non-small-cell lung cancer: The NVALT-4 study. *J Clin Oncol,* 29: 4320–6.

70 Koch A, Bergman B, Holmberg E, *et al.* (2011) Effect of celecoxib on survival in patients with advanced non-small cell lung cancer: A double blind randomised clinical phase III trial (CYCLUS study) by the Swedish Lung Cancer Study Group. *Eur J Cancer,* 47: 1546–55.

71 Altorki N, Lane ME, Bauer T, *et al.* (2010) Phase II proof-of-concept study of pazopanib monotherapy in treatment-naive patients with stage I/II resectable non-small-cell lung cancer. *J Clin Oncol,* 28: 3131–7.

72 Nikolinakos PG, Altorki N, Yankelevitz D, *et al.* (2010) Plasma cytokine and angiogenic factor profiling identifies markers associated with tumor shrinkage in early-stage non-small cell lung cancer patients treated with pazopanib. *Cancer Res,* 70: 2171–9.

73 Dautzenberg B, Benichou J, Allard P, *et al.* (1990) Failure of the perioperative PCV neoadjuvant polychemotherapy in resectable bronchogenic non-small cell carcinoma. Results from a randomized phase II trial. *Cancer,* 65: 2435–41.

74 Liao ML, Zhou YZ, Ding JA, *et al.* (2003) The study of peri-operative chemotherapy in stage I-IIIa NSCLC. *Zhonghua Yi Xue Za Zhi,* 83: 962–6.

75 Li Q, Song YH, Zheng ZY (2005) Clinical evaluation of preoperative short course chemotherapy in treatment of stage III non-small cell lung cancer. *Chin J Cancer Prev Treat,* 10: 505–7.

76 Yao K, Xiang MZ, Min JX (2004) A randomized clinical trial of preoperative neoadjuvant chemotherapy in the treatment of stage III non-small cell lung cancer. *J Clin Oncol China,* 31: 611–13.

CHAPTER 20

Image-Guided Radiation Therapy

Kenneth E. Rosenzweig and Sonal Sura
Department of Radiation Oncology, Icahn School of Medicine at Mount Sinai, New York, NY, USA

Introduction

There are two major treatment techniques for non-small cell lung cancer (NSCLC): stereotactic body radiation therapy (SBRT) for early stage disease and chemoradiation for locally advanced NSCLC.

The clinical efficacy of SBRT has been definitively established by the Radiation Therapy Oncology Group (RTOG) 0236, a Phase II multicenter study that demonstrated a 3-year rate of local tumor control of 97.6% for patients with medically inoperable stage I NSCLC [1]. SBRT typically involves the use of high dose per fraction radiation treatment. A dose of 18 Gy per fraction (correcting for density heterogeneity) given at least every other day was used in RTOG 0236. Due to this large dose and the relatively few treatments (3–5 fractions), many centers use IGRT to insure that the treatment is accurately delivered.

For locally advanced NSCLC, local control and survival continue to be a major challenge when fractionated and protracted radiation therapy is used. Even with newer techniques such as three-dimensional conformal radiation therapy (3D-CRT) and intensity modulated radiation therapy (IMRT) [2–8], 2-year local failure rates have been reported between 22–50% [4, 7]. Recently, the RTOG 0617 reported its preliminary results of a study comparing 60 Gy to 74 Gy(A) and concurrent chemotherapy with or without cetaximab. The 74 Gy experimental arm showed poor over all survival and inferior local control compared to 60 Gy standard dose arm. The local failure rate was 34% in 74 Gy Arm and 25% in 60 Gy Arm [9].

Traditional imaging used for identifying tumor size and location, and geometry and patient anatomy has been through fluoroscopy, or more recently, static computed tomography (CT) scans done prior to treatment planning. However, conventional imaging modalities such as CT may be inadequate for visualization of disease. One strategy to improve tumor delineation has been the incorporation of fludeoxyglucose (FDG)-PET scanning into the treatment planning process. This provides both anatomic and metabolic imaging of the tumor.

Another challenge in planning and delivering radiation to treat tumors in the thorax is tumor and surrounding normal organ motion during respiration. This motion may change the exact location of the tumor during each treatment, from the time of the planning scan and the time of actual treatment and during a course of radiation treatment.

IGRT involves the production of images in the radiation therapy treatment room prior to the initiation of treatment. The images are either three-dimensional (3D) images by CT or two-dimensional (2D) images by x-rays that are aided with bony, anatomical or fiducial markers in, or near, the tumor [10]. There are a number of techniques that are able to provide these images.

Lung Cancer, Fourth Edition. Edited by Jack A. Roth, Waun Ki Hong and Ritsuko U. Komaki.

Conventional versus CT-based simulation

In the modern era there has been a paradigm shift in the radiation oncology field from 2D treatment planning to 3D treatment planning with the incorporation of CT simulation into the treatment planning process. Chen *et al.* reviewed the SEER database looking at stage III non-small cell lung cancer patients treated with definitive radiation therapy. They reported a rapid adoption of 3D-CRT: in 1994, it was used in 2.4% of patients undergoing definitive RT in this cohort, in 2000, it was 34% and by the end of the study period, 2005, its use had increased to 77.4%. Controlling for demographic and clinical characteristics, CT simulation was associated with lower risk of death ($P < 0.01$) when compared with conventional simulation [11].

PET and PET-CT in radiation treatment planning

A crucial component of lung cancer radiation treatment planning is accurate tumor delineation. Often patients present with locally advanced disease that is not detected by CT alone or have abnormalities on PET that do not represent areas of cancer. PET scans have been compared to thoracotomy and mediastinoscopy for detecting mediastinal lymphadenopathy and determining stage. In two meta-analyses the sensitivity and specificity of PET for nodal staging in NSCLC ranged from 84% to 88% and 89% to 92% respectively [12, 13]. PET scans have been shown to have a good negative predictive value ranging from 87% to 100% [14–16] and less notable positive predictive values reported as < 80% in several studies [14, 16, 17]. In a multicenter study by Li *et al.* pre-operative FDG PET-CT were performed in 200 lung cancer patients. In regards to lymph nodes, PET-CT findings were confirmed with histopathological examination. PET-CT demonstrated a specificity of 83% and negative predictive value of 91% for presence of mediastinal lymph node metastases. The conclusion of this study was that a negative PET-CT for mediastinal nodal metastases was sufficient evidence to justify treating the primary tumor alone with SBRT [18].

The effect of FDG-PET imaging on radiation treatment planning has been investigated (Figure 20.1) To assess the adequacy of coverage of RT fields planned with CT or X-ray data, Kiffer *et al.* retrospectively performed a graphical co-registration of PET and AP simulator images using coordinates measured from the carina. In 4/15 patients, they found inadequate coverage by the AP portals due to abnormal mediastinal nodes detected on PET but not CT [19]. Munley *et al.* found that PET data increased target volumes (expressed in terms of beam apertures) by up to 15 mm in 34% of patients in their series, using the union of PET and CT-defined volumes [20]. Nestle *et al.* performed a retrospective evaluation of AP/PA portal sizes as altered by PET data. Thirty-five percent of cases

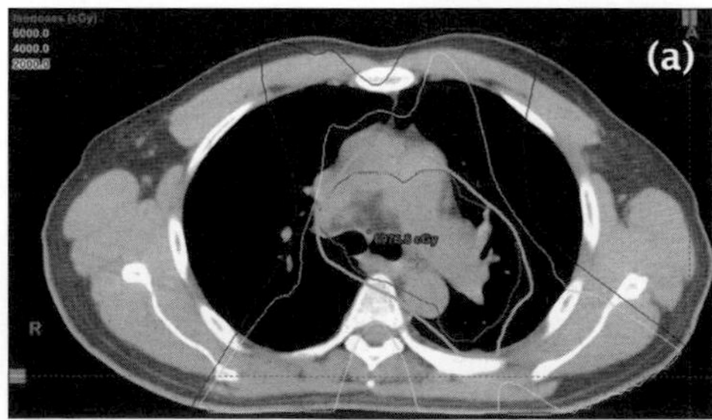

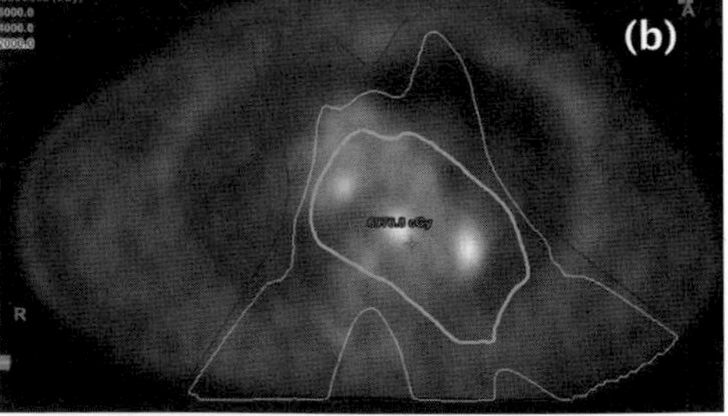

Figure 20.1 A 62-year-old male with inoperable Stage IIIB NSCLC. 60 Gy in 30 fractions was delivered to this site safely. Treatment planning was done using PET-CT registration. a: A CT scan slice from the treatment planning simulation with the planning target volume outlined in red. b: The FDG-PET image of the corresponding slice. The 6000 cGy, 4000 cGy and 2000 cGy isodose curves are shown in green, cyan and blue respectively. (For a color version, see the color plate section.)

had a change in the size or shape of the original CT portals, mostly a reduction in size, and mostly in patients with atelectasis [21]. Schmuecking *et al.* report decreases in the PTV of up to 21% due to distinction of atelectasis from tumor after integrating PET data, with subsequent decreases in the volume of normal lung irradiated (V20) [22]. Hellwig *et al.* showed that PET-CT can also change the radiation field significantly by the inclusion of FDG avid nonenlarged metastatic lymph nodes within the treatment field. While the sensitivity of CT for mediastinal node metastases detection was 56%, for PET-CT it was 83% for all stages, 91% when the CT scan shows enlarged lymph nodes, and 70% for normal-sized lymph nodes [23]. A review article regarding the use of PET-CT in radiation planning for NSCLC further highlighted the role of PET-CT in more accurate radiation treatment planning [24].

The use of software registered PET/CT images in radiation treatment planning has also been studied. Caldwell *et al.* evaluated 30 patients who were to be treated with definitive RT for NSCLC who had features of atelectasis on CT scan. The majority of the patients had smaller PTVs when contoured using fused PET and CT images as compared with volumes generated from CT alone, resulting in decreases of dose to normal lung and spinal cord [24]. In a study of 11 patients with NSCLC, Erdi *et al.* found that registered PET/CT altered the PTV that had previously been contoured on CT images in all cases. Increases in volume were due to inclusion of positive lymph nodes not detected on CT and decreases were due to exclusion of atelectatic lung [26]. Bradley *et al.* studied differences in GTVs contoured with CT data alone versus PET/CT fusion images. The addition of PET information altered the inclusion of tumor and/or nodal regions in 14 of 24 patients receiving 3D-CRT. Two of these were decreases due to atelectasis distinguished from tumor by PET. In such cases, parameters calculated to predict for normal tissue toxicity such as mean lung dose (MLD), mean esophageal dose (MED) and the volume of lung receiving > 20 Gy (V20) were decreased as well, theoretically decreasing the risk of radiation pneumonitis or esophagitis [27]. Giraud *et al.* reported results consistent with these studies using PET images from dual-head coincidence (CDET) gamma cameras fused with simulation CT images by use of external fiducial markers [28]. The above findings suggest that the use of PET data can potentially improve patient outcomes, both by identifying areas of disease that would not have been contoured on CT alone, and by decreasing the amount of normal lung tissue included in the target volume and thus the volume at risk for pulmonary toxicity.

Similarly, in patient with limited stage SCLC Shirvani *et al.* studied dose escalation in PET-CT avid regions with omission of elective nodal irradiation. Sixty-two patients were treated with IMRT based on PET-CT findings with the treatment plan omitting areas if they were PET-CT negative. By planning the target volume based on PET-CT, 45 Gy was delivered in 30 twice-daily fractions. Upon review, only 1 of 62 patients had recurrence in an unirradiated elective nodal region. Most recurrences were either distant or within the high-dose volume and not in the initially PET negative elective nodal regions. This suggests that PET-CT-based radiation therapy planning may obviate elective nodal irradiation even in small-cell lung cancer. However the authors did suggest that, although PET-defined mediastinal radiotherapy fields appear to be safe, because of a false-positive rate of approximately 30%, ideally pathological confirmation of PET-positive mediastinal nodes should be obtained [29].

Due to the promising results of the initial studies of the incorporation of PET imaging in lung cancer treatment planning, the RTOG initiated a trial to further investigate its utility. RTOG 0515 was a Phase II prospective trial that investigated the impact of PET scanning on radiation therapy treatment plans. Each of the 47 evaluable patients had two gross tumor volumes generated: one using just a CT data set and one utilizing PET-CT. The differences between these two datasets was quantified by the size of the GTV, number of involved nodes, nodal station, mean lung dose (MLD), volume of lung exceeding 20 Gy (V20), and mean esophageal dose (MED). The GTV was significantly smaller for PET/CT-derived volumes and the mean lung dose was slightly lower. The other measures were not significantly different. Nodal contours were altered in 51% of patients. This trial demonstrates that the use of PET scanning does alter GTVs in the majority of patients and that they tend to be smaller [30].

The use of adaptive radiation treatment with the use of mid-treatment PET-CT scans stems from the head and neck literature but has started to gain some popularity in the treatment of lung cancer. Two studies investigating mid-treatment PET scan after 5 to 6 weeks of radiation and assessed the volume changes, with the goal of reduced volume high-dose boost. These studies have demonstrated reductions in full-dose radiation target volume by 20% to 44%, although the benefit in normal tissue complications averaged approximately 2% [31, 32].

Tumor motion

Managing respiratory motion during radiation treatments is an important aspect of treating thoracic malignancies. For patients who are medically unfit for surgery or whose tumors are inoperable based on stage and/or location, radiotherapy is the primary treatment option often in conjunction with chemotherapy [33]. Organ motion during respiration can limit the accuracy with which radiation can be delivered to the tumor volume. Some investigators have shown underdosing as high as 30% with conventional radiation therapy techniques [34]. Stevens *et al.* and others have reported that lung tumors move during free breathing from 5 to 10 mm and in some cases as much as 4.5 cm [35]. To account for these inaccuracies larger margins are added to the gross target volume (GTV) to create a planning target volume (PTV). The increase in volume may limit dose escalation to tumoricidal doses based on predictors of normal tissue toxicity, such as the V20 [36].

Lymph nodes are also susceptible to motion during respiration. Donnelly *et al.* showed that mediastinal and hilar lymph nodes also move during respiration by an average of 2.5–5.2 mm, but as much as 14.4 mm [37]. In a similar study, Pantarotto *et al.* evaluated the motion of 100 lymph nodes and reported motion of 6.8 mm (range, 1.7–16.4 mm) [38]. Both studies demonstrated that lymph nodes in the lower mediastinum moved significantly more than in the upper mediastinum. Therefore, limiting the effects of organ and tumor motion during treatment planning and delivery may help in increasing accuracy and allow for further dose escalation and more favorable survival outcomes while maintaining an acceptable toxicity profile.

Two distinct techniques have been used to reduce the effects of respiratory motion. The first involves confining radiation delivery to a specified phase in the breathing cycle by gating the linear accelerator while the patient breathes freely. Breathing is monitored with devices that trigger radiation delivery during specific phases of the patient's respiratory cycle [39]. In the second approach, breathing is controlled either voluntarily by the patient or by using an occlusion valve, such as the active breathing control (ABC) developed by Wong *et al.* [40, 41] or the deep inspiration breath hold (DIBH) technique [42].

STIC 2003 was a comparative, nonrandomized, multicenter prospective study based in France [43]. It compared conformal radiation therapy to respiratory-gated conformal radiation therapy in 401 patients with NSCLC. They reported a decrease in dose to the heart, lung and esophagus with respiratory-gated treatment. In addition, treatment toxicity to the lung, esophagus and heart was significantly reduced, especially with deep inspiration techniques. Some practitioners have advocated using respiratory gating only with image guidance since there are interfraction baseline shifts which cannot be accounted for by respiratory gating [44].

Another approach uses images obtained during inspiration and expiration to create an internal target volume (ITV). This ITV would therefore theoretically account for the full extent of organ motion during the entire treatment [45]. There are multiple ways of determining an ITV. One common method is to perform a respiratory correlated CT scan. In this technique, a CT scan is obtained while simultaneously, an external postion-sensitive monitor records respiration. Infrafractional tumor motion can then be obtained and tumor volumes adjusted accordingly [46]. Another method uses the maximum intensity projection from either a CT scan or a PET scan to determine the ITV [47]. Multiple commercial systems are available to monitor patient's breathing.

Image guided radiation therapy

The use of stereotactic body radiation therapy (SBRT) has demonstrated previously unprecedented local control rates of 98% [1]. SBRT typically involves extremely high dose per fraction treatment, such as 1200–2400 cGy per treatment. Day to day changes in organ motion, tumor shape, and patient position can lead to variability in tumor location while patients are being treated. IGRT attempts to account for this variability, which can lead to more accurate treatment. In addition, due to the increased precision of the radiation therapy treatment plan, and radiation doses and fraction sizes not conventionally delivered, such as 5400 cGy in three 1800 cGy fractions, can now be safely delivered (Figure 20.2).

Although many of the initial studies of SBRT did not use IGRT for daily set-up verification, most large centers with extensive experience in SBRT use IGRT. Five top academic centers throughout the world recently pooled their experience into a large cohort. Each center used daily CBCT to ensure correct patient position [48]. There are numerous commercially available technical solutions for IGRT in the treatment room. They include cone beam CT, tomotherapy, orthogonal kV x-rays and CT scanning in the treatment room.

Cone-beam CT

Newer therapies, such as IMRT, have high-dose gradients that make it particularly important to verify accurate treatment. Currently, most patient treatments are verified using two-dimensional portal imaging using anatomic structures such as bones or air cavities. Cone-beam CT (CBCT) is a method to assess tumor position for patients on the treatment table. There are two technologies available for producing cone beam images. The first uses the linear accelerator's megavoltage (MV) beam to produce the image. This is called megavoltage cone beam CT (MVCBCT). The other, more

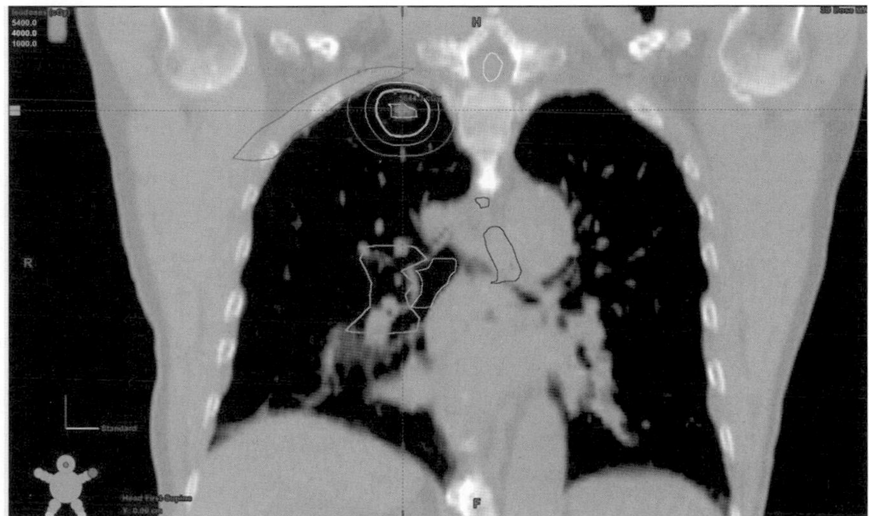

Figure 20.2 An 89-year-old male with medically inoperable early stage NSCLC. 54 Gy in three fractions was delivered to this site safely. The yellow contour represents the gross tumor volume. The green, white and blue isodose curves represent 1000 cGy, 4000 cGy and 5400 cGy respectively. The normal structures which need to have their radiation dose minimized include the chest wall (magenta), spinal cord (yellow), esophagus (blue), bronchial tree (orange and blue). (For a color version, see the color plate section.)

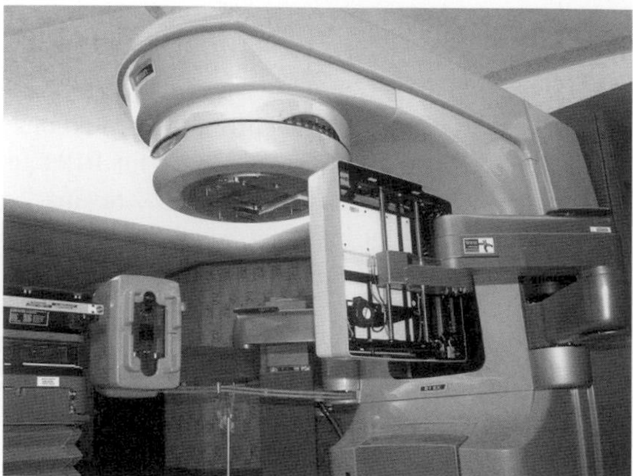

Figure 20.3 Varian kV Imaging system (OBI). The kV source, kV detector, and MV detector are all mounted on robotic arms.

popular method uses a separate imaging source with kilovoltage energy to produce the images (kV CBCT, Figure 20.3). Although there are several CBCT technologies available [49–57], the basic concept behind the CBCT system is that the ability to obtain information about anatomy and tumor location immediately before each treatment may lead to more accurate delivery of radiation. By monitoring these daily changes, treatment plans can be tailored for each fraction [58].

With CBCT, a 3D image can be acquired in the treatment position immediately prior to each treatment without having to reposition the patient on a different imaging machine, which further minimizes the variation in the planned versus actual target position. Increased precision in target localization with image guidance in the form of CBCT can also allow for reduction in the safety margin added to the GTV [59]. Therefore, cone-beam CT facilitates the use of high dose radiotherapy for the treatment of NSCLC by accounting for both inter- and intrafractional tumor motion and improving treatment accuracy [60].

Tomotherapy

The helical tomotherapy unit is an innovative device used for radiation delivery that combines a linear accelerator and a helical CT scanner allowing for the targeted region to be imaged before, during, and after each treatment. This allows for improved tumor localization and can help account for target motion during and between treatments. CT scans provide improved soft tissue resolution over the standard port films, thereby providing increased anatomical detail. With tomotherapy the concept of "adaptive radiotherapy" can be implemented allowing for daily adjustments in radiation delivery based on changes in tumor position and size [61, 62]. By using information obtained during previous fractions to modify an ongoing treatment, errors in dose and tumor location can be better accounted [63, 64]. Another concept that is equally important in radiotherapy for lung cancer is "conformal avoidance" which emphasizes the importance of protecting normal structures from radiation damage. With the use of tomotherapy both conformal radiotherapy and "conformal avoidance" can be achieved by daily imaging of target motion and changes in size and position [61, 65, 66].

The unit is designed to deliver IMRT treatments using a binary multi-leaf collimator but has the ability to deliver radiation along every possible gantry angle. This translates into higher degrees of freedom when compared to linac-based IMRT. Clinical results have shown that helical tomotherapy is well tolerated and provides adequate local control for patients with lung cancer [67].

Markers and respiratory gating

Fiducial markers provide another way to localize lung tumors. These markers are placed within the lung tumor or external to the tumor and monitored during all aspects of radiotherapy. The markers are radio-opaque and can be a simple gold seed or more complex, such as a coil. The role of the marker is to act as a surrogate for the tumor's location.

BrainLab (Munich, Germany) has developed a system that allows for image guidance and respiratory gating using the Exactrac Adaptive Gating system (Version 4.5, Gating Version 1). The system itself consists of an infrared camera, 2 amorphous silicon plates, and 2 kilovoltage (kV) X-ray tubes and uses a combination of X-ray and optical tracking to monitor internal target motion. Signals are sent to the linear accelerator to turn on the beam when the target is located at the machine's isocenter. For thoracic tumors, this system can be used to track tumor motion by X-ray localization of internal fiducials along with optical tracking of external landmarks [68–70]. The system works by allowing the placement of internal fiducials as surrogate for tumor location. X-rays are then used to determine the location of the internal target to the linac isocenter and displacement of the internal target is corrected by optical tracking. These X-rays are registered to digitally reconstructed images from the treatment-planning CT. This gating system has been shown to have an accuracy of 1.7 mm for tumor localization with motion up to 2 cm in the anteroposterior and superoinferior directions [71].

The Cyberknife system (Accuray, Sunnyvale, CA) is another system that allows for imaging of tumor motion and variation by monitoring gold seeds placed near the tumor. The system consists of a linear accelerator radiation source that is mounted on a robotic arm and through the use of image-guided cameras can precisely track tumor motion during the treatment. Also with the addition of the Synchrony™ respiratory tracking system, dynamic radiosurgery during respiration is possible. By recording the breathing movements of a patient's chest the Synchrony option combines that information with sequential X-ray pictures of the fiducials to facilitate delivery of radiation during any point in the respiratory cycle. This allows further precision during radiation delivery and reduces normal tissue exposure [72, 73]. Some patients have lung tumors that are visible without fiducial markers through the use of the Xsight® Lung Tracking System [74]. Clinical results with Cyberknife have been favorable with high tolerance and excellent local control.

Orthogonal kV X-rays

The use of orthogonal kV X-rays provides another method of onboard imaging allowing for daily target localization while exposing the patient to lower doses of radiation as compared to MV radiographs [75]. Similar to the kV CBCT system, the kV X-ray source and two fluoroscopic imaging systems (one for the kV X-ray beam and the other for the MV beam) are installed on a linear accelerator. The kV X-ray beam is mounted orthogonally to the MV treatment beam and the two fluoroscopic systems are placed perpendicular to the corresponding beam axis. Three-dimensional target localization is then assessed by measurements of 2D shifts in four orthogonal images (anteroposterior, posteroanterior, and right and left lateral images). Each image provides a way of measuring shifts of the tumor relative to the treatment machine isocenter and simulation films. The benefit of using a kV imaging X-ray system may be that it exposes the patient to less radiation because of its lower imaging dose thereby allowing for more routine use of 2D imaging for daily tumor localization when compared to MV radiographs [76].

In-room CT

Many systems have been developed that incorporate use in-room CT scanners but the basic steps and concepts are the same. First the patient is positioned by aligning the initial setup marks with the treatment positioning lasers. Then the table is rotated 180 degrees to obtain a CT scan of the patient that is limited to the treatment area. Finally the planning CT scan is compared with the CT just obtained to determine if a shift in patient position is necessary and adjustments can be made accordingly.

An example of a system that incorporates the in-room CT with a linear accelerator is a CT-on-Rails. The system consists of a CT scanner that slides on rails in the floor so the patient doesn't have to move between the time of the scan and treatment. It slides over the patient's treatment table and then is pushed out of the way during treatment. The system allows for corrections to be made based on changes in the patient's daily positioning between treatments to assure the accurate delivery of radiation [77].

The role of image guidance in stereotactic body radiotherapy (SBRT)

Standard techniques used in SBRT to reduce respiration-related organ motion include frames, belts, and active breathing control which requires patients to hold their breath at different points during the treatment [78, 79]. However, often times these patients are unable to tolerate frames or have poor baseline pulmonary function and are unable to hold their breath long enough. Another method of image guidance in hypofractionated radiotherapy involves fusing the clinical target volumes (CTV) derived from CT scans from different phases of respiration to represent the internal target volume (ITV) which would then account for the effects of respiratory motion. Onimaru *et al.* implemented this method of analyzing tumor motion through CT scans at inspiration, expiration, and while the patient was breathing normally. CTV was defined for each respiratory cycle and then fused together when determining the PTV. This method was thought to account for the effects of respiratory motion [80]. A similar technique for PTV definition through fusion of CTV's derived from CT scans taken at different phases of respiration was applied by Fukumoto *et al.* when treating patients with NSCLC with SBRT [81].

Conclusions

The definitive role of IGRT for lung cancer treatment has yet to be established. With local control as the main goal of radiotherapy, precision and accuracy through all parts of the treatment process, including initial staging, treatment planning, and treatment delivery, remains a challenge. Image guidance, whether through PET-CT fusion for staging or MV CBCT, orthogonal kV X-rays and CT-based SBRT for treatment may change how patients with thoracic malignancies are treated in the future.

References

1 Timmerman R, Paulus R, Galvin J, *et al.* (2010) Stereotactic body radiation therapy for inoperable early stage lung cancer. *JAMA*, 303: 1070–6.

2 Armstrong JG, Burman C, Leibel SA, *et al.* (1993) Three-dimensional conformal radiation therapy may improve the therapeutic ratio of high dose radiation therapy for lung cancer. *Int J Radiat Oncol Biol Phys*, 26: 685–9.

3 Hayman JA, Martel MK, Ten Haken RK, *et al.* (2001) Dose escalation in non-small cell lung cancer using three-dimensional conformal radiation therapy: Update of a phase I trial. *J Clin Oncol*, 19: 127–36.

4 Narayan S, Henning GT, Randall TK, *et al.* (2004) Results following treatment to doses of 92.4 or 102.9 Gy on a phase I dose escalation study for non-small cell lung cancer. *Lung Cancer*, 44: 79–88.

5 Rosenzweig KE, Mychalzhak B, Fuks Z, *et al.* (2000) Final report of the 70.2-Gy and 75.6-Gy dose levels of a phase I dose escalation study using three-dimensional conformal radiotherapy in the treatment of inoperable non-small cell lung cancer. *Cancer*, 6: 82–7.

6 Rosenzweig KE, Fox JL, Leibel SA, *et al.* (2005) Results of a phase I dose-escalation study using three-dimensional conformal radiotherapy in the treatment of inoperable nonsmall cell lung carcinoma. *Cancer*, 103: 2118–27.

7 Bradley J, Graham MV, Winter K, *et al.* (2005) Toxicity and outcome results of RTOG 9311: A phase I-II dose-escalation study using three-dimensional conformal radiotherapy in patients with inoperable non-small-cell lung carcinoma. *Int J Radiat Oncol Biol Phys*, 61: 318–28.

8 Schwarz M, Alber M, Lebesque LV, *et al.* (2005) Dose heterogeneity in the target volume and intensity-modulated radiotherapy to escalate the dose in the treatment of non-small-cell lung cancer. *Int J Radiat Oncol Biol Phys*, 62(2): 561–70.

9 Bradley JD, Paulus R, Komaki R, *et al.* (2013) A randomized phase III comparison of standard-Dose (60 Gy) versus high-dose (74 Gy) conformal chemoradiotherapy +/− cetuximab for stage IIIA/IIIB non-small cell lung cancer: Preliminary findings on radiation dose in RTOG 0617. *2013 ASCO Annual Meeting; May 28–31, 2013*, Chicago. Abstract #7501.

10 Grau C, Hoyer M, Lindegaard J, Overgaard J (2006) The emerging evidence for stereotactic body radiotherapy. *Acta Oncologia*, 45: 771–4.

11 Chen, AB, Neville BA, Sher DJ (2011) Survival outcomes after radiation therapy for stage III non-small-cell lung cancer after adoption of computed tomography-based simulation. *J Clin Oncol*, Jun 10; 29(17): 2305–11 (http://www.ncbi.nlm.nih.gov/pubmed/21537034).

12 Toloza E, Harpole L, McCrory DC (2003) Noninvasive staging of non-small cell lung cancer: A review of the current evidence. *Chest*, 123: 137S–146S.

13 Reske SN and Kotzerke J. (2001) FDG-PET for clinical use Results of the 3rd German Interdisciplinary Consensus Conference. *Eur J Nucl Med*, 28: 1707–1723.

14 Vansteenkiste JF, Stroobants SG, Dupont PJ *et al.* (1998) The Leuven Lung Cancer Group, FDG-PET scan in potentially operable non-small cell lung cancer Do anatometabolic PET-CT fusion images improve the localization of regional lymph node metastases? *Eur J Nucl Med*, 25: 1495–1501.

15 Steinert HC, Hauser M, Allemann F, *et al.* (1997) Non-small cell lung cancer Nodal staging with FDG PET versus CT with correlative lymph node mapping and sampling. *Radiology*, 202: 441–6.

16 Pieterman RM, van Putten JW, Meuzelaar JJ, *et al.* (2000) Preoperative staging of non-small-cell lung cancer with positron-emission tomography. *N Engl J Med*, 203: 254–61.

17 Poncelet AJ, Lonneux M, Coche E, *et al.* (2001) PET-FDG scan enhances but does not replace preoperative surgical staging in non-small cell lung carcinoma. *Eur J Cardiothorac Surg*, 20: 468–75.

18 Li X, Zhang H, Xing L *et al.* (2012) Mediastinal lymph nodes staging by 18F-FDG PET/CT for early stage non-small cell lung cancer: A multicenter study. *Radiother Oncol*, Feb; 102(2): 246–50.

19 Kiffer JD, Berlangieri SU, Scott AM, *et al.* (1998) The contribution of 18F-fluoro-2-deoxy-glucose positron emission tomographic imaging to radiotherapy planning in lung cancer. *Lung Cancer*, 19: 167–77.

20 Munley MT, Marks LB, Scarfone C, *et al.* (1999) Multimodality nuclear medicine imaging in three-dimensional radiation treatment planning for lung cancer: challenges and prospects. *Lung Cancer*, 23: 105–14.

21 Nestle U, Hellwig D, Schmidt S, *et al.* (2002) 2-Deoxy-2-[18F]fluoro-D-glucose positron emission tomography in target volume definition for radiotherapy of patients with non-small-cell lung cancer. *Mol Imaging Biol*, 4: 257–63.

22 Schmucking M, Baum RP, Bonnet R, *et al.* (2005) Correlation of histologic results with PET findings for tumor regression and survival in locally advanced non-small cell lung cancer after neoadjuvant treatment. *Pathologe*, 26: 178–89.

23 Hellwig D, Baum RP, Kirsch C *et al.* (2009) Review FDG-PET, PET/CT and conventional nuclear medicine procedures in the evaluation of lung cancer: a systematic review. *Nuklearmedizin*, 48(2): 59–69, quiz N8–9.

24 MacManus MP, Hicks RJ, *et al.* (2012) The role of positron emission tomography/computed tomography in radiation therapy planning for patients with lung cancer. *Seminars in Nuclear Medicine*, Sep; 42(5): 308–19.

25 Caldwell, CB, Mah, K, Ung, YC, Danjoux, CE, Blaogh, JM, Ganguli, SN, Ehrlich, LE (2001) Observer variation in contouring gross tumor volume in patients with poorly defined non-small-cell lung tumors on CT: the impact of 18FDG-hybrid PET fusion. *Int J Radiat Oncol Biol Phys*, 51(4): 923–31

26 Erdi YE, Rosenzweig K, Erdi AK, *et al.* (2002) Radiotherapy treatment planning for patients with non-small cell lung cancer using positron emission tomography (PET). *Radiother Oncol*, 62: 51–60.

27 Bradley J, Thorstad WL, Mutic S, *et al.* (2004) Impact of FDG-PET on radiation therapy volume delineation in non-small-cell lung cancer. *Int J Radiat Oncol Biol Phys*, 59: 78–86.

28 Giraud P, Grahek D, Montravers F, *et al.* (2001) CT and (18)F-deoxyglucose (FDG) image fusion for optimization of conformal radiotherapy of lung cancers. *Int J Radiat Oncol Biol Phys*, 49: 1249–57.

29 Shirvani SM, Komaki R, Stewart DJ, *et al.* (2010) PET/CT-guided involved-field intensity modulated radiation therapy for limited-stage small cell lung cancer. *Int. J Radiat Oncol Biol Phys*, 78: S34–S35.

30 Bradley J, Bae K, Choi N, *et al.* (2012) A phase II comparative study of gross tumor volume definition with or without PET/CT fusion in dosimetric planning for non-small-cell lung cancer (NSCLC): primary analysis of Radiation Therapy Oncology Group (RTOG) 0515. *Int J Radiat Oncol Biol Phys*, 82: 435–41.

31 Feng M, Kong FM, Gross M, *et al.* (2009) Using fluorodeoxyglucose positron emission tomography to assess tumor volume during radiotherapy for non-small-cell lung cancer and its potential impact on adaptive dose escalation and normal tissue sparing. *Int J Radiat Oncol Biol Phys*, 73(4): 1228–34.

32 Gillham C, Zips D, Ponisch F, *et al.* (2008) Additional PET/CT in week 5–6 of radiotherapy for patients with stage III non-small cell lung cancer as a means of dose escalation planning? *Radiother Oncol*, 88(3): 335–41.

33 Vora SA, Daly B, Blaszkowsky L, *et al.* (2000) High dose radiation therapy and chemotherapy as induction treatment for Stage III non-small cell lung carcinoma RTOG 7311. *Cancer,* 89(9): 1946–52.

34 Ross CS, Hussey DH, Pennington EC, Stanford W, Doornbos JF (1990) Analysis of movement of intrathoracic neoplasms using ultrafast computerized tomography. *Int J Radiation Oncology Biol Phys,* 18: 671–7

35 Stevens CW, Munden RF, Forster KM, *et al.* (2001) Respiratory-driven lung tumor motion is independent of time size, tumor location, and pulmonary function. *Int J Radiat Oncol Biol Phys,* 51: 62.

36 Bradley, J, Graham, MV, Winter, K, Purdy, JA, Komaki, R, Roa, WH, Ryu, JK, Bosch, W, Emami, B (2005) Toxicity and outcome results of RTOG 9311: a phase I-II dose-escalation study using three-dimensional conformal radiotherapy in patients with inoperable non-small cell lung carcinoma. *Int J Radiat Oncol Biol Phys,* 61: 318–28.

37 Donnelly ED, Parikh PJ, Lu W, *et al.* (2007) Assessment of intrafraction mediastinal and hilar lymph node movement and comparison to lung tumor motion using four-dimensional CT. *Int J Radiat Oncol Biol Phys,* 69: 580–8.

38 Patarotto JR, Piet AH, Vincent A, *et al.* (2009) Motion analysis of 100 mediastinal lymph nodes: Potential pitfalls in treatment planning and adaptive strategies. *Int J Radiat Oncol Biol Phys,* 74: 1092–9.

39 Kubo HD, Hill BC (1996) Respiration gated radiotherapy treatment: A technical study. *Phys Med Biol,* 41: 83–91.

40 Wong JW, Sharpe MB, Jaffray DA, *et al.* (1997) The use of active breathing control (ABC) to minimize breathing motion during radiation therapy. *Int J Radiat Oncol Biol Phys,* 39(suppl 2): 164 (abstract).

41 Stromberg JS, Sharpe MB, Kini VR, *et al.* (1998) Active breathing control (ABC) for Hodgkin's disease: Reduction in normal tissue irradiation with deep inspiration and implication for treatment. *Int J Radiat Oncol Biol Phys,* 42(1S): 140 (abstract).

42 Rosenzweig KE, Hanley J, Mah D, *et al.* (2000) The deep inspiration breath-hold technique in the treatment of ioperable non-small cell lung cancer. *Int J Radiat Oncol Biol Phys,* 48: 81 (abstract).

43 Giraud P, Morvan E, Claude L, *et al.* (2011) Respiratory gating techniques for optimization of lung cancer radiotherapy. *J Thor Oncol,* 6(12): 2058–68.

44 Korreman SS, Juhler-Nøttrup T, Boyer AL (2009) Respiratory gated beam delivery cannot facilitate margin reduction, unless combined with respiratory correlated image guidance. *Radiother Oncol,* 86(1): 61–8.

45 Liu H, Koch N, Starkschall G, *et al.* (2004) Evaluation of internal lung motion for respiratory-gated radiotherapy using MRI: Part II – margin reduction of internal target volume. *Int J Radiat Oncol Biol Phys,* 60(5): 1473–83.

46 Mageras GS, Pevsner A, Yorke ED, *et al.* (2004) Measurement of lung tumor motion using respiration-correlated CT. *Int J Radiat Oncol Biol Phys,* 60: 933–41.

47 Lamb JM, Robinson C, Bradley J, *et al.* (2011) Generating lung tumor internal target volumes from 4D-PET maximum intensity projections. *Med Phys,* 38: 5732–7.

48 Grills IS, Hope AJ, Guckenberger M (2012) A collaborative analysis of stereotactic lung radiotherapy outcomes for early-stage non-small-cell lung cancer using daily online cone-beam computed tomography image-guided radiotherapy. *Thor Oncol,* 7(9): 1382–93.

49 Ma CM, Paskalev K (2006) In-room CT techniques for image-guided radiation therapy. *Med. Dosim,* 31: 30–9.

50 Wong JR, Cheng CW, Grimm L, *et al.* (2001) Clinical implementation of the world's first Primatom, a combination of CT scanner and linear accelerator, for precise tumor targeting and treatment. *Med Phys,* 17: 271–6.

51 Jaffray DA, Siewerdsen JH, Wong JW, *et al.* (2002) Flat-panel cone-beam computed tomography for image-guided radiation therapy. *Int. J. Radiat. Oncol. Biol. Phys,* 53: 1337–49.

52 Oelfke U, Tucking T, Nill S, *et al.* (2006) Linac-integrated KV cone-beam CT technical features and first applications. *Med. Dosim,* 31: 62–70.

53 Sorensen SP, Chow E, Kriminski S, *et al.* (2006) Image guided radiotherapy using a mobile kilovoltage x-ray device. *Med Dosim,* 31: 40–50.

54 Sillanpaa J, Chang J, Mageras G, *et al.* (2005) Developments in megavoltage cone beam CT with an amorphous silicon EPID Reduction of exposure and synchronization with respiratory gating. *Med Phys,* 32: 819–29.

55 Pouliot J, Bani-Hashemi A, Chen J, *et al.* (2005) Low-dose megavoltage cone-beam CT for radiation therapy. *Int. J. Radiat. Oncol. Biol. Phys,* 61: 552–60.

56 Gildersleve J, Dearnaley DP, Evans PM, *et al.* (1994) A randomised trial of patient repositioning during radiotherapy using a megavoltage imaging system. *Radiother Oncol,* 31: 161–8.

57 Evans PM, Gildersleve JQ, Rawlings C, *et al.* (1993) Technical note: The implementation of patient position correction using a megavoltage imaging device on a linear accelerator. *Br. J. Radiol,* 66: 833–8.

58 Morin O, Gillis A, Chen J, *et al.* (2006) Megavoltage cone-beam CT: System description and clinical applications. *Med Dosim*, 31(1): 51–61.

59 Guckenberger M, Meyer J, Wilbert J, *et al.* (2006) Cone-beam CT based image-guidance for extracranial stereotactic radiotherapy of intrapulmonary tumors. *Acta Oncologica*, 45: 897–906.

60 Sidhu K, Ford EC, Spirou S, *et al.* Optimization of conformal thoracic radiotherapy using cone-beam CT imaging for treatment verification. *Int J Radiat Oncol Biol Phys*, 55(3): 757–67.

61 Welsh JS, Patel R, Ritter MA, *et al.* (2002) Helical tomotherapy: An innovative technology and approach to radiation therapy. *Technology in Cancer Research & Treatment*, 1(4): 311–16.

62 Ruchala KJ, Olivera GH, Kapatoes JM, *et al.* (2000) Megavoltage CT image reconstruction during tomotherapy treatments. *Phys Med. Biol*, 45: 3545–62.

63 Olivera GH, Shepard DM, Ruchala KJ, *et al.* (1999) Tomotherapy. In: Van Dyk J (ed.), *Modern Technology of Radiation Oncology*. Madison, Wisconsin: Medical Physics Publishing. Chapter 15, pp. 521–87.

64 Mackie TR (1997) Tomotherapy: Rethinking the process of radiotherapy. In: Leavitt DD, Starkshall G (eds), *XII International Conference on the Use of Computers in Radiation Therapy*. Salt Lake City, Utah, USA: Medical Physics Publishing, pp. 329–31.

65 Kapatoes JM, Olivera GH, Ruchala KJ, *et al.* (2001) On the verification of the incident energy fluence in tomotherapy IMRT. *Phys Med Biol*, 46: 2953–65.

66 Yan D, Ziaga E, Jaffray D, *et al.* (1998) The use of adaptive radiation therapy to reduce set-up error: A prospective clinical study. *Int J Radiat Oncol Biol Phys*, 41: 715–20.

67 Marcenaro M, Vagge S, Belgioia L, *et al.* (2013) Ablative or palliative stereotactic body radiotherapy with helical tomotherapy for primary or metastatic lung tumor. *Anticancer Res*, 33(2): 655–60.

68 Meeks SL, Tome WA, Willoughby TR, *et al.* (2005) Optically guided patient positioning techniques. *Semin Radiat Oncol*, 15: 192–201.

69 Medin PM, Solberg TD, De Salles AA, *et al.* (2002) Investigations of a minimally invasive method for treatment of spinal malignancies with LINAC stereotactic radiation therapy: Accuracy and animal studies. *Int J Radiat Oncol Biol Phys*, 52: 1111–22.

70 Krupelian PA, Willoughby TR, Meeks SL, *et al.* (2005) Intraprostatic fiducials for localization of the prostate gland: Monitoring intermarker distances during radiation therapy to for the marker stability. *Int J Radiat Oncol Biol Phys*, 62: 1291–6.

71 Willoughby TR, Forbes AR, Buchholz D, *et al.* (2006) Evaluation of an infrared camera and X-ray system using implanted fiducials in patients with lung tumors for gated radiation therapy *Int J Radiat Oncol Biol Phys*, 66(2): 568–75.

72 Whyte RI, Crownover R, Murphy MJ, *et al.* (2003) Stereotactic radiosurgery for lung tumors: Preliminary report of a phase I trial. *Ann Thorac Surg*, 75: 1097–1101.

73 El-Sherif A, Luketich JD, Landreneau RJ, *et al.* (2005) New therapeutic approached for early stage non-small cell lung cancer. *Surigal Oncol*, 14(1): 27–32.

74 Bibault JE, Prevost B, Dansin E, *et al.* (2012) Image-guided robotic stereotactic radiation therapy with fiducial-free tumor tracking for lung cancer. *Radiat Oncol*, 24(7): 102.

75 Jaffray DA, Chawla K, Yu C, *et al.* (1995) Dual-beam imaging for online verification of radiotherapy field placement. *Int J Radiat Oncol Biol Phys*, 33: 1273–80.

76 Pisani L, Lockman D, Jaffray D, *et al.* (2000) Set-up error in radiotherapy: on-line correction using electronic kilovoltage and megavoltage radiographs. *Int J Radiat Oncol Biol Phys*, 47(3): 825–39.

77 Mah D (2006) IGRT: In-room technologies. *Medical Imaging*, 21: 26–9.

78 Uematsu M, Shioda A, Tahara K, *et al.* (1998) Focal, high dose, and fractionated modified stereotactic radiation therapy for lung carcinoma patients. *Cancer*, 82: 1062–70.

79 Blomgren H, Lax I, Naslund I, Svanstrom R (1995) Stereotactic high dose fraction radiation therapy of extracranial tumors using an accelerator. *Acta Oncol*, 34: 861–70.

80 Onimaru R, Shirato H, Shimizu S, *et al.* (2003) Tolerance of organs at risk in small-volume, hypofractionated, image-guided radiotherapy for primary and metastatic lung cancers. *Int J Radiat Oncol Biol Phys*, 56(1): 126–35.

81 Fukumoto S, Shirato H, Shimzu S, *et al.* (2002) Small-volume image-guided radiotherapy using hypofractionated, coplanar, and noncoplanar multiple fields for patients with inoperable stage I non-small cell lung carcinomas. *Cancer*, 95(7): 1546–53.

CHAPTER 21

Stereotactic Ablative Radiotherapy for Lung Cancer

Puneeth Iyengar[1] *and Robert D. Timmerman*[2]

[1]Department of Radiation Oncology, University of Texas Southwestern, Medical Center, Dallas, TX, USA

[2]Department of Radiation Oncology and Neurosurgery, University of Texas Southwestern, Medical Center, Dallas, TX, USA

Introduction

Stereotactic ablative radiotherapy (SABR), historically known as Stereotactic Body Radiation Therapy (SBRT), has rather quickly emerged as an important cancer treatment strategy that challenges dogmas associated with conventional fractionated radiation therapy (CFRT) [1]. Whereas CFRT is typically administered in daily doses, or fractions, in the range of 1.8–2.0 Gy to total doses of 60–70 Gy or so, with SABR much higher doses per fraction are applied, generally in the range of 10–20 Gy per fraction, in an abbreviated, hypofractionated regimen of 5 or fewer fractions. Such high doses per treatment were unthinkable in the past because of limitations in treatment delivery technology that raised concerns about potential toxicity if large volumes of normal tissues were exposed to so much radiation each treatment.

SABR has clearly been facilitated by recent refinements in technology including image-guided techniques, motion assessment and control techniques, and advanced treatment planning dosimetry. This technology has allowed what was previously unattainable, namely, the delivery of very large or ablative dose treatments without necessarily resulting in unacceptable late toxicity. Careful, disciplined analyses of the results of well-designed clinical trials of SABR have led to new understandings of the nuances of normal tissue responses to high-dose ionizing radiation. As clinician-researchers at more institutions become familiar with the principles and adept in the application of SABR, this new treatment paradigm will likely become an established alternative in numerous clinical indications.

Interestingly, SABR has been most commonly applied in either early stage cancer or in metastatic cancer with few indications for intermediate stage cancer [2]. As a primary therapy for early stage lung cancer, for example, SABR offers an elegantly noninvasive and highly efficient treatment option. And for patients with metastatic disease, SABR can serve as a physically targeted systemic cytoreductive agent, envisioned as complementary to novel biologically targeted agents that retard cancer growth generally but provide low response rates in sites of gross disease. In the latter indication, the conceptual approach is aligned with the Norton-Simon hypothesis of cancer growth within a host, whereby it is proposed that reductions in systemic disease burden will render cancers more susceptible to systemic therapy by increasing the proportion of cells within more sensitive phases of the *cell* cycle.

While mostly used in frail medically inoperable patients with lung cancer, SABR should still be

Lung Cancer, Fourth Edition. Edited by Jack A. Roth, Waun Ki Hong and Ritsuko U. Komaki.

viewed as a most potent treatment against gross tumor deposits. Local control with SABR has been shown to be dramatically superior to historical controls using CFRT for early stage lung cancer. Indeed, local control with SABR rivals surgical resection for most indications. Limitations definitely exist as will be discussed in this review. With careful clinical testing, SABR is finding a prominent place within the cancer treatment arsenal.

History of SABR

The negative effects suffered by normal tissue related to very large dose per fraction treatment are well known. Soon after the discovery of radiation at the turn of the last century, large dose per treatment irradiations were performed against accessible tumors. Responses were impressive and hopes were high for a true cancer cure. Unfortunately, late toxic effects appeared months and even years after therapy that were severe. This late toxicity associated with large dose per fraction treatment appeared mostly to affect the normal tissue stroma such as soft tissues, connective tissues, and bone. The toxicity was sclerosing and tissues had definite signs of reduced vasculature. The experience led to an abandonment of using limited numbers of large dose treatments in favor of what became CFRT.

CFRT exploited inherent differences between normal and neoplastic tissues. In particular, neoplastic tissues were noted to allocate much of the cellular machinery to proliferation (via a characteristic called clonogenicity). On the other hand, normal tissues have potential for proliferation, but relatively more capability to repair life's day to day injuries. CFRT gives small multiple small daily doses of radiation resulting in injury to both normal tissues and tumors. On a given day, the normal tissues with greater repair capability will fix relatively more of this modest damage than tumor tissues as shown in Figure 21.1. Over the course of very many days (e.g., 30 or more treatments), the cumulative damage to the tumor is greater than the cumulative damage to the normal tissues. Hence, there is a therapeutic benefit as was first explained decades ago by Coutard and Baclesse. This is very different

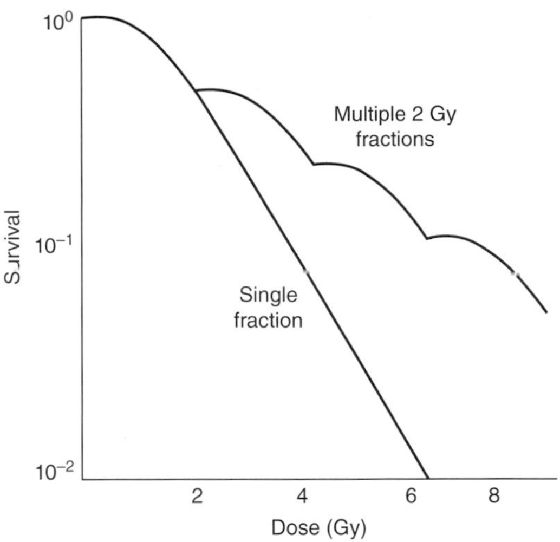

Figure 21.1 Total dose versus log of survival probability (retained ability to form colonies, clonogenicity) for idealized treatments given in a single fraction and for similar doses given in multiple fractions.

than SABR where all tissues exposed to the high prescription doses, whether normal tissue or tumor, are equally and irreversibly destroyed.

The problem with CFRT as demonstrated throughout the modern era of oncology is that even after many days and large cumulative doses of radiation, some populations of tumor clonogens still survive. This puts the patient at substantial risk of local, regional, and distance tumor recurrence with associated morbidity in addition to shortened survival. Oncologists have tried to overcome this inherent radioresistance to CFRT by adding "sensitizers" like chemotherapy or by using CFRT as an adjunct to surgery. While gains have been made, considerable room for improvement remains for many cancer presentations.

The success of brain radiosurgery pioneered by Swedish neurosurgeon Lars Leksell forms the basis of SABR [3]. Leksell broke from the perceived wisdom of CFRT by using large dose single sessions of radiation delivery in, of all places, the radio-intolerant CNS. Although a single large dose radiation treatment was historically intolerable, Leksell's approach defied conventional wisdom by its technology and conduct. Unlike CFRT which often irradiates much larger volumes of normal tissue to the prescription dose than the tumor itself,

Leksell's stereotactic radiosurgery (SRS) went to great lengths to avoid delivering high dose to nontargeted tissues. Whatever normal tissue was included, either by being adjacent to the target or by inferior dosimetry, was likely damaged. However, if this damaged tissue was small in volume or noneloquent, the patient did not suffer clinically apparent toxicity, even as a late event. On the other hand, it is undeniable that the large dose per fraction treatments are biologically extremely potent by overwhelming repair mechanisms. The net result was a convenient and effective treatment.

The earliest examples of treatments mimicking the SRS treatments outside of the brain were reported for treating spine tumors by Hamilton and colleagues [4]. These treatments employed the same rigid immobilization principles of SRS by screwing a frame to the spinous processes. While reports were encouraging, the conduct of the treatment was not as gratifying as natural and inherent motion confounded accuracy. The brain can be practically immobilized by immobilizing the skull. Once the skull is immobilized, targets within the brain have very little additional movement. Such is not the case outside of the skull. Tumors in the body may be displaced as a function of time by forces exerted by muscle contraction, breathing, gastrointestinal peristalsis, cardiac activity, and many other important physiological processes. We cannot eliminate or *account* for all of these forces. As such, SABR is inherently less accurate than SRS.

Not to be dissuaded, researchers again from Sweden, Ingmar Lax and Henric Blomgren, constructed a body frame that would both comfortably immobilize the patient's torso as well as dampen the internal motion relating to respiration [5]. Subsequently, they treated patients with localized tumors using dosimetry plans that mimicked SRS. The dosimetry was constructed using multiple noncoplanar beams with aperture dimensions on the order of the target dimensions. Each of the many beams carried relatively lower weight than with CFRT such that the target dose at the convergence could be dramatically escalated. The team treated patients with mostly metastases initially. Local tumor control was better than expected leading them to treat more limited stage cancer patients. Blomgren and Lax shared their results via publications and eventually trained others in this new technique [6].

Nearly simultaneously with the work carried out by Blomgren and Lax, investigators from Japan were exploring radiosurgery-like treatments in the chest. Shirato and colleagues pioneered investigation into characterization and accounting of respiratory motion [7]. While initially they did not use dose schedules similar to current SABR regimens, the understanding of target motion control was very important for the ultimate feasibility of SABR as it currently exists. Uematsu and colleagues again from Japan worked in the early 1990s on developing technologies for delivering multiple focused beams of radiation for extracranial targets [8]. In addition, Uematsu's group started treating patients with lung tumors and following their outcomes.

With acquisition of more sophisticated technology, the groups at University of Heidelberg, University of Wuerzburg, Kyoto University, and Indiana University refined and broadened their approach for extracranial treatments and began formalized prospective testing [9–12]. Initially, dose escalation toxicity studies were carried out in the liver and lung trying to find the most potent dose schedules for typically radioresistant primary and metastatic tumors. These prospective trials are still following patients long-term and will add a wealth of understanding for the use of SABR. It already has been determined that local tumor control is higher with SABR than has been observed with CFRT. However, true rates of tumor control will require years of follow-up on all treated patients and such data is still maturing. Furthermore, toxicity from large dose per fraction radiation schedules often appears quite "late" from time of treatment. Therefore, it is unlikely that all serious toxicity has yet been observed from prospective trials with less than 10 years follow-up.

Radiobiology of SABR tumor biology

Classical understanding of radiobiology of tumor and normal tissue response was mostly derived from the administration of attainable dose per fraction. SABR involves the administration of very high individual radiation doses. Because many of the fundamental tenets of classical radiobiology were derived and refined over decades through the study of small radiation doses, does SABR stretch traditional radiation dose – response relationship concepts beyond their limits of applicability?

The most widely accepted means of describing the relationship between radiation dose and cell survival is the linear-quadratic (LQ) formula. Although this formula had served the field of radiobiology quite well for decades, Guerrero and Li have questioned whether it is applicable in the range of high doses applied with SABR [13]. These authors have proposed modifying the linear-quadratic formula by incorporating features of the so-called lethal – potentially lethal (LPL) model [14]. The LPL model differs from the LQ model primarily insofar as it accounts for ongoing radiation repair processes that occur *during* the radiation exposure. The net result is a substantial difference in the predicted tumor cell kill at SABR-level doses. For example, for a dose of approximately 20 Gy, the LQ model would predict several orders of magnitude greater cell kill than the LPL model [13].

This debate has practical clinical implications, because it is possible that different available techniques of SABR will deliver the radiation at noticeably different dose rates, over quite variable lengths of total time. This problem of variable treatment delivery time for cranial radiosurgery has been evaluated experimentally by Benedict and colleagues, who evaluated clonogenic survival in vitro doses in the range of 12–18 Gy, using a glioma cell line [15]. For a dose of 18 Gy, increasing the length of treatment from approximately 1/2 to 2 hours corresponded to an order of magnitude decrement in cytotoxicity. Fowler and colleagues have reviewed this topic of loss of biological effect with length of individual treatment delivery and concluded that any treatment administration that lasts more than half an hour might be associated with a clinically significant loss of cytotoxicity [16].

Normal tissue biology and tolerance

Within the lung itself, there are a variety of tissues that possess unique radiation tolerance characteristics, namely, the airways (both large and small functioning as serial structures), vascular trunks and pedicles following similar routes as the bronchial tree (functioning as serial structures), and the alveoli/capillary complexes (functioning as parallel structures) [17, 18]. In addition, the thoracic cavity includes the serially functioning esophagus, serially functioning nerve tissue (e.g., phrenic nerves, brachial plexus, etc.), heart, pericardium, and pleura (all difficult to categorize as parallel or serial), and the bones and musculature of the chest wall. All of these structures will have a unique mechanism of injury and tolerance after SABR.

Conventional radiotherapy commonly causes large serially functioning airway irritation, such as cough, but rarely dose limiting toxicity. In contrast, high-dose SABR schemes may cause significant large airway damage by both mucosal injury and ultimate collapse of the airway. Along the routes of bronchial airways, a similar injury is experienced by blood vessels following a similar route. Altogether, this collective radiation injury appears to mostly affect oxygenation parameters including diffusing capacity for carbon monoxide (DLCO), arterial oxygen tension (pressure) on room air ($P0_2$), and supplemental oxygen requirements ($FI0_2$) [12]. Decline in spirometry indices, including FEV_1 and FVC, are less commonly observed. Because the degree of this airway injury toxicity is related to the proximity of the target to proximal trunks of the branching tubular lung structure, great care should be taken when considering treatment to tumors near the hilum or central chest.

While acute and sometimes severe esophageal toxicity is commonly seen after conventionally fractionated radiation for lung cancer, most of the injury is self-limiting and resolves after treatment. After high dose SABR, esophageal strictures may form as a late effect. Another more unique toxicity from stereotactic ablative radiation therapy relates to pericardial injury. Pericardial effusions may result after treatment for tumors treated adjacent to the heart. Probably by a similar mechanism, pleural effusions commonly develop after SABR treatment of tumors treated adjacent to the chest wall. Usually these fluid collections will reabsorb without intervention after several months of follow-up. Rarely, such fluid collections will need to be drained via thoracentesis in patients symptomatic with shortness of breath, pleurisy, or hypoxia.

Most reports of stereotactic ablative radiation therapy do not include long-term follow-up data. As such, there may be unexpected toxicities that need to be recognized, monitored, and evaluated. Particularly with large doses per fraction there may be unexpected injury related to nerve tissue and vascular tissue. Ideally, dose to brachial plexus, spinal cord, phrenic nerves, and intercostal nerves will be kept low via prudent treatment planning. Furthermore, avoiding large blood vessels in the *central* chest would be reasonable as well. Neurovascular calamities including aneurysms, fistulas with bleeding, or neuropathies (including phrenic or vagal nerve palsies) have rarely *been* reported but may only manifest after many years of follow-up.

Lung toxicity is correlated to target volume. Toxicity related to serially functioning tissues is more predominant in the central chest. Ideally, SABR should demonstrate a high degree of conformality between the prescription dose and the target. Lung within the target exceeds tolerance and is no longer functional after high dose SABR. A dose fall-off region exists outside of the target, the volume of which depends on the size of the target, the location of the target within the chest, the quality of the radiation dosimetry (e.g., number of beams, beam arrangements, radiation energy, etc.), and the type of radiation (e.g., photon versus proton, etc.). This dose fall-off region, also called the gradient region, constitutes unintended radiation exposure and should be kept as small as possible.

Defining SABR

In 2004 after several years of planning, the lung committee of the Radiation Therapy Oncology Group (RTOG) finalized plans to carry out a multicenter trial of SABR in patients with medically inoperable non-small cell lung cancer (NSCLC). As this was the first multicenter trial of its kind, the first step was to define the therapy. Previously, a working group from the American College of Radiology and American Society for Therapeutic Radiology and Oncology had formulated guidelines for the conduct of SBRT [1]. The guidelines described the following essential components collectively unique to its conduct:

1 Secure immobilization avoiding patient movement for the typical long treatment sessions.

2 Accurate repositioning of the patient from planning sessions to each of the treatment sessions.

3 Proper accounting of inherent internal organ motion including breathing motion consistently between planning and treatment.

4 Construction of dose distributions confidently covering tumor and yet falling off very rapidly to surrounding normal tissues. The dosimetry must be extremely conformal in relation to the prescription isodose line compared to the target outline but may allow very heterogeneous target dose ranges.

5 Registration of the patient's anatomy, constructed dosimetry, and treatment delivery to a 3D coordinate system as referenced to fiducials. Fiducia are "markers" whose position can be confidently correlated both to the tumor target and the treatment delivery device. A "stereotactic" treatment is one directed by such fiducial references. SABR treatment deliveries can also be guided and directed by volumetric image data sets.

6 Biologically potent dose prescriptions using a few (i.e., 1–5) fractions of very high dose (e.g., generally a minimum of 6 Gy per fraction but often as high as 20–30 Gy per fraction).

This therapy is used to treat well demarcated visible gross disease up to 5–7 cm in dimension. It is not used for prophylactic (adjuvant) treatment as the intent is to totally disrupt clonogenicity and likely disrupt all cellular functioning of the target tissues (i.e., the definition of an ablative therapy).

Effectively, SABR is a treatment that can ablate or totally destroy that to which it is aimed. Such a treatment, properly directed would constitute a most potent form of cancer therapy. In turn, if misdirected or used too liberally, SABR could lead to debilitating toxicity. Whether the potent SABR dose can truly be placed primarily within tumor using stereotactic targeting, motion control, ideal immobilization and specialized dosimetry techniques remains to be proven in all clinical circumstances. At any rate, SABR is not similar to CFRT in its conduct, toxicity, or ability to control cancer.

Immobilization and target motion issues related to SABR

The geometry and dose distribution from the radiation therapy treatment plan should be a reasonably true characterization of what is actually delivered to the patient. With the typical large volume of treatment and homogeneous dose distributions characteristic of CFRT, such an emphasis on the proper correlation of the treatment plan and actual treatment is probably not so critical. However, for SABR, claims regarding accuracy of equipment, quality of dose distributions, and dose tolerance should not be made based on the virtual computer simulation of the treatment plan; rather, on actual delivery of dose to treated patients. This is particularly true for predicting normal tissue toxicity from SABR where both heterogeneous dose and differential volume effects may equally affect outcome.

Consistent and reproducible immobilization is one option for improving treatment accuracy. Body frames, vacuum pillows, thermal plastic restraints, and other equipment have been used to try to achieve relocalization similar to the position of simulation [19–32]. Other systems will effectively relocate a reference position within the patient prior to each treatment without the aid of frames or other immobilization devices (i.e., "frameless" systems) [33–36]. Both approaches have advantages and disadvantages and no clearly superior method has been identified in clinical practice. In the end, it is most critical to be practical. SABR treatment sessions are longer than CFRT sessions. Hence, it is important that the positioning system be comfortable and avoid awkward positions or positions fighting against gravity. In addition, the system employed must be properly utilized. As such, staff training and properly administered quality assurance programs are more essential than using a particular brand of equipment.

Motion control devices fall into three general categories: (a) dampening, (b) gating, and (c) chasing. Within the category of dampening includes the systems of abdominal compression aimed at decreasing one of the largest contributors to respiratory motion related to the diaphragm [22, 25, 26, 28, 29, 32]. Also included in this category are the systems employing breath hold maneuvers to "freeze" the tumor in a reproducible stage of the respiratory cycle (e.g., deep inspiration) [37–40]. Gating systems follow the respiratory cycle using a surrogate and employ an electronic beam activation trigger allowing irradiation to only occur during a specific segment (e.g., end expiration) [34, 41–43]. Tracking systems literally move the radiation beam along the same path as the tumor from the beam's eye view [44,47]. Tracking may be accomplished by moving the entire accelerator, the aperture (e.g., with the multi-leaf collimator), or moving the patient on the couch counter to the motion of the tumor. In the case of gating and breath hold, the beam is triggered on and off constituting a duty cycle avoided by the other systems. In any case, the acquisition of planning information must include the same consideration for motion accounting as the treatment in order to achieve accuracy. Despite available motion control equipment, some uncertainty continues to require that planning treatment volume (PTV) be larger than gross tumor volume (GTV). In general for typical dose prescriptions, this enlargement should not be greater than 1.0 cm in the cranial caudal plane and 0.5 cm in the axial plane.

Physics and dosimetry of SABR

SABR requires extremely conformal dose distributions that fall off very rapidly, ideally in all directions, and generally requires the use of multiple shaped beams [48–50]. Highly shaped beams are desired because high dose is best eliminated in normal tissues by sharp collimation of primary beam fluence attenuation outside of the target from the beam's-eyeview. Conversely, smaller nonshaped beams may be used to treat successive regions of the target [51]. Scatter dose is less easily controlled, even by highly shaped beams. Most modern SABR treatments for lung and liver targets use around 10–12 highly collimated beams. In order to avoid overlap dose between entrance and exit trajectories, these beams are ideally nonopposing and have as large hinge angles between them as possible. In addition and in an effort to assure dose gradients fall off rapidly in all directions, the beams should generally be noncoplanar. Coplanar treatments such as is commonly utilized in CFRT particularly with IMRT results in low and intermediate dose "spillage" that surrounds the tumor in an annular fashion. Ideally, this spillage dose would be distributed in a geometry potentially capable of treating occult microscopic extension of tumor. Except perhaps for targets in the vertebral bodies of the spine, there is no reason based on anatomy, tissue function, or known patterns of tumor spread to construct such a predominantly axial dose distribution around the target. Collisions between the patient and accelerator head or the couch and accelerator head will limit the ability to create truly isotropically decreasing dose gradients around targets, but effort should be made to mimic such ideal distributions as much as possible [52, 53].

For SABR, it is assumed that the GTV is nearly identical to the clinical target volume (CTV) for conduct of the treatment. Because of target motion and setup inaccuracies, an additional margin must encompass the GTV/CTV target in order to avoid missing the intended target during part or all of the treatment session. This expanded target called the PTV constitutes the final target for high-dose conformal coverage. In addition to the PTV and its contents, ablation is likely to occur in the shell of normal tissue immediately outside of the target in the regions of intermediate to high dose. As such, side effects will or will not occur depending on: (1) how essential this inner shell of tissue is for normal function of the organ, and (2) the thickness or volume of this shell as it relates to the quality of the dosimetry. This *high dose spillage* is likely the culprit in most of the toxicity related to serially functioning tissues like tubular structures in the lung, GI tract, and liver causing obliteration of the lumen and subsequent downstream effects. Furthermore, the quality of the dose distribution will affect the volume and geometry of low to intermediate dose distributions. This *intermediate dose spillage* is characterized by the maximum dose at a defined distance away from the target (e.g., 2–3 cm) or by the volume of tissue encompassed by an intermediate isodose line (e.g., the 50% of prescription isodose line). *Intermediate dose spillage* can affect the organ more globally, similar to the historically large fields associated with CFRT damaging parallel functioning tissues, but may also cause focal organ injury if the prescription dose is high enough.

Prescription isodose conformality to the target volume is generally assessed by a conformality index. This index is the ratio of the prescription isodose volume to the PTV volume. Generally, this ratio should be kept below 1.2. Achieving this degree of conformality is easier with larger targets. While CFRT results in mostly homogeneous target dose distributions, SABR may have dramatic heterogeneity of dose. It must be insured that regions within the PTV target is not underdosed relative to the minimum prescription dose; however, overdosage is probably of no consequence and may even be advantageous in centrally hypoxic tumors. It is critical, however, that high dose "hot spots" associated with this dose heterogeneity are not physically located outside of the PTV. This would be an extreme form of *high dose spillage* and can generally be avoided by using additional highly shaped beams with unique entrance angles.

Organ exposure limits must be respected with SABR. It has been known that radiation tolerance of specific organs is related to total dose (and fractionation), volume, and inherent radiosensitivity. However, most quoted tolerances are generally quantified as essentially dose limits. Such characterization is clearly inadequate for SABR where toxicity is more often related to exceeding a specified volume of tissue receiving a given dose than the absolute dose level itself. Data are accumulating for dose – volume tolerances for specific organs affected by SABR. At the present time, however, such tolerances are not available. Instead, most

Table 21.1 Normal tissue dose constraints for 3 fraction SABR treatments to the lung

Organ	Volume	Dose (cGy)
Spinal cord esophagus	Any point	18 Gy (6 Gy per fraction)
Ipsilateral brachial	Any point	27 Gy (9 Gy per fraction)
Plexus	Any point	24 Gy (8 Gy per fraction)
Heart/pericardium	Any point	30 Gy (10 Gy per fraction)
Trachea and ipsilateral bronchus	Any point	30 Gy (10 Gy per fraction)
Skin	Any point	24 Gy (8 Gy per fraction)

investigators are using limits converted from CFRT using linear quadratic modeling or applying limits based on limited experience in treated patients. Since volume effects are poorly understood, absolute point limits were implemented for critical organs like the spinal cord, esophagus, and major bronchial airways. These limits are subject to modification after further evaluation but the limits used in the RTOG lung cancer 3 fraction protocols are listed for reference in Table 21.1. These were implemented as part of a protocol that uses 60 Gy total in 3 fractions (20 Gy per fraction) for target prescription and would not necessarily apply to different fractionation schedules.

Many potential targets for SABR will require beams to travel through tissues of variable electronic density en route to the target. Ideally, then, the planning system would include algorithms for accurate accounting of tissue heterogeneity effects as it relates to dose deposition from both attenuation and scattering events. Some planning systems do a good job of modeling these effects; however, some do a very poor job. Indeed, published reports show that using a primitive heterogeneity correction algorithm may lead to greater inaccuracies of dose representation at the edge of the PTV than using no correction at all [54]. As such, it seems most reasonable that either sophisticated heterogeneity corrections be implemented (e.g., collapsed cone) or that no heterogeneity corrections should be used for SABR treatments in or near the lungs.

An example of typical SABR dosimetry for treating a primary lung cancer is shown in Figure 21.2. The beam angles were chosen by first considering the realm of attainable beam angles for a tumor in this location avoiding collisions with the accelerator head. Within this subset of attainable beam angles, a beam weight optimization algorithm was used to select these particular 10 angles using the RTOG tolerances to construct avoidance structures. In the end, the beams are noncoplanar, nonopposing, and are separated by fairly large hinge angles. Beam weights are divided fairly equal between all beams so as to spread out entrance dose.

Treatment experience in non-small cell lung cancer

Medically inoperable stage I patients

Early experience using SABR for NSCLC consisted of mostly uncontrolled retrospective reports as mentioned above in section under history. These experiences showed that tumor shrinkage early after therapy was very likely after SABR, even with more modest dose prescriptions. There was wide variability of both the number of fractions and the dose prescribed per fraction, even within a single institution experience. Some reports had very small numbers followed short periods of time, yet made strong conclusions regarding adequacy of dose and late effects. Tumor recurrence after an effective therapy will occur much later than after an ineffective therapy due to population growth kinetics. Furthermore, toxicity of high dose per fraction therapy will likely occur quite late after therapy. Therefore, it is most rational to investigate the role of SABR in NSCLC using clearly defined selection, consistent treatment, strict quality assurance measures, and uniform follow-up policy. In addition, follow-up should make mandatory that all patients are assessed and published reports await mature evaluation of outcome data. Such constraints can only be met by regimented prospective testing.

Using the treatment process described above, researchers at Indiana University performed a

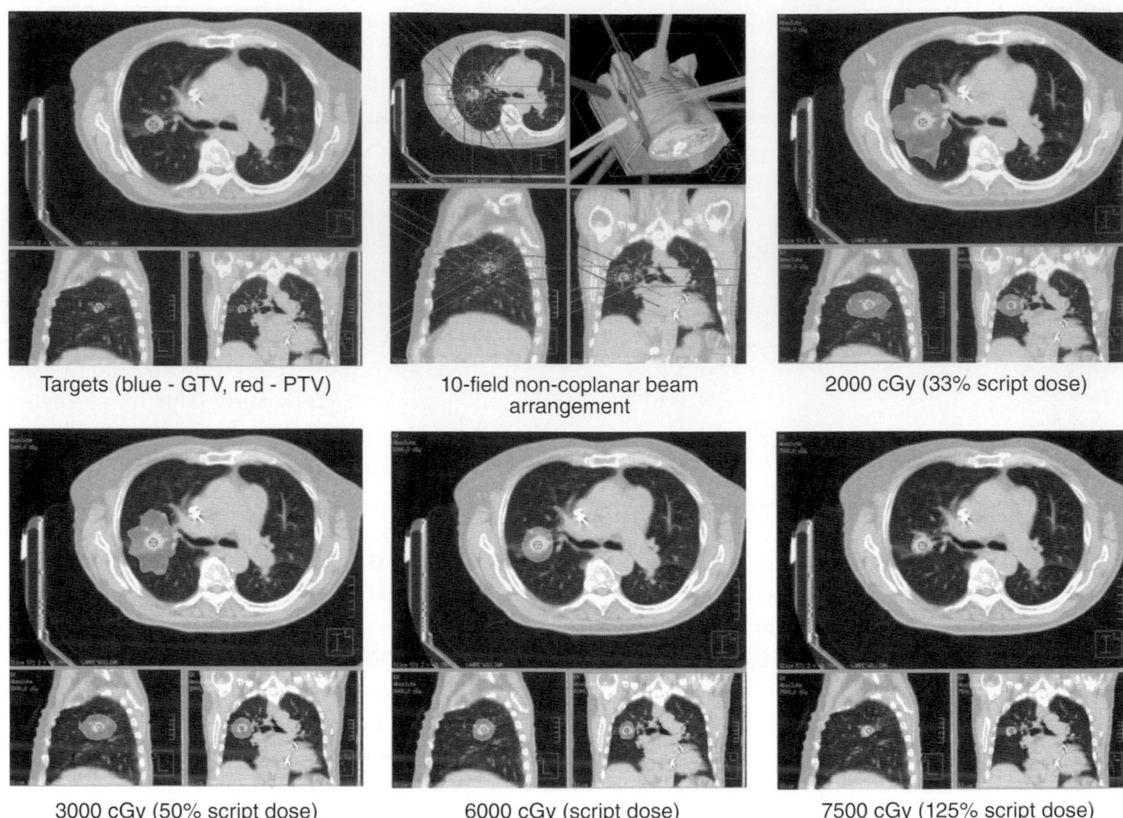

Figure 21.2 Targeting and dose construction for a typical SBRT treatment in the lung. Ten nonopposing and noncoplanar beams deliver radiation fluence to the demarcated tumor target with high dose delivery to the tumor and margin and rapid falloff in all directions.

formal phase I dose escalation toxicity study with 47 patients with medically inoperable non-small cell lung cancer, T1-T2, N0 [12,55]. The starting dose was 8 Gy per fraction times three, 24 Gy total. All patients were treated with 3 fractions at all dose levels. Independent dose escalation trials were carried out in three separate patient groups: T_1 tumor patients, T_2 tumor <5 cm patients, and T_2 tumor 5–7 cm patients. There was no restriction regarding the location of the tumor in the lung as both central and peripheral tumors were treated. A total of seven dose levels were tested. The maximum tolerated dose (MTD) was never reached for T_1 tumors and T_2 tumors less than 5 cm despite reaching 60–66 Gy in 3 fractions. For the largest tumors, dose was escalated all the way to 72 Gy in 3 fractions which proved to be too toxic. A characteristic tumor response for a patient is shown in Figure 21.3. Dose limiting toxicity in that subset included pneumonia and pericardial effusion. Therefore, the MTD for tumors 5–7 cm in diameter was 66 Gy in 3 fractions while the MTD for smaller tumors lies at an undetermined level beyond this dose. Classic radiation pneumonitis (fever, chest pain, shortness of breath, dry cough, and infiltrative X-ray findings), which had been erroneously predicted to be the dose-limiting toxicity, only occurred sporadically.

At the lower doses (i.e., 24–36 Gy in 3 fractions), very impressive tumor responses with little normal tissue effects were observed by 3 months. Unfortunately many of these patients ultimately had tumor recurrence. As the dose was escalated

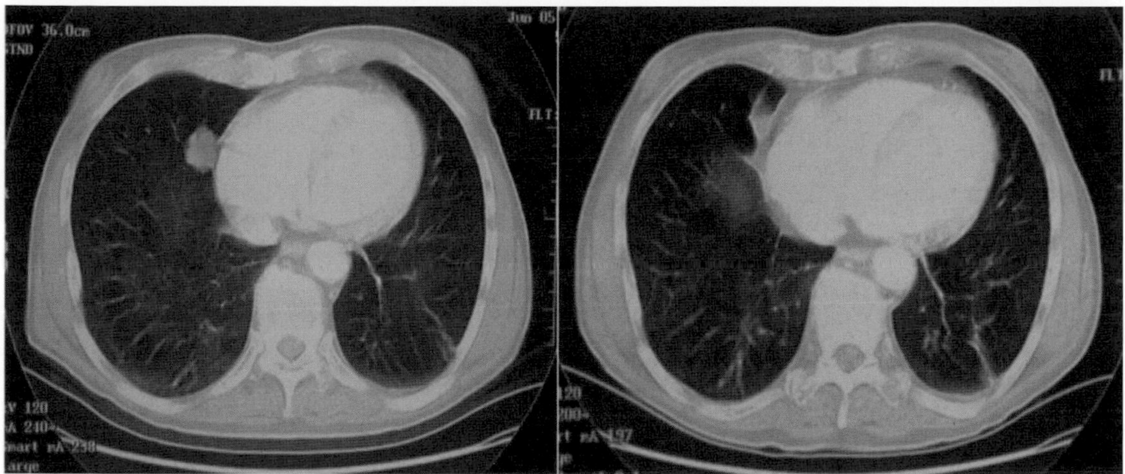

Figure 21.3 Patient with a solitary pulmonary nodule before and 2 years after treatment with SABR. The tumor has dramatically reduced in size, but a remnant remains. The lung shows some focal fibrosis and the nearby pericardium is thicker in the posttreatment scan.

beyond 42–48 Gy, striking imaging changes began to appear near the treated tumor by around 6–12 months. This seemed to be related to a bronchial toxicity, which was not commonly described with CFRT. Radiographic changes by themselves were not considered dose limiting, and most of these imaging changes were asymptomatic. In many cases the radiographic changes mimic tumor recurrence. With no salvage therapy in this population, patients were followed without treatment. Repeat PET scans and biopsies showed no evidence of tumor recurrence in the large majority of patients treated at the higher dose levels. In the end, a dose of 60–66 Gy in 3 fractions was determined to be reasonably safe for enrolled medically inoperable NSCLC patients.

Upon completion of the phase I study finding a clearly potent dose for SABR, the Indiana group embarked on a 70-patient phase II study in the same population. The phase II study was aimed at validating toxicity in a larger patient population and determining efficacy (local control or survival) using a total dose of 60 Gy in 3 fractions for the small tumors and 66 Gy in 3 fractions for the large tumors (35 patients for each group). The target control rate for the statistical power calculation was 80% which is dramatically higher than the typical 30–45% control seen with CFRT. All high-grade adverse events (e.g., emergency room visits, surgical procedures, hospitalizations, and deaths) were reviewed by an independent data safety monitoring panel to determine if the event was treatment related (i.e., treatment-related toxicity). In addition, this panel was responsible for final scoring of efficacy such as determining local recurrence.

The principal results of this phase II trial are in Timmerman *et al.* [56]. The actuarial 2-year local control for this potent dose regimen was 95%, and isolated hilar or mediastinal nodal relapse was extremely rare despite clinical staging. The overall 2-year survival for this frail population was poor at 56% with most of the deaths related to comorbid illness rather than disease progression or toxicity. The protocol placed no time limits on scoring treatment-related toxicity and many late toxic events have been recorded. Fewer than 20% of patients have experienced high-grade toxicity confirming the phase I model. However, interim analysis showed that severe toxicity (grade 3–5) was significantly more likely in patients treated for tumors in the regions around the proximal bronchial tree or central chest region. In fact, the risk of severe toxicity is two times greater when treating central tumors as compared to peripheral tumors.

Table 21.2 Local control in early-stage non-small cell lung cancer

Author	Treatment	Local control	Single fraction equivalent dose (ref. [62])	Reference
North America/Europe				
Timmerman, 2010	20 Gy × 3	91% (3 yr)	56 Gy	[67]
Timmerman, 2006	20–22 Gy × 3	95% (2+ yr)	56–62 Gy	[56]
Baumann, 2006	15 Gy × 3	80% (3 yr)	41 Gy	[57]
Fritz, 2006	30 Gy × 1	80% (3 yr)	30 Gy	[58]
Nyman, 2006	15 Gy × 3	80% (crude)	41 Gy	[59]
Zimmermann, 2005	12.5 Gy × 3	87% (3 yr)	43.5 Gy	[60]
Timmerman, 2003	18–24 Gy × 3	90% (2 yr)	50–68 Gy	[12, 55]
Asia				
Xia, 2006	5 Gy × 10	95% (3 yr)	32 Gy	[64]
Hara, 2006	30–34 Gy × 1	80% (3 yr)	30–34 Gy	[65]
Nagata, 2005	12 Gy × 4	94% (3 yr)	42 Gy	[63]

Similar experiences have been reported in Europe and Japan. Active groups from Sweden, Denmark, Germany, the Netherlands, and Italy have reported rates of local control and toxicity similar to the Indiana experience at similar dose levels [57–60]. A variety of dose and fractionation schemes have been used, however, generally fewer than 5 total fractions have been employed. As with the Indiana group, Wulf and colleagues from Wurzburg have demonstrated a clear dose response relationship with better control at higher dose levels [61]. As shown in Table 21.2, clinical results are generally better with similar dose potency in Japan as opposed to North America/Europe [62–65].

As an example, Nagata and colleagues from Kyoto University published a series of 45 patients treated with a dose of 48 Gy in 4 fractions to the isocenter [63]. This dose is biologically less potent than the dose fractionation schemes used in prospective North American trials (60–66 Gy in 3 fractions) or roughly equivalent to European trials (45 Gy in 3 fractions). Still, Nagata reported effectively no in-field local failures (100% local control) with this dose which is in contrast to the results published from North America and Europe where local control is only 70–80% with dose prescriptions in the this range. The techniques used by Nagata and colleagues for immobilization, targeting, dosimetry, and treatment conduct are essentially identical to what was used at Indiana University. This same dose prescription piloted at Kyoto University was tested in the larger Japan Clinical Oncology Group 0403 phase II trial for operable peripheral T1N0 stage 1 patients [66]. Preliminary results from this study, in abstract form, demonstrated an 86% 3-year primary tumor control and 76% 3-year overall survival rate for patients with a median age of 79 years, in line with surgical series. A clue, however, to the likely explanation for these conflicting results between experienced centers in North America and Asia may be found in the overall survival results. Two-year overall survival in the Nagata series was over 80% in striking contrast to the Indiana phase II study and European experiences where only around 50% of patients are alive. Indeed, the Nagata series survival for medically inoperable patients is quite comparable to series describing operable patients in North America. As such, it appears these are different populations indicating a striking difference in patient selection.

In 2004, after several years of planning, the lung committee of the RTOG finalized plans to carry out a multicenter trial of SABR in patients with medically inoperable NSCLC. The results of RTOG 0236 using SABR for medically inoperable lung cancer in patients with peripherally situated tumors was published in *JAMA* in 2010 [67]. This trial was based on the preliminary data from Indiana University using 60 Gy in 3 fractions for T1, T2, and peripheral T3 tumors less than 5 cm in diameter. Extensive accreditation, conduct, and dosimetry constraints were developed in the RTOG Lung, Physics, and Image-Guided Therapy Committees in order to form a basis for meaningful quality assurance and consistent treatment for a multicenter trial. Three toxicity analyses were performed during the trial which showed no excessive toxicity warranting trial closure. RTOG 0236 accrued 55 patients, 44 with T_1 lesions and 11 with T_2. With a median follow-up of 2.9 years, 3-year tumor control was 98%, 3-year local control was 91%, the rate of distant metastases was 22%, and median overall survival was four years [67]. At three years, disease free survival was 48% and overall survival was 56%, similar to surgical outcomes. No deaths from treatment related toxicity was reported. This study has set the practice pattern for treatment of medically inoperable, early stage NSCLC with SABR. Of note, for RTOG 0236 as well as the Indiana University institutional lead up studies, doses to 60–66 Gy in 3 fractions were planned and delivered without heterogeneity corrections.

In addition to the practice changing results from RTOG 0236, large population based studies may also have shed light on the role of SABR for medically inoperable patients. A cohort based population study out of David Palma's group from the Netherlands used national records to demonstrate changes in lung cancer treatment practice patterns over three chronological eras. For early stage, medically inoperable NSCLC patients, the first era had no use of SABR, followed by gradual acceptance in some centers during the second era, and more wide appeal in the most recent era. There was a fundamental improvement in survival within this population of patients from the first thru third eras that could only be ascribed to increasing use of SABR. Other than prospective clinical trials, these population based cohort studies can provide some correlative evidence demonstrating the increasing relevance and benefit of specific treatment modalities, in this case SABR [68].

RTOG 0236 has logically been followed by RTOG 0813, a phase I/II trial attempting to identify a maximum tolerated dose for medically inoperable patients treated with SABR for centrally located lesions. Five fraction regimens have been used, starting at 50 Gy, with the study now evaluating a larger cohort of patients at 60 Gy. The study has very recently finished accruing its target number of patients at the highest 60 Gy dose cohort. Several other single institution efforts have suggested fractionation and total dose schemes that may offer safe and effective means of treating centrally located tumors with SABR [69, 70]. Interestingly, future studies with centrally located tumors may employ protons, as retrospective and dose evaluation studies have demonstrated a superiority with protons versus photons with respect to normal tissue toxicity [71].

Along with location and operability being an important variable in SABR usage, total dose and fractionation are also important questions. RTOG 0915 is a large, phase II cooperative group study aimed at determining control and toxicity rates between two fractionation schemes – 12 Gy × 4 and 34 Gy × 1, for peripherally located lesions. The more optimal of the two fractionations will be compared to 18 Gy × 3 (with heterogeneity corrections). Accrual for this study has been completed and data analysis of results soon to be reported.

Finally, several trials have been proposed for giving adjuvant systemic therapy along with SABR in an effort to reduce the risk of patients at higher risk of systemic relapse – very relevant in light of the rate of distant metastases seen in RTOG 0236 patients. The goal will be to use the systemic agents to help with regional and distant control, while the SABR will be used to promote local control. The combination therapy may hold the greatest promise for even greater disease free intervals and even improved overall survival.

Operable stage I patients

Patients deemed healthy enough for surgery have been treated with SABR based on the patient's preference to avoid surgery. Most of the work in this population has been carried out in Japan. Onishi and colleagues performed a large retrospective chart review of patients treated at several Japanese centers using SABR in early stage NSCLC [72]. While dose and number of fractions varied considerably, all patients were treated with small volumes under stereotactic guidance. This report included a large number of operable patients that were analyzed separately. For such patients who received dose levels such that the biological effective dose (BED) was greater than 100 [73], local control and survival rivaled best surgical series according to the authors. The 3-year overall survival in this group was 88%. This report has formed the basis for enrolling patient with operable tumors onto a separate arm of the Japan Clinical Oncology Group 0403 trial for peripheral T1N0 stage I patients.

In the United States, very few patients with operable stage I NSCLC have been treated on clinical trials. That situation may change after the resuls of RTOG 0618 for operable patients are published. RTOG 0618 has completed accrual of patients with documented NSCLC who are medically suitable for surgical anatomical resection but treated with SABR. This is a dramatic departure from previous trials in North America where only frail medically inoperable patients were enrolled onto SABR trials. This trial, patterned after RTOG 0236, included an early assessment for surgical salvage in people with less than ideal response. As such, SABR is being studied in broader populations with early stage NSCLC building on the existing prospective testing. Based on best surgical literature, it will be required that SABR attain a local control rate of 90% or better in order to compete with lobectomy [74]. Consequently, very potent dose prescriptions will be required. As noted above, it is likely that higher dose levels will be required in the United States as opposed to Asian series in order to attain this high rate of local control. RTOG 0618 is modeled after RTOG 0236 except eligibility is for healthier patients capable of tolerating thoracotomy. The prescription dose is 60 Gy in 3 fractions and frequent tumor status assessments are made in order to identify failure early and attempt surgical salvage. Preliminary data from RTOG 0618 was recently presented at the American Society of Clinical Oncology Annual Meeting 2013. Twenty-six of 33 patients were evaluable with 23 having T1 disease and the other three having T2 disease. There were no grade 4–5 toxicity and only four patients had grade 3 toxicities attributable to SABR. With a median follow-up of 25 months, an estimated 2-year primary tumor failure rate was 7.7%. Progression free survival and overall survival at 2 years was estimated at 65.4% and 84.4%, respectively, suggesting a high rate of primary tumor control and relative equivalence with historical surgical outcomes [75].

While waiting on RTOG 0618 data to be finalized in paper form, a study initiated in the United States may offer very important clues as to the equivalence between SABR and resection. The ACOSOG (Z4099)/RTOG (1021) randomized phase III study has recently begun to accrue high risk, early stage T1/T2 N0 NSCLC patients (tumors less than or equal to 3 cm) to either sublobar resection or SABR to 54 Gy in three fractions. These patients are considered at high risk for significant toxicity associated with lobectomy and thus are randomized to lesser resections +/− brachytherapy versus SABR. This study will provide important data on toxicity profiles and local and distant control rates with the use of the two key treatment modalities.

SABR for lung cancer metastases, multiple primary lung tumors, and recurrent lung cancer

For late stage NSCLC, systemic therapy has traditionally been the mainstay of treatment. Failure rates are generally high in this setting and overall survival is low. Recent efforts have been employed to identify newer paradigms to improve both progression free survival and overall survival in the stage IV setting [76, 77]. Over the last several years, SABR has been used in the treatment of isolated pulmonary metastases in medically inoperable patients from a number of primary disease sites. Several institutions have also used SABR to treat limited or oligometastatic disease to many body sites (lung, mediastinum, liver, bone, adrenal) in the stage IV NSCLC setting to aid in PFS with promising outcomes [78]. As a means of debulking active disease to make tumor more amenable to systemic agents, in line with the Norton-Simon hypothesis, Kavanagh, Timmerman, and colleagues opened a Phase II study for stage IV NSCLC patients who have failed first line chemotherapy. These patients, as long as they had only up to six sites of metastatic disease extracranially, were treated with SABR to all sites of known disease and concurrently given Erlotinib. Twenty-four of 24 planned patients have been accrued to the trial. Results appear very encouraging but are still under review. From an early look at the study outcomes, these stage IV NSCLC patients have a far greater PFS and OS than the historical findings for systemic therapy use alone in a second line setting [79].

SABR has also been indicated for two other patient populations with promise for future therapeutic intervention – those with multiple early stage primaries and patients with recurrent disease after previous radiation. SABR appears to be a viable alternative to multiple or larger resections for patients with several smaller primary lung cancers [80, 81]. It can also be used safely and effectively in patients who have recurred locally after conventionally fractionated thoracic radiation for their primary NSCLCs [82].

Summary

The technological developments surrounding the implementation of SABR were the product of mostly engineering and physics research. However, they facilitate the exploitation of the more important biological determinants of local control [83]. Ablation of tumor using total dose or dose per fraction well beyond conventional radiation promises in the end to serve to improve outcome. This necessary collaboration between technical resource development and biological innovation holds considerable promise for patients with lung cancer.

As systemic treatments become more effective, radiotherapy will be used more selectively to target isolated deposits of gross disease [2]. Currently limited to treatment with curative intent in stage I–III disease, radiotherapy will likely be used more often in stage IV disease either as a measure for consolidation or to ablate cancer deposits resistant to systemic therapy. With exploitation of technology and biological understanding, this is an ideal role for SABR as an efficacious and cost effective modality for local control of gross disease.

The goal of technical, biological, and clinical research in radiation oncology as well as in collaboration with surgical and medical oncologists is to facilitate "adaptive" therapy [84–86]. In this paradigm, pretreatment diagnostic information including imaging, staging, tissue samples (proteomic, genomics, etc.), and other predictive assays will be integrated to make therapy selection. Having chosen the correct approach, the patient is started on therapy while monitoring progress. Early assessments relating to accuracy of delivery, tumor response, metabolic changes, tolerance, and others can be used to change the therapy appropriately during therapy [87–89]. Soon after treatment, imaging and metabolic assessment may direct the need for adjuvant therapies or avoid toxicity. Rather than a "one size fits all" cancer therapy, the adaptive process uses a tailored approach that constantly re-evaluates and responds to redirect the therapy toward a better outcome. Until this goal is achieved, patients will continue to be enrolled onto well-designed prospective trials such that SABR might be refined to its optimal potential.

References

1 Potters L, Steinberg M, Rose C, *et al.*, for American Society for Therapeutic Radiology and Oncology; American College of Radiology (2004) American Society for Therapeutic Radiology and Oncology and American College of Radiology practice guideline for the performance of stereotactic ablative radiation therapy. *Int J Radiat Oncol Biol Phys*, Nov 15, 60(4): 1026–32.

2 Timmerman R, Papiez L. Review of Song *et al.* (2004) Stereotactic ablative radiation therapy: rationale, techniques, applications, and optimization of an emerging technology. *Oncology*, 18(4): 474–7.

3 Leksell L (1951) The stereotaxic method and radiosurgery of the brain. *Acta Chir Scand*, 102: 316–19.

4 Hamilton AJ, Lulu BA, Fosmire H, Stea B, Cassady JR (1995) Preliminary clinical experience with

linear accelerator-based spinal stereotactic radiosurgery. *Neurosurgery*, 36(2): 311–19.

5 Lax I, Blomgren H, Naslund I, Svanstrom R (1994) Stereo-tactic radiotherapy of extracranial targets. *Z Med Phys*, 4: 112–13.

6 Blomgren H, Lax I, Naslund I, Svanstrom R (1995) Stereo-tactic high dose fraction radiation therapy of extracranial tumors using an accelerator. *Acta Oncol*, 34(6): 861–70.

7 Shirato H, Shimizu S, Tadashi S, Nishioka T, Miyasaka K (1999) Real time tumour-tracking radiotherapy. *Lancet*, 353: 1331–2.

8 Uematsu M, Shioda A, Tahara K, *et al.* (1998) Focal, high dose, and fractionated modified stereotactic radiation therapy for lung carcinoma patients: a preliminary experience. *Cancer*, Mar 15, 82(6): 1062–70.

9 Herfarth KK, Debus J, Lohr F, *et al.* (2001) Stereotactic single-dose radiation therapy of liver tumors: Results of a phase PH trial. *J Clin Onc*, Jan 1, 19(1): 164–70.

10 Wulf J, Hadinger U, Oppitz U, Thiele W, NessDourdoumas R, Flentje M (2001) Stereotactic radiotherapy of targets in the lung and liver. *Strahlenther Onkol Dec*, 177(12): 645–55.

11 Nagata Y, Negoro V, Aoki T *et al.* (2002) Clinical outcomes of 3D conformal hypofractionated single high-dose radiotherapy for one or two lung tumors using a stereotactic ablative frame. *Int J Radiat Oncol Biol Phys*, Mar 15, 52(4): 1041–6.

12 Timmerman R, Papiez L, McGarry R *et al.* (2003) Extracranial stereotactic radioablation: Results of a phase I study in medically inoperable stage I non-small cell lung cancer. *Chest*, Nov; 124(5): 1946–55.

13 Guerrero M, Li X (2004) Extending the linear – quadratic model for large fraction doses pertinent to stereotactic radiotherapy. *Phys Med Biol*, 49: 4825–35.

14 Curtis SB (1986) Lethal and potentially lethal lesions induced by radiation – a unified repair model. *Radiat Res*, 106: 252–70.

15 Benedict SH, Lin PS, Zwicker RD, *et al.* (1997) The biological effectiveness of intermittent irradiation as a function of overall treatment time: development of correction factors for linac-based stereotactic radiotherapy. *Int J Radiat Oncol Biol Phys*, 37: 765–9.

16 Fowler IF, Welsh JS, Howard SE (2004) Loss of biological effect in prolonged fraction delivery. *Int J Radiat Oncol Biol Phys*, May 1, 59(1): 242–9.

17 Wolbarst AB, Chin LM, Svensson GK (1982) Optimization of radiation therapy: integral-response of a model biological system. *Int J Radiat Oncol Biol Phys*, 8: 1761–9.

18 Yeas RJ, Kalend A (1988) Local stem cell depletion model for radiation myelitis. *Int J Radiat Oncol Biol Phys*, 14: 1247–59.

19 Nevinny-Stickel M, Sweeney RA, Bale RJ, Posch A, Auberger T, Lukas P (2004) Reproducibility of patient positioning for fractionated extracranial stereotactic radiotherapy using a double-vacuum technique. *Strahlenther Onkol*, Feb, 180(2): 117–22.

20 Fuss M, Salter J, Rassiah P, Cheek D, Cavanaugh SX, Herman TS (2004) Repositioning accuracy of a commercially available double-vacuum whole body immobilization system for stereotactic ablative radiation therapy. *Technol Cancer Res Treat*, Feb; 3(1): 59–67.

21 Hof H, Herfarth KK, Munter M, Essig M, Wannenmacher M, Debus J (2003) The use of the multislice CT for the determination of respiratory lung tumor movement in stereotactic single-dose irradiation. *Strahlenther Onkol*, Aug; 179(8): 542–7.

22 Nagata Y, Negoro Y, Aoki T *et al.* (2001) Three-dimensional conformal radiotherapy for extracranial tumors using a stereotactic ablative frame. *Igaku Butsuri*, 2: 28–34.

23 Fairclough-Tompa L, Larsen T, Jaywant SM (2001) Immobilization in stereotactic radiotherapy: The head and neck localizer frame. *Med Dosim*, Fall; 26(3): 267–73.

24 Albeit H, Dornfeld S, Dawel M *et al.* (2001) Patient position reproducibility in fractionated stereotactically guided conformal radiotherapy using the BrainLab mask system. *Strahlenther Onkol*, May; 177(5): 264–8.

25 Negoro Y, Nagata Y, Aoki T *et al.* (2001) The effectiveness of an immobilization device in conformal radiotherapy for lung tumor: reduction of respiratory tumor movement and evaluation of the daily setup accuracy. *Int J Radiat Oncol Biol Phys*; 50(4): 889–98.

26 Wulf J, Hadinger U, Oppitz U, Olshausen B, Flentje M (2000) Stereotactic radiotherapy of extracranial targets: CT-simulation and accuracy of treatment in the stereotactic ablative frame. *Radiother Onc*, Nov; 57(2): 225–36.

27 Takacs H, Kishan A, Deogaonkar M, *et al.* (1999) Respiration induced target drift in spinal stereotactic radiosurgery: Evaluation of skeletal fixation in a porcine model. *Stereotact Funct Neurosurg*, 73(1–4): 70.

28 Herfarth KK, Debus J, Lehr F, *et al.* (2000) Extracranial stereo-tactic radiation therapy: Set-up accuracy of patients treated for liver metastases. *Int J Radiat Oncol Biol Phys*, Jan 15; 46(2): 329–35.

29 Lohr F, Debits J, Frank C, *et al.* (1999) Noninvasive patient fixation for extracranial stereotactic radiotherapy. *Int J Radiat Oncol Biol Phys*, Sep 1; 45(2): 521–7.

30 Bale RI, Sweeney R, Vogele M, *et al.* (1998) Noninvasive head fixation for external irradiation of tumors of the head–neck area. *Strahlenther Onkol*, Jul; 174(7): 350–4.

31 Lax I, Blomgren H, Larson D, Naslund I (1998) Extracranial stereotactic radiosurgery of localized targets. *I Radiosurg;* 1(2): 135–48.

32 Lax I, Blorngren H, Naslund I, Svanstrom R (1994) Stereo-tactic radiotherapy of malignancies in the abdomen: Methodological aspects. *Ada Onc*, 33(6): 677–83.

33 Takai Y, Mituya M, Ncmoto K, *et al.* (2001) Simple method of stereotactic radiotherapy without stereotactic ablative frame for extracranial tumors. *Nippon Igaku Hoshasen Gakkai Zasshi*, Jul; 61(8): 403–7.

34 Wang LT, Solberg TD, Medin PM, Boone R (2001) Infrared patient positioning for stereotactic radiosurgery of extracranial tumors. *Comput Biol Med*, Mar; 31(2): 101–11.

35 Uematsu M, Shioda A, Suda A, *et al.* (2000) Intrafractional tumor position stability during computed tomography (CT)-guided frameless stereotactic radiation therapy for lung or liver cancers with a fusion of CT and linear accelerator (FOCAL) unit. *Int J Radiat Oncol Biol Phys*, Sep I; 48(2): 443–8.

36 Uematsu M, Sonderegger M, Shioda A, *et al.* (1999) Daily positioning accuracy of frameless stereotactic radiation therapy with a fusion of computed tomography and linear accelerator (focal) unit: Evaluation of z-axis with a z-marker. *Radiother Onc*, 50(3): 337–9.

37 Kimura T, Hirokawa Y, Murakami Y, *et al.* (2004) Reproducibility of organ position using voluntary breath-hold method with spirometer for extracranial stereo-tactic radiotherapy. *Int J Radiat Oncol Biol Phys*, Nov 15; 60(4): 1307–13.

38 O'Dell WG, Schell MC, Reynolds ll, Okunieff R (2002) Dose broadening due to target position variability during fractionated breath-held radiation therapy. *Med Phys*, Jul; 29(7): 1430–7.

39 Murphy MJ, Martin D, Whyte R, Hai I, Ozhasoght C, Le QT (2002) The effectiveness of breath-holding to stabilize lung and pancreas tumors during radiosurgery. *Int J Radiat Oncol Biol Phys*, Jun 1; 53(2): 475–82.

40 Yin F. Kim JG, Haughton C, *et al.* (2001) Extracranial radiosurgery: Immobilizing liver motion in dogs using high-frequency jet ventilation and total intravenous anesthesia. *Int J Radiat Oncol Biol Phys*, Jan 1; 49(1): 211–16.

41 Kini VR, Vedam SS, Keall PJ, Patil S, Chen C, Mohan R (2003) Patient training in respiratory-gated radiotherapy. *Med Dosim*, Spring; 28(1): 7–11.

42 Vedam SS, Keall PJ, Kini VR, Mohan R (2001) Determining parameters for respiration-gated radiotherapy. *Med Phys*, Oct; 28(10): 2139–46.

43 Hara R, Itarni J, Aruga T, *et al.* (2002) Development of stereotactic irradiation system of body tumors under respiratory gating. *Nippon Igaku Hoshasen Gakkai Zasshi*, Mar; 62(4): 156–60.

44 Kuriyama K, Onishi H, Saito N, *et al.* (2003) A new irradiation unit constructed of self-moving gantry-CT and linac. *Int J Radiat Oncol Biol Phys*, Feb 1; 55(2): 428–35.

45 Kitamura K, Shirai H, Seppenwoolde Y *et al.* (2003) Tumor location, cirrhosis, and surgical history contribute to tumor movement in the liver, as measured during stereotactic irradiation using a real-time tumor-tracking radiotherapy system. *Int J Radiat Oncol Biol Phys*, May 1; 56(1): 221–8.

46 Sharp GC, Jiang SB, Shimizu S, Shirato H (2004) Prediction of respiratory tumour motion for real-time image-guided radiotherapy. *Phys Med Biel*, Feb 7; 49(3): 425–40.

47 Schweikard A, Shiomi H, Adler J (2004) Respiration tracking in radiosurgery. *Med Phys*, Oct; 31(10): 2738–41.

48 Papiez L, Timmerman R, DesRosiers C, Randall M (2003) Extracranial stereotactic radioablation: Physical principles. *Acta Onc*; 42(8): 882–94.

49 Liu R, Wagner TH, Buatti JM, Modrick J, Dill J, Meeks SL (2004) Geometrically based optimization for extracranial radiosurgery. *Phys Med Biol*, Mar 21; 49(6): 987–96.

50 Cardinale RM, Wu Q, Benedict SH, Kavanagh BD, Bump F, Mohan R (1999) Determining the optimal block margin on the planning target volume for extracranial stereotactic radiotherapy. *Int J Radiat Onc Biol Phys*, Sep 1; 45(2): 515–20.

51 Papiez L (2000) On the equivalence of rotational and concentric therapy. *Phys Med Biol*, Feb; 45(2): 399–409.

52 Hadinger U, Thiele W, Wulf J (2002) Extracranial stereotactic radiotherapy: evaluation of PTV coverage and dose conformity. *Z Med Phys*, 12(4): 221–9.

53 Papiez L, Moskvin V, Timmerman R (2005) Dosimetry of stereotactic ablative radiation therapy treatments. In: *Stereotactic Ablative Radiation Therapy*. Baltimore, MD: Lippincott, Williams and Wilkins, pp. 57–68.

54 Mayer R, Williams A, Frankel T, *et al.* (1997) Two-dimensional film dosimetry application in

heterogeneous materials exposed to megavoltage photon beams. *Med Phys*, 24(3): 455–60.

55 McGarry RC, Papiez L, Williams M, *et al.* (2005) Stereotactic ablative radiation therapy of early-stage non-small-cell lung carcinoma: Phase I study. *Int J Radiat Oncol Biol Phys*, 63: 1010–15.

56 Timmerman R, McGarry R, Yannoutsos C, *et al.* (2006) Excessive toxicity when treating central tumors in a phase II study of stereotactic ablative radiation therapy for medically inoperable early-stage lung cancer. *J Clin Onc*; 24: 4833–9.

57 Baumann P, Nyman J. Lax T, *et al.* (2006) Factors important for efficacy of stereotactic ablative radiotherapy of medically inoperable stage I lung cancer. A retrospective analysis of patients treated in the Nordic countries. *Acta Onc*, 45: 787–95.

58 Fritz P, Kraus HJ, Muhlnickel W *et al.* (2006) Stereotactic, single-dose irradiation of stage 1 non-small cell lung cancer and lung metastases. *Radiat Onc*, 1: 30.

59 Nyman J, Johansson KA, Hulten U (2006) Stereotactic bypofractionated radiotherapy for stage I non-small cell lung cancer – mature results for medically inoperable patients. *Lung Cancer*, 51: 97–103.

60 Zimmermann F, Geinitz H, Schill S, *et al.* (2005) Stereotactic hypofractionated radiation therapy for stage I non-small cell lung cancer. *Lung Cancer*, 48: 107–14.

61 Wulf J, Baler K, Mueller G, *et al.* (2005) Dose–response in stereotactic irradiation of lung tumors. *Radiother Onc*, 77: 83–7.

62 Timmerman RD, Park C, Kavanagh BD (2007) The North American experience with stereotactic ablative radiation therapy in non-small *cell* lung cancer. *J Thorac Oncol*, Jul; 2(7, Suppl 3): S101–12.

63 Nagata Y, Takayama K, Matsuo Y, *et al.* (2005) Clinical out comes of a phase I/II study of 48 Gy of stereotactic body radiotherapy in 4 fractions for primary lung cancer using a stereotactic ablative frame. *Int J Radiat Oncol Biol Phys*, 63: 1427–31.

64 Xia T, Li H, Sun Q, *et al.* (2006) Promising clinical outcome of stereotactic ablative radiation therapy for patients with inoperable Stage I/II non-small-cell lung cancer. *Int J Radiat Oncol Biol Phys*, 66: 117–25.

65 Hara R, Bann J, Kondo T, *et al.* (2006) Clinical outcomes of single-fraction stereotactic radiation therapy of lung tumors. *Cancer*, 106: 1347–52.

66 Nagata Y, Hiraoka M, Shibata T, Onishi H, Kokubo M, Karasawa K, *et al.* (2010) A phase II trial of stereotactic body radiation therapy for operable T1N0M0 non-small cell lung cancer: Japan Clinical Oncology Group (JCOG0403) [Abstract]. *Int J Radiat Oncol Biol Phys*, 78: s27–8.

67 Timmerman R, Paulus R, Galvin J, *et al.* (2010) Stereotactic body radiation therapy for inoperable early stage lung cancer. *JAMA*, 303: 1070–6.

68 Palma D, Visser O, Lagerwaard FJ, Belderbos J, Slotman BJ, Senan S (2010) Impact of introducing stereotactic lung radiotherapy for elderly patients with stage I non-small-cell lung cancer: A population-based time-trend analysis. *J Clin Oncol*, 28: 5153–9.

69 Chang JY, Balter PA, Dong L, Yang Q, Liao Z, Jeter M, Bucci MK, McAleer MF, Mehran RJ, Roth JA, Komaki R (2008) Stereotactic body radiation therapy in centrally and superiorly located stage I or isolated recurrent non-small-cell lung cancer. *Int J Radiat Oncol Biol Phys*, Nov 15; 72(4): 967–71.

70 Lagerwaard F, Haasbeek C, Smit E, Slotman B, Senan S (2008) Outcomes of risk-adapted fractionated stereotactic radiotherapy for stage I non-small-cell lung cancer. *Int J Radiat Oncol Biol Phys*, 70: 685–92.

71 Register SP, Zhang X, Mohan R, Chang JY (2011) Proton stereotactic body radiation therapy for clinically challenging cases of centrally and superiorly located stage I non-small-cell lung cancer. *Int J Radiat Oncol Biol Phys*, Jul 15; 80(4): 1015–22.

72 Onishi H, Araki T, Shirato H, *et al.* (2004) Stereotactic hypofractionated high-dose irradiation for stage I non-small cell lung carcinoma: clinical outcomes in 245 subjects in a Japanese multiinstitutional study. *Cancer*, 101: 1623–31.

73 Fowler JF (1989) The linear-quadratic formula and progress in fractionated radiotherapy. *Br J Radiat*, 62: 679–94.

74 Ginsberg RJ, Rubinstein LV (1995) Randomized trial of lobectomy versus limited resection for T1 NO non-small *cell* lung cancer. *Ann Thorac Surg*, 60: 615–23.

75 Timmerman RD, Paulus R, Pass HI, *et al.* (2013) RTOG 0618: Stereotactic body radiation therapy (SBRT) to treat operable early-stage lung cancer patients. *J Clin Oncol*, 31 (suppl; abstr 7523).

76 Milano MT, Katz AW, Schell MC, *et al.* (2008) Descriptive analysis of oligometastatic lesions treated with curative-intent stereotactic body radiotherapy. *Int J Radiat Oncol Biol Phys*, 72: 1516.

77 Milano MT, Philip A, Okunieff P (2009) Analysis of patients with oligometastases undergoing two or more curative-intent stereotactic radiotherapy courses. *Int J Radiat Oncol Biol Phys*, 73: 832.

78 Salama JK, Hasselle MD, Chmura SJ, Malik R, Mehta N, Yenice KM, Villaflor VM, Stadler WM, Hoffman PC, Cohen EE, Connell PP, Haraf DJ, Vokes EE, Hellman S,

Weichselbaum RR (2012) Stereotactic body radiotherapy for multisite extracranial oligometastases: Final report of a dose escalation trial in patients with 1 to 5 sites of metastatic disease. *Cancer*, Jun 1; 118(11): 2962–70.

79 Iyengar P, Kavanagh BD, Smith I, *et al.* (2013) A phase II trial of second-line erlotinib in combination with stereotactic body radiation therapy (SBRT) for patients with metastatic non-small cell lung cancer (NSCLC). *J Clin Oncol*, 31 (Suppl; abstr 8074).

80 Chang JY, Liu YH, Zhu Z, Welsh JW, Gomez DR, Komaki R, Roth JA, Swisher SG (2013) Stereotactic ablative radiotherapy: A potentially curable approach to early stage multiple primary lung cancer. *Cancer*, Jun 24. doi: 10.1002/cncr.28217.

81 Kelly P, Balter PA, Rebueno N, Sharp HJ, Liao Z, Komaki R, Chang JY (2010) Stereotactic body radiation therapy for patients with lung cancer previously treated with thoracic radiation. *Int J Radiat Oncol Biol Phys*, Dec 1; 78(5): 1387–93.

82 Liu H, Zhang X, Vinogradskiy YY, Swisher SG, Komaki R, Chang JY (2012) Predicting radiation pneumonitis after stereotactic ablative radiation therapy in patients previously treated with conventional thoracic radiation therapy. *Int J Radiat Oncol Biol Phys*, Nov 15; 84(4): 1017–23. doi: 10.1016/j.ijrobp.2012.02.020. Epub 2012 Apr 27.

83 Timmerman RD, Story M (2006) Stereotactic ablative radiation therapy: A treatment in need of basic biological re search. *Cancer J*, Jan–Feb; 12(1): 19–20.

84 Martinez AA, Yan D, Lockman D, *et al.* (2001) Improvement in dose escalation using the process of adaptive radiotherapy combined with three-dimensional conformal or intensity-modulated beams for prostate cancer. *Int J Radiat Oncol Biol Phys*, Aug 1; 50(5): 1226–34.

85 Bortfeld T, Paganetti H (2006) The biologic relevance of daily dose variations in adaptive treatment planning. *Int J Radiat Oncol Biol Phys*, Jul 1; 65(3): 899–906.

86 Song W, Schaly B, Bauman G, Battista J, Van Dyk J (2005) Image-guided adaptive radiation therapy (IGART): Radiobiological and dose escalation considerations for localized carcinoma of the prostate. *Med Phys*, Jul; 32(7): 2193–2203.

87 Yan D, Lockman D, Brabbins D, Tyburski L, Martinez A (2000) An off-line strategy for constructing *a* patient-specific planning target volume in adaptive treatment process for prostate cancer. *Int J Radiat Onc Biol Phys*, Aug 1; 48(1): 289–302.

88 Wu C, Jeraj R, Olivera GH, Mackie TR (2002) Re-optimization in adaptive radiotherapy. *Phys Med Biel*, Sep; 47(17): 3181–95.

89 Brahine A (2003) Biologically optimized 3-dimensional in vivo predictive assay-based radiation therapy using positron emission tomography-computerized tomography imaging. *Acta Oncol*, 42(2): 123–36.

CHAPTER 22

Proton Therapy

Joe Y. Chang and James D. Cox
Department of Radiation Oncology, The University of Texas MD Anderson Cancer Center, Houston, TX, USA

Introduction

Non-small cell lung cancer (NSCLC) accounts for 80% of all lung cancer cases. Only 20–25% of patients with NSCLC present with early-stage disease that can be surgically resected, and a substantial proportion of those patients are considered unable to tolerate surgery because of comorbid conditions. For such patients, photon (X ray)-based radiotherapy has been the standard treatment. Approximately 50% of patients with NSCLC present with locally advanced disease that requires multimodality treatment, including radiotherapy. For patients with stage I disease, radiotherapy can provide effective locoregional control of small primary tumors for up to about 2 years when conventional doses of radiotherapy are used [1–3]. For patients with stage III disease, however, locoregional control with radiotherapy and chemotherapy ranges from 50% to 60%, with median survival times of only 15–17 months and 5-year survival rates of 10–15% [4].

Uncontrolled locoregional disease is a major source of continuous seeding to distant organs and is the eventual cause of treatment failure; thus, its eradication is essential for cure. Substantial clinical evidence exists to suggest a radiation dose–response relationship in both survival and local control in patients with NSCLC [5–8]. However, higher radiation doses are associated with higher toxicity, particularly when radiotherapy is given concurrently with chemotherapy [4].

The current standard dose of photon radiation for lung cancer, 60–66 Gy, is based on findings from the Radiation Therapy Oncology Group (RTOG) 73-01 trial, which showed survival benefits from doses >60 Gy [9]. However, doses ranging from 60 to 66 Gy are still substantially lower than the anticipated dose needed to achieve local control rates in excess of 50%. The RTOG 83-11 trial, led by Cox *et al.* [10], showed that radiotherapy alone to a dose of 69.6 Gy given in 1.2 Gy fractions led to higher survival rates. However, the RTOG 94-10 trial indicated that treatment with 69.6 Gy and concurrent chemotherapy, compared with treatment with 60 Gy and concurrent chemotherapy, resulted in greater toxicity and no survival advantage. More recent findings from RTOG 0617 indicate that escalation of the (photon) radiation dose to 74 Gy with concurrent chemotherapy led to increased toxicity and was associated with worse survival than the conventional (photon) radiation dose of 60 Gy [11].

Advances in diagnostic imaging in the 1980s prompted the development of more individualized radiation therapy based on the specific anatomy of individual patients rather than on anatomic atlases. Computed tomography (CT) and other tomographic scanning technologies permitted the three-dimensional (3D) display of tumors in relation to the surrounding normal anatomy. Accurate

Lung Cancer, Fourth Edition. Edited by Jack A. Roth, Waun Ki Hong and Ritsuko U. Komaki.

3D radiation dose computations were developed, as were multileaf collimators for use within linear accelerators. These tools permitted a "beams-eye" view of tumors and conformal delivery of radiation to them.

Commercially available treatment-planning systems allowed the introduction of 3D conformal radiation therapy (CRT) by the early 1990s. Computer simulations of dose distributions clearly showed that using 3D CRT could allow higher total doses to be delivered to the gross tumor volume than were possible with two-dimensional (2D) treatment. Also with 3D CRT, normal tissues could be avoided or at least exposed to much lower doses than with 2D treatment. The rapid adoption of 3D CRT was based entirely on computer-generated treatment plans that showed a reduced volume of normal tissue irradiated with this method compared with 2D treatment plans and delivery. Indeed, 3D CRT allowed the radiation dose to be escalated from 63 to 74 Gy with concurrent chemotherapy for patients with stage III NSCLC [12, 13].

The delivery of small X-ray beams with different intensities permitted further shaping of the high-dose volume. Physicists optimized the different intensities, and with use of dynamic multileaf collimators, *intensity-modulated radiation therapy* (IMRT) was fully realized. In contrast to the rather rapid adoption of 3D CRT, IMRT was appreciated and introduced into practice more slowly. Physicians, physicists, and dosimetrists had to devote much more time and effort to treatment planning with IMRT, but the ability to achieve reduced toxicity with this therapy was a worthy goal that has been realized. Such precision in radiation delivery requires more careful target delineation, treatment planning, and quality assurance. Moreover, because of the risk of missing tumors that may move between daily fractions or during treatments (e.g., during respiration), imaging is needed with each treatment. As such, the term *image-guided radiotherapy* encompasses daily imaging as well as 3D CRT and IMRT.

Although 3D CRT or IMRT have the potential to reduce normal tissue toxicity, the relatively high exit dose of photon X-ray therapy limits the possibility of dose escalation or acceleration. A proton beam, on the other hand, is made up of charged particles that have a well-defined range of penetration into tissues. As the proton beam penetrates the body, the particles slow down and deposit a large fraction of their energy near the end of their range. The resultant central axis depth dose distribution is known as the Bragg peak. By modulating the Bragg peak in both energy and time (the so-called "spread-out Bragg peak" [SOBP]), a full, localized, uniform dose can be delivered to the target while sparing the surrounding normal tissues. Proton beam treatment is ideal when organ preservation is a priority, particularly for patients with lung cancer [14, 15]. In this chapter, we review the rationale for and aspects of treatment planning and delivery of proton therapy for patients with lung cancer and emerging information on clinical outcomes after such treatment.

Relative biologic effectiveness and biological research on protons

Charged particle radiotherapy (i.e., that with high-energy particles such as protons or carbon nuclei) is directly ionizing because, by virtue of their charge, the accelerated particles can interact with atomic electrons via Coulomb forces. Consequently, charged particles, unlike photons, are associated with high linear energy transfer (LET) – that is, their interaction with tissues is characterized by both direct damage to cellular DNA and a dense mobilization of secondary electrons along the particle track that results in a high local concentration of free radicals, which also cause DNA damage. In clinical systems involving use of SOBPs, cellular damage is considered to be nearly constant across the plateau phase of the depth-dose curve, but in reality, the degree of cellular damage may vary along the particle track.

Although the various nuclei used in charged particle radiotherapy may be similar with respect to the general shape of their depth-dose curve, their ultimate radiobiological effects depend on the specific LET of the particle that is used. Thus, the shape of the SOBP is useful for determining the dose distribution, but the extent of radiobiological damage to the target tumor depends on a different property – the relative biological effectiveness (RBE) of the radiation. This quantity is defined as the ratio of the dose of photons to the dose of charged particles necessary to achieve the same biological effect in a specified test system. If the RBE for a specific particle is high, then that particle exerts a significant amount of damage per absorbed unit of energy and is said to have high quality. Notably, the RBE also varies in different tissues, varies with the rate of cellular proliferation, and varies with dose (RBE increases as the dose decreases).

Protons have nearly the same RBE as photons. Paganetti *et al.* summarized the available data from numerous experiments with protons and concluded that the RBE of protons is approximately 1.1 [16]. This means that protons are radiobiologically similar to photons and offer a 10% improvement in radiation quality, whereas heavy nuclei have considerably greater biological effects. For example, the RBE for carbon ions is approximately 3, similar to the RBE for neutrons. Although the higher RBE of carbon ions would seem advantageous for control of hypoxic tumors, it is disadvantageous for normal tissues.

Other radiobiological phenomena deserve mention with regard to the relative advantages of charged particle radiotherapy. In photon radiobiology, the radiosensitivity of a tumor cell can be diminished by the absence of oxygen or by the cell's being in a radioresistant phase of the cell cycle (e.g., S phase). In both cases, the altered radiosensitivity is attributable to the cell's ability to repair the radiation-induced damage to the DNA, and that ability is enhanced by hypoxia and the presence of sister chromatids and DNA repair enzymes in certain cell cycle phases. However, the single-track, double-strand break is a subtype of DNA injury that is difficult to repair even in the presence of these radiobiological modifiers. Because high-quality particles (*e.g.*, those with heavy nuclei such as carbon ions) are more likely to induce this type of injury, tumor oxygenation and cell cycle effects become less important. This ability of heavy ion particles to overcome these intrinsic mechanisms of radioresistance gives them a major theoretical advantage over photons. In fact, this difference in radiobiology is the main feature that distinguishes heavy ions from protons, the radiobiological quality of which is similar to that of photons. However, the RBE of protons can vary according to tumor histology and dose/fractionation regimen [17, 18]. For practical reasons, treatment modeling does not at present take these RBE variations into account. However, as the use of charged particle therapy increases over time, accounting for this variability in specific circumstances may become necessary.

Another potential advantage of the use of protons in radiotherapy is that they may preferentially target cancer stem cells, the presence of which is thought to lead to local recurrence and distant metastasis. A recent preclinical study indicated that protons effectively targeted and killed cancer stem cells in treatment-resistant NSCLC cell lines to a greater extent than did photons of the same dose (RBE), but this cell-killing effect was not seen in a normal bronchial epithelium cell line [19]. These findings suggest that protons may be more effective than photons for preventing local recurrence or distant metastasis resulting from the presence of treatment-resistant cancer stem cells, but clinical studies are needed to confirm this hypothesis. Future research in molecular biology to address mechanisms of DNA damage/repair and signal transduction induced by proton treatment will help in identifying the optimal regimens for proton therapy [20]. In addition, the interactions among proton treatment, chemotherapy, and molecular targeted therapy may well open a new field of research to further improve therapeutic ratio [21].

Rationale for proton therapy

As described in the previous section, the primary advantage from the use of protons in cancer therapy is their highly localized dose distribution, rather than an enhanced biological effect. A high dose of therapeutic proton beams can be safely delivered to the tumor/target volume while sparing adjacent normal tissues that are vulnerable to radiation injury, particularly those tissues that are distal to the target volume in the beam direction. When similar complexities have been considered and similar treatment-delivery techniques have been used, protons have typically deposited one half or less of the integral dose that X-rays deposit to uninvolved normal tissues [22]. Higher doses should result in an increased probability of local tumor control.

The fundamental property of proton beams that provides a substantial advantage over X-ray beams is that protons can be made to stop within a few millimeters past the distal surface of the target volume, whereas X-rays deposit their dose in the healthy tissues and organs that lie in the beam path beyond the target volume and then exit the patient on the side opposite to the beam entrance. In addition, protons deposit a lower dose than do X-rays to normal tissues and organs that lie in the beam path between the surface of the patient and the target volume. For a given level of normal tissue toxicity, the maximum tolerated dose of proton radiotherapy is probably higher than that of conventional photon radiotherapy because of the physical characteristics of the proton beam (i.e., its Bragg peak). Therefore, proton radiotherapy may have an advantage over conventional photon therapy, including IMRT, in attaining local tumor control and improving survival rates [14, 15].

Proton treatment planning and delivery

Physical characteristics of proton beams

As is true for all heavy charged particles (helium and carbon ions, negative pi-mesons, etc.), protons have a unique depth dose distribution, commonly referred to as the Bragg peak. The depth dose is characterized by a low entrance dose (about 30–40% of the maximum dose), followed by a relatively flat dose plateau, which rises sharply to a narrow peak (the Bragg peak) and then falls rather rapidly to zero dose immediately after the maximum dose is reached. The depth of the Bragg peak depends on the composition of the material being penetrated and the energy of the proton. A typical Bragg peak is shown in Figure 22.1a.

The width of the Bragg peak is too narrow to allow treatment of any but the smallest of clinical targets, which typically range up to 20 cm deep. Generally, range modulation, i.e., adding Bragg peaks of sequentially lower energies and smaller weights (time duration), is used to produce an extended region of dose uniformity in depth called the SOBP (Figure 22.1b). SOBPs can be achieved by placing either a range modulation wheel (for dynamic modulation) or a ridge filter (for passive modulation) in the beam or by changing the energy in the accelerator or energy-selection system while adjusting the weight (time duration) of each individual Bragg peak. By appropriately selecting the range pullback and weight of each pristine Bragg peak, depth uniformity can be achieved that covers the tumor. To achieve lateral uniformity in the tumor target, the beam must also be spread laterally, either by a passive, double scattering system or by magnetically scanning a small spot beam in a uniform pattern. In general, SOBPs can be produced with different widths, customized to individual target volumes. Notably, as the width of the SOBP increases, the surface dose increases. Proton therapy requires a source of protons in an energy range of about 70 to 230–250 MeV to achieve penetration in the patient from 7 to 30–37 cm. Dose rates should be approximately 2 Gy/min.

Passive scattering systems

Until recently, passive scattering systems were the standard method for spreading the proton beam laterally for therapeutic applications. In this system, the proton beam is passed through a range-modulating wheel, which is often part of the first scatterer, a second scattering device, a range shifter, an aperture for shaping the beam laterally, and a customized compensator before it enters the patient. The double scattering system (use of the range-modulating wheel as the first scatterer with a second scattering device) creates a broad flattened beam at the final aperture. The range shifter determines the maximum depth penetrated by the protons. The range-modulating wheel spreads the narrow Bragg peak, forming a uniform dose distribution that covers the target while sparing the surrounding normal tissue (the SOBP). The customized range compensator tailors the distal surface of the dose distribution to match

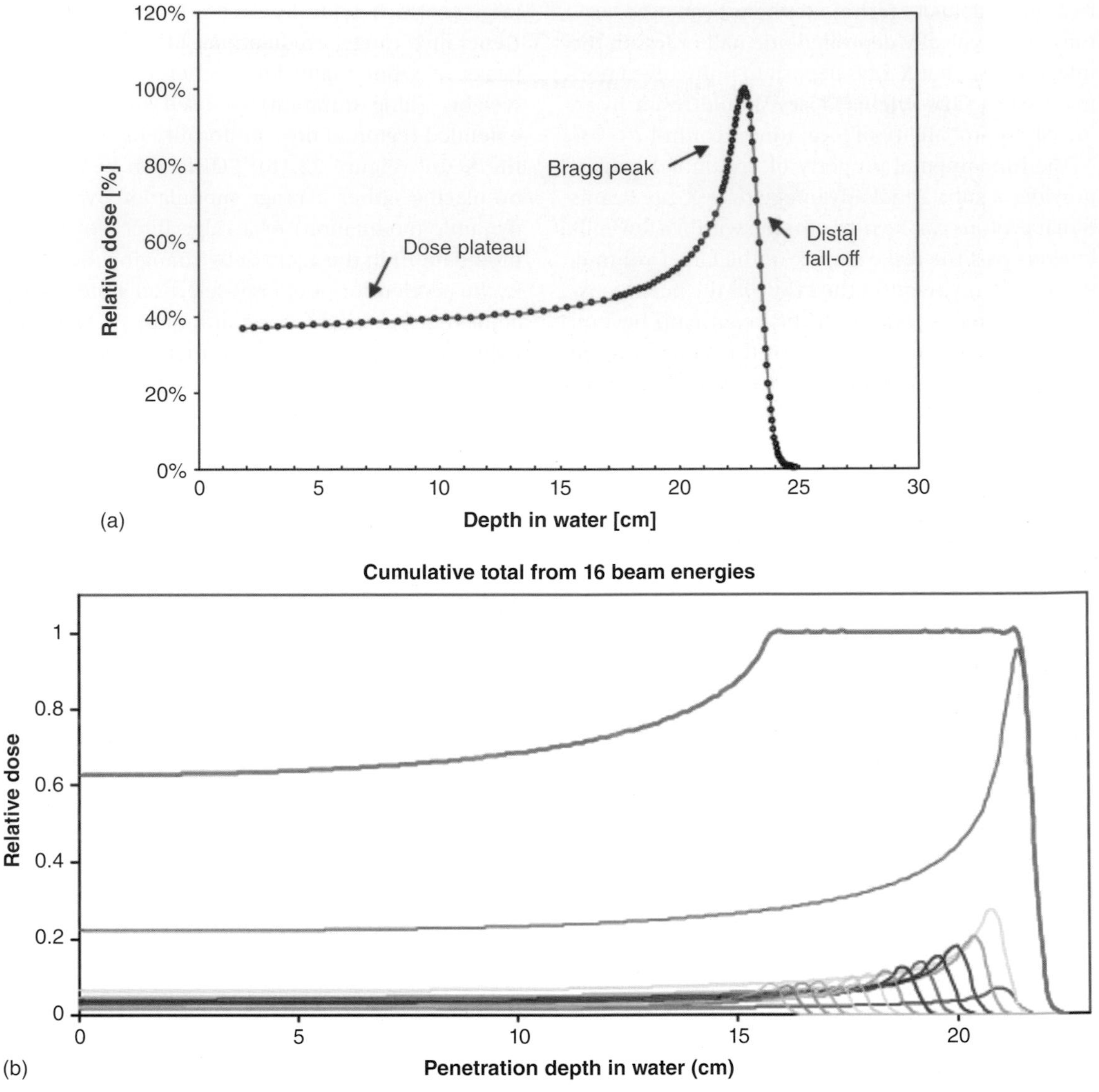

Figure 22.1 a: A typical proton dose distribution for a Bragg peak. b: Spread-out Bragg peak.

the distal shape of the target volume, with necessary margins and lateral smearing to account for possible small misalignment of the compensator with the patient's anatomy. In the design of the range compensator, the treatment planning system calculates the water equivalent path-lengths between the patient surface and the distal planning volume, thereby calculating the thickness of each point of the range compensator to correct for the shape of the patient surface, all inhomogeneities between the patient surface and the planning target volume, and the shape of distal surface of the planning target volume. The beam number and angle are important for passive scattering proton therapy to cover the target while minimizing dose exposure to critical structures. Typically beam number and angle used in lung cancer is shown in Figure 22.2.

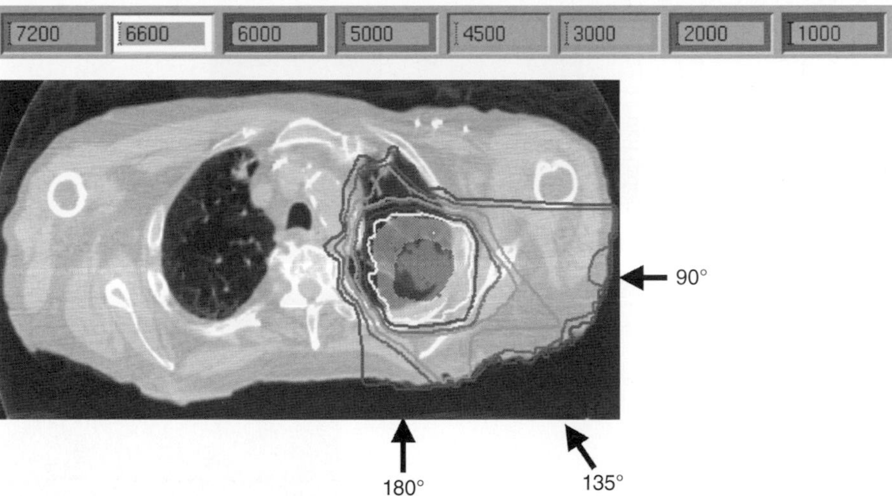

Figure 22.2 Typical beam arrangement for a passive scattering proton therapy plan. The internal gross tumor volume (iGTV) is shown in maroon; the surrounding clinical target volume (CTV) in khaki (green); and the planning target volume (PTV) in aqua. Arrows indicate beam angles. The numbers at top indicate isodoses in cGy, as represented by the respective colors.

The advantages of passive scattering systems are their safety, simplicity, and lesser sensitivity to the time structure of the accelerator. Although these systems have well served their intended purpose, they also have several disadvantages, the most serious being their efficiency, which at 20–40% wastes large numbers of protons in the scattering system and in the beam-limiting aperture. This substantial loss of protons can pose a problem for synchrotron-based proton therapy systems, in which the dose rate is more limited than in cyclotrons. Passive scattering systems also tend to be sensitive to variations in the beam position. Furthermore, when protons are stopped in the scattering system and aperture, they produce secondary neutrons, which can contribute to the whole-body dose of the patient. Neutrons have a high RBE and are thought to be the source of secondary cancers in some patients [23]. Another disadvantage of this system is that it produces a single SOBP for the entire target volume; thus, during treatment of large irregular target volumes with notable differences in their thickest and thinnest depths, the high-dose region is pulled back into normal tissues. For this reason, the dose-shaping properties of passive scattering techniques are often described as "2.5-dimensional." The solution to the disadvantages of passive scattering systems is found in dynamic spot scanning systems, which are described further below.

Dynamic spot scanning systems

In dynamic spot scanning, a narrow beam entering the treatment nozzle is magnetically scanned across the target cross-section and in depth to achieve the intended dose pattern. The beam can be either scanned continuously or stopped at predetermined positions for a specified time until the desired dose is delivered. In discrete spot scanning, the beam is then turned off and the currents in the magnets are adjusted so as to move the next beam spot to the desired position [24]. The deepest layer is scanned by selecting the appropriate energy, and when scanning of that layer is completed, the energy is decreased and the next layer is scanned. In this manner, the entire target volume can be irradiated either to deliver a uniform dose distribution for each field, much like the passive scattering method, or to deliver a nonuniform dose distribution for each field in such a way that when the doses from all fields are summed, the total dose distribution is uniform. This is called *intensity-modulated proton therapy* (IMPT). Figure 22.3 shows a typical dynamic

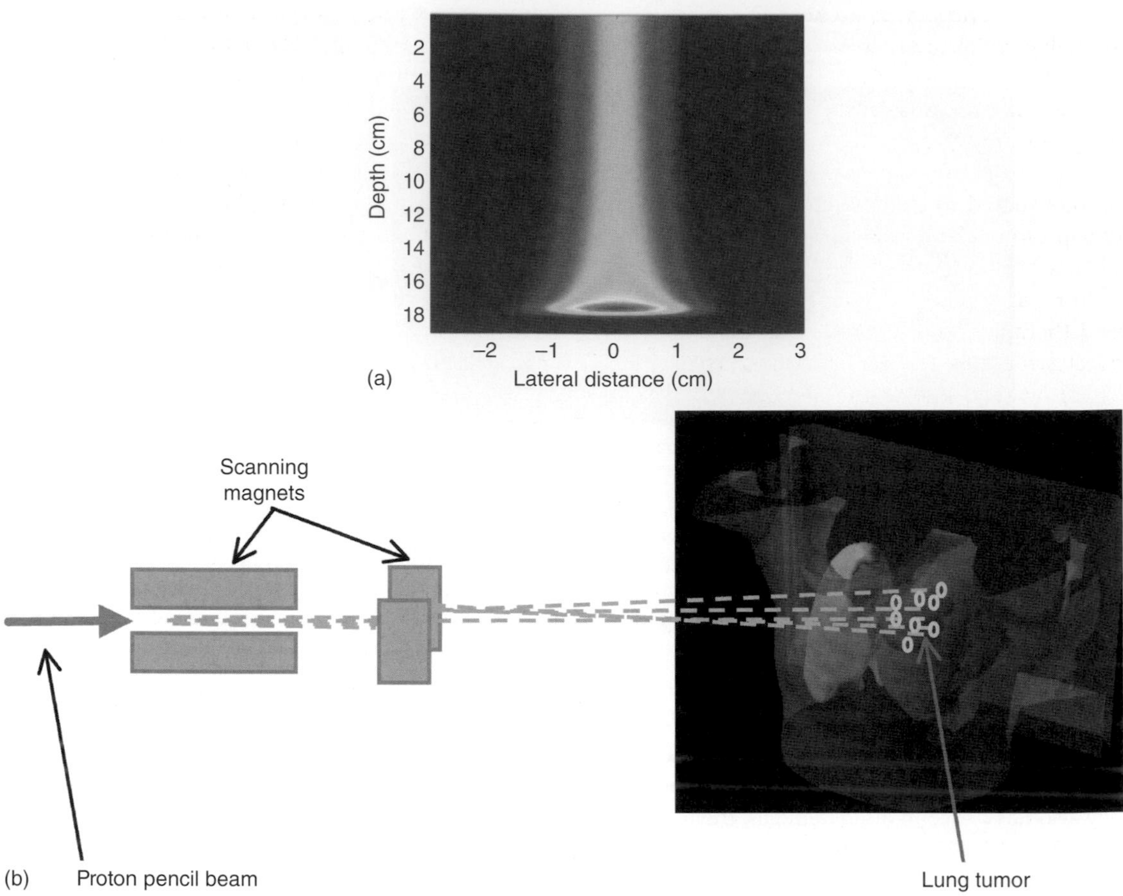

Figure 22.3 a: Typical dynamic spot scanning beam. b: Illustration of scanning beam dose painting.

spot scanning system. With continuous scanning, the intensity of the beam can be varied as the spot is moved to produce a nonuniform dose distribution. With discrete spot scanning, the time that the spot remains at each "voxel" can be varied to produce the nonuniform dose distribution.

Dynamic spot scanning has several advantages: it provides full shaping of the dose distribution to the target volume; no devices such as dose-limiting apertures and range compensators are required; the efficiency is high because very few protons are wasted; and very few neutrons are produced. One disadvantage of dynamic spot scanning is the difficulty in delivering a desired dose to tumors that move during irradiation; however, beam gating techniques such as respiratory-gated proton beam radiotherapy (described in the section on "Tumor Motion Considerations") should reduce the uncertainty in such treatments. Another way to reduce the effect of target motion is to scan each layer several times; the dose error due to target motion decreases and/or increase fractionations as the number of scans increases and/or fractionation increased, although there is a practical limit to the number of times a layer can be rescanned. The time required to deliver IMPT should be comparable to that required for X-ray IMRT.

Planning proton therapy versus photon therapy

As is true for treatments with X-rays and electrons, treatments with protons use multiple treatment fields, often noncoplanar, to keep the skin dose at reasonable limits and to spare normal tissues in the beam path. However, treatment-planning strategies involving protons can be quite different from those involving X-rays and electrons because of the particular properties of proton beams. For example, in proton-based treatments, the rapid distal falloff of the proton dose distribution permits the planner to aim a proton beam directly at a critical normal structure, as opposed to X-ray–based and electron-based therapies, which may deliver toxic doses to critical structures because of the significant exit doses. However, some uncertainty exists regarding the distal edge of the proton dose and possibly increased RBE toward the end of the SOBP. These sources of uncertainty must be taken into consideration.

Proton-based therapies thus require a more critical understanding of uncertainties associated with the proton beam. Specifically, uncertainties associated with the exact stopping point of the proton beam caused by errors in the CT data or in the treatment planning and delivery process, can result in either the beam being stopped too quickly (thereby underdosing the target) or the beam's being delivered for too long (thereby overdosing a critical structure). A correlation between CT Hounsfield units and proton mass stopping powers, based on measurements of materials of known stopping powers on the CT scanner, is used to calculate proton ranges in tissue [25]. As noted previously, uncertainty of RBE is another concern. Preliminary evaluations indicate that the RBE of s proton beam depends on tissue specificity, dose, dose rate, energy, and depth of penetration [16] but does not vary significantly from its nominal value.

Another important difference between X-ray- and proton-based treatment planning is the use of margins to expand the clinical target volume to the planning target volume. Proton beams have essentially three edges, the two lateral penumbras resulting from Coulomb multiple scattering and the distal falloff resulting from range straggling. Since both multiple scattering and range straggling depend on range (energy), proton dose distributions have three sides, with depth-dependent dose gradients. Also, the depth dependence of the lateral penumbra is stronger than that of X-rays for water equivalent depths greater than about 17 cm; for shallower depths the proton lateral penumbra is generally smaller than that for X-rays. In general, each treatment beam must have its own margins that depend on the distance traveled by the beam in tissue. Therefore, expanding the clinical target volume to the planning target volume is not a straightforward process and depends strongly upon the beam direction. Indeed, the concept of the planning target volume is not useful for proton treatment planning.

The most severe limitation of the proton therapy plans for passive scattering arises from the uniform width of the SOBP throughout the target volume, which results in some high-dose spillover into adjacent normal tissues. However, this problem is greatly reduced by the use of multiple beams and is reduced still further by the use of spot scanning techniques and intensity-modulated treatment planning. With the advent of dynamic spot scanning techniques, proton therapy has taken an important step forward. As stated earlier in this chapter, spot scanning allows the application of intensity-modulated techniques in treatment planning and delivery, which substantially improves the proton dose distribution, as has been the case for IMRT in X-ray therapy.

IMPT plans are optimized with an "inverse" treatment-planning system, which is similar to the inverse planning for IMRT [26, 27]. However, there is additional complexity in IMPT because the energy of each proton pencil beam, in addition to the intensity and dose of each beam, can be varied, which increases the number of degrees of freedom for optimization and the dose-shaping potential of the IMPT plans, but at the cost of both computational and treatment complexity.

For treatment plans of equivalent complexity, the IMPT plans will always be superior to IMRT plans, especially in the sparing of normal tissues if motion uncertainty has been resolved [28]. The coverage of the target volume can be quite similar for IMPT and IMRT (Figure 22.4). On average, IMRT plans have twice the integral dose of IMPT plans, which results in substantial sparing of critical tissues and organs with the IMPT plans [23, 28].

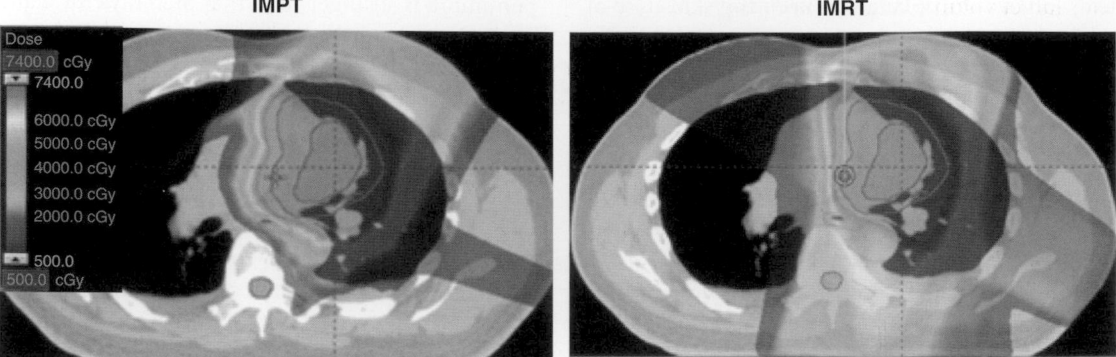

Figure 22.4 Comparison of dose distributions from intensity-modulated (photon) radiation therapy (IMRT) and those from intensity-modulated proton therapy (IMPT) for stage III NSCLC.

Image-guided proton delivery

Proton dose distributions are highly localized because of the SOBP high-dose region that is followed by an abrupt falloff of the dose to a zero value. However, much of this advantage (compared with X-rays) can be lost if the treatment-planning process, patient setup, or delivery is not optimized, appropriate, and accurate. An error in the calculated range of the proton beam can cause either a portion of the distal target volume to receive no dose (if the range is too short) or an overdose to a critical structure (if the range is too long). The accuracy of the patient setup for treatment and of the treatment delivery is usually ensured by the use of onboard imaging and extensive monitoring and by the quality assurance of the beam-delivery process.

Most proton treatment delivery systems contain three orthogonal imaging systems (X-ray tubes and flat-panel imagers), image analysis systems, and computerized couches with six degrees of freedom. More modern proton delivery systems will be guided by on-board volumetric imaging with cone-beam CT or CT on-rails systems. These technologies allow stereotactic techniques to be used to accurately position the patient, correct for misalignments, and verify the treatment setup daily for each treatment field.

Tumor motion considerations

Proton radiotherapy for lung cancer is complicated by several issues. Among the most challenging of these issues is the need to account for respiration-related tumor motion during treatment. The beating of the heart also causes tumor motion, but the magnitude is relatively small compared with the motion caused by respiration. Development of multislice detectors and faster imaging reconstruction has made it possible to obtain images from patients in real time, while they breathe, and to assess the extent of tumor and organ motion by using four-dimensional (4D) CT.

A more interesting and challenging application of 4D CT imaging is in planning 4D treatment, in which the actual dose distributions for free-breathing treatment can be calculated [29, 30]. In this process, the dose distributions are calculated for each phase of the breathing cycle and then added by deformable image registration. Such composite dose distributions and dose-volume histograms can demonstrate the actual dose that the patient receives from the treatment if the patient breathes in the same way as shown in the 4D CT images.

To ensure that all of the cancer cells are adequately covered by the proton beam, investigators at MD Anderson [29] and Massachusetts General Hospital [30] have used 4D CT-based treatment planning to evaluate the proton dose-volume distribution in the target and in the surrounding normal tissues. These plans involved generating an internal target volume by combining the gross tumor volumes at different phases of the respiratory cycle. The MD Anderson group used the internal gross target volume created with maximal intensity projection density to design the necessary compensators [30]. This approach produced dose distributions similar to those that were actually delivered. Compared with the use of a large smearing margin for highly mobile lung tumors, as proposed by Moyers *et al.* [31], our internal gross tumor volume-maximal intensity approach achieved similar target coverage while sparing more normal tissue, because no uniformly large smearing margin was used. Instead, individualized internal gross tumor volumes that were based on actual tumor motion were used for the compensator design [30]. This approach may slightly overtreat the normal tissues behind the tumor when the tumor moves out of the field, but it ensures that the entire tumor is treated adequately, no matter where it moves during the different breathing phases.

IMPT is more sensitive to motion than is IMRT or passive scattering proton therapy. In current clinical practice, the recommendation is that tumors that move by less than 1 cm be treated with IMRT or passive scatter proton therapy. Tumors that are to be treated with IMPT, by contrast, should move no more than 5 mm so as to minimize the motion uncertainty. About 50% lung cancers move about 5 mm, 30–40% move about 5–10 mm, and about 10% move more than 1 cm during respiration [32]. Managing tumor motion through the use of techniques such as respiratory-gated radiotherapy is particularly crucial in proton therapy for tumors that move significantly during respiration.

Adaptive proton therapy

In addition to the movement of tumors within fractions (intrafraction motion), proton therapy is also sensitive to tumor motion and anatomic changes between fractions. Investigators have recently begun to examine the effect of interfractional motion and anatomic changes on dose distribution in proton therapy. In one study, Hui, Chang, and others [33] acquired weekly 4D CT scans from 8 patients with locally advanced NSCLC being treated with IMRT. A conformal passive scattering proton plan was generated for each patient and compared with the IMRT plan over the 7-week course of radiotherapy. For one of these patients, the normal tissue doses were found to be increased and coverage of the clinical target volume was significantly compromised (with a decrease in approximately 8%) over the course of treatment if proton therapy were used, but these changes over time were much less significant in the IMRT plan. The conclusion was that interfractional adaptive planning is indicated for at least some patients undergoing proton therapy. A subsequent clinical study from the same group showed that about 20% of patients with stage III NSCLC being treated with proton radiation [to 74 Gy(RBE) in 37 fractions] in combination with paclitaxel and carboplatin need adaptive proton therapy because of anatomic changes over time that would compromise coverage of the target volume or violate dose constraints [34]. Adaptive planning can reduce normal tissue doses and prevent target misses, particularly for patients with large tumors that shrink substantially during therapy. Adaptive plans seem to have acceptable toxicity and achieve similar local, regional, and distant control and overall survival rates than those achieved with nonadaptive plans, even for patients with larger tumors.

Normal-tissue doses from proton therapy versus other forms of radiation therapy

Protons produce lower normal tissue doses than 3D CRT, IMRT, or SBRT

As noted earlier in this chapter, escalation of radiation doses is crucial for local disease control in lung cancer. The advent of 3D CRT was a major step forward in reducing the inadvertent exposure of normal tissues compared with 2D radiotherapy. IMRT may also offer the benefit of dose escalation without causing greater toxicity to surrounding normal tissue in some patients with lung cancer [35–37]. However, the use of IMRT for treating lung cancer has been delayed because of concerns that IMRT may deliver low but damaging doses to larger volumes of normal lung tissue than would be affected by other treatments. Respiration-induced motion of tumors introduces another level of complexity to both the dosimetry and the technique used to deliver IMRT [38, 39]. Indeed, in one study IMRT was associated with an increase in the volume of lung exposed to 5 Gy or more (V_5) in half of the patients tested compared with 3D CRT [35, 36]. Nevertheless, IMRT may allow greater dose escalation than 3D CRT without significantly increasing the incidence of adverse effects in at least some patients with locally advanced disease [35–37, 40, 41].

Reasoning that proton therapy may be better able to spare critical structures than 3D CRT or IMRT, we compared DVHs from patients with either stage I or stage IIIA/B NSCLC that had been treated with standard-dose 3D CRT or IMRT or with simple 3D passive scattering proton therapy, without intensity modulation, at standard or escalated doses [14]. This comparison indicated that proton therapy spared 15–17% more of the total lung and 19–23% more of the contralateral lung, from exposure to 5 Gy or more compared with IMRT. This reduced exposure would be expected to substantially reduce lung toxicity. Proton therapy also significantly reduced the dose to esophagus, spinal cord, and heart, even with dose escalation, compared with standard-dose photon therapy. In addition, proton therapy produced absolute improvements in the nontarget integral dose of 33–60%. These reductions were greatest in early-stage disease and in exposure of the contralateral lung. The apparent ability of proton therapy to minimize the dose to the heart and spinal cord may translate to better quality of life and survival and opens the possibility of using proton therapy for re-irradiation. Again, the expectation is that sparing critical normal structures with proton therapy will allow further dose escalation, acceleration, or both in the treatment of lung cancer that may translate to better local control and survival rates without increasing treatment-related toxicity. The development of IMRT optimization and autoplanning has significantly improved the conformality of IMRT over the past 5 years. Nevertheless, passive scattering proton therapy still spares significantly more heart, spinal cord, and ipsilateral and contralateral lung. However, improvements in lung V_{20}, total mean lung dose, and esophageal dosimetric values from passive scattering proton therapy (and presumably the reduction in toxic effects associated with these improvements) may not be evident in all cases, especially those that are challenging anatomically, e.g., when the contralateral hilum or supraclavicular nodes are involved or the tumors are adjacent to the esophagus or spinal cord. Because passive scattering proton therapy is limited in the numbers of treatment fields that can be used and requires significant margins to address uncertainties, delivering ablative doses to targets of complicated shape or location, such as tumors curved around sensitive critical structures, can be very difficult. Such cases may require a compromise in dose coverage to avoid damaging critical normal tissue structures. A more effective alternative may be IMPT, in which scanning beam therapy can simultaneously optimize the intensities and the energies of all pencil beams using an objective function that takes into account targets as well as normal tissue constraints. Zhang, Chang, and others compared the DVHs of IMPT with those of IMRT and passive scattering proton therapy for the treatment of stage IIIB NSCLC, with the goal of exploring the possibility of individualized radical radiotherapy [28]. In that comparison, IMPT spared more lung, heart, spinal cord, and esophagus, even with dose escalation from 63 Gy to 83.5 Gy, than did IMRT, with a mean maximum tolerated dose of 74 Gy. Compared with passive scattering proton therapy, IMPT allowed further dose escalation from 74 Gy to a mean maximum tolerated dose 84.4 Gy (range, 79.4-88.4 Gy) while maintaining or reducing the extent of normal tissue exposure. IMPT further eliminated the need for lower-dose target coverage of complicated tumors. Clinical implementation of IMPT for lung cancer is ongoing at MD Anderson Cancer Center, but at this time the technique remains investigational owing to uncertainties associated with tumor motion and the complexity of treatment planning and quality assurance.

Proton therapy may also produce less toxicity than stereotactic ablative radiotherapy, another photon-based technique used for centrally or superiorly located stage I lung tumors, because most of the energy of protons is deposited at end of the range of the proton beam. MD Anderson investigators also used treatment plans to compare the relative benefits of passive scattering proton therapy and with those of stereotactic ablative radiotherapy for such cases [42]. The conclusion was that proton therapy, particularly IMPT, could deliver ablative doses to the target volume with significantly lesser doses to the surrounding normal tissues compared with photon-based stereotactic ablative radiotherapy.

Clinical trials

Several clinical trials of proton radiotherapy for NSCLC have been conducted. Early trials focused on dose-escalated or accelerated proton therapy for early-stage disease and showed promising clinical results that were comparable to surgical resection in stage IA cases. Bush *et al.* [43] studied 68 patients with clinical stage I disease treated with 51 cobalt Gray equivalents (CGE) in 10 fractions over 2 weeks or with 60 CGE in 10 fractions over 2 weeks. No cases of symptomatic radiation pneumonitis or late esophageal or cardiac toxicity were seen. The 3-year local control and disease-specific survival rates were 74% and 72%. Significant improvements in local tumor control were noted for T1 (87%) and T2 (49%) tumors, with a trend toward improved survival rates as well. Local tumor control seemed to be better than that achieved with conventional radiotherapy in historical control subjects, with good disease-specific survival rates expected at 3 years after treatment. Shioyama *et al.* [44] described 51 patients with NSCLC who were treated with proton therapy to a median dose of 76 Gy and a median fraction size of 3.0 Gy. The 5-year overall survival rates were 70% for 9 patients with stage IA disease and 16% for 19 patients with stage IB disease ($p < 0.05$). The 5-year in-field local control rate was higher among patients with stage IA disease (89%) than among those with stage IB disease (39%). Forty-seven patients (92%) experienced acute lung toxicity of grade ≤ 1; three had grade 2, one had grade 3, and none experienced grade 4 or higher toxicity. Patients in this study showed very little late toxicity. Nihei *et al.* [45] subsequently reported the results from their preliminary study of 37 patients with stage I NSCLC who received 70–94 CGE delivered in 20 fractions. The 2-year progression-free survival and overall survival rates were 80% and 84%, respectively. The 2-year locoregional relapse-free survival rates were 79% for patients with stage IA disease and 60% for those with stage IB disease. No serious acute toxicity was observed, and only three patients developed grade 2 or 3 chronic lung toxicity. More recently, Chang and colleagues [46] reported findings from a phase I/II prospective study targeting patients with centrally or superiorly located stage IA-II NSCLC. Early results from that study (median follow-up time, 16.3 months) showed that proton radiotherapy to a total dose of 87.5 CGE at 2.5 CGE per fraction produced grade 2 dermatitis in 67% of patients, grade 2 fatigue in 44%, grade 2 pneumonitis in 11%, grade 2 esophagitis in 6%, and grade 2 chest wall pain in 6% of patients. No grade 4 or 5 toxic effects were observed, and the local control rate was 88.9%. These findings were similar to those of Shioyama and colleagues in the aforementioned study [44], in which the local control rate at 5 years was 89% for patients with stage IA disease, and one case of grade 3 acute toxicity was observed.

These clinical studies indicate that proton therapy can be safe and effective for early-stage NSCLC. However, the optimal regimen has not been well defined. In addition, simple 3D proton therapy was used in these studies; optimized proton therapy such as IMPT was not available, and image-guided radiotherapy was not strictly applied. At this time, clinical data on proton therapy for patients with stage III NSCLC, the most common stage requiring radiotherapy, remain sparse. In a retrospective review of 35 patients with stage II or III NSCLC who underwent proton therapy without concurrent chemotherapy (median dose delivered 78.3 CGE, range, 67.1–91.3 CGE), Nakayama and colleagues [47] found overall survival and local progression-free survival rates of 81.8% and 93.3% at 1 year and 58.9% and 65.9% at 2 years. Surprisingly, no grade 3 or higher toxic effects were observed. Sejpal and colleagues [48] also analyzed 62 patients with locally advanced NSCLC who underwent proton therapy with concurrent platinum- or taxane-based chemotherapy and compared their outcomes with those of patients who had had photon-based therapy (3D CRT or IMRT) in previous eras. The median total radiation dose was 74 CGE for the proton therapy group and 63 Gy in both photon therapy groups. Rates of pneumonitis, esophagitis, and hematologic toxicity were lower in the patients given proton therapy than in did the patients given photon therapy despite the higher proton doses. Finally, Chang and colleagues completed a phase II study of 44 patients with stage III NSCLC who received 74 CGE via conventional fractionation (2 CGE per fraction) with weekly concurrent carboplatin and paclitaxel [49]. Despite the intensity of this treatment, few patients experienced grade 3 toxic effects: five patients had grade 3 esophagitis, five patients had grade 3 dermititis, and only one patient had grade 3 pneumonitis. No grade 4 or 5 toxic effects were observed. The local control rate was 80%, and the overall survival duration was 29.4 months. Collectively, these studies indicate that proton therapy can reduce adverse effects, which in turn could not only lead to better quality of life but may also extend survival for some patients with locally advanced lung cancer.

The results of other ongoing trials are eagerly awaited. One such trial is a randomized phase II study comparing IMRT with proton therapy (74 Gy(RBE) with concurrent chemotherapy) for stage III NSCLC; another is a randomized trial comparing stereotactic ablative photon radiotherapy with stereotactic ablative proton therapy for centrally located or recurrent NSCLC. Other ongoing projects include a joint effort by MD Anderson Cancer Center and Massachusettes General Hospital, supported by the US National Institutes of Health, to study the optimization of proton therapy with the appropriate management of uncertainties, particularly gated proton therapy and IMPT.

References

1 Kaskowitz L, Graham M, Emami B, Halverson K, Rush C (1993) Radiation therapy alone for stage I non-small cell lung cancer. *Int Radiat Oncol Biol Phys,* 27: 517–23.

2 Dosoretz D, Kann M, Blitzer P, *et al.* (1996) Medically inoperable lung carcinoma: the role of radiation therapy. *Semin Radiat Oncol,* 6: 98–104.

3 Dosoretz D, Galmarini D, Rubenstein J, *et al.* (1993) Local control in medically inoperable lung cancer: an analysis of its importance in outcome and factors determining the probability of tumor eradication. *Int J Radiat Oncol Biol Phys,* 27: 507–16.

4 Curran WJ, Paulus R, Langer CJ, *et al.* (2011) Sequential vs. concurrent chemoradiation for stage III non-small cell lung cancer: Randomized phase III trial RTOG 9410. *J Natl Cancer Inst,* 103(19): 1452–60.

5 Rosenman J, Halle J, Socinski M, *et al.* (2002) High-dose conformal radiotherapy for treatment of stage IIIA/IIIB non-small-cell lung cancer: technical issues and results of a phase I/II trial. *Int J Radial Oncol Biol Phys,* 54(2): 348–56.

6 Kong E, Ten Haken R, Schipper M, *et al.* (2005) High-dose radiation improved local tumor control and overall survival in patients with inoperable/unresectable nonsmall-cell lung cancer: long-term results of a radiation dose escalation study. *Int J Radial Once! Biol Phys,* 63(2): 324–33.

7 Choi N, Doucette J (1981) Improved survival of patients with unresectable non-small-cell bronchogenic carcinoma by an innovated high-dose en-bloc radiotherapeutic approach. *Cancer,* 48: 101–9.

8 Machtay M, Bae K, Movsas B, *et al.* (2012) Higher biologically effective dose of radiotherapy is associated with improved outcomes for locally advanced Non-Small Cell Lung Carcinoma treated with chemoradiation: An analysis of the Radiation Therapy Oncology Group. *Int J Radiat Oncol Biol Phys,* 82(1): 425–34.

9 Perez C, Bauer M, Edelstein S, Gillespie B, Birch R (1986) Impact of tumor control on survival in carcinoma of the lung treated with irradiation. *Int J Radiat Oncol Biol Phys,* 12: 539–47.

10 Cox J, Azarnia N, Byhardt R, Shin K, Emami B, Pajak T (1990) A randomized phase I/II trial of hyperfractionated radiation therapy with total doses of 60.0 Gy to 79.2 Gy: Possible survival benefit with greater than or equal to 69.6 Gy in favorable patients with Radiation Therapy Oncology Group stage III non-small-cell lung carcinoma: report of Radiation Therapy Oncology Group 83-11. *J Clin Oncol,* 8(9): 1543–55.

11 Bradley JD, Paulus R, Komaki R, *et al.* (2011) Randomized phase III comparison of standard-dose (60 Gy) versus high-dose (74 Gy) conformal chemoradiotherapy ± cetuximab for stage IIIA/IIIB non-small cell lung cancer: Preliminary findings on radiation dose in RTOG 0617. Presented at the 53rd Annual Meeting of the American Society for Radiation Oncology (ASTRO), Miami, FL, October 3, 2011.

12 Schild S, McGinnis W, Graham D, *et al.* (2006) Results of a phase I trial of concurrent chemotherapy and escalating doses of radiation for unresectable non-smallcell

lung cancer. *Int J Radiat Oncol Biol Phys*, 65(4): 1106–11.

13 Belderbos J, Heemsbergen W, De Jaeger K, Baas P, Lebesque J (2006) Final results of a phase I/II dose escalation trial in non-small-cell lung *cancer* using three-dimensional conformal radiotherapy. *Int Radial Oncol Biol Phys*, 66(1): 126–34.

14 Chang JY, Zhang X, Wang X, *et al.* (2006) Significant reduction of normal tissue dose by proton radiotherapy compared with three-dimensional conformal or intensity-modulated radiation therapy in stage I or stage III non-small-cell lung cancer. *Int J Radiat Oncol Biol Phys*, 65: 1087–96.

15 Ruysscher DK, Chang JY (2013) Proton therapy for thoracic tumors. *Semin Radiat Oncol*, 23(3): 115–19.

16 Paganetti H, Niemierko A, Ancukiewicz M, *et al.* (2002) Relative biological effectiveness (RBE) values for proton beam therapy. *Int J Radiat Oncol Biol Phys*, 53(2): 407–21.

17 Carabe A, Moteabbed M, Depauw N, Schuemann J, Paganetti H (2012) Range uncertainty in proton therapy due to variable biological effectiveness. *Phys Med Biol*, 57(5): 1159–72.

18 Paganetti H (2002) Nuclear interactions in proton therapy: Dose and relative biological effect distributions originating from primary and secondary particles. *Phys Med Biol*, 47(5): 747–64.

19 Zhang X, Lin SH, Fang B, Gillin M, Mohan R, Chang JY. (2013) Therapy-resistant cancer stem cells have differing sensitivity to photon versus proton beam radiation. *J Thorac Oncol*, 8(12): 1484–91.

20 Halperin E (2006) Particle therapy and treatment of cancer. *Lancet Oncol*, 7(8): 676–85.

21 Baumann M (2006) Keynote comment: radiotherapy in the age of molecular oncology. *Lancet Oncol*, 7: 786–7.

22 Lomax A, Bortfeld T, Goitein G, *et al.* (1999) A treatment planning inter-comparison of proton and intensity modulated photon radiotherapy. *Radiother Oncol*, 51(3): 257–71.

23 Hall E (2006) Intensity-modulated radiation therapy, protons, and the risk of second cancers. *Int I Radiat Oncol Biel Phys*, 65(1): 1–7.

24 Kanai T, Kawachi K, Kumamoto Y, *et al.* (1980) Spot scanning system for proton radiotherapy. *Med Phys*, 7(4): 365–9.

25 Schneider U, Pedroni E, Lomax A (1996) The calibration of CT Hounsfield units for radiotherapy treatment planning. *Phys Med Biol*, 41: 111–24.

26 Oelfke U, Bortfeld T (2001) Inverse planning for photon and proton beams. *Med Dosim*, 26(2): 113–24.

27 Bortfeld T (1997) An analytical approximation of the Bragg curve for therapeutic proton beams. *Med Phys*, 24: 2024–33.

28 Zhang X, Li Y, Pan X, *et al.* (2009) Intensity-modulated proton therapy reduces the dose to normal tissue compared with intensity-modulated radiation therapy or passive scattering proton therapy and enables individualized radical radiotherapy for extensive stage IIIB non-small-cell lung cancer: a virtual clinical study. *Int J Radiat Oncol Biol Phys*, 77(2): 357–66.

29 Kang Y, Zhang X, Chang JY, *et al.* (2007) 4D Proton treatment planning strategy for mobile lung tumors. *Int J Radiat Oncol Biol Phys*, 67(3): 906–14.

30 Engelsman M, Rietzel E, Kooy HM (2006) Four-dimensional proton treatment planning for lung tumors. *Int J Radiat Oncol Biol Phys*, 64(5): 1589–95.

31 Moyers M, Miller D, Bush D, Slater J (2001) Methodologies and tools for proton beam design for lung tumors. *Int J Radiat Oncol Biol Phys*, 49(5): 1429–38.

32 Chang JY, Dong L, Liu H, *et al.* (2008) Image-guided radiation therapy for non-small cell lung cancer. *J Thorac Oncol*, 3: 177–86.

33 Hui Z, Zhang X, Starkschall G, *et al.* (2008) Effects of interfractional motion and anatomic changes on proton therapy dose distribution in lung cancer. *Int J Radiat Oncol Biol Phys*, 72(5): 1385–95.

34 Koay EJ, Lege D, Mohan R, Komaki R, Cox JD, Chang JY (2012) Adaptive/nonadaptive proton radiation planning and outcomes in a phase II trial for locally advanced non-small cell lung cancer. *Int J Radiat Oncol Biol Phys*, 84(5): 1093–1100.

35 Murshed H, Liu H, Liao Z, *et al.* (2004) Dose and volume reduction for normal lung using intensity-modulated radiotherapy for advanced-stage non-small-cell lung cancer. *Int J Radial Oncol Biol Phys*, 58(4): 1258–67.

36 Liu H, Wang X, Dong L, *et al.* (2004) Feasibility of sparing lung and other thoracic structures with intensity-modulated radiotherapy for non-small-cell lung cancer. *Int. J Radiat Oncol Biol Phys*, 58(4): 1268–79.

37 Grills I, Yan D, Martinez A, Vicini F, Wong J, Kestin L (2003) Potential for reduced toxicity and dose escalation in the treatment of inoperable non-small-cell lung cancer: A comparison of intensity-modulated radiation therapy (1MRT), 3D conformal radiation, and elective nodal irradiation. *Int Radial – Oncol Biol Phy*, 57(3): 875–90.

38 Chul C, Yorke B, Hong L (2003) The effects of intrafraction organ motion on the delivery of intensity-modulated field with a multileaf collimator. *Med Phys*, 30(7): 4736–46.

39 Bortfeld T, Jokivarsi K, Goitein M, Kung J, Jiang S (2002) Effects of intra-fraction motion on IMRT dose delivery: Statistical analysis and simulation. *Phys Med Biol*, 47(13): 2203–20.

40 Yom SS, Liao Z, Liu HH, *et al.* (2007) Initial evaluation of treatment-related pneumonitis in advanced-stage non-small-cell lung cancer patients treated with concurrent chemotherapy and intensity-modulated radiotherapy. *Int J Radiat Oncol Biol Phys*, 68(1): 94–102.

41 Jiang ZQ, Yang K, Komaki R, *et al.* (2012) Long-term clinical outcome of intensity-modulated radiotherapy for inoperable non-small cell lung cancer: The MD Anderson experience. *Int J Radiat Oncol Biol Phys*, 83(1): 332–9.

42 Register SP, Zhang X, Mohan R, Chang JY (2011) Proton stereotactic body radiation therapy for clinically challenging cases of centrally and superiorly located stage I non-small-cell lung cancer. *Int J Radiat Oncol Biol Phys*, 80(4): 1015–22.

43 Bush D, Slater J, Shin B, Cheek G, Miller D, Slater J (2004) Hypofractionated proton beam radiotherapy for stage I lung cancer. *Chest*, 126(4): 1198–1203.

44 Shioyama Y, Tokuuye K, Okumura T, *et al.* (2003) Clinical evaluation of proton radiotherapy for non-small-cell lung cancer. *Int J Radiat Oncol Biol Phys*, 56(1): 7–13.

45 Nihei K, Ogino T, Ishikura S, Nishimura H (2006) High-dose proton beam therapy for stage I non-small-cell lung cancer. *Int J Radiat Oncol Biol Phys*, 65(1): 107–11.

46 Chang JY, Komaki R, Wen HY, *et al.* (2011) Toxicity and patterns of failure of adaptive/ablative proton therapy for early-stage, medically inoperable non-small cell lung cancer. *Int J Radiat Oncol Biol Phys*, 80(5): 1350–7.

47 Nakayama H, Satoh H, Sugahara S, *et al.* (2011) Proton beam therapy of stage II and III non-small-cell lung cancer. *Int J Radiat Oncol Biol Phys*, 81(4): 979–84.

48 Sejpal S, Komaki R, Tsao A, *et al.* (2011) Early findings on toxicity of proton beam therapy with concurrent chemotherapy for nonsmall cell lung cancer. *Cancer*, 117(13): 3004–13.

49 Chang JY, Komaki R, Lu C, *et al.* (2011) Phase 2 study of high-dose proton therapy with concurrent chemotherapy for unresectable stage III nonsmall cell lung cancer. *Cancer*, 117(20): 4707–13.

CHAPTER 23

Combinations of Radiation Therapy and Chemotherapy for Non-small Cell and Small-Cell Lung Carcinoma

Daniel Gomez,[1] Zhongxing Liao,[1] Pierre Saintigny,[2] and Ritsuko U. Komaki[1]
[1]Department of Radiation Oncology, The University of Texas MD Anderson Cancer Center, Houston, TX, USA
[2]Department of Thoracic/Head and Neck Medical Oncology, The University of Texas MD Anderson Cancer Center, Houston, TX, USA

Introduction

Many patients with locally advanced non-small-cell lung cancer (NSCLC) are unable to undergo surgical resection with curative intent. In such cases, one viable option is to combine chemotherapy and radiation, given either in sequence or concurrently. Numerous studies done over the past two decades to assess and compare these approaches have demonstrated varying rates of toxicity and efficacy based on factors such as patient characteristics, radiation dose, systemic therapy regimen, and the respective timing of chemotherapy and radiation. Collectively, the results of these trials have led to the establishment of concurrent chemoradiation therapy as the current standard of care for inoperable NSCLC.

This chapter describes the rationale for combining chemotherapy with radiation therapy (RT) and reviews relevant studies that have shaped the current paradigm for the treatment of lung cancer. Also reviewed are aspects of the various forms of toxicity associated with combined chemoradiation as well as the long-term prognosis for patients so treated.

Rationale for combining radiation therapy and chemotherapy

Traditionally the rationale for combining RT and chemotherapy to improve the therapeutic effect has been based on four principles: toxicity independence, normal tissue protection, spatial cooperation, and tumor response enhancement. Of these principles, only spatial cooperation and tumor response enhancement hold true for the treatment of NSCLC [1]. The virtues of spatial cooperation (i.e., radiation therapy for the local-regional tumor and chemotherapy for metastases) are obvious; those of tumor response enhancement are less so. Because terms such as *radiation sensitization* may have different meanings for different investigators, we prefer to use the terminology suggested by Steel and Peckham [1].

An excellent review of the rationale for combining chemotherapy with radiation was recently provided by Eberhardt and colleagues [2]. To summarize the key points of this review, ionizing radiation works to destroy tumor cells through the formation of free radicals in addition to the related

Lung Cancer, Fourth Edition. Edited by Jack A. Roth, Waun Ki Hong and Ritsuko U. Komaki.

processes of necrosis and apoptosis [3]. Similarly, systemic therapy works by disrupting signaling pathways involving cell death and reduced proliferative potential [4]. When given sequentially, chemotherapy and RT can theoretically work through complementary mechanisms, with radiation acting to control locoregional disease and chemotherapy providing systemic control of micrometastatic malignant cells. Because each modality can be given at higher doses when delivered sequentially, this complementarity could be more effective in that context.

In contrast, when chemotherapy and RT are delivered concurrently, not only can the distinct but related cell-killing processes act on the same cells, presumably increasing efficacy, but they can also act on different cells to cause DNA damage, kill specific cells, and reduce the rapidity of proliferation [1, 5]. As Eberhardt and colleagues stated, "theoretically, supra-additive effects could be achieved by optimally scheduled inhibition of repair processes of the two modalities, thus making the treatments complementary in their antineoplastic potential" [1,2, 5]. For example, cell cycle synchronization can lead to increased cell kill by means of ionizing damage from radiation.

Nevertheless, despite the theoretical differences in these approaches, death for most patients with unresectable NSCLC is caused by inadequate treatment of a local tumor. This observation is supported by strong clinical evidence. First, the occurrence of tumor persistence or progression within the irradiated field is associated with poorer survival among patients who receive RT only as opposed to patients who receive RT after local tumor control has been achieved [6, 7]. Second, patients who receive only palliative RT or single-agent chemotherapy more often die from intrathoracic disease than from extrathoracic metastasis [8], especially if the tumor is a squamous cell carcinoma. Third, many more patients with localized but unresectable NSCLC treated with a few large fractions of radiation die from local intrathoracic tumor complications than from distant metastasis (72% vs. 15%) [9]. In contrast, Perez *et al.* [10] found that improved local tumor control was associated with an *increased* incidence of distant metastasis. Finally, other groups have shown that concurrent chemotherapy and RT improves local tumor control, which in turn improves survival [11].

Sequential chemotherapy and radiation therapy

As alluded to in the previous section, the approach of giving induction chemotherapy before RT has two attractive features. First, it permits the most immediate attack on all components of the tumor, both those that are evident clinically and those that are presumed to be present at subclinical levels. Second, if systemic chemotherapy elicits a response, then its continuation during or after RT is justified. Although overall survival rates in several prospective randomized clinical trials have been mixed, overall survival was found to be favorable in three trials of cisplatin-based chemotherapy and RT to total doses of 60 Gy or more (Table 23.1) [12–16].

The most well known of these three trials was reported by the Cancer and Leukemia Group B and showed a clear survival advantage for induction chemotherapy. Called CALGB 8433 [17], this trial compared two treatment regimens, one consisting of induction therapy with cisplatin (100 mg/m^2 on days 1 and 29) and vinblastine (5 mg/m^2 weekly for 5 weeks) followed by RT (2.0 Gy/fraction, 5 days/week, to a total dose of 60 Gy) beginning on day 50, and the other consisting of RT only beginning on day 1. This trial was closed before the planned accrual was reached when the induction chemotherapy approach demonstrated superior median survival times and 5-year survival rates, benefits that continued on long-term follow-up [13]. The encouraging results of the CALGB trial were validated by a second trial of 353 patients reported by Le Chevalier and colleagues [14, 18, 19]. As was true in the earlier CALGB trial, patients were randomly assigned to undergo either induction chemotherapy followed by RT or RT alone. Those in the induction chemotherapy group received 3 monthly cycles of vindesine (1.5 mg/m^2 on days 1–2), cyclophosphamide (200 mg/m^2 on days 2–4), cisplatin (100 mg/m^2 on day 2), and lomustine (75 mg/m^2 on day 3) followed by RT (daily 2.5-Gy fractions, 4 days/week, to a total dose

Table 23.1 Trials of sequential chemotherapy and radiation therapy for locally advanced non-small cell lung cancer

First author, year (reference)	No. of patients	RT (Gy)	CT	MST (mo)	LRC (%)		OS (%)	
					3-yr	5-yr	3-yr	5-yr
Dillman *et al.*, 1996 [13]	77	60	—	9.7	6	5	11	7
	79	60	PV	13.8	18	6 ($P = 0.026$)	23	19 ($P = 0.012$)
Brodin *et al.*, 1996 [12]	164	56 (SC)	—	N/R	N/R	3 (4-yr)	6	1.4
	163	56 (SC)	CE	N/R	N/R	7 (4-yr) ($P = 0.07$)	13	3 ($P = 0.16$)
Morton *et al.*, 1991 [15]	58	60	—	9.6	N/R	N/R	N/R	7
	56	60	MACC	10.4	N/R	N/R	N/R	5
Le Chevalier *et al.*, 1992 [14]	177	65	—	10.0	17 (1-yr)	N/R	4	3
	176	65	VCPC	12.0	15 (1-yr)	N/R	12	6 ($P < 0.02$)
Sause *et al.*, 2000 [16]	149	60	—	11.4	N/R	N/R	11	5
	151	60	PV	13.2	N/R	N/R	17	8
	152	69.6 (bid)	—	12	N/R	N/R	14	6 ($P = 0.04$)

bid, 1.2 Gy twice daily; CT, chemotherapy; MACC, methotrexate, doxorubicin, cyclophosphamide, lomustine; MST, median surivival time; LRC, local-regional control; N/R, not reported; OS, overall survival; PV, cisplatin, vinblastine; RT, radiation therapy; SC, split course; VCPC, vindesine, cyclophosphamide, cisplatin, lomustine.

of 65 Gy) beginning on day 75–80; those in the other group received only RT. Again, survival was better in the group given induction chemotherapy; moreover, the incidence of distant metastasis was significantly reduced, although no improvement in local tumor control was found. In fact, because the French cooperative group investigators routinely used fiberoptic bronchoscopy and biopsy at the site of the original lesions 3 months after the start of treatment, they were able to demonstrate high treatment failure rates at tumor sites (>80%) in both treatment groups and no advantage for induction chemotherapy in terms of local control.

These results led the Radiation Therapy Oncology Group (RTOG) and the Eastern Cooperative Oncology Group (ECOG) to conduct a cooperative three-armed trial (RTOG 88–08, also known as ECOG 4588) to compare survival rates after standard RT, sequential chemoradiation therapy (i.e., the CALGB regimen), and hyperfractionated radiotherapy (to a total dose of 69.6 Gy) for NSCLC [16, 20]. Sequential chemoradiation therapy was found to be superior to both standard RT and hyperfractionated RT, whereas standard RT and hyperfractionated RT were found to produce essentially similar effects. In a subsequent analysis of failure patterns among the patients in this trial [21], Komaki *et al.* found that control of distant metastasis improved only for those patients who had squamous cell carcinoma and chemotherapy had no influence on the local tumor [22], a finding consistent with that of the French trial.

After the CALGB trial was completed, Dillman and associates [13, 17] later conducted a retrospective quality-control review of the trial data and found that, in a relatively large proportion of cases (23%), radiation fields had failed to completely encompass the primary tumor. In addition, all of the above trials of induction chemotherapy followed by RT used two-dimensional (2D) RT for treatment planning, which is now considered substandard practice.

Several assumptions can be made based on the findings from these trials. First, when feasible, sequential chemotherapy plus radiation is preferred over RT alone. Second, chemotherapy can indeed control the distant metastatic spread of squamous cell carcinoma, at least in some cases, an observation that is consistent with preclinical findings. Finally, primary tumor control within the field of irradiation is poorer than was originally thought, and induction chemotherapy offers no further benefit in that regard.

Concurrent chemotherapy and radiation therapy

Further efforts to improve local control and reduce distant metastasis have led investigators to pursue other strategies including concurrent cisplatin-based chemotherapy and RT, combinations of chemotherapy and hyperfractionated RT, and combinations of new chemotherapeutic and molecular targeting agents with RT. The specific rationale for adding a single chemotherapeutic agent to RT is to increase local tumor control.

The first RTOG trial of concurrent combination chemotherapy and RT was reported by Byhardt *et al.* [23]. Designated RTOG 90–15, this trial combined the cisplatin-vinblastine regimen from the CALGB 8433 trial with a regimen of hyperfractionated RT (69.6 Gy delivered in 1.2-Gy fractions twice daily, 5 days/week) that had been chosen for its superiority in light of a dose-seeking study by Cox *et al.* [24]. Although few patients in the RTOG 90–15 trial had favorable prognostic factors, the median survival time was an encouraging 12.2 months [23]. Notably, while the RTOG 90–15 trial was ongoing, this hyperfractionated RT regimen was simultaneously being compared with standard fractionation in the RTOG 88–08/ECOG4588 trial.

A successor trial to RTOG 90–15, designated RTOG 91–06, had the same design but tested the hypothesis that oral etoposide given daily during much of the RT period would be more effective than vinblastine when given with cisplatin [25]. In brief, cisplatin (75 mg/m^2 IV on days 1 and 29) and etoposide (50 mg PO twice daily on days 1–14 and days 29–43) were given with hyperfractionated RT, also beginning on day 1. The toxicity of this combined regimen, especially to the esophagus, was considerable. However, its effect on survival was remarkable: for patients with favorable prognostic factors, the median survival time was 21 months and the 2-year survival rate was 42%. Corroborative results were obtained in a subsequent trial, reported by Reboul *et al.* from Avignon [26], that had a similar chemotherapy regimen but a more standard RT fractionation schedule.

To reduce the severity of the RTOG 91–06 regimen's acute effects, the chemotherapy schedule was slightly modified for use in a subsequent phase I/II trial designated RTOG 92–04 [27]. In brief, etoposide (50 mg PO) was omitted on the weekends, when RT was not given, thus reducing from 28 to 20 the total number of days on which etoposide was administered. The results of this schedule were mixed. Although use of the modified chemotherapy regimen reduced the incidence of chemotherapy-induced nonhematologic toxicity, it did so at the price of higher in-field tumor progression rates. Moreover, median survival and 1-year survival rates did not significantly improve (15.5 vs. 14.1 months and 65% vs. 58%, respectively).

Numerous studies have been done to assess the role of concurrent chemoradiation vs. radiation alone in NSCLC. A Cochrane meta-analysis of 19 randomized trials of concurrent chemoradiation vs. RT alone for NSCLC (2728 participants) indicated that concurrent chemoradiation significantly improved overall survival, progression-free survival, and locoregional progression–free survival. Moreover, concurrent chemoradiation was not associated with higher rates of grade ≥3 radiation pneumonitis or late lung or esophageal toxicity compared with RT alone. However, concurrent chemotherapy was associated wth worse acute esophagitis and hematologic toxicity such as neutropenia and anemia. Finally, a subgroup analysis revealed that the benefit of concurrent chemoradiation was evident in the subgroup given once-daily fractionation but not in those given twice-daily fractionation [28].

Sequential versus concurrent chemoradiation therapy

Several studies have compared sequential vs. concurrent chemoradiation for locally advanced NSCLC to determine the optimal timing of treatment. As noted previously, potential benefits of sequential treatment include lesser toxicity and the ability to often deliver higher systemic doses of chemotherapy when delivered alone. Concurrent treatment, on the other hand, allows radiosensitization by chemotherapy through complementary mechanisms and thus could theoretically improve the probability of controlling disease. In all, at least seven clinical trials have directly compared sequential vs. concurrent chemoradiation in terms of progression-free and overall survival [29–35]. These trials used a variety of chemotherapy regimens, with virtually all being platin-based, as well as different radiation regimens. Overall, the findings from these trials showed that concurrent chemoradiation leads to improved survival outcomes, albeit at the cost of increased toxicity. For example RTOG 94–10 compared three chemoradiation regimens ((1) sequential treatment with cisplatin and vinblastine followed by RT at 1.8 Gy once daily to 63 Gy; (2) concurrent chemoradiation with cisplatin and vinblastine with RT at 1.8 Gy fractions once daily to 63 Gy; and (3) concurrent cisplatin and etoposide with RT at 1.2 Gy twice daily to 69.6 Gy). The median survival time was better in group 2 (17 months) than in groups 1 and 3 (14.6 and 15.2 months), but twice-daily concurrent RT was associated with greater toxicity [29]. Similarly, a study from France found that concurrent cisplatin and etoposide with RT followed by consolidation cisplatin and vinorelbine was superior to sequential cisplatin and vinorelbine followed by RT in terms of both median survival times (16.3 months vs. 14.5 months) and 2- to 4-year overall survival rates. Esophageal toxicity was more common with concurrent chemotherapy.

Two other trials of sequential versus concurrent chemotherapy and RT investigated the more novel drug combination of carboplatin and paclitaxel [34, 35]. Neither trial showed any significant improvement in overall survival from concurrent therapy. However, the trial reported by Huber *et al.* suggested possibly improved median survival, and the trial reported by Belani *et al.* trial suggested that upfront concurrent chemotherapy improved median survival time by 3 months compared with that in the other treatment groups.

In two different meta-analyses, Auperin *et al.* [36] and O'Rourke *et al.* [28, 37] assessed differences in survival and toxicity in six phase III randomized trials of concurrent vs. sequential chemoradiation. These analyses showed that concurrent chemoradiation produced a statistically significant benefit in overall survival, with a hazard ratio (HR) of 0.74 [95% confidence interval (CI) 0.62–0.89], with absolute benefits of 5.7% (from 18.1% to 23.8%) at 3 years and 4.5% at 5 years Concurrent treatment was further shown to reduce locoregional progression but not distant metastasis, suggesting that this survival benefit resulted from improved locoregional control (Figure 23.1). Concurrent doublet or triplet chemotherapy seemed to produce a larger improvement in progression-free survival than did concurrent single-agent chemotherapy (HR = 0.83, 95% CI 0.72–0.95 vs. HR = 1.15, 95% CI 0.90–1.48; $p = 0.02$]. The number of treatment-related deaths was greater for those receiving concurrent therapy (4% vs. 2% for those given sequential therapy), although this apparent difference was not statistically significant. In contrast, the risk of high-grade esophagitis was substantially increased with concurrent treatment (relative risk 4.96, 95% CI 2.17–11.37) [28].

Together, the evidence from these multicenter clinical trials warrants use of concurrent chemoradiation therapy that include a cisplatin-based combination chemotherapy regimen as the treatment of choice for patients with locally advanced NSCLC. This approach gives the best 5-year survival results and is a curative treatment option for patients with inoperable stage IIIA or IIIB NSCLC.

Concurrent chemoradiation therapy followed by surgical resection

Another concurrent approach of interest is induction chemoradiation followed by surgical resection. This approach makes sense for patients whose disease might be considered resectable by one group of thoracic surgeons but unresectable by another and for patients who are willing to accept the risks associated with surgery. Unfortunately, most trials involving this approach have not clearly defined which subsets of stage IIIA N2 NSCLC might be amenable to this approach, nor have they clearly defined eligibility criteria. Heterogeneity has been significant in the size and number of lymph nodes involved, and some trial results suggest that patients with minimal mediastinal nodal involvement might be best treated with preoperative

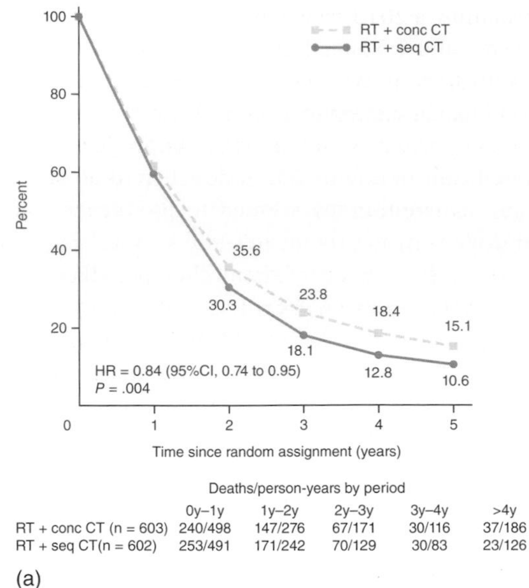

Deaths/person-years by period	0y–1y	1y–2y	2y–3y	3y–4y	>4y
RT + conc CT (n = 603)	240/498	147/276	67/171	30/116	37/186
RT + seq CT(n = 602)	253/491	171/242	70/129	30/83	23/126

(a)

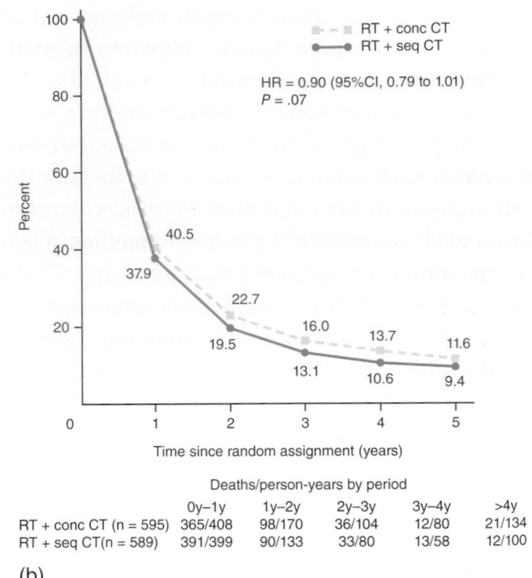

Deaths/person-years by period	0y–1y	1y–2y	2y–3y	3y–4y	>4y
RT + conc CT (n = 595)	365/408	98/170	36/104	12/80	21/134
RT + seq CT(n = 589)	391/399	90/133	33/80	13/58	12/100

(b)

Figure 23.1 Overall and progression-free survival curves for patients in a meta-analysis of concurrent vs. sequential chemoradiation for locally advanced non-small cell lung cancer. *Source*: From Auperin A, Le Pechoux C, Rolland E *et al.* (2010) Meta-analysis of concomitant versus sequential radiochemotherapy in locally advanced non-small-cell lung cancer. *J Clin Oncol*, 28: 2181–90 [36]. Reproduced with permission of American Society of Clinical Oncology.

chemotherapy [38]. This heterogeneity has limited the applicability of trial results to wider clinical practice.

The Southwest Oncology Group, in their phase II study SWOG 8805 [39], evaluated concurrent chemoradiation followed by resection in 126 carefully selected patients with stage IIIA or IIIB tumors and documented mediastinal lymph node metastasis (by biopsy or percutaneous fine-needle aspiration). The trial regimen consisted of combination chemotherapy with cisplatin (50 mg/m^2 on days 1, 8, 29, and 36) and intravenous etoposide (50 mg/m^2 on days 1–5 and 29–33) and concurrent RT (45 Gy in 1.8-Gy fractions, 5 days/week) for 5 weeks, followed 2–4 weeks later by thoracotomy and resection. The median survival time was 15 months, and the 2-year survival rate was 40%. More than 50% of the cases that were staged as N2 disease before chemoradiation therapy were downstaged to N0 afterward; yet almost 40% of patients experienced local recurrence, and most patients experienced distant metastasis. The overall 3-year survival rate was 27%, but that rate was significantly better among patients who had had mediastinal disease eradicated after chemoradiation therapy than among those who had not (44% vs 18%).

These encouraging results led to a randomized trial comparing surgery versus combination chemotherapy and RT for patients with stage N2 disease, the final results of which were published in 2005 (INT 0139, also known as RTOG 93–09 and ECOG/SWOG 9336) [40]. All patients underwent a 5-week regimen of induction chemotherapy with RT similar to that used in the SWOG 8805 study. At that time half of the patients were randomly assigned to undergo surgical exploration after an interval of 2–4 weeks, and the other half were randomly assigned to continue the chemoradiation uninterrupted (total dose of 61.0 Gy in 33 fractions). Progression-free survival times were found to be slightly longer in the surgical group (12.8 months vs. 10.5 months, $p = 0.017$), but the median survival time was no different between groups (23.6 months vs. 22.2 months, $p = 0.24$). Eight percent of the surgical group experienced treatment-related death compared with 2% of the nonsurgical group. Finally, exploratory analyses revealed that overall survival was better for patients who underwent lobectomy than for those with chemoradiation only, but not for patients who received pneumonectomy [41]. Based on the results of this study, either definitive concurrent chemoradiation (ideally delivered in a concurrent fashion), or induction chemotherapy with or without RT followed by surgical resection, are acceptable regimens for patients with locally advanced disease. At MD Anderson Cancer Center, cases such as these are reviewed by a multidisciplinary panel, and generally patients with high performance status, adequate pulmonary function, nonbulky lymph nodes, and single-lymph node station involvement who will not require a pneumonectomy are referred for definitive surgery. These criteria are also consistent with the 2012 guidelines from the National Comprehensive Cancer Network [42].

Radiation therapy

The importance of radiation dose in local tumor control

As noted previously, a major pattern of treatment failure after definitive chemoradiation for locally advanced NSCLC is local tumor recurrence [13, 16]. Local recurrence ultimately develops in up to 90% of patients; however, these local failures are visible on radiography in only about 45–52% of cases but biopsy findings suggest that failures are present in as many as 85% of cases [13, 43, 44].

Locoregional disease control is important because uncontrolled local tumors can cause severe symptoms including obstructive pneumonia, hemoptysis, pain, and, in many cases, death. The benefit of improved locoregional disease control seems to translate to improved long-term survival among patients treated with concurrent chemoradiation [36]. One way of improving local tumor control is to intensify locoregional treatment; for patients whose tumors cannot be removed surgically, radiation dose escalation is a logical approach. Although many individual studies have not shown a definitive survival benefit from radiation dose escalation, a 2012 review of seven prospective trials of concurrent chemoradiation conducted by the RTOG demonstrated a strong association between locoregional tumor control and the probability of overall survival (Figure 23.2a) [44]. In that review, locoregional control was defined in one of two ways: as freedom from local-regional progression, which assumed that all patients had locoregional control at the date of randomization; or as "response mandatory," meaning that the primary tumor had to show at least a partial response on imaging. If no partial response was noted, then those patients were considered as having locoregional failure at the date of randomization. Only 46% of patients achieved a partial response immediately after treatment. Locoregional control rates decreased over time to 28% at 1 year, 17% at 2 years, and to 8% at 5 years (Figure 23.2b). Furthermore, receipt of higher biologically effective doses (BED) of radiation was strongly associated with both locoregional control and survival ($p < 0.0001$) (Figure 23.2c). In that analysis of almost 1400 patients treated with concurrent chemotherapy and radiation therapy to 60–69.6 Gy, a time-adjusted increase in BED intensity of 1 Gy was associated with an approximately 4% relative improvement in survival and a 3% relative improvement in locoregional control [44]. This evidence support the hypothesis that high-dose radiation has the potential to improve locoregional control and overall survival after fractionated therapy.

However, the importance of high-dose radiation in terms of survival was called into question by early results from RTOG 0617, which was originally designed as a phase III randomized trial of concurrent chemotherapy and radiation at doses of 60 Gy or 74 Gy, given with or without the epidermal growth factor receptor inhibitor cetuximab, for stage III NSCLC. A planned interim analysis in June 2011 showed that survival among the two treatment groups (high-dose vs. low-dose radiation) had crossed a futility boundary, meaning that it was highly unlikely that high-dose radiation would result in better survival compared with the lower-dose radiation. When this chapter was written, no differences in toxicity had become evident between the two treatment groups, and the reason

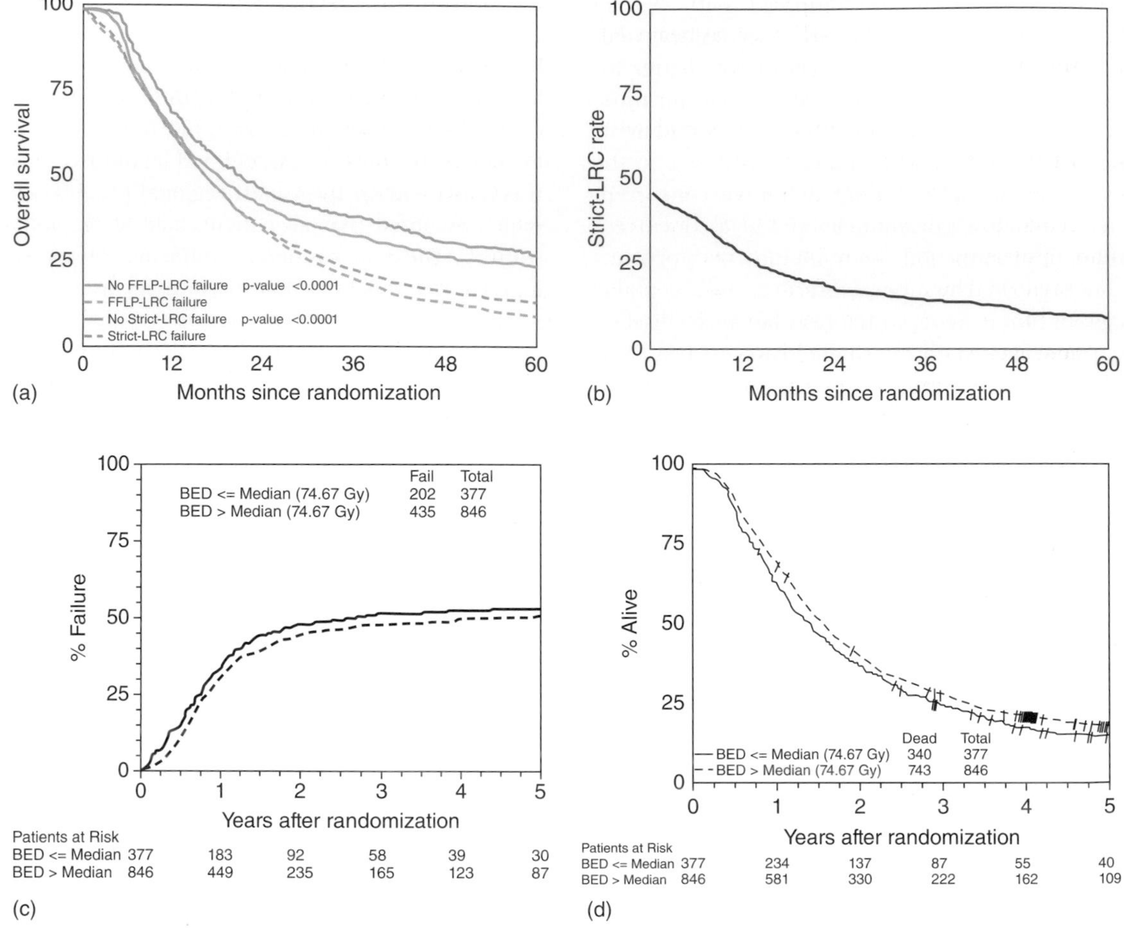

Figure 23.2 a: Improvement of locoregional control translating to a benefit in overall survival in patients treated with definitive radiation therapy. b: Declining rates of locoregional control (LRC) over time for 1390 patients, from 46% immediately after treatment to 8% at 5 years. FFLP, freedom from locoregional progression. c: Decreased rates of treatment failure and improved rates of overall survival with increased intensity of radiation therapy. *Source*: From Machtay M, Paulus R, Moughan J *et al.* (2012) Defining local-regional control and its importance in locally advanced non-small cell lung carcinoma. *J Thorac Oncol*, 7: 716–22 [44]. Reproduced with permission of Elsevier.

for the lack of survival difference with high-dose therapy remained to be determined. Investigations of the differences in the high-dose vs. standard-dose groups are ongoing and will likely clarify these results.

Designing the radiation volume and configuration

Several factors determine the volume to be treated and the configuration of the radiation portals to be used in treating NSCLC. These factors include the size and location of the primary tumor, the areas of lymphatic drainage in the hila and mediastinum, the histologic tumor type, and the equipment and beam energy available. Historically, treatment portals have been designed with large margins, to encompass appropriate fields. However, with the advent of highly conformal techniques, we recommend that conformal approaches be used rather than conventional methods.

Elective nodal irradiation

In many respects, surgery and external-beam RT have similar roles in the treatment of lung cancer. The intent of both modalities is local control within the treated field. Thus, for many years and with only a few exceptions [45–50], standard RT practice in the United States was to deliver 40–50 Gy to selected regional lymph nodes (e.g., ipsilateral hilum, ipsilateral and contralateral mediastinum, supraclavicular fassa) and an additional 20 Gy to the primary tumor through reduced fields. The major argument against this practice of elective nodal irradiation (ENI) is the high rate of local recurrence within previously irradiated tumor volumes. If gross disease cannot be controlled with radiation, then why enlarge the irradiated volumes to include areas that might harbor microscopic disease? However, this concern has largely been allayed by several major changes in lung cancer therapy since the standards for radiation doses and volumes were first established by the RTOG 73–01 trial, specifically the use of chemotherapy with RT, the advent of three-dimensional (3D) conformal RT, and the incorporation of positron emission tomography into the staging process for NSCLC.

Several recent trials have shown that rates of failure in electively treated nodes are low, and thus when modern methods are used for diagnosis, staging, and radiation delivery, irradiating areas outside of known disease is not beneficial in terms of disease control. For example, one review of failure patterns after definitive RT for early-stage NSCLC indicated that isolated regional failure occurred in no more than 15% of cases [51], suggesting that localized radiation fields could be effective without using ENI.

In one trial, Zhang and colleagues [45] observed 3-year and 5-year overall survival rates of 55% and 32% for selected patients with bronchogenic carcinoma whose primary tumors were irradiated but whose lymphatics were not. In another trial, Dosoretz and associates [50] observed no correlation between field size and treatment outcome, even after stratifying their data according to tumor size. In a third trial, Krol and colleagues [48] reported 3-year and 5-year overall survival rates of 31% and 15% for 108 patients with stage I lung cancer who underwent definitive RT encompassing the primary tumor but no ENI. Notably, the 3-year and 5-year cancer-specific survival rates in this study were 42% and 31%. These results are comparable to results achieved in trials of RT encompassing both traditional fields and regional lymphatics. They have also been confirmed by Senan and colleagues [46], who reported similarly low failure rates in untreated elective nodal areas in patients with stage III disease.

Additional studies have further corroborated these findings of low elective nodal failure rates. Rosenzweig *et al.* published several studies on the incidence of elective nodal failure in patients treated with 3D conformal RT and found those rates to be 5–10% [47, 52]. Yuan *et al.* reported a randomized trial of 200 patients with inoperable stage III NSCLC treated with 4–6 cycles of cisplatin-based chemotherapy and 3D conformal RT. Patients were randomly assigned to receive radiation to involved fields, to a total dose of 68–74 Gy in 1.8- to 2.0-Gy fractions, versus ENI to 60–64 Gy. The elective nodal field included the primary tumor, ipsilateral hilum, bilateral mediastinum, and supraclavicular fossa if the patients had superior mediastinal metastases. Rates of overall survival were higher, and rates of radiation pneumonitis lower, for the patients given involved-field radiation [53]. Caveats for interpreting the results of this trial include variations in radiation doses in the two treatment groups and the uncertainty engendered by allowing induction chemotherapy. Nevertheless, the authors of a recent multi-institutional consensus editorial on ENI suggested that clinicians tailor the approach for individual patients based on factors such as staging studies and safely achievable dose, such that ENI could be considered in some cases [54]. At least two explanations are possible for the lower-than-expected elective nodal failure rates observed in trials of ENI. First, the incidental doses to the ipsilateral hilar, paratracheal, and subcarinal nodes approach 40–50 Gy even when these regions are not intentionally irradiated [55]. Second, patients with lung cancer often face several competing causes of death (e.g., local failure, distant failure, or intercurrent illness) that may kill them without elective nodal failures ever being detected.

Three-dimensional conformal radiation therapy

Three-dimensional conformal RT has several significant advantages over traditional RT techniques: improved delineation of tumor and normal tissue; image segmentation and display; accurate dose calculation; and the ability to manipulate beam geometry and weighting through forward planning. The importance of improved target delineation cannot be overemphasized. Once the patient is immobilized and can undergo computed tomography in the treatment position, radiation oncologists can delineate the tumor and adjacent tissues in three dimensions; choose beam angles that maximize tumor coverage, minimize the amount of normal tissue exposed to radiation, or both; alter beam weighting; and perhaps alter couch angles for noncoplanar beam delivery. This conformal technique also enables the fusion of complementary imaging modalities, such as positron emission tomography to aid in tumor delineation and single photon emission computed tomography to choose beam angles.

Planning for 3D conformal RT in NSCLC has benefitted substantially from the application of target-defining guidelines published by the International Commission on Radiation Units [56]. According to these guidelines, the gross tumor volume (GTV) is defined as the primary tumor and any grossly involved lymph nodes. The clinical tumor volume (CTV) is defined as the anatomically defined area thought to harbor micrometastases (hilar or mediastinal lymph nodes or a margin around the grossly visible disease). The planning target volume (PTV) accounts for physiologic organ motion during treatment and the uncertainties of daily setup for fractionated therapy. When 3D treatment planning is done with the goals of conformal high-dose irradiation of the GTV and minimal irradiation of surrounding normal organs (especially lungs), unique portals, beam arrangements, and beam weights result.

It is extremely important when applying 3D conformal RT to not exceed the maximum doses tolerated by sensitive tissue structures, which for lung cancer include the normal lung, esophagus, spinal cord, and heart. Unfortunately, partial-volume normal tissue tolerances are not well understood. Special care should be taken to restrict the radiation dose to normal lung tissue (e.g., to no more than 20 Gy, uncorrected for inhomogeneity) whenever possible. Dose-volume histograms (DVHs) for all normal thoracic organs should be generated and analyzed for the dose and volume of irradiation. Although DVH analysis is still considered to be under development, it can be useful for predicting complications such as pneumonitis and for improving treatment planning [55, 57–59]. Figure 23.3 shows typical radiographic images used in IMRT for a stage T2N2 squamous cell carcinoma of the right upper lung.

Minimizing radiation-induced toxicity to normal tissues

For the past decade, partial-volume organ tolerances for irradiation have been defined according to variables established by a task force designated by the US National Cancer Institute [60], which reviewed the literature and solicited the opinions of experienced clinical radiation oncologists. When the task force report was published in 1991, many clinicians were still using probabilities of complications at 5 years to estimate tolerance doses (e.g., toxicity endpoints for irradiated tissue were set at probabilities of a 5% rate of complications at 5 years ($TD_{5/5}$) or a 50% rate of complications at 5 years ($TD_{50/5}$)). However, the task force acknowledged that these endpoints, especially those regarding normal thoracic tissues, were based on "less than adequate" information that had been compiled in an era before the advent of biological modifiers, concurrent chemotherapy, or 3D conformal radiation.

Significant strides have been made since that time in understanding normal toxicity, as summarized in a series of consensus papers published in 2010 called the *Quantitative Analyses of Normal Tissue Effects in the Clinic* (QUANTEC). These papers collectively summarize the available literature and offer recommendations on dose constraints for a variety of normal structures. The studies reported provide well-established, evidence-based dose constraints for the clinical treatment of lung cancer (Table 23.2) [61–65]. The development of dose constraints for the lung and esophagus are described further below.

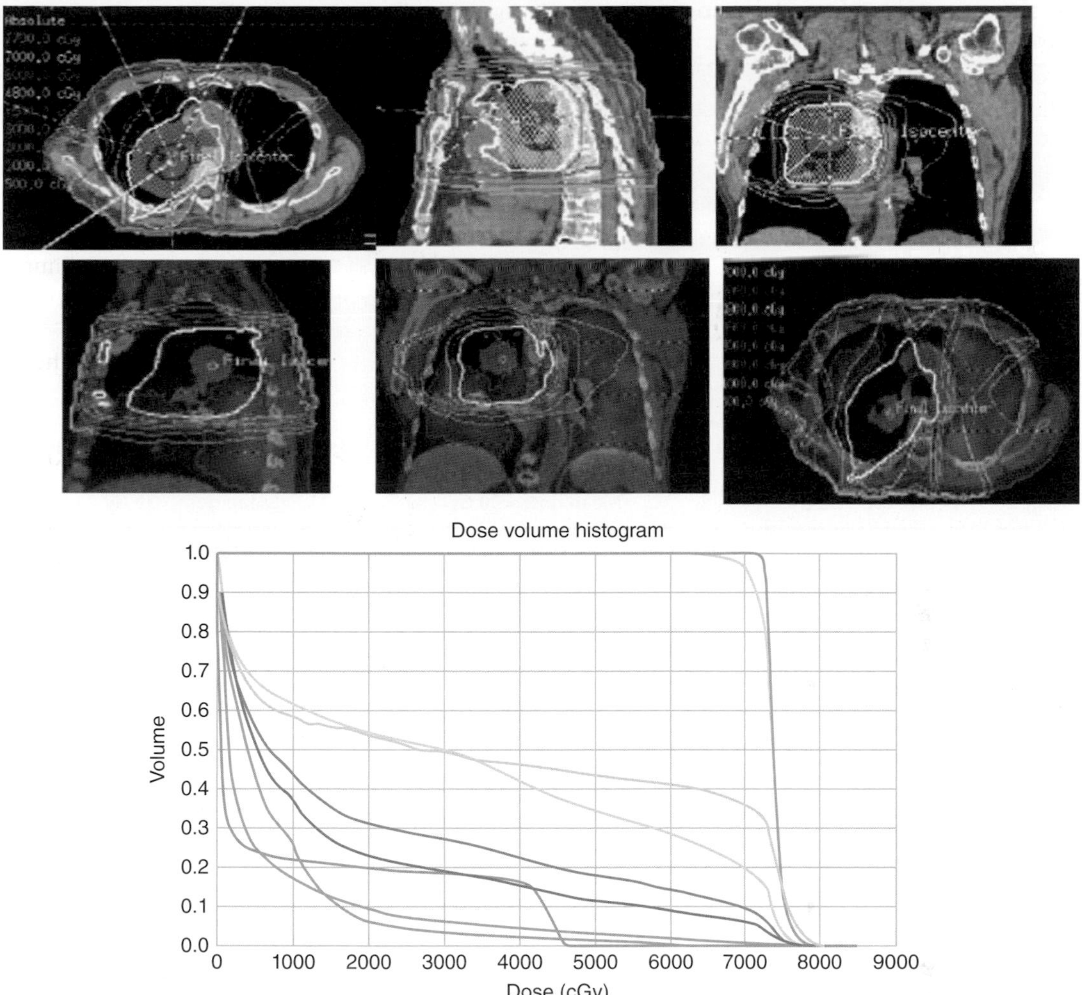

Figure 23.3 Typical dose-distribution images and dose-volume histograms for use in planning treatment of stage III non-small cell lung cancer (NSCLC). Upper panel, intensity-modulated radiation therapy (IMRT) plan based on CT images; middle panel, IMRT plan based on lung single positron emission computed tomography images; lower panel, a typical dose-volume histogram. Different colors in the histogram indicate different organ structures. (For a color version, see the color plate section.)

Lung

Radiation-induced lung injury is related to both dose and volume effects. The acute/subacute complication of radiation-induced lung injury is radiation pneumonitis, and the late complication is lung fibrosis. Both complications can be severely debilitating and even fatal.

The reported incidence of pneumonitis ranges from 13% to 44%; the breadth of this range reflects inconsistencies in criteria used, heterogeneity in patient populations, and differences in treatment regimens and RT techniques used [59, 66–70]. Clinical factors thought to predict pneumonitis include poor performance status [71], poor pulmonary function before RT, concurrent cigarette smoking [72, 73], chronic obstructive pulmonary disease [74], lower-lobe tumors [75], concurrent chemotherapy [75], high total radiation dose, and

Table 23.2 Suggested radiation dose constraints for thoracic malignancies using conventionally fractionated radiation (i.e., fractions of <3 Gy each) (derived from QUANTEC recommendations [61–64])

	RT alone	Chemo and RT	Chemo and RT before surgery
Spinal cord[1]	D_{max} <45 Gy	D_{max} <45 Gy	D_{max} <45 Gy
Lung[2]	MLD ≤20 Gy	MLD ≤20 Gy	MLD ≤20 Gy
	V_{20} ≤40%	V_{20} ≤35%	V_{20} ≤30%
		V_{10} ≤45%	V_{10} ≤40%
		V_5 ≤65%	V_5 ≤55%
Heart	V_{30} ≤45%	V_{30} ≤45%	V_{30} ≤45%
	Mean dose <26 Gy	Mean dose <26 Gy	Mean dose <26 Gy
Esophagus	D_{max} ≤80 Gy	D_{max} ≤80 Gy	D_{max} ≤80 Gy
	V_{70} <20%	V_{70} <20%	V_{70} <20%
	V_{50} <50%	V_{50} <40%	V_{50} <40%
	Mean dose <34 Gy	Mean dose <34 Gy	Mean dose <34 Gy
Kidney[3]	20 Gy to <32% of bilateral kidney	20 Gy to <32% of bilateral kidney	20 Gy < 32% of bilateral kidney
Liver	V_{30} ≤40%	V_{30} ≤40%	V_{30} ≤40%
	Mean dose <30 Gy	Mean dose <30 Gy	Mean dose <30 Gy

D_{max}, maximum dose; MLD, mean lung dose; RT, radiation therapy; V_x, volume (percentage) of the organ exposed to radiation dose x.

high radiation dose per fraction. Dosimetric factors thought to predict pneumonitis include mean lung dose (MLD) [74, 76–78] and the volume (percentage) of lung receiving more than a threshold dose (V_{dose}) [57, 70, 72, 76, 78–80]. Predictive dosimetric parameters range from the simple to the complex. MLD is both simple and clinically useful, as are the volume of total lung irradiated to doses of 20 Gy or more (V_{20}) [81]. Indeed, the QUANTEC group recommended limiting the V_{20} to no more than 30–35% and the MLD to 20 Gy (for radiation delivered in conventional fractionation), as many studies have demonstrated relationships between these two variables and risk of pneumonitis. Using these constraints should reduce the risk of pneumonitis to no more than 20% in patients with definitively treated NSCLC. Other variables that involve more complicated calculations include DVH reduction (reduction of the DVH of an organ to a single effective uniform dose), effective lung dose (V_{eff}), normal tissue complication probability models [82–84], and Niemierko's functional subunit model [85].

One key question in treating NSCLC and in evaluating dose constraints is what is more predictive of lung toxicity: high doses delivered to small regions or low doses delivered to large regions (otherwise stated as "a little to a lot or a lot to a little") [86]. In general, the answer seems to be that a collection of parameters are important in analyzing DVH data. For example, Graham et al. assessed DVH data from 99 patients treated definitively for inoperable NSCLC, all treated with 3D conformal therapy, and found that both the V_{20} and the MLC were statistically relevant to the development of grade ≥2 radiation pneumonitis [57]. However, in another DVH analysis, 49 patients were treated with thoracic 3D conformal RT (48 with chemotherapy), 18 of whom ultimately developed pneumonitis. The radiation dose levels were defined as low (≤10 Gy), moderate (10–40 Gy), and high (>40 Gy), and the lung dose was analyzed as both a single unit and as separate organs (ipsilateral and contralateral). In this analysis, the authors found that higher doses were most imporatant, such that doses exceeding 10 Gy increased the risk of pneumonitis from approximately 10% to more than 50%. Studies such as these provide further support for the combination of constraints such as use of V_{10}, V_{20}, and MLD as the standard dose constraints in treating patients with NSCLC.

Esophagus

The radiotherapeutic management of thoracic malignancies often exposes the esophagus to high levels of ionizing radiation. After 2–3 weeks of conventionally fractionated RT, patients often experience unpleasant acute reactions such as dysphagia, odynophagia, or both. These reactions can cause significant morbidity from dehydration and weight loss, and can necessitate interruption of treatment. Late reactions of the esophagus to radiation generally involve fibrosis, which can lead to stricture. Patients may experience various degrees of dysphagia and may require endoscopic dilation. In rare instances, acute and late responses can both involve esophageal perforation or obstruction.

Clinical and dosimetric predictors of acute and late esophagitis have been intensely studied over the past decade. Several of the factors shown to be important in increasing the risk of esophagitis include the volume of the esophagus irradiated, whether the entire circumference of the esophagus is in the radiation field, the fractionation regimen used (once daily vs. twice daily, and the dose per day), having a history of esophageal comorbidities such as esophageal stricture, maximum esophageal dose, mean dose, and the involvement of mediastinal lymph nodes [87–93].

We recently published results of an analysis of 652 patients who underwent RT for NSCLC to assess predictors of grade ≥3 esophagitis. In this analysis, we used the Lyman-Kutcher-Berman model to analyze radiation esophagitis as a function of the esophageal DVH per fraction, and included various clinical factors as dose-modifying factors. We found that high doses to small volumes were more predictive of toxicity than the mean dose to the entire esophagus, and that inclusion of concurrent chemotherapy as a dose-modifying factor significantly improved the predictiveness of the model. We also found a trend suggesting receipt of concurrent taxanes may increase the risk of esophagitis [94].

The QUANTEC group also published several consensus recommendations regarding the risk of radiation esophagitis. First, they acknowledged that esophageal infections (e.g., candidiasis or herpes simplex virus) can resemble esophagitis, and recommended that clinicians keep this similarity in mind when treating patients. Second, they emphasized that conditions such as gastroesophageal reflux disease can exacerbate the symptoms of radiation esophagitis. Third, treatment of lower-lobe lung tumors should consider the risk of radiation gastritis as well as esophagitis, because portions of the stomach may be in the radiation field. Fourth, and perhaps most important, is the potential for substantial variation in scoring esophagitis symptoms because some of the criteria depend on decisions made by treating physicians. For example, the Common Terminology Criteria for Adverse Events considers the need for intravenous fluids to indicate grade 2 esophagitis and the need for hospital admission for management to indicate grade 3 esophagitis. As a result, esophagitis in two patients with similar symptom burdens could potentially be given different grades. Hence the QUANTEC group concluded that more robust scoring systems, perhaps based on quality of life or molecular endpoints, are needed. Finally, the authors of the QUANTEC analysis acknowledged that "at present, it is not possible to identify a single best threshold volumetric parameter for esophageal irradiation, particularly because a wide range of percentage of lung volume receiving more than a threshold dose parameters correlate significantly with severe acute esophagitis." The dose constraints at used MD Anderson (mean esophageal dose <34 Gy, esophageal V_{70} <20%, and maximum dose ≤80 Gy) are based in part on reported outcomes from other studies [95]. Also, as is true for estimates of lung toxicity, several models are used to predict esophageal toxicity, including the normal tissue complication probability model, the Lyman-Kutcher-Berman model, and the relative seriality model. Given this choice in predictive algorithms, the QUANTEC authors recommend that clinicians and investigators use the model with which their institution has the most experience. They further emphasize that any novel components of these analyses should be tested in retrospective or prospective studies.

In some cases, irradiation of the esophagus is unavoidable in RT for NSCLC, particularly for patients with central disease or significant mediastinal lymphadenopathy. For such patients, investigators at Dana-Farber Cancer Institute/Brigham and Women's Hospital proposed a new parameter, "esophagus-in-field" ($Esoph_{in}$), for predicting the risk of eosphagitis. In their retrospective analysis of 109 patients with locally advanced NSCLC treated with concurrent chemoradiation in

2000–2006, they found that this parameter correlated well with the development of esophageal stricture. Specifically, a V_{55} <50% for the $Esoph_{in}$ was the best cutoff point for predicting the development of esophagitis [96]. Further studies such as these will be useful for developing appropriate and individualized dose constraints.

Novel radiation delivery techniques

Intensity-modulated radiation therapy

Intensity-modulated radiation therapy (IMRT) has become more prevalent for the treatment of NSCLC over the past decade. The technical advantages of IMRT over 3D conformal RT include the ability to use inverse treatment planning and dynamic multileaf collimators, which allow clinicians to set standards with respect to tumor coverage and normal tissue constraints before beam arrangement, as well as the ability to vary the fluence of the radiation beam to create highly conformal plans with sharp high-dose fall-off. Investigators at MD Anderson have demonstrated the dose superiority of IMRT over that of 3D conformal RT in several studies involving comparison of treatment plans. In one such study, IMRT was found to produce lower lung V_{20} and MLD than 3D conformal RT in stage I-III NSCLC in all cases studied. However, values of V_5 and V_{10} were higher for IMRT than for 3D conformal RT because of the use of multiple beams to achieve conformality [97]. Another study at William Beaumont Hospital showed that IMRT was particularly beneficial for patients with NSCLC and lymph node involvement, and the investigators emphasized that dose escalation above 70 Gy may be possible only with techniques that offer the conformality of IMRT [98].

Perhaps the most comprehensive analysis done to date on the clinical benefit of IMRT over 3D conformal RT came from MD Anderson, where investigators retrospectively analyzed almost 500 patients, 318 of whom had been treated with 3D conformal RT without accounting for respiratory motion, and the remainder with IMRT with treatment planning that accounted for respiratory-induced tumor motion. In that study, use of IMRT with image-guided planning reduced the rate of high-grade radiation pneumonitis from 25% to 10% as well as producing a benefit in overall survival [99]. IMRT with image-guided planning (incorporating respiratory motion) is now the standard for definitive RT for lung cancer at MD Anderson.

Proton beam therapy

During the past 5–10 years, proton beam therapy (PBT) has been increasingly used to treat several types of cancer, including NSCLC. The dosimetric benefit of PBT stems from the favorable dose distribution of proton particles, specifically the "Bragg peak" that allows minimal dose proximal and distal to the target of interest. Several dosimetric studies involving comparisons of treatment-planning images have demonstrated the benefit of PBT over that of 3D conformal RT or IMRT. Specifically, investigators from MD Anderson assessed normal tissue variables in both early-stage and locally advanced NSCLC and found that PBT offered substantial dosimetric improvements with respect to lung V_5, V_{10}, and V_{20} as well as doses to the esophagus, spinal cord, and heart [100]. Dosimetric analyses from other institutions have further confirmed this potential benefit of PBT [101, 102].

Newer studies have also begun to show that this potential dosimetric advantage does translate to clinical benefit. In one such study, Sejpal and others demonstrated that PBT led to lower rates of radiation pneumonitis and esophagitis than did 3D conformal RT or IMRT, even with delivery of higher radiation doses to the target volume [103]. Chang and others reported a phase II study of 44 patients with stage III NSCLC, all of whom were treated with high-dose PBT (74 Gy) and concurrent chemotherapy consisting of weekly paclitaxel and carboplatin. At a median follow-up interval of 19.7 months, the median overall survival time was 29.4 months [104], which was much longer than for previous phase III trials involving a similar regimen with photon-based therapy. Both the incidence and severity of toxicity were considered reasonable, with only five patients experiencing grade 3 esophagitis and one experiencing grade 2 pneumonitis. When this chapter was written, a multi-institutional phase III trial of PBT vs. IMRT and concurrent chemotherapy was underway for patients with locally advanced NSCLC. Accrual to this trial, which has the endpoints of radiation pneumonitis and locoregional control, is expected to be reached in July 2013.

Chemoradiation for small-cell lung cancer

Systemic therapy is a critical component in the treatment of both limited-stage and extensive-stage SCLC. More than 20 years ago, a landmark meta-analysis showed that the addition of chemotherapy for limited-stage SCLC produced a 5% benefit in overall survival at 3 years (20% vs. 15%, $p < 0.05$) and a 25% improvement in local control compared with RT alone [105]. Thus, chemoradiation has been the standard of care in limited-stage SCLC for some time except for rare cases of T1-T2N0 lesions, for which surgery followed by systemic therapy is recommended. Most of the discussion that follows focuses on chemoradiation for limited-stage disease, i.e., disease that is confined to only one lung, with possible extension to the mediastinum or ipsilateral lymph nodes.

Sequencing of radiation and chemotherapy for limited-stage disease

Four to six cycles of systemic therapy are usually used in the treatment of limited-stage SCLC. The two options in terms of the sequence of chemotherapy and RT are "early RT," in which radiation is delivered concurrent with the beginning of systemic treatment, and "late RT," in which RT is delivered after several cycles of chemotherapy and often sequentially. Each approach has theoretical advantages. With early RT, the overall treatment time is shorter, which in theory would improve patient compliance and reduce the accelerated repopulation of the tumor. As is true for NSCLC, this approach could increase the treatment intensity and even involve synergism between the two modalities. Late RT would be less toxic, if the chemotherapy and radiation were delivered sequentially, and perhaps would reduce the volume of tissue requiring RT in the event that the tumor responds to the chemotherapy. Finally, delays in the delivery of RT allow the response to chemotherapy to be assessed, which may influence the choice of further local treatment, which can evoke further toxicity.

Several comparisons of early and late RT have produced conflicting results. In one study by the National Cancer Institute of Canada Clinical Trials Group, 308 patients were randomly assigned to early RT, defined as RT concurrent with the first cycle of chemotherapy, or late RT, defined as RT given with the final cycle of chemotherapy. The chemotherapy consisted of cyclophosphamide, doxorubicin, and vincristine alternating with etoposide and cisplatin. The radiation dose was 40 Gy in 15 fractions, and all patients received prophylactic cranial irradiation (PCI). Early RT produced superior progression-free survival ($p = 0.036$) and overall survival ($p = 0.008$) [106]. However, an almost identical trial by the London Lung Cancer Group, in which patients received the same chemotherapy regimens, the same RT doses, and early vs. late RT (defined as concurrent with the second vs. sixth cycle) revealed no benefit from early RT versus late RT [107].

Although individual clinical trials have produced conflicting results, recommendations arising from meta-analyses have helped to guide decisions with regard to caring for patients with SCLC. These meta-analyses have consistently reported a small but discernible benefit from early vs. late RT, albeit at the cost of increased toxicity. Two notable studies from Fried *et al.* in 2004 [108] and de Ruysscher *et al.* in 2006 [109] reported improvements from the use of twice-daily radiation and platinum-based chemotherapy. The 2012 NCCN guidelines of the National Comprehensive Cancer Network currently consider early RT for limited-stage SCLC as being supported by category 1 evidence. Early findings from a phase III trial presented at the 2012 meeting of the American Society of Clinical Oncology indicated no difference in overall survival when RT (52.5 Gy once daily in 2.1-Gy fractions) was begun either with the first cycle of systemic therapy (cisplatin 70 mg/m^2 and etoposide 100 mg/m^2) or with the third cycle, although patients who began RT with the third cycle had lower rates of febrile neutropenia [110]. The current practice at MD Anderson is to begin RT no later than the third cycle of systemic treatment in most patients.

Chemotherapy regimens

Currently the standard systemic therapy given for SCLC is a platinum-based regimen with etoposide (for limited-stage disease) or with etoposide or irinotecan (for extensive-stage disease). This regimen was chosen based on findings from several studies showing greater toxicity but analogous efficacy with other, more aggressive regimens that include alkylators or anthracyclines [111, 112]. The combination of irinotecan and cisplatin became an option for extensive-stage disease after a randomized trial in Japan demonstrated that irinotecan and cisplatin produced better overall survival and progression-free survival than did etoposide and cisplatin [113], but subsequent randomized trials did not show a significant benefit [114, 115]. Indeed, a SWOG trial that enrolled larger numbers of patients showed higher rates of severe gastrointestinal toxicity (with less hematologic toxicity) than in the Japanese study [115] (Figure 23.4). Notably, the SWOG trial also involved population-related pharmacogenomics sttudies that revealed molecular predictors of irinotecan-cisplatin–related diarrhea and neutropenia that could be useful in future studies.

At this time, either carboplatin or cisplatin can be used as the platin in the systemic therapy regimen. Typically cisplatin carries a higher risk of gastrointestinal toxicity (nausea), peripheral neuropathy, and renal side effects, and carboplatin has a higher risk of myelosuppression. The comparative effectiveness of these two agents has been investigated in several small clinical trials, but one recent meta-analysis of almost 700 patients in four randomized trials demonstrated similar overall survival and progression-free survival from the two regimens (Figure 23.5), with the toxicity profiles matching those noted above [116].

Radiation dose and fractionation schedule

Three common radiation regimens are used in conjunction with chemotherapy for limited-stage SCLC, each supported by its own studies and high-level evidence. The most common regimen

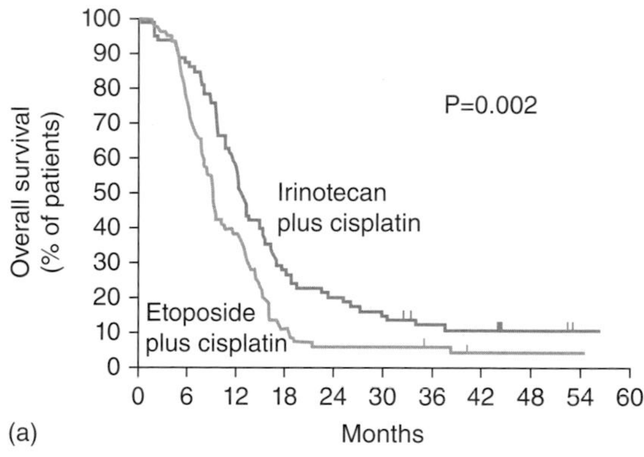

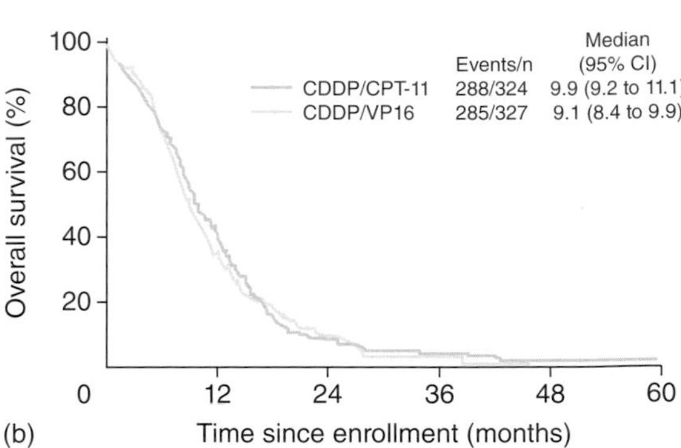

Figure 23.4 Findings from two phase III trials of irinotecan and cisplatin (IP) versus etoposide and cisplatin (EP) for extensive-stage small-cell lung cancer. A study from Japan demonstrated higher overall survival and disease-free survival with IP than with EP (panel a), but a larger trial by the Southwest Oncology Group did not demonstrate any advantage (panel b). Currently, National Comprehensive Cancer Network considers either chemotherapy couplet an option for extensive-stage disease.
Source: Panel (a): Noda 2002 [113]. Reproduced with permission of the Massachusetts Medical Society. Panel (b): Lara 2009 [115]. Reproduced with permission of the American Society of Clinical Oncology.

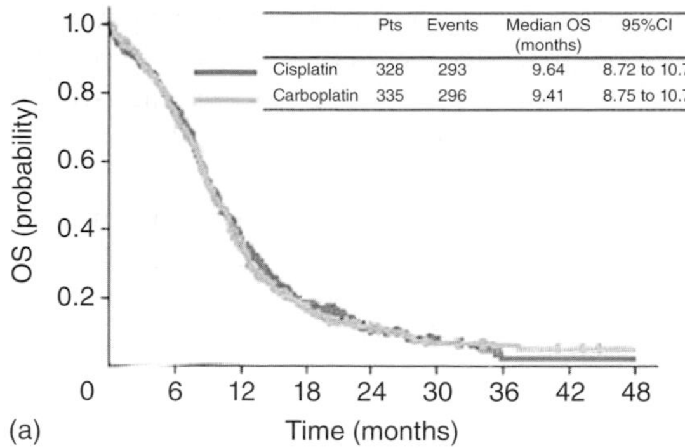

Figure 23.5 The comparative effectiveness of carboplatin versus cisplatin in chemotherapy regimens for small cell lung cancer. A meta-analysis of four randomized trials involving 663 patients revealed no differences in overall survival (panel a) or progression-free survival (panel b) for the two agents, although their toxicity profiles are different (see text).
Source: Rossi 2012 [116]. Reproduced with permission of the American Society of Clinical Oncology.

involves 45 Gy delivered twice daily in 1.5-Gy fractions. Evidence in support of this regimen comes from INT-0096, a randomized trial published by Turrisi *et al.* in which patients were assigned to receive concurrent sisplatin-etopiside chemotherapy with either this regimen or 45 Gy delivered once daily in 1.8-Gy fractions. Survival rates at 2 years were 26% for patients given twice-daily RT and 16% for those given once-daily RT ($p < 0.05$). Not surprisingly, the twice-daily regimen was associated with much higher rates of high-grade (grade ≥3) esophagitis (27% vs. 11%, $p < 0.001$) [117].

The second regimen was derived from from a CALGB study reported by Berger *et al.*, who analyzed 63 patients with limited-stage SCLC given concurrent chemotherapy and thoracic RT. The chemotherapy consisted of 2 cycles of induction paclitaxel and topotecan, followed by 3 cycles of carboplatin and etoposide with thoracic RT. PCI was offered to patients who experienced a complete or partial response. This regimen produced a 2-year overall survival rate of 48% and a 2-year progression-free survival rate of 31%, with comparable rates of hematologic toxicity and lower rates of esophagitis than in the INT-0096 trial (21% vs. 32%) [118].

The third regimen arose from RTOG 97–12, in which 64 patients received four cycles of cisplatin (60 mg/m^2) and etoposide (120 mg/m^2, subsequently changed to 240 mg/m^2), with early concurrent thoracic RT beginning on day 1. A dose escalating scheme was used in which radiation therapy was given at 1.8 Gy/fraction daily to the entire CTV, followed by twice-daily fractions to the GTV for the remaining treatment days, beginning at 3 days and escalating to 5, 7, 9, and 11 days (corresponding to total doses of 50.4 Gy, 54.0 Gy, 57.6 Gy, 61.2 Gy, and 64.8 Gy, respectively). The maximum tolerated dose was found to be 61.2 Gy, given over a period of 5 weeks, and the 18-month survival rate was 82% [119].

The reasonable efficacy and toxicity of these three regimens led to a phase III randomized study, begun in 2008, to compare these three RT regimens (CALGB 30610/RTOG 0538). All patients are to receive early RT (beginning either at the beginning of chemotherapy or after one cycle), with systemic therapy regimen of cisplatin 80 mg/m^2 and etoposide 100 mg/m^2 every 21 days for four cycles. PCI is offered to all patients who experience a complete or near-complete response, and the primary endpoint is overall survival. As of December 2012, this protocol was continuing to accrue well nationally, and the results will provide level 1 evidence regarding the optimal radiation approach or approaches in this context.

Radiation target volumes and dose constraints

As was true in the treatment of NSCLC, before the advent of modern 3D or 4D imaging techniques, large radiation fields were used to treat SCLC. For example, in the INT-0096 trial, the RT fields encompassed the parenchymal tumor (if applicable), the bilateral mediastinum, ipsilateral hilar lymph nodes, and 5 cm below the carina if the subcarinal lymph nodes were involved [117]. Over the past several years, however, the use of more sensitive imaging modalities, such as positron emission/computed tomography scans, has improved staging [120] and allowed the RT target to be reduced to an involved-field approach. This transition is reflected by the requirements of the aforementioned CALGB 30610/RTOG 0538 study for 3D conformal planning and defines the CTV as the GTV plus a margin of not less than 1.0 cm if 4D RT planning is used. However, the only elective nodal basins treated as part of this protocol are those of the ipsilateral hilum. This general approach of irradiating involved nodes, with strong consideration of treatment of the ipsilateral hilum, is currently used at MD Anderson.

The radiation dose constraints used for thoracic RT for SCLC are similar to those used for NSCLC, with a couple of notable exceptions related to twice-daily irradiation. First, the dose to the spinal cord is restricted to no more than 36 Gy. Second, the threshold dose to the esophagus dose has not been established, but the esophageal dose requires particular attention given the high rates of severe esophagitis reported. Although target coverage should not be compromised, patients should be made aware of the risk of severe treatment-related symptoms, and feeding tube placement should be considered based on the dose to the esophagus and the patient's performance status.

Consolidative thoracic radiation for extensive-stage disease

Evidence from phase III trials supports the use of thoracic RT for patients with extensive-stage disease who experience a good response to chemotherapy. In one such trial reported by Jeremic *et al.*, 210 patients were treated with three cycles of cisplatin (80 mg/m^2) and etoposide (80 mg/m^2). Patients who experienced a complete response at both local and distant sites, or a partial response locally and a complete response distantly, were then randomly assigned to hyperfractionated thoracic RT (54 Gy in 36 fractions delivered twice daily) with concurrent carboplatin and etoposide, followed by two further cycles of cisplatin/etoposide, versus four more cycles of cisplatin/etoposide. The median survival time was significantly longer among patients given consolidative thoracic RT (17 months vs. 11 months, $p = 0.041$) but no difference was seen in distant metastasis–free survival [121].

At MD Anderson, we typically recommend consolidative thoracic RT for patients who meet the response criteria noted above. In 2009, the RTOG opened a randomized phase II study in which patients with extensive-stage SCLC are given 4–6 cycles of platin-based therapy followed by either PCI plus consolidative RT to systemic sites, including the thorax, or PCI alone (RTOG 0937). The findings from this trial will help to clarify the role of comprehensive RT for extensive-stage disease.

Prophylactic cranial irradiation

Many trials have been conducted over the past several decades to assess the role of PCI in both limited-stage and extensive-stage SCLC. From these studies, a few key analyses have established PCI as being appropriate for specific patient subpopulations for reducing intracranial metastases and improving overall survival. With regard to limited-stage SCLC, the key study was a meta-analysis reported by Auperin et al. that assessed findings from 1000 patients in seven randomized trials comparing PCI vs. no PCI for patients experiencing a complete response to prior therapy. Receipt of PCI led to a 5.4% increase in overall survival rate and to reductions in the risk of recurrence and the cumulative incidence of brain metastases [122]. For extensive-stage SCLC, the key trial was reported by Slotman *et al.*, in which patients who had experienced at least a partial response to 4–6 cycles of chemotherapy were randomly assigned to receive PCI to various doses versus no PCI. PCI led to an increase in median overall survival time (from 5.4 to 6.7 months) and an increase in overall survival rates at 1 year (from 13.3% to 27.1%) ($p < 0.05$). PCI also reduced the rate of intracranial metastases and extended disease-free survival times as well [123].

The optimal dose for PCI, particularly for patients who are also being treated with whole-brain radiation therapy but have no discernible evidence of disease, has been debated for some time because of the risk of potentially serious side effects. The findings from an important multi-cooperative group study may help to resolve some of the uncertainty. In this analysis, 720 patients with limited-stage SCLC who experienced a complete response were randomly assigned to receive PCI at one of two dosages, 10 fractions of 2.5 Gy each or 18 fractions of 2.0 Gy each. No difference in outcomes were found between the two dosage groups, but five serious adverse events were noted in the high-dose group (one death with neurological deterioration, one generalized seizure, one cerebrovascular event, one bilateral cataract, and one death from generalized seizure), with none in the standard-dose group. Toxic effects such as headache, fatigue, and nausea were also more prevalent in the high-dose group [124]. In a subsequent follow-up analysis, assessments of neurologic outcomes and quality of life revealed mild deteriorations over time in communication, intellectual deficit, and memory. Although the incidence of severe deterioration was low, but the authors emphasized that patients who are considering PCI should be made aware of the risk of these side effects, particularly those of advanced age or those with existing cognitive impairment [125].

Conclusions

The successes achieved to date by combining chemotherapy with RT for NSCLC, albeit somewhat modest, warrant continuation of this strategy. Major issues still to be addressed include the role of surgery for the treatment marginally resectable tumors, the selection of novel systemic agents, and the incorporation of improved radiation techniques. Progress in treating NSCLC continues to be hampered by the rush to follow up phase I studies of toxicity with phase II trials rather than with comparative phase III trials. Moving newer and more effective drugs more quickly from phase I to phase III studies should help to increase the pace of progress in treating NSCLC while at the same time providing the basis for appropriate general standards for comparison and clinical practice.

As for SCLC, significant advances have included establishing the relative efficacy and toxicity of various chemotherapy regimens, determining the optimal timing of chemotherapy and RT, and clarifying the role of PCI for both limited- and extensive-stage disease. Further studies are needed to identify the most effective RT fractionation regimen and the role of consolidative RT to systemic sites for the purposes of local control in extensive-stage SCLC. As is true for NSCLC, advances in molecular therapy will be key in achieving substantial progress in survival outcomes for patients with SCLC and for the ability to predict which patients will experience particular toxicities, so that treatment approaches can be truly personalized to individual patients.

References

1 Steel GG, Peckham MJ (1979) Exploitable mechanisms in combined radiotherapy-chemotherapy: the concept of additivity. *Int J Radiat Oncol Biol Phys*, Jan; 5(1): 85–91.

2 Eberhardt W, Pottgen C, Stuschke M (2006) Chemoradiation paradigm for the treatment of lung cancer. *Nat Clin Pract Oncol*, Apr; 3(4): 188–99.

3 Weichselbaum RR, Beckett MA, Vokes EE, Brachman DG, Haraf D, Hallahan D, *et al.* (1995) Cellular and molecular mechanisms of radioresistance. *Cancer Treat Res*, 74: 131–40.

4 Chabner BA (1993) Biological basis for cancer treatment. *Ann Intern Med*, Apr 15; 118(8): 633–7.

5 Tannock IF (1996) Treatment of cancer with radiation and drugs. *J Clin Oncol*, Dec; 14(12): 3156–74.

6 Perez CA, Bauer M, Edelstein S, Gillespie BW, Birch R (1986) Impact of tumor control on survival in carcinoma of the lung treated with irradiation. *Int J Radiat Oncol Biol Phys*, Apr; 12(4): 539–47.

7 Eisert DR, Cox JD, Komaki R (1976) Irradiation for bronchial carcinoma: reasons for failure. I. Analysis of local control as a function of dose, time, and fractionation. *Cancer*, Jun; 37(6): 2665–70.

8 Cox JD, Byhardt R, Komaki R, Wilson JF, Libnoch JA, Hansen R (1979) Interaction of thoracic irradiation and chemotherapy on local control and survival in small cell carcinoma of the lung. *Cancer Treat Rep*, Aug; 63(8): 1251–5.

9 Saunders MI, Barltrop MA, Rassa PM, Anderson PJ, Dische S (1984) The relationship between tumor response and survival following radiotherapy for carcinoma of the bronchus. *Int J Radiat Oncol Biol Phys*, Apr; 10(4): 503–8.

10 Perez CA, Pajak TF, Rubin P, Simpson JR, Mohiuddin M, Brady LW, *et al.* (1987) Long-term observations of the patterns of failure in patients with unresectable non-oat cell carcinoma of the lung treated with definitive radiotherapy. Report by the Radiation Therapy Oncology Group. *Cancer*, Jun 1; 59(11): 1874–81.

11 Schaake-Konning C, Van Den Bogaert W, Dalesio O, Festen J, Hoogenhout J, Van Houtte P, *et al.* (1992) Effects of concomitant cisplatin and rediotherapy on inoperable non-small-cell lung cancer. *New England Journal of Medicine*, 326(8): 524–30.

12 Brodin O, Nou E, Mercke C, Linden CJ, Lundstrom R, Arwidi A, *et al.* (1996) Comparison of induction chemotherapy before radiotherapy with radiotherapy only in patients with locally advanced squamous cell carcinoma of the lung. The Swedish Lung Cancer Study Group. *Eur J Cancer*, Oct; 32A(11): 1893–1900.

13 Dillman RO, Herndon J, Seagren SL, Eaton WL, Green MR (1996) Improved survival in stage III non-small-cell lung cancer: Seven-year follow-up of cancer and leukemia group B (CALGB) 8433 trial. *Journal of the National Cancer Institute*, 88(17): 1210–15.

14 Le Chevalier T, Arriagada R, Tarayre M, Lacombe-Terrier MJ, Laplanche A, Quoix E, *et al.* (1992) Significant effect of adjuvant chemotherapy on survival in locally advanced non-small-cell lung carcinoma. *J Natl Cancer Inst*, Jan 1; 84(1): 58.

15 Morton RF, Jett JR, McGinnis WL, Earle JD, Therneau TM, Krook JE, *et al.* (1991) Thoracic radiation therapy alone compared with combined chemoradiotherapy for locally unresectable non-small cell lung cancer. A randomized, phase III trial. *Ann Intern Med*, Nov 1; 115(9): 681–6.

16 Sause W, Kolesar P, Taylor SI, Johnson D, Livingston R, Komaki R, *et al.* (2000) Final results of phase III trial in regionally advanced unresectable non-small cell lung cancer: Radiation Therapy Oncology Group, Eastern Cooperative Oncology Group, and Southwest Oncology Group. *Chest*, Feb; 117(2): 358–64.

17 Dillman RO, Seagren SL, Propert KJ, Guerra J, Eaton WL, Perry MC, *et al.* (1990) A randomized trial of induction chemotherapy plus high-dose radiation versus radiation alone in stage III non-small-cell lung cancer [see comments]. *New England Journal of Medicine*, 323(14): 940–5.

18 Arriagada R, Le Chevalier T, Quoix E, Ruffie P, de Cremoux H, Douillard JY, *et al.* (1991) ASTRO (American Society for Therapeutic Radiology and Oncology) plenary: Effect of chemotherapy on locally advanced non-small cell lung carcinoma: a randomized study of 353 patients. GETCB (Groupe d'Etude et Traitement des Cancers Bronchiques), FNCLCC (Federation Nationale des Centres de Lutte contre le Cancer) and the CEBI trialists. *Int J Radiat Oncol Biol Phys*, Jun; 20(6): 1183–90.

19 Le Chevalier T, Arriagada R, Quoix E, Ruffie P, Martin M, Tarayrek M, *et al.* (1991) Radiotherapy alone versus combined chemotherapy and radiotherapy in nonresectable non-small-cell lung cancer: First analysis of a randomized trial in 353 patients. *Journal of National Cancer Institute*, 83: 417–23.

20 Sause WT, Scott C, Taylor S, Johnson D, Livingston R, Komaki R, *et al.* (1995) Radiation Therapy Oncology Group (RTOG) 88–08 and Eastern Cooperative Oncology Group (ECOG) 4588: Preliminary results of a phase III trial in regionally advanced, unresectable non-small-cell lung cancer. *Journal of the National Cancer Institute*, 87(3): 198–205.

21 Komaki R, Scott CB, Sause WT, Johnson DH, Taylor SGt, Lee JS, *et al.* (1997) Induction cisplatin/vinblastine and irradiation vs. irradiation in unresectable squamous cell lung cancer: failure patterns by cell type in RTOG 88–08/ECOG 4588. Radiation Therapy Oncology Group. Eastern Cooperative Oncology Group [see comments]. *International Journal of Radiation Oncology, Biology, Physics*, 39(3): 537–44.

22 Komaki R, Scott CB, Sause WT, Johnson DH, Taylor SGt, Lee JS, *et al.* (1997) Induction cisplatin/vinblastine and irradiation vs. irradiation in unresectable squamous cell lung cancer: failure patterns by cell type in RTOG 88–08/ECOG 4588. Radiation Therapy Oncology Group. Eastern Cooperative Oncology Group. *Int J Radiat Oncol Biol Phys*, Oct 1; 39(3): 537–44.

23 Byhardt RW, Scott CB, Ettinger DS, Curran WJ, Doggett RL, Coughlin C, *et al.* (1995) Concurrent

hyperfractionated irradiation and chemotherapy for unresectable nonsmall cell lung cancer. Results of Radiation Therapy Oncology Group 90–15. *Cancer*, May 1; 75(9): 2337–44.

24 Cox JD, Azarnia N, Byhardt RW, Shin KH, Emami B, Pajak TF (1990) A randomized phase I/II trial of hyperfractionated radiation therapy with total doses of 60.0 Gy to 79.2 Gy: possible survival benefit with greater than or equal to 69.6 Gy in favorable patients with Radiation Therapy Oncology Group stage III non-small-cell lung carcinoma: report of Radiation Therapy Oncology Group 83–11. *Journal of Clinical Oncology*, 8(9): 1543–55.

25 Lee JS, Scott C, Komaki R, Fossella FV, Dundas GS, McDonald S, *et al.* (1996) Concurrent chemoradiation therapy with oral etoposide and cisplatin for locally advanced inoperable non-small-cell lung cancer: Radiation therapy oncology group protocol 91–06. *Journal of Clinical Oncology*, 14(4): 1055–64.

26 Reboul F, Brewer Y, Vincent P, Chauvet B, Faure CF, Taulelle M (1996) Concurrent cisplatin, etoposide, and radiotherapy for unresectable stage III nonsmall cell lung cancer: A phase II study. *Int J Radiat Oncol Biol Phys*, May 1; 35(2): 343–50.

27 Komaki R, Scott C, Ettinger D, Lee JS, Fossella FV, Curran W, *et al.* (1997) Randomized study of chemotherapy/radiation therapy combinations for favorable patients with locally advanced inoperable nonsmall cell lung cancer: Radiation Therapy Oncology Group (RTOG) 92–04. *Int J Radiat Oncol Biol Phys*, Apr 1; 38(1): 149–55.

28 O'Rourke N, Roque IFM, Farre Bernado N, Macbeth F (2010) Concurrent chemoradiotherapy in nonsmall cell lung cancer. *Cochrane Database Syst Rev*, 6: CD002140.

29 Curran WJ (2000) Sequential versus concurrent chemoradiation in unresected stage III NSCLC: RTOG 94–10 initial report. *Journal of Clinical Oncology*, 19: 484a.

30 Fournel P, Robinet G, Thomas P, Souquet PJ, Lena H, Vergnenegre A, *et al.* (2005) Randomized phase III trial of sequential chemoradiotherapy compared with concurrent chemoradiotherapy in locally advanced non-small-cell lung cancer: Groupe Lyon-Saint-Etienne d'Oncologie Thoracique-Groupe Francais de Pneumo-Cancerologie NPC 95–01 Study. *J Clin Oncol*, Sep 1; 23(25): 5910–17.

31 Rao CZ (2007) Study of concurrent versus sequential chemoradiotherapy with vinorelbine and cisplatin in stage III non-small cell lung cancer. *Chinese Journal of Cancer Prevention and Treatment*, 14(12): 942–3.

32 Reinfuss MS, Kowalska T, Glinski B, Dymek P, Walasek T (2005) Evaluation of efficacy of combined chemoradiotherapy in locoregional advanced, inoperable non-small cell lung cancer. *Nowotwory*, 55(3): 200–6.

33 Zatloukal P, Petruzelka L, Zemanova M, Havel L, Janku F, Judas L, *et al.* (2004) Concurrent versus sequential chemoradiotherapy with cisplatin and vinorelbine in locally advanced non-small cell lung cancer: A randomized study. *Lung Cancer*, 46(1): 87–98.

34 Belani CP, Choy H, Bonomi P, Scott C, Travis P, Haluschak J, *et al.* (2005) Combined chemoradiotherapy regimens of paclitaxel and carboplatin for locally advanced non-small-cell lung cancer: A randomized phase II locally advanced multi-modality protocol. *J Clin Oncol*, Sep 1; 23(25): 5883–91.

35 Huber RM, Flentje M, Schmidt M, Pollinger B, Gosse H, Willner J, *et al.* (2006) Simultaneous chemoradiotherapy compared with radiotherapy alone after induction chemotherapy in inoperable stage IIIA or IIIB non-small-cell lung cancer: Study CTRT99/97 by the Bronchial Carcinoma Therapy Group. *J Clin Oncol*, Sep 20; 24(27): 4397–4404.

36 Auperin A, Le Pechoux C, Rolland E, Curran WJ, Furuse K, Fournel P, *et al.* (2010) Meta-analysis of concomitant versus sequential radiochemotherapy in locally advanced non-small-cell lung cancer. *J Clin Oncol*, May 1; 28(13): 2181–90.

37 O'Rourke N, Macbeth F (2010) Is concurrent chemoradiation the standard of care for locally advanced non-small cell lung cancer? A review of guidelines and evidence. *Clin Oncol (R Coll Radiol)*, Jun; 22(5): 347–55.

38 Andre F, Grunenwald D, Pignon JP, Dujon A, Pujol JL, Brichon PY, *et al.* (2000) Survival of patients with resected N2 non-small-cell lung cancer: evidence for a subclassification and implications. *J Clin Oncol*, Aug; 18(16): 2981–9.

39 Albain KS, Rusch VW, Crowley JJ, Rice TW, Turrisi AT, 3rd, Weick JK, *et al.* (1995) Concurrent cisplatin/etoposide plus chest radiotherapy followed by surgery for stages IIIA (N2) and IIIB non-small-cell lung cancer: mature results of Southwest Oncology Group phase II study 8805. *J Clin Oncol*, Aug 1, 13(8): 1880–92.

40 Albain K, Swann R, Rusch V, Turrisi A, Shepherd F, Smith C, *et al.* (2005) Phase III study of concurrent chemotherapy and radiotherapy (CT/RT) vs CT/RT followed by surgical resection for stage IIIA(pN2) non-small cell lung cancer (NSCLC):

Outcomes update of North American Intergroup 0139 (RTOG 9309). *Proceedings of American Society of Clinical Oncology*, 23(16s): 624s.

41 Albain KS, Swann RS, Rusch VW, Turrisi AT, 3rd, Shepherd FA, Smith C, *et al.* (2009) Radiotherapy plus chemotherapy with or without surgical resection for stage III non-small-cell lung cancer: A phase III randomised controlled trial. *Lancet*, Aug 1; 374(9687): 379–86.

42 National Comprehensive Cancer Network guidelines, www.nccn.org, 2012.

43 Kong FM, Ten Haken RK, Schipper MJ, Sullivan MA, Chen M, Lopez C, *et al.* (2005) High-dose radiation improved local tumor control and overall survival in patients with inoperable/unresectable non-small-cell lung cancer: long-term results of a radiation dose escalation study. *Int J Radiat Oncol Biol Phys*, Oct 1; 63(2): 324–33.

44 Machtay M, Paulus R, Moughan J, Komaki R, Bradley JE, Choy H, *et al.* (2012) Defining local-regional control and its importance in locally advanced non-small cell lung carcinoma. *J Thorac Oncol*, Apr; 7(4): 716–22.

45 Zhang HX, Yin WB, Zhang LJ, Yang ZY, Zhang ZX, Wang M, *et al.* (1989) Curative radiotherapy of early operable non-small cell lung cancer. *Radiother Oncol*, Feb; 14(2): 89–94.

46 Senan S, Burgers S, Samson MJ, van Klaveren RJ, Oei SS, van Sornsen de Koste J, *et al.* (2002) Can elective nodal irradiation be omitted in stage III non-small-cell lung cancer? Analysis of recurrences in a phase II study of induction chemotherapy and involved-field radiotherapy. *Int J Radiat Oncol Biol Phys*, Nov 15; 54(4): 999–1006.

47 Rosenzweig KE, Sim SE, Mychalczak B, Braban LE, Schindelheim R, Leibel SA (2001) Elective nodal irradiation in the treatment of non-small-cell lung cancer with three-dimensional conformal radiation therapy. *Int J Radiat Oncol Biol Phys*, Jul 1; 50(3): 681–5.

48 Krol AD, Aussems P, Noordijk EM, Hermans J, Leer JW (1996) Local irradiation alone for peripheral stage I lung cancer: Could we omit the elective regional nodal irradiation? *Int J Radiat Oncol Biol Phys*, Jan 15; 34(2): 297–302.

49 Dosoretz DE, Katin MJ, Blitzer PH, Rubenstein JH, Galmarini DH, Garton GR, *et al.* (1996) Medically inoperable lung carcinoma: The role of radiation therapy. *Seminars in Radiation Oncology*, 6(2(April)): 98–104.

50 Dosoretz DE, Galmarini D, Rubenstein JH, Katin MJ, Blitzer PH, Salenius SA, *et al.* (1993) Local control in medically inoperable lung cancer: an analysis of its importance in outcome and factors determining the probability of tumor eradication. *Int J Radiat Oncol Biol Phys*, Oct 20; 27(3): 507–16.

51 Jeremic B, Casas F, Wang L, Perin B (2010) Radiation therapy for early stage (I/II) non-small cell lung cancer. *Front Radiat Ther Oncol*, 42: 87–93.

52 Rosenzweig KE, Sura S, Jackson A, Yorke E (2007) Involved-field radiation therapy for inoperable non small-cell lung cancer. *J Clin Oncol*, Dec 10; 25(35): 5557–61.

53 Yuan S, Sun X, Li M, Yu J, Ren R, Yu Y, *et al.* (2007) A randomized study of involved-field irradiation versus elective nodal irradiation in combination with concurrent chemotherapy for inoperable stage III non-small cell lung cancer. *Am J Clin Oncol*, Jun; 30(3): 239–44.

54 Belderbos JS, Kepka L, Kong FM, Martel MK, Videtic GM, Jeremic B (2009) Elective nodal irradiation (ENI) in locally advanced non-small-cell lung cancer (NSCLC): Evidence versus opinion? *Int J Radiat Oncol Biol Phys*, May 1; 74(1): 322; author reply -3.

55 Martel MK, Strawderman M, Hazuka MB, Turrisi AT, Fraass BA, Lichter AS (1997) Volume and dose parameters for survival of non-small cell lung cancer patients. *Radiother Oncol*, Jul; 44(1): 23–9.

56 International Commission on Radiation Units and Measurements (ICRU), www.icru.org, 2012.

57 Graham M, Purdy J, Emami B, Harms W, Bosch W, Lockett M (1999) Clinical dose-volume histogram analysis for pneumonitis after 3D treatment for non-small cell lung cancer (NSCLC). *Int J Radiat Oncol*, 45: 323–9.

58 Graham MV, Matthews JW, Harms WB, Sr., Emami B, Glazer HS, Purdy JA (1994) Three-dimensional radiation treatment planning study for patients with carcinoma of the lung. *Int J Radiat Oncol Biol Phys*, Jul 30; 29(5): 1105–17.

59 Martel M, Ten Haken R, Hazuka M (1994) Dose-volume histogram and 3-D treatment planning evaluation of patients with pneumonitis. *Int J Radiat Oncol*, 28: 575–81.

60 Emami B, Lyman J, Brown A, Coia L, Goitein M, Munzenrider JE, *et al.* (1991) Tolerance of normal tissue to therapeutic irradiation. *Int J Radiat Oncol Biol Phys*, May 15; 21(1): 109–22.

61 Kirkpatrick JP, van der Kogel AJ, Schultheiss TE (2010) Radiation dose-volume effects in the spinal cord. *Int J Radiat Oncol Biol Phys*, Mar 1; 76(3 Suppl): S42–9.

62 Werner-Wasik M, Yorke E, Deasy J, Nam J, Marks LB (2010) Radiation dose-volume effects in the esophagus. *Int J Radiat Oncol Biol Phys*, Mar 1; 76(3 Suppl): S86–93.

63 Marks LB, Bentzen SM, Deasy JO, Kong FM, Bradley JD, Vogelius IS, *et al.* (2010) Radiation dose-volume effects in the lung. *Int J Radiat Oncol Biol Phys*, Mar 1; 76(3 Suppl): S70–6.

64 Gagliardi G, Constine LS, Moiseenko V, Correa C, Pierce LJ, Allen AM, *et al.* (2010) Radiation dose-volume effects in the heart. *Int J Radiat Oncol Biol Phys*. Mar 1; 76(3 Suppl): S77–85.

65 Bentzen SM, Constine LS, Deasy JO, Eisbruch A, Jackson A, Marks LB, *et al.* (2010) Quantitative Analyses of Normal Tissue Effects in the Clinic (QUANTEC): An introduction to the scientific issues. *Int J Radiat Oncol Biol Phys*, Mar 1; 76(3 Suppl): S3–9.

66 Oetzel D, Schraube P, Hensley F, Sroka-Perez G, Menke M, Flentje M (1995) Estimation of pneumonitis risk in three-dimensional treatment planning using dose-volume histogram analysis. *Int J Radiat Oncol*, 1995/9/30; 33(2): 455–60.

67 Marks LB, Munley MT, Bentel GC, Zhou S-M, Hollis D, Scarfone C, *et al.* (1997) Physical and biological predictors of changes in whole-lung function following thoracic irradiation. *Int J Radiat Oncol*, 1997/10/1; 39(3): 563–70.

68 Armstrong J, Raben A, Zelefsky M, Burt M, Leibel S, Burman C, *et al.* (1997) Promising survival with three-dimensional conformal radiation therapy for non-small cell lung cancer. *Radiotherapy and Oncology*, 44: 17–22.

69 Kwa S, Lebesque J, Theuws J, Marks L, Munley M, Bentel GC, *et al.* (1998) Radiation pneumonitis as a function of mean lung dose: an analysis of pooled data of 540 patients. *Int J Radiat Oncol*, 42: 1–9.

70 Fu X, Huang H, Bentel G, Clough R, Jirtle R, Kong F, *et al.* (2001) Predicting the risk of symptomatic radiation-induced lung injury using both the physical and biologic parameters V(30) and transforming growth factor beta. *Int J Radiat Oncol*, 50: 899–908.

71 Robnett TJ, Machtay M, Vines EF, McKenna MG, Algazy KM, McKenna WG (2000) Factors predicting severe radiation pneumonitis in patients receiving definitive chemoradiation for lung cancer. *Int J Radiat Oncol*, 2000/08/01; 48(1): 89–94.

72 Hernando ML, Marks LB, Bentel GC, Zhou S-M, Hollis D, Das SK, *et al.* (2001) Radiation-induced pulmonary toxicity: A dose-volume histogram analysis in 201 patients with lung cancer. *Int J Radiat Oncol*, 2001/11/01; 51(3): 650–9.

73 Johansson S, Bjermer L, Franzen L, Henriksson R (1998) Effects of ongoing smoking on the development of radiation-induced pneumonitis in breast cancer and oesophagus cancer patients. *Radiotherapy and Oncology*, 1998/10; 49(1): 41–7.

74 Rancati T, Ceresoli GL, Gagliardi G, Schipani S, Cattaneo GM (2003) Factors predicting radiation pneumonitis in lung cancer patients: a retrospective study. *Radiotherapy and Oncology*, 2003/06; 67(3): 275–83.

75 Yamada M, Kudoh S, Hirata K, Nakajima T, Yoshikawa J (1998) Risk factors of pneumonitis following chemoradiotherapy for lung cancer. *European Journal of Cancer*, 1998/01; 34(1): 71–5.

76 Claude L, PerolPérol D, Ginestet C, Falchero L, Arpin D, Vincent M, *et al.* (2004) A prospective study on radiation pneumonitis following conformal radiation therapy in non-small-cell lung cancer: clinical and dosimetric factors analysis. *Radiotherapy and Oncology*, 2004/05/01; 71(2): 175–81.

77 Kim TH, Cho KH, Pyo HR, Lee JS, Zo JI, Lee DH, *et al.* (2005) Dose-volumetric parameters for predicting severe radiation pneumonitis after three-dimensional conformal radiation therapy for lung cancer. *Radiology*, April 1, 2005; 235(1): 208–15.

78 Willner J, Jost A, Baier K, Flentje M (2003) A little to a lot or a lot to a little? An analysis of pneumonitis risk from dose-volume histogram parameters of the lung in patients with lung cancer treated with 3-D conformal radiotherapy. *Strahlentherapie Onkologie*, 179: 548–56.

79 Armstrong J, Zelefsky M, Leibel S, Burman C, Han C, Harrison L, *et al.* (1995) Strategy for dose escalation using 3-dimensional conformal radiation therapy for lung cancer. *Annals of Oncology*, 6: 693–7.

80 Tsujino K, Hirota S, Endo M, Obayashi K, Kotani Y, Satouchi M, *et al.* (2003) Predictive value of dose-volume histogram parameters for predicting radiation pneumonitis after concurrent chemoradiation for lung cancer. *Int J Radiat Oncol*, 55: 110–15.

81 Munley MT, Lo JY, Sibley GS, Bentel GC, Anscher MS, Marks LB (1999) A neural network to predict symptomatic lung injury. *Physics in Medicine and Biology*, Sep; 44(9): 2241–9.

82 Seppenwoolde Y, Lebesque J, De Jaeger K, Belderbos J, Boersma L, Schilstra C, *et al.* (2003) Comparing different NTCP models that predict the incidence of radiation pneumonitis. *Int J Radiat Oncol*, 55(3): 724–35.

83 Lyman JT (1985) Complication probability as assessed from dose-volume histograms. *Radiat Res Suppl*, 8: S13–19.

84 Kutcher GJ, Burman C (1989) Calculation of complication probability factors for non-uniform normal tissue irradiation: The effective volume method. *Int J Radiat Oncol Biol Phys*, Jun; 16(6): 1623–30.

85 Niemierko A (1997) Reporting and analyzing dose distributions: A concept of equivalent uniform dose. *Med Phys*, Jan; 24(1): 103–10.

86 Willner J, Jost A, Baier K, Flentje M (2003) A little to a lot or a lot to a little? An analysis of pneumonitis risk from dose-volume histogram parameters of the lung in patients with lung cancer treated with 3-D conformal radiotherapy. *Strahlenther Onkol*, Aug; 179(8): 548–56.

87 Ahn SJ, Kahn D, Zhou S, Yu X, Hollis D, Shafman TD, *et al.* (2005) Dosimetric and clinical predictors for radiation-induced esophageal injury. *Int J Radiat Oncol Biol Phys*, Feb 1; 61(2): 335–47.

88 Bradley J, Deasy JO, Bentzen S, El-Naqa I (2004) Dosimetric correlates for acute esophagitis in patients treated with radiotherapy for lung carcinoma. *Int J Radiat Oncol Biol Phys*, Mar 15; 58(4): 1106–13.

89 Kim TH, Cho KH, Pyo HR, Lee JS, Han JY, Zo JI, *et al.* (2005) Dose-volumetric parameters of acute esophageal toxicity in patients with lung cancer treated with three-dimensional conformal radiotherapy. *Int J Radiat Oncol Biol Phys*, Jul 15; 62(4): 995–1002.

90 Maguire PD, Sibley GS, Zhou SM, Jamieson TA, Light KL, Antoine PA, *et al.* (1999) Clinical and dosimetric predictors of radiation-induced esophageal toxicity. *Int J Radiat Oncol Biol Phys*, Aug 1; 45(1): 97–103.

91 Takeda K, Nemoto K, Saito H, Ogawa Y, Takai Y, Yamada S (2005) Dosimetric correlations of acute esophagitis in lung cancer patients treated with radiotherapy. *Int J Radiat Oncol Biol Phys*, Jul 1; 62(3): 626–9.

92 Wei X, Liu HH, Tucker SL, Liao Z, Hu C, Mohan R, *et al.* (2006) Risk factors for acute esophagitis in non-small-cell lung cancer patients treated with concurrent chemotherapy and three-dimensional conformal radiotherapy. *Int J Radiat Oncol Biol Phys*, Sep 1; 66(1): 100–7.

93 Werner-Wasik M, Pequignot E, Leeper D, Hauck W, Curran W (2000) Predictors of severe esophagitis include use of concurrent chemotherapy, but not the length of irradiated esophagus: A multivariate analysis of patients with lung cancer treated with nonoperative therapy. *Int J Radiat Oncol Biol Phys*, Oct 1; 48(3): 689–96.

94 Gomez DR, Tucker SL, Martel MK, Mohan R, Balter PA, Lopez Guerra JL, *et al.* (2012) Predictors of high-grade esophagitis after definitive three-dimensional conformal therapy, intensity-modulated radiation therapy, or proton beam therapy for non-small cell lung cancer. *Int J Radiat Oncol Biol Phys*, 84(4): 1010–6.

95 Singh AK, Lockett MA, Bradley JD (2003) Predictors of radiation-induced esophageal toxicity in patients with non-small-cell lung cancer treated with three-dimensional conformal radiotherapy. *Int J Radiat Oncol Biol Phys*, Feb 1; 55(2): 337–41.

96 Caglar HB, Othus M, Allen AM (2010) Esophagus in-field: a new predictor for esophagitis. *Radiother Oncol*. Oct; 97(1): 48–53.

97 Liu HH, Wang X, Dong L, Wu Q, Liao Z, Stevens CW, *et al.* (2004) Feasibility of sparing lung and other thoracic structures with intensity-modulated radiotherapy for non-small-cell lung cancer. *Int J Radiat Oncol Biol Phys*, Mar 15; 58(4): 1268–79.

98 Grills IS, Yan D, Martinez AA, Vicini FA, Wong JW, Kestin LL (2003) Potential for reduced toxicity and dose escalation in the treatment of inoperable non-small-cell lung cancer: a comparison of intensity-modulated radiation therapy (IMRT), 3D conformal radiation, and elective nodal irradiation. *Int J Radiat Oncol Biol Phys*, Nov 1; 57(3): 875–90.

99 Liao ZX, Komaki RR, Thames HD, Jr., Liu HH, Tucker SL, Mohan R, *et al.* (2010) Influence of technologic advances on outcomes in patients with unresectable, locally advanced non-small-cell lung cancer receiving concomitant chemoradiotherapy. *Int J Radiat Oncol Biol Phys*, Mar 1; 76(3): 775–81.

100 Chang JY, Zhang X, Wang X, Kang Y, Riley B, Bilton S, *et al.* (2006) Significant reduction of normal tissue dose by proton radiotherapy compared with three-dimensional conformal or intensity-modulated radiation therapy in Stage I or Stage III non-small-cell lung cancer. *Int J Radiat Oncol Biol Phys*, Jul 15; 65(4): 1087–96.

101 Nichols RC, Huh SN, Henderson RH, Mendenhall NP, Flampouri S, Li Z, *et al.* (2012) Proton radiation therapy offers reduced normal lung and bone marrow exposure for patients receiving dose-escalated radiation therapy for unresectable stage iii non-small-cell lung cancer: a dosimetric study. *Int J Radiat Oncol Biol Phys*, 83(1): 158–63. doi: 10.1016/j.ijrobp.2011.05.045. Epub 2012 Jan 13.

102 Vogelius IR, Westerly DC, Aznar MC, Cannon GM, Korreman SS, Mackie TR, *et al.* (2011) Estimated radiation pneumonitis risk after photon versus proton therapy alone or combined with chemotherapy for lung cancer. *Acta Oncol*. Aug; 50(6): 772–6.

103 Sejpal S, Komaki R, Tsao A, Chang JY, Liao Z, Wei X, *et al.* (2011) Early findings on toxicity of proton beam therapy with concurrent chemotherapy for nonsmall cell lung cancer. *Cancer*, Jul 1; 117(13): 3004–13.

104 Chang JY, Komaki R, Lu C, Wen HY, Allen PK, Tsao A, *et al.* (2011) Phase 2 study of high-dose proton therapy with concurrent chemotherapy for unresectable stage III nonsmall cell lung cancer. *Cancer*, Oct 15; 117(20): 4707–13.

105 Pignon JP, Arriagada R, Ihde DC, Johnson DH, Perry MC, Souhami RL, *et al.* (1992) A meta-analysis of thoracic radiotherapy for small-cell lung cancer. *N Engl J Med*, Dec 3; 327(23): 1618–24.

106 Murray N, Coy P, Pater JL, Hodson I, Arnold A, Zee BC, *et al.* (1993) Importance of timing for thoracic irradiation in the combined modality treatment of limited-stage small-cell lung cancer. The National Cancer Institute of Canada Clinical Trials Group. *J Clin Oncol*, Feb; 11(2): 336–44.

107 Spiro SG, James LE, Rudd RM, Trask CW, Tobias JS, Snee M, *et al.* (2006) Early compared with late radiotherapy in combined modality treatment for limited disease small-cell lung cancer: A London Lung Cancer Group multicenter randomized clinical trial and meta-analysis. *J Clin Oncol*, Aug 20; 24(24): 3823–30.

108 Fried DB, Morris DE, Poole C, Rosenman JG, Halle JS, Detterbeck FC, *et al.* (2004) Systematic review evaluating the timing of thoracic radiation therapy in combined modality therapy for limited-stage small-cell lung cancer. *J Clin Oncol*, Dec 1; 22(23): 4837–45.

109 De Ruysscher D, Pijls-Johannesma M, Bentzen SM, Minken A, Wanders R, Lutgens L, *et al.* (2006) Time between the first day of chemotherapy and the last day of chest radiation is the most important predictor of survival in limited-disease small-cell lung cancer. *J Clin Oncol*, Mar 1; 24(7): 1057–63.

110 Park KS, Kim S-W, Ahn M-j, Ahn JS, Lee DH, Cheolwon S, Ahn YC, Pyo H, Choi EK, Song SY, Lee SH, Lee JS (2012) Phase III trial of concurrent thoracic radiotherapy (TRT) with either the first cycle or the third cycle of cisplatin and etoposide chemotherapy to determine the optimal timing of TRT for limited-disease small cell lung cancer. *J Clin Oncol*, suppl; abstr 7005.

111 Laurie SA, Logan D, Markman BR, Mackay JA, Evans WK (2004) Practice guideline for the role of combination chemotherapy in the initial management of limited-stage small-cell lung cancer. *Lung Cancer*, Feb; 43(2): 223–40.

112 Sundstrom S, Bremnes RM, Kaasa S, Aasebo U, Hatlevoll R, Dahle R, *et al.* (2002) Cisplatin and etoposide regimen is superior to cyclophosphamide, epirubicin, and vincristine regimen in small-cell lung cancer: Results from a randomized phase III trial with 5 years' follow-up. *J Clin Oncol*, Dec 15; 20(24): 4665–72.

113 Noda K, Nishiwaki Y, Kawahara M, Negoro S, Sugiura T, Yokoyama A, *et al.* (2002) Irinotecan plus cisplatin compared with etoposide plus cisplatin for extensive small-cell lung cancer. *N Engl J Med*, Jan 10; 346(2): 85–91.

114 Hanna N, Bunn PA, Jr., Langer C, Einhorn L, Guthrie T, Jr., Beck T, *et al.* (2006) Randomized phase III trial comparing irinotecan/cisplatin with etoposide/cisplatin in patients with previously untreated extensive-stage disease small-cell lung cancer. *J Clin Oncol*, May 1; 24(13): 2038–43.

115 Lara PN, Jr., Natale R, Crowley J, Lenz HJ, Redman MW, Carleton JE, *et al.* (2009) Phase III trial of irinotecan/cisplatin compared with etoposide/cisplatin in extensive-stage small-cell lung cancer: Clinical and pharmacogenomic results from SWOG S0124. *J Clin Oncol*, May 20; 27(15): 2530–5.

116 Rossi A, Di Maio M, Chiodini P, Rudd RM, Okamoto H, Skarlos DV, *et al.* (2012) Carboplatin- or cisplatin-based chemotherapy in first-line treatment of small-cell lung cancer: The COCIS meta-analysis of individual patient data. *J Clin Oncol*, May 10; 30(14): 1692–8.

117 Turrisi AT, 3rd, Kim K, Blum R, Sause WT, Livingston RB, Komaki R, *et al.* (1999) Twice-daily compared with once-daily thoracic radiotherapy in limited small-cell lung cancer treated concurrently with cisplatin and etoposide. *N Engl J Med*, Jan 28; 340(4): 265–71.

118 Bogart JA, Herndon JE, 2nd, Lyss AP, Watson D, Miller AA, Lee ME, *et al.* (2004) 70 Gy thoracic radiotherapy is feasible concurrent with chemotherapy for limited-stage small-cell lung cancer: Analysis of Cancer and Leukemia Group B study 39808. *Int J Radiat Oncol Biol Phys*, Jun 1; 59(2): 460–8.

119 Komaki R, Swann RS, Ettinger DS, Glisson BS, Sandler AB, Movsas B, *et al.* (2005) Phase I study of thoracic radiation dose escalation with concurrent chemotherapy for patients with limited small-cell lung cancer: Report of Radiation Therapy Oncology Group (RTOG) protocol 97–12. *Int J Radiat Oncol Biol Phys*, Jun 1; 62(2): 342–50.

120 Bradley JD, Dehdashti F, Mintun MA, Govindan R, Trinkaus K, Siegel BA (2004) Positron emission tomography in limited-stage small-cell lung cancer: a prospective study. *J Clin Oncol*, Aug 15; 22(16): 3248–54.

121 Jeremic B, Shibamoto Y, Nikolic N, Milicic B, Milisavljevic S, Dagovic A, *et al.* (1999) Role of radiation therapy in the combined-modality treatment of patients with extensive disease small-cell lung cancer: A randomized study. *J Clin Oncol,* Jul; 17(7): 2092–9.

122 Auperin A, Arriagada R, Pignon JP, Le Pechoux C, Gregor A, Stephens RJ, *et al.* (1999) Prophylactic cranial irradiation for patients with small-cell lung cancer in complete remission. Prophylactic Cranial Irradiation Overview Collaborative Group. *N Engl J Med,* Aug 12; 341(7): 476–84.

123 Slotman B, Faivre-Finn C, Kramer G, Rankin E, Snee M, Hatton M, *et al.* (2007) Prophylactic cranial irradiation in extensive small-cell lung cancer. *N Engl J Med,* Aug 16; 357(7): 664–72.

124 Le Pechoux C, Dunant A, Senan S, Wolfson A, Quoix E, Faivre-Finn C, *et al.* (2009) Standard-dose versus higher-dose prophylactic cranial irradiation (PCI) in patients with limited-stage small-cell lung cancer in complete remission after chemotherapy and thoracic radiotherapy (PCI 99–01, EORTC 22003–08004, RTOG 0212, and IFCT 99–01): A randomised clinical trial. *Lancet Oncol,* May; 10(5): 467–74.

125 Le Pechoux C, Laplanche A, Faivre-Finn C, Ciuleanu T, Wanders R, Lerouge D, *et al.* (2011) Clinical neurological outcome and quality of life among patients with limited small-cell cancer treated with two different doses of prophylactic cranial irradiation in the intergroup phase III trial (PCI99–01, EORTC 22003–08004, RTOG 0212 and IFCT 99–01). *Ann Oncol,* May; 22(5): 1154–63.

CHAPTER 24

Individualized Radiotherapy by Dose Escalation and Altered Fractionation in Non-small Cell Lung Cancer

Heath D. Skinner, Ritsuko U. Komaki, Joe Y. Chang, and James D. Cox
Department of Radiation Oncology, The University of Texas MD Anderson Cancer Center, Houston, TX, USA

Introduction

Radiotherapy has been used in the management of lung cancer, as either definitive or adjuvant therapy for decades. Technology has significantly evolved during that time, allowing clinicians to improve tumor control rates while minimizing normal tissue toxicity. The link between local tumor control and increased survival in patients with non-small cell lung cancer (NSCLC) was confirmed in two recent meta-analyses [1, 2]. In many cases, improved local control has been achieved by either accelerated fractionation, dose escalation, or both. However, recent studies have called into question the benefits of dose escalation for NSCLC. This chapter focuses primarily on medically inoperable or surgically unresectable, locally advanced NSCLC and reviews the historical precedents for both radiation dose escalation and accelerated fractionation. Some recent technological advances that facilitate safe dose escalation and some recent trials involving these advanced applications in dose escalation are briefly discussed, and the chapter concludes with a discussion of individualized dose escalation involving still more sophisticated forms of imaging, dose delivery, and biological targeting.

History of radiation dose escalation and altered fractionation

In the 1960s, the common practice for treating medically inoperable or surgically unresectable NSCLC was to prescribe radiation as monotherapy to doses of 40 Gy in 20 fractions with 2 Gy delivered daily using 2-dimensional treatment planning. Unfortunately this approach produced disappointingly poor results [3]. At that time, individual investigators began to explore the possibility of increasing the total dose to 50 or 60 Gy, whereas others advocated the use of hypofractionated split-course radiotherapy [4]. These conflicting viewpoints led to a randomized trial by the Radiation Therapy Oncology Group, RTOG 73-01, which compared four treatment groups: those given 40 Gy, 50 Gy, or 60 Gy in 2-Gy daily fractions and a separate group given 40 Gy in 10 fractions of 4 Gy each, with a planned 2-week break in the middle of the treatment [5]. The local-regional failure rate at 3 years in the hypofractionated, split-course arm was 44% as compared with 52%, 42% and 33% in the corresponding conventional fractionation groups; a similar stepwise increase in survival was noted with

Lung Cancer, Fourth Edition. Edited by Jack A. Roth, Waun Ki Hong and Ritsuko U. Komaki.

increasing radiation dose. Although any survival benefit from dose escalation disappeared after several years of follow-up, these results were considered promising with regard to a possible benefit from dose escalation when radiation alone was given in standard fractionation. Long-term follow-up of these patients revealed acceptable normal tissue toxicity rates, specifically rates of grade 3 pneumonitis or esophagitis of <15% [6].

During the 1970s, attention was turned to highly hypofractionated radiotherapy for the management of locally advanced NSCLC [7–9]. This approach was taken primarily to augment the radiosensitizing effects of misonidazole and culminated in an RTOG phase III trial in which large, 6-Gy fractions were given twice a week, to a total dose of 36 Gy, for locally advanced NSCLC [7]. Not only did this trial show no benefits in terms of local control or survival from the misonidazole, it also showed significantly higher rates of grade 3 toxicity (17%) relative to the <15% rate in the 60 Gy group of RTOG 73-01 and no commensurate improvement in outcome.

Based on the less than optimal results of hypofractionation in these early studies and the positive results of RTOG 73-01, 60 Gy in 2-Gy daily fractions was adopted as the standard radiotherapeutic regimen for locally advanced NSCLC, specifically within the RTOG and generally in the United States. Further trials from this group and others focused primarily on the twin goals of dose escalation and the addition of systemic agents. The addition of chemotherapy to radiotherapy in NSCLC is discussed elsewhere in other chapters; the evolution of dose escalation and altered fractionation is described further here.

After the publication of RTOG 73-01, much attention was given to safer dose escalation, with one possibility being the use of hyperfractionation. Because toxicity was thought to be – and still is – the primary limiting factor for giving higher doses in the treatment of lung cancer, hyperfractionation was investigated with the goal of exploiting tumor radiobiology. Theoretically, hyperfractionation would allow repair of normal tissues to take place while still being cytotoxic to the tumor. The initial phase I trial of this approach, RTOG 81-08, showed the feasibility and safety of using hyperfractionated radiotherapy for dose escalation to a maximum of 74.4 Gy, given in 1.2-Gy fractions delivered twice daily, for locally advanced NSCLC [10]. This trial was followed by RTOG 83-11, a randomized phase I/II dose-escalation trial in which hyperfractionation was used to achieve a stepwise increase in total radiation dose [11]. In that trial, patients with locally advanced NSCLC were treated with a total radiation dose that was escalated from the standard 60 Gy in 4.8-Gy stepwise intervals to a maximum of 79.2 Gy; all radiation was delivered in 1.2-Gy fractions given twice daily with a 6 hour interfraction interval. Among patients with good performance status, a median survival time of 13.7 months was observed in the group given 69.6 Gy, which was significantly longer than that observed in the lower-dose groups, but no benefit was observed for dose escalation beyond 69.6 Gy. Moreover, no significant differences were noted among groups in grade ≥3 toxicity, with the 69.6 Gy group having had a total grade ≥3 treatment-related toxicity rate of 8.5%. These outcomes compared favorably to those of a contemporary cohort of patients treated with radiotherapy alone to 60 Gy in 30 daily fractions as well as to outcomes of the Cancer and Leukemia Group B (CALGB) trial 84-33, a trial of induction chemotherapy followed by conventional radiotherapy for NSCLC [12, 13].

A similar concept was introduced with the so-called "CHART" schedule (short for Continuous, Hyperfractionated, Accelerated Radiation Treatment) [14–16]. In the pilot study of this regimen, 23 patients with locally advanced NSCLC were treated with radiotherapy alone to 50.4 Gy in 1.4-Gy fractions three times a day [14]. When this regimen was found to produce tolerable results in terms of toxicity, the dose was increased to 54 Gy, given in 1.5-Gy fractions three time a day. When the 1-year survival rate was found to be 64%, a randomized trial was done to compare CHART (54 Gy) with conventional radiotherapy to 60 Gy [15, 16]. In that trial, the 2-year overall survival rate was significantly higher in the CHART group than in the conventional-treatment group (30% vs. 21%), but the rates of acute esophagitis at 3 months (19% vs. 3%) and symptomatic pneumonitis at 3 months (19% vs. 10%) were also higher in the CHART group than in the conventional-fractionation group [15].

These findings suggesting improved survival for dose escalated, hyperfractionated radiotherapy as well as promising findings from other trials involving chemotherapy led to the conduct of RTOG 88-08 [17]. RTOG 88-08 was a phase III trial comparing three treatment conditions: standard 60 Gy given in 2-Gy once-daily fractions, either alone or after induction cisplatin and vinblastine, or 69.6 Gy given in 1.2-Gy twice-daily fractions. In that trial, survival was significantly improved by the addition of chemotherapy, but the median survival time in the 69.6-Gy group was considered to be reasonable at 12 months.

After RTOG 88-08, two separate studies addressed the known benefit of both induction chemotherapy and hyperfractionation [18, 19]. An initial pilot study (RTOG 90-15) and a larger phase II trial (RTOG 91-06) examined the addition of chemotherapy to hyperfractionated radiotherapy to 69.6 Gy. Outcomes from these studies seemed to indicate a survival advantage from the addition of chemotherapy over hyperfractionated radiotherapy alone (median survival times 18.9 months vs. 10.6 months), but at the cost of significant toxicity, with nearly 60% of patients developing grade 4 hematologic toxicity and a treatment-related death rate of 3.9% [19]. This fractionation schedule proved particularly toxic to the esophagus, with a grade ≥3 esophagitis rate of 53%. However, because of the encouraging survival outcomes, this hyperfractionated regimen was incorporated into several further trials [20,21]. In addition to addressing the optimal sequencing of chemotherapy and radiation, RTOG 94-10 specifically compared 63 Gy delivered in conventional daily fractionation versus hyperfractionated radiation to 69.6 Gy, with both groups including concurrent chemotherapy. In that trial, no significant differences in survival were observed between the fractionation regimens, but the rates of severe esophagitis were significantly higher in the hyperfractionated group compared to the conventional fractionation group:45% vs. 22%, respectively. Several additional trials found nearly equivalent survival outcomes using conventional fractionation to similar doses [22, 23]. Interestingly, in a separate trial of the hyperfractionation regimen used by the RTOG, albeit with a smaller number of patients, the addition of chemotherapy to this regimen greatly improved survival outcome (median survival times 22 vs. 14 months) with no significant increase in toxicity [24]. However, a more contemporary trial comparing 60 Gy delivered daily in 6 weeks versus 60 Gy given twice daily in 3 weeks with or without concurrent chemotherapy showed no differences in survival outcome between these two fractionation regimens [25]. Esophageal toxicity was again substantially higher in the hyperfractionated group.

The addition of chemotherapy to radiotherapy for locally advanced NSCLC added a layer of complexity to trials addressing either dose escalation or accelerated fraction (Table 24.1), mainly because of concerns regarding toxicity. However, since the publication of the findings from these trials, the advent of several technological advances has reduced the toxicity associated with dose escalation, as described below.

Advances in technology and conformality

Several technological advances occurring over the past two or three decades have allowed much greater conformality in radiotherapy planning and delivery for lung cancer. Although these advances are explored in more depth in other chapters, several are particularly important in the context of effective dose escalation, especially image-guided planning and delivery. With the advent of computed tomography (CT), radiation treatments could truly be planned in 3 dimensions, leading to more conformal radiotherapy plans that could spare uninvolved lung and esophagus as well as notably improving local control in NSCLC [26]. Image-based radiotherapy planning has progressed still further to the development of 4-dimensional CT, which can account for respiratory motion as well as techniques for visualizing tumor motion in real time, such as implanted fiducial markers, and techniques for limiting tumor motion during treatment, such as breath-hold and respiratory gating

Table 24.1 Phase III trials of dose escalation and hyperfractionation in locally advanced non-small cell lung cancer

Trial and reference	No. of patients	Inclusion criteria	Comparison	Chemotherapy	Outcome	Toxicity
RTOG 73-01 (4)	447	Stage III	Arm 1: 40 Gy split course Arm 2: 40 Gy/2 Gy QD Arm 3: 50 Gy/2 Gy QD Arm 4: 60 Gy/2 Gy QD	None	LRF rate improved in Arm 4 (33%) No differences in survival in longer follow-up	15% grade ≥3 pneumonitis and esophagitis
RTOG 83–11 (11)	884	Stage II-IV (no distant metastasis), KPS >50%	All doses delivered 1.2 Gy BID Arm 1: 60 Gy Arm 2: 64.8 Gy Arm 3: 69.6 Gy Arm 4: 74.4 Gy Arm 5: 79.2 Gy	None	Survival improved in Arm 3 versus in Arms 1 & 2	~ 10% grade ≥3 toxicity in each arm
CHART (14–16)	563	Inoperable disease, PS 0–1	Arm 1: 60 Gy/2 Gy QD Arm 2: 54 Gy/1.5 Gy TID	None	Survival improved in Arm 2	19% rate of severe esophagitis and pneumonitis in Arm 2
RTOG 88–08 (17)	458	Stage II, IIIA-B, KPS>70%, weight loss <5%	Arms 1 & 2: 60Gy/2 Gy QD Arm 3: 69.6 Gy/1.2 Gy BID	Induction cisplatin+vinblastine (only in Arm 2)	Survival improved in Arm 2	No difference between arms
Jeremic et al. (24)	131	Stage III, KPS >50	Arms 1 & 2: 69.6 Gy/1.2 Gy BID	Concurrent carboplatin + etoposide (Arm 2)	Survival improved with chemo (24 mos)	No difference between arms
RTOG 94–10 (21)	610	Stage II-III, KPS >70%, weight loss <5%	Arms 1 & 2: 63 Gy 1.8/2 Gy QD Arm 3: 69.6 Gy/1.2 Gy BID	Cisplatin+vinblastine either sequential (Arm 1) or concurrent (Arms 2 & 3)	Survival significantly improved in Arms 2 & 3 (17 mos. & 15.2 mos)	Acute toxicity significantly worse with concurrent chemo
Australian (25)	204	Inoperable disease, PS 0–1	2×2 design, 60 Gy in 2 Gy QD vs. 2 Gy BID ± chemotherapy	Carboplatin	No difference between arms, but higher in QD with chemo (20.3 mos)	Severe esophageal toxicity worse for BID dosing
RTOG-0617 (51)	423	Stage IIIA-B, PS 0–1, FEV1 ≥1.2 L/s	2×2 design, 60 Gy/2 Gy QD vs. 74 Gy 2 Gy/QD	Carboplatin + paclitaxel ± cetuximab	Crossed futility on interim analysis for 74 Gy, arm closed	No significant difference between arms

BID, twice a day; KPS, Karnofsky performance status score; LRF, local-regional failure; PS, performance status;.QD, once a day; TID, three times a day.

[27–29]. When the location of the tumor target is known throughout the respiratory cycle, radiotherapy plans can be generated with smaller target margins and, hence, lower incidental exposures to normal tissues [30].

During treatment, techniques for ensuring that the position of the patient remains consistent over multiple treatment sessions have advanced from the previous standard of MV port films to daily onboard image guidance with either high-quality kV imaging or CT. Techniques such as these can allow still further reductions in target margins and normal tissue irradiated.

Finally, the technology for delivery of radiotherapy has also advanced significantly. The advent of intensity-modulated radiotherapy (IMRT) represents an opportunity for additional sparing of normal tissues in the thorax. In retrospective reviews, the use of IMRT seems to offer advantages in terms of both dosimetry and toxicity [31–34]. Although prospective comparisons of IMRT with other forms of radiation delivery are somewhat sparse at this time, the use of IMRT for NSCLC, and cancer at other sites, has become common based on these findings. Further, several investigators have begun to publish their experiences with using proton radiotherapy in this disease site. A phase II trial of proton radiotherapy with concurrent chemotherapy for locally advanced NSCLC showed that rates of grade ≥3 toxicity after treatment to 74 Gy (RBE) were lower than those observed in a separate cohort of patients treated to 63 Gy by using photon (X-ray) based therapy [35].

All of these advances can help to minimize dose to uninvolved structures. Moreover, specific dosimetric parameters have been linked with the risk of acute and long-term toxicity [36,37]. Values such as lung V_{20} (the percentage of lung volume receiving at least 20 Gy) and mean lung dose are invaluable for assessing radiotherapy plans in the modern era and are also useful when considering dose escalation, chiefly because they allow selection of modalities and patients for whom dose escalation is feasible and carries a reasonably low risk of toxicity.

In short, numerous opportunities exist in the modern era for limiting the toxicity of radiotherapy for locally advanced NSCLC, which again raises the question of whether dose escalation is feasible and safe for such patients. This issue is explored further in the section that follows.

Modern studies of dose-escalation for locally advanced disease

Given the successes of previous trials using the CHART approach as well as the development of novel technologies that allow greater conformality, several studies have attempted to incorporate chemotherapy into the CHART regimen. Unfortunately, to date accrual to these trials has been slow, leading to premature closure. The Eastern Cooperative Oncology Group in their ECOG 2597 trial compared CHART with conventional fractionation after induction chemotherapy. Although the median survival time was considered promising and the rate of severe radiation-related toxicity low in the CHART group (20.3 months and 10%), this study was not powered to detect an improvement in outcome [23]. A separate trial in which induction chemotherapy was given before CHART showed a median survival time of 25 months and acceptable toxicity; however, this trial closed after accruing only 43 patients [38]. Additionally, the CHARTWEL trial examined a similar dose and fractionation scheme in a randomized fashion [39]. Although no benefit in local control was seen for the study population, unplanned subset analysis did show improved local control for this regimen in patients with higher tumor and nodal stages or following chemotherapy. Unfortunately, acute toxicity due to radiotherapy was significant higher in the experimental arm.

Because of the apparent lack of benefit and associated toxicity, enthusiasm for the hyperfractionated and accelerated approach seems to have waned at this time, most probably because of concerns about the toxicity associated with adding concurrent chemotherapy to this regimen.

Conversely, dose escalation given in standard radiation fractionation has become increasingly more common, with many institutions treating patients with locally advanced NSCLC to doses near or beyond 70 Gy. This practice was thought to be reasonable if treatment plans could be generated that did not violate known dose constraints and thus were unlikely to produce significant radiation-associated toxicity [36, 37]. Further, retrospective analyses seemed to indicate a survival advantage for patients with locally advanced NSCLC treated to doses higher than 67–74 Gy [40–43]. These retrospective observations were tested in a phase I/II trial conducted at the University of North Carolina for patients with locally advanced NSCLC treated with induction and concurrent chemotherapy [44, 45]. In that trial, the total radiotherapy dose was escalated from the standard 60 Gy in conventional fractionation to 74 Gy in four stepwise increases in dose. The rate of grade ≥3 esophagitis in this trial was only 8%, and the median survival time was 24 months. An additional phase I study by the same group investigated further dose escalation to 90 Gy for locally advanced NSCLC [46]. In that study, the rate of severe esophagitis was 16%, but two patients died of hemoptysis; moreover, the 24-mnth median survival time was no longer than that in the previous study. A subsequent review of these trials urged caution, because despite a median survival time of nearly 25 months among patients treated to >66 Gy in these trials, the rate of severe late complications was 24% [47].

The improvement in survival outcome and the manageable acute toxicity seen in these trials prompted a phase I/II trial by the RTOG examining the safety of delivering 74 Gy, in conventional fractionation, with concurrent chemotherapy [48, 49]. In the initial phase I component, the maximum tolerated dose was found to be 74 Gy, similar to the findings from the initial phase I/II trial at the University of North Carolina [44, 45, 48]. Thereafter a total of 55 patients were treated to 74 Gy in the combined phase I/II portion of the trial; the median survival time was 25.9 months, the rate of grade ≥3 pneumonitis was 22%, and the overall rate of severe nonhematologic toxicity was 61%. Similar findings were observed in CALGB 30105, a randomized phase II trial designed to compare two chemotherapeutic regimens but with both groups receiving 74 Gy as well [50]. In that trial, the addition of gemcitabine was found to add significant toxicity and in fact led to the premature closure of that arm. Although the median survival time was nearly 25 months, toxicity was again a concern, with rates of 16% for both severe pneumonitis and severe esophagitis in the standard-therapy group. Nevertheless, despite the higher rates of toxicity, the survival outcomes from that study were thought to warrant further examination, and the RTOG undertook a phase III trial comparing 60 Gy and 74 Gy, both given in conventional fractionation with conventional systemic therapy, with the added question of the efficacy of adding cetuximab to the systemic therapy [51]. In that trial, RTOG 0617, 500 patients with stage III NSCLC were projected to be enrolled in one of four treatment groups: 60 Gy in 30 fractions, 74 Gy in 37 fractions, or either radiation dose with the addition of cetuximab. All patients received concurrent weekly carboplatin and paclitaxel chemotherapy. After 423 patients had been accrued, this trial was closed prematurely because it crossed a futility boundary (90 events in the high-dose group). Moreover, the 1-year survival rate was found to be better in the low-dose group (81% vs. 74%). When this chapter was written, the low-dose arms of this trial remained open, but no further patients were to be accrued to the high-dose arm.

RTOG 0617 has left lingering questions for the radiation oncology community. Although answers to some questions will not be available until full publication of this study, examining the data that are available at this time is also important. For example, even though no significant differences in treatment-related toxicity were observed between the high-dose versus low-dose groups, 7 patients died of treatment-related toxicity in the high-dose group but only 3 died in the low-dose group. This finding has led to considerable speculation regarding the relationship between the known greater toxicity of high-dose radiotherapy and the observed outcome of this trial.

Interpretation of these findings is further complicated by the results of two recent meta-analyses of available data from trials of radiotherapy for NSCLC, both of which demonstrated a benefit from dose escalation [52, 53]. Specifically,

Partridge and colleagues examined 16 clinical trials in NSCLC of all stages with available data and found a significant dose–response relationship after the dose was converted to the biologically equivalent dose (BED) [52]. In another analysis of 1356 patients with locally advanced NSCLC in RTOG trials treated with radiotherapy and some form of chemotherapy (induction, concurrent or both), Machtay and colleagues demonstrated that BED was associated with survival as well as local-regional control [53]. Specifically, for each increase of 1 BED, survival increased by approximately 4% and local-regional control increased by 3%. These large datasets offer a powerful counter-balance to the negative results of RTOG 0617; however, at the time of publication, the current standard dose schedule in RTOG trials is 60 Gy in 30 fractions, the same schedule as that used in RTOG 88-08.

Individualized radiation treatment planning

At this point, future investigations of dose escalation, altered fractionation, or combinations of both must take into account the significant toxicity associated with concurrent chemoradiotherapy. As we have seen, normal tissue toxicity from radiotherapy has generally increased with each successive trial reviewed in this chapter, culminating in a negative trial of dose escalation (RTOG 0617). So what does the future hold for this therapeutic approach?

As noted previously, the technology that has become available for the radiation-based treatment of NSCLC is constantly improving on ways that allow ever more conformal and individualized radiotherapy. With the wide adoption of improved image-based planning techniques and image-guided delivery of radiotherapy, the hope is that greater normal tissue sparing can be achieved on a routine basis, with commensurate decreases in the rates of treatment-related toxicity. Moreover, as the use of advanced forms of radiotherapy delivery (IMRT and proton radiotherapy) becomes more standard, tailored and still more individualized radiotherapy plans will become more common. The hope is that this would lead to commensurate decreases in treatment-related toxicity and allow safer escalation of radiation doses.

Another advance, adaptive planning, could allow true individualization of dose escalation in radiotherapy for NSCLC. Adaptive planning involves repeated imaging of the tumor during radiotherapy, with the goal of reducing the size of the radiotherapy fields as the tumor shrinks while still maintaining adequate tumor coverage. At present, adaptive planning can be based on either CT or positron emission tomography (PET), typically with ^{18}F-florodeoxyglucose, and can improve the dose distribution, particularly for tumors that are close to critical structures [54]. For example, repeated FDG-PET imaging has shown that substantial tumor responses can be observed in many patients after as little as 45 Gy is delivered in conventional fractionation [55]. With this information, adaptive plans are being generated that take into account PET response [56]. In fact, this approach is the subject of RTOG 1106, an ongoing randomized phase II trial incorporating FDG-PET–based re-planning midway through treatment for the experimental treatment group. In this trial, the total tumor dose will be escalated up to 85.5 Gy based on PDG-PET response, if dosimetric constraints can be met. This trial should yield interesting results.

Finally, significant interest has been expressed in biologically driven dose escalation. This approach acknowledges that not all regions of a tumor are radioresponsive, particularly areas of significant hypoxia. Thus, if a particular area of a tumor is known to be radioresistant and this area can be visualized, that region of the tumor could be targeted for dose escalation, again minimizing the region to which high radiation doses is to be delivered and, presumably, leading to lower rates of toxicity. For example, higher standardized uptake values (SUVs) within a tumor as visualized by PET seem to be associated with radioresistance and tumor recurrence [57]; if such areas could targeted with a higher dose, then the benefits of dose escalation could be realized without increased toxicity. Other imaging markers, primarily markers of hypoxia, have been proposed for use in a similar fashion, and deserve further investigation [58].

Conclusions

Radiation dose escalation and altered fractionation in the treatment of NSCLC have been investigated for several decades, with several advances and, recently, a notable setback. For future efforts, it is important to acknowledge the significant normal tissue toxicity of this therapy while simultaneously seeking to leverage further advances in imaging and biological targeting for dose escalation, to find the balance between efficacy and toxicity.

References

1 Aupérin A, Le Péchoux C, Rolland E, Curran WJ, Furuse K, Fournel P, *et al.* (2010) Meta-analysis of concomitant versus sequential radiochemotherapy in locally advanced non-small-cell lung cancer. *J. Clin. Oncol*, May 1; 28(13): 2181–90.

2 O'Rourke N, Roqué I, Figuls M, Farré Bernadó N, Macbeth F (2010) Concurrent chemoradiotherapy in non-small cell lung cancer. *Cochrane Database Syst Rev*, 6: CD002140.

3 Roswit B, Patno ME, Rapp R, Veinbergs A, Feder B, Stuhlbarg J, *et al.* (1968) The survival of patients with inoperable lung cancer: a large-scale randomized study of radiation therapy versus placebo. *Radiology*, Apr; 90(4): 688–97.

4 Lee RE, Carr DT, Childs DS Jr (1976) Comparison of split-course radiation therapy and continuous radiation therapy for unresectable bronchogenic carcinoma: 5 year results. *AJR Am J Roentgenol*, Jan; 126(1): 116–22.

5 Perez CA, Pajak TF, Rubin P, Simpson JR, Mohiuddin M, Brady LW, *et al.* (1987) Long-term observations of the patterns of failure in patients with unresectable non-oat cell carcinoma of the lung treated with definitive radiotherapy. Report by the Radiation Therapy Oncology Group. *Cancer*, Jun 1; 59(11): 1874–81.

6 Kong F-M, Hayman JA, Griffith KA, Kalemkerian GP, Arenberg D, Lyons S, *et al.* (2006) Final toxicity results of a radiation-dose escalation study in patients with non-small-cell lung cancer (NSCLC): predictors for radiation pneumonitis and fibrosis. *Int. J. Radiat. Oncol. Biol. Phys*, Jul 15; 65(4): 1075–86.

7 Simpson JR, Bauer M, Wasserman TH, Perez CA, Emami B, Wiegensberg I, *et al.* (1987) Large fraction irradiation with or without misonidazole in advanced non-oat cell carcinoma of the lung: A phase III randomized trial of the RTOG. Radiation Therapy Oncology Group. *Int. J. Radiat. Oncol. Biol. Phys*, Jun; 13(6): 861–7.

8 Jakobsson M, Taskinen PJ, Kylmämaa T (1987) Misonidazole combined with radiotherapy in the treatment of non-small cell lung cancer. A randomized double-blind trial. *Strahlenther Onkol*, Feb; 163(2): 90–3.

9 Panduro J, Kjaer M, Wolff-Jensen J, Hansen HH (1983) Misonidazole combined with radiotherapy in the treatment of inoperable squamous cell carcinoma of the lung. A double-blind randomized trial. *Cancer*, Jul 1; 52(1): 20–4.

10 Cox JD, Pajak TF, Herskovic A, Urtasun R, Podolsky WJ, Seydel HG (1991) Five-year survival after hyperfractionated radiation therapy for non-small-cell carcinoma of the lung (NSCCL): Results of RTOG protocol 81-08. *Am. J. Clin. Oncol*, Aug; 14(4): 280–4.

11 Cox JD, Azarnia N, Byhardt RW, Shin KH, Emami B, Pajak TF (1990) A randomized phase I/II trial of hyperfractionated radiation therapy with total doses of 60.0 Gy to 79.2 Gy: Possible survival benefit with greater than or equal to 69.6 Gy in favorable patients with Radiation Therapy Oncology Group stage III non-small-cell lung carcinoma: Report of Radiation Therapy Oncology Group 83-11. *J. Clin. Oncol*, Sep; 8(9): 1543–55.

12 Dillman RO, Herndon J, Seagren SL, Eaton WL Jr, Green MR (1996) Improved survival in stage III non-small-cell lung cancer: seven-year follow-up of cancer and leukemia group B (CALGB) 8433 trial. *J. Natl. Cancer Inst*, Sep 4; 88(17): 1210–15.

13 Scott C, Sause WT, Byhardt R, Marcial V, Pajak TF, Herskovic A, *et al.* (1997) Recursive partitioning analysis of 1592 patients on four Radiation Therapy Oncology Group studies in inoperable non-small cell lung cancer. *Lung Cancer*, Jun; 17(Suppl 1): S59–74.

14 Saunders MI, Dische S (1990) Continuous, hyperfractionated, accelerated radiotherapy (CHART) in non-small cell carcinoma of the bronchus. *Int. J. Radiat. Oncol. Biol. Phys*, Nov; 19(5): 1211–15.

15 Saunders M, Dische S, Barrett A, Harvey A, Gibson D, Parmar M (1997) Continuous hyperfractionated accelerated radiotherapy (CHART) versus conventional radiotherapy in non-small-cell lung cancer: A randomised multicentre trial. CHART Steering Committee. *Lancet*, Jul 19; 350(9072): 161–5.

16 Saunders M, Dische S, Barrett A, Harvey A, Griffiths G, Palmar M (1999) Continuous, hyperfractionated, accelerated radiotherapy (CHART) versus conventional radiotherapy in non-small cell lung cancer: Mature data from the randomised multicentre trial. CHART Steering committee. *Radiother Oncol*, Aug; 52(2): 137–48.

17 Sause W, Kolesar P, Taylor S IV, Johnson D, Livingston R, Komaki R, *et al.* (2000) Final results of phase III trial in regionally advanced unresectable non-small cell lung cancer: Radiation Therapy Oncology Group, Eastern Cooperative Oncology Group, and Southwest Oncology Group. *Chest*, Feb; 117(2): 358–64.

18 Byhardt RW, Scott CB, Ettinger DS, Curran WJ, Doggett RL, Coughlin C, *et al.* (1995) Concurrent hyperfractionated irradiation and chemotherapy for unresectable nonsmall cell lung cancer. Results of Radiation Therapy Oncology Group 90-15. *Cancer*, May 1; 75(9): 2337–44.

19 Komaki R, Scott C, Lee JS, Urtasun RC, Byhardt RW, Emami B, *et al.* (1997) Impact of adding concurrent chemotherapy to hyperfractionated radiotherapy for locally advanced non-small cell lung cancer (NSCLC): Comparison of RTOG 83-11 and RTOG 91-06. *Am. J. Clin. Oncol*, Oct; 20(5): 435–40.

20 Komaki R, Scott C, Ettinger D, Lee JS, Fossella FV, Curran W, *et al.* (1997) Randomized study of chemotherapy/radiation therapy combinations for favorable patients with locally advanced inoperable nonsmall cell lung cancer: Radiation Therapy Oncology Group (RTOG) 92-04. *Int. J. Radiat. Oncol. Biol. Phys*, Apr 1; 38(1): 149–55.

21 Curran WJ, Scott CB, Langer CJ, Komaki R, Lee JS, Hauser S, *et al.* (2003) Long-term benefit is observed in a phase III comparison of sequential vs concurrent chemo-radiation for patients with unresected stage III NSCLC: RTOG 9410. *Proceedings of the American Society of Clinical Oncology, 2003*; Abstract #2499.

22 Furuse K, Fukuoka M, Kawahara M, Nishikawa H, Takada Y, Kudoh S, *et al.* (1999) Phase III study of concurrent versus sequential thoracic radiotherapy in combination with mitomycin, vindesine, and cisplatin in unresectable stage III non-small-cell lung cancer. *J. Clin. Oncol*, Sep; 17(9): 2692–9.

23 Belani CP, Choy H, Bonomi P, Scott C, Travis P, Haluschak J, *et al.* (2005) Combined chemoradiotherapy regimens of paclitaxel and carboplatin for locally advanced non-small-cell lung cancer: A randomized phase II locally advanced multi-modality protocol. *J. Clin. Oncol*, Sep 1; 23(25): 5883–91.

24 Jeremic B, Shibamoto Y, Acimovic L, Milisavljevic S (1996) Hyperfractionated radiation therapy with or without concurrent low-dose daily carboplatin/etoposide for stage III non-small-cell lung cancer: A randomized study. *J. Clin. Oncol*, Apr; 14(4): 1065–70.

25 Ball D, Bishop J, Smith J, O'Brien P, Davis S, Ryan G, *et al.* (1999) A randomised phase III study of accelerated or standard fraction radiotherapy with or without concurrent carboplatin in inoperable non-small cell lung cancer: Final report of an Australian multi-centre trial. *Radiother Oncol*, Aug; 52(2): 129–36.

26 Fang LC, Komaki R, Allen P, Guerrero T, Mohan R, Cox JD (2006) Comparison of outcomes for patients with medically inoperable Stage I non-small-cell lung cancer treated with two-dimensional vs. three-dimensional radiotherapy. *International Journal of Radiation Oncology Biology Physics*, Sep 1; 66(1): 108–16.

27 Nehmeh SA, Erdi YE, Pan T, Pevsner A, Rosenzweig KE, Yorke E, *et al.* (2004) Four-dimensional (4D) PET/CT imaging of the thorax. *Med Phys*, Dec; 31(12): 3179–86.

28 Rosenzweig KE, Hanley J, Mah D, Mageras G, Hunt M, Toner S, *et al.* (2000) The deep inspiration breath-hold technique in the treatment of inoperable non-small-cell lung cancer. *Int. J. Radiat. Oncol. Biol. Phys*, Aug 1; 48(1): 81–7.

29 Ramsey CR, Scaperoth D, Arwood D, Oliver AL (1999) Clinical efficacy of respiratory gated conformal radiation therapy. *Med Dosim*, 24(2): 115–19.

30 Chang JY, Dong L, Liu H, Starkschall G, Balter P, Mohan R, *et al.* (2008) Image-guided radiation therapy for non-small cell lung cancer. *J Thorac Oncol*, Feb; 3(2): 177–86.

31 Yom SS, Liao Z, Liu HH, Tucker SL, Hu C-S, Wei X, *et al.* (2007) Initial evaluation of treatment-related pneumonitis in advanced-stage non-small-cell lung cancer patients treated with concurrent chemotherapy and intensity-modulated radiotherapy. *Int. J. Radiat. Oncol. Biol. Phys*, May 1; 68(1): 94–102.

32 Liao ZX, Komaki RR, Thames HD Jr, Liu HH, Tucker SL, Mohan R, *et al.* (2010) Influence of technologic advances on outcomes in patients with unresectable, locally advanced non-small-cell lung cancer receiving concomitant chemoradiotherapy. *Int. J. Radiat. Oncol. Biol. Phys*, Mar 1; 76(3): 775–81.

33 Bezjak A, Rumble RB, Rodrigues G, Hope A, Warde P (2012) Intensity-modulated radiotherapy in the treatment of lung cancer. *Clin Oncol (R Coll Radiol)*, Sep; 24(7): 508–20.

34 Govaert SLA, Troost EGC, Schuurbiers OCJ, De Geus-Oei L-F, Termeer A, Span PN, *et al.* (2012) Treatment outcome and toxicity of intensity-modulated (chemo) radiotherapy in stage III non-small cell lung cancer patients. *Radiat Oncol*, 7: 150.

35 Chang JY, Komaki R, Lu C, Wen HY, Allen PK, Tsao A, *et al.* (2011) Phase 2 study of high-dose proton therapy with concurrent chemotherapy for unresectable stage III nonsmall cell lung cancer. *Cancer*, Oct 15; 117(20): 4707–13.

36 Marks LB, Yorke ED, Jackson A, Ten Haken RK, Constine LS, Eisbruch A, *et al.* (2010) Use of normal tissue complication probability models in the clinic. *Int. J. Radiat. Oncol. Biol. Phys*, Mar 1; 76(3 Suppl): S10–19.

37 Marks LB, Bentzen SM, Deasy JO, Kong F-MS, Bradley JD, Vogelius IS, *et al.* (2010) Radiation dose-volume effects in the lung. *Int. J. Radiat. Oncol. Biol. Phys*, Mar 1; 76(3 Suppl): S70–76.

38 Hatton M, Nankivell M, Lyn E, Falk S, Pugh C, Navani N, *et al.* (2011) Induction chemotherapy and continuous hyperfractionated accelerated radiotherapy (chart) for patients with locally advanced inoperable non-small-cell lung cancer: the MRC INCH randomized trial. *Int. J. Radiat. Oncol. Biol. Phys*, Nov 1; 81(3): 712–18.

39 Baumann M, Herrmann T, Koch R, Matthiessen W, Appold S, Wahlers B, *et al.* (2011) Final results of the randomized phase III CHARTWEL-trial (ARO 97-1) comparing hyperfractionated-accelerated versus conventionally fractionated radiotherapy in non-small cell lung cancer (NSCLC). *Radiother Oncol*, Jul; 100(1): 76–85.

40 Rengan R, Rosenzweig KE, Venkatraman E, Koutcher LA, Fox JL, Nayak R, *et al.* (2004) Improved local control with higher doses of radiation in large-volume stage III non-small-cell lung cancer. *Int. J. Radiat. Oncol. Biol. Phys*, Nov 1; 60(3): 741–7.

41 Bradley JD, Ieumwananonthachai N, Purdy JA, Wasserman TH, Lockett MA, Graham MV, *et al.* (2002) Gross tumor volume, critical prognostic factor in patients treated with three-dimensional conformal radiation therapy for non-small-cell lung carcinoma. *Int. J. Radiat. Oncol. Biol. Phys*, Jan 1; 52(1): 49–57.

42 Kong F-M, Ten Haken RK, Schipper MJ, Sullivan MA, Chen M, Lopez C, *et al.* (2005) High-dose radiation improved local tumor control and overall survival in patients with inoperable/unresectable non-small-cell lung cancer: Long-term results of a radiation dose escalation study. *Int. J. Radiat. Oncol. Biol. Phys*, Oct 1; 63(2): 324–33.

43 Wang L, Correa CR, Zhao L, Hayman J, Kalemkerian GP, Lyons S, *et al.* (2009) The effect of radiation dose and chemotherapy on overall survival in 237 patients with Stage III non-small-cell lung cancer. *Int. J. Radiat. Oncol. Biol. Phys*, Apr 1; 73(5): 1383–90.

44 Socinski MA, Rosenman JG, Halle J, Schell MJ, Lin Y, Russo S, *et al.* (2001) Dose-escalating conformal thoracic radiation therapy with induction and concurrent carboplatin/paclitaxel in unresectable stage IIIA/B nonsmall cell lung carcinoma: A modified phase I/II trial. *Cancer*, Sep 1; 92(5): 1213–23.

45 Rosenman JG, Halle JS, Socinski MA, Deschesne K, Moore DT, Johnson H, *et al.* (2002) High-dose conformal radiotherapy for treatment of stage IIIA/IIIB non-small-cell lung cancer: Technical issues and results of a phase I/II trial. *Int. J. Radiat. Oncol. Biol. Phys*, Oct 1; 54(2): 348–56.

46 Socinski MA, Morris DE, Halle JS, Moore DT, Hensing TA, Limentani SA, *et al.* (2004) Induction and concurrent chemotherapy with high-dose thoracic conformal radiation therapy in unresectable stage IIIA and IIIB non-small-cell lung cancer: A dose-escalation phase I trial. *J. Clin. Oncol*, Nov 1; 22(21): 4341–50.

47 Lee CB, Stinchcombe TE, Moore DT, Morris DE, Hayes DN, Halle J, *et al.* (2009) Late complications of high-dose (>/ = 66 Gy) thoracic conformal radiation therapy in combined modality trials in unresectable stage III non-small cell lung cancer. *J Thorac Oncol*, Jan; 4(1): 74–9.

48 Bradley JD, Moughan J, Graham MV, Byhardt R, Govindan R, Fowler J, *et al.* (2010) A phase I/II radiation dose escalation study with concurrent chemotherapy for patients with inoperable stages I to III non-small-cell lung cancer: phase I results of RTOG 0117. *Int. J. Radiat. Oncol. Biol. Phys*, Jun 1; 77(2): 367–72.

49 Bradley JD, Bae K, Graham MV, Byhardt R, Govindan R, Fowler J, *et al.* (2010) Primary analysis of the phase II component of a phase I/II dose intensification study using three-dimensional conformal radiation therapy and concurrent chemotherapy for patients with inoperable non-small-cell lung cancer: RTOG 0117. *J. Clin. Oncol*, May 10; 28(14): 2475–80.

50 Socinski MA, Blackstock AW, Bogart JA, Wang X, Munley M, Rosenman J, *et al.* (2008) Randomized phase II trial of induction chemotherapy followed by concurrent chemotherapy and dose-escalated thoracic conformal radiotherapy (74 Gy) in stage III non-small-cell lung cancer: CALGB 30105. *J. Clin. Oncol*, May 20; 26(15): 2457–63.

51 Bradley JD, Paulus R, Komaki R, Masters G, Forster K, Schild SE, *et al.* (2011) A randomized phase III

comparison of standard-dose (60 Gy) versus high-dose (74 Gy) conformal chemoradiotherapy +/− cetuximab for stage IIIa/IIIb non-small cell lung cancer: Preliminary findings on radiation dose in RTOG 0617. *Int J Radiat Oncol Biol Phys*, Dec 1; 81(5 (Supplement)).

52 Partridge M, Ramos M, Sardaro A, Brada M. (2011) Dose escalation for non-small cell lung cancer: analysis and modelling of published literature. *Radiother Oncol*, Apr; 99(1): 6–11.

53 Machtay M, Bae K, Movsas B, Paulus R, Gore EM, Komaki R, *et al.* (2012) Higher biologically effective dose of radiotherapy is associated with improved outcomes for locally advanced non-small cell lung carcinoma treated with chemoradiation: An analysis of the Radiation Therapy Oncology Group. *Int. J. Radiat. Oncol. Biol. Phys*, Jan 1; 82(1): 425–34.

54 Sonke J-J, Belderbos J (2010) Adaptive radiotherapy for lung cancer. *Semin Radiat Oncol*, Apr; 20(2): 94–106.

55 Kong F-MS, Frey KA, Quint LE, Ten Haken RK, Hayman JA, Kessler M, *et al.* (2007) A pilot study of [18F]fluorodeoxyglucose positron emission tomography scans during and after radiation-based therapy in patients with non small-cell lung cancer. *J. Clin. Oncol*, Jul 20; 25(21): 3116–23.

56 Feng M, Kong F-M, Gross M, Fernando S, Hayman JA, Ten Haken RK (2009) Using fluorodeoxyglucose positron emission tomography to assess tumor volume during radiotherapy for non-small-cell lung cancer and its potential impact on adaptive dose escalation and normal tissue sparing. *Int. J. Radiat. Oncol. Biol Phys*, Mar 15; 73(4): 1228–34.

57 Klopp AH, Chang JY, Tucker SL, Sulman EP, Balter PA, Liu HH, *et al.* (2007) Intrathoracic patterns of failure for non-small-cell lung cancer with positron-emission tomography/computed tomography-defined target delineation. *Int. J. Radiat. Oncol. Biol. Phys*, Dec 1; 69(5): 1409–16.

58 Bollineni VR, Wiegman EM, Pruim J, Groen HJM, Langendijk JA (2012) Hypoxia imaging using Positron Emission Tomography in non-small cell lung cancer: implications for radiotherapy. *Cancer Treat. Rev*, Dec; 38(8): 1027–32.

CHAPTER 25

Molecular Target Treatment for Personalized Radiotherapy in Lung Cancer

Steven H. Lin and Ritsuko U. Komaki
Department of Radiation Oncology, The University of Texas MD Anderson Cancer Center, Houston, TX, USA

Technologic improvements in radiation delivery enhances therapeutic ratio

Technological advances have significantly enhanced radiotherapy effectiveness. Conventional radiation using older techniques did not have good outcomes due to the inability to deliver adequate tumoricidal doses given the constraints of normal tissue dose limitations [1]. Advances in radiation technology and delivery, particularly the use of conformal treatments such as 3-dimensional conformal radiation, Intensity Modulated Radiation Therapy (IMRT) and proton beam, enables the delivery of much higher doses of radiation while minimizing exposure of adjacent tissues to the damaging effects of radiation [2]. Such advances have already enhanced cure rates in early stage lung cancers using Stereotactic Body Radiation Therapy (SBRT) since it is more effective compared to conventionally fractionated radiation. Substantial amounts of clinical experience and prospective clinical trials have shown SBRT to exert excellent local control rates (>95%) with survival that appears to be mainly dictated by comorbidities of the patient and distant metastatic rates, which are similar to surgically resected patient at about 25–30% [3, 4]. Definitive phase III trials comparing SBRT to lobectomy in operable patients are currently being conducted throughout the world to determine the equipoise of SBRT in clinical efficacy compared to surgery. In resected stage III-N2 NSCLC the incorporation of conformal postoperative radiation therapy can also increase survival because of the improved morbidity/mortality of treatment when compared to older techniques [1]. However in small cell and locally advanced (stage II-III medically or technically unresectable) NSCLC, radiation and chemotherapy is the mainstay of treatment. The extent of disease in these patients usually precludes the use of SBRT, and conventionally-fractionated radiation is needed over the course of 6–7 weeks. While metastatic recurrence is the predominant form of recurrence and is the cause of most cancer deaths, enhancing local control of nonmetastatic stage III-N2 lung cancer can impact overall survival. This is based on the seminal study of RTOG 7301 which showed that higher dose of radiation (60 Gy) improved local control and overall survival compared to lower doses of radiation. To further improve upon these results by counteracting the accelerated repopulation of tumor

Lung Cancer, Fourth Edition. Edited by Jack A. Roth, Waun Ki Hong and Ritsuko U. Komaki.

cells, CHART (continuous hyperfractionated accelerated radiation therapy, which is three-times-daily radiation administered continuously 7 days a week) was studied in comparison to conventionally fractionated radiation, both done without chemotherapy [5]. CHART improved local control and overall survival; however, this has not impacted clinical practice in the United States because of the difficulty to administer CHART in the standard clinical practice. The introduction of chemotherapy with radiation in the treatment of lung cancer made the largest impact. Several randomized trials conducted in the 1980s demonstrated improved survival outcomes with the addition of sequential chemotherapy to conventionally fractionated radiotherapy [6]. Additional important studies were conducted that compared sequential chemotherapy with concurrent chemotherapy, with the demonstration of improved overall survival with concurrent chemotherapy, at the expense of added toxicity [7].

Overcoming the plateau of radiation efficacy

While cytotoxic chemotherapy given concurrently with radiation enhanced radiation effects and improved outcomes over radiation alone, there has not been significant advances beyond this point. So far, there are minimal differences between the different types of chemotherapy given concurrently with radiation therapy, with little to no advantage (sometimes even detrimental) with the addition of induction or consolidation chemotherapy [8, 9]. Altered fractionated radiation therapy combined with chemotherapy (CHART-WEL) compared to standard chemoradiation had comparable outcomes at the cost of increased acute toxicities [10]. Phase I/II dose-escalated trials using modern delivery techniques have shown feasibility and promise in the improvement of local control and possibly survival [11–13]. However, results of the phase III randomized trial comparing standard dose (60 Gy) to high dose (74 Gy) with concurrent chemotherapy demonstrated worse local control and overall survival outcomes in the high dose arm [14]. Therefore despite decades of research and advances in radiation therapy, disease outcomes for locally advanced lung cancer remains poor, with a median survival on the order of 17–24 months, and a 5 year overall survival of 15–20%. At this point it appears we are at a standstill and have reached a threshold on further improving on the outcomes of lung cancer treatment using current approaches (Figure 25.1a). Raising the therapeutic threshold may need biologic innovations which will result in a leftward shift in the therapeutic ratio curve (Figure 25.1b). The biologic effect must be specific for the tumor cells with minimal effect on the normal tissues. This occurs since genetic defects of the tumor cell make them susceptible to the drugs that synergizes with the biologic effects of radiation on these cells. Adding targeted drugs to current standard therapies, with radiation or with chemoradiation, may further improve the efficacy of radiation, although promising data has only so far come from single arm phase II trials.

Targeted therapy with radiotherapy: past successes and failures

Cytotoxic chemotherapy acts in synergy with radiation to kill tumor cells; however, because of the unselective nature of both therapies, toxicity is also enhanced in normal tissue. Several strategies have been used to combine molecularly targeted therapies with radiotherapy in order to enhance radiation effects on tumor cells. These strategies leverage on the tumor or microenvironment characteristics that allow selective targeting of tumors with radiotherapy. The strategies that have been well studied in the past are those that target tumor hypoxia, tumor vasculature, and the Epidermal Growth Factor Receptor pathway.

Hypoxia targeting

Hypoxia targeting has been a long time strategy in radiation oncology for several decades. It is well established that hypoxia contributes significantly to radiation resistance [15]. Tumors often outgrow the vascular supply and have abnormal proangiogenic

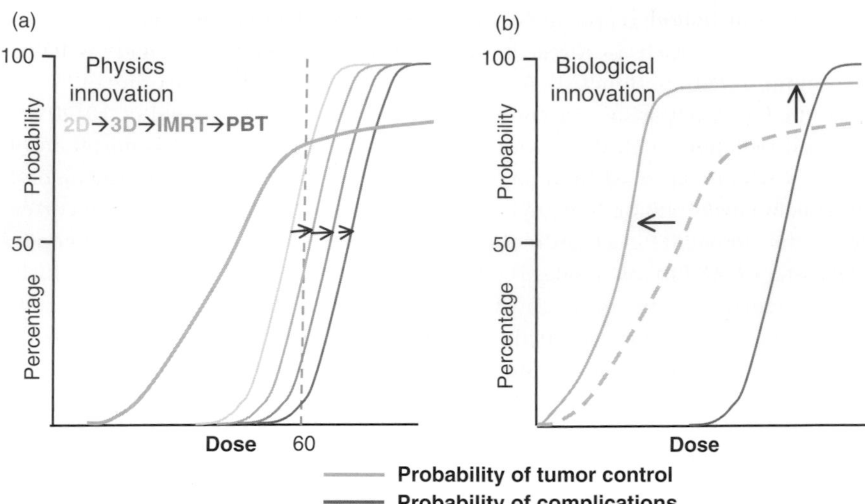

Figure 25.1 Improving outcomes in lung cancer requires both physics and biological innovations. The figure represents therapeutic index curves, with the theoretical incremental improvements in therapeutic ratio with each successive improvements in technologic innovations. However, while toxicities improve with these advancements, the biologic efficacy has reached a threshold. To enhance disease outcomes will require a leftward shift in the biologic curve by combining molecularly targeted agents with radiation therapy.

and anti-angiogenic homeostasis, and therefore necrosis and hypoxic regions within the tumor are commonly seen in most tumor types. Cure rates are attenuated by hypoxia, both in preclinical models and in clinical situations [16, 17]. There are two main reasons responsible for this effect. For one, the cytotoxic effect of radiation is critically dependent on the chemical fixation of molecular oxygen on DNA. Second, tumors can be rendered resistant to both chemotherapy and radiotherapy by the cytoprotection mediated by the hypoxia-inducible factor HIF1, a master transcription factor that induces many hypoxia-inducible genes and renders the cell resistant to hypoxic stress [18]. Several clinical strategies have been employed to counteract the effects of hypoxia, such as the use of bioreductive agents [19], hypoxic cell toxin such as tirapazamine [20], or HIF1 alpha antagonist [21], but most of these efforts have been focused on radiotherapy for head and neck cancers, and either have had some promise [19] or have not had mature clinical development [21]. The only hypoxia-targeting strategy that has had at least some clinical experience in lung cancer is the use of carbogen to increase oxygen delivery to the tumor. Carbogen, which is 95% oxygen and 5% CO_2, enhances tumor's effect to radiation by increasing the oxygen concentration in the blood when it is inhaled before and after each session of radiotherapy. Preclinical studies have shown that this is an effective strategy to enhance the radiation response, particularly when administered with nicotinamide (vitamin B3) which enhances tumor perfusion and reoxygenation through microvascular changes [22]. The phase III ARCON trial (Accelerated Radiotherapy plus Carbogen and Nicotinamide) in lung cancer was closed early to poor accrual, and showed no evidence of improvement with ARCON over conventional radiotherapy [23]. The only positive trial was the phase III ARCON trial in cT2-4 squamous cell laryngeal cancer that compared accelerated radiotherapy to ARCON [24]. A total of 345 patients were accrued. While local control was no different, the regional control rate was significantly better with ARCON (93% vs. 86%, $p = 0.04$). More importantly, this benefit was largely confined to hypoxic tumors and not to well-oxygenated tumors (100% vs. 55%, p = 0.01). There was an equal level of toxicity in the two groups. Since this trial used accelerated radiotherapy as the standard arm, the benefit of combining Carbogen/Nicotinamide with chemotherapy and radiation for the treatment of H&N cancer is not known. Since the current standard is concurrent chemoradiation, it is uncertain whether adding Carbogen will ever affect the standard of care, particularly in lung cancer therapy.

Vascular targeting

Along with the importance of oxygenation for anti-tumor effects by radiation, adequate perfusion of the tumor is an important factor in therapeutic effectiveness. Tumors are known to have abnormal and disorganized vascular architecture due to dysregulated pro- and anti-angiogenic factors [25]. Anti-angiogenic agents such as bevacizumab can help normalize tumor vasculature and improve chemotherapy deliver and oxygenation of tumors. This "vascular normalization" enhances radiation response in tumors. Although a number of mechanisms may be responsible for the effects seen, it is clear that combining anti-angiogenic agents with radiation is a promising approach for cancer therapy [26, 27]. Preclinical studies in vivo using various vascular targeting drugs have demonstrated vascular normalization effects, but the therapeutic enhancement of radiation has not been consistent given differences in the timing and sequence of when these agents are given with the combination of radiation [26, 28]. A number of trials have been conducted in various cancers, including GI, head and neck, rectal, pancreatic cancers, with promising phase I/II results showing clinical responses [29]. However, the incidence of GI hemorrhage and perforation seen from numerous drug combination trials (~6–7%) has led to careful monitoring of any combination trials using any anti-angiogenic agents. In NSCLC, the addition of Bevacizumab to carboplatin/taxol as first line therapy for stage IIIB-IV NSLC in a randomized phase III trial also demonstrated fatal hemoptysis in some patients, particularly those with central or squamous carcinoma cancers, leading to the exclusion of this treatment for these patients [30]. The combination with chemoradiation with this class of agents has been even more concerning. In a phase II study in limited stage SCLC combining Bevacizumab with chemoradiation, the study closed early after accrual of 29 patients due to the report of 2 patients with tracheoesophageal fistula (TEF) and 1 patient with fatal aerodigestive bleeding. In a separate phase II trial in locally advanced NSCLC treated with concurrent Bevacizumab with chemoradiation, the study was closed after enrolling 5 patients when 2 patients were reported to develop TEF. Socinski and colleagues recently reported combining bevacizumab and erlotinib with concurrent chemotherapy and high-dose radiotherapy (74 Gy), delivered with 2-dimensional radiotherapy techniques, and elective nodal irradiation, for stage III NSCLC [31]. The clinical outcomes of this study were disappointing, with severe toxicity (29% grade 3 or 4 esophagitis, with one grade 3 TEF) and no improvement in survival. This study again showed that it is not safe to combine bevacizumab with radiotherapy. With the report of these toxicities, developing these agents with concurrent radiotherapy in NSCLC need to proceed with particular caution and requires continued research [32]. It is not known whether other classes of vascular-targeting drugs (such as endostatin, currently being developed in China in combination with chemoradiation for LA-NSCLC) will have a different toxicity profile. Ongoing research is much needed to understand how best to combine these class of agents with radio- or chemoradiotherapy.

EGFR targeting

The EGFR receptor family (ERBB1-4) is an important growth factor receptor tyrosine kinase (RTK) involved in tumor growth and survival. It is overexpressed in nearly 100% head and neck cancers, and in numerous other cancers, including NSCLC. Various subtypes of these RTKs may be more important in one cancer over another, such as ERBB1 in H&N and NSCLC, and ERBB2/Her2 in breast and upper GI cancers. Activation of these receptors activates multiple intracellular signaling pathways including the RAS and PI3K pathways to stimulate growth, enhance DNA damage repair, and block apoptosis [33,34]. The RTKs are excellent targets for drug development, as both antibody-based therapy that binds to the extracellular domain to inhibit receptor activation (e.g., cetuximab → ERBB1/EGFR, Herceptin → ERBB2/Her2) and ATP-competitive antagonists to inhibit kinase activation (e.g., erlotinib, lapatinib) are efficacious as single agents [35]. Moreover, targeting becomes even more specific and efficacious depending on how dependent the tumor is on the RTKs, either through oncogenic addiction conferred by activating mutations of EGFR in NSCLC or by gene amplification. EGFR targeting has been shown to be effective as radiation sensitizers. The best known example is cetuximab combined with radiation therapy in H&N cancer cell lines, as established by key studies by Harari *et al.* [36] and Ang *et al.* in the 1990s [37]. These preclinical studies led to the pivotal trial that demonstrated a 10% OS benefit of adding cetuximab with radiation compared to radiation alone in the treatment of H&N cancers [38]. Unfortunately, the benefit of cetuximab seemed to vanish when chemoradiotherapy was combined with cetuximab-radiotherapy in RTOG 0522 [39]. The role of cetuximab when combined with chemoradiation was first studied as a phase II study in RTOG 0324. In this single arm study, the median survival was 22.7 months, and the 24-month overall survival was 49.3% [40]. However, RTOG 0617 tested the benefit of cetuximab in the phase III randomized trial in a 2X2 factorial design randomizing to either standard dose (60 Gy) or high dose (74 Gy) +/− cetuximab found no survival benefit of adding cetuximab (HR 0.99, p = 0.4838) [41]. Overall, grade 3 to 5 toxicities were worse for patients on the cetuximab arm. When tumors were stained for EGFR expression (hybrid score, or H-score), high H-score tumors were significantly more likely to benefit from cetuximab than tumor with low H-score (p = 0.02) [41]. Another strategy of targeting EGFR is the use of small molecule EGFR-targeting TKI. A phase II trial at MD Anderson combined erlotinib with chemoradiation in stage III NSCLC was recently reported, showing a median OS of 34.1 months and a 2-year OS of 68%, without grade 4 or 5 AEs [42]. Unfortunately, all of these studies were conducted in unselected patients, so it is possible that surrogate biomarkers for EGFR activation could help select for patient benefit for these therapies, as the RTOG 0617 trial seems to indicate. Biomarker-based trials in EGFR targeting with concurrent CRT are lacking, although RTOG 1306 is a phase III trial testing the role of induction erlotinib or crizotinib followed by CRT in EGFR mutant or EML4-ALK translocation NSCLC, respectively.

Guidelines for incorporating novel targeted agents in combination with radiation in lung cancer

Conventional therapies have mostly treated NSCLC as a single disease, and only more recently has the adoption of differing chemotherapy strategies depended on the tumor's histology, whether it is an adenocarcinoma (pemetrexed) or a squamous cell carcinoma (gemcitabine) [43]. However, through high-throughput genome sequencing efforts of lung cancers have revealed the genetic heterogeneity of NSCLC [44,45], and that adenocarcinomas largely differ from squamous cell carcinomas in the set of oncogenic alterations [46]. It is a fact that NSCLC is not one disease but a series of diseases that differ based on the oncogenetic profile [46,47]. About 60% of NSCLC have causative genetic mutations that could be targetable with drugs, but a substantial proportion of tumors do not have known or targetable genetic alterations. While genetic alterations in EGFR, ALK, or ROS1 genes implicate a direct therapeutic opportunity, it is less clear how other more common mutations such as TP53, LKB1, KRAS could be targeted. There is also a paucity of targetable mutations in SCLC that have yet to be identified. In order to bring advances to the field, particularly to help improve cure rates in unresectable NSCLC and SCLC requires continued efforts to combine molecularly targeted agents with radiation therapy. Agents that can enhance both chemotherapy and radiotherapy selectively for tumor cells would lead to substantial improvement in the cure rates of these cancers. However, a systematic approach is needed so that efforts are not expended on poorly designed clinical trials.

Several recent reviews have outlined strategies to best combine targeted therapies with radiation. I will refer the reader to these excellent guidelines [48–50]. We provide a general summary of the strategies in how best to combine molecularly targeted agents with radiation.

Potential targeted agents to combine with radiation therapy

There are a number of pathways that confer radiation protection when activated by radiation during the reparative process or by oncogenic pathway activation. There are theoretical advantages of tumor cell kill when combining drugs that inhibit these pathways with radiation. Many of these approaches have been supported by evidence from preclinical studies and are summarized below (Figure 25.2a).

DNA damage repair targeting drugs

Since single and double-strand DNA (dsDNA) breaks are the main mechanisms for radiation cytotoxicity, and enhancing DNA damage repair (DDR) is a most direct way for the cell to counteract the effects of radiation. DDR pathway proteins often belong to large signaling pathways emanating from the onset of a dsDNA breakage event that affects cell cycle progression and DNA repair kinetics [51]. Depleting these proteins in the cell using knockdown strategies are effective means to sensitize cells to the effects of radiation. Since many of these proteins are in the PI3Kinase family of proteins, numerous drugs have been developed that inhibit these pathways. These include PARP, ATM/ATR, and DNA-PK inhibitors. A number of these agents, particularly the PARP inhibitors, have shown potent preclinical efficacy of cell kill when combined with radiation in both in vitro and in vivo models [52, 53]. Currently, many of these agents

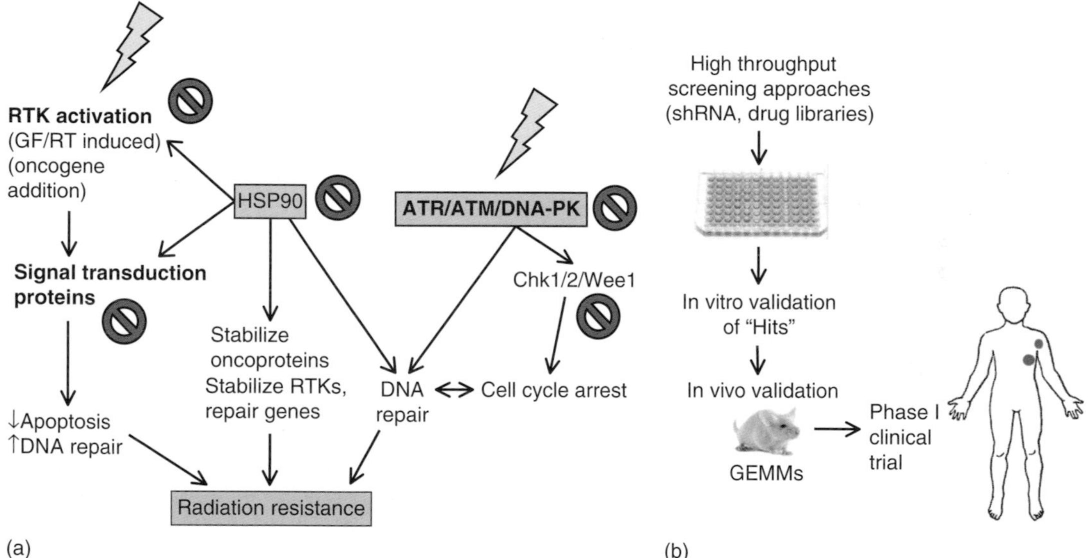

Figure 25.2 Approaches to identify the targeted agents to bring forward into clinical testing. a: Pathway-based approach of rational understanding of the interplay of DDR and cellular pathway activation after irradiation will allow the prioritizing candidates for clinical testing. These pathways represent a small example of pathways that have been shown preclinically to have important interactions with the radiation response. Red circles with a diagonal line indicate known inhibitors that can radiosensitize cells to the damaging effects of radiation. b: Screening approach to identify the genes or drugs that are synthetically lethal with radiation. In vitro discovery and downstream validation are necessary steps prior to clinical testing. GEMM, Genetically Engineered Mouse Models.

are in early phase clinical trial testing. ABT888, the PARP inhibitor from Abbott, is the earliest drug in this class of drugs, is the most advanced in clinical testing in combination with chemoradiation in a number of tumor sites, including NSCLC. A current SWOG phase I/II trial (S1206) tests the safety and preliminary efficacy of adding ABT-888 to CRT in unresectable stage III NSCLC. ATM and DNA-PK inhibitors have been developed and are currently being evaluated in small early phase clinical trials. The potential for the clinical development of these agents may best be seen in particular subgroups of patients with tumors that harbor mutations that make these tumors more susceptible for radiation killing in combination with these drugs. This is an example of synthetic lethality, and several clinical trials have demonstrated that PARP inhibitors are particularly efficacious in BRCA1 or 2 tumors since these tumors are defective in homologous recombination repair [54, 55].

Cell cycle checkpoint inhibitors

DNA damage induced by radiation is deleterious to the cell if it goes unrepaired. Repair occurs if the cell is arrested during cell cycle progression orchestrated by a series of signaling transduction events that impacts cell cycle and mitotic spindle proteins. Transducing signals from ATM/ATR to Chk1/2, and phosphatases or cyclin-dependent kinases induces cell cycle arrest in the G1/S and G2/M phase. P53 is a critical protein that mediates cell cycle arrest through induction of WAF1/P21 which directly inhibit cyclin-CDK2 to result in G1/S arrest. Other proteins, mediated through protein kinases such as Chk1/2 and Wee1, regulates entry into mitosis by placing a block at the G2/M checkpoint. The mitotic checkpoint, mediated by the likes of polo-like kinases and aurora kinases, is another critical point in the cell cycle that regulates progression through mitosis. Any perturbance of these checkpoints during cellular stress such as DNA damage will cause the cells to enter mitosis not having had the time to undergo adequate DDR, resulting in cell death due to mitotic catastrophe. These pathways present a therapeutic opportunity for cancer treatment with radiation [56]. Preclinical studies have demonstrated the efficacy of these agents when combined with radiation, particularly in TP53 deficient tumors. Cells with TP53 defects cannot undergo G1/S arrest during cellular stress, and therefore rely on G2/M or mitotic arrest for DNA damage repair. A number of drugs that inhibit Chk1 (AZD7762), Wee1 (MK1775), and aurora kinase A inhibitors (MLN8237, VX-680) have been shown to selectively enhance chemotherapy and radiotherapy cytotoxicity in TP53 mutated tumors [56, 57, 59–61]. Early phase trials are ongoing to combine these agents with chemotherapy in advanced tumor types. However, combining these agents with radiotherapy is clearly an exciting area for clinical development.

Signal transduction inhibitors

Signal transduction cascades through activated GF receptors or oncogenic pathways are critical to help the cell maintain survival of cells by enhancing repair and resist apoptosis. Such inhibitors may act downstream of the signaling of a number of potential RTKs or GPCRs, and therefore have a more general anti-cancer action. The use of these drugs as single agents are being tested in chemotherapy or single agent trials in a number of phase I-III drug trials. As mentioned above, a phase II trial combining erlotinib with chemoradiation in unselected stage III NSCLC has completed accrual and showed a promising 2 year overall survival of 66%. A number of other inhibitors to PI3K, AKT, mTOR, MEK have demonstrated radiation sensitization in preclinical studies. It will be important to bring these agents into clinical testing.

Epigenetic agents

Aberrant gene expression due to aberrant epigenetic alterations due to methylation or chromatin assembly is a characteristic of cancer. Demethylating agents have been shown to have clinical efficacy in hematologic malignancies, but have limited success in solid tumors. HDAC inhibitors such as vorinostat is FDA approved for refractory cutaneous T-cell lymphoma and have been tested in numerous clinical trials in combination with chemotherapy in solid tumors, with variable success, however none has become a standard of care in the treatment of solid tumors compared to standard chemotherapy.

Preclinical studies have shown potent radiation sensitizing effects with the combination of epigenetic agents [62–64], but the mechanism of these actions are rather nonspecific due to both DNA damaging and gene expression effects [65]. No trials combining radiation and HDAC inhibitors in lung cancer are known, although a couple of trials have gone through phase I testing for palliative pelvic radiotherapy for metastatic GI cancers with Vorinostat [66] and as a phase II trial in GBM using valproic acid and radiation (NCT00302159).

HSP90 inhibitors

Heat Shock Proteins are a large class of proteins collectively known as molecular chaperones that function in the folding and unfolding of proteins. They are upregulated during cellular stress, such as heat shock, that enables the cell to survive the cytotoxic effects of misfolded proteins. HSP90 is a highly conserved molecular chaperone that helps facilitate the maturation of over 200 proteins, called client proteins, many of which are oncoproteins that are mutated in the tumor cell and are critical to maintain the malignancy state. Therefore targeting HSP90 is a potent target for general cancer therapy [67]. These agents have been shown in numerous reports to exhibit potent radiation sensitizing effects, by enhancing apoptosis and induce mitotic catastrophe [68]. Despite potent anti-cancer actions of these agents, the clinical development of these agents, namely 17-AAG and NVP-AUY922, has been limited by hepatic and ocular toxicities, respectively. A promising agent, STA-9090, is a second generation HSP90 inhibitor that appears to have reduced toxicities compared to 17-AAG and lacks the ocular toxicities as seen so far in phase I/II clinical trials [69]. These agents will be exciting agents to develop in combination with radiation.

Immunotherapy

A critical component of tumor survival is related to the ability of tumor cells to evade the immune system. The immunosuppressive microenvironment of the tumor inhibits the appropriate activation of the cytotoxic T cells against tumor cells [70]. Using antibodies to block immune checkpoint molecules such as CTLA [71] or to infuse patients with activated autologous immune cells [72] have shown improved overall survival in patients with advanced melanoma or prostate cancers, respectively, and have won FDA approvals using these approaches. Currently, other checkpoint blockade inhibitors using monoclonal antibodies against PD-1, PD-L1, and other molecules, are being explored in early phase clinical trials in advanced cancers, including NSCLC. Several early phase trials have demonstrated significant and durable responses in heavily-pretreated advanced NSCLC, with overall responses in the range of 14–28% [73,74]. It is expected that many of these therapies will eventually be approved for use in multiple tumor types, and combining immunotherapies that have distinct mechanisms may be promising to further enhance tumor responses [75]. With the number of known and yet to be discovered genes involved in immunologic regulation, there is much research needed to identify the best combinations to enhance tumor kill and to minimize the potentially lethal allergic and autoimmunity that can be induced with such therapies.

It is also known that radiation-induced killing of cells is also dependent on CD8+ cells, as depleting CD8+ cells or treating tumor cells in immunocompromised animals has an attenuated effect over tumors treated with radiation in wild-type animals [76]. The interaction of radiation-induced cytotoxicity and the immune system creates the abscopal effect, in that tumor lysis due to radiation damage can induce a generalized immune response so that a systemic effect towards cancer cells is elicited. The abscopal effect has been recognized in patients receiving radiotherapy but it has been controversial since the response is neither robust nor reproducible in the past [77]. It has been demonstrated preclinically that the response is a CD8-T cell mediated process, and the effect can be unmasked by combining immunotherapies with radiotherapy [78]. A small number of studies have recently shown that this effect could be recapitulated in patients receiving either immune-checkpoint blockade or cytokine therapy [79,80]. It is therefore a promising approach to help enhance the effect of immunotherapies in stage IV cancers by combining with ablative radiotherapy, or to improve cancer cure rates in localized tumors receiving SBRT in early stage tumors or definitive chemoradiation in locally advanced disease. The best combination of immunotherapy with radiotherapy will be fruitful research for the future.

Considerations for bringing agents into clinical testing

The synthetic lethality effect with radiation

With so many agents being developed for cancer therapy, identifying the agents to be brought forth into clinical testing with radiation is a challenge. To determine which class of agents would be suitable to bring forward may require two approaches. The first is a rationally-designed approach, which would require a detailed evaluation of the pathways that may impact radiation effects, either by counteracting cellular protective mechanisms to DNA damaging effects of radiation or those that are synthetically lethal in genetically susceptible cells (i.e., PARP inhibitors in BRCA1/2 mutants), and identifying drugs that act on these pathways. Some of this is illustrated in Figure 25.2a. However, there will likely be other agents that possess radiation sensitizing effects for which the mechanism of action is still not well established. Therefore a second approach of target identification using high throughput screening approaches to identify genes that may be important for radiation sensitizing effects as well as functional screens of drug libraries to identify new targets and unveil novel pathways that may synergize with radiation (Figure 25.2b). Both of these approaches could be utilized to identify agents that can be brought into clinical testing.

Prioritizing agents for clinical development

Among the numerous agents with potential radiation sensitizing effects, there will only be a few that will ultimately be developed for clinical use. This is due to a number of factors, namely safety profile, systemic efficacy, and economic factors involved in the development of the agent. While the latter is difficult to predict, the former factors are important to consider when an agent is being considered for clinical development. Fortunately, many drugs have already gone through phase I/II trials in multiple cancers with established dose and safety profile, as well as systemic activity, both as single agents and in combination with various cytotoxic chemotherapies.

Preclinical studies in the disease site of interest

Since most of the available drugs were developed for systemic efficacy, there needs to be some preclinical evidence to suggest the drug's synergy with radiation. This should be demonstrated, at a minimum, in cell lines of the disease site of interest (e.g., lung cancer, breast cancer, pancreatic cancer, etc). Clonogenic survival assay is the gold standard assay for producing this type of data [81]. Data from in vitro culture experiments does not adequately reflect tumors grown in an intact organism, so it is preferable that drugs be tested in appropriate tumor models. While there may be certain advantages of one tumor model over another, none fully recapitulate the human condition quite like the actual patient. Therefore, while most of the guidelines recommend testing the drug in combination with radiation in at least 2 cell lines in vitro and at least 1 animal model experiment.

Biomarkers for patient selection

Targeted drug therapies appear to be most efficacious when used in patients harboring specific mutations that activate oncogenic pathways. Patient selection based on predictive biomarkers enriches for patients who will derive the greatest benefit from the drug of interest. The same consideration needs to be made when selecting agents to combine with radiation. There are a number of drugs that target downstream of RAS such as PI3K and MEK inhibitors may have some selectivity for RAS mutants [82, 83]. MEK inhibitors for KRAS mutant lung cancers as demonstrated in a recent phase II trial of combining docetaxel with AZD6244 demonstrated superior progression free survival compared to docetaxel alone [84]. TP53 mutations could help predict for efficacy for cell cycle drugs such as Chk1, Wee1, Aurora Kinase A, and PLK1 inhibitors [85]. Tumors harboring EGFR mutation or EML4-ALK translocation could be used to select patients to receive erlotinib or crizotinib in combination with radiation, either concurrently or sequentially. However, for agents where predictive biomarkers are not available, biomarker development should be integrated into clinical trials as exploratory aims utilizing biospecimens collected during these trials. Developing validated biomarkers that could predict for clinical response (or lack thereof) could help enrich patients who could optimally benefit from these therapies. These biomarkers could be used for patient selection or stratification factors in subsequent large phase III trials.

Design of clinical trials

Phase I testing must ensure the safety of combining these drugs with radiation. Since some agents may have overlapping toxicities, such as mucositis/esophagitis, or pneumonitis, it is important that compounds are tested for each site of interest, and not necessarily the disease of interest (i.e., pelvic cancers vs. thoracic cancers). Typical dose escalation studies combining current conventional therapies (radiation or chemoradiation) and escalating doses of the drug of interest establishes the maximum tolerated dose (MTD) of the drug with standard therapy. The dose limited toxicities (DLT) that help define the MTD need to be evaluated within a window of time that is suitable for assessing acute/intermediate term toxicities, such as esophagitis during treatment and pneumonitis post-treatment. Most radiation trials allow at least 10 weeks from the start of therapy to the first follow-up appointment after completion of radiation to assess for DLTs, but this is only for pragmatic reasons. Certainly toxicities such as TE fistulas, pneumonitis, and esophageal strictures, may not happen until much later. Therefore it is imperative to consider the fact that while the traditional 3+3 trial designs can be adopted for these types of trials, allowing a continuous assessment strategy such as TiTE CRM may ensure trials to be conducted more efficiently and safely.

The conduct of phase I trial in potentially curative patients is an ethical concern. Since the combination of agents with radiation has not been tested, potential dose limiting toxicities could limit the delivery of full dose therapy in an otherwise curative patient. Therefore the patient cohort must be carefully chosen to initiate for these types of studies, in that the potential benefit outweigh the potential risk that such treatment may pose. For example, drug therapy combined with radiation should target patients who would likely benefit, such as patients harboring certain mutations where there is a direct inhibitor (i.e., erlotinib for EGFR mutants, MEK inhibitors for KRAS mutants). Targeting these patients with investigational agents is an unmet need, and therefore may justify the risk that such therapies may pose. However, considerations need to be made to incorporate early phase studies in a palliative setting combining targeted agents with radiation alone. However, this is unlikely an ideal setting for long term drug development but rather as an in-human clinical validation of the synergistic effect of the drug with radiotherapy, and evaluate the toxicity of the combination. It provides preliminary data to further develop the drug in the curative setting.

In a classic 3+3 phase I design, 3–6 patients are usually enrolled at a particular dose level and observed for toxicity. Because of the longer evaluation period necessary to evaluate radiation toxicities, the trial halts accrual until toxicity is fully assessed at a particular dose level. This may be adequate for single institution studies where accrual may be slow, but this is particularly inefficient for multi-institutional studies where accrual could be faster. A more efficient design would be one that evaluates multiple agents simultaneously using a "master template." Different informed consents are given to patients depending on the drug group that the patient is enrolled on. This can be done as a "ping-pong" or "flip-flop" type of trial [86], where patients are enrolled into one group or another depending on the timing of the trial (Figure 25.3a). Depending on the number of agents, a "rolling" design will enroll patients into different drug groups at random depending if there are more than one drug groups to fill. This design will allow

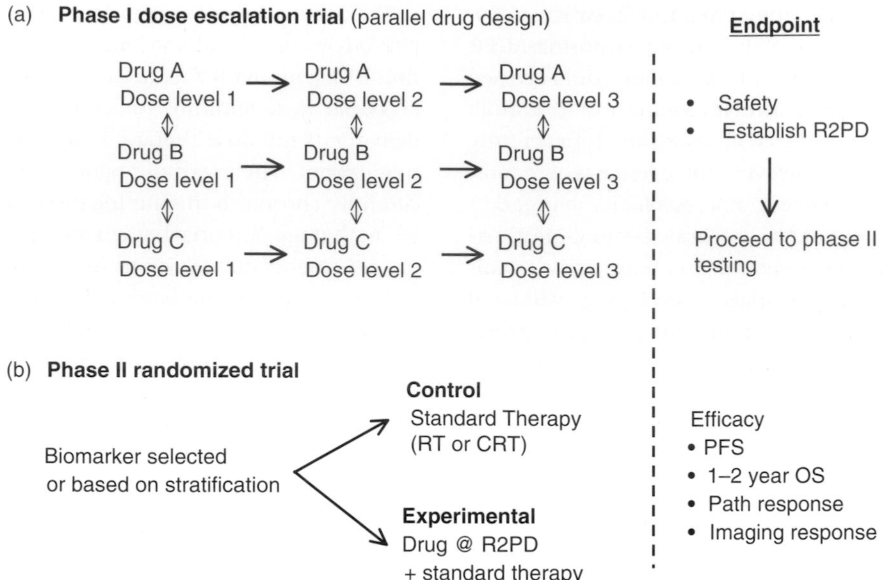

Figure 25.3 Phase I/II trial designs for bringing targeted agents into clinical testing with radiation therapy. a: Concept of a phase I trial determine the maximum tolerated dose (MTD) with a certain drug X in combination with radiation. In a classic 3+3 dose escalation design, 3 patients are enrolled at any one time to each drug X, and flip-flops to other drugs in the pipeline. This parallel drug trial design will allow the use of a "master" template. b: After determining the MTD of drug X, patients are enrolled into a phase II trial, that could select patients based on a particular validated biomarker or stratified based on a marker of interest, and randomized to either the control or the experimental (drug X + radiation) groups. The primary endpoints commonly employed are progression free survival, 1–2 year overall survival rates, pathologic or imaging responses.

continual accrual of patients in a parallel fashion while still maintaining the safety of a 3+3 trial design.

For drugs that have minimal added toxicities when combined with radiation or chemoradiation, the recommended phase II dosing (RP2D) should be guided by drug alone trials, or the maximal dose achievable based on the biologic effect of the drug on an effectiveness surrogate, such as phosphorylation of a protein within the tumor for a kinase inhibitor trial. This may be easier for some disease sites where the tumors are more assessable with a needle biopsy but may be difficult to implement for thoracic cancer trials given the difficulty to obtain multiple biopsies before, during, and after completion of radiation.

Once the MTD has been established for the drug of interest in combination with radiation, the phase II trial will provide some evidence for the efficacy of treatment while continuing the safety evaluation (Figure 25.3b). A commonly used primary endpoint for phase II testing is progression free survival, with overall survival usually as secondary exploratory endpoints. Response rate is typically not a useful endpoint to use in radiation trials given the high rates of clinical response seen with radiation or chemoradiation alone, the uncertainty of the optimal time to assess response given the differences in tumor growth kinetics, and the difficulty to discriminate inflammatory changes from residual disease. Besides progression free survival, other surrogate endpoints could be 1-yr local control rates or 1- or 2-year survival rates as compared to historical data in patients treated using standard of care, image response markers (such as FDG-PET response) or pathologic response (if surgery is done after neoadjuvant radiation therapy). Since the existence of historical data is unlikely to be available for these end points, it is recommended that future phase II trials testing novel radiation combinations be done as randomized-controlled trials. This is because historical controls (which are traditionally used for single arm phase II trials) are often inadequate controls since they often do not accurately account for factors not related to treatment, such as better staging and technologic improvements. This has plagued some phase II studies which had demonstrated superior outcomes compared to historical data, but to yield negative results in the phase III setting when compared to randomized control group [87].

Challenges and opportunities for the clinical development of targeted agents with radiation therapy

A main challenge to accelerate the development of drugs in combination with radiation is overcoming the tradition of how drug trials were conducted in the past. The traditional approach has been the testing of single agents for safety and response, and then combining them with approved cytotoxic chemotherapy in phase II/III testing. These types of trials are typically done in the palliative setting, usually in stage IV patients after multiple lines of failed therapies. Although some drugs have demonstrated improved disease outcomes, which ultimately leads to the coveted FDA approval, but often these long and tedious trials yield modest results with small improvement in disease free survival or overall survival. Pharmaceutical companies, including governmental regulatory agencies, should realize and invest in the potential of using these drugs in curative settings with radiation. Once these drugs demonstrate systemic activity, either as single agents or in combination with chemotherapy, and show preclinical evidence of sensitizing radiation therapy, there is the great potential that combining these targeted drugs and radiation can improve all disease outcome endpoints. There will likely be an improvement in locoregional control and reduced distant metastatic recurrences since the drug has only the burden to control invisible micrometastatic disease not visualized by staging studies. This will likely result in a much larger survival benefit compared to current standard approaches, thereby reducing the number of patients that are needed to show such survival differences. This also makes economic sense, since many drugs used in the metastatic setting often fail to meet cost effectiveness analysis given the small improvements in outcomes (sometimes only a few weeks detectable in large clinical trials) seen for the enormous expense of administering such therapies. So one could argue that drugs brought forward into clinical testing from the palliative setting into the curative setting will actually accelerate the development and approval of drugs. Using surrogate endpoints such as imaging or pathologic response may be helpful to expedite drug approval [88].

Conclusion

As radiation technology improves, the ability to bring drugs to combine with radiation becomes more feasible. Toxicities are likely related to the added effects of the combination therapy to the high dose regions, and not due to indiscriminate scatter of poorly positioned radiation dose. Given the enormous investments that pharmaceutical companies have made for drug development, there are numerous drugs with differing potency and safety profile that can target nearly every pathway in the cancer cell. Inhibiting these pathways often synergize with the damaging effect of radiation, and mutually may also help stave off the development of cross resistance if the therapies were administered alone. Concerted efforts to develop the preclinical evidence to support radiation sensitizing effects of these drugs, and to bring these drugs into early phase I/II clinical testing will be critical steps to improve disease outcomes in locally advanced lung cancer. Pharmaceutical companies and regulatory agencies should see the benefit that such trials will bring to the development of these drugs. With such efforts, a large improvement in survival outcomes may finally become a reality in the treatment of locally advanced lung cancers.

References

1 Liao ZX, Komaki RR, Thames Jr HD, *et al.* (2010) Influence of technologic advances on outcomes in patients with unresectable, locally advanced non-small-cell lung cancer receiving concomitant chemoradiotherapy. *International Journal of Radiation Oncology Biology Physics* 76(3): 775–81.

2 Berman AT, Rengan R (2008) New approaches to radiotherapy as definitive treatment for inoperable lung cancer. *Seminars in Thoracic and Cardiovascular Surgery*, 20(3): 188–97.

3 Onishi H, Shirato H, Nagata Y, *et al.* (2007) Hypofractionated stereotactic radiotherapy (HypoFXSRT) for stage I non-small cell lung cancer: Updated results of 257 patients in a Japanese multi-institutional study. *Journal of Thoracic Oncology*, 2(7 suppl.3): S94–S100.

4 Timmerman R, Paulus R, Galvin J, *et al.* (2010) Stereotactic body radiation therapy for inoperable early stage lung cancer. *JAMA*, 303(11): 1070–6.

5 Saunders M, Dische S, Barrett A, Harvey A, Griffiths G, Parmar M (1999) Continuous, hyperfractionated, accelerated radiotherapy (CHART) versus conventional radiotherapy in non-small cell lung cancer: Mature data from the randomised multicentre trial. *Radiotherapy and Oncology*, 52(2): 137–48.

6 Dillman RO, Seagren SL, Propert KJ, *et al.* (1990) A randomized trial of induction chemotherapy plus high-dose radiation versus radiation alone in Stage III non-small-cell lung cancer. *New England Journal of Medicine*, 323(14): 940–5.

7 Curran Jr WJ, Paulus R, Langer CJ, *et al.* (2011) Sequential vs concurrent chemoradiation for stage iii non-small cell lung cancer: Randomized phase III trial RTOG 9410. *Journal of the National Cancer Institute*, 103(19): 1452–60.

8 Vokes EE, Herndon Ii JE, Kelley MJ, *et al.* (2007) Induction chemotherapy followed by chemoradiotherapy compared with chemoradiotherapy alone for regionally advanced unresectable stage III non-small-cell lung cancer: Cancer and leukemia group B. *Journal of Clinical Oncology*, 25(13): 1698–1704.

9 Yamamoto S, Tsujino K, Ando M, *et al.* (2012) Is consolidation chemotherapy after concurrent chemoradiotherapy beneficial for locally advanced non-small cell lung cancer? A pooled analysis of the literature. *J Clin Oncol*, 30(suppl; abstr 7000).

10 Baumann M, Herrmann T, Koch R, *et al.* (2011) Final results of the randomized phase III CHARTWEL-trial (ARO 97-1) comparing hyperfractionated-accelerated versus conventionally fractionated radiotherapy in non-small cell lung cancer (NSCLC). *Radiotherapy and Oncology*, 100(1): 76–85.

11 Belderbos JSA, De Jaeger K, Heemsbergen WD, *et al.* (2003) First results of a phase I/II dose escalation trial in non-small cell lung cancer using three-dimensional conformal radiotherapy. *Radiotherapy and Oncology*, 66(2): 119–26.

12 Kong FM, Ten Haken RK, Schipper MJ, *et al.* (2005) High-dose radiation improved local tumor control and overall survival in patients with inoperable/unresectable non-small-cell lung cancer: Long-term results of a radiation dose escalation study. *International Journal of Radiation Oncology Biology Physics*, 63(2): 324–33.

13 Bradley JD, Moughan J, Graham MV, *et al.* (2010) A phase I/II radiation dose escalation study with concurrent chemotherapy for patients with inoperable stages I to III non-small-cell lung cancer: Phase I results of RTOG 0117. *International Journal of Radiation Oncology Biology Physics*, 77(2): 367–72.

14 Bradley J, Paulus R, Komaki R, *et al.* (2011) A randomized phase III comparison of standard-dose (60 Gy) versus high-dose (74 Gy) conformal chemoradiotherapy +/− Cetuximab for Stage IIIA/IIIB non-small cell lung cancer: Preliminary findings on radiation dose in RTOG 0617 *Proceedings of the American Society for Radiation Oncology Annual Meeting.* PL 01.

15 Vaupel P, Mayer A (2007) Hypoxia in cancer: Significance and impact on clinical outcome. *Cancer and Metastasis Reviews*, 26(2): 225–39.

16 Brizel DM, Sibley GS, Prosnitz LR, Scher RL, Dewhirst MW (1997) Tumor hypoxia adversely affects the prognosis of carcinoma of the head and neck. *International Journal of Radiation Oncology Biology Physics*, 38(2): 285–9.

17 Nordsmark M, Overgaard M, Overgaard J (1996) Pretreatment oxygenation predicts radiation response in advanced squamous cell carcinoma of the head and neck. *Radiotherapy and Oncology*, 41(1): 31–9.

18 Carmeliet P, Dor Y, Herber JM, *et al.* (1998) Role of HIF-1α in hypoxiamediated apoptosis, cell proliferation and tumour angiogenesis. *Nature*, 394(6692): 485–90.

19 Overgaard J, Hansen HS, Overgaard M, *et al.* (1998) A randomized double-blind phase III study of nimorazole as a hypoxic radiosensitizer of primary radiotherapy in supraglottic larynx and pharynx carcinoma. Results of the Danish Head and Neck Cancer Study (DAHANCA) Protocol 5-85. *Radiotherapy and Oncology*, 46(2): 135–46.

20 Rischin D, Peters LJ, O'Sullivan B, *et al.* (2010) Tirapazamine, cisplatin, and radiation versus cisplatin and radiation for advanced squamous cell carcinoma of the head and neck (TROG 02.02, headstart): A phase III trial of the trans-tasman radiation oncology group. *Journal of Clinical Oncology*, 28(18): 2989–95.

21 Schwartz DL, Powis G, Thitai-Kumar A, *et al.* The selective hypoxia inducible factor-1 inhibitor PX-478 provides in vivo radiosensitization through tumor stromal effects. *Molecular Cancer Therapeutics*, 8(4): 947–58.

22 Chaplin DJ, Horsman MR, Trotter MJ (1990) Effect of nicotinamide on the microregional heterogeneity of oxygen delivery within a murine tumor. *Journal of the National Cancer Institute*, 82(8): 672–6.

23 Bernier J, Denekamp J, Rojas A, *et al.* (1999) ARCON: Accelerated radiotherapy with carbogen and nicotinamide in non small cell lung cancer: A phase I/II study by the EORTC. *Radiotherapy and Oncology*, 52(2): 149–56.

24 Janssens GO, Rademakers SE, Terhaard CH, *et al.* (2012) Accelerated radiotherapy with carbogen and nicotinamide for laryngeal cancer: Results of a phase III randomized trial. *Journal of Clinical Oncology*, 30(15): 1777–83.

25 Jain RK (2005) Normalization of tumor vasculature: An emerging concept in antiangiogenic therapy. *Science*, 307(5706): 58–62.

26 Mauceri HJ, Hanna NN, Beckett MA, *et al.* (1998) Combined effects of angiostatin and ionizing radiation in antitumour therapy. *Nature*, 394(6690): 287–91.

27 Lee CG, Heijn M, Di Tomaso E, *et al.* (2000) Anti-vascular endothelial growth factor treatment augments tumor radiation response under normoxic or hypoxic conditions. *Cancer Research*, 60(19): 5565–70.

28 Williams KJ, Telfer BA, Brave S, *et al.* (2004) ZD6474, a potent inhibitor of vascular endothelial growth factor signaling, combined with radiotherapy: Schedule-dependent enhancement of antitumor activity. *Clinical Cancer Research*, 10(24): 8587–93.

29 Ranpura V, Hapani S, Wu S (2011) Treatment-related mortality with bevacizumab in cancer patients: A meta-analysis. *JAMA*, 305(5): 487–94.

30 Sandler A, Gray R, Perry MC, *et al.* (2006) Paclitaxel-carboplatin alone or with bevacizumab for non-small-cell lung cancer. *New England Journal of Medicine*, 355(24): 2542–50.

31 Socinski MA, Stinchcombe TE, Moore DT, *et al.* (2012) Incorporating bevacizumab and erlotinib in the combined-modality treatment of stage III non-small-cell lung cancer: Results of a phase I/II trial. *Journal of Clinical Oncology*, 30(32): 3953–9.

32 Spigel DR, Hainsworth JD, Yardley DA, *et al.* (2010) Tracheoesophageal fistula formation in patients with lung cancer treated with chemoradiation and bevacizumab. *Journal of Clinical Oncology*, 28(1): 43–8.

33 Normanno N, De Luca A, Bianco C, *et al.* (2006) Epidermal growth factor receptor (EGFR) signaling in cancer. *Gene*, 366(1): 2–16.

34 Mendelsohn J, Baselga J (2006) Epidermal growth factor receptor targeting in cancer. *Seminars in Oncology*, 33(4): 369–85.

35 Ciardiello F, Tortora G (2008) Drug therapy: EGFR antagonists in cancer treatment. *New England Journal of Medicine*, 358(11): 1160–74, 1096.

36 Harari PM, Huang SM (2001) Head and neck cancer as a clinical model for molecular targeting of therapy: Combining EGFR blockade with radiation. *International Journal of Radiation Oncology Biology Physics*, 49(2): 427–33.

37 Milas L, Mason K, Hunter N, *et al.* (2000) In vivo enhancement of tumor radioresponse by C225 antiepidermal growth factor receptor antibody. *Clinical Cancer Research*, 6(2): 701–8.

38 Bonner JA, Harari PM, Giralt J, *et al.* (2010) Radiotherapy plus cetuximab for locoregionally advanced head and neck cancer: 5-year survival data from a phase 3 randomised trial, and relation between cetuximab-induced rash and survival. *Lancet Oncology*, 11(1): 21–8.

39 Numico G, Franco P, Cristofano A, *et al.* (2013) Is the combination of Cetuximab with chemo-radiotherapy regimens worthwhile in the treatment of locally advanced head and neck cancer? A review of current evidence. *Critical Reviews in Oncology /Hematology*, 85(2): 112–20.

40 Blumenschein Jr GR, Paulus R, Curran WJ, *et al.* (2011) Phase II study of cetuximab in combination with chemoradiation in patients with stage IIIA/B non-small-cell lung cancer: RTOG 0324. *Journal of Clinical Oncology*, 29(17): 2312–18.

41 Bradley J, Masters G, Hu C, *et al.* (2013) An intergroup randomized phase III comparison of standard-dose (60 Gy) vs high-dose (74 Gy) chemoradiotherapy (CRT) +/− cetuximab (cetux) for stage III non-small cell lung cancer (NSCLC): results on cetux from RTOG 0617. *J Thorac Oncol*, 8(suppl. 2).

42 Komaki R, Allen PK, Wei X, *et al.* (2013) Value of adding erlotinib to thoracic radiation therapy with chemotherapy for stage III non-small cell lung cancer: a prospective phase II study. *J Thorac Oncol*, 8(suppl. 2).

43 Scagliotti GV, Parikh P, Von Pawel J, *et al.* (2008) Phase III study comparing cisplatin plus gemcitabine

with cisplatin plus pemetrexed in chemotherapy-naive patients with advanced-stage non-small-cell lung cancer. *Journal of Clinical Oncology*, 26(21): 3543–51.

44 Lee W, Jiang Z, Liu J, *et al.* (2010) The mutation spectrum revealed by paired genome sequences from a lung cancer patient. *Nature*, 465(7297): 473–7.

45 Gerlinger M, Rowan AJ, Horswell S, *et al.* (2012) Intratumor heterogeneity and branched evolution revealed by multiregion sequencing. *New England Journal of Medicine*, 366(10): 883–92.

46 Weir BA, Woo MS, Getz G, *et al.* (2007) Characterizing the cancer genome in lung adenocarcinoma. *Nature*, 450(7171): 893–8.

47 Govindan R, Ding L, Griffith M, *et al.* (2012) Genomic landscape of non-small cell lung cancer in smokers and never-smokers. *Cell*, 150(6): 1121–34.

48 Harrington KJ, Billingham LJ, Brunner TB, *et al.* (2011) Guidelines for preclinical and early phase clinical assessment of novel radiosensitisers. *British Journal of Cancer*, 105(5): 628–39.

49 Lawrence YR, Vikram B, Dignam JJ, *et al.* (2013) NCI-RTOG translational program strategic guidelines for the early-stage development of radiosensitizers. *Journal of the National Cancer Institute*, 105(1): 11–24.

50 Lin SH, George T, Ben-Josef E, *et al.* (2013) Opportunities and challenges in the era of molecularly targeted agents and radiation therapy. *Journal of the National Cancer Institute*. In press.

51 Hall EJ (ed.) (2012) *Radiobiology for the Radiologist*, 7th edn. Lippincott/Williams & Wilkins.

52 Veuger SJ, Curtin NJ, Richardson CJ, Smith GCM, Durkacz BW (2003) Radiosensitization and DNA repair inhibition by the combined use of novel inhibitors of DNA-dependent protein kinase and poly(ADP-ribose) polymerase-1. *Cancer Research*, 63(18): 6008–15.

53 Donawho CK, Luo Y, Penning TD, *et al.* (2007) ABT-888, an orally active poly(ADP-ribose) polymerase inhibitor that potentiates DNA-damaging agents in preclinical tumor models. *Clinical Cancer Research*, 13(9): 2728–37.

54 Farmer H, McCabe H, Lord CJ, *et al.* (2005) Targeting the DNA repair defect in BRCA mutant cells as a therapeutic strategy. *Nature*, 434(7035): 917–21.

55 Fong PC, Boss DS, Yap TA, *et al.* (2009) Inhibition of poly(ADP-ribose) polymerase in tumors from BRCA mutation carriers. *New England Journal of Medicine*, 361(2): 123–34.

56 Luo Y, Leverson JD (2005) New opportunities in chemosensitization and radiosensitization: Modulating the DNA-damage response. *Expert Review of Anticancer Therapy*, 5(2): 333–42.

57 Bridges KA, Hirai H, Buser CA, *et al.* (2011) MK-1775, a novel wee1 kinase inhibitor, radiosensitizes p53-defective human tumor cells. *Clinical Cancer Research*, 17(17): 5638–48.

58 Li J, Wang Y, Sun Y, Lawrence TS (2002) Wild type TP53 inhibits G2-phase checkpoint abrogation and radiosensitization induced by PD0166285 a WEE1 kinase inhibitor. *Radiation Research*, 157(3): 322–30.

59 Chen Z, Xiao Z, Gu WZ, *et al.* (2006) Selective Chk1 inhibitors differentially sensitize p53-deficient cancer cells to cancer therapeutics. *International Journal of Cancer*, 119(12): 2784–94.

60 Moretti L, Niermann K, Schleicher S, *et al.* (2011) MLN8054, A small molecule inhibitor of Aurora kinase A, sensitizes androgen-resistant prostate cancer to radiation. *International Journal of Radiation Oncology Biology Physics*, 80(4): 1189–97.

61 Wan XB, Fan XJ, Chen MY, *et al.* (2009) Inhibition of Aurora-A results in increased cell death in 3-dimensional culture microenvironment, reduced migration and is associated with enhanced radiosensitivity in human nasopharyngeal carcinoma. *Cancer Biology and Therapy*, 8(15).

62 Zhang F, Zhang T, Teng ZH, Zhang R, Wang JB, Mei QB (2008) Sensitization to γ-irradiation-induced cell cycle arrest and apoptosis by the histone deacetylase inhibitor trichostatin A in non-small cell lung cancer (NSCLC) cells. *Cancer Biology and Therapy*, 8(9): 823–31.

63 Zhang Y, Jung M, Dritschilo A (2004) Enhancement of radiation sensitivity of human squamous carcinoma cells by histone deacetylase inhibitors. *Radiation Research*, 161(6): 667–74.

64 Brieger J, Mann SA, Pongsapich W, Koutsimpelas D, Fruth K, Mann WJ (2012) Pharmacological genome demethylation increases radiosensitivity of head and neck squamous carcinoma cells. *International Journal of Molecular Medicine*, 29(3): 505–9.

65 Zhu WG, Hileman T, Ke Y, *et al.* (2004) 5-Aza-2′-deoxycytidine Activates the p53/p21 Waf1/Cip1 Pathway to Inhibit Cell Proliferation. *Journal of Biological Chemistry*, 279(15): 15161–6.

66 Ree AH, Dueland S, Folkvord S, *et al.* (2010) Vorinostat, a histone deacetylase inhibitor, combined with pelvic palliative radiotherapy for gastrointestinal carcinoma: The Pelvic Radiation and Vorinostat (PRAVO) phase 1 study. *Lancet Oncology*, 11(5): 459–64.

67 Isaacs JS, Xu W, Neckers L (2003) Heat shock protein 90 as a molecular target for cancer therapeutics. *Cancer Cell,* 3(3): 213–17.

68 Camphausen K, Tofilon PJ (2007) Inhibition of Hsp90: A multitarget approach to radiosensitization. *Clinical Cancer Research,* 13(15): 4326–30.

69 Ying W, Du Z, Sun L, *et al.* (2012) Ganetespib, a unique triazolone-containing Hsp90 inhibitor, exhibits potent antitumor activity and a superior safety profile for cancer therapy. *Molecular Cancer Therapeutics,* 11(2): 475–84.

70 Pardoll DM (2012) Immunology beats cancer: A blueprint for successful translation. *Nature Immunology,* 13(12): 1129–32.

71 Hodi FS, O'Day SJ, McDermott DF, *et al.* (2010) Improved survival with ipilimumab in patients with metastatic melanoma. *New England Journal of Medicine,* 363(8): 711–23.

72 Kantoff PW, Higano CS, Shore ND, *et al.* (2010) Sipuleucel-T immunotherapy for castration-resistant prostate cancer. *New England Journal of Medicine,* 363(5): 411–22.

73 Topalian SL, Hodi FS, Brahmer JR, *et al.* (2012) Safety, activity, and immune correlates of anti-PD-1 antibody in cancer. *New England Journal of Medicine,* 366(26): 2443–54.

74 Brahmer JR, Tykodi SS, Chow LQM, *et al.* (2012) Safety and activity of anti-PD-L1 antibody in patients with advanced cancer. *New England Journal of Medicine,* 366(26): 2455–65.

75 Wolchok JD, Kluger H, Callahan MK, *et al.* (2013) Nivolumab plus Ipilimumab in advanced melanoma. *New England Journal of Medicine,* 369(2): 122–33.

76 Lee Y, Auh SL, Wang Y, *et al.* (2009) Therapeutic effects of ablative radiation on local tumor require CD8+ T cells: changing strategies for cancer treatment. *Blood,* 114: 589–95.

77 Kaminski JM, Shinohara E, Summers JB, Niermann KJ, Morimoto A, Brousal J (2005) The controversial abscopal effect. *Cancer Treatment Reviews,* 31(3): 159–72.

78 Demaria S, Ng B, Devitt ML, *et al.* (2004) Ionizing radiation inhibition of distant untreated tumors (abscopal effect) is immune mediated. *International Journal of Radiation Oncology Biology Physics,* 58(3): 862–70.

79 Postow MA, Callahan MK, Barker CA, *et al.* (2012) Immunologic correlates of the abscopal effect in a patient with melanoma. *New England Journal of Medicine,* 366(10): 925–31.

80 Seung SK, Curti BD, Crittenden M, *et al.* (2012) Phase 1 study of stereotactic body radiotherapy and interleukin-2: Tumor and immunological responses. *Science Translational Medicine,* 4(137).

81 Franken NAP, Rodermond HM, Stap J, Haveman J, van Bree C (2006) Clonogenic assay of cells in vitro. *Nature Protocols,* 1(5): 2315–19.

82 Wee S, Jagani Z, Kay KX, *et al.* (2009) PI3K pathway activation mediates resistance to MEK inhibitors in KRAS mutant cancers. *Cancer Research,* 69(10): 4286–93.

83 Williams TM, Flecha AR, Keller P, *et al.* (2012) Cotargeting MAPK and PI3K signaling with concurrent radiotherapy as a strategy for the treatment of pancreatic cancer. *Molecular Cancer Therapeutics,* 11(5): 1193–1202.

84 Jänne PA, Shaw AT, Pereira JR, *et al.* (2013) Selumetinib plus docetaxel for KRAS-mutant advanced non-small-cell lung cancer: A randomised, multicentre, placebo-controlled, phase 2 study. *Lancet Oncology,* 14(1): 38–47.

85 Sur S, Pagliarini R, Bunz F, *et al.* (2009) A panel of isogenic human cancer cells suggests a therapeutic approach for cancers with inactivated p53. *Proceedings of the National Academy of Sciences of the United States of America,* 106(10): 3964–9.

86 Choy H, Jain AK, Moughan J, *et al.* (2009) RTOG 0017: A phase I trial of concurrent gemcitabine/carboplatin or gemcitabine/paclitaxel and radiation therapy ("ping-pong trial") followed by adjuvant chemotherapy for patients with favorable prognosis inoperable stage IIIA/B non-small cell lung cancer. *Journal of Thoracic Oncology,* 4(1): 80–6.

87 Hanna N, Neubauer M, Yiannoutsos C, *et al.* (2008) Phase III study of cisplatin, etoposide, and concurrent chest radiation with or without consolidation docetaxel in patients with inoperable stage III non-small-cell lung cancer: The Hoosier Oncology Group and U.S. Oncology. *Journal of Clinical Oncology,* 26(35): 5755–60.

88 Pazdur R (2008) Endpoints for assessing drug activity in clinical trials. *Oncologist,* 13(suppl. 2): 19–21.

CHAPTER 26

EGFR Tyrosine Kinase Inhibitors and Monoclonal Antibodies: Clinical Trial Review

Kathryn F. Mileham,[1] Edward S. Kim,[1] and William N. William Jr[2]

[1]Solid Tumor Oncology, Levine Cancer Institute, Carolinas HealthCare System, Charlotte, NC, USA

[2]Department of Thoracic/Head and Neck Medical Oncology, The University of Texas MD Anderson Cancer Center, Houston, TX, USA

Background

In 1962, Stanley Cohen isolated a novel protein from mice that demonstrated increased growth of incisors and eyelids in newborn animals [1]. In 1986, Cohen was awarded a Nobel Prize for the discovery of what we now call epidermal growth factor (EGF). The importance of EGF and its family of related receptors to cancer development and proliferation has since become increasing evident. Drugs that target the EGF signaling pathway are now widely utilized.

There are two classes of anti-epidermal growth factor receptor (EGFR) agents that have been tested extensively in patients with non-small cell lung cancer (NSCLC): the low molecular weight tyrosine kinase inhibitors (TKIs) and the monoclonal antibodies (mAbs). TKIs such as gefitinib, and erlotinib have been approved for treatment in patients with advanced NSCLC.

In this chapter, we will review the main clinical trials that have evaluated the role of EGFR-targeted agents for treatment of recurrent/metastatic NSCLCs, including front-line (in combination with chemotherapy, sequentially with chemotherapy, or as single-agent), maintenance and salvage therapy, as well as novel drugs related to the EGFR axis.

Front-line therapy: combination anti-EGFR therapy and chemotherapy for molecularly unselected NSCLC patients

Front-line erlotinib in combination with platinum-doublet chemotherapy for treatment of advanced NSCLC has been evaluated in two large multicenter, randomized placebo-controlled clinical trials.

In the phase III TRIBUTE trial, patients with advanced NSCLC were randomized to either erlotinib 150 mg/day or placebo combined with up to six cycles of carboplatin-paclitaxel, followed by continuation of erlotinib or placebo [2]. In the 1059 patients assessed, the median overall survival (mOS) (primary endpoint) as well as the objective response rate (ORR) and time to progression (secondary endpoints) were not statistically different between the two groups (mOS 10.6 vs 10.5 months in erlotinib vs placebo, respectively; HR,

Lung Cancer, Fourth Edition. Edited by Jack A. Roth, Waun Ki Hong and Ritsuko U. Komaki.

0.99; CI 0.86–1.16; p = 0.95). However, because of emerging data regarding efficacy of EGFR-TKIs in never-smokers, the statistical plan of TRIBUTE was revised prior to unblinding to review the overall survival in this population based on previously collected smoking history screening case report forms. Patients who reported to be never-smokers experienced a prolonged median overall survival if treated on the erlotinib arm (22.5 vs 10.1 months in 72 vs 44 patients, respectively) independent of tumor histology [2].

TALENT was a phase III, randomized, double-blind, placebo-controlled, multicenter trial that evaluated the efficacy and safety of erlotinib 150 mg/day or placebo in combination with up to six cycles of cisplatin-gemcitabine followed by maintenance erlotinib or placebo as first-line treatment for advanced NSCLC [3]. Of note, upon disease progression, patients could continue with study treatment (erlotinib or placebo) with or without second-line therapy or receive second-line therapy alone. There were no differences in overall survival (primary endpoint) or time to progression, response rate, duration of response, or quality of life (secondary endpoints). The median overall survival was 43 weeks versus 44.1 weeks in the erlotinib and placebo groups, respectively (HR 1.06). A retrospective evaluation of patients enrolled in TALENT that never smoked (N = 18) had an increased overall survival and progression free survival when treated with erlotinib, mirroring the observations from TRIBUTE.

As seen with erlotinib in combination with platinum-doublet chemotherapy in TRIBUTE and TALENT, no clinical benefit with gefitinib in combination with platinum-doublet chemotherapy was identified in phase III trials [4, 5]. In the two multinational, randomized, double-blind, placebo-controlled INTACT-1 and INTACT-2 trials, more than 2100 chemo-naive patients were randomized to cisplatin-gemcitabine (INTACT-1) or carboplatin-paclitaxel (INTACT 2) plus gefitinib 250 mg/day or plus gefitinib 500 mg/day or plus placebo. The progression free survival in INTACT-1 was 5.8 months versus 5.5 months versus 6.0 months, respectively (p = 0.76). The progression free survival in INTACT-2 was 5.3 months versus 4.6 months versus 5.0 months, respectively (p = 0.06). Neither trial revealed statistically significant improvements in overall response rate or median overall survival.

Taken together, TRIBUTE, TALENT, INTACT-1, and INTACT-2 do not demonstrate any clinical benefit with concurrent use of erlotinib or gefitinib with chemotherapy in unselected patients, and this combination regimen is not recommended for front-line treatment of advanced NSCLC.

Cetuximab is a chimeric monoclonal IgG1 antibody that blocks EGFR signaling. Two phase III studies investigated the efficacy of cetuximab in combination with platinum-based chemotherapy in advanced NSCLC.

FLEX was a multinational, multicenter, open-label, phase III trial in patients with EGFR-expressing advanced NSCLC treated front-line with either cisplatin-vinorelbine plus cetuximab or cisplatin-vinorelbine alone [6]. Chemotherapy was administered for up to six cycles, and cetuximab was continued weekly until disease progression or unacceptable toxicities. In the intention-to-treat analysis of 1125 randomized patients, mOS (primary endpoint) was prolonged in those treated with cisplatin-vinorelbine plus cetuximab compared with those treated with chemotherapy alone (11.3 months vs 10.1 months; HR, 0.871; CI 0.762–0.996; p = 0.044).

The randomized, phase III BMS099 trial was a multicenter, open-label study enrolling 676 patients without restrictions on histology or EGFR expression/mutation for front-line treatment of advanced NSCLC with either taxane-carboplatin plus cetuximab or taxane-carboplatin alone [7]. The use of paclitaxel or docetaxel was at the discretion of the investigator. As seen with FLEX, chemotherapy was administered for up to six cycles, and cetuximab was continued weekly until disease progression or unacceptable toxicities. ORR was significantly improved with the addition of cetuximab to taxane-carboplatin (25.7% versus 17.2%, p = 0.007); however this was a secondary endpoint. Progression free survival, the primary endpoint, as assessed by independent radiologic review committee (IRRC), was not significantly different with the addition of cetuximab. The mPFS-IRRC was 4.40 months with cetuximab plus chemotherapy versus

4.24 months with chemotherapy alone (HR, 0.902; CI 0.761–1.069; p = 0.236). Median overall survival favored cetuximab however this was not statistically significant (9.69 months vs 8.39 months; HR, 0.890; CI 0.754–1.051; p = 0.169). Notably, the results were similar in magnitude to the significant overall survival improvement from FLEX.

Although BMS099 did not meet its endpoint of PFS, BMS099 and FLEX had similar outcomes. Both revealed statistically significance increases in ORR with the addition of cetuximab to chemotherapy, and both demonstrated about a 1.3 month increase in mOS, although BMS099 lacked power to detect a statistically significant difference of this magnitude. These results contrast those found with EGFR-TKIs when combined with chemotherapy, which may be attributed to the different mechanism of action of the monoclonal antibody. Despite the positive FLEX results, cetuximab has not been approved by regulatory agencies for treatment of NSCLCs.

The combination of two monoclonal antibodies – bevacizumab against VEGF and cetuximab against EGFR – showed promising results in SWOG 0536 [8]. In this safety and efficacy phase II single arm study, around 100 patients with advanced NSCLC were treated front-line with carboplatin, paclitaxel, bevacizumab, and cetuximab. Chemotherapy was administered for up to 6 cycles, while bevacizumab and cetuximab were continued until progression. The feasibility endpoint was met. Secondary endpoints included ORR, PFS, OS, and toxicity. The ORR was 53%; PFS was 7 months, and OS was 14 months. These results have led to the large and currently ongoing phase III SWOG 0819 trial of carboplatin-paclitaxel and bevacizumab (in eligible patients) with or without cetuximab in patients with advanced NSCLC.

Front-line therapy: chemotherapy and intermittent anti-EGFR therapy

Because preclinial data suggested potential antagonism from TKI-induced cell cycle arrest reducing phase-specific activity of chemotherapy [9–11], sequential administration of chemotherapy and EGFR-TKIs was tested as another means of combining therapies in the front-line setting.

FAST-ACT was a randomized phase II study testing this concept [12]. After receiving gemcitabine-platinum chemotherapy on days 1 and 8, 154 patients received either erlotinib 150 mg/day or placebo on days 15–28 every four weeks. Responding patients continued to receive erlotinib or placebo until progression or unacceptable toxicities. The primary endpoint was nonprogression rate (NPR: CR+PR+SD) at eight weeks using RECIST. The NPR at eight weeks was 80.3% in the erlotinib arm and 76.9% in the placebo arm. Because PFS was significantly improved with the addition of erlotinib (29.4 weeks vs 23.4 weeks; adjusted HR 0.47; p = 0.0002), a large randomized phase III clinical trial with sequential use of erlotinib after chemotherapy called FAST-ACT II was launched. This 451-patient placebo-controlled, double-blinded study confirmed a significantly prolonged PFS (primary endpoint) in those randomized to receive erlotinib over placebo with a median PFS of 7.6 versus 6.0 months, respectively (HR 0.57, 95% CI 0.46–0.70, p < 0.0001) [13]. The ORR was also significantly improved with erlotinib compared with placebo (42.9% versus 17.8%, p<0.0001). Overall survival was another secondary endpoint, however these results may be confounded by the 73% crossover rate from placebo to second-line erlotinib. Biomarker analysis of 283 patients revealed that EGFR mutation positive patients experienced the strongest PFS benefit with intercalated erlotinib and front-line chemotherapy [14].

Another trial did not have promising results when utilizing erlotinib sequentially with chemotherapy [15]. In this randomized phase II trial, 143 patients were assigned to either erlotinib 150 mg/day or carboplatin-paclitaxel chemotherapy followed by erlotinib 150 mg/day on days 2–15 every three weeks for four cycles followed by erlotinib until disease progression. The six-month PFS rates (primary endpoint) were 26% for chemotherapy plus erlotinib followed by erlotinib versus 31% for erlotinib alone. Median PFS was 4.57 and 2.69 months, respectively. This smaller phase II trial did not support to use of sequential EGFR-TKIs with chemotherapy.

Front-line therapy: anti-EGFR single agent

Several phase II trials evaluated the efficacy of single-agent TKIs as front-line treatment for advanced NSCLC because of encouraging findings in second- and third-line management. The results from these studies on molecularly unselected patient populations were not overwhelmingly promising [16, 17]. However, when responses were evaluated further based on EGFR mutation status, findings suggested that those with EGFR-mutant tumors achieved better clinical outcomes [17–20]. Additional phase II trials investigated single-agent TKIs as front-line treatment in poor performance patients, again unselected for EGFR-mutated lung cancers. Response rates were low, and PFS and mOS were not significantly prolonged [21, 22].

The phase III TOPICAL study [23] randomized 670 chemotherapy-naïve patients deemed unsuitable for chemotherapy (because of poor performance status or presence of several comorbidities) to receive erlotinib versus placebo. Median overall survival (the primary endpoint of the study) did not differ between the two treatment arms (3.7 versus 3.6 months for erlotinib and placebo, respectively, HR 0.94, 95% CI 0.81–1.10, p = 0·46).

These phase II and III studies indicated no evidence to support the use of EGFR TKIs as front-line treatment for unselected patients not candidates for chemotherapy.

There are also studies in unselected EGFR populations evaluating single-agent TKIs as front-line treatment in elderly. One trial was a phase II, open-label, multicenter study evaluating erlotinib 150 mg/day in chemotherapy-naïve patients at least age 70 with advanced NSCLC [24]. Eighty patients were treated. The median OS (primary endpoint) was 10.9 months while one- and two-year survival rates (also primary endpoints) were 46% and 19%, respectively. The presence of an EGFR mutation correlated with disease control, prolonged time to progression, as well as survival. The authors concluded that this monotherapy was active and well-tolerated. These findings were contrasted with those from INVITE which was also a phase II, open-label, multicenter study evaluating a TKI in chemotherapy-naïve patients at least age 70 with advanced NSCLC [25]. This trial differed in that it was randomized to a chemotherapy arm (vinorelbine) and the TKI utilized was gefitinib (250 mg/day) rather than erlotinib. The primary endpoint was PFS and was 2.7 months in the gefitinib group versus 2.9 months in the vinorelbine group (HR 1.19; CI, 0.85–1.65; p = 0.310). There was no improvement in RR or OS, however the quality of life assessment and toxicity profile favored gefitinib.

TORCH was an international, multicenter, open-label randomized phase III trial conducted in Italy and Canada designed for patients with advanced NSCLC to evaluate whether front-line erlotinib followed at progression by cisplatin-gemcitabine was non-inferior in OS compared with the reverse standard sequence [26]. When this trial was planned, erlotinib was registered for unselected patients based on the efficacy of erlotinib across all patients in BR.21, so no clinical or biologic factors were applied to patient population selection. At the first planned interim analysis, erlotinib followed by chemotherapy was inferior to chemotherapy followed by erlotinib, so the study was terminated. Median OS was 11.6 months in the standard group and 8.7 months in the experimental group. The unadjusted HR of death for the experimental arm was 1.22 (95% CI, 1.03–1.44).

Thus, the current data suggest that within an unselected population, even those with reduced performance or advanced age, single agent EGFR-TKIs in the front-line setting do not provide clinical benefit in RR, PFS, or OS.

As trial results matured and information about EGFR-mutations and tyrosine kinase inhibition evolved, it became more apparent that subsequent trials needed more tailoring to achieve better RR, PFS, and OS with EGFR TKIs. Studies using single-agent TKIs for treatment of advanced NSCLC in second- and third-line therapy compared with best supportive care care [27, 28] or standard chemotherapy [29] were promising. Subgroups of responders were identified including women, never-smokers, Asian origin, and adenocarcinoma histology [30]. Ultimately, additional studies revealed a high incidence of EGFR mutations in these patients and subsequent studies concluded that front-line therapy with EGFR-TKIs resulted in improved objective response rates and progression-free survival in patients with these mutations [31, 32].

By December 2010, four randomized phase III trials comparing front-line gefitinib to platinum-based chemotherapy in patients with advanced NSCLC were reported or published. These include IPASS, First-SIGNAL, WJTOG3405, and NEJ002 [33–36].

IPASS was designed to study a select population of advanced NSCLC patients (never or former light smokers with adenocarcinoma histology) to receive front-line treatment with either carboplatin-paclitaxel or gefitinib in a 1:1 randomization [40]. In this 1217 patient open-labeled, randomized phase III trial in East Asia, gefitinib was not only noninferior to carboplatin-paclitaxel based on primary endpoint of PFS (5.7 vs 5.8 months, HR, 0.741, 95% CI 0.651–0.845; $p < 0.0001$) but also was superior to the chemotherapy arm with a 12-month rate of progression-free survival of 24.9% with gefitinib and 6.7% with carboplatin-paclitaxel (HR, 0.74; $P < 0.0001$). EGFR mutation data were evaluated in 437 (35.9%) of the patients and 261 (59.7%) were positive. Of these, 140 had deletions at exon 19, 111 had mutations at exon 21 (L858R), 11 had mutations at exon 20 (T790M), 10 had other mutations, and 11 had multiple mutations. The presence of the EGFR mutation correlated with a better outcome with gefitinib treatment. The PFS was significantly longer among those who were mutation positive and treated with gefitinib (HR, 0.48; 95% CI, 0.36–0.64; $p < 0.0001$); and the PFS was significantly shorter among those who were mutation negative and treated with gefitinib (HR, 2.85; 95% CI, 2.05–3.98, $p < 0.0001$). Also in this EGFR mutation subgroup, the response rate was 71.2% for gefitinib versus 47.3% for carboplatin-paclitaxel ($p = 0.0001$). Quality of life was also significantly improved in those treated with gefitinib. Toxicities were tolerable. Overall, IPASS highlighted the distinct nature of EGFR-mutant lung cancer and its selected response to TKI intervention.

Following IPASS, First-SIGNAL, NEJ002 and WJTOG3405 are three additional phase III studies utilizing gefitinib versus chemotherapy as front-line treatment for EGFR-mutated advanced NSCLC patients (Table 26.1). First-SIGNAL was a randomized phase III trial trial of 313 Korean never-smokers with advanced lung adenocarcinoma treated front-line with either gefitinib 250 mg/day or gemcitabine-cisplatin chemotherapy [34]. Overall survival (primary endpoint) was similar between treatment groups, failing to show hypothesized superiority of gefitinib to chemotherapy (22.3 months for gefitinib vs 22.9 months for gemcitabine-cisplatin, HR, 0.932; 95% CI, 0.716–1.213; $p = 0.604$). However, response rates were higher with gefitinib (55% versus 46%) and the one-year PFS rates were higher with gefitinib (16.7% versus 2.8%) [37]. In First-SIGNAL, EGFR mutation status was only known in 96 patients with only 42 of whom were positive. Within this subset, median PFS was longer for patients treated with gefitinib (8.4 months versus 6.7 months; HR, 0.613; 95% CI, 0.308–1.221; $p = 0.084$) [34].

Both randomized phase III trials conducted by Japanese institutions comparing gefitinib to chemotherapy in front-line treatment of advanced NSCLC showed statistically significant and clinically relevant increased PFS in patients with EGFR mutations treated with gefitinib. NEJ002 study compared gefitinib with carboplatin-paclitaxel as front-line treatment for Japanese patients with EGFR-mutated advanced NSCLC [36]. A significant benefit in PFS was demonstrated in favor of gefitinib at a planned interim analysis, so the study stopped accrual at 230 patients. At the final analysis of 228 patients, median PFS was 10.8 months with gefitinib and 5.4 months with carboplatin-paclitaxel (HR 0.30; 95% CI 0.22–0.41; $p < 0.001$). Overall response rate was also significantly higher with gefitinib (73.7% versus 30.7%; $p < 0.001$). Subsequent analysis updated the survival data and no significant difference was seen in overall survival between the two treatment groups [38]. This finding is possibly due to extensive crossover with 96% of patients treated with chemotherapy subsequently receiving gefitinib and 90% of those treated with gefitinib switching to carboplatin-paclitaxel in second-line. The median OS was 27.7 months with gefitinib and 26.6 months with carboplatin-paclitaxel (HR 0.887; 95% CI 0.634–1.241; $p = 0.483$). No

Table 26.1 Phase III trials of EGFR TKIs versus chemotherapy in front-line NSCLC with EGFR mutations

Trial	Location	EGFR TKI	Chemotherapy	Number of Patients	Median PFS (Months)	HR	Response Rate (%)
IPASS (Mok 2009)	East Asia	gefitinib	carboplatin-paclitaxel	261	9.5 vs. 6.3	0.48 (0.36–0.64) $p < 0.0001$	71.2% vs. 47.3%
First-SIGNAL (Lee 2009)	Korea	gefitinib	cisplatin-gemcitabine	42	8.4 vs. 6.7	0.61 (0.31–1.22) $p = 0.084$	84.6% vs. 37.5%
NEJ002 (Maemondo 2010)	Japan	gefitinib	carboplatin-paclitaxel	230	10.8 vs. 5.4	0.30 (0.22–0.41) $p < 0.001$	73.7% vs. 30.7%
WJTOG3405 (Mitsudomi 2010)	Japan	gefitinib	cisplatin-docetaxel	177	9.2 vs. 6.3	0.49 (0.34–0.71) $p < 0.0001$	62.1% vs. 32.2%
EURTAC (Rosell 2012)	Spain, France, and Italy	erlotinib	cisplatin-docetaxel cisplatin-gemcitabine carboplatin-docetaxel carboplatin-gemcitabine	173	9.7 vs. 5.2	0.37 (0.25–0.54) $p < 0.0001$	58% vs. 15%
OPTIMAL (Zhou 2011)	China	erlotinib	carboplatin-gemcitabine	165	13.1 vs. 4.6	0.16 (0.1–0.26) $p < 0.0001$	83% vs. 36%

significant difference in OS was defined based on subset analyses.

The open-label WJTOG3405 phase III study involved 177 chemotherapy-naive Japanese patients with advanced NSCLC and EGFR mutations (exon 19 deletion or L858R point mutation) [35]. Due to molecular selection, the study population was more than two-thirds women in both arms, more than two-thirds never-smokers in both arms, and a large majority of adenocarcinoma. Eligible patients were randomized to either gefitinib 250 mg/day or cisplatin-docetaxel. The study reached its primary endpoint of progression free survival. Of the 172 patients included in survival analyses, the gefitinib arm showed significantly longer PFS compared with the cisplatin-docetaxel arm (9.2 months versus 6.3 months; HR, 0.489; 95% CI, 0.336–0.710; $p < 0.0001$).

Two phase III trials have been conducted to test the efficacy of erlotinib as front-line treatment of patients with EGFR-mutant positive advanced NSCLC. EURTAC, performed by the Spanish Lung Cancer Group, is a prospective, randomized phase III trial comparing front-line erlotinib versus platinum-based chemotherapy in advanced NSCLC patients with EGFR mutations [39]. Ninety-nine percent of the 173 patients were Caucasian. Permitted chemotherapy regimens including cisplatin-docetaxel, cisplatin-gemcitabine, carboplatin-docetaxel, and carboplatin-gemcitabine were administered every three weeks for four cycles. Erlotinib was superior to chemotherapy for PFS (primary endpoint) in this patient population (9.7 months vs 5.2 months; HR, 0.37; 95% CI, 0.25–0.54; $p < 0.0001$). Response rate was also improved with erlotinib (58% vs 15%) but mOS was not significantly different (22.9 months vs 18.8 months; HR, 0.80; $p = 0.42$).

OPTIMAL is an open-labeled, randomized phase III trial in China comparing efficacy as well as tolerability of front-line erlotinib versus gemcitabine-carboplatin in advanced NSCLC patients with EGFR mutations [40]. Although the design was similar to that of EURTAC, this patient population included 165 Asians. Treatment with erlotinib resulted in significantly longer PFS (primary endpoint) compared with chemotherapy (13.1 months vs 4.6 months; HR, 0.16; 95% CI, 0.1–0.26; $p < 0.0001$). Erlotinib was also superior in response rate (83% vs 36%).

Collectively, the results of the aforementioned trials demonstrate that testing for EGFR mutations is the best way to identify patients who would benefit from first-line EGFR TKI treatment. There is consistent benefit across the studies in terms of improvement of progression-free survival, response rates and quality of life in favor of erlotinib/gefitinib compared to chemotherapy. None of the studies demonstrated an overall survival benefit, likely because of the high cross over rates to the alternative therapy at the time of disease progression. Based on these data, it has become common practice to assess EGFR mutation status in treatment-naïve patients with recurrent/metastatic disease; patients with mutant tumors are preferentially treated with EGFR TKIs; patients with wild-type tumors should not receive an EGFR TKI first-line.

The addition of erlotinib to first-line carboplatin and paclitaxel was also evaluated in treatment-naïve patients who were never or light former smokers [41]. The primary endpoint of PFS was similar in 81 patients assigned to erlotinib alone versus 100 patients assigned to chemotherapy plus erlotinib (5.0 vs 6.6 months, $p = 0.1988$). Patients with EGFR mutations had better outcomes in both arms. As such, there does not seem to be an advantage of adding chemotherapy to first-line EGFR TKIs in patients selected by demographical or mutation criteria.

Maintenance therapy

The double-blind, randomized phase III SATURN study was initiated to evaluate erlotinib as maintenance therapy after first-line platinum-based chemotherapy in patients with advanced NSCLC [42]. Patients with no evidence of progression after four cycles of chemotherapy were randomized either to erlotinib 150 mg/day or placebo until progression or toxicity. The primary endpoint was PFS and a second primary endpoint was PFS in those with EGFR mutations. In both arms, there were almost equal percentages of adenocarcinoma and squamous cell carcinoma represented. The study met both primary endpoints. The PFS for all patients was significantly prolonged with erlotinib versus placebo (HR, 0.71; 95% CI 0.62–0.82; $p < 0.0001$). PFS was also significantly prolonged in those with an EGFR mutation (HR, 0.10, 95% CI 0.04–0.25; $p<0.0001$) or without an EGFR mutation (HR, 0.78, 95% CI 0.63–0.96; $p = 0.0185$).

ATLAS was a randomized, double-blind, placebo-controlled phase IIIb trial that compared bevacizumab alone with or without erlotinib after completion of platinum-containing doublet chemotherapy plus bevacizumab [43]. The trial was closed after the second planned interim analysis, when the endpoint of PFS was achieved. Median PFS was 4.8 months for those treated with bevacizumab plus erlotinib versus 3.7 months for those treated with bevacizumab alone (HR, 0.722; 95% CI 0.592–0.881; $p = 0.0012$). Thus ATLAS concluded that patients with advanced NSCLC treated front-line with chemotherapy plus bevacizumab, maintenance bevacizumab plus erlotinib resulted in significant prolongation of PFS with a typical and anticipated side effect profile.

Erlotinib has been approved by regulatory agencies to be used as maintenance therapy in patients that have a CR, PR, or SD to first-line therapy (in the United States), or in patients that have SD to first-line therapy (in Europe).

Salvage therapy

The NCIC CTG BR.21 phase III randomized trial compared erlotinib with placebo in advanced NSCLC patient who had failed first- or second-line chemotherapy [27]. The 731 patients were randomized in a 2:1 fashion to receive either erlotinib 150 mg/day versus placebo. The ORR was higher in the erlotinib group at 8.9% versus <1% in the placebo group ($p < 0.001$). The median duration of response was 7.9 months and 3.7 months, respectively; and the progression free survival was 2.2 months and 1.8 months, respectively (HR, 0.61, $p < 0.001$). The OS favored erlotinib (6.7 months vs 4.7 months; HR, 0.70; $p < 0.001$). Subgroup analyses revealed a greater response to erlotinib in women, nonsmokers, Asians, and adenocarcinoma. The most common toxicities associated with erlotinib including rash and diarrhea were manageable, especially since cancer symptoms and quality of life were better controlled when treated with erlotinib over placebo [27].

Based on promising results from the IDEAL-1 and IDEAL-2 phase II trials [44, 45], the Iressa Survival Evaluation in Lung Cancer (ISEL) was launched. ISEL was a placebo-controlled phase III study investigating the effect on survival of gefitinib as second-line or third-line treatment in patients with advanced NSCLC [30]. In the planned two–to-one assignment, 1129 patients were randomized to 250 mg/day of gefitinib and 563 to placebo. The primary endpoint was survival in the overall population of patients and those with adenocarcinoma. At the 7.2-month median follow up, median OS was not significantly different in the overall population (5.6 months vs 5.1 months; HR, 0.89; CI, 0.77–1.02; $p = 0.087$) or in the 812 adenocarcinoma patients (6.3 months vs 5.4 months; HR, 0.84; CI, 0.68–1.03; $p = 0.089$). In preplanned subgroup analyses, there were significantly longer survival outcomes in never-smokers and Asian patients [30, 46].

The results of BR.21 and ISEL have been reviewed in concert. Gefitinib and erlotinib had similar response rates (8% versus 9%). However, erlotinib demonstrated a survival benefit for all patients enrolled whereas gefitinib only showed a survival benefit in those with adenocarcinoma or never-smokers. Interestingly, in the ISEL trial, 45% of those treated with gefitinib had progressed and 18% had responded to their most recent chemotherapy but 28% of those treated with erlotinib had progressed and 38% had responded to their most recent chemotherapy. This raises some questions as to whether or not these differences influence the efficacy of gefitinib and erlotinib in the ISEL and BR.21 studies, respectively [47].

INTEREST compared gefitinib directly with docetaxel in advanced NSCLC patients previously treated with platinum-based chemotherapy. Findings in 1433 patients established non-inferiority of gefitinib versus docetaxel in mOS (7.6 months vs 8.0 months; HR, 1.020; CI, 0.905–1.150) [8]. As a part of a preplanned analysis, tumor biopsies were analyzed for relationships between biomarkers and clinical outcomes. Patients with EGFR mutations treated with gefitinib had prolonged PFS and increased ORR compared with those treated with docetaxel. The PFS among patients with EGFR mutation-positive tumors was 7.0 months with gefitinib and 4.1 months with docetaxel (HR, 0.16; 95% CI, 0.05–0.49; p = 0.001). The RR in this patient population was 42.1% with gefitinib and 21.1% with docetaxel (p = 0.04) [48].

TITAN also compared the efficacy of an EGFR TKI (erlotinib) versus chemotherapy in the second-line setting. TITAN accrued patients that were screened for the maintenance SATURN study and progressed after four cycles of front-line platinum doublet chemotherapy. Patients were randomized to receive docetaxel or pemetrexed versus erlotinib [49]. The primary endpoint was overall survival in the intention-to-treat population. The trial closed sooner than anticipated due to slow enrollment. With 424 patients, the results were underpowered. Still, the results revealed that erlotinib was comparable to chemotherapy as regards to mOS (5.3 months with erlotinib versus 5.5 months with chemotherapy). Once it was clear that squamous cell histology should not be managed with pemetrexed, a separate analysis was conducted excluding the 30 patients with squamous cell carcinomas who received pemetrexed. However, this did not significantly alter the results. These results corroborate the findings from INTEREST, supporting the concept that EGFR inhibitor is not an inferior second line therapy compared with standard chemotherapy as regards to OS in unselected patients.

Given that benefits from EGFR TKIs are more pronounced in patients with an EGFR mutation, a phase III study was launched to investigate the efficacy of erlotinib versus docetaxel in individuals with EGFR wild-type NSCLCs previously treated with chemotherapy (TAILOR study). Final results of TAILOR describing the primary endpoint of OS are not available yet, but on interim analysis, the secondary endpoint of PFS was longer for the chemotherapy-treated patients compared to erlotinib (HR 0.70; 95% CI 0.53–0.94; p = 0.016). These results suggest that chemotherapy might be favored over EGFR TKIs for salvage therapy of patients with wild-type NSCLCs [50].

The SELECT trial tested the effect of cetuximab with chemotherapy in patients who were previously treated. This multicenter, open label, randomized phase III trial, combined either pemetrexed or docetaxel with cetuximab. The primary objective was PFS for cetuximab-pemetrexed versus pemetrexed by Independent Review Committee assessment. 938 patients comprised the intent-to-treat population, of which 605 were in the pemetrexed group (301 cetuximab-pemetrexed; 304 pemetrexed). Median PFS was 2.9 months with cetuximab-pemetrexed and 2.8 months with pemetrexed alone (HR, 1.03; 95% CI 0.87–1.21; p = 0.76). Median overall survival was 6.9 months with cetuximab-pemetrexed compared with 7.8 months with pemetrexed alone (HR, 1.01; 95% CI 0.86–1.20; p = 0.86). Objective response rate for cetuximab-pemetrexed was 6.6% and for pemetrexed was 4.3% (OR, 1.59; 95% CI 0.78–3.26; p = 0.20). No statistically significant differences in efficacy based on histology, EGFR immunohistochemistry staining intensity, or histoscore (H-score) were observed. More serious/nonserious adverse events were observed with cetuximab-pemetrexed mainly due to skin toxicities, gastrointestinal symptoms (diarrhea/stomatitis), and hypomagnesemia. Similar results were observed with docetaxel. The addition of cetuximab to pemetrexed did not improve efficacy in this population [51].

Other TKIs and MAbs

Active research is now focusing on mechanisms of resistance to EGFR TKIs identified as amplification of the MET oncogene and secondary mutations in EGFR. The T790M mutation is the most common mechanism of acquired resistance, accounting for more than 50% of these cases. Irreversible EGFR inhibitors, targeted therapies against MET, and dual-pathway blockades have activity.

Dacomitinib (PF-00299804) is a pan-HER inhibitor that binds irreversibly to the adenosine triphosphate (ATP) domain of EGFR, HER2 and HER4 whereas erlotinib alters signaling through competitive, reversible binding at the tyrosine kinase domain of EGFR. In cell lines harboring L858R and T790M mutations, dacomitinib has shown EGFR inhibition [52, 53]. In a global, multicenter, randomized, open-label phase II study, 188 patients were randomized to either dacomitinib 45 mg orally daily or erlotinib 150 mg orally daily after progression with chemotherapy. PFS (primary endpoint) was improved with dacomitinib (2.86 months vs 1.91 months, HR, 0.66; 95% CI, 0.47–0.91; p = 0.012) [54]. This is the first randomized data on irreversible EGFR TKIs in patients with lung cancer without previous TKI exposure. The results suggest another potential option for those patients with advanced NSCLC, especially with a more complete inhibition of HER signaling.

D019/XL647 is a small-molecule TKI that targets EGFR, VEGFR-2, HER2, and Ephrin type B receptor 4. In a phase II study evaluating two dosing regimens, the response rate was 20% and the PFS was 5.3 months. In patients with EGFR mutations, the response rate was 57% and the PFS was 9.3 months [55]. This is a compound that will continue clinical evaluation.

Afatinib (BIBW 2992) is an irreversible ErbB family blocker. It differs from the reversible EGFR-TKIs gefitinib and erlotinib such that after it enters the cell, it covalently binds to the cysteine residue of EGFR providing longer inhibition of EGFR. Afatinib also has activity against HER2, HER3, and HER4 as well as the EGFR-resistant T790M mutation.

A Phase II trial of afatinib in patients with advanced NSCLC who were previously treated with erlotinib or gefitinib was conducted in Japan. The primary end point was objective tumor response. Afatinib was deemed efficacious based on 69% disease control rate of greater than 8 weeks and median PFS of 4.4 months [56].

In another trial, the combination of afatinib and cetuximab was used in patients with EGFR mutations whose disease progressed on erlotinib. Disease control was observed in all 22 patients treated with the 40mg dose of afatinib, with tumor size reduction up to 76% [57].

LUX-Lung 2 was a phase II study confirming efficacy of afatinib in patients with EGFR mutation positive lung adenocarcinoma. In the 61 patients who received front-line afatinib, PFS was 12 months. In those with Del19 and L858R mutations, the PFS was prolonged to 13.7 months [58].

Based on these results, LUX-Lung 3 was designed as a randomized, open-label, phase III study of afatinib versus the highly effective and well-tolerated cisplatin-pemetrexed regimen as front-line therapy for patients with advanced lung adenocarcinoma harboring EGFR-activating mutations. The study met its primary endpoint (by independent review), demonstrating prolonged PFS in those treated with afatinib (mPFS 11.1 months vs 6.9 months; HR, 0.58; p = 0.0004) [59]. The hazard ratio was less than one for PFS among all subgroups including gender, age, race, EGFR mutation category, ECOG performance status, and smoking history (except for current or ex-smokers with HR 1.04). The preplanned analysis of the 308 patients with the common EGFR mutations (Del19 or L858R) revealed a mPFS of 13.6 months with afatinib and 6.9 months with cisplatin-pemetrexed chemotherapy. The objective response rate was also significantly higher in the afatinib group (56.1% versus 22.6%, p < 0.001 in all patients and 60.8% versus 22.1%, p < 0.0001 in patients with common mutations). There was also improved disease control such that at 12 months, 47% of patients who had received afatinib had not progressed while 22% of patients who had received chemotherapy had not progressed. Asian patients had a slightly longer PFS. The most frequent related adverse events were diarrhea and rash, although no patients discontinued afatinib for rash. There were three patients with interstitial lung disease-like events. Tolerability overall was milder in non-Asian patients. Based on patients' symptoms and questionnaires, cancer related symptoms were delayed and quality of life was improved with afatinib over chemotherapy.

Necitumumab (IMC-11F8) is another fully humanized IgG monoclonal antibody inhibiting EGFR that has been evaluated in clinical trial. In February 2011, the phase III INSPIRE trial comparing cisplatin-pemetrexed with or without necitumumab in front-line metastatic nonsquamous NSCLC was stopped due to rates of thromboembolism in the necitumumab arm

[60]. The phase I and II trials did not report any thromboembolic events [61].

A number of agents targeting parallel/downstream signaling of the EGFR pathway are in development for the treatment of NSCLC. MET inhibitors are among these that are further in advancement. The rationale for dual inhibition of EGFR and MET for treatment of NSCLC is based on evidence that MET is associated with resistance to erlotinib and gefinitib; preclinical and clinical data suggest additive or synergistic antitumor activity which may overcome resistance [62–64].

Tivantinib (ARQ 197) is an oral, selective, non-ATP competitive inhibitor of MET receptor tyrosine kinase. A global randomized, double-blind, placebo controlled Phase II trial compared erlotinib plus ARQ 197 with erlotinib plus placebo in previously treated EGFR inhibitor-naïve patients with advanced NSCLC. In this 167 patient trial, median PFS (primary endpoint) was prolonged with combination therapy (16.1 weeks vs 9.7 weeks; HR, 0.81; CI, 0.57–1.15; p = 0.23). PFS was particularly improved among patients with nonsquamous histology, KRAS mutations, and EGFR wild-type status [65]. Based on this promising data, the MARQUEE trial was designed as a phase III, randomized, double-blind study of tivantinib plus erlotinib versus placebo plus erlotinib in previously treated patients with advanced non-squamous NSCLC. The primary objective is to evaluate overall survival in the intent-to-treat population [66].

Onartuzumab (OAM4558) is a recombinant humanized monvalent monoclonal antibody that specifically binds to the extracellular domain of MET. A global randomized, double-blind, placebo-controlled Phase II study compared erlotinib plus onartuzumab with erlotinib plus placebo in the second- or third-line management of advanced NSCLC. The addition of MetMAb to erlotinib in these patients significantly improved PFS and OS in patients who had high expression of MET in their tumors, resulting in a near 2-fold reduction in the risk of disease progression and a 3-fold reduction in the risk of death [67]. This is being followed by the MetLung study which is a randomized, phase III, multicenter, double-blind, placebo-controlled study in patients with advanced NSCLC and MET positive tumors who have failed at least one but no more than two prior lines of platinum-based chemotherapy. The primary endpoint is overall survival [68].

Lapatinib is an oral, reversible, dual tyrosine kinase inhibitor of EGFR and EGFR-2 (HER2). EGFR can signal via homodimers and heterodimers with HER2 dual inhibition of both receptors may provide clinical benefit beyond that achieved with inhibitors of EGFR alone. One multicenter, open-label, parallel-group, randomized phase II study evaluated patients with advanced NSCLC with two schedules of lapatinib as first- or second-line monotherapy. Although well-tolerated, lapatinib failed to provide a predetermined response rate in a target population. A portion of patients were able to maintain stable disease for less than or equal to 24 weeks. In this setting, single agent lapatinib had minimal activity at these doses based on response rate [69].

Conclusions

Utilizing the EGFR pathway in the treatment of non-small cell lung cancer has evolved. The reversible EGFR TKIs erlotinib and gefitinib have demonstrable activity in patients with advanced NSCLC, especially those harboring EGFR mutations. Resistance, both primary and acquired, is a developing concern. Novel therapies with irreversible EGFR TKIs and monoclonal antibodies are being developed and evaluated. This evolution has defined a standard of molecular profiling in the management of NSCLC.

References

1 Cohen S (1962) Isolation of a mouse submaxillary gland protein accelerating incisor eruption and eyelid opening in the new born animal. *J Biol Chem*, 237: 1555–62.

2 Herbst RS, Prager D, Hermann R, *et al.* (2005) TRIBUTE: a phase III trial of erlotinib hydrochloride (OSI-774) combined with carboplatin and paclitaxel chemotherapy in advanced non-small-cell lung cancer. *J Clin Oncol*, 23: 5892–9.

3 Gatzemerier U, Pluzanska A, Szczesna A, *et al.* (2007) Phase III study of erlotinib in combination with

cisplatin and gemcitabine in advanced non-small-cell lung cancer: the Tarceva Lung Cancer Investigation Trial. *J Clin Oncol*, 25: 1545–52.

4 Giaccone G, Herbst RS, Manegold C, *et al.* (2004) Gefitinib in combination with gemcitabine and cisplatin in advanced non-small-cell lung cancer: A phase III trial – INTACT 1. *J Clin Oncol*, 22: 777–84.

5 Herbst RS, Giaccone G, Schiller JH, *et al.* (2004) Gefitinib in combination with paclitaxel and carboplatin in advanced non-small-cell lung cancer: A phase III trial – INTACT 2. *J Clin Oncol*, 22: 785–94.

6 Pirker R, Pereira JR, Szczesna A, *et al.* (2009) Cetuximab plus chemotherapy in patients with advanced non-small-cell lung cancer (FLEX): An open-label randomized phase III trial. *Lancet*, 373: 1525–31.

7 Lynch TJ, Patel T, Dreisbach L, *et al.* (2010) Cetuximab and first-line taxane/carboplatin chemotherapy in advanced non-small-cell lung cancer: results of the randomized multicenter phase III trial BMS099. *J Clin Oncol*, 28: 911–17.

8 Kim E, Herbst RS, Moon J, *et al.* (2008) SWOG 0536: Phase II trial of carboplatin, paclitaxel, cetuximab and bevacizumab followed by cetuximab and bevacizumab in advanced non-small cell lung cancer. *J Thor Oncol*, 3: S266.

9 Tracy S, Mukohara T, Hansen M, *et al.* (2004) Gefitinib induces apoptosis in the EGFRL858R non-small-cell lung cancer cell line H3255. *Cancer Res*, 64: 7241–4.

10 Gumerlock PH, Pryde BJ, Kimura T, *et al.* (2003) Enhanced cytotoxicity of docetaxel OSI-774 combination in non-small cell lung carcinoma (NSCLC). *Proc Am Soc Clin Oncol*, 662 (abstr 2661).

11 Solit DB, She Y, Lobo J, *et al.* (2005) Pulsatile administration of the epidermal growth factor receptor inhibitor gefitinib is significantly more effective than continuous dosing for sensitizing tumors to paclitaxel. *Clin Cancer Res*, 11: 1983–9.

12 Mok TS, Wu YL, Yu CJ, *et al.* (2009) Randomized, placebo-controlled, phase II study of sequential erlotinib and chemotherapy as first-line treatment for advanced non-small-cell lung cancer. *J Clin Oncol*, 27: 5080–7.

13 Mok TS, Wu YL, Thongprasert S, *et al.* (2012) A randomized placebo-controlled phase III study of intercalated erlotinib with gemcitabine-platinum in first-line advanced non-small cell lung cancer (NSCLC): FASTACT-II. *J Clin Oncol*, 30(suppl): Abstr 7519.

14 Mok TS, Lee JS, Zhang L, *et al.* (2012) Biomarker analyses and overall survival (OS) from the randomized, placebo-controlled, phase 3, FASTACT-2 study of intercalated erlotinib with first-line chemotherapy in advanced non-small-cell lung cancer. *ESMO*, Abstr 1023.

15 Hirsch FR, Kabbinavar F, Eisen T, *et al.* (2011) A randomized, phase II, biomarker-selected study comparing erlotinib to erlotinib intercalated with chemotherapy in first-line therapy for advanced non-small cell lung cancer. *J Clin Oncol*, 29: 3567–73.

16 Reck M, Buchholz E, Romer KS, *et al.* (2006) Gefitinib monotherapy in chemotherapy-naive patients with inoperable stage III/IV non-small-cell lung cancer. *Clin Lung Cancer*, 7: 406–11.

17 Niho S, Kubota K, Goto K, *et al.* (2006) First-line single agent treatment with gefitinib in patients with advanced non-small-cell lung cancer: A phase II study. *J Clin Oncol*, 24: 64–9.

18 Giaccone G, Gallegos RM, Le Chevalier T, *et al.* (2006) Erlotinib for frontline treatment of advanced non-small cell lung cancer: a phase II study. *Clin Cancer Res*, 12: 6049–55.

19 Lee DH, Kim SW, Suh C, *et al.* (2011) Phase II study of erlotinib for chemotherapy-naïve patients with advanced or metastatic non-small cell lung cancer who are ineligible for platinum doublets. *Cancer Chemother Pharmacol*, 67: 35–9.

20 Yang CH, Yu CJ, Shih JY, *et al.* (2008) Specific EGFR mutations predict treatment outcome of stage IIIB/IV patients with chemotherapy-naive non-small-cell lung cancer receiving first-line gefitinib monotherapy. *J Clin Oncol*, 26: 2745–53.

21 Hesketh PJ, Chansky K, Wozniak AJ, *et al.* (2008) Southwest Oncology Group phase II trial (S0341) of erlotinib (OSI-774) in patients with advanced non-small cell lung cancer and a performance status of 2. *J Thorac Oncol*, 3: 1026–31.

22 Goss G, Ferry D, Wierzbicki R, *et al.* (2009) Randomized phase II study of gefitinib compared with placebo in chemotherapy-naïve patients with advanced non-small-cell lung cancer and poor performance status. *J Clin Oncol*, 27: 2253–60.

23 Lee SM, Khan I, Upadhyay S, *et al.* (2012) First-line erlotinib in patients with advanced non-small-cell lung cancer unsuitable for chemotherapy (TOPICAL): A double-blind, placebo-controlled, phase 3 trial. *Lancet Oncol*, 13(11): 1161–70.

24 Jackman DM, Yeap BY, Linderman NI, *et al.* (2007) Phase II clinical trial of chemotherapy-naïve patients > = 70 years of age treated with erlotinib for advanced non-small cell lung cancer. *J Clin Oncol*, 25: 760–6.

25 Crino L, Cappuzzo F, Zatloukal P, *et al.* (2008) Gefitinib versus vinorelbine in chemotherapy-naive elderly patients with advanced non-small-cell lung cancer

(INVITE): A randomized, phase II study. *J Clin Oncol*, 26: 4253–60.

26 Gridelli C, Ciardiello F, Gallo C, *et al.* (2012) First-line erlotinib followed by second-line cisplatin-gemcitabine chemotherapy in advanced non-small-cell lung cancer: the TORCH randomized trial. *J Clin Oncol*, 30: 3002–11.

27 Shepherd FA, Pereira J, Ciuleanu TE, *et al.* (2004) A randomized placebo-controlled trial of erlotinib in patients with advanced non-small cell lung cancer (NSCLC) following failure of 1st line or 2nd line chemotherapy. A National Cancer Institute of Canada Clinical Trials Group (NCIC CTG) trial. *J Clin Oncol*, 22: 622s.

28 Shepherd FA, Rodrigues PJ, Cieleanu TE, *et al.* (2005) Erlotinib in previously treated non-small-cell lung cancer. *N Engl J Med*, 353: 123–32.

29 Kim ES, Hirsh V, Mok T, *et al.* (2008) Gefitinib versus docetaxel in previously treated non-small-cell lung cancer (INTEREST): A randomised phase III trial. *Lancet*, 372: 1809–18.

30 Thatcher N, Chang A, Parikh P, *et al.* (2005) Gefitinib plus best supportive care in previously treated patients with refractory advanced non-small cell lung cancer: results from a randomised, placebo-controlled, multicentre study (Iressa Survival Evaluation in Lung Cancer). *Lancet*, 366: 1527–37.

31 Inoue A, Suzuki T, Fukuhara T, *et al.* (2006) Prospective phase II study of gefitinib for chemotherapy-naive patients with advanced non-small-cell lung cancer with epidermal growth factor receptor gene mutations. *J Clin Oncol*, 24: 3340–6.

32 Sequist LV, Martins RG, Spigel D, *et al.* (2008) First-line gefitinib in patients with advanced non-small-cell lung cancer harboring somatic EGFR mutations. *J Clin Oncol*, 26: 2442–9 (Erratum in: *J Clin Oncol*, 26: 3472).

33 Mok TS, Wu YL, Thongprasert S, *et al.* (2009) Gefitinib or carboplatin-paclitaxel in pulmonary adenocarcinoma. *N Engl J Med*, 361: 947–57.

34 Lee JS, Park K, Kim SW, *et al.* (2009) Presented at World Conference on Lung Cancer. A randomized phase III study of gefitinib (IRESSA) versus standard chemotherapy (gemcitabine plus cisplatin) as a first-line treatment for never-smokers with advanced or metastatic adenocarcinoma of the lung [abstract PRS.4].

35 Mitsudomi T, Morita S, Yatabe Y, *et al.* (2010) Gefitinib versus cisplatin plus docetaxel in patients with non-small-cell lung cancer harbouring mutations of the epidermal growth factor receptor (WJTOG3405): An open label, randomized phase 3 trial. *Lancet Oncol*, 11: 121–8.

36 Maemondo M, Inoue A, Kobayashi K, *et al.* (2010) Gefitinib or chemotherapy for non-small-cell lung cancer with mutated EGFR. *N Engl J Med*, 362: 2380–8.

37 Han JY, Park K, Kim SW, *et al.* (2012) First-SIGNAL: first-line single-agent iressa versus gemcitabine and cisplatin trial in never-smokers with adenocarcinoma of the lung. *J Clin Oncol*, 30: 1122–8.

38 Inoue A, Kobayashi K, Maemondo M, *et al.* (2013) Updated overall survival results from a randomized phase III trial comparing gefitinib with carboplatin-paclitaxel for chemo-naïve non-small cell lung cancer with sensitive EGFR gene mutations (NEJ002). *Ann Oncol*, 24(1): 54–9.

39 Rosell R, Carcereny E, Gervais R, *et al.* (2012) Erlotinib versus standard chemotherapy as first-line treatment for European patients with advanced EGFR mutation-positive non-small-cell lung cancer (EURTAC): A multicenter, open-label-randomised phase 3 trial. *Lancet Oncol*, 13: 239–46.

40 Zhou C, Wu YL, Chen G, *et al.* (2011) Erlotinib versus chemotherapy as first-line treatment for patients with advanced EGFR mutation-positive non-small-cell lung cancer (OPTIMAL, CTONG-0802): A multicenter, open-label, randomized, phase 3 study. *Lancet Oncol*, 12: 735–42.

41 Jänne PA, Wang X, Socinski MA, *et al.* (2012) Randomized phase II trial of erlotinib alone or with carboplatin and paclitaxel in patients who were never or light former smokers with advanced lung adenocarcinoma: CALGB 30406 trial. *J Clin Oncol*, 30(17): 2063–9.

42 Cappuzzo, F, Ciuleanu T, Stelmakh L, *et al.* (2010) Erlotinib as maintenance treatment in advanced non-small-cell lung cancer: a multicentre, randomised, placebo-controlled phase 3 study. *Lancet Oncol*, 11: 521–9.

43 Miller VA, O'Connor P, Soh C, *et al.* (2009) A randomized, double-blind, placebo-controlled, phase IIIb trial (ATLAS) comparing bevacizumab (B) therapy with or without erlotinib (E) after completion of chemotherapy with B for first-line treatment of locally advanced, recurrent, or metastatic non-small cell lung cancer (NSCLC). *J Clin Oncol*, 27: 18s: LBA8002.

44 Fukuoka M, Yano S, Giaccone G, *et al.* (2003) Multi-institutional randomized phase II trial of gefinitib for previously treated patients with advanced non-small-cell lung cancer. *J Clin Oncol*, 21: 2237–46.

45 Kris MG, Natale RB, Herbst RS, *et al.* (2003) Efficacy of gefitinib, an inhibitor of the epidermal growth factor receptor tyrosine kinase, in symptomatic patients with non-small cell lung cancer: A randomized trial. *JAMA*, 290: 2149–58.
46 Hirsch FR, Varella-Garcia M, Bunn PA, Jr., *et al.* (2006) Molecular predictors of outcome with gefitinib in a phase III placebo-controlled study in advanced non-small cell lung cancer. *J Clin Oncol*, 24: 5034–42.
47 Wang Y, Schmid-Bindert, Zhou C (2011) Erlotinib in the treatment of advanced non-small cell lung cancer: An update for clinicians. *Ther Adv Med Oncol*, 4: 19–29.
48 Douillard JY, Shepherd FA, Hirsh V, *et al.* (2010) Molecular predictors of outcome with gefitinib and docetaxel in previously treated non-small-cell lung cancer: data from the randomized phase III INTEREST trial. *J Clin Oncol*, 28: 744–52.
49 Ciuleanu T, Stelmakh L, Cicenas S, *et al.* (2012) Efficacy and safety of erlotinib versus chemotherapy in second-line treatment of patients with advanced, non-small-cell lung cancer with poor prognosis (TITAN): A randomised multicentre, open-label, phase 3 study. *Lancet Oncol*, 13: 300–8.
50 Garassino MC, Martelli O, Bettini A, *et al.* (2012) TAILOR: A phase III trial comparing erlotinib with docetaxel as the second-line treatment of NSCLC patients with wild-type (wt) EGFR. *J Clin Oncol*, 30(suppl): Abstr LBA7501.
51 Kim ES, Neubauer MA, Cohn AL, *et al.* (2012) SELECT: Randomized phase III study of docetaxel (D) or pemetrexed (P) with or without cetuximab (C) in recurrent or progressive non-small cell lung cancer (NSCLC) after platinum-based therapy. *J Clin Oncol*, 30(suppl): Abstr 7502.
52 Engelman JA, Zejnullahu K, Gale CM, *et al.* (2007) PF00299804, an irreversible pan-ERBB inhibitor, is effective in lung cancer models with EGFR and ERBB2 mutations that are resistant to gefitinib. *Cancer Res*, 67: 11924–32.
53 Gonzales AJ, Hook KE, Althaus IW, *et al.* (2008) Antitumor activity and pharmacokinetic properties of PF-00299804, a second-generation irreversible pan-erbB receptor tyroside kinase inhibitor. *Mol Cancer Ther*, 7: 1880–9.
54 Ramalingam SS, Blackhall F, Krzakowski M, *et al.* (2012) Randomized phase II study of dacomitinib (PF-00299804), an irreversible pan-human epidermal growth factor receptor inhibitor, versus erlotinib in patients with advanced non-small cell lung cancer. *J Clin Oncol*, 30: 3337–44.
55 Pietanza MC, Gadgeel SM, Dowlati A, *et al.* (2012) Phase II study of the multitargeted tyroside kinase inhibitor XL647 in patients with non-small-cell lung cancer. *J Thorac Oncol*, 7: 856–65.
56 Yamamoto N, Katakami N, Atagi S, *et al.* (2011) A phase II trial of afatinib (BIBW 2992) in patients (pts) with advanced non-small cell lung cancer previously treated with erlotinib (E) or gefitinib (G). *J Clin Oncol*, 29(suppl): Abstr 7524.
57 Janijigian YY, Groen HJ, Horn L, *et al.* (2011) Activity and tolerability of afatinib (BIBW 2992) and cetuximab in NSCLC patients with acquired resistance to erlotinib or gefitinib. *J Clin Oncol*, 29(suppl): Abstr 7525.
58 Yang JC, Shih JY, Su WC, *et al.* (2012) Afatinib for patients with lung adenocarcinoma and epidermal growth factor receptor mutations (LUX-Lung 2): A phase 2 trial. *Lancet Oncol*, 13: 539–48.
59 Yang JC, Schuler MH, Yamamoto N, *et al.* (2012) LUX-Lung 3: A randomized, open-label, phase III study of afatinib versus pemetrexed and cisplatin as first-line treatment for patients with advanced adenocarcinoma of the lung harboring EGFR-activating mutations. *J Clin Oncol*, 30(suppl): Abstr LBA7500.
60 Lilly, Bristol-Myers Squibb stop enrollment in one of two phase III lung cancer trials of necitumumab (2012) [press release]. Bristol-Myers Squibb website. http://bms.newshq.businesswire.com/press-release/rd-news/lilly-bristol-myers-squibb-stop-enrollment-one-two-phase-iii-lung-cancer-trial.
61 Tabernero J, Cervantes A, Delaunoit T, *et al.* (2009) A phase 2 study of IMC-11F8, a monoclonal antibody directed against the EGFR, in combination with mFOLFOX-6 chemotherapy in the first-line treatment of advanced or metastatic colorectal carcinoma. *Ann Oncol*, 20: 18–19.
62 Merchant M, Zhang YW, Su Y, *et al.* (2008) Combination efficacy with MetMAb and erlotinib in a NSCLC tumor model highlight therapeutic opportunities for c-Met inhibitors in combination with EGFR inhibitors. *Proceedings of the 99th Annual Meeting of the American Association for Cancer Research; April 12–16*; San Diego, CA, USA; Abstract 1336.
63 Janne PA, Wax M, Leach JW, *et al.* (2008) Targeting MET with XL184 to reverse EGFR tyrosine kinase inhibitor (TKI) resistance in NSCLC: Impact of preclinical studies on clinical trial design. *EJC*, 6(Suppl): Abstr 174.
64 Wakelee HA, Gettinger SN, Engelman JA, *et al.* (2010) A phase Ib/II study of XL184 (BMS 907351) with and without erlotinib (E) in patients (pts) with non-small

cell lung cancer (NSCLC). *J Clin Oncol*, 28(suppl): Abstr 3017.

65 Schiller JH, Akerley WL, Brugger W, *et al.* (2010) Results from ARQ 197–209: A global randomized placebo-controlled phase II clinical trial of erlotinib plus ARQ 197 versus erlotinib plus placebo in previously treated EGFR inhibitor-naive patients with locally advanced or metastatic non-small cell lung cancer (NSCLC). *J Clin Oncol*, 28(suppl): Abstr LBA7502.

66 Scagliotti GV, Novello S, Schiller JH, *et al.* (2012) Rationale and design of MARQUEE: A phase III, randomized, double-blind study of tivantinib plus erlotinib versus placebo plus erlotinib in previously treated patients with locally advanced or metastatic, nonsquamous, non-small-cell lung cancer. *Clin Lung Cancer*, 13: 391–5.

67 Spigel DR, Ervin TJ, Ramlau R, *et al.* (2011) Final efficacy results from OAM4558g, a randomized phase II study evaluating MetMAb or placebo in combination with erlotinib in advanced NSCLC. *J Clin Oncol*, 29(suppl): Abstr 7505.

68 Spigel DR, Edelman MJ, Mok T, *et al.* (2012) The MetLUNG study: A randomized, double-blind, phase III study of onartuzumab (MetMAb) plus erlotinib versus placebo plus erlotinib in patients with advanced, MET-positive non-small cell lung cancer (NSCLC). *J Clin Oncol*, 30(suppl): Abstr TPS7616.

69 Ross HJ, Blumenschein GR, Aisner J, *et al.* (2010) Randomized phase II multicenter trial of two schedules of lapatinib as first- or second-line monotherapy in patients with advanced or metastatic non-small cell lung cancer. *Clin Cancer Res*, 16: 1938–49.

CHAPTER 27

Mechanisms of Resistance to Epidermal Growth Factor Receptor (EGFR) in Non-small Cell Lung Cancer

Erminia Massarelli
Department of Thoracic Head and Neck Medical Oncology, The University of Texas MD Anderson Cancer Center, Houston, TX, USA

Introduction

Lung cancer is the leading cause of cancer death in the United States [1]. Screening for lung cancer in high-risk populations has only recently been approved [2], and unfortunately, the majority of non-small cell lung cancer (NSCLC) cases continue to be diagnosed at an advanced stage. A change in the treatment paradigm of NSCLC followed the discovery of activating epidermal growth factor receptor (*EGFR)* mutations in patients who responded to EGFR tyrosine kinase inhibitors (EGFR TKIs) such as gefitinib or erlotinib [3–5] as these drugs are now FDA-approved for first-line therapy in advanced NSCLC.

The EGFR family contains 4 members: EGFR, human epidermal growth factor receptor 2 (HER2), HER3, and HER4. Ligand binding to the extracellular binding region initiates receptor homo- and heterodimerization and activates the cytoplasmic tyrosine kinase-stimulating intracellular signaling pathways, including the Ras/mitogen-activated protein kinase (MAPK) pathway, the phosphatidylinositol-3-kinase (PI3K)/v-Akt murine thymoma viral oncogene (AKT) pathway, and signal transducers and activators of transcription signaling pathways [6]. The recognition that mutations in the region of the *EGFR* gene encoding the tyrosine kinase domain are associated with dramatic responses to EGFR TKIs led to better characterization of the types of mutations as well as their functional significance.

EGFR mutations occur in about 15% of Caucasian patients with NSCLC and 30% of Asian patients with NSCLC, and these mutations are strongly associated with adenocarcinoma histology, female sex, and nonsmoking status [7]. The most common *EGFR* -activating mutations are point mutations in exon 18 (6%), insertions or deletions in exon 19 (6%), insertions/duplications and point mutations in exon 20 (9%), and point mutations in exon 21 (39%) [7]. These mutations destabilize the equilibrium between the active and inactive states of EGFR kinase activity and promote enzyme activation, resulting in an "oncogene addiction" to EGFR that translates into tumor growth and survival advantages [7, 8]. The best-characterized mutations that confer sensitivity to EGFR TKI therapy are located in exon 19 (deletions, particularly E746-A750del) and exon 21 (L858R). Patients with these mutations

Lung Cancer, Fourth Edition. Edited by Jack A. Roth, Waun Ki Hong and Ritsuko U. Komaki.

have high response rates (up to 70%) when treated with EGFR TKIs and longer median survival than patients with wild-type *EGFR* (up to 27 months) [9, 10].

Primary resistance to EGFR TKIs is typically caused by mutations in the *EGFR* gene that are not associated with sensitivity to first-generation EGFR TKIs, such as insertion mutations in exon 20, or by other somatic mutations in genes that have an impact on the EGFR signaling pathway, such as *KRAS* [11, 12]. Primary resistance also may be due to the *de-novo* presence of EGFR TKI-resistant or non-activating *EGFR* mutations. Clinical data about the use of erlotinib and gefitinib in patients with NSCLC whose tumors harbor activating *EGFR* mutations indicate that these tumors eventually develop resistance to reversible EGFR TKIs, which may result from secondary acquired *EGFR* mutations or other mechanisms not directly related to the *EGFR* genotype, such as alternative signaling pathways.

The engagement of alternative signaling pathways can lead to either primary or acquired resistance to EGFR inhibitors. These alternative pathways include PI3K/AKT [13], insulin-like growth factor 1 receptor [14], and c-mesenchymal-epithelial transition factor (c-MET) [15, 16]. *MET* gene amplification can mediate both *de novo* and acquired resistance. In addition, multiple mechanisms of resistance could coexist in any given patient owing to tumor heterogeneity.

This chapter will describe the known mechanisms of primary and acquired EGFR TKI resistance in patients with NSCLC.

Primary resistance to EGFR TKIs

Figure 27.1 illustrates the frequency and mechanisms of primary resistance in *EGFR*-mutated NSCLC, including *EGFR*-resistant mutations, mutation or amplifications in other members of the *ErbB* family receptors, and mutation in other genes responsible for activating escape pathways such as v-Ki-ras2 Kirsten rat sarcoma viral oncogene homolog *(KRAS)*, proto-oncogene B-Raf (*BRAF*), phosphatidylinositol-4,5-bisphosphate 3-kinase catalytic subunit alpha (*PIK3CA*), and phosphatase and tensin homolog (PTEN) loss [7, 10, 11, 13, 17–23].

EGFR-resistant mutations

In-frame insertion mutations in *EGFR* exon 20 account for about 1–10% of the total number of *EGFR* mutations, with the majority of these exon 20 insertions likely conferring resistance to EGFR TKIs [12]. Table 27.1 shows a comprehensive list of primary resistant mutations. Exon 20 insertions add residues within the N-terminal positions or at the opposite end of the C-helix. Although crystal structures have not been reported, effects on kinase domain function have been postulated [24]. Insertion mutations are restricted to a spectrum of residues at the N-lobe of *EGFR* after the C-helix (M766 to C775) and their preferential location following the C-helix (A767 to C775), and have a critical role in the catalytic activity of the EGFR tyrosine kinase [25]. This might indicate the importance of this region in orienting the kinase into a state that controls adenosine-5′-triphosphate and EGFR TKI binding [6] and may indeed push the C-helix, and therefore the kinase domain conformation, into an active position [26]. Some C-helix exon 20 insertions have been reported to affect E762 to Y764 residues inducing EGFR activation [7, 13, 27, 28]. In one study, two patients with tumors harboring Y764_V765insHH or M766_A767insA had prolonged periods of disease control with reversible EGFR TKIs, suggesting at least intermediate sensitivity [29].

Insertion mutations such as D770_N771 (insNPG), D770_(insSVQ), D770_(insG), N771T-(30), and H773_V774insH [31] appear to confer *de-novo* resistance to clinically achievable doses of gefitinib and erlotinib. In a study characterizing *EGFR* mutations in patients of African-American descent with NSCLC [32], two exon 20 insertion mutations (N771GY_delN771insGY and A767-V769dup) conferring increased kinase activity and resistance to erlotinib were identified. A767_V769dupASV has been verified as a resistance mutation in two other studies [31, 33]. Q787R transfectants showed lower sensitivity *in vitro* to gefitinib than L858R transfectants, and the double

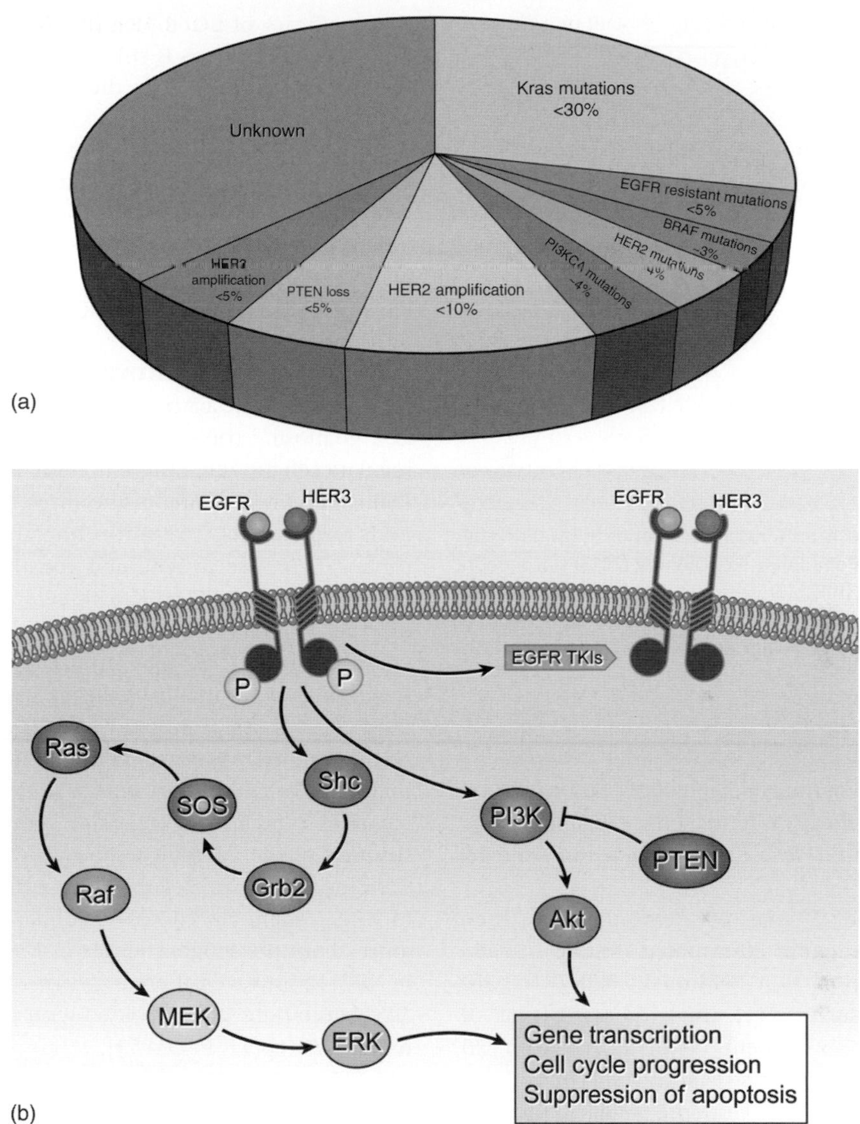

Figure 27.1 Mechanisms of primary resistance to EGFR TKIs. a: The spectrum and relative frequency of known oncogenic drivers of primary resistance to EGFR inhibition therapy in lung cancer. b: The activation of EGFR downstream molecules and the other ErbB family member receptor tyrosine kinases bypasses EGFR inhibition signaling by EGFR TKIs and induces primary resistance to EGFR TKIs.

transfectant Q787R plus L858R demonstrated intermediate sensitivity [17].

Results with oral irreversible inhibitors of EGFR and HER2 (neratinib [HKI-272], afatinib [BIBW2992], and dacomitinib [PF00299804]) show that tumors with A767_V769dupASV, D770_N771insNPG, delN771insGY, and H773_V774insH mutations have IC_{50} responses to these compounds in dose ranges similar to those of T790M transfectant models, on average, 100 times less sensitive than the classic L858R transfectants, and exon 19 deletions. Therefore, it would be

Table 27.1 Exon 20 *EGFR* primary resistant mutations

Insertions and deletions	Point mutations
D770_N771 ins NPG/D770_N771insNPG	A763V
N771GY delN771insGY	K806E
N771dupN	
A767_V769dupASV	L777G
H773_V774insH/M/dup H	P772R
DelA767_V769	S784F
770_771ins VDSVDNP	V769L/M
S768_V769EinsVAS	V774M
V769D770delinsGI	Y801C
V768D770dupSVD	
M766V769insWPA	
S768D770dupSVD	
A767S768insSVR	

Source: Adapted from Massarelli E, Johnson FM, Erickson HS, Wistuba, II, Papadimitrakopoulou V (2013) Uncommon Epidermal Growth Factor Receptor mutations in non-small cell lung cancer and their mechanisms of EGFR tyrosine kinase inhibitors sensitivity and resistance. *Lung Cancer*, Feb 25.

expected that afatinib and PF00299804 would be less clinically effective in this setting than in tumors with sensitive *EGFR* mutations (L858R or exon 19 deletions).

In a phase 2 trial of neratinib, the three patients with exon 20-mutated NSCLC (S768_D770dupSVD, H773_V774dupHV, delN771insGF) had no responses [34]. In a phase I trial of PF00299804, six patients with *EGFR* exon 20 insertions were included and only one (with delA770insGY) had a response [35]. A phase 2 trial of afatinib (BIBW2992) enrolled 11 patients with *EGFR* exon 20 insertions, and only one had a partial response; progression-free survival for these patients was short [36, 37]. Heat-shock protein 90 inhibitors have been investigated in EGFR-mutated advanced NSCLC, as mutated oncoproteins, including EGFR, may rely on heat-shock protein 90 chaperones more than their wild-type counterparts [38]. A phase II trial of the heat-shock protein 90 inhibitor IPI-504 in 76 patients with advanced NSCLC demonstrated modest activity in EGFR-mutated patients (response rate = 4%) [39].

The efficacy of EGFR TKIs in patients with multiple EGFR mutations is still unclear in most cases and depends on whether the types of mutations involved are similar to those in patients with single mutations [40, 41]. However, patients with G719S plus L858R have shown poor outcomes with gefitinib [40, 42–45], while the complex mutations L858R plus D761Y, L858R plus L747S, and L858R plus T854A [16, 46, 47] show patterns of resistance less pronounced than in L858R plus T790M [48].

KRAS and *BRAF* mutations

RAS genes encode a family of membrane-bound 21-kDa guanosine triphosphate-binding proteins that regulate cell growth, differentiation, and apoptosis. Point mutations of one of the three *Ras* genes (*H-RAS, K-RAS, N-RAS*) result in impaired guanosine triphosphate -ase activity and constitutive activation of the RAS-RAF-MEK-ERK cytoplasmic kinase cascade.

KRAS and *EGFR* gene mutations have been reported to be mutually exclusive in several studies [7, 11, 49]. *KRAS* mutations occur in 20–30% of NSCLC tumors, mainly in patients with adenocarcinoma (30%) and in smokers (17%) [50]. The most common mutation of the *KRAS* gene is the substitution of the guanine residue in codon 12 with thymine, which causes the constitutive activation of *KRAS*. There are controversial data in the literature about the prognostic role of *KRAS* mutations in NSCLC; however, there is growing evidence that *KRAS* mutations are associated with poor response to EGFR TKIs [11, 17, 51–53].

BRAF mutations are detected in only 2–3% of NSCLC tumors, are mutually exclusive of *RAS* and *EGFR* mutations, and are seen predominantly in current or former smokers [21]. The incidence of *BRAF* mutations other than V600E substitutions is significantly higher in lung cancer than in other tumor types (i.e., melanoma) [21]. Patients whose tumors harbor *BRAF* mutations have a poor prognosis [22].

PIK3CA mutations and *PTEN* loss

The PI3K/AKT signaling cascade is another EGFR-activated pathway that is pivotal to cell growth and survival [54, 55]. Activating mutations in *PIK3CA* (the gene that encodes the p110 subunit of PI3K) and the loss of *PTEN* tumor-suppressor gene function lead to the stimulation of this oncogenic pathway. *PTEN* loss occurs through a variety of mechanisms, including germ-line mutations (such as the autosomal dominant Cowden's syndrome) [56], sporadic mutations causing allele loss at the Cowden gene location on chromosome 10q [57], gene silencing through promoter hypermethylation [58], and upregulation of a specific micro-RNA that promotes gene silencing [59]. These diverse mechanisms of gene silencing and protein inactivation lead to methodological constraints when assessing PTEN tumor status. The expressions of *PI3K* and *PTEN* have been related to EGFR TKI resistance in preclinical models [60–62].

PIK3CA encodes the p110α isoform, the main catalytic subunit of PI3K, and is mutated in 3–4%, and amplified in 12–20%, of lung squamous cell cancers [63–65]. *PIK3CA* mutations are not mutually exclusive of *EGFR* or *KRAS* mutations [64–66]. *PIK3CA* mutations have been observed in patients with *EGFR* mutations without prior exposure to EGFR TKIs [64, 67]. In one study, all four patients with *PIK3CA* mutations had coexisting *EGFR* mutations, and the *PIK3CA* mutations were found in exons 9 and 20 [67]. However, mutations in the main catalytic subunit of PI3K (PIK3CA) have also been observed as a mechanism of acquired resistance to EGFR TKIs *in vitro* [68] and in two *EGFR* mutation-positive patients after disease progression while on EGFR TKI therapy [69].

PTEN loss has been suggested as a potential mechanism of EGFR TKI resistance in NSCLCs that have activating *EGFR* mutations [13] and has been associated with poor overall survival in gefitinib-treated patients [70]. In *EGFR* wild-type tumors, the combination of *PTEN* loss by gene copy number and *PI3KCA* mutation predicted a far worse outcome in gefitinib-treated patients [18].

ErbB family members: mutation and amplification

Other ErbB family members, including HER2, HER3, and HER4, play important roles in the resistance to EGFR TKIs because EGFR forms homo- or heterodimers with other ErbB family members in response to ligand binding. Somatic mutations of the *HER2* gene, which are mutually exclusive with those of *EGFR*, have been identified in a very small fraction of lung adenocarcinomas (up to 4%) [7, 19, 71] and are mostly found in females, nonsmokers, East Asians, and adenocarcinoma patients. Most types of *HER2* mutations are in-frame insertion mutations in exon 20 that lead to constitutive activation of the HER2 kinase [7, 19, 71].

HER2 amplification recently has been detected in a subset of EGFR TKI–resistant lung cancers in the absence of *EGFR* T790M mutation [20]. However, the association between *HER2* amplification and sensitivity to EGFR TKIs remains a controversial field [72–75].

Acquired resistance to EGFR TKIs

Acquired resistance to EGFR TKIs can develop from secondary acquired *EGFR* mutations, most commonly T790M in exon 20, or from activation of alternative pathways that rescue the cell from the "oncogene addiction" state. *MET* amplification, hepatocyte growth factor (HGF) overexpression, and IGF-1R signaling are the most commonly found escaping mechanisms indirectly related to the EGFR pathway activation. Another emerging mechanism of resistance is histological transformation, most frequently to small cell lung cancer [69]. Figure 27.2 summarizes the frequency and the mechanisms of acquired EGFR TKI resistance [20, 69, 76, 77].

Acquired *EGFR* mutations

T790M is the most frequent acquired resistance mutation [78–80]. T790M is located in the EGFR adenosine-5′-triphosphate-binding pocket of the catalytic region to which EGFR TKIs bind and its presence causes a higher affinity to adenosine-5′-triphosphate and a relatively lower affinity to EGFR TKIs [25].

The *EGFR* T790M mutation occurs in a position analogous to that of the imatinib-resistant mutation in the kinase domains of *BCR-ABL1*, *KIT*, and *PDGFR A* (a point mutation in T315 to isoleucine

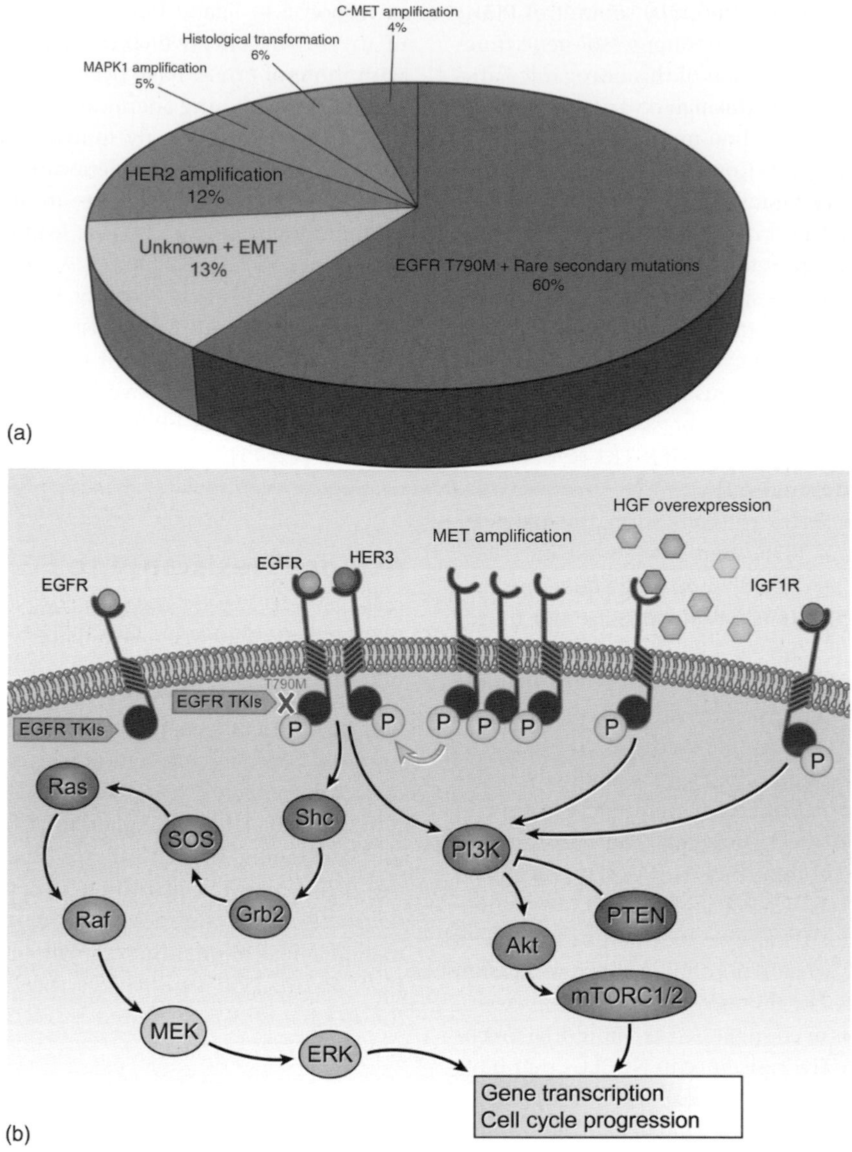

Figure 27.2 Mechanisms of acquired resistant to EGFR TKIs. a: The spectrum and relative frequency of known oncogenic drivers of acquired resistance to EGFR inhibition therapy in lung cancer. b: Schematic representation of pathways to EGFR inhibitor acquired resistance. The secondary T790M mutation of EGFR leads to a decrease in the affinity to EGFR TKIs. MET or IGFR activation induces activation of the PI3K/Akt pathway, independent of EGFR activation.

[I] in *ABL1*, T670I in *KIT*, and T764I in *PDGFR A*) [81, 82].

The well-conserved threonine residue is located near the kinase active site, and its mutation leads to the stabilization of the active conformation of the EGFR tyrosine kinase [83]. Clinical specimens from patients with acquired resistance to EGFR TKIs were used to demonstrate that the T790M mutation is present in approximately 50% of lung adenocarcinoma tissues [84]. It has been shown that in some patients T790M is present in a small number of tumor cells at diagnosis [13] and that during treatment with first-generation EGFR TKIs, clonal selection allows the expansion of the tumor cells bearing T790M, which then become the predominant cells in the tumor mass [85, 86].

In vitro, the T790M-containing cells show a growth disadvantage in the presence of erlotinib and the irreversible EGFR inhibitor BIBW2992 versus their EGFR TKI-sensitive parental counterparts [87]. It has been reported in the literature that these differential growth kinetics may be partly responsible for the "flare" and "re-response" phenomenon observed in some patients with acquired resistance, suggesting that resistant tumors are likely a mixed population of TKI-sensitive and TKI-resistant cells [80]. Upon withdrawal of the selective pressure (TKI), previously arrested TKI-sensitive cells can repopulate more quickly than resistant cells, and tumors may regain sensitivity to EGFR TKI. In patients with acquired resistance, T790M has also been found to be associated with a more indolent phenotype. T790M testing on biopsy specimens from 93 patients with *EGFR*-mutant lung cancer and acquired resistance to TKI showed that those with T790M-mediated resistance had a better prognosis [88]. The indolent nature of T790M-mediated resistance means that these patients can sometimes do well for months on continued single-agent TKI despite progression [89]; the eventual development of more aggressive growth suggests a molecular "third hit," the biology of which requires further characterization. The favorable prognosis associated with the presence of T790M on biopsy suggests a valuable clinical role for biopsy in the assessment of treatment response in these patients.

Other less commonly acquired mutations that do not show sensitivity to EGFR TKIs are L747S, D761Y, and T854A [16, 46, 48]. D761Y in exon 19 has been shown to decrease the sensitivity of the EGFR L858R mutant to EGFR TKIs as described in a patient with brain metastasis [46]. L747S secondary mutation affects the catalytic cleft of the EGFR; this has been described in a patient with prolonged response to single-agent gefitinib who eventually developed this mutant allele [6, 30]. The pattern of resistance with L747S was less pronounced than with L858R-T790M. More recently, the T854A mutation was identified in a patient undergoing prolonged treatment with gefitinib and erlotinib. This mutation to the hydrophobic alanine residue may increase the size of the selectivity pocket, with an eventual negative impact on TKI binding; this finding was equally supported by *in vitro* and *in vivo* data [16, 90].

HER2 amplification

Recently, *HER2* amplification by fluorescence in-situ hybridization has been found in 12% of tumors with acquired resistance versus in only 1% of untreated lung adenocarcinomas [20]. Notably, *HER2* amplification and *EGFR* T790M were mutually exclusive. These results reveal a previously unrecognized mechanism of resistance to EGFR TKIs and provide a rationale to assess the status of and possibly target HER2 in *EGFR*-mutant tumors with acquired resistance to EGFR TKIs.

MAPK1 amplification

In one tumor specimen from erlotinib-treated NSCLC patient who had developed drug resistance a *de novo MAPK1* gene amplification was found that was not present in the pretreatment tumor specimen [76]. The resistant tumors also lacked the more common drug-resistance mechanism *EGFR* T790M or *MET* amplification [76].

MET amplification

c-*MET* amplification is responsible for acquired EGFR TKI resistance in approximately 20% of all patients with *EGFR* mutations and in only 3% of patients with untreated NSCLC with *EGFR* mutation [15, 16]. In tumors that contain the *MET* gene amplification, stimulation of the tumor occurs via the co-receptor HER3, resulting in activation of the PI3K signaling pathway, thereby circumventing the effects of EGFR TKIs [15]. Approximately 50% of patients with *MET* amplification also have the T790M mutation, and it is unclear whether c-*MET*-amplified clones are preferentially selected in the presence of gefitinib or erlotinib therapy. In two more recent studies, *MET* amplification by fluorescence in-situ hybridization was high in 3% [77] and 5% [69] of the reported cases. The lower prevalence of *MET* amplification in these recent studies may be due to the difficulty in identifying this genetic alteration in clinical specimens. The original studies used several methods to assess for amplification [15, 16], including array comparative genomic hybridization, quantitative real-time polymerase chain reaction, and fluorescence in-situ hybridization.

The analysis of 16 clinical specimens from NSCLC patients with acquired resistance revealed that *MET* amplification was present in 25% [4 of 16] of the tumor specimens after gefitinib treatment, although an extremely low level (< 1%) of *MET* amplification was detected in these four cases before gefitinib treatment. Moreover, in all 4 of these cases, a higher expression of HGF was observed after gefitinib treatment than before treatment. These results indicate that HGF accelerates the expansion of the tumor cells with *MET* amplification.

HGF overexpression

HGF overexpression in the absence of *MET* amplification has been reported as a mechanism of EGFR TKI resistance [91]. In cancer tissues from patients with lung adenocarcinoma who showed resistance to gefitinib, high expression levels of HGF were observed in the lung cancer cells that did not harbor the T790M mutation or *MET* amplification. Overexpression of HGF was shown to induce resistance to gefitinib or erlotinib in lung adenocarcinoma cells harboring the EGFR TKI-sensitive mutations [91]. Overexpression of HGF stimulates the PI3K/AKT pathway through MET phosphorylation, independent of ErbB3 phosphorylation. *In vitro* experiments showed that gefitinib-sensitive lung cancer cells became resistant to gefitinib when co-cultured with HGF-producing fibroblasts [92]. Furthermore, the resistance induced by fibroblast-derived HGF was abolished by anti-HGF antibodies or HGF antagonists, such as NK4 [92]. It was suggested that such HGF inhibitors could be used to overcome the resistance to EGFR TKIs.

IGF-1R signaling and other pathways

Other parallel signaling pathways may contribute to the development of resistance to EGFR TKIs, such as the vascular endothelial growth factor receptor (VEGFR) and IGF-1R. Exposing NSCLC cell lines to anti-EGFR antibodies results in a fourfold upregulation of vascular endothelial growth factor (VEGF) [93]. Activation of the VEGF pathway can co-stimulate the tumor cells. Similarly, IGF-1R can activate downstream targets in the EGFR pathway, thereby bypassing cell dependency on the EGFR [14]. In NSCLC cell lines that have been continuously exposed to a first-generation TKI, increased activation of IGF-1R has led to cell growth [94].

Histological transformation

Sequist *et al.* [69] recently reported on a cohort of 37 patients with advanced NSCLC who underwent repeat biopsy at the time of progression on an EGFR TKI. Five of the 37 patients underwent a histological transformation to a small cell lung cancer phenotype. These transformed cancers responded to traditional small cell lung cancer chemotherapy regimens.

Epithelial-mesenchymal transition (EMT)

EMT is observed in several types of epithelial cancers, including NSCLC. EMT is associated with the loss of cell adhesion proteins, such as E-cadherin, and increased invasion, migration, and cell proliferation [95]. Preclinical and clinical data suggest that EMT markers may be associated with limited response to EGFR inhibitors, whereas the retention of an epithelial phenotype is associated with response, even in patients without *EGFR* mutations [96]. Among the several markers that have been associated with EMT, the receptor tyrosine kinase Axl has emerged as a potential target for the identification of EGFR TKI resistance [97].

Pharmacologic interactions

Pharmacologic interactions can also affect EGFR TKI plasma concentrations. As it has been reported for erlotinib and concomitant therapy with cytochrome P450 3A4 (CYP3A4) inducers such as fenofibrate, pharmacologic interactions can cause suboptimal drug exposure and may also result in the lack of an antitumor effect [98]. Cigarette smoking decreases plasma EGFR TKI concentrations. In a Phase 3 NSCLC trial, current smokers achieved erlotinib steady-state trough plasma concentrations which were approximately 2-fold less than the former smokers or patients who had never smoked [99]. This effect was accompanied by a 24% increase in apparent erlotinib plasma clearance due to induction of cytochrome P450 (CYP) 1A isoforms by cigarette smoke [99]. In a separate study which evaluated the single-dose pharmacokinetics of erlotinib in healthy volunteers, current smokers cleared the drug faster than former smokers or volunteers who had never smoked [100]. The area under the curve (AUC)0-infinity in smokers was about 1/3 to 1/2 of that in never/former smokers. In another study which was conducted in NSCLC patients (N = 35) who were current smokers, pharmacokinetic analyses at steady-state indicated a dose-proportional increase in erlotinib exposure when the erlotinib dose was increased from 150 mg to 300 mg. However, the exact dose to be recommended for patients who currently smoke is unknown.

Tumor heterogeneity

Intratumoral heterogeneity may play an important role in EGFR TKI resistance [101]. In fact, in a recent study, 30% of the patients studied had intratumoral heterogeneity, and the *EGFR* mutant content was correlated with response to EGFR TKIs and prognosis [101].

Another challenge for studying acquired resistance to EGFR TKI is that tumor tissue is not always available to confirm the presence of a sensitizing *EGFR* mutation. Current clinical trials are testing optimal strategies and timing for treatment, prevention, or delay of resistance, taking tumor heterogeneity into account.

Conclusions

In conclusion, *EGFR* mutations define a distinct clinical entity of NSCLC with available approved targeted agents such as EGFR TKIs. However, the greatest challenge is to overcome primary and acquired resistance to EGFR TKIs. Confirmation of EGFR TKI resistance should be obtained before altering therapy, and biopsy of a resistant tumor should preferentially guide subsequent therapeutic approaches.

References

1 Siegel R, Naishadham D, Jemal A. (2013) Cancer statistics, 2013. *CA Cancer J Clin*, Jan; 63(1):11–30.

2 Aberle DR, Adams AM, Berg CD, Black WC, Clapp JD, Fagerstrom RM, *et al.* (2011) Reduced lung-cancer mortality with low-dose computed tomographic screening. *N Engl J Med*, Aug 4; 365(5): 395–409.

3 Lynch TJ, Bell DW, Sordella R, Gurubhagavatula S, Okimoto RA, Brannigan BW, *et al.* (2004) Activating mutations in the epidermal growth factor receptor underlying responsiveness of non-small-cell lung cancer to gefitinib. *N Engl J Med*, May 20; 350(21): 2129–39.

4 Paez JG, Janne PA, Lee JC, Tracy S, Greulich H, Gabriel S, *et al.* (2004) EGFR mutations in lung cancer: correlation with clinical response to gefitinib therapy. *Science*, Jun 4; 304(5676): 1497–1500.

5 Pao W, Miller V, Zakowski M, Doherty J, Politi K, Sarkaria I, *et al.* (2004) EGF receptor gene mutations are common in lung cancers from "never smokers" and are associated with sensitivity of tumors to gefitinib and erlotinib. *Proc Natl Acad Sci USA*, Sep 7; 101(36): 13306–11.

6 Kumar A, Petri ET, Halmos B, Boggon TJ (2008) Structure and clinical relevance of the epidermal growth factor receptor in human cancer. *J Clin Oncol*, Apr 1; 26(10): 1742–51.

7 Shigematsu H, Lin L, Takahashi T, Nomura M, Suzuki M, Wistuba, II, *et al.* (2005) Clinical and biological features associated with epidermal growth factor receptor gene mutations in lung cancers. *J Natl Cancer Inst*, Mar 2; 97(5): 339–46.

8 Gazdar AF, Minna JD (2008) Deregulated EGFR signaling during lung cancer progression: mutations, amplicons, and autocrine loops. *Cancer Prev Res (Phila)*, Aug; 1(3): 156–60.

9 Costa DB, Kobayashi S, Tenen DG, Huberman MS (2007) Pooled analysis of the prospective trials of gefitinib monotherapy for EGFR-mutant non-small cell lung cancers. *Lung Cancer*, Oct; 58(1): 95–103.

10 Sequist LV, Martins RG, Spigel D, Grunberg SM, Spira A, Janne PA, *et al.* (2008) First-line gefitinib in patients with advanced non-small-cell lung cancer harboring somatic EGFR mutations. *J Clin Oncol*, May 20; 26(15): 2442–9.

11 Pao W, Wang TY, Riely GJ, Miller VA, Pan Q, Ladanyi M, *et al.* (2005) KRAS mutations and primary resistance of lung adenocarcinomas to gefitinib or erlotinib. *PLoS Med*, Jan; 2(1): e17.

12 Yasuda H, Kobayashi S, Costa DB. EGFR exon 20 insertion mutations in non-small-cell lung cancer: preclinical data and clinical implications. *Lancet Oncol*, Jan; 13(1): e23–31.

13 Sos ML, Koker M, Weir BA, Heynck S, Rabinovsky R, Zander T, *et al.* (2009) PTEN loss contributes to erlotinib resistance in EGFR-mutant lung cancer by activation of Akt and EGFR. *Cancer Res*, Apr 15; 69(8): 3256–61.

14 Guix M, Faber AC, Wang SE, Olivares MG, Song Y, Qu S, *et al.* (2008) Acquired resistance to EGFR tyrosine kinase inhibitors in cancer cells is mediated by loss of IGF-binding proteins. *J Clin Invest*, Jul; 118(7): 2609–19.

15 Engelman JA, Zejnullahu K, Mitsudomi T, Song Y, Hyland C, Park JO, *et al.* (2007) MET amplification leads to gefitinib resistance in lung cancer by activating ERBB3 signaling. *Science*, May 18; 316(5827): 1039–43.

16 Bean J, Riely GJ, Balak M, Marks JL, Ladanyi M, Miller VA, *et al.* (2008) Acquired resistance to epidermal growth factor receptor kinase inhibitors associated with a novel T854A mutation in a patient with EGFR-mutant lung adenocarcinoma. *Clin Cancer Res*, Nov 15; 14(22): 7519–25.

17 Tam IY, Chung LP, Suen WS, Wang E, Wong MC, Ho KK, *et al.* (2006) Distinct epidermal growth factor receptor and KRAS mutation patterns in non-small cell lung cancer patients with different tobacco exposure and clinicopathologic features. *Clin Cancer Res*, Mar 1; 12(5): 1647–53.

18 Fidler MJ, Morrison LE, Basu S, Buckingham L, Walters K, Batus M, *et al.* (2011) PTEN and PIK3CA gene copy numbers and poor outcomes in non-small cell lung cancer patients with gefitinib therapy. *Br J Cancer*, Dec 6; 105(12): 1920–6.

19 Sasaki H, Shimizu S, Endo K, Takada M, Kawahara M, Tanaka H, *et al.* (2006) EGFR and erbB2 mutation status in Japanese lung cancer patients. *Int J Cancer*, Jan 1; 118(1): 180–4.

20 Takezawa K, Pirazzoli V, Arcila ME, Nebhan CA, Song X, de Stanchina E, *et al.* (2012) HER2 amplification: a potential mechanism of acquired resistance to EGFR inhibition in EGFR-mutant lung cancers that lack the second-site EGFRT790M mutation. *Cancer Discov*, Oct; 2(10): 922–33.

21 Paik PK, Arcila ME, Fara M, Sima CS, Miller VA, Kris MG, *et al.* (2011) Clinical characteristics of patients with lung adenocarcinomas harboring BRAF mutations. *J Clin Oncol*, May 20; 29(15): 2046–51.

22 Marchetti A, Felicioni L, Malatesta S, Grazia Sciarrotta M, Guetti L, Chella A, *et al.* (2011) Clinical features and outcome of patients with non-small-cell lung cancer harboring BRAF mutations. *J Clin Oncol*, Sep 10; 29(26): 3574–9.

23 Cappuzzo F, Toschi L, Domenichini I, Bartolini S, Ceresoli GL, Rossi E, *et al.* (2005) HER3 genomic gain and sensitivity to gefitinib in advanced non-small-cell lung cancer patients. *Br J Cancer*, Dec 12; 93(12): 1334–40.

24 Pao W, Chmielecki J (2010) Rational, biologically based treatment of EGFR-mutant non-small-cell lung cancer. *Nat Rev Cancer*, Nov; 10(11): 760–74.

25 Yun CH, Mengwasser KE, Toms AV, Woo MS, Greulich H, Wong KK, *et al.* (2008) The T790M mutation in EGFR kinase causes drug resistance by increasing the affinity for ATP. *Proc Natl Acad Sci USA*, Feb 12; 105(6): 2070–5.

26 Eck MJ, Yun CH (2010) Structural and mechanistic underpinnings of the differential drug sensitivity of EGFR mutations in non-small cell lung cancer. *Biochim Biophys Acta*, Mar; 1804(3): 559–66.

27 Linardou H, Dahabreh IJ, Bafaloukos D, Kosmidis P, Murray S (2009) Somatic EGFR mutations and efficacy of tyrosine kinase inhibitors in NSCLC. *Nat Rev Clin Oncol*, Jun; 6(6): 352–66.

28 Murray S, Dahabreh IJ, Linardou H, Manoloukos M, Bafaloukos D, Kosmidis P (2008) Somatic mutations of the tyrosine kinase domain of epidermal growth factor receptor and tyrosine kinase inhibitor response to TKIs in non-small cell lung cancer: an analytical database. *J Thorac Oncol*, Aug; 3(8): 832–9.

29 Yasuda H, Kobayashi S, Costa DB (2012) EGFR exon 20 insertion mutations in non-small-cell lung cancer: preclinical data and clinical implications. *Lancet Oncol*, 13(1): e23–e31.

30 Greulich H, Chen TH, Feng W, Janne PA, Alvarez JV, Zappaterra M, *et al.* (2005) Oncogenic transformation by inhibitor-sensitive and -resistant EGFR mutants. *PLoS Med*, Nov; 2(11): e313.

31 Yuza Y, Glatt KA, Jiang J, Greulich H, Minami Y, Woo MS, *et al.* (2007) Allele-dependent variation in the

relative cellular potency of distinct EGFR inhibitors. *Cancer Biol Ther*, May; 6(5): 661–7.

32 Harada T, Lopez-Chavez A, Xi L, Raffeld M, Wang Y, Giaccone G (2011) Characterization of epidermal growth factor receptor mutations in non-small-cell lung cancer patients of African-American ancestry. *Oncogene*, Apr 14; 30(15): 1744–52.

33 Engelman JA, Zejnullahu K, Gale CM, Lifshits E, Gonzales AJ, Shimamura T, *et al.* (2007) PF00299804, an irreversible pan-ERBB inhibitor, is effective in lung cancer models with EGFR and ERBB2 mutations that are resistant to gefitinib. *Cancer Res*, Dec 15; 67(24): 11924–32.

34 Sequist LV, Besse B, Lynch TJ, Miller VA, Wong KK, Gitlitz B, *et al.* (2010) Neratinib, an irreversible pan-ErbB receptor tyrosine kinase inhibitor: results of a phase II trial in patients with advanced non-small-cell lung cancer. *J Clin Oncol*, Jun 20; 28(18): 3076–83.

35 Janne PA, Boss DS, Camidge DR, Britten CD, Engelman JA, Garon EB, *et al.* (2011) Phase I dose-escalation study of the pan-HER inhibitor, PF299804, in patients with advanced malignant solid tumors. *Clin Cancer Res*, Mar 1; 17(5): 1131–9.

36 Shih J, Yu CJ, Su W (2011) Activity of BIBW 2992, an irreversible EGFR/HER1 TKI, in lung adenocarcinoma patients harboring less common EGFR mutations. *Ann Oncol*, 21(Suppl 8): 415.

37 Yang CH, Shih J, Chao T (eds) (2008) Use of BIBW 2992, a novel irreversible EGFR/HER2 TKI to induce regression in patients with adenocarcinoma of the lung and activating EGFR mutations preliminary results of a single-arm phase II clinical trial. *Proc Am Soc Clin Oncol*, 26(15S) (May 20 Supplement): 8026.

38 Shimamura T, Lowell AM, Engelman JA, Shapiro GI (2005) Epidermal growth factor receptors harboring kinase domain mutations associate with the heat shock protein 90 chaperone and are destabilized following exposure to geldanamycins. *Cancer Res*, Jul 15; 65(14): 6401–8.

39 Sequist LV, Gettinger S, Senzer NN, Martins RG, Janne PA, Lilenbaum R, *et al.* (2010) Activity of IPI-504, a novel heat-shock protein 90 inhibitor, in patients with molecularly defined non-small-cell lung cancer. *J Clin Oncol*, Nov 20; 28(33): 4953–60.

40 Wu SG, Chang YL, Hsu YC, Wu JY, Yang CH, Yu CJ, *et al.* (2008) Good response to gefitinib in lung adenocarcinoma of complex epidermal growth factor receptor (EGFR) mutations with the classical mutation pattern. *Oncologist*, Dec; 13(12): 1276–84.

41 Zhang GC, Lin JY, Wang Z, Zhou Q, Xu CR, Zhu JQ, *et al.* (2007) Epidermal growth factor receptor double activating mutations involving both exons 19 and 21 exist in Chinese non-small cell lung cancer patients. *Clin Oncol (R Coll Radiol)*, Sep; 19(7): 499–506.

42 Chou TY, Chiu CH, Li LH, Hsiao CY, Tzen CY, Chang KT, *et al.* (2005) Mutation in the tyrosine kinase domain of epidermal growth factor receptor is a predictive and prognostic factor for gefitinib treatment in patients with non-small cell lung cancer. *Clin Cancer Res*, May 15; 11(10): 3750–7.

43 Hata A, Yoshioka H, Fujita S, Kunimasa K, Kaji R, Imai Y, *et al.* (2010) Complex mutations in the epidermal growth factor receptor gene in non-small cell lung cancer. *J Thorac Oncol*, Oct; 5(10): 1524–8.

44 Jiang J, Greulich H, Janne PA, Sellers WR, Meyerson M, Griffin JD (2005) Epidermal growth factor-independent transformation of Ba/F3 cells with cancer-derived epidermal growth factor receptor mutants induces gefitinib-sensitive cell cycle progression. *Cancer Res*, Oct 1; 65(19): 8968–74.

45 Mitsudomi T, Yatabe Y (2007) Mutations of the epidermal growth factor receptor gene and related genes as determinants of epidermal growth factor receptor tyrosine kinase inhibitors sensitivity in lung cancer. *Cancer Sci*, Dec; 98(12): 1817–24.

46 Balak MN, Gong Y, Riely GJ, Somwar R, Li AR, Zakowski MF, *et al.* (2006) Novel D761Y and common secondary T790M mutations in epidermal growth factor receptor-mutant lung adenocarcinomas with acquired resistance to kinase inhibitors. *Clin Cancer Res*, Nov 1; 12(21): 6494–6501.

47 Costa DB, Schumer ST, Tenen DG, Kobayashi S (2008) Differential responses to erlotinib in epidermal growth factor receptor (EGFR)-mutated lung cancers with acquired resistance to gefitinib carrying the L747S or T790M secondary mutations. *J Clin Oncol*, Mar 1; 26(7): 1182–4; author reply 4–6.

48 Costa DB, Halmos B, Kumar A, Schumer ST, Huberman MS, Boggon TJ, *et al.* (2007) BIM mediates EGFR tyrosine kinase inhibitor-induced apoptosis in lung cancers with oncogenic EGFR mutations. *PLoS Med*, Oct; 4(10): 1669–79; discussion 80.

49 Janne PA, Engelman JA, Johnson BE (2005) Epidermal growth factor receptor mutations in non-small-cell lung cancer: Implications for treatment and tumor biology. *J Clin Oncol*, May 10; 23(14): 3227–34.

50 Graziano SL, Gamble GP, Newman NB, Abbott LZ, Rooney M, Mookherjee S, *et al.* (1999) Prognostic significance of K-ras codon 12 mutations in patients with resected stage I and II non-small-cell lung cancer. *J Clin Oncol*, Feb; 17(2): 668–75.

51 Eberhard DA, Johnson BE, Amler LC, Goddard AD, Heldens SL, Herbst RS, *et al.* (2005) Mutations in the epidermal growth factor receptor and in KRAS are predictive and prognostic indicators in patients with non-small-cell lung cancer treated with chemotherapy alone and in combination with erlotinib. *J Clin Oncol*, Sep 1; 23(25): 5900–9.

52 Massarelli E, Varella-Garcia M, Tang X, Xavier AC, Ozburn NC, Liu DD, *et al.* (2007) KRAS mutation is an important predictor of resistance to therapy with epidermal growth factor receptor tyrosine kinase inhibitors in non-small-cell lung cancer. *Clin Cancer Res*, May 15; 13(10): 2890–6.

53 Zhu CQ, da Cunha Santos G, Ding K, Sakurada A, Cutz JC, Liu N, *et al.* (2008) Role of KRAS and EGFR as biomarkers of response to erlotinib in National Cancer Institute of Canada Clinical Trials Group Study BR.21. *J Clin Oncol*, Sep 10; 26(26): 4268–75.

54 Cantley LC (2002) The phosphoinositide 3-kinase pathway. *Science*, May 31; 296(5573): 1655–7.

55 Osaki M, Oshimura M, Ito H (2004) PI3K-Akt pathway: Its functions and alterations in human cancer. *Apoptosis*, Nov; 9(6): 667–76.

56 Di Cristofano A, Pesce B, Cordon-Cardo C, Pandolfi PP (1998) Pten is essential for embryonic development and tumour suppression. *Nat Genet*, Aug; 19(4): 348–55.

57 Frayling IM, Bodmer WF, Tomlinson IP (1997) Allele loss in colorectal cancer at the Cowden disease/juvenile polyposis locus on 10q. *Cancer Genet Cytogenet*, Aug; 97(1): 64–9.

58 Goel A, Arnold CN, Niedzwiecki D, Carethers JM, Dowell JM, Wasserman L, *et al.* (2004) Frequent inactivation of PTEN by promoter hypermethylation in microsatellite instability-high sporadic colorectal cancers. *Cancer Res*, May 1; 64(9): 3014–21.

59 Meng F, Henson R, Wehbe-Janek H, Ghoshal K, Jacob ST, Patel T (2007) MicroRNA-21 regulates expression of the PTEN tumor suppressor gene in human hepatocellular cancer. *Gastroenterology*, Aug; 133(2): 647–58.

60 Janmaat ML, Kruyt FA, Rodriguez JA, Giaccone G (2003) Response to epidermal growth factor receptor inhibitors in non-small cell lung cancer cells: limited antiproliferative effects and absence of apoptosis associated with persistent activity of extracellular signal-regulated kinase or Akt kinase pathways. *Clin Cancer Res*, Jun; 9(6): 2316–26.

61 Engelman JA, Janne PA, Mermel C, Pearlberg J, Mukohara T, Fleet C, *et al.* (2005) ErbB-3 mediates phosphoinositide 3-kinase activity in gefitinib-sensitive non-small cell lung cancer cell lines. *Proc Natl Acad Sci USA*, Mar 8; 102(10): 3788–93.

62 Yamasaki F, Johansen MJ, Zhang D, Krishnamurthy S, Felix E, Bartholomeusz C, *et al.* (2007) Acquired resistance to erlotinib in A-431 epidermoid cancer cells requires down-regulation of MMAC1/PTEN and up-regulation of phosphorylated Akt. *Cancer Res*, Jun 15; 67(12): 5779–88.

63 Hiles ID, Otsu M, Volinia S, Fry MJ, Gout I, Dhand R, *et al.* (1992) Phosphatidylinositol 3-kinase: structure and expression of the 110 kd catalytic subunit. *Cell*, Aug 7; 70(3): 419–29.

64 Kawano O, Sasaki H, Endo K, Suzuki E, Haneda H, Yukiue H, *et al.* (2006) PIK3CA mutation status in Japanese lung cancer patients. *Lung Cancer*, Nov; 54(2): 209–15.

65 Kawano O, Sasaki H, Okuda K, Yukiue H, Yokoyama T, Yano M, *et al.* (2007) PIK3CA gene amplification in Japanese non-small cell lung cancer. *Lung Cancer*, Oct; 58(1): 159–60.

66 Okudela K, Suzuki M, Kageyama S, Bunai T, Nagura K, Igarashi H, *et al.* (2007) PIK3CA mutation and amplification in human lung cancer. *Pathol Int*, Oct; 57(10): 664–71.

67 Sun Y, Ren Y, Fang Z, Li C, Fang R, Gao B, *et al.* (2010) Lung adenocarcinoma from East Asian never-smokers is a disease largely defined by targetable oncogenic mutant kinases. *J Clin Oncol*, Oct 20; 28(30): 4616–20.

68 Engelman JA, Mukohara T, Zejnullahu K, Lifshits E, Borras AM, Gale CM, *et al.* (2006) Allelic dilution obscures detection of a biologically significant resistance mutation in EGFR-amplified lung cancer. *J Clin Invest*, Oct; 116(10): 2695–2706.

69 Sequist LV, Waltman BA, Dias-Santagata D, Digumarthy S, Turke AB, Fidias P, *et al.* (2011) Genotypic and histological evolution of lung cancers acquiring resistance to EGFR inhibitors. *Sci Transl Med*, Mar 23; 3(75): 75ra26.

70 Buckingham LE, Coon JS, Morrison LE, Jacobson KK, Jewell SS, Kaiser KA, *et al.* (2007) The prognostic value of chromosome 7 polysomy in non-small cell lung cancer patients treated with gefitinib. *J Thorac Oncol*, May; 2(5): 414–22.

71 Stephens P, Hunter C, Bignell G, Edkins S, Davies H, Teague J, *et al.* (2004) Lung cancer: intragenic ERBB2 kinase mutations in tumours. *Nature*, Sep 30; 431(7008): 525–6.

72 Cappuzzo F, Varella-Garcia M, Shigematsu H, Domenichini I, Bartolini S, Ceresoli GL, *et al.* (2005)

Increased HER2 gene copy number is associated with response to gefitinib therapy in epidermal growth factor receptor-positive non-small-cell lung cancer patients. *J Clin Oncol*, Aug 1; 23(22): 5007–18.

73 Cappuzzo F, Bemis L, Varella-Garcia M (2006) HER2 mutation and response to trastuzumab therapy in non-small-cell lung cancer. *N Engl J Med*, Jun 15; 354(24): 2619–21.

74 Cappuzzo F, Ligorio C, Toschi L, Rossi E, Trisolini R, Paioli D, *et al.* (2007) EGFR and HER2 gene copy number and response to first-line chemotherapy in patients with advanced non-small cell lung cancer (NSCLC). *J Thorac Oncol*, May; 2(5): 423–9.

75 Daniele L, Macri L, Schena M, Dongiovanni D, Bonello L, Armando E, *et al.* (2007) Predicting gefitinib responsiveness in lung cancer by fluorescence in situ hybridization/chromogenic in situ hybridization analysis of EGFR and HER2 in biopsy and cytology specimens. *Mol Cancer Ther*, Apr; 6(4): 1223–9.

76 Ercan D, Xu C, Yanagita M, Monast CS, Pratilas CA, Montero J, *et al.* (2012) Reactivation of ERK signaling causes resistance to EGFR kinase inhibitors. *Cancer Discov*, Oct; 2(10): 934–47.

77 Arcila ME, Oxnard GR, Nafa K, Riely GJ, Solomon SB, Zakowski MF, *et al.* (2011) Rebiopsy of lung cancer patients with acquired resistance to EGFR inhibitors and enhanced detection of the T790M mutation using a locked nucleic acid-based assay. *Clin Cancer Res*, Mar 1; 17(5): 1169–80.

78 Pao W, Miller VA, Politi KA, Riely GJ, Somwar R, Zakowski MF, *et al.* (2005) Acquired resistance of lung adenocarcinomas to gefitinib or erlotinib is associated with a second mutation in the EGFR kinase domain. *PLoS Med*, Mar; 2(3): e73.

79 Kobayashi S, Boggon TJ, Dayaram T, Janne PA, Kocher O, Meyerson M, *et al.* (2005) EGFR mutation and resistance of non-small-cell lung cancer to gefitinib. *N Engl J Med*, Feb 24; 352(8): 786–92.

80 Kosaka T, Yatabe Y, Endoh H, Yoshida K, Hida T, Tsuboi M, *et al.* (2006) Analysis of epidermal growth factor receptor gene mutation in patients with non-small cell lung cancer and acquired resistance to gefitinib. *Clin Cancer Res*, Oct 1; 12(19): 5764–9.

81 Azam M, Seeliger MA, Gray NS, Kuriyan J, Daley GQ (2008) Activation of tyrosine kinases by mutation of the gatekeeper threonine. *Nat Struct Mol Biol*, Oct; 15(10): 1109–18.

82 Carter TA, Wodicka LM, Shah NP, Velasco AM, Fabian MA, Treiber DK, *et al.* (2005) Inhibition of drug-resistant mutants of ABL, KIT, and EGF receptor kinases. *Proc Natl Acad Sci USA*, Aug 2; 102(31): 11011–16.

83 Raben D, Helfrich B, Chan DC, Ciardiello F, Zhao L, Franklin W, *et al.* (2005) The effects of cetuximab alone and in combination with radiation and/or chemotherapy in lung cancer. *Clin Cancer Res*, Jan 15; 11(2 Pt 1): 795–805.

84 Suda K, Onozato R, Yatabe Y, Mitsudomi T (2009) EGFR T790M mutation: A double role in lung cancer cell survival? *J Thorac Oncol*, Jan; 4(1): 1–4.

85 Inukai M, Toyooka S, Ito S, Asano H, Ichihara S, Soh J, *et al.* (2006) Presence of epidermal growth factor receptor gene T790M mutation as a minor clone in non-small cell lung cancer. *Cancer Res*, Aug 15; 66(16): 7854–8.

86 Maheswaran S, Sequist LV, Nagrath S, Ulkus L, Brannigan B, Collura CV, *et al.* (2008) Detection of mutations in EGFR in circulating lung-cancer cells. *N Engl J Med*, Jul 24; 359(4): 366–77.

87 Chmielecki J, Foo J, Oxnard GR, Hutchinson K, Ohashi K, Somwar R, *et al.* (2011) Optimization of dosing for EGFR-mutant non-small cell lung cancer with evolutionary cancer modeling. *Sci Transl Med*, Jul 6; 3(90): 90ra59.

88 Oxnard GR, Arcila ME, Sima CS, Riely GJ, Chmielecki J, Kris MG, *et al.* (2011) Acquired resistance to EGFR tyrosine kinase inhibitors in EGFR-mutant lung cancer: distinct natural history of patients with tumors harboring the T790M mutation. *Clin Cancer Res*, Mar 15; 17(6): 1616–22.

89 Mok TS (2010) Living with imperfection. *J Clin Oncol*, Jan 10; 28(2): 191–2.

90 Avizienyte E, Ward RA, Garner AP (2008) Comparison of the EGFR resistance mutation profiles generated by EGFR-targeted tyrosine kinase inhibitors and the impact of drug combinations. *Biochem J*, Oct 15; 415(2): 197–206.

91 Yano S, Wang W, Li Q, Matsumoto K, Sakurama H, Nakamura T, *et al.* (2008) Hepatocyte growth factor induces gefitinib resistance of lung adenocarcinoma with epidermal growth factor receptor-activating mutations. *Cancer Res*, Nov 15; 68(22): 9479–87.

92 Wang W, Li Q, Yamada T, Matsumoto K, Matsumoto I, Oda M, *et al.* (2009) Crosstalk to stromal fibroblasts induces resistance of lung cancer to epidermal growth factor receptor tyrosine kinase inhibitors. *Clin Cancer Res*, Nov 1; 15(21): 6630–8.

93 Viloria-Petit A, Crombet T, Jothy S, Hicklin D, Bohlen P, Schlaeppi JM, *et al.* (2001) Acquired resistance to the antitumor effect of epidermal growth factor

receptor-blocking antibodies in vivo: a role for altered tumor angiogenesis. *Cancer Res*, Jul 1; 61(13): 5090–6101.

94 Nguyen KS, Kobayashi S, Costa DB (2009) Acquired resistance to epidermal growth factor receptor tyrosine kinase inhibitors in non-small-cell lung cancers dependent on the epidermal growth factor receptor pathway. *Clin Lung Cancer*, Jul; 10(4): 281–9.

95 Thiery JP, Acloque H, Huang RY, Nieto MA (2009) Epithelial-mesenchymal transitions in development and disease. *Cell*, Nov 25; 139(5): 871–90.

96 Yauch RL, Januario T, Eberhard DA, Cavet G, Zhu W, Fu L, *et al.* (2005) Epithelial versus mesenchymal phenotype determines in vitro sensitivity and predicts clinical activity of erlotinib in lung cancer patients. *Clin Cancer Res*, Dec 15; 11(24 Pt 1): 8686–98.

97 Zhang Z, Lee JC, Lin L, Olivas V, Au V, LaFramboise T, *et al.* (2012) Activation of the AXL kinase causes resistance to EGFR-targeted therapy in lung cancer. *Nat Genet*, Aug; 44(8): 852–60.

98 Mir O, Blanchet B, Goldwasser F (2011) Drug-induced effects on erlotinib metabolism. *N Engl J Med*, Jul 28; 365(4): 379–80.

99 Hamilton M, Wolf JL, Rusk J, Beard SE, Clark GM, Witt K, *et al.* (2006) Effects of smoking on the pharmacokinetics of erlotinib. *Clin Cancer Res*, Apr 1; 12(7 Pt 1): 2166–71.

100 Clark GM, Zborowski DM, Santabarbara P, Ding K, Whitehead M, Seymour L, *et al.* (2006) Smoking history and epidermal growth factor receptor expression as predictors of survival benefit from erlotinib for patients with non-small-cell lung cancer in the National Cancer Institute of Canada Clinical Trials Group study BR.21. *Clin Lung Cancer*, May; 7(6): 389–94.

101 Bai H, Wang Z, Wang Y, Zhuo M, Zhou Q, Duan J, *et al.* (2013) Detection and clinical significance of intratumoral EGFR mutational heterogeneity in Chinese patients with advanced non-small cell lung cancer. *PLoS One*, 8(2): e54170.

CHAPTER 28

Predictive Tumor Biomarkers for EGFR Inhibitors

Lucia Kim,[1] *Geoffrey Liu,*[2] *and Ming-Sound Tsao*[3]

[1]Department of Pathology, Inha University School of Medicine, Incheon, South Korea
[2]Department of Medicine, Medical Biophysics, and Epidemiology, University of Toronto, Toronto, ON, Canada
[3]Department of Laboratory Medicine and Pathobiology, University of Toronto, Toronto, ON, Canada

Oncogenesis involves the stepwise acquisition of activating mutations in the oncogenes and inactivating mutations in the tumor suppressor genes. In several types of cancer, it has now been established that tumor cells are "addicted" to specific oncogenic mutations (driver mutations) and are dependent on their continued effects for the maintenance of their malignant phenotype. Consequently, the inhibition of these mutant gene products can result in massive apoptosis and tumor shrinkage without any ill effects on the normal cells [1]. The concept of oncogene addiction shifts the paradigm of cancer treatment from cytotoxic chemotherapy toward a personalized therapy targeting specific protein product of driver oncogenes.

Epidermal growth factor receptor (EGFR) is commonly highly expressed in various types of epithelial cancers including non-small cell lung cancer (NSCLC). Mutations in the tyrosine kinase (TK) domain of *EGFR* have been found almost exclusively in NSCLC, especially adenocarcinoma [2–5]. The *EGFR* gene is often also amplified [6, 7]. The targeted inhibition of EGFR pathway may cause massive cancer cell death and dramatic clinical response [3, 8]. EGFR has been selected as a target molecule for NSCLC treatment and clinical effectiveness of small molecule EGFR-tyrosine kinase inhibitors (TKIs), such as gefitinib and erlotinib, and EGFR specific monoclonal antibodies, such as cetuximab have been studied extensively. However, in unselected NSCLC patient populations, the efficacy of EGFR inhibitors was not superior to cytotoxic chemotherapeutic drugs [9, 10], and only a subset of NSCLC patients showed dramatic response to EGFR inhibitors. Females, having a non-smoking history, being East Asian and having an adenocarcinoma histology have been associated with greater response rates to EGFR inhibitor therapies [11, 12]. Although *EGFR* mutation is the strongest biomarker for predicting sensitivity to the EGFR inhibitors [3, 8, 13], patient responses to treatment vary considerably. A small proportion of *EGFR* mutant patients show primary resistance to EGFR inhibitor therapy, while *EGFR* mutation-independent responses have also been identified. In order to successfully treat NSCLC with EGFR-inhibitors, it is critical to identify which patients are likely to respond to treatment. Therefore understanding of biologic processes related to the sensitivity to these drugs and exploring predictive biomarkers for response to EGFR inhibitors is important, not only for patients selection, but also for progress of therapeutic strategies. Here we review the molecular abnormalities

Lung Cancer, Fourth Edition. Edited by Jack A. Roth, Waun Ki Hong and Ritsuko U. Komaki.

associated with EGFR pathway in NSCLC and their clinical relevance to EGFR inhibitors and potential value as predictive biomarkers to guide to therapy with EGFR-inhibitors.

EGFR

EGFR is a member of the receptor tyrosine kinase (RTK) family which includes EGFR (ERBB1/HER1), HER2 (ERBB2), HER3 (ERBB3) and HER4 (ERBB4). The *EGFR* gene is located on the short arm of chromosome 7 (7p11.2). EGFR protein is composed of four functional domains; an extracellular ligand-binding domain, a transmembrane domain, an intracellular TK domain, and a C-terminal regulatory domain. The TK domain contains an ATP binding pocket formed between the N-lobe and C- lobe. Binding of specific ligands such as EGF, transforming growth factor (TGF)-alpha or amphiregulin to the extracellular domain of EGFR induces the formation of homodimers between two EGFRs or heterodimers between EGFR and one of the other family members. Receptor dimerization activates the intrinsic TK through binding of ATP and promotes autophosphorylation of tyrosine residues in the cytoplasmic domain including TK domains. Phosphorylated tyrosine residues serve as docking sites for multiple adaptor molecules, which in turn, activate downstream signaling pathways, including RAS/RAF/MAPK, PI3K/AKT and STAT pathways, which regulate cell proliferation, apoptosis, motility, differentiation and adhesion. There is accumulating evidence that selected blocking of EGFR or downstream molecules is an effective therapeutic option against cancers. Tumor response or resistance to TKIs may be influenced by many factors, including type of mutation on the *EGFR* gene, *EGFR* gene copy number changes, *KRAS* mutations, and others (Figure 28.1).

EGFR mutation

EGFR mutations are distributed across exons 18 through 21, specifically around the ATP binding pocket [3, 8]. The ATP binding pocket is involved in the activation of the receptor and is also the binding site for EGFR-TKIs, which compete with ATP. *EGFR* mutations destabilize the inactive conformation, promote the active conformation of the kinase [14], and induce ligand-independent activation and autophosphorylation of the tyrosine residues in the cytoplasmic domain of the receptor [15, 16]. This results in selective activation of downstream AKT and STAT pathways, which then promote cell survival [17]. They also enhance the oncogenicity and transformation ability of tumor cells [15, 16]. The dependency of NSCLC tumors on mutated EGFR is essential for initiation and maintenance of the malignant phenotype [1]. EGFR mutated tumors exhibit increased affinity for EGFR-TKIs [15], and treatment with EGFR-TKIs induce a temporary imbalance in pro-survival and pro-apoptotic signals resulting in apoptotic cell death [18].

Sensitizing *EGFR* mutations

The commonly identified sensitizing mutations in NSCLC are in-frame deletions on exon 19, and point mutation on exon 21 (L858R) [3, 8, 19]. An exon 19 deletion centered around codon 746 to 750 and a substitution mutation of leucine with arginine at codon 858 (L858R) represent approximately 85–90% of the sensitizing (classical) *EGFR* mutations [3, 8, 20, 21]. The prevalence of *EGFR* mutations in NSCLC among clinical responders to EGFR-TKIs is very high, with more than 70% in most studies, compared with less than 10% in NSCLC patients who are refractory to EGFR-TKIs [22]. In clinical trials, 60–80% of chemotherapy naïve patients with sensitizing mutations respond to EGFR-TKIs, whereas only approximately 10% of patients with wild type *EGFR* shows response (Table 28.1) [4, 5, 7, 21–28].

EGFR mutated tumors represent a specific subset of NSCLC that shows distinct clinicopathologic features similar to EGFR-TKI responders. *EGFR* mutations preferentially but not exclusively affect females, nonsmokers, East Asians, and patients with an adenocarcinoma histology [3, 4, 21]. Preference of *EGFR* mutation in female and nonsmokers suggests that *EGFR* mutations are associated with other carcinogenic mechanisms that are unrelated to cigarette smoking. In East Asian populations, about 30–50% of NSCLC patients

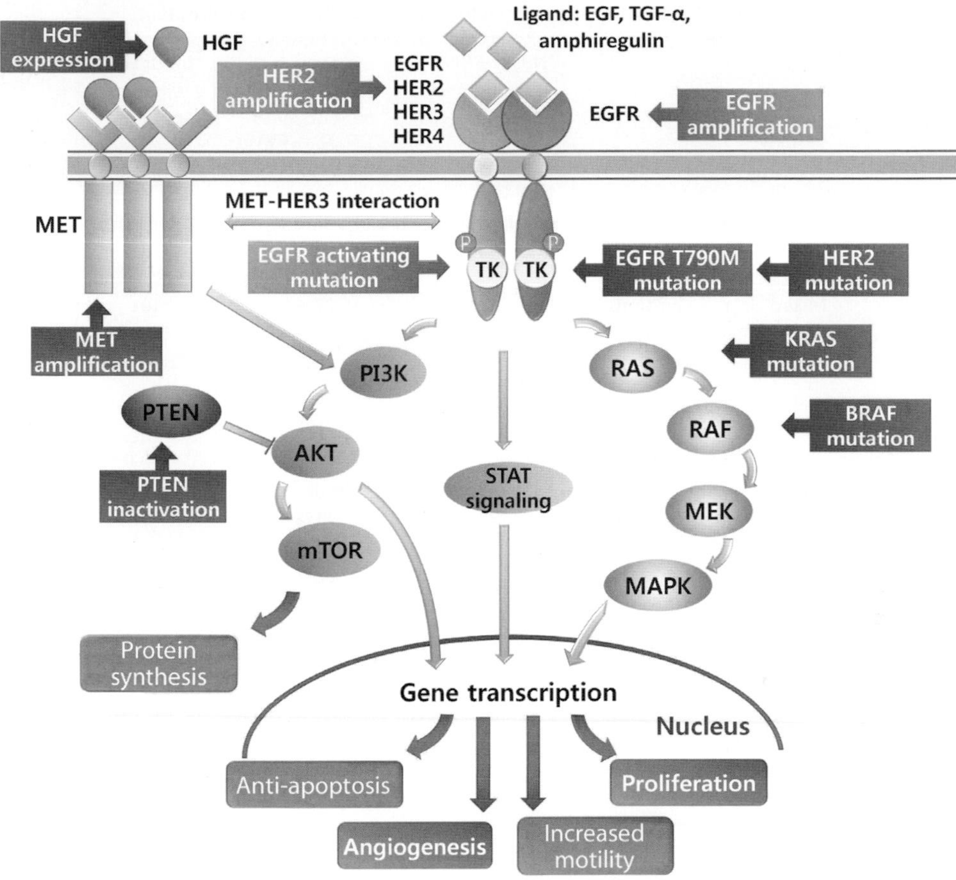

Figure 28.1 Signaling pathway of EGFR and related molecules. Binding of ligand to EGFR induce the receptors to form homodimers or heterodimers, which activate the intrinsic intracellular TK by autophosphorylation of tyrosine residues. The activation of EGFR drives signaling cascades involving downstream RAS, PI3K/AKT and STAT pathways and eventually results in cellular response such as proliferation, anti-apoptosis, increased cell motility and angiogenesis. *MET* amplification triggers HER3-dependent activation of PI3K/AKT pathway bypassing EGFR, which results in acquired resistance in *EGFR* mutant tumors. Genetic and epigenetic abnormalities targeting EGFR and downstream molecules which are associated with sensitivity (blue box) or resistance (red box) to EGR-TKIs are indicated. (For a color version, see the color plate section.)

harbor *EGFR* mutations, whereas, in Caucasian populations, only 10–20% of patients harbor *EGFR* mutations in their tumors [4, 24, 29]. However, there is no significant differences in the type and locations of *EGFR* mutations between the tumors of East Asian and non-East Asian and predominantly Caucasian patients [30]. In terms of tumor histology, *EGFR* mutations are associated with adenocarcinomas that show lepidic, papillary or acinar histology [2] and most demonstrate immunoreactivity for thyroid transcription factor-1 (TTF-1). This latter association has led to the hypothesis that *EGFR* mutant tumors represent terminal respiratory unit type adenocarcinoma [31].

In East Asian populations, relatively higher proportions of squamous cell carcinoma harbor *EGFR* mutations [32–34] and some *EGFR* mutated squamous cell carcinomas also show focal adenocarcinomatous differentiation as revealed by immunohistochemistry (IHC)-based marker studies [34, 35]. As some *EGFR* mutated squamous cell carcinomas diagnosed with biopsies might

Table 28.1 Response rate to EGFR-TKIs in chemotherapy naïve or previously treated patients

Trials	Patient ethnicity	EGFR-TKI	No. of *EGFR* sensitizing mutant patients evaluable for TKI response	Percent of *EGFR* mutant patients with response* to TKI	No. of *EGFR* wild type patients evaluable for TKI response	Percent of *EGFR* wild type patients with response to TKI
			One or more previous chemotherapy (second-line or more)			
IDEAL (Bell *et al.*, 2005) [5]	Mixed	Gefitinib	13	46%	61	10%
BR.21 (Zhu *et al.*, 2008) [23]	Mixed	Gefitinib	15	27%	101	7%
ISEL (Hirsch *et al.*, 2006) [7]	Mixed	Gefitinib	16	38%	116	3%
INTEREST (Douillard *et al.*, 2010) [4]	Mixed	Gefitinib	19	42%	106	7%
			No previous chemotherapy (first-line)			
IPASS (Mok *et al.* 2009) [24]	East-Asian	Gefitinib	132	71%	91	1%
WJTOG3405 (Mitsudomi *et al.* 2010) [25]	Japanese	Gefitinib	58	62%	NA	NA
NEJ002 (Maemondo *et al.* 2010) [26]	Japanese	Gefitinib	114	74%	NA	NA
OPTIMAL (Zhou *et al.*, 2011) [27]	Chinese	Erlotinib	82	83%	NA	NA
EURTARC (Rosell *et al.*, 2012) [28]	Caucasian	Erlotinib	77	64%	NA	NA

*Response: complete response or partial response; NA: data not available.

represent incompletely sampled adenosquamous carcinoma or poorly differentiated adenocarcinoma mimicking squamous morphology, the real prevalence of *EGFR* mutations in pure squamous cell carcinoma is likely low [35, 36]. However, a recent study from Japan [34] reported that using a highly sensitive mutation assay, EGFR mutation could be found in 13% of 249 patients. The Cancer Genome Atlas (TCGA) project also reported the identification of only 2 EGFR mutated tumors among 176 squamous cell carcinomas sequenced, and both had the less common L861Q mutation [36, 37]. EGFR-TKIs also seem to be less effective in patients with *EGFR* mutated squamous cell carcinomas than in patients with *EGFR* mutated adenocarcinomas [34, 37]. Similarly, *EGFR* mutations are very rarely found in small cell lung carcinomas, and most of these patients are never-smokers and have an adenocarcinoma component. EGFR-TKIs also seem to be less effective in these patients [38, 39].

Resistant *EGFR* mutations

All NSCLC patients harboring *EGFR* mutations, who initially respond to TKIs treatment, invariably progress due to the development of drug resistance. Substitution mutation of threonine with methionine at codon 790 (T790M) of exon 20 has been found in approximately 50% of the tumors of *EGFR* mutant patients who progress when being treated by EGFR-TKIs [40, 41]. The T790M mutation is always present in *cis* arrangement with a sensitizing *EGFR* mutation [40], and has shown synergistic kinase activity and transformation potential when they occur [15, 42]. The T790M mutation increases affinity of the receptor for ATP back to the level of the wild type and decreases the potency of EGFR-TKIs resulting in resistance [41, 43, 44]. Paradoxically, patients who develop resistance due to T790M mutation may have a better overall outcome than those who fail to EGFR-TKI therapy without this mutation [41]. The newer generations of EGFR-TKIs are being developed to overcome this resistance, and results are pending.

The T790M mutation has been very rarely identified with direct sequencing in patients who are naïve to EGFR-TKI therapy [40]. However, using highly sensitive detection methods, it can be detected up to 38% of NSCLC patients with *EGFR* sensitizing mutations [45–48]. This suggests that the very small subpopulation of T790M tumor cells may be present in the primary tumors and, during TKI treatment, the T790M mutant cells are selectively enriched under TKI pressure and causes drug resistance (Figure 28.2) [45, 46]. Identification of pretreatment T790M mutation reveals significant association with a shorter progression free survival (PFS) in patients treated with EGFR-TKIs and is a negative predictor of response to EGFR-TKI treatment [45, 47]. However, in early stage NSCLC patients harboring *EGFR* mutations, who were not treated with EGFR-TKIs, T790M mutation was associated with relatively favorable prognosis [48].

Other rare mutations

G719X and L861Q mutations occur less commonly in NSCLC, and occupy 3–5% of all types of *EGFR* mutations. They exist alone or with other *EGFR* mutations forming complex mutations [20]. The mutations on G719 and L861 are less sensitive to EGFR-TKIs compared with classical mutations [14, 16, 20]. *EGFR* exon 19 insertions showing 18-base pair insertion are newly reported EGFR-TKI sensitive mutations in lung adenocarcinoma [49] Small insertions or duplications on exon 20 which are restricted to a spectrum of residues from A767 to C775 represent 3–4% of the *EGFR* TK domain mutations and are associated with primary resistance to TKI therapy [16, 50]. Secondary mutations such as L747S, D761Y and T854A rarely occur in tumors with acquired resistance to EGFR-TKIs [51–53]. Other rarely identified *EGFR* mutations may occur solitary or together with sensitizing mutations such as L858R, G719X and L861Q [54, 55]; these complex mutations have shown attenuated responses to EGFR-inhibitors as compared with G719X or L858R alone [20, 52–55].

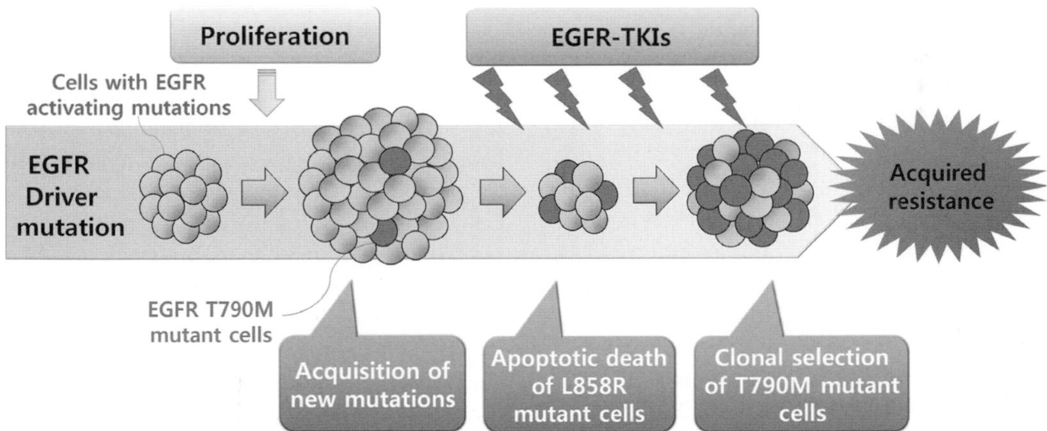

Figure 28.2 The overview of acquired resistance mechanism induced by *EGFR* T790M mutation. Proliferation of tumor cells induces emergence of mixed population of clones with diverse genetic abnormalities and a small number of tumor cells harboring T790M mutation appear in it. Under the influence of EGFR-TKIs, tumor cells with *EGFR* sensitizing mutations undergo apoptosis, while the T790M mutant cells continue to proliferate with selective pressure, which causes drug resistance. (For a color version, see the color plate section.)

Role of *EGFR* mutations in clinical settings

The overall response rate of *EGFR* mutants to EGFR-TKIs does not appear to be different based on ethnicity, but may be influenced by whether the patients have had previous chemotherapy (Table 28.1). However, the data may be biased as those for chemotherapy naïve patients mainly originated from clinical trials conducted in East Asian patients, while data for previously chemotherapy treated patients were mainly from clinical trials conducted in the Western countries with mixed ethnicity populations (Table 28.1) [4, 5, 7, 23–28]. Phase III clinical trials in both East Asian and Caucasian comparing EGFR-TKIs and conventional chemotherapy as a first-line therapy demonstrated that patients harboring *EGFR* mutations showed significantly longer PFS when TKIs were given first (Table 28.2) [24–28, 56]. More importantly, in studies that included both *EGFR* mutant and wild type patients, it is clear that wild type *EGFR* patients had better PFS when treated with chemotherapy first as compared to TKI first, both in East Asian and Caucasian populations [24, 57]. However, for all phase III studies with a relatively higher proportion of *EGFR* mutant patients, the overall survival was similar regardless of the drug sequence. The postulated reason was due to extensive crossover to the alternative treatment after progression (Table 28.2) [13, 25, 27, 28, 58]. The results of these studies have firmly established *EGFR* mutation status as a predictive marker for response to EGFR-TKI therapy, especially in the first-line setting. For patients with *EGFR* mutation positive test results, TKIs are the choice for the first-line treatment. If the *EGFR* mutation test is negative, conventional chemotherapy is preferred [13, 57]. Significant PFS benefits from erlotinib and gefitinib compared to placebo have also been demonstrated in the clinical setting of maintenance therapy after first-line chemotherapy [59, 60]. SATURN trial, but not INFORM trial, additionally found an overall survival benefit of TKI as maintenance therapy regardless of tumor histology or *EGFR* status [59, 61]. Unlike EGFR-TKIs, *EGFR* mutation status was not found to be a predictive biomarker for cetuximab efficacy [62].

The type of *EGFR* mutations determines a different sensitivity of the tumor to EGFR-TKIs. Exon 19 deletion mutations showed higher response rates to EGFR-TKIs (63–100%) than those with exon 21 mutations (50–67%) [63–65]. However, patients' survivals were not significantly different. There is currently limited data to compare the efficacy of erlotinib versus gefitinib [63, 66, 67]. While patients harboring *EGFR* sensitizing mutations most likely experience no significant difference in survival outcome with either agent, in patients with wild-type *EGFR*, erlotinib treatment may have greater benefit than gefitinib treatment [23, 59, 66, 67]. Additionally, erlotinib might provide limited benefit in some patients who failed to respond to gefitinib therapy [68].

Although acquired resistance typically occurs in NSCLC patients who have sensitizing mutations and have initially responded to EGFR-TKIs, a subset of patients demonstrated disease flares after stopping TKI therapy [69, 70]. Patients who develop recurrence following the discontinuation of TKIs usually do not harbor T790M mutation and may respond to TKI retreatment. Therefore, restarting with EGFR-TKIs has been proposed as a treatment option in patients with *EGFR*-mutant lung cancer who recur after discontinuation of TKI therapy [71].

Mutation detection methods

In many clinical trials, it has been reported that a small proportion of patients who do not have detectable *EGFR* mutation have responded to EGFR-TKIs therapy. One explanation offered has been the low sensitivity of detection methods, although other genetic abnormalities as a cause have not been ruled out. The standard method for the detection of *EGFR* mutation is direct sequencing (Figure 28.3a). It can detect all types of mutations, is accurate and cost-effective. However, its low sensitivity is problematic because most NSCLC tissues are infiltrated extensively by non-neoplastic cells, including inflammatory cells, stromal fibroblasts, endothelial cells, etc. Direct sequencing requires ≥40% of mutation-harboring tumor cells for detection [72]. The diagnosis in patients with advanced

Table 28.2 Survival outcomes in randomized phase III trials of EGFR-TKIs

Trials	Patient selection	Patient randomized	Treatment arms	Progression free survival		Overall survival	
				HR (95% CI)	P value	HR (95% CI)	P value
At least one previous chemotherapy (second-line or more)							
BR.21 (Shepherd *et al.*, 2005) [11]	None	731	Erlotinib vs Placebo	0.61 (0.51–0.74)	<0.001	0.70 (0.58–0.85)	<0.001
ISEL (Hirsch *et al.*, 2006) [7]	None	1692	Gefitinib vs Placebo	NA	NA	0.89 (0.77–1.02)	0.087
INTEREST (Douillard *et al.*, 2010) [4]	None	1433	Gefitinib vs Docetaxel	1.04 (0.93–1.18)	0.47	1.02 (0.91–1.15)	NS
LUX–Lung1 (Miller *et al.*, 2012) [119]	Progression after E/G Therapy	585	Afatinib vs. Placebo	0.38 (0.31–0.48)	<0.0001	1.08 (0.86–1.35)	0.74
No previous chemotherapy (first-line)							
IPASS (Mok *et al.*, 2009; Fukuoka *et al.*, 2011) [13, 24]	ADC; Non-smokers	1217	Gefitinib vs. Carboplatin/ paclitaxel	0.74 (0.65–0.85)	<0.001	0.90 (0.79–1.02)	0.11
WJTOG3405 (Mitsudomi *et al.*, 2010) [25]	*EGFR* Mutation	175	Gefitinib vs. Cisplatin/ docetaxel	0.49 (0.34–0.71)	<0.0001	1.64 (0.75–3.58)	0.211
NEJ002 (Inoue *et al.*, 2013) [58]	*EGFR* Mutation	224	Gefitinib vs. Carboplatin/ paclitaxel	0.32 (0.24–0.44)	<0.001	0.89 (0.63–1.24)	0.483
EURTARC (Rosell *et al.*, 2012) [28]	*EGFR* Mutation	173	Erlotinib vs Plastinum doublets	0.37 (0.25–0.54)	<0.0001	1.04 (0.65–1.68)	0.87
OPTIMAL (Zhou *et al.*, 2011) [27]	*EGFR* Mutation	165	Erlotinib vs. Carboplatin/ gemcitabine	0.16 (0.10–0.26)	<0.0001	1.04 (0.69–1.58)	0.69
LUX-Lung3 (Yang *et al.*, 2012) [56]	*EGFR* Mutation	345	Afatinib vs. Cisplatin/ pemetrexed	0.58 (0.43–0.78)	0.0004	NA	NA
TORCH (Gridelli *et al.*, 2012)[§] [57]	None	760	Erlotinib vs Cisplatin/ gemcitabine	1.21 (1.04–1.42)	NS	1.24 (1.04–1.47)[§]	NS
Chemotherapy followed by TKI (maintenance)							
SATURN (Cappuzzo *et al.*, 2010) [59]	No progression after CTx	884	Erlotinib vs. Placebo	0.71 (0.62–0.82)	<0.0001	0.81 (0.70–0.95)	0.009
INFORM (Zhang *et al.*, 2012) [60]		296	Gefitinib vs. Placebo	0.42 (0.33–0.55)	<0.0001	0.86 (0.62–1.14)	0.26

[§]This trial is the crossover study evaluating first-line chemotherapy followed by second-line erlotinib versus the opposite order.
ADC: adenocarcinoma histology; CTx: chemotherapy; E/G: erlotinib or gefitinib; NA: data not available at the time of writing; NS: not significant.

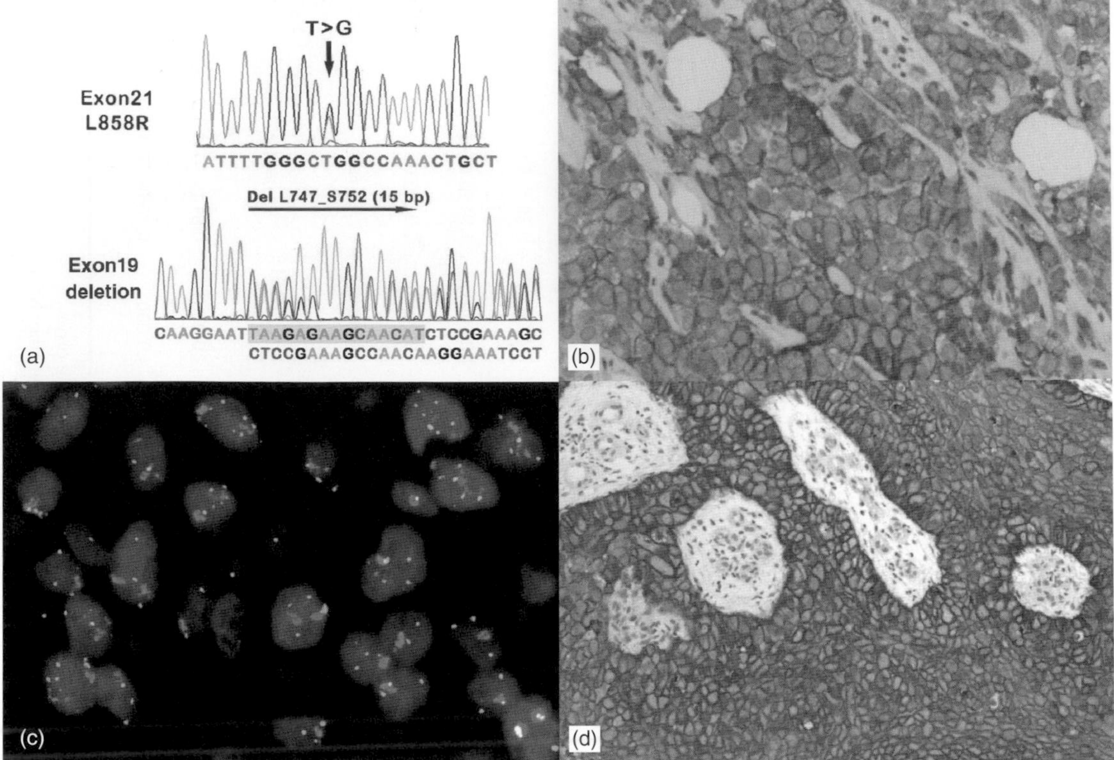

Figure 28.3 Common detection methods for *EGFR* mutation, gene copy number change, and protein expression. a: Direct sequencing results of *EGFR* L858R point mutation and Exon 19 deletion mutation. b: Immunohistochemistry with *EGFR* L858R mutation-specific antibody shows distinct membranous and cytoplasmic staining pattern in *EGFR* mutant tumor cells. c: *EGFR* amplification detected by fluorescence in situ hybridization. (Red signals, *EGFR* gene probe; green signals, chromosome 7 centromere probe.) d: EGFR protein expression assessed by immunohistochemistry shows distinct membranous staining pattern in the lung squamous cell carcinoma cells. (For a color version, see the color plate section.)

lung cancer is usually performed with small biopsies or cytology samples and the number of tumor cells in the context of contaminating nontumor cells present might not be sufficiently abundant to detect the mutant *EGFR* gene sequences. Therefore many detection methods with greater sensitivities capable of detecting 1–5% tumor cells have been developed, such as Scorpion amplification refractory mutation system (ARMS) [45, 73], length analysis with fluorescence-labeled PCR products and TaqMan assay [74], restriction fragment length polymorphism [40, 75], high resolution melting curve analysis [76], mutation-enriched PCR [46], partially denaturing high-performance liquid chromatography [77], etc. Each method has its own advantages and disadvantages, and the efforts to develop new techniques that can detect all possible mutations with high sensitivity and low cost are ongoing.

Recently, IHC with mutation-specific monoclonal antibodies which can detect *EGFR* mutant proteins was developed (Figure 28.3b) [78]. These antibodies can identify L858R and the exon 19 mutant with the common 15bp deletion, respectively. Although the *EGFR* exon 19 mutation-specific antibody demonstrated reduced sensitivity for exon 19 mutants other than the 15bp deletion [79], it may assess the *EGFR* mutation status directly on tumor cells which are not sufficient for DNA extraction for molecular tests [78]. Therefore, mutant-specific EGFR IHC may be used as initial screening methods or for patients in whom molecular testing cannot be performed.

EGFR gene copy number

The methods for detecting *EGFR* gene copy number (GCN) change and dosage are fluorescent in situ hybridization (FISH), silver in situ hybridization (SISH) and real-time quantitative PCR. FISH is the commonly used detection method and copy number change of *EGFR* with FISH has mostly been assessed using the University of Colorado classification system [80]. When FISH result demonstrates either amplification (presence of tight *EGFR* gene clusters and an *EGFR* genes/chromosome 7 ratio of ≥ 2 or ≥ 15 copies of *EGFR* per cell in ≥ 10% of analyzed tumor cells) or high polysomy (≥4 copies of the gene in ≥ 40% of cells), it is interpreted as high *EGFR* GCN (Figure 28.3c). The incidence of NSCLC patients harboring high *EGFR* GCN is variable and ranged from 22% to 70%, depending on the study design and the population involved [7]. In Non-Asian populations, 22–48% showed high GCN, whereas, in East Asian populations, 42–70% had tumors with high GCN [6, 13, 61]. *EGFR* amplification is closely associated with *EGFR* mutation in lung adenocarcinoma, as up to 80% of patients with high *EGFR* GCN had coexisting *EGFR* mutations [7, 13, 23, 81]. High GCN putatively generates increased transcription of mutant allele and gene activity [81,82]. Through this mechanism, the tumors with *EGFR* mutations and high GCN may be more dependent on EGFR signaling pathway and are more likely to respond dramatically to targeted therapies [83]. While *EGFR* mutations are known to be involved in the initiation of lung cancer and is present in precancerous lesion or early stage lung adenocarcinoma [31], *EGFR* amplification is involved in the later stage of adenocarcinoma progression and is heterogeneously distributed within tumors [82, 84].

There have been conflicting results regarding the clinical significance of *EGFR* high GCN in NSCLC patients. Placebo-controlled studies demonstrated that high *EGFR* GCN was associated with higher response rates and significantly prolonged OS from EGFR-TKI treatment [7, 23]. However, these observations have not been reproduced in clinical trials where the conventional chemotherapy was the comparator [4, 13]. Additionally, the beneficial role of high *EGFR* GCN for EGFR-TKI therapy might be limited in Caucasian patients, but not in East Asian patients [6, 85]. At present, *EGFR* GCN analysis is not recommended routinely for the selection of patients for EGFR-TKI therapy.

EGFR protein expression

EGFR protein expression is easily detected by IHC (Figure 28.3d) and is present in about 60–80% of NSCLC patients [4, 7, 61, 86]. EGFR protein expression as determined by IHC was not correlated with *EGFR* sensitizing mutations, high *EGFR* GCN, nor clinical features [88]. In most studies, the performed assays, the applied antibodies and the scoring systems were different, which resulted in high discordance rate between studies [85]. There have been inconsistent clinical data on the role of EGFR protein expression as a predictive marker for EGFR-TKIs therapy [4, 13, 29, 59, 61]. FLEX study demonstrated high EGFR expression (IHC–score ≥ 200) can predict survival benefit from the addition of cetuximab to first-line chemotherapy in patients with advanced NSCLC [87]. In this study, they proposed IHC scoring system assessing membrane staining intensity of tumor cells (on a scale of 0–3) and the percentages of staining cells at each intensity. While EGFR protein expression by IHC is not yet optimal for selection of candidates responsive to EGFR-TKI therapy it could be a good predictive biomarker for decision of addition of cetuximab to the chemotherapy, pending additional prospective validation.

Germline polymorphisms of *EGFR*

The efficacy of EGFR inhibitor treatment could vary according to patient's genetic polymorphic variations. The first intron of the *EGFR* gene has a highly polymorphic CA repeat close to a downstream enhancer sequence and increasing numbers of CA repeat is associated with decreased transcriptional activity and low EGFR expression [89]. Patients with a short length of CA repeats of *EGFR* were more likely to have better response and longer survival time than were patients with longer CA repeats when treated with EGFR inhibitors [90–92], but the results of clinical trials evaluating its role as a predictive marker for the response to EGFR inhibitors did not support this finding [61, 93]. Further studies are needed to clarify whether germline polymorphisms are independently predictive with EGFR-TKI therapy, or are simply coupling with other molecular or clinical parameters [85].

KRAS mutations

KRAS gene encodes GTP binding protein, a member of EGFR downstream RAS/RAF/MAPK pathway. In NSCLC, *KRAS* mutations involve codon 12, 13, or rarely codon 61 [94], and the most common mutation type is G12C (43%) [95]. Mutant RAS proteins are insensitive to the action of GTPase activating protein which inactivates RAS-GTP, leading to constitutive activation of RAS protein independent on upstream ligand-kinase interaction. *KRAS* mutations are found in about 10–30% of NSCLC and are more common in patients with adenocarcinomas, especially mucinous type, and Caucasian [96, 97]. *KRAS* mutations are found at a higher rate in smokers and have different spectrum of mutations. *KRAS* transition mutations (G→A) are more common in never-smokers whereas transversion mutations (G→T or G→C) are more common in smokers.

The response rates to EGFR-TKIs for patients with *KRAS* mutation and wild type *KRAS* were 3% and 26% respectively [97]. Although *KRAS* mutation status may serve as a negative predictive marker for response to EGFR-TKIs therapy [94], its role as a predictive marker of differential survival has been inconclusive [4, 9, 23, 61]. *KRAS* and *EGFR* mutations are usually mutually exclusive [7, 94], and there is a large proportion of nonresponders among *KRAS* wild-type patients, while the survival is not different between patients with *KRAS* mutant/*EGFR* wild-type and *KRAS* wild-type/*EGFR* wild-type NSCLC [64, 97]. Currently, *KRAS* mutation testing for selection of patients to EGFR-TKIs therapy is not recommended, although it may be helpful to identify a subgroup of patients who are highly unlikely to respond to EGFR-TKIs.

Recent studies demonstrated that different *KRAS* mutation types were related to different activation of cell signaling pathways [98], and different patient outcome for EGFR-TKI treatment [99], for other targeted therapies [98], and for the adjuvant chemotherapy [100]. The G12C *KRAS* mutation group receiving EGFR-TKI therapy showed significantly worse PFS than non-G12C mutation group, but overall survival was not different [99]. In BATTLE trial testing treatment effects with erlotinib, vandetanib, bexarotene and erlotinib or sorafenib, patients with either G12C or G12V *KRAS* mutations had worse PFS than other *KRAS* mutations or wild-type *KRAS* [98]. NSCLC patients with *KRAS* codon 13 mutations had significantly poorer outcomes with adjuvant chemotherapy [100]. Although the small number of *KRAS* mutation-positive patients was included in these studies, these results are provocative and the significance of *KRAS* mutation type as a predictive marker need to be validated.

Other biomarkers

HER2 is a preferred dimerization partner to EGFR, and heterodimers with HER2 produce stronger signals than other dimers [101]. The proportion of patients with high *HER2* GCN detected by FISH ranges 2–23% of NSCLC patients, and are commonly encountered in patients with adenocarcinoma, in females and in nonsmokers [101, 102]. High *HER2* GCN increases gefitinib sensitivity in patients with EGFR positive tumors, although this effect is confined to double EGFR/HER2 positive tumors [102]. *HER2* mutation is very rarely encountered as driver mutations of NSCLC. It is commonly identified in nonsmokers and patients with adenocarcinomas [101, 103]. Most *HER2* mutations are exon 20 insertion mutations involving tyrosine kinase domain [103]. Mutant HER2 generates more potent catalytic and transforming activity and suppresses apoptosis than wild type HER2. Additionally, most tumors harboring *HER2* mutations are resistant to EGFR-TKIs but sensitive to novel agents that simultaneously inhibit HER2 and EGFR [104]. Therefore, the dual inhibition of EGFR and HER2 may be an attractive target for new treatments for NSCLC. However, it is difficult to verify their predictive role in prospective clinical trials due to the very low frequency of *HER2* mutations in NSCLC.

There are efforts trying to classify a serum proteomic profile to predict the response to EGFR-TKI therapy. Taguchi *et al.* developed a predictive algorithm detected by matrix-assisted laser desorption ionization (MALDI) mass spectrometry analysis and identified subgroup of NSCLC patients based on eight protein expression profiles for their clinical benefit from EGFR-TKI treatment [105]. This serum proteomic test 'VeriStrat®' has been shown to be able to differentiate NSCLC patients into two groups with good or poor outcome after treatment with EGFR-TKIs or with combination of EGFR and VEGF inhibitors [105–107]. However, its predictive potential for survival benefit was not confirmed in the BR.21 trial in which only prognostic value are shown [108]. Therefore, prospective randomized controlled studies are needed to validate its value as a predictive marker.

EGFR testing in the clinical setting

Current evidence from clinical trials [13, 24–26] has established the need to test advanced NSCLC patients for *EGFR* mutation status routinely to select those who are most likely to benefit from first-line EGFR-TKI therapy [109, 110]. Clinical parameters, such as gender, ethnicity or smoking history, could not be used as sole markers for selection of EGFR-TKI treatment [24]. At present, *EGFR* GCN analyses with FISH and EGFR protein expression status with IHC are not recommended to direct treatment [109, 110]. *KRAS* testing is also not recommended for routine testing at this time, as the results have little value in current clinical decision making. However, this is likely to change in the near future with the new MEK inhibitors showing preliminary efficacy in *KRAS* mutated patients [111].

EGFR mutation testing should be performed for all advanced NSCLCs that have an adenocarcinoma component [112, 113] and not for pure squamous cell carcinomas, small cell carcinomas or neuroendocrine carcinomas. In cases where subtyping of NSCLCs is difficult on histological examination, application of IHC markers, such as TTF-1, p63 or p40, CK5/6 and mucin may be performed to establish the presence of adenocarcinoma features. For patients whose tumors do not exhibit adenocarcinoma histology but have clinical features associated with higher prevalence of *EGFR* mutations, e.g., never-smokers, *EGFR* mutation test should be performed (Figure 28.4) [112].

As 90% of *EGFR* mutations that are sensitive to EGFR-TKIs are composed of exon 19 deletions and exon 21 L858R mutations, routine testing should minimally include these two groups of mutations. Testing for less common sensitizing mutations such as L861Q, G719X and E709X are also desirable if adequate tumor material is available. As the T790M mutation is uncommonly detected in TKI naïve tumor samples and its presence does not exclude the initial use of first generation TKIs, such as gefitinib or erlotinib, its inclusion in routine testing is optional. However, the detection of T790M mutation may provide the rationale to select the irreversible inhibitors that are effective against this mutation as the primary inhibitors to use (Table 28.3).

The *EGFR* mutation testing paradigm has established the need to obtain sufficient tissue for not only diagnosis and histologic subtyping, but also molecular testing. The specimens should be handled properly and ancillary IHC studies should be kept to what are necessary for making the diagnosis and subtyping, such that enough materials for molecular analyses can be reserved [113]. Although tissue samples are preferred over cytology [110, 114], sometimes, cytologic samples might be the only available samples. The amount of tumor cells as well as preservation state and quality of DNA are the major issues for cytology samples. All mutations detected in the histological material can also be identified in the cytologic samples and a cytology cell block is an excellent substitute for molecular testing because microscopic examination of the presence and percentage of tumor cells is possible [115]. In cases where the biopsy or cytologic samples cannot be obtained, the patient's plasma may also be another option. While sensitivity of testing using plasma samples require improvement, a

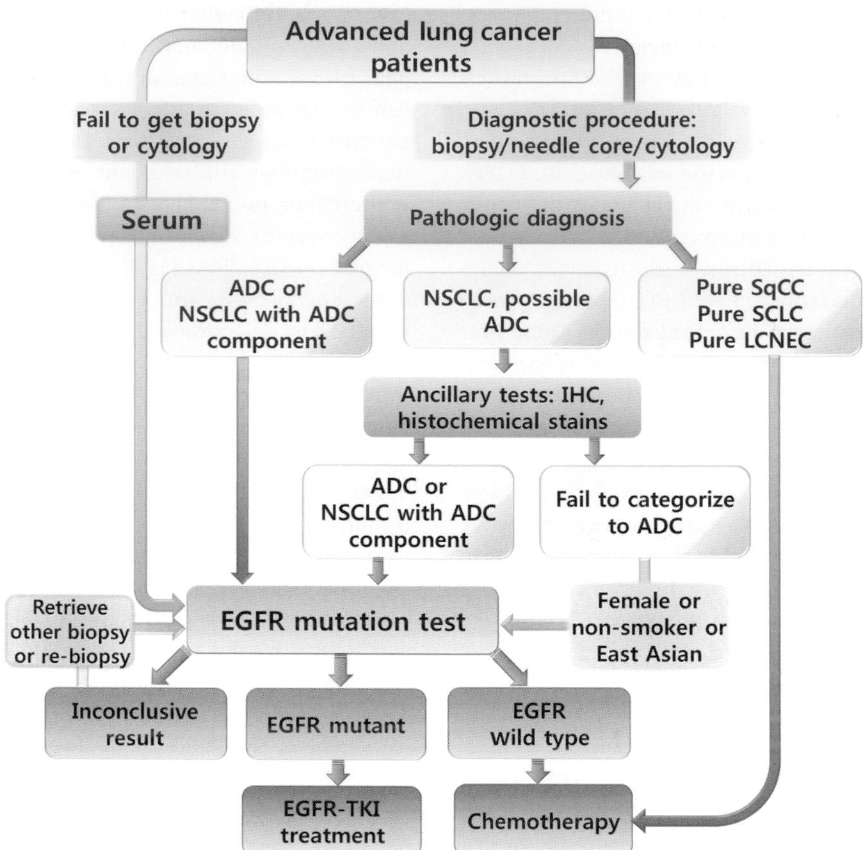

Figure 28.4 Decision-making algorithm for patients with newly diagnosed advanced NSCLC regarding *EGFR* mutation tests for directing first-line EGFR-TKI therapy. (For a color version, see the color plate section.)

Table 28.3 Predictive biomarkers and their response to EGFR-TKIs in non-small cell lung cancer patients

Biomarkers	Frequency	Closely related subpopulations	Response to EGFR-TKIs	Efficacy on routine clinical practice
EGFR Sensitizing mutation	30–50% in East Asian/ 10–20% in non-Asian	East Asian, Female, non-smokers, ADC	Sensitive	Recommended for the first-line EGFR-TKIs therapy
EGFR T790M mutation	50% in patients with acquired resistance	Patients with *EGFR* sensitizing mutations	Resistant	For patients with acquired resistance
EGFR high GCN	42–70% in East Asian/ 22–48% in non-Asian	Closely associated with *EGFR* mutations	Sensitive	Not recommended
EGFR protein expression	60–80%	More common in SqCC	Inconclusive	Not recommended
KRAS mutation	10–30%	ADC, smokers, Caucasian	Resistant	Supportive
HER2 amplification	2–23%	Female, non-smokers, ADC	Sensitive	Need more validation
HER2 mutation	~2%	Non-smokers, ADC	Resistant	Need more validation

ADC: adenocarcinoma histology; SqCC: squamous cell carcinoma histology.

recent study reported that isolation of circulating tumor cells using special high efficiency devices may increase the sensitivity to clinically acceptable levels [45]. However the clinical significance of the results of *EGFR* mutation tests using plasma or circulating tumor cells is yet to be established [45, 116].

The clinical significance of genomic heterogeneity in lung cancer remains to be fully evaluated. The genetic profiles of metastases can be similar to or different from that of the primary tumor and between different metastatic tumors [113]. The important clinical considerations for selecting samples for molecular tests include which samples are more easily accessible, immediately fixed and have adequate amount of tumor cell contents [114, 117]. Any sample that meets the requirements for tumor cell contents and quality can be selected for the tests and the choice should be performed by the experienced pathologists. Immediate fixation with appropriate fixatives is very important for DNA preservation. Fresh frozen, formalin-fixed paraffin embedded or alcohol-fixed samples are suitable for molecular analysis. The use of acidic or heavy metal fixatives or decalcifying solution for the tissue should be avoided, as they may result in DNA degradation. The ideal sample would have a high proportion of malignant cells and minimal amount of necrosis or mucin. Usually at least 50% of tumor cell contents is recommended for direct sequencing [114] but histologically more than 40% is possible [72]. For cases showing lower tumor cell contents, manual microdissection for tumor cell enrichment is recommended to improve accuracy on the heterogeneous samples.

For the patients with advanced stage disease, rapid diagnosis in time is important. Turn-around time (TAT) means the period from receipt of specimen in the molecular pathology lab to the reporting the final results to the clinicians. Five working days is an ideal TAT for *EGFR* mutation tests and the maximum TAT should not exceed 10 working days [112, 114]. Treatment with EGFR-TKI can be recommended within 3 days after the results are released [112]. To avoid potentially lengthy TAT, some institutions have instituted "reflex" molecular testing at the time of initial diagnosis. This trend is likely to increase as high throughput multiplex testing methods that allow simultaneous assessment of large number of mutations are being developed. For detecting mutations in specimens with low tumor cell content, more sensitive methods should be available in laboratories where only direct sequencing is performed. For selection of appropriate detection methods, we should consider the sensitivity and specificity of the tests, the spectrum of detectable mutations, and TAT. Any method that meets the requirements of each institute may be chosen and the validation for the method should be performed.

Perspectives for future development of the biomarkers

Since the discovery of the role of *EGFR* mutation as a promising predictive marker for response to *EGFR*-inhibitors, *EGFR* has been one of the most intensively studied molecules. New mechanisms of insensitivity to *EGFR*-inhibitors in a small proportion of *EGFR* mutants and sensitivity in patients with *EGFR* wild-type tumor remain to be investigated; the clinical implications of new biomarkers continue to be explored. Further searches for other driver mutations and new biomarkers for selection of responders to other drugs for targeted therapy will continue. Additionally, the development of a rapid, low-cost mutation assay that can detect all possible mutations at the necessary sensitivity for *EGFR* is needed. For personalized therapy, the development of more advanced screening systems that can test for multiple mutations in various genes including *EGFR* simultaneously is ongoing and will be applied for clinical use [118]. The techniques that can easily isolate circulating cancer cells from the blood of lung cancer patients with low-cost could monitor changes of biomarker status and make the adjustment of patients' treatment regimens possible over the course of their disease [45].

Acquisition of resistance during drug treatment is a major obstacle against the success of personalized therapy. Through considerable efforts to reveal the biological mechanisms of drug resistance, a variety of genetic and epigenetic processes have been proposed (see Chapter 27, 'Mechanisms of

Resistance to Epidermal Growth Factor Receptor in Non-small Cell Lung Cancer'). Lung cancer is a histologically and genetically heterogeneous tumor which is composed of populations of cells showing mixed drug sensitivity. Like the cases showing acquired resistance through *EGFR* T790M mutation (Figure 28.2), presence of rare, resistance-inducing genetic abnormalities in cancer cell population selected during drug treatment might be a major obstacle. Clinical implication of the tumor heterogeneity associated with responsiveness and resistance to the drugs should be clarified, and how to control the genetic heterogeneity to overcome resistance to targeted therapy might be a main problem that will require resolutions.

References

1 Weinstein I (2002) Addiction to oncogenes – the Achilles heel of cancer. *Science*, 297: 63–4.

2 Yatabe Y (2010) EGFR mutations and the terminal respiratory unit. *Cancer Metastasis Rev*, 29: 23–36.

3 Paez JG, Janne PA, Lee JC, *et al.* (2004) EGFR mutations in lung cancer: correlation with clinical response to gefitinib therapy. *Science*, 304: 1497–1500.

4 Douillard JY, Shepherd FA, Hirsh V, *et al.* (2010) Molecular predictors of outcome with gefitinib and docetaxel in previously treated non-small-cell lung cancer: data from the randomized phase III INTEREST trial. *J Clin Oncol*, 28: 744–52.

5 Bell DW, Lynch TJ, Haserlat SM, *et al.* (2005) Epidermal growth factor receptor mutations and gene amplification in non-small-cell lung cancer: molecular analysis of the IDEAL/INTACT gefitinib trials. *J Clin Oncol*, 23: 8081–92.

6 Dahabreh IJ, Linardou H, Kosmidis P, *et al.* (2011) EGFR gene copy number as a predictive biomarker for patients receiving tyrosine kinase inhibitor treatment: a systematic review and meta-analysis in non-small-cell lung cancer. *Ann Oncol*, 22: 545–52.

7 Hirsch FR, Varella-Garcia M, Bunn PA, Jr., *et al.* (2006) Molecular predictors of outcome with gefitinib in a phase III placebo-controlled study in advanced non-small-cell lung cancer. *J Clin Oncol*, 24: 5034–42.

8 Lynch TJ, Bell DW, Sordella R, *et al.* (2004) Activating mutations in the epidermal growth factor receptor underlying responsiveness of non-small-cell lung cancer to gefitinib. *N Engl J Med*, 350: 2129–39.

9 Kim ES, Hirsh V, Mok T, *et al.* (2008) Gefitinib versus docetaxel in previously treated non-small-cell lung cancer (INTEREST): A randomised phase III trial. *Lancet*, 372: 1809–18.

10 Giaccone G, Herbst RS, Manegold C, *et al.* (2004) Gefitinib in combination with gemcitabine and cisplatin in advanced non-small-cell lung cancer: a phase III trial-INTACT 1. *J Clin Oncol*, 22: 777–84.

11 Shepherd FA, Rodrigues Pereira J, Ciuleanu T, *et al.* (2005) Erlotinib in previously treated non-small-cell lung cancer. *N Engl J Med*, 353: 123–32.

12 Vincent MD, Kuruvilla MS, Leighl NB, *et al.* (2012) Biomarkers that currently affect clinical practice: EGFR, ALK, MET, KRAS. *Curr Oncol*, 19: S33–44.

13 Fukuoka M, Wu YL, Thongprasert S, *et al.* (2011) Biomarker analyses and final overall survival results from a phase III, randomized, open-label, first-line study of gefitinib versus carboplatin/paclitaxel in clinically selected patients with advanced non-small-cell lung cancer in Asia (IPASS). *J Clin Oncol*, 29: 2866–74.

14 Yun CH, Boggon TJ, Li Y, *et al.* (2007) Structures of lung cancer-derived EGFR mutants and inhibitor complexes: Mechanism of activation and insights into differential inhibitor sensitivity. *Cancer Cell*, 11: 217–27.

15 Mulloy R, Ferrand A, Kim Y, *et al.* (2007) Epidermal growth factor receptor mutants from human lung cancers exhibit enhanced catalytic activity and increased sensitivity to gefitinib. *Cancer Res*, 67: 2325–30.

16 Greulich H, Chen TH, Feng W, *et al.* (2005) Oncogenic transformation by inhibitor-sensitive and -resistant EGFR mutants. *PLoS Med*, 2: e313.

17 Sordella R, Bell DW, Haber DA, *et al.* (2004) Gefitinib-sensitizing EGFR mutations in lung cancer activate anti-apoptotic pathways. *Science*, 305: 1163–7.

18 Sharma SV, Gajowniczek P, Way IP, *et al.* (2006) A common signaling cascade may underlie "addiction" to the Src, BCR-ABL, and EGF receptor oncogenes. *Cancer Cell*, 10: 425–35.

19 Gazdar AF (2009) Activating and resistance mutations of EGFR in non-small-cell lung cancer: role in clinical response to EGFR tyrosine kinase inhibitors. *Oncogene*, 28(Suppl 1): S24–31.

20 Wu JY, Yu CJ, Chang YC, *et al.* (2011) Effectiveness of tyrosine kinase inhibitors on "uncommon" epidermal growth factor receptor mutations of unknown

clinical significance in non-small cell lung cancer. *Clin Cancer Res*, 17: 3812–21.

21 Riely GJ, Politi KA, Miller VA, *et al.* (2006) Update on epidermal growth factor receptor mutations in non-small cell lung cancer. *Clin Cancer Res*, 12: 7232–41.

22 Sequist LV, Bell DW, Lynch TJ, *et al.* (2007) Molecular predictors of response to epidermal growth factor receptor antagonists in non-small-cell lung cancer. *J Clin Oncol*, 25: 587–95.

23 Zhu CQ, da Cunha Santos G, Ding K, *et al.* (2008) Role of KRAS and EGFR as biomarkers of response to erlotinib in National Cancer Institute of Canada Clinical Trials Group Study BR.21. *J Clin Oncol*, 26: 4268–75.

24 Mok TS, Wu YL, Thongprasert S, *et al.* (2009) Gefitinib or carboplatin-paclitaxel in pulmonary adenocarcinoma. *N Engl J Med*, 361: 947–57.

25 Mitsudomi T, Morita S, Yatabe Y, *et al.* (2010) Gefitinib versus cisplatin plus docetaxel in patients with non-small-cell lung cancer harbouring mutations of the epidermal growth factor receptor (WJTOG3405): an open label, randomised phase 3 trial. *Lancet Oncol*, 11: 121–8.

26 Maemondo M, Inoue A, Kobayashi K, *et al.* (2010) Gefitinib or chemotherapy for non-small-cell lung cancer with mutated EGFR. *N Engl J Med*, 362: 2380–8.

27 Zhou C, Wu YL, Chen G, *et al.* (2011) Erlotinib versus chemotherapy as first-line treatment for patients with advanced EGFR mutation-positive non-small-cell lung cancer (OPTIMAL, CTONG-0802): A multicentre, open-label, randomised, phase 3 study. *Lancet Oncol*, 12: 735–42.

28 Rosell R, Carcereny E, Gervais R, *et al.* (2012) Erlotinib versus standard chemotherapy as first-line treatment for European patients with advanced EGFR mutation-positive non-small-cell lung cancer (EURTAC): A multicentre, open-label, randomised phase 3 trial. *Lancet Oncol*, 13: 239–46.

29 Tsao MS, Sakurada A, Cutz JC, *et al.* (2005) Erlotinib in lung cancer – molecular and clinical predictors of outcome. *N Engl J Med*, 353: 133–44.

30 Pao W, Chmielecki J (2010) Rational, biologically based treatment of EGFR-mutant non-small-cell lung cancer. *Nat Rev Cancer*, 10: 760–74.

31 Yatabe Y, Kosaka T, Takahashi T, *et al.* (2005) EGFR mutation is specific for terminal respiratory unit type adenocarcinoma. *Am J Surg Pathol*, 29: 633–9.

32 Park SH, Ha SY, Lee JI, *et al.* (2009) Epidermal growth factor receptor mutations and the clinical outcome in male smokers with squamous cell carcinoma of lung. *J Korean Med Sci*, 24: 448–52.

33 An SJ, Chen ZH, Su J, *et al.* (2012) Identification of enriched driver gene alterations in subgroups of non-small cell lung cancer patients based on histology and smoking status. *PLoS One*, 7: e40109.

34 Hata A, Katakami N, Yoshioka H, *et al.* (2013) How sensitive are epidermal growth factor receptor-tyrosine kinase inhibitors for squamous cell carcinoma of the lung harboring EGFR gene-sensitive mutations? *J Thorac Oncol*, 8: 89–95.

35 Rekhtman N, Paik PK, Arcila ME, *et al.* (2012) Clarifying the spectrum of driver oncogene mutations in biomarker-verified squamous carcinoma of lung: lack of EGFR/KRAS and presence of PIK3CA/AKT1 mutations. *Clin Cancer Res*, 18: 1167–76.

36 Hammerman PS, Sos ML, Ramos AH, *et al.* (2012) Comprehensive genomic characterization of squamous cell lung cancers. *Nature*, 489: 519–25.

37 Shukuya T, Takahashi T, Kaira R, *et al.* (2011) Efficacy of gefitinib for non-adenocarcinoma non-small-cell lung cancer patients harboring epidermal growth factor receptor mutations: a pooled analysis of published reports. *Cancer Sci*, 102: 1032–7.

38 Shiao TH, Chang YL, Yu CJ, *et al.* (2011) Epidermal growth factor receptor mutations in small cell lung cancer: a brief report. *J Thorac Oncol*, 6: 195–8.

39 Tatematsu A, Shimizu J, Murakami Y, *et al.* (2008) Epidermal growth factor receptor mutations in small cell lung cancer. *Clin Cancer Res*, 14: 6092–6.

40 Pao W, Miller VA, Politi KA, *et al.* (2005) Acquired resistance of lung adenocarcinomas to gefitinib or erlotinib is associated with a second mutation in the EGFR kinase domain. *PLoS Med*, 2: e73.

41 Oxnard GR, Arcila ME, Sima CS, *et al.* (2011) Acquired resistance to EGFR tyrosine kinase inhibitors in EGFR-mutant lung cancer: distinct natural history of patients with tumors harboring the T790M mutation. *Clin Cancer Res*, 17: 1616–22.

42 Godin-Heymann N, Bryant I, Rivera MN, *et al.* (2007) Oncogenic activity of epidermal growth factor receptor kinase mutant alleles is enhanced by the T790M drug resistance mutation. *Cancer Res*, 67: 7319–26.

43 Yoshikawa S, Kukimoto-Niino M, Parker L, *et al.* (2013) Structural basis for the altered drug sensitivities of non-small cell lung cancer-associated mutants of human epidermal growth factor receptor. *Oncogene*, 32(1): 27–38.

44 Yun CH, Mengwasser KE, Toms AV, *et al.* (2008) The T790M mutation in EGFR kinase causes drug

resistance by increasing the affinity for ATP. *Proc Natl Acad Sci USA*, 105: 2070–5.

45 Maheswaran S, Sequist LV, Nagrath S, *et al.* (2008) Detection of mutations in EGFR in circulating lung-cancer cells. *N Engl J Med*, 359: 366–77.

46 Inukai M, Toyooka S, Ito S, *et al.* (2006) Presence of epidermal growth factor receptor gene T790M mutation as a minor clone in non-small cell lung cancer. *Cancer Res*, 66: 7854–8.

47 Rosell R, Molina MA, Costa C, *et al.* (2011) Pretreatment EGFR T790M mutation and BRCA1 mRNA expression in erlotinib-treated advanced non-small-cell lung cancer patients with EGFR mutations. *Clin Cancer Res*, 17: 1160–8.

48 Fujita Y, Suda K, Kimura H, *et al.* (2012) Highly sensitive detection of EGFR T790M mutation using colony hybridization predicts favorable prognosis of patients with lung cancer harboring activating EGFR mutation. *J Thorac Oncol*, 7: 1640–4.

49 He M, Capelletti M, Nafa K, *et al.* (2012) EGFR exon 19 insertions: a new family of sensitizing EGFR mutations in lung adenocarcinoma. *Clin Cancer Res*, 18: 1790–7.

50 Yasuda H, Kobayashi S, Costa DB (2012) EGFR exon 20 insertion mutations in non-small-cell lung cancer: preclinical data and clinical implications. *Lancet Oncol*, 13: e23–31.

51 Bean J, Riely GJ, Balak M, *et al.* (2008) Acquired resistance to epidermal growth factor receptor kinase inhibitors associated with a novel T854A mutation in a patient with EGFR-mutant lung adenocarcinoma. *Clin Cancer Res*, 14: 7519–25.

52 Balak MN, Gong Y, Riely GJ, *et al.* (2006) Novel D761Y and common secondary T790M mutations in epidermal growth factor receptor-mutant lung adenocarcinomas with acquired resistance to kinase inhibitors. *Clin Cancer Res*, 12: 6494–6501.

53 Massarelli E, Johnson FM, Erickson HS, *et al.* (2013) Uncommon Epidermal Growth Factor Receptor mutations in non-small cell lung cancer and their mechanisms of EGFR tyrosine kinase inhibitors sensitivity and resistance. *Lung Cancer*, 80: 235–41.

54 Tam IY, Leung EL, Tin VP, *et al.* (2009) Double EGFR mutants containing rare EGFR mutant types show reduced in vitro response to gefitinib compared with common activating missense mutations. *Mol Cancer Ther*, 8: 2142–51.

55 Kancha RK, von Bubnoff N, Peschel C, *et al.* (2009) Functional analysis of epidermal growth factor receptor (EGFR) mutations and potential implications for EGFR targeted therapy. *Clin Cancer Res*, 15: 460–7.

56 Yang JC, Shih JY, Su WC, *et al.* (2012) Afatinib for patients with lung adenocarcinoma and epidermal growth factor receptor mutations (LUX-Lung 2): A phase 2 trial. *Lancet Oncol*, 13: 539–48.

57 Gridelli C, Ciardiello F, Gallo C, *et al.* (2012) First-line erlotinib followed by second-line cisplatin-gemcitabine chemotherapy in advanced non-small-cell lung cancer: the TORCH randomized trial. *J Clin Oncol*, 30: 3002–11.

58 Tsao MS, Sakurada A, Ding K, *et al.* (2011) Prognostic and predictive value of epidermal growth factor receptor tyrosine kinase domain mutation status and gene copy number for adjuvant chemotherapy in non-small cell lung cancer. *J Thorac Oncol*, 6: 139–47.

59 Cappuzzo F, Ciuleanu T, Stelmakh L, *et al.* (2010) Erlotinib as maintenance treatment in advanced non-small-cell lung cancer: a multicentre, randomised, placebo-controlled phase 3 study. *Lancet Oncol*, 11: 521–9.

60 Zhang L, Ma S, Song X, *et al.* (2012) Gefitinib versus placebo as maintenance therapy in patients with locally advanced or metastatic non-small-cell lung cancer (INFORM; C-TONG 0804): A multicentre, double-blind randomised phase 3 trial. *Lancet Oncol*, 13: 466–75.

61 Brugger W, Triller N, Blasinska-Morawiec M, *et al.* (2011) Prospective molecular marker analyses of EGFR and KRAS from a randomized, placebo-controlled study of erlotinib maintenance therapy in advanced non-small-cell lung cancer. *J Clin Oncol*, 29: 4113–20.

62 Khambata-Ford S, Harbison CT, Hart LL, *et al.* (2010) Analysis of potential predictive markers of cetuximab benefit in BMS099, a phase III study of cetuximab and first-line taxane/carboplatin in advanced non-small-cell lung cancer. *J Clin Oncol*, 28: 918–27.

63 Jackman DM, Yeap BY, Sequist LV, *et al.* (2006) Exon 19 deletion mutations of epidermal growth factor receptor are associated with prolonged survival in non-small cell lung cancer patients treated with gefitinib or erlotinib. *Clin Cancer Res*, 12: 3908–14.

64 Jackman DM, Miller VA, Cioffredi LA, *et al.* (2009) Impact of epidermal growth factor receptor and KRAS mutations on clinical outcomes in previously untreated non-small cell lung cancer patients: Results of an online tumor registry of clinical trials. *Clin Cancer Res*, 15: 5267–73.

65 Mitsudomi T, Kosaka T, Endoh H, *et al.* (2005) Mutations of the epidermal growth factor receptor gene predict prolonged survival after gefitinib treatment in

patients with non-small-cell lung cancer with postoperative recurrence. *J Clin Oncol*, 23: 2513–20.

66 Cho BC, Im CK, Park MS, *et al.* (2007) Phase II study of erlotinib in advanced non-small-cell lung cancer after failure of gefitinib. *J Clin Oncol*, 25: 2528–33.

67 Wu WS, Chen YM, Tsai CM, *et al.* (2012) Erlotinib has better efficacy than gefitinib in adenocarcinoma patients without EGFR-activating mutations, but similar efficacy in patients with EGFR-activating mutations. *Exp Ther Med*, 3: 207–13.

68 Vasile E, Tibaldi C, Chella A, *et al.* (2008) Erlotinib after failure of gefitinib in patients with advanced non-small cell lung cancer previously responding to gefitinib. *J Thorac Oncol*, 3: 912–14.

69 Riely GJ, Kris MG, Zhao B, *et al.* (2007) Prospective assessment of discontinuation and reinitiation of erlotinib or gefitinib in patients with acquired resistance to erlotinib or gefitinib followed by the addition of everolimus. *Clin Cancer Res*, 13: 5150–5.

70 Chaft JE, Oxnard GR, Sima CS, *et al.* (2011) Disease flare after tyrosine kinase inhibitor discontinuation in patients with EGFR-mutant lung cancer and acquired resistance to erlotinib or gefitinib: implications for clinical trial design. *Clin Cancer Res*, 17: 6298–6303.

71 Oxnard GR, Janjigian YY, Arcila ME, *et al.* (2011) Maintained sensitivity to EGFR tyrosine kinase inhibitors in EGFR-mutant lung cancer recurring after adjuvant erlotinib or gefitinib. *Clin Cancer Res*, 17: 6322–8.

72 Warth A, Penzel R, Brandt R, *et al.* (2012) Optimized algorithm for Sanger sequencing-based EGFR mutation analyses in NSCLC biopsies. *Virchows Arch*, 460: 407–14.

73 Newton CR, Graham A, Heptinstall LE, *et al.* (1989) Analysis of any point mutation in DNA: The amplification refractory mutation system (ARMS). *Nucleic Acids Res*, 17: 2503–16.

74 Molina-Vila MA, Bertran-Alamillo J, Reguart N, *et al.* (2008) A sensitive method for detecting EGFR mutations in non-small cell lung cancer samples with few tumor cells. *J Thorac Oncol*, 3: 1224–35.

75 Kawada I, Soejima K, Watanabe H, *et al.* (2008) An alternative method for screening EGFR mutation using RFLP in non-small cell lung cancer patients. *J Thorac Oncol*, 3: 1096–1103.

76 Do H, Dobrovic A (2009) Limited copy number-high resolution melting (LCN-HRM) enables the detection and identification by sequencing of low level mutations in cancer biopsies. *Mol Cancer*, 8: 82.

77 Chin TM, Anuar D, Soo R, *et al.* (2007) Detection of epidermal growth factor receptor variations by partially denaturing HPLC. *Clin Chem*, 53: 62–70.

78 Yu J, Kane S, Wu J, *et al.* (2009) Mutation-specific antibodies for the detection of EGFR mutations in non-small-cell lung cancer. *Clin Cancer Res*, 15: 3023–8.

79 Brevet M, Arcila M, Ladanyi M (2010) Assessment of EGFR mutation status in lung adenocarcinoma by immunohistochemistry using antibodies specific to the two major forms of mutant EGFR. *J Mol Diagn*, 12: 169–76.

80 Cappuzzo F, Hirsch FR, Rossi E, *et al.* (2005) Epidermal growth factor receptor gene and protein and gefitinib sensitivity in non-small-cell lung cancer. *J Natl Cancer Inst*, 97: 643–55.

81 Soh J, Okumura N, Lockwood WW, *et al.* Oncogene mutations, copy number gains and mutant allele specific imbalance (MASI) frequently occur together in tumor cells. *PLoS One*, 4: e7464.

82 Sholl LM, Yeap BY, Iafrate AJ, *et al.* (2009) Lung adenocarcinoma with EGFR amplification has distinct clinicopathologic and molecular features in never-smokers. *Cancer Res*, 69: 8341–8.

83 Gazdar AF, Minna JD (2008) Deregulated EGFR signaling during lung cancer progression: Mutations, amplicons, and autocrine loops. *Cancer Prev Res (Phila)*, 1: 156–60.

84 Yatabe Y, Takahashi T, Mitsudomi T (2008) Epidermal growth factor receptor gene amplification is acquired in association with tumor progression of EGFR-mutated lung cancer. *Cancer Res*, 68: 2106–11.

85 John T, Liu G, Tsao MS (2009) Overview of molecular testing in non-small-cell lung cancer: Mutational analysis, gene copy number, protein expression and other biomarkers of EGFR for the prediction of response to tyrosine kinase inhibitors. *Oncogene*, 28(Suppl 1): S14–23.

86 Hirsch FR, Varella-Garcia M, Bunn PA, Jr., *et al.* (2003) Epidermal growth factor receptor in non-small-cell lung carcinomas: Correlation between gene copy number and protein expression and impact on prognosis. *J Clin Oncol*, 21: 3798–3807.

87 Pirker R, Pereira JR, von Pawel J, *et al.* (2012) EGFR expression as a predictor of survival for first-line chemotherapy plus cetuximab in patients with advanced non-small-cell lung cancer: analysis of data from the phase 3 FLEX study. *Lancet Oncol*, 13: 33–42.

88 Pinter F, Papay J, Almasi A, *et al.* (2008) Epidermal growth factor receptor (EGFR) high gene copy number and activating mutations in lung

adenocarcinomas are not consistently accompanied by positivity for EGFR protein by standard immunohistochemistry. *J Mol Diagn*, 10: 160–8.

89 Gebhardt F, Burger H, Brandt B (2000) Modulation of EGFR gene transcription by secondary structures, a polymorphic repetitive sequence and mutations-a link between genetics and epigenetics. *Histol Histopathol*, 15: 929–36.

90 Nie Q, Wang Z, Zhang GC, *et al.* (2007) The epidermal growth factor receptor intron1 (CA) n microsatellite polymorphism is a potential predictor of treatment outcome in patients with advanced lung cancer treated with Gefitinib. *Eur J Pharmacol*, 570: 175–81.

91 Han SW, Jeon YK, Lee KH, *et al.* (2007) Intron 1 CA dinucleotide repeat polymorphism and mutations of epidermal growth factor receptor and gefitinib responsiveness in non-small-cell lung cancer. *Pharmacogenet Genomics*, 17: 313–19.

92 Liu G, Gurubhagavatula S, Zhou W, *et al.* (2008) Epidermal growth factor receptor polymorphisms and clinical outcomes in non-small-cell lung cancer patients treated with gefitinib. *Pharmacogenomics J*, 8: 129–38.

93 Liu G, Cheng D, Ding K, *et al.* (2012) Pharmacogenetic analysis of BR.21, a placebo-controlled randomized phase III clinical trial of erlotinib in advanced non-small cell lung cancer. *J Thorac Oncol*, 7: 316–22.

94 Riely GJ, Marks J, Pao W (2009) KRAS mutations in non-small cell lung cancer. *Proc Am Thorac Soc*, 6: 201–5.

95 Roberts PJ, Stinchcombe TE (2013) KRAS mutation: Should we test for it, and does it matter? *J Clin Oncol*, 31: 1112–21.

96 Finberg KE, Sequist LV, Joshi VA, *et al.* (2007) Mucinous differentiation correlates with absence of EGFR mutation and presence of KRAS mutation in lung adenocarcinomas with bronchioloalveolar features. *J Mol Diagn*, 9: 320–6.

97 Mao C, Qiu LX, Liao RY, *et al.* (2010) KRAS mutations and resistance to EGFR-TKIs treatment in patients with non-small cell lung cancer: a meta-analysis of 22 studies. *Lung Cancer*, 69: 272–8.

98 Ihle NT, Byers LA, Kim ES, *et al.* (2012) Effect of KRAS oncogene substitutions on protein behavior: Implications for signaling and clinical outcome. *J Natl Cancer Inst*, 104: 228–39.

99 Fiala O, Pesek M, Finek J, *et al.* (2013) The dominant role of G12C over other KRAS mutation types in the negative prediction of efficacy of epidermal growth factor receptor tyrosine kinase inhibitors in non-small cell lung cancer. *Cancer Genet*, 206: 26–31.

100 Shepherd FA, Domerg C, Hainaut P, *et al.* (2013) Pooled analysis of the prognostic and predictive effects of KRAS mutation status and KRAS mutation subtype in early-stage resected non-small-cell lung cancer in four trials of adjuvant chemotherapy. *J Clin Oncol*, 31(17): 2173–81.

101 Swanton C, Futreal A, Eisen T (2006) Her2-targeted therapies in non-small cell lung cancer. *Clin Cancer Res*, 12: 4377s–83s.

102 Cappuzzo F, Varella-Garcia M, Shigematsu H, *et al.* (2005) Increased HER2 gene copy number is associated with response to gefitinib therapy in epidermal growth factor receptor-positive non-small-cell lung cancer patients. *J Clin Oncol*, 23: 5007–18.

103 Arcila ME, Chaft JE, Nafa K, *et al.* (2012) Prevalence, clinicopathologic associations, and molecular spectrum of ERBB2 (HER2) tyrosine kinase mutations in lung adenocarcinomas. *Clin Cancer Res*, 18: 4910–18.

104 Wang SE, Narasanna A, Perez-Torres M, *et al.* (2006) HER2 kinase domain mutation results in constitutive phosphorylation and activation of HER2 and EGFR and resistance to EGFR tyrosine kinase inhibitors. *Cancer Cell*, 10: 25–38.

105 Taguchi F, Solomon B, Gregorc V, *et al.* (2007) Mass spectrometry to classify non-small-cell lung cancer patients for clinical outcome after treatment with epidermal growth factor receptor tyrosine kinase inhibitors: A multicohort cross-institutional study. *J Natl Cancer Inst*, 99: 838–46.

106 Kuiper JL, Lind JS, Groen HJ, *et al.* (2012) VeriStrat((R)) has prognostic value in advanced stage NSCLC patients treated with erlotinib and sorafenib. *Br J Cancer*, 107(11): 1820–5.

107 Akerley W, Boucher K, Rich N, *et al.* (2012) A phase II study of bevacizumab and erlotinib as initial treatment for metastatic non-squamous, non-small cell lung cancer with serum proteomic evaluation. *Lung Cancer*, 79(3): 307–11.

108 Carbone DP, Ding K, Roder H, *et al.* (2012) Prognostic and predictive role of the VeriStrat plasma test in patients with advanced non-small-cell lung cancer treated with erlotinib or placebo in the NCIC Clinical Trials Group BR.21 trial. *J Thorac Oncol*, 7: 1653–60.

109 Keedy VL, Temin S, Somerfield MR, *et al.* (2011) American Society of Clinical Oncology provisional clinical opinion: epidermal growth factor receptor (EGFR) Mutation testing for patients with advanced non-small-cell lung cancer considering first-line EGFR tyrosine kinase inhibitor therapy. *J Clin Oncol*, 29: 2121–7.

110 Ellis PM, Blais N, Soulieres D, *et al.* (2011) A systematic review and Canadian consensus recommendations on the use of biomarkers in the treatment of non-small cell lung cancer. *J Thorac Oncol,* 6: 1379–91.

111 Janne PA, Shaw AT, Pereira JR, *et al.* (2013) Selumetinib plus docetaxel for KRAS-mutant advanced non-small-cell lung cancer: A randomised, multicentre, placebo-controlled, phase 2 study. *Lancet Oncol,* 14: 38–47.

112 Salto-Tellez M, Tsao MS, Shih JY, *et al.* (2011) Clinical and testing protocols for the analysis of epidermal growth factor receptor mutations in East Asian patients with non-small cell lung cancer: A combined clinical-molecular pathological approach. *J Thorac Oncol,* 6: 1663–9.

113 Travis WD, Brambilla E, Noguchi M, *et al.* (2011) International Association for the Study of Lung Cancer/American Thoracic Society/European Respiratory Society international multidisciplinary classification of lung adenocarcinoma. *J Thorac Oncol,* 6: 244–85.

114 Pirker R, Herth FJ, Kerr KM, *et al.* (2010) Consensus for EGFR mutation testing in non-small cell lung cancer: results from a European workshop. *J Thorac Oncol,* 5: 1706–13.

115 da Cunha Santos G, Saieg MA, Geddie W, *et al.* (2011) EGFR gene status in cytological samples of nonsmall cell lung carcinoma: Controversies and opportunities. *Cancer Cytopathol,* 119: 80–91.

116 Brevet M, Johnson ML, Azzoli CG, *et al.* (2011) Detection of EGFR mutations in plasma DNA from lung cancer patients by mass spectrometry genotyping is predictive of tumor EGFR status and response to EGFR inhibitors. *Lung Cancer,* 73: 96–102.

117 Gately K, O'Flaherty J, Cappuzzo F, *et al.* (2012) The role of the molecular footprint of EGFR in tailoring treatment decisions in NSCLC. *J Clin Pathol* 65: 1–7.

118 Su Z, Dias-Santagata D, Duke M, *et al.* (2011) A platform for rapid detection of multiple oncogenic mutations with relevance to targeted therapy in non-small-cell lung cancer. *J Mol Diagn,* 13: 74–84.

119 Miller VA, Hirsh V, Cadranel J, *et al.* (2012) Afatinib versus placebo for patients with advanced, metastatic non-small-cell lung cancer after failure of erlotinib, gefitinib, or both, and one or two lines of chemotherapy (LUX-Lung 1): A phase 2b/3 randomised trial. *Lancet Oncol,* 13: 528–38.

CHAPTER 29
Immunologic Approaches to Lung Cancer Therapy

Jay M. Lee,[1] *Steven M. Dubinett,*[2] *and Sherven Sharma*[2]
[1]Division of Thoracic Surgery, Jonsson Comprehensive Cancer Center, David Geffen School of Medicine at UCLA, Los Angeles, CA
[2]Division of Pulmonary and Critical Care Medicine, Department of Medicine, UCLA Lung Cancer Research Program, David Geffen School of Medicine at UCLA, Los Angeles, CA, USA

Cancer immunotherapy

In contrast to melanoma and renal cell carcinoma, early attempts of immune stimulation for treatment of thoracic malignancies have not proven to be reliably effective suggesting that thoracic malignancies are nonimmunogenic and will not be amenable to immunologic interventions. However the identification of tumor associated antigens (TAA), advances in cellular and molecular immunology and an improved understanding of tumor immunity has facilitated the development of promising immune based strategies. While there has been a multitude of lung cancer immunotherapy studies, clinical trials focused on inducing a specific antitumor immune response can be categorized into (1) mAb mediated blockade of immune inhibitory checkpoints, (2) tumor protein and peptide vaccines, (3) dendritic cell vaccines, (4) modified tumor cell vaccines, (5) immune adjuvant vaccines, and (6) gene delivery vaccines. In this chapter we will discuss immunotherapy approaches that are most advanced in their clinical development for the treatment of NSCLC and summarize the most recent data from clinical studies of these approaches.

Targeting immune regulatory checkpoints for lung cancer therapy

Tumors use immune inhibitory mechanisms to evade the immune system. One such immune inhibitory pathway that holds promise for the treatment of lung cancer is mediated by the expression of programmed death ligand-1 (PD-L1) on tumors that binds to PD-1 on T cells and prevents T cells from detecting the tumor and evoking the immune system to attack. Treatment of cancer patients with MAbs that block either PD-1 or PD-L1 lead to tumor shrinkage and improvement in long term survival [1].

Despite the large number of tumor antigens induced by genetic and epigenetic alterations found in all cancers, tumors resist immune attack by inducing tolerance among tumor specific T cells and by expressing ligands that engage inhibitory receptors and dampen T-cell functions within the tumor microenvironment. The rationale for the targeting of regulatory T-cells and negative regulatory molecules has been to circumvent immune tolerance. In both preclinical studies and early clinical

Lung Cancer, Fourth Edition. Edited by Jack A. Roth, Waun Ki Hong and Ritsuko U. Komaki.

trials, inhibitory antibodies to components of the B7 family, including the negative regulatory receptor, cytotoxic T-lymphocyte antigen-4 (CTLA-4) and programmed death-1 receptor (PD-1), expressed on activated T-cells, have proven promising targets for immunotherapy. PD-1 is a T-cell co-inhibitory receptor with a structure similar to that of CTLA-4 but with a distinct biologic function and ligand specificity [2]. PD-1 has two known ligands, PD-L1 (B7-H1) [3] and PD-L2 (B7-DC) [4, 5]. In contrast to CTLA-4 ligands, CD80 (B7-1) and CD86 (B7-2), PD-L1 is selectively expressed on many tumors and cells within the tumor microenvironment in response to inflammatory stimuli. Blockade of the interaction between PD-1 and PD-L1 potentiates immune responses in vitro [6] and mediates preclinical antitumor activity [7, 8]. PD-L1 is the primary PD-1 ligand that is up-regulated in solid tumors, where it can inhibit cytokine production and the cytolytic activity of PD-1+, tumor-infiltrating CD4+ and CD8+ T cells [7, 9, 10]. These properties make PD-L1 a potentially promising target for cancer immunotherapy.

BMS-936559 is a high-affinity, fully human, PD-L1–specific, IgG4 (S228P) monoclonal antibody that inhibits the binding of PD-L1 to both PD-1 and CD80. This antibody was evaluated in a multicenter phase 1 trial, as intravenous administration to patients with selected advanced cancers. Anti–PD-L1 antibody was administered every 14 days in 6-week cycles for up to 16 cycles or until the patient had a complete response or confirmed disease progression. The results of this study demonstrated that antibody-mediated blockade of PD-L1 induced durable tumor regression (objective response rate of 6–17%) and prolonged stabilization of disease (rates of 12–41% at 24 weeks) in patients with advanced cancers, including non-small-cell lung cancer, melanoma, and renal-cell cancer [1]. The objective response in 5 of 49 patients (10%) with advanced non-small-cell lung cancer who received anti-PD-L1 was quite unexpected. Although melanoma and renal-cell cancer are responsive to cancer immunotherapy (e.g., interleukin-2 and anti–CTLA-4), non-small-cell lung cancer has been considered to be nonimmunogenic and poorly responsive to immune-based therapies. Another important feature of anti–PD-L1 therapy was the durability of response across multiple tumor types. This was particularly notable given the advanced stage of disease and previous treatments of patients in the study. This durability appeared to be greater than that observed with most chemotherapy and kinase inhibitors used in these diseases, although no direct comparisons have been performed [11]. The patient response rate with the anti-PD-1 trial in lung cancer was 14 of 76. Objective responses were observed across non-small-cell histologic types: in 6 of 18 patients (33%) with squamous tumors, 7 of 56 (12%) with nonsquamous tumors, and 1 of 2 with tumors of unknown type. The most common side effects of treatment included fatigue, rash, and diarrhea. Other less-common side effects, such as fever, were consistent with the activation of the immune system. Five percent of patients in the trial targeting PD-1, and 6% in the trial targeting PD-L1 trial, stopped receiving treatment because of severe side effects, and three patients who received the PD-1 targeted drug died of uncontrolled lung inflammation caused by the treatment [1]. The therapeutic potential of these inhibitory pathways that places the brake on the immune system from recognizing cancers has been realized and additional phase II trials of the PD-1 targeted agent are under way, and phase III trials involving patients with melanoma, non-small cell lung cancer, and kidney cancer are being planned. PD-1 pathway targeted agents are also top priority agents for clinical trials that will be conducted by researchers in NCI's Immunotherapy Clinical Trials Network.

Tumor protein and peptide vaccines

Activated proto-oncogenes, inactivated tumor suppressor genes, and genetic mutations have been linked to molecular events involved in lung cancer tumorigenesis and have led to the identification of tumor associated antigens ideal for the development of vaccines. Proteins and peptides are processed via MHC molecules and presented by

APC on the cell surface to T lymphocytes resulting in the generation of a specific immune response [12]. Only a short segment of peptide sequences from the original tumor protein are immunogenic, and these peptide sequences, called epitopes, are presented by MHC molecules according to a complex set of cellular rules [12]. Peptides are smaller than proteins, readily produced, and generate reproducible immune responses by readily available immune assays. However, peptides are restricted to specific HLA types for presentation, which may not allow universal application to all patients [12]. Therapeutic peptide cancer vaccines aim at inducing strong CD8 and CD4 T-cell responses and require the involvement of host antigen presenting cells (APC) to efficiently present the peptide antigens for the activation of the respective T cell subsets. The rationale for the use of peptide vaccines is based on extensive preclinical studies that demonstrated the requirement of T-lymphocytes for the eradication of solid tumors. Cytotoxic T-lymphocytes (CTLs) or CD8 T cells represent the primary effector cells involved in tumor-specific immune-mediated destruction of cancer cells. CTLs recognize, engage and destroy targets cells through the tri-molecular interaction of the antigen-specific receptor (TCR) on the CTL and peptides that are presented by the target cell to the CTL in the context of class I major histocompatibility complex antigens [(MHC) also referred to as human leukocyte antigens or HLA]. All somatic cells express HLA molecules on their surfaces and use them to present antigens to T cells. Whole proteins within the cell are processed into small peptide fragments (8–10 amino acids in length) that are displayed on the cell surface in the context of HLA molecules. The HLA-peptide molecular complex enables CTLs to recognize tumor-associated antigens and results in the targeted destruction of the cancer cell expressing these antigens by the CTL. Many primary cancers express adequate HLA molecules and are capable of being recognized and destroyed by TAA-specific CTLs. The identification and reintroduction of tumor associated specific peptides in increased concentration to the immune system via vaccination activates and deploys the appropriate CTLs to destroy cancer cells. The use of a single peptide antigen or a few peptide antigens in the therapeutic cancer vaccine is based on the assumption that the initial induced antitumor response to one or few antigens will eventuate into a broad immune response to a multitude of TAAs after uptake of dying tumor cells and presentation by host APC.

The expression of the melanoma-associated antigen (MAGE) genes is silent in all normal cells except germ cells [13]. There has been more than 50 related MAGE genes identified thus far, and have been shown to play an important role physiologically and pathologically during embryogenesis, germ cell development, cell cycle progression, and apoptosis [13]. Nearly 75% of small cell lung cancers (SCLC) and approximately 40% of NSCLC express MAGE-3 and as a result this testis cancer antigen has received attention as an immunotherapy target. Atanackovic *et al.* reported on the successful induction of humoral and specific cell mediated immunity in early stage NSCLC (I and II) patients vaccinated with MAGE-3 protein [14]. Seventeen patients with MAGE-3 expressing NSCLC were analyzed in two groups, one receiving MAGE-3 protein alone and the other receiving MAGE-3 protein with adjuvant AS02B [14]. Of the 9 patients in the first cohort, 3 patients developed marginal Ab titers and another patient had a CD8 T cell response to HLA-A2-restricted peptide MAGE-3 271–279 [14]. In contrast, of 8 patients from the second cohort vaccinated with MAGE-3 protein and adjuvant, 7 patients developed antibody high titers to MAGE-3, and 4 had a strong concomitant CD4 T cell response to HLA-DP4-restricted peptide 243–258 [14]. One patient simultaneously developed CD8 T cells to HLA-A1-restricted peptide 168–176 [14]. Although the clinical relevance of the immune responses was not addressed, this study demonstrated the importance of CD4 T cell mediated immunity that correlated with antibody production following vaccination, in addition to the traditionally understood involvement of antigen specific CD8 T cell response. Moreover, this study provides the foundation for further evaluating integrated humoral and cell mediated immune responses in vaccine strategies and also to pursue the relevance of this approach in clinical outcomes. GlaxoSmithKline's specific vaccine against the MAGE 3 expressing non-small cell lung cancer consists of purified MAGE-A3 recombinant protein in liposomal formulation containing the AS02B immunoadjuvant system. Based on early studies of this vaccine in patients with non-small cell lung cancer a large clinical trial is underway testing this vaccine (called the Phase III MAGRIT trial). Many centers around the world are participating in this trial for post-surgical patients being conducted worldwide at this time. The study is powered for disease free survival as the primary endpoint in the total population and in the cohort without postoperative chemotherapy [15].

After a long developmental phase, mucin 1 (MUC1) peptide vaccine candidate in NSCLC patients has demonstrated increased survival in phase II clinical trials [16, 17] that provided the rationale for the initiation of phase III trials in large cohorts of lung cancer patients. The vaccine targets MUC1, an antigen widely expressed in lung carcinomas. The BLP25 liposomal vaccine (L-BLP25) approach for lung cancer is a peptide liposomal vaccine to target the exposed core peptide of MUC1 tumor-associated antigen in lung cancer. MUC1 is a cell membrane glycoprotein overexpressed in many types of cancers including NSCLC, breast, colorectal, prostate, pancreatic, ovarian, and multiple myeloma. MUC 1 expression in tumors promotes growth and survival and is associated with disease progression and poor prognosis. The relevance of MUC1 as an antitumor target is based on preclinical and clinical studies. MUC 1 expression pattern in tumor cells is different from normal cells. More than 80% of the tumor cells express MUC1 with greater than 60% of NSCLCs express MUC1 [18]. The BLP25 lipopeptide vaccine consists of a 25-amino acid MUC1 sequence (STAPPAHGVTSAPDTRPAPGSTAPP) that provides MUC1 specificity. It is slightly larger than one tandem repeat of MUC1 protein and contains a palmitoyl lysine residue at the carboxy terminal to enhance the incorporation of the lipopeptide into the liposome particle. The vaccine is a lyophilized preparation consisting of BLP25 lipopeptide, immunoadjuvant monophosphoryl lipid A, and three lipids (cholesterol, dimyristoyl phosphatidylglycerol, and dipalmitoyl phosphatidylcholine). The lipids serve as adjuvants, to enhance the immunogenicity of the peptide MUC1 vaccine. The monophosphoryl lipid A is the toll-like receptor-4 agonist that activates DC and macrophages. The liposomal delivery system is designed to facilitate uptake by APC such that the lipopeptide is delivered into the intracellular space for presentation by MHC molecules to activate specific T-cells that will identify and target cancer cells expressing MUC1. It is encouraging to see that the L-BLP25 cancer vaccine is currently being evaluated in a phase III trial for the treatment of unresectable, stage III NSCLC (Emepepimut-S for non-small cell lung cancer). There is much optimism for this vaccine based on the favorable toxicity profile in patients treated with this drug and the benefit in survival in patients with local and regional stage III non-small cell lung cancer. In studies described to date on the L-BLP25 vaccine there has not been adequate immune monitoring of vaccination responses. The studies lack data on immune responses to the vaccine component through quantification of the frequency of MUC1 specific CTL pre and post vaccination in PBMCs and how it correlates with overall performance of the patients. Hopefully the omission in quantification of immune responses will be improved as the studies progress.

Dendritic cell vaccines

The predominant mechanism of antitumor immunity is a cell (T lymphocyte) mediated destruction of tumor cells. Specifically, the expansion of cytotoxic T lymphocytes (CTL) capable of recognizing antigens on cancerous cells presented in association with MHC molecules is the goal of most immunotherapy strategies. Antigen presenting cells (APC) appear to play a central role in T cell activation by presenting tumor antigens and providing essential co-stimulatory signals necessary for the production of CTL. In optimal circumstances, APC can migrate and gain access to the tumor microenvironment, and overcome tumor-induced obstacles to have effective function. T cell activation results in the generation of CTL capable of recognizing and destroying cancer cells, and the production of cytokines, such as IFN-γ and TNFα, which can suppress both tumor cell proliferation and induction of angiogenesis [19, 20]. CTL can cause lysis of tumor cells mediated by perforin and/or Fas [19, 21]. Therefore, therapeutic efforts have focused on identifying tumor antigens, providing the antigens in immunogenic contexts, manipulating T cell responses to increase the number of CTL, and thus augmenting their effector functions.

Dendritic cells (DC) are extremely potent APC that present tumor-associated antigens to T cells and thereby initiate tumor-specific immunity [22–24]. DC are bone marrow-derived leukocytes characterized by a high level of expression of MHC and co-stimulatory molecules [25]. As a result, they are capable of capturing antigens and producing large numbers of immunogenic MHC-peptide complexes [25] and they migrate to secondary lymphoid organs to select and stimulate antigen-specific T cells. With the application of appropriate cytokines, one can generate large quantities of DC. Human DC may be generated from proliferating CD34+ cells or from nonproliferating CD14+ progenitor cells. The production of DC from CD34+ cells requires GM-CSF and tumor necrosis factor alpha (TNF-α), whereas CD14+ cells require stimulation with GM-CSF and interleukin-4 (IL-4) to produce sufficient quantities of DC.

Because of the importance of DC in tumor immunity a variety of strategies have been used to exploit activated DC in cancer immunotherapy [26,27] and numerous clinical trials are addressing the feasibility and safety of DC-based strategies [28–32]. DC have been investigated as a delivery mechanism for tumor-associated antigens. Both whole cell and peptide strategies have been reported. Hirschowitz *et al.* used autologous DC pulsed with apoptotic bodies of an allogeneic non-small cell lung cancer (NSCLC) cell line that overexpressed 5 known antigens (Her2/*neu*, CEA, WT1, Mage2, and survivin) [31]. Kontani *et al.* studied autologous DC pulsed with either MUC-1 peptides in patients with MUC-1 positive tumors (9) or autologous tumor lysates in patients with MUC-1 negative tumors (5) in a total of 14 patients with locally advanced or metastatic lung (8 patients) or breast cancer (6 patients) [32]. Antonia *et al.* reported on a vaccination strategy that entailed autologous DC transfected with an adenovirus containing wild-type p53 [30].

Insights into cellular and molecular events that lead to recruitment and activation of immune cells suggest that obstacles present in the tumor might be bypassed and tumor immunity initiated by providing selected cytokines and/or chemokines in the solid tumors. Expression of molecules such as secondary lymphoid-tissue chemokine from gene modified DC and intratumoral administration have shown efficacy in preclinical murine tumor models [33–35]. Based on the pre-clinical model systems, a clinical trial was initiated at University of California Los Angeles (in collaboration with the National Cancer Institute – Rapid Access to Intervention Development program) in patients with advanced stage NSCLC. This trial is a dose-escalation of DC-AdCCL21 administered intratumorally in patients with advanced NSCLC. A GMP grade AdCCL21 replication deficient virus [36] was made available through the RAID program to conduct the Phase I clinical trial. Human DCs transduced with advenovirus-CCL21 produce CCL21 to attract T cells and DCs. Preliminary findings demonstrate tumor specific systemic immune responses as assessed by the IFN-γ T cell ELISPOT. Multiplex assessment of plasma cytokines before and after therapy in these patients revealed induction of IL-2, IFN-γ, IL-12 and CXCL10. Immunohistochemistry of post tumor biopsies revealed an influx of CD4 expressing tumor infiltrating lymphocytes.

Modified tumor cell vaccines

Tumors differ fundamentally from their normal cell counterparts in antigenic makeup and biologic behavior, and a defining component of carcinogenesis is genetic instability [37]. The culmination of genetic mutations in cancer cells is the generation of new antigens as tumors develop and progress [37]. As a result, autologous and allogeneic tumors are a rich source for tumor antigens in vaccine trials.

The advantage of autologous tumor vaccines is the ability to generate patient specific immune responses and avoidance of identifying the tumor cell antigenic phenotype. However, this is weighed by the limitation in availability and amount of the patient's own tumor, and vaccine trials based on this concept are restricted to enrolling patients undergoing surgical resection. The utility of gene modified tumor cell vaccines has been well established from several preclinical tumor models. The cytokine GM-CSF promotes immune memory, and prevents tumor recurrence and metastasis. GM-CSF is a mediator of proliferation, maturation, and migration of DC and enhances antitumor immunity. Autologous, irradiated NSCLC cells engineered to secrete GM-CSF were tested in patients with metastatic NSCLC in a Phase I clinical trial [38]. In an effort to remove the need for viral transduction of autologous tumors, a vaccine (GVAX) composed of the combination of autologous tumor cells and an allogeneic GM-CSF secreting cell line has been utilized in clinical trials [39, 40]. Due to the lack of efficacy from GVAX in advanced NSCLC, this vaccine has transferred its use to other malignancies.

Allogeneic antigens are attractive sources of tumor antigens in vaccine trials given that they eliminate the need for patient tumor procurement. Tumor cell lines can serve as an allogeneic whole cell vaccine. Malignant cells often change the cell surface phenotype by lacking costimulatory signals required for the generation of effective antitumor immunity [41]. The most critical molecules involved in co-stimulation are CD80/CD86 and CD40L [41]. Lung cancer cells downregulate MHC molecule expression on the cell surface. As a result, several studies have embarked on genetic manipulation of tumor cell lines to express necessary co-stimulatory and MHC molecules necessary for induction of antitumor immunity [42, 43]. Raez *et al.* who conducted a phase I trial in stage IIIB and IV NSCLC patients with a vaccine therapy comprised of a human lung adenocarcinoma cell line transfected with B7.1 (CD80) and HLA A1 or A2 (MHC I molecules) [43]. Although allogeneic cell lines provide a convenient alternative to autologous patient tumors, a major limitation with the use of this strategy is the fundamental assumption that lung tumor antigens expressed on the cell line are common with the patient's unique tumor and this antigenic phenotype is also shared among different patients.

Immune adjuvant vaccines

Transforming growth factor-β (TGF-β) is a protein that inhibits proliferation and induces apoptosis in normal and neoplastic cells classifying it as a tumor suppressor gene, and regulates angiogenesis [44–46]. The accumulation of mutations in the TGF-β receptor or Smad genes inactivates the TGF-β receptor-Smad pathway favoring tumor growth [44, 45]. All human tumors overproduce TGF-β whose actions promote tumor cell invasiveness and metastasis, and thus induce EMT [44]. TGF-β suppresses the proliferation and differentiation of lymphocytes including cytolytic T cells, natural killer cells, macrophages, and dendritic cells providing a mechanism of tumor mediated immune evasion [44, 46]. Elevated TGF-β2 levels have been linked to immunosuppression in cancer patients, and TGF-β2 levels have inversely correlated to prognosis of patients with NSCLC. Nemunaitis *et al.* performed a Phase II study of belagenpumatucel-L, a TGF-β2 antisense gene-modified allogeneic tumor cell line vaccine, in patients with stages II-IV NSCLC [47]. The study showed that belagenpumatucel-L was well tolerated, and the survival advantage justified pursuit for a phase III evaluation. Given that upregulation of the immune responses correlated to favorable clinical outcomes, this trial supports the concept that correct selection of allogeneic tumor cell lines that have shared immunodominant tumor antigens with the patient's tumor may be an effective antitumor strategy. Combining this approach with targeting the TGF pathway may add to this beneficial effect.

Anti-idiotypic monoclonal antibodies (Mab) can mimic both protein and non-protein antigenic epitopes and induce immune responses against tumor antigens. Anti-idiotypic antibody based vaccines are ideal when the antigen is not readily available in sufficient quantities or when the antigen is not a protein. Small cell lung cancer (SCLC) is of neuroectodermal origin, and as a result, has a unique number of differentiation antigens as potential immune targets due to its specific embryonic basis [48]. Bec2 is an anti-idiotypic antibody that mimics GD3, a ganglioside antigen of neuroectodermal origin expressed on the surface of tumor cells, and are involved in numerous functions including cell-cell recognition, cell matrix attachment, and cell differentiation [48, 49]. Giaccone *et al.* conducted a phase III trial immunizing Bec2 in combination with Bacille Calmette-Guerin (BCG), in patients with limited-disease SCLC after a major response to chemotherapy and chest radiation [49]. Five hundred and fifteen patients were randomly assigned to receive five vaccinations of Bec2/BCG vaccine over a 10-week period or follow-up [49]. The primary toxicities of immunization were transient skin ulcerations and mild flu-like symptoms [49]. In the patients who received the vaccine, there was no improvement in survival, progression-free survival, or quality of life [49]. The median survival from randomization was 16.4 and 14.3 months in the observation and vaccination arms ($P = 0.28$), respectively [49]. In summary, this study revealed that vaccination with Bec2/BCG had no impact on clinical outcome of patients with limited-disease SCLC responding to chemotherapy and radiation therapy. The anti-idiotypic antibody vaccine is the only phase III study in lung cancer. A series of other trials have established the immunogenicity of several keyhole limpet hemocyanin conjugate vaccines relevant to SCLC, including GM2, Globo H, fucosyl GM1, and polysialic acid [48].

Gene delivery vaccines

Gene transfer vectors have been utilized as drug delivery systems to provide high level expression of a protein of interest intracellularly or secretion into the local milieu of the tumor [50, 51]. MUC1 is a glycoprotein normally found on the surface of mucin secreting epithelial cells, and its expression has been shown to be increased in breast, lung, ovary, and colon carcinomas suggesting that MUC1 aberrant expression is common to adenocarcinomas. A humoral response to this protein in NSCLC patients has found to have a prognostic significance [52]. Mennecier *et al.* reported a phase II trial with TG4010, a recombinant vaccinia vector (MVA) containing DNA sequences for the human MUC1 antigen and interleukin-2 (IL-2), in advanced NSCLC cancer patients [53]. A multicenter randomized trial was conducted in 65 stage IIIB and IV patients with either upfront TG4010 in combination with cisplatin and vinorelbine (arm 1) or TG4010 alone followed by both chemotherapeutic agents upon disease progression [53]. In arm 1, a partial response was seen in 68% (24/35) patients [53]. In arm 2, two patients had stable disease, and in subsequent combination with chemotherapy, a partial response was seen in 3 of 14 patients [53]. TG4010 was well tolerated with the injection site reaction being the most common drug related adverse event [53]. In this preliminary report, the combination of TG4010 with standard chemotherapy for NSCLC demonstrated encouraging results.

Conclusion

The challenge for immunotherapy is to use advances in cellular and molecular immunology to develop strategies that effectively and safely augment antitumor responses. This can be achieved by understanding the complex issues surrounding cancer immunosurveillance, cancer immuno-editing, complicity of host cellular networks in lung tumorigenesis, tumor mediated immunosuppression and immune regulatory check points that control T cell activities. The numerous challenges that pose obstacles to cancer vaccine efficacy include (1) correct identification of optimal antigens and immune adjuvants, (2) determination of the appropriate immune response to be generated, (3) elicitation of long-term antitumor memory, and (4) tumor induced immunosuppression and immune evasion. When developing immune based strategies, the requirements for (1) immune cell activation, homing, and accumulation at tumor sites, (2) disruption of the regulatory mechanisms that limit immune responses, and (3) the ability to direct a coordinated and effective attack against tumors engaging multiple components of the immune system should evolve in parallel. It is clear that effective antitumor responses require the complex interaction of APC, lymphocyte, and NK cells and down regulation of immune suppressor activities and immune regulatory check points. As we unravel and elucidate the mechanisms that dampen antitumor immune activity there will be additional opportunity for exploitation of targets for effective immunotherapy for lung cancer.

References

1 Brahmer JR, Tykodi SS, Chow LQ, Hwu WJ, Topalian SL, Hwu P, *et al.* (2012) Safety and activity of anti-PD-L1 antibody in patients with advanced cancer. *New England Journal of Medicine*, Jun 28; 366(26): 2455–65. PubMed PMID: 22658128. Pubmed Central PMCID: 3563263.

2 Okazaki T, Honjo T (2007) PD-1 and PD-1 ligands: From discovery to clinical application. *International Immunology*, Jul; 19(7): 813–24. PubMed PMID: 17606980.

3 Freeman GJ, Long AJ, Iwai Y, Bourque K, Chernova T, Nishimura H, *et al.* (2000) Engagement of the PD-1 immunoinhibitory receptor by a novel B7 family member leads to negative regulation of lymphocyte activation. *Journal of Experimental Medicine*, Oct 2; 192(7): 1027–34. PubMed PMID: 11015443. Pubmed Central PMCID: 2193311.

4 Tseng SY, Otsuji M, Gorski K, Huang X, Slansky JE, Pai SI, *et al.* (2001) B7-DC, a new dendritic cell molecule with potent costimulatory properties for T cells. *Journal of Experimental Medicine*, Apr 2; 193(7): 839–46. PubMed PMID: 11283156. Pubmed Central PMCID: 2193370.

5 Latchman Y, Wood CR, Chernova T, Chaudhary D, Borde M, Chernova I, *et al.* (2001) PD-L2 is a second ligand for PD-1 and inhibits T cell activation. *Nature Immunology*, Mar; 2(3): 261–8. PubMed PMID: 11224527.

6 Fife BT, Pauken KE, Eagar TN, Obu T, Wu J, Tang Q, *et al.* (2009) Interactions between PD-1 and PD-L1 promote tolerance by blocking the TCR-induced stop signal. *Nature Immunology*, Nov; 10(11): 1185–92. PubMed PMID: 19783989. Pubmed Central PMCID: 2778301.

7 Dong H, Strome SE, Salomao DR, Tamura H, Hirano F, Flies DB, *et al.* (2002) Tumor-associated B7-H1 promotes T-cell apoptosis: A potential mechanism of immune evasion. *Nature Medicine*, Aug; 8(8): 793–800. PubMed PMID: 12091876.

8 Iwai Y, Ishida M, Tanaka Y, Okazaki T, Honjo T, Minato N (2002) Involvement of PD-L1 on tumor cells in the escape from host immune system and tumor immunotherapy by PD-L1 blockade. *Proceedings of the National Academy of Sciences of the United States of America*, Sep 17; 99(19): 12293–7. PubMed PMID: 12218188. Pubmed Central PMCID: 129438.

9 Hino R, Kabashima K, Kato Y, Yagi H, Nakamura M, Honjo T, *et al.* (2010) Tumor cell expression of programmed cell death-1 ligand 1 is a prognostic factor for malignant melanoma. *Cancer*, Apr 1; 116(7): 1757–66. PubMed PMID: 20143437.

10 Taube JM, Anders RA, Young GD, Xu H, Sharma R, McMiller TL, *et al.* (2012) Colocalization of inflammatory response with B7-h1 expression in human melanocytic lesions supports an adaptive resistance mechanism of immune escape. *Science Translational Medicine*, Mar 28; 4(127): 127ra37. PubMed PMID: 22461641.

11 Holt GE, Podack ER, Raez LE (2011) Immunotherapy as a strategy for the treatment of non-small-cell lung cancer. *Therapy*, Jan; 8(1): 43–54. PubMed PMID: 21359153. Pubmed Central PMCID: 3042692.

12 Ribas A, Butterfield LH, Glaspy JA, Economou JS (2003) Current developments in cancer vaccines and cellular immunotherapy. *Journal of Clinical Oncology*, Jun 15; 21(12): 2415–32. PubMed PMID: 12805342.

13 Tsai JR, Chong IW, Chen YH, Yang MJ, Sheu CC, Chang HC, *et al.* (2007) Differential expression profile of MAGE family in non-small-cell lung cancer. *Lung Cancer*, May; 56(2): 185–92. PubMed PMID: 17208331.

14 Atanackovic D, Altorki NK, Stockert E, Williamson B, Jungbluth AA, Ritter E, *et al.* (2004) Vaccine-induced CD4+ T cell responses to MAGE-3 protein in lung cancer patients. *Journal of Immunology*, Mar 1; 172(5): 3289–96. PubMed PMID: 14978137.

15 GSK1572932A Antigen-specific cancer immunotherapeutic as adjuvant therapy in patients with non-small cell lung cancer [Internet]. 2013 [cited March 24, 2011]. Available from: http://www.clinicaltrials.gov/ct2/show/NCT00480025?term=MAGE-A3&rank=8

16 Butts C, Murray N, Maksymiuk A, Goss G, Marshall E, Soulieres D, *et al.* (2005) Randomized phase IIB trial of BLP25 liposome vaccine in stage IIIB and IV non-small-cell lung cancer. *J Clin Oncol*, 23(27): 6674–81.

17 Sangha R, Butts C (2007) L-BLP25: a peptide vaccine strategy in non small cell lung cancer. *Clin Cancer Res*, 13(15 Pt 2): s4652-4.

18 Vlad AM, Kettel JC, Alajez NM, Carlos CA, Finn OJ (2004) MUC1 immunobiology: From discovery to clinical applications. *Adv Immunol*, 82: 249–93.

19 Peng L, Krauss JC, Plautz GE, Mukai S, Shu S, Cohen PA (2000) T cell-mediated tumor rejection displays diverse dependence upon perforin and IFN-gamma mechanisms that cannot be predicted from in vitro

T cell characteristics. *Journal of Immunology*, Dec 15; 165(12): 7116–24. PubMed PMID: 11120842.

20 Poehlein CH, Hu HM, Yamada J, Assmann I, Alvord WG, Urba WJ, *et al.* (2003) TNF plays an essential role in tumor regression after adoptive transfer of perforin/IFN-gamma double knockout effector T cells. *Journal of Immunology*, Feb 15; 170(4): 2004–13. PubMed PMID: 12574370.

21 Seki N, Brooks AD, Carter CR, Back TC, Parsoneault EM, Smyth MJ, *et al.* (2002) Tumor-specific CTL kill murine renal cancer cells using both perforin and Fas ligand-mediated lysis in vitro, but cause tumor regression in vivo in the absence of perforin. *Journal of Immunology*, Apr 1; 168(7): 3484–92. PubMed PMID: 11907109.

22 Aragoneses-Fenoll L, Corbi AL (2007) Dendritic cells: still a promising tool for cancer immunotherapy. *Clinical & Translational Oncology*, Feb; 9(2): 77–82. PubMed PMID: 17329218.

23 Fong L, Engleman EG (2000) Dendritic cells in cancer immunotherapy. *Annual Review of Immunology*, 18: 245–73. PubMed PMID: 10837059.

24 Banchereau J, Palucka AK (2005) Dendritic cells as therapeutic vaccines against cancer. *Nature Reviews Immunology*, Apr; 5(4): 296–306. PubMed PMID: 15803149.

25 Pardoll DM (2002) Spinning molecular immunology into successful immunotherapy. *Nature Reviews Immunology*, Apr; 2(4): 227–38. PubMed PMID: 12001994.

26 Banchereau J, Steinman RM (1998) Dendritic cells and the control of immunity. *Nature*, Mar 19; 392(6673): 245–52. PubMed PMID: 9521319.

27 Timmerman JM, Levy R (1999) Dendritic cell vaccines for cancer immunotherapy. *Annual Review of Medicine*, 50: 507–29. PubMed PMID: 10073291.

28 Nair SK, Hull S, Coleman D, Gilboa E, Lyerly HK, Morse MA (1999) Induction of carcinoembryonic antigen (CEA)-specific cytotoxic T-lymphocyte responses in vitro using autologous dendritic cells loaded with CEA peptide or CEA RNA in patients with metastatic malignancies expressing CEA. *International Journal of Cancer*, Jul 2; 82(1): 121–4. PubMed PMID: 10360830.

29 Sharma S, Miller P, Stolina M, Zhu L, Huang M, Paul R, *et al.* (1997) Multi-component gene therapy vaccines for lung cancer: Effective eradication of established murine tumors *in vivo* with Interleukin 7/Herpes Simplex Thymidine Kinase-transduced autologous tumor and *ex vivo*-activated dendritic cells. *Gene Therapy*, 4: 1361–70.

30 Antonia SJ, Mirza N, Fricke I, Chiappori A, Thompson P, Williams N, *et al.* (2006) Combination of p53 cancer vaccine with chemotherapy in patients with extensive stage small cell lung cancer. *Clinical Cancer Research*, Feb 1; 12(3 Pt 1): 878–87. PubMed PMID: 16467102.

31 Hirschowitz EA, Foody T, Kryscio R, Dickson L, Sturgill J, Yannelli J (2004) Autologous dendritic cell vaccines for non-small-cell lung cancer. *Journal of Clinical Oncology*, Jul 15; 22(14): 2808–15. PubMed PMID: 15254048.

32 Kontani K, Taguchi O, Ozaki Y, Hanaoka J, Sawai S, Inoue S, *et al.* (2003) Dendritic cell vaccine immunotherapy of cancer targeting MUC1 mucin. *International Journal of Molecular Medicine*, Oct; 12(4): 493–502. PubMed PMID: 12964025.

33 Yang SC, Hillinger S, Riedl K, Zhang L, Zhu L, Huang M, *et al.* (2004) Intratumoral administration of dendritic cells overexpressing CCL21 generates systemic antitumor responses and confers tumor immunity. *Clinical Cancer Research*, Apr 15; 10(8): 2891–2901. PubMed PMID: 15102698.

34 Yang SC, Batra RK, Hillinger S, Reckamp KL, Strieter RM, Dubinett SM, *et al.* (2006) Intrapulmonary administration of CCL21 gene-modified dendritic cells reduces tumor burden in spontaneous murine bronchoalveolar cell carcinoma. *Cancer Research*, Mar 15; 66(6): 3205–13. PubMed PMID: 16540672.

35 Sharma S, Stolina M, Luo J, Strieter RM, Burdick M, Zhu LX, *et al.* (2000) Secondary lymphoid tissue chemokine mediates T cell-dependent antitumor responses in vivo. *Journal of Immunology*, May 1; 164(9): 4558–63. PubMed PMID: 10779757.

36 Baratelli F, Takedatsu H, Hazra S, Peebles K, Luo J, Kurimoto PS, *et al.* (2008) Pre-clinical characterization of GMP grade CCL21-gene modified dendritic cells for application in a phase I trial in non-small cell lung cancer. *J Transl Med*, Jul 22; 6(1): 38. PubMed PMID: 18644162.

37 Pardoll D (2003) Does the immune system see tumors as foreign or self? *Annual Review of Immunology*, 21: 807–39. PubMed PMID: 12615893.

38 Salgia R, Lynch T, Skarin A, Lucca J, Lynch C, Jung K, *et al.* (2003) Vaccination with irradiated autologous tumor cells engineered to secrete granulocyte-macrophage colony-stimulating factor augments antitumor immunity in some patients with metastatic non-small-cell lung carcinoma. *Journal of Clinical Oncology*, Feb 15; 21(4): 624–30. PubMed PMID: 12586798.

39 Nemunaitis J, Sterman D, Jablons D, Smith JW, 2nd, Fox B, Maples P, *et al.* (2004) Granulocyte-

macrophage colony-stimulating factor gene-modified autologous tumor vaccines in non-small-cell lung cancer. *Journal of the National Cancer Institute*, Feb 18; 96(4): 326–31. PubMed PMID: 14970281.

40 Nemunaitis J, Jahan T, Ross H, Sterman D, Richards D, Fox B, *et al.* (2006) Phase 1/2 trial of autologous tumor mixed with an allogeneic GVAX vaccine in advanced-stage non-small-cell lung cancer. *Cancer Gene Therapy*, Jun; 13(6): 555–62. PubMed PMID: 16410826.

41 Singh NP, Yolcu ES, Taylor DD, Gercel-Taylor C, Metzinger DS, Dreisbach SK, *et al.* (2003) A novel approach to cancer immunotherapy: tumor cells decorated with CD80 generate effective antitumor immunity. *Cancer Research*, Jul 15; 63(14): 4067–73. PubMed PMID: 12874008.

42 Raez LE, Cassileth PA, Schlesselman JJ, Padmanabhan S, Fisher EZ, Baldie PA, *et al.* (2003) Induction of CD8 T-cell-Ifn-gamma response and positive clinical outcome after immunization with gene-modified allogeneic tumor cells in advanced non-small-cell lung carcinoma. *Cancer Gene Therapy*, Nov; 10(11): 850–8. PubMed PMID: 14605671.

43 Raez LE, Cassileth PA, Schlesselman JJ, Sridhar K, Padmanabhan S, Fisher EZ, *et al.* (2004) Allogeneic vaccination with a B7.1 HLA-A gene-modified adenocarcinoma cell line in patients with advanced non-small-cell lung cancer. *Journal of Clinical Oncology*, Jul 15; 22(14): 2800–7. PubMed PMID: 15254047.

44 Pardali K, Moustakas A (2007) Actions of TGF-beta as tumor suppressor and pro-metastatic factor in human cancer. *Biochimica et biophysica acta*, Jan; 1775(1): 21–62. PubMed PMID: 16904831.

45 Levy L, Hill CS (2006) Alterations in components of the TGF-beta superfamily signaling pathways in human cancer. *Cytokine & Growth Factor Reviews*, Feb–Apr; 17(1–2): 41–58. PubMed PMID: 16310402.

46 Gajewski TF, Meng Y, Harlin H (2006) Immune suppression in the tumor microenvironment. *Journal of Immunotherapy*, May–Jun; 29(3): 233–40. PubMed PMID: 16699366.

47 Nemunaitis J, Dillman RO, Schwarzenberger PO, Senzer N, Cunningham C, Cutler J, *et al.* (2006) Phase II study of belagenpumatucel-L, a transforming growth factor beta-2 antisense gene-modified allogeneic tumor cell vaccine in non-small-cell lung cancer. *Journal of Clinical Oncology*. Oct 10; 24(29): 4721–30. PubMed PMID: 16966690.

48 Krug LM (2004) Vaccine therapy for small cell lung cancer. *Seminars in Oncology*, Feb; 31(1 Suppl 1): 112–6. PubMed PMID: 14981589.

49 Giaccone G, Debruyne C, Felip E, Chapman PB, Grant SC, Millward M, *et al.* (2005) Phase III study of adjuvant vaccination with Bec2/bacille Calmette-Guerin in responding patients with limited-disease small-cell lung cancer (European Organisation for Research and Treatment of Cancer 08971-08971B; Silva Study). *Journal of Clinical Oncology*, Oct 1; 23(28): 6854–64. PubMed PMID: 16192577.

50 Toloza EM, Morse MA, Lyerly HK (2006) Gene therapy for lung cancer. *Journal of Cellular Biochemistry*, Sep 1; 99(1): 1–22. PubMed PMID: 16767697.

51 Hege KM, Carbone DP (2003) Lung cancer vaccines and gene therapy. *Lung Cancer*, Aug; 41(Suppl 1): S103–13. PubMed PMID: 12867069.

52 Hirasawa Y, Kohno N, Yokoyama A, Kondo K, Hiwada K, Miyake M (2000) Natural autoantibody to MUC1 is a prognostic indicator for non-small cell lung cancer. *American Journal of Respiratory and Critical Care Medicine*, Feb; 161(2 Pt 1): 589–94. PubMed PMID: 10673204.

53 Mennecier B, Ramlau R, Rolski J (2006) Phase II study evaluating clinical efficacy of TG 4010 (MVA - MUC1 - IL 2) in association with cisplatin and binorelbine in a patient with non small cell lung cancer. In: Roth JA, Cox JD, Hong WK (eds). *Lung Cancer*: Chichester, UK: John Wiley & Sons, Ltd.

CHAPTER 30

Novel and Emerging Agents in NSCLC

Anne S. Tsao[1] *and Jack A. Roth*[2]

[1]Department of Thoracic/Head and Neck Medical Oncology, The University of Texas MD Anderson Cancer Center, Houston, TX, USA

[2]Department of Thoracic and Cardiovascular Surgery, The University of Texas MD Anderson Cancer Center, Houston, TX, USA

Introduction

The emergence of rapid DNA sequencing technology has led to a paradigm shift in oncology. Both gene therapy and pharmaco-development of novel targeted agents are evolving fields in oncology. The following chapter is divided into two sections and will review the impact of novel targeted agents and gene therapy in non-small cell lung cancer (NSCLC) treatment. In the targeted therapies section, each class of drug will examine the scientific rationale behind the target and provide an update on agents' clinical development. The different classes of agents reviewed target the following molecules or pathways: hsp90, MET/HCF, MEK, PI3K/AKT/mTOR, PARP, NOTCH/Hedgehog pathway, and mitosis. The gene therapy section will focus on the science and background behind p53 gene replacement, review the clinical trial studies completed to date, and discuss the clinical trial results of FUS1 replacement with DOTAP.

Novel targeted agents

HSP 90 inhibitors

Heat-shock protein 90 (Hsp90) is an ATP-dependent molecular chaperone. It is presumed to be overexpressed in cancer cells and works thru a multi-chaperone complex that stabilizes proteins and promotes activation. Hsp90 is assumed to preferentially support mutated proteins especially from amplified oncogenes. It is presumed that inhibiting Hsp90 leads to degradation of potentially multiple oncoproteins and several signaling pathways. Several Hsp90 inhibitors are under investigation.

Published results from a phase II trial of IPI-504 (retaspimycin hydrochloride, Infinity Pharmaceuticals) in 76 NSCLC patients who had failed any line of prior chemotherapy showed promising activity, especially in the EML4 ALK positive translocation patients. Three patients with the ALK translocation were included and 2 had partial responses and 1 had disease stabilization with a 24% tumor reduction. The treatment was well tolerated with the most common side effects of grade 1–2 fatigue, nausea, and diarrhea. Grade 3 and higher liver function abnormalities were seen in 11.8% of patients [1]. Retaspimycin HCl is in clinical development in trials studying the combination with docetaxel and also in ALK translocated patients.

Ganetespib (STA-9090) is a second-generation Hsp90 inhibitor that has a different structure than the first-generation ansamycin class of drug. Ganetespib has single agent activity in several tumor type phase 1 trials and has for the most common adverse events mild to moderate diarrhea. Most importantly, there is no dose-limiting hepatic or ocular toxicities, which have been reported

Lung Cancer, Fourth Edition. Edited by Jack A. Roth, Waun Ki Hong and Ritsuko U. Komaki.

in other Hsp90 inhibitor trials. A phase II trial of ganetespib [2] reported activity in ALK translocated patients, four of four responders on the trial (n = 76) had ALK translocations. Six of the eight patients with ALK-positive tumors had tumor shrinkage. Ongoing studies are combining ganetespib with docetaxel (GALAXY trial), and as monotherapy in ALK translocated patients.

Met inhibitors/HCF inhibitors

The *MET* (N-methyl-*N′*-nitro-*N*-nitrosoguanidine) gene is located on chromosome 7 and encodes for a transmembrane receptor. Hepatocyte growth factor (HGF) is the sole ligand to the c-MET receptor and leads to dimerization and subsequent activation of downstream signaling pathways important for wound healing and embryonic development. In abnormal or dysregulated phenotypes, activation of c-MET can occur by several mechanisms, including *MET* mutations, protein overexpression by gene amplification or copy number gain, and diminished receptor degradation. Met gene amplification has been associated with a poor prognosis in NSCLC and has also been implicated in resistance to EGFR tyrosine kinase inhibitors [3].

There have been several approaches to target the MET and HGF pathway. Onartuzumab (OAM4558g, MetMAb; Genentech, Inc. San Francisco, California), an anti-MET single-armed humanized 5D5 antibody, has been evaluated in a prior phase II trial evaluating salvage NSCLC patients with erlotinib with or without onartuzumab demonstrated no significant difference in the intent to treat population; however, in the Met diagnostic positive patients, the combination of erlotinib and onartuzumab led to a progression-free and overall survival benefit [4]. The definition of Met diagnostic positive was ≥50% of tumor cells with moderate or strong staining intensity by immunohistochemistry. Patients who were Met diagnostic negative had a worse progression free and overall survival when treated with the combination over erlotinib alone. This positive result for the Met diagnostic positive patients was not driven by EGFR mutations or by fluorescent in situ hybridation (FISH) results. The most common side effects from the combination of erlotinib and onartuzumab included rash, diarrhea, fatigue, nausea, anorexia, peripheral edema, and anemia. Additional ongoing phase II onartuzumab trials are underway in front-line non-squamous NSCLC and front-line squamous cell NSCLC. A randomized phase III trial in pre-treated NSCLC patients (second or third-line therapy) who are Met diagnostic positive administers erlotinib (150 mg daily) with or without onartuzumab (15 mg/kg IV every 3 weeks).

Tivantinib (ARQ197, ArQule and Daiichi Sankyo, Woburn, MA), an oral non-ATP competitive small molecule inhibitor that targets c-Met receptor tyrosine kinase, is under evaluation in a phase III study of erlotinib with and without tivantinib in patients with nonsquamous NSCLC who received less than 2 lines of prior therapy (MARQUEE, NCT01377376). A prior phase II trial of erlotinib with or without tivantinib (720 mg daily) showed a nonstatistically significant improvement in survival in 167 pre-treated unselected NSCLC patients [5]. The median PFS was 3.8 months with the combination compared to 2.3 months with erlotinib alone (HR 0.81, 95% CI 0.57–1.16, p = 0.24). The median overall survival was also improved with the combination at 8.5 months compared to 6.9 months (HR 0.87, 95% CI 0.44–1.27, 0 = 0.47). In the subgroup analysis, patients who had *KRAS* mutations (n = 15) and received the combination of tivantinib and erlotinib had a significant impro vement in PFS (HR 0.18, 95% CI 0.05–0.70, p < 0.01) and OS (HR 0.43, 95% CI 0.12–1.5, p = 0.17). The most common side effects experienced with tivantinib and erlotinib in this trial were rash, anemia, and diarrhea. The combination of erlotinib-tivantinib is also under investigation in a phase II trial of pre-treated *KRAS* mutation positive NSCLC (NCT01395758).

Carbozantinib (XL184, Exelixis, Inc. San Francisco, CA) is a small molecular c-Met, RET, and VEGFR2 tyrosine kinase inhibitor. Carbozantinib has received FDA approval in November 2012 for the treatment of medullary thyroid cancer. A phase IB/II trial of carbozantinib with or without erlotinib in pretreated NSCLC patients is ongoing. Ficlatuzumab (AV-299, AVEO, Cambridge, MA) is a humanized anti-HGF IgG1 monoclonal antibody that inhibits ligand-receptor binding. A randomized phase II of gefitinib with or without ficlatuzumab (20 mg/kg) in Asian NSCLC patients with never or minimal smoking histories released preliminary results suggesting benefit in patients with the *EGFR* mutation but low c-Met expression and in those patients with high stromal HGF [6].

MEK inhibitors

The mitogen-activated protein (MAPK)/extracellular signal-regulated kinase (ERK) pathway communicates signaling from growth factors. MAPK kinase or MEK is an enzyme immediately downstream of RAS and RAF. Often, genetic mutations in RAS or RAF lead to abnormal signaling of the RAS/RAF/MEK/ERK pathway, dysregulation, and tumorigenesis. Direct inhibition of MEK leads to reduction of the MAPK/ERK signaling and subsequent cell growth. MEK inhibitors have recently achieved greater scrutiny after preclinical studies demonstrated sensitivity of BRAF or RAS gene mutated cell lines to MEK inhibitors [7]. A randomized phase II trial in unselected pretreated NSCLC patients compared oral selumetinib (AZD6244, ARRY-142886, AstraZeneca/Array BioPharma) to pemetrexed and showed no difference in survival [8]. This trial and the preclinical studies prompted selumetinib drug development to be focused on the mutated RAS and RAF populations. Selumetinib blocks both MEK1 and MEK2 isoforms of the enzyme.

A subsequent phase II trial of oral selumetinib in pre-treated NSCLC patients with confirmed *KRAS* mutations demonstrated significant benefit [9]. This trial compared docetaxel with and without selumetinib (75 mg twice daily) and reported a benefit in response rate (35% vs 0%, $p < 0.001$) and 6-mont h PFS rate ($p = 0.0158$) in the combination arm. The main side effects to the selumetinib and docetaxel were rash, asthenia, neutropenia, and febrile neutropenia [9]. Selumetinib is also being developed further in phase I trials for *BRAF* mutants. Numerous additional allosteric inhibitors and small molecule inhibitors to MEK 1/2 are under development and include trametinib (GSK1120212, GlaxoSmithKline), PD325901 (Pfizer), MEK162 (Novartis), and GDC-0973/XL518 (Genentech).

PI3K/AKT/mTOR pathway inhibitors

The phosphatidylkinosital 3-kinase (PI3K)/protein kinase B (AKT)/mammalian target of rapamycin (mTOR) pathway has been highly investigated in NSCLC therapy due to its role in regulating apoptosis. In oncology, it is one of the most commonly dysregulated pathways seen in solid tumors [10]. The PI3K/AKT/mTOR pathway is an intracellular signaling pathway activated by multiple transmembrane receptor kinases that respond to extracellular growth factors. Aberrant signaling can result from upstream gene mutations or amplifications (i.e., RAS mutations, ErbB2 overexpression), gene mutations leading to deficiency in pathway regulators/inhibitors (i.e., PTEN deficiency) or PI3K/AKT gene amplifications or mutations [10–12].

The PI3K family consists of lipid kinases which are organized into 3 unique classes with differing lipid byproducts and target specificity. The lipid products function as second messengers to activate cell proliferation, differentiation, apoptosis, and glucose homeostasis [12]. The most common aberration is found in the Class IA PI3Ks, which are heterodimeric proteins with a p110 catalytic subunit that phosphorylates lipid substrates [10, 12]. There are several PI3K small molecule inhibitors (pan-PI3K or isoform specific) ongoing in phase I and II NSCLC trials; as well as dual PI3K-mTOR inhibitors in phase I studies.

BKM120 (Novartis) is an oral pan-class I PI3K inhibitor that is under investigation in several phase I trials, and is an agent that may be more beneficial against tumors with *PI3KCA* gene mutations [13]. *PI3KCA* encodes for the human p110α protein, which is the class I PI3K catalytic subunit. The main toxicities associated with BKM-120 are pruritus, skin rash, mucositis, nausea, anorexia, diarrhea, fatigue, hyperglycemia, and altered mood [14]. BKM-120 is being combined with carboplatin-pemetrexed in nonsquamous NSCLC and in combination with erlotinib in *EGFR*-mutated NSCLC previously treated with EGFR tyrosine kinase inhibitors.

GDC-0941 (Genentech) is an ATP-competitive inhibitor with selective binding to the PI3K isoform p100α and p100δ. A phase I trial of carboplatin-paclitaxel-GDC-0941 +/− bevacizumab was conducted and preliminary toxicity analysis showed grade 1-2 alopecia, asthenia, nausea, stomatitis, anorexia, neutropenia, paresthesia, epistaxis, arthralgia, peripheral neuropathy and rash [15]. There was also grade 3 and 4 neutropenia seen but this did not lead to dose-limitations. In the subgroup analysis, patients with squamous cell carcinoma had a higher overall response rate compared to nonsquamous cell carcinoma (71% vs 38%). A phase II trial of carboplatin-paclitaxel-GDC0941 is underway in squamous cell carcinoma NSCLC patients.

PX-866 (Oncothyreon) is an oral irreversible pan-class I PI3K inhibitor that covalently binds to the $PI3K_{\alpha,\beta,\delta,\gamma}$ isoforms. A phase I trial in solid tumors reported the most common side effects seen with the agent are nausea, vomiting, diarrhea, and reversible liver enzyme elevation [16]. Although not statistically significant, patients with PIKCA mutations had a longer duration of disease stability on the trial. A phase II trial of PX-866 and docetaxel is ongoing in patients with pretreated metastatic NSCLC or head and neck squamous cell carcinoma.

AKT, also known as protein kinase B, is a serine-threonine specific protein kinase. Three isoforms exist, but AKT 1 and 2 are implicated in oncogenesis. AKT 1 has a significant role in cell survival and AKT 2 is required in glucose transport for the insulin signaling pathway. AKT inhibitors include both ATP mimetics and noncatalytic site inhibitors. The allosteric inhibitors bind to the AKT protein in the pleckstrin-homology domain, induce a conformational change, and prevent localization of AKT to the plasma membrane where it would normally be activated. The agent furthest along is MK-2206 (Merck), a first-in-class oral allosteric $AKT_{1,2,3}$ inhibitor. Preclinical models of MK-2206 have shown that it can augment EGFR tyrosine kinase inhibitor activity and also resensitize NSCLC cell lines with MET-refractory phenotypes. A phase I trial [17] reported that the dose-limiting toxicity was a generalized erythematous nonblistering maculopapular rash. The main side effects included rash, nausea, vomiting, diarrhea, and hyperglycemia. In this trial, a patient with both *PTEN* loss and *KRAS* G12D mutation had significant tumor shrinkage for 24 weeks' duration. Two additional neuroendocrine patients had tumor shrinkage and duration of response for 32 weeks [17]. Several phase II trials are ongoing and include combinations of MK-2206 and AZD6244 (MEK inhibitor) in KRAS mutation patients and also MK-2206 – erlotinib in erlotinib refractory NSCLC patients. Additional AKT inhibitors under investigation in phase I trials include GSK2141795 and GSK2110183 (GlaxoSmithKline), GDC-0068 (Genentech), LY2780301 (Eli Lilly).

mTOR, mammalian target of rapamycin, is encoded for by the *FRAP1* gene. mTOR is a serine/threonine protein kinase with regulatory effects on proliferation, motility, and apoptosis. The mTOR protein forms a complex mTOR Complex 1 (mTORC1) which controls protein synthesis and targets p70-S6 Kinase 1 (S6K1) and 4E-BP1 (eukaryotic initiation factor 4E binding protein 1). S6K1 also provides a positive feedback loop to mTORC1. mTOR also complexes into mTORC2 (consists of mTOR, Rictor, GBL, mSIN1) and regulates AKT phosphorylation at serine residue S473 and the cytoskeleton via F-actin stress fibers, paxillin, CDC42, and protein kinase Cα.

Several mTOR inhibitors have been developed. Everolimus and temsirolimus have been Food and Drug Administration approved for several tumor types, but not NSCLC. To date, everolimus has not demonstrated significant clinical benefit in unselected NSCLC patients either as monotherapy or in combination with chemotherapy or novel agents [18–22]. Temsirolimus has limited efficacy as a single agent in NSCLC [23]. Temsirolimus has also been evaluated in extensive stage SCLC as maintenance therapy but showed no clinical benefit [24]. Ridaforolimus (MK-8669, Merck) is a small molecule inhibitor under investigation in NSCLC in combination with cetuximab and in a phase II NSCLC trial where all patients have *KRAS* mutations.

BEZ235 (Novartis) is an oral imidazoquinoline deritive that is a pan-PI3K inhibitor and inhibits both mTORC1 and mTORC2 [25]. In the first phase I trial, the main side effects encountered were nausea, vomiting, diarrhea, fatigue, anemia, and anorexia [26]. An additional phase I trial (NCT01343498) is ongoing and is evaluating the twice daily dosing schedule [27]. A separate phase I trial in solid tumors is evaluating the combination of BEZ235 with everolimus based on a preclinical trial demonstrating synergistic activity [28]. Some additional mTORC1/2 inhibitors include INK128 (Intellikine), OSI-027 (OSI Pharmaceuticals) and AZD8055 (AstraZeneca).

PARP inhibitors

Poly-adenosine diphosphate-ribose polymerase (PARP) consists of several proteins which regulate DNA repair and apoptosis. The main role of the PARP enzyme is to identify single strand DNA breaks and initiate the base excision repair mechanisms via DNA ligase III, DNA polymerase beta, and scaffolding proteins X-ray cross-complementing gene 1 (XRCC1). In cells with significant DNA damage, PARP can deplete the cell of ATP in an effort to repair the DNA, and thereby induce cell lysis and death. PARP is also involved in programmed cell death [29].

When PARP is inhibited, cells with single strand DNA nicks occur, which eventually lead to double strand breaks during cell replication. In cancer cells with existing genetic mutations (BRCA 1 or BRCA2), PARP inhibitors can induce multiple DNA strand breaks and ultimately lead to cell death. In addition, PARP inhibitors will bind PARP to the DNA and the complexes are toxic to cells as they obstruct replication forks [30].

Several PARP inhibitors are under evaluation as monotherapy and in combination with other agents in NSCLC. Veliparib (ABT-888, Abbott, Abbott Park, IL) is currently being evaluated in a phase II trial of carboplatin-paclitaxel with or without veliparib in unselected NSCLC patients. A phase I trial combining veliparib and a cyclin-dependent kinase inhibitor SCH727965 in *BRCA* proficient tumors is also underway. The SWOG phase I trial (NCI8811) combining carboplatin-paclitaxel-veliparib and radiation in stage III NSCLC is also ongoing. Olaparib (AZD2281, AstraZeneca, London, England) is an oral agent that has been highly investigated in BRCA-mutated breast cancer and in ovarian cancers (BRCA1/2 mutated or wild-type) [31, 32]. The most common side effects experienced by patients treated with olaparib in these trials included nausea, vomiting, fatigue, and anemia. For NSCLC, the Spanish Lung Group is conducting an ongoing phase IB/II trial of gefitinib with and without olaparib in patients with *EGFR* mutations.

Notch and hedgehog inhibitors

Cancer stem cells are pluripotent and self-renewing and are believed to be responsible for cancer recurrence or disease progression after effective therapy. Notch and Hedgehog are critical signaling pathways involved in continued proliferation of cancer stem cells [33]. Notch receptors (1–4) are single-pass transmembrane receptors activated by 5 ligands (Delta-like-1 (DLL1), DLL3, DLL4, Jagged 1 and Jagged 2) that are located on a neighboring cell [34, 35]. The Notch signaling pathway is one of most highly conserved pathways in multicellular organisms [36]. Once the Notch receptor and ligand bind, the extacellular domain is cleaved from the membrane by ADAM-family metalloprotease TACE (tumor necrosis factor alpha coverting enzyme). Subsequently, gamma-secretase enzyme cleaves the intracellular portion of the receptor next to the inner leaflet of the cell membrane and enables Notch to traverse to the nucleus to activate transcription factor CSL and regulate gene expression [34–36].

To date, most inhibitors of the notch signaling pathway are gamma-secretase inhibitors. One agent REGN421 (Regeneron) is a human monoclonal antibody to Delta 4-ligand and is under investigation in a phase I trial. Inhibitors of gamma-secretase increase polyadenosine diphosphate ribose polymerase cleavage and induce apoptosis in cells. A phase I/II trial in NSCLC is combining RO4929097 with erlotinib in pre-treated patients. RO4929097 is also under investigation in the maintenance setting after front-line therapy. An additional gamma-secretase inhibitor PF-03084014 is being assessed in a phase I trial in solid tumors [37].

The hedgehog pathway is a main regulator of development in mammals and is involved in regulating adult stem cells. There are 2 transmembrane receptors that initiate the hedgehog signaling pathway – Patched homologue -1 (PTCH1) and Patched homologue-2 (PTCH2). Hedgehog protein is secreted by cells and attaches to PTCH1 and/or 2 on neighboring cells. PTCH1 inhibits Smoothened homologue (SMO), a 7-transmembrane protein that prevents glioma-associated oncogene homologue (GLI) activation. GLI activation leads to transcriptional regulation of hedgehog target genes and subsequent cell proliferation and survival [38]. In basal cell carcinoma, either PTCH1 or SMO gene mutations can be identified [39, 40]. Vismodegib (GDC-0449, Genentech, South San Francisco, CA) was FDA approved for use in basal cell carcinomas in January 2012. The main side effects associated with vismodegib are taste loss, hair loss, and muscle cramps [40]. Vismodegib is under investigation in ECOG1508 a randomized phase II study of cisplatin-etoposide with or without vismodegib or IMC-A12 (insulin-like growth factor receptor) in patients with chemo-naïve extensive stage small cell lung cancer.

Mitotic inhibitors

There are several different approaches to mitosis inhibition, but four methods are under aggressive pharmacologic development: microtubulin binders, microtubulin enzyme inhibitors, mitosis enzyme inhibitors, and the mitosis checkpoint inhibitors. Microtubulin binder agents stabilize microtubules and prevent disassociation by attaching to the αβ-tubulin heterodimer subunit. Microtubulin enzyme inhibitors or mitotic kinesins prevent spindle function and cause mitotic arrest and cell death. Mitotic enzyme inhibitors target aurora kinase and polo-like kinase (PLK) which are serine-theronine kinases that regulate cell division with some redunancy. Mitosis checkpoint inhibitors are sensitizers to DNA damage – in normal cells, activation of checkpoint 1 (Chk1) leads to cell cycle arrest and is crucial for adequate DNA repair. Most checkpoint inhibitors are intravenous but an oral agent is under development.

Several agents that are microtubulin binders already have FDA approval in breast cancer and lung cancer. Some common microtubulin binders are paclitaxel (lung and breast cancer approved), epothilone, abraxane (lung and breast cancer approved), erbulin (breast cancer approved) and ixabepilone (breast cancer approved). Erbulin is a synthetic analog of halichondrin B that suppresses microtubule polymerization and sequesters tubulin into nonfunctional aggregates. A phase Ib of eribulin with carboplatin in solid tumors showed the main toxicities as neutropenia, thrombocytopenia, fatigue and nausea. A number of NSCLC studies combining eribulin with standard chemotherapy and erlotinib are ongoing. Ixabepilone, a microtubule stabilizing epothilone B analog, has anti-tumor activity in βIII-tubulin (β3T) expressing, taxane-resistant metastatic breast cancer. In NSCLC, high β3T levels was a poor prognostic factor in advanced NSCLC patients treated with taxanes [41]. Unfortunately, a randomized phase II study of ixabepilone or paclitaxel with carboplatin, with β3T expression stratification failed to show a survival difference [42]. Abraxane, a nanoparticle albumin-bound paclitaxel (NAB-paclitaxel) is an albumin-bound formulation of paclitaxel. A phase III study [43] of abraxane and carboplatin in chemo-naive NSCLC patients showed superior response rates especially in squamous cell carcinoma patients when compared to carboplatin-paclitaxel. Abraxane was FDA approved for non-small cell lung cancer in October 2012.

There are 3 subtypes of aurora kinases (A, B, C), but only aurora kinase A and B are potential therapeutic targets. Aurora kinase A inhibition leads to mitotic delay, monopolar spindles, and chromosomal segregation errors whereas aurora kinase B inhibition causes dysfunctional cytokinesis, polyploidy, and apoptosis. There are several aurora kinase inhibitors under investigation. For aurora kinase A inhibitors, ENMD-0276 (Entremed) and MLN8237 (Millenium) are under investigation in phase I and II trials. Preliminary results suggest dose limiting toxicity to be myelosuppression and mucositis. Aurora kinase B inhibitors, GSK1070916A (GlaxoSmithKline) and AZD1152 (AstraZeneca) are also under investigation in phase I and II trials in solid tumors and AML. Several additional phase I and II trials of pan-aurora kinase inhibitor trials are underway. To date, there are no aurora kinase inhibitor trials that are specific to NSCLC and their role in NSCLC therapy is unknown.

Polo-like kinase (PLK) is involved in all cell cycle steps but is expressed in primarily in M-phase. PLK-1 is overexpressed in higher stage NSCLC disease with higher histologic grading and is correlated to chromosome instability and aneuploidy. Preclinical NSCLC murine xenograft models have suggested that PLK-1 inhibition by siRNA leads to a reduction in liver metastases and tumor cell growth [44]. BI6727 (Boehringer Ingelheim) targets the PLK-1 ATP binding pocket and disrupts the spindle assembly leading to cell arrest and apoptosis. A phase I trial (n = 65) of BI6727 in solid tumors reported dose limiting toxicity to be myelosuppression. A 3-arm phase II trial in salvage NSCLC randomizes patients to monotherapy BI6727, monotherapy pemetrexed, or the combination is ongoing primarily in Canada (planned n = 150, primary endpoint PFS).

Kinesin protein inhibitors are early in development. As a class of agent, they cause neutropenia, fatigue, anemia, nausea, rash, and hyponatremia. Ispinesib, (SB-715992, GlaxoSmithKline) targets mitotic kinesin spindle protein (KSP) Eg5 and has the additional toxicity of hyperglycemia but no neuropathy. LY-2523355 (Eli Lilly) is an allosteric inhibitor of Eg5 and is in a phase II trial in small cell lung cancer. SB-743921 (GlaxoSmithKline) targets KSP Eg5 and is under evaluation in a phase II trial with small cell lung cancer and non-small cell lung cancer.

Most checkpoint inhibitors are presumed to function better with DNA damaging agents such as chemotherapy. Checkpoint kinase 1 inhibitor LY2603618 (Eli Lilly/Array BioPharma) was shown in preclinical models to have synergistic activity with pemetrexed, especially in p53 mutant tumor cells. A single-arm phase II trial of LY2603618-pemetrexed in metastatic NSCLC is ongoing in internationally and include pharmacogenomics analysis. A phase I/II trial of LY2603618 in combination with cisplatin-pemetrexed is also underway and will focus the phase II portion in nonsquamous NSCLC (primary objective PFS). AZD7762 (AstraZeneca) is an ATP-competitive inhibitor of checkpoint 1/2 and is in phase 1 trials.

Conclusion and future directions for novel targeted agents

The targeted therapies discussed in this section are not inclusive of all the new agents or classes of drugs that are under development. The pathways and agents selected were highlighted as they are furthest along in clinical development and have the potential for additional progress in the field of NSCLC therapeutics. It is anticipated that as a greater understanding of the cancer cell biology occurs, there will be future advances in novel drug development. Ultimately, it is anticipated that patients with NSCLC will have identified driver mutations which will dictate their initial treatment plan. Subsequently, at the time of their disease progression, the tumors will be re-biopsied and additional mutations or pathway dysregulation will be found and will direct salvage targeted therapy. This new paradigm of personalized medicine has been illustrated in the other chapters focused on *EGFR* mutated, EML-4ALK translocated, and *BRAF* mutated NSCLC.

Targeted gene therapy for lung cancer

Studies over the past 20 years have established a genetic basis for lung cancer. Genes that suppress tumors and repair DNA can be inactivated and growth regulatory genes can be activated by the more than 100 carcinogens contained in tobacco smoke [45]. Histologically normal bronchial mucosa from people with a smoking history shows multiple genetic lesions. Approximately 15% of lung cancer cases occur in individuals without a smoking history and the genetic profile of those cancers are distinct [46]. Whole genome sequencing discussed elsewhere in this book has uncovered many oncogenes with driver mutations resulting in continuous activation. Small molecule drugs blocking oncogene activation can result in dramatic although short-lived responses; however, individual gene mutations are detected in fewer than 10% of lung cancer patients [47]. The most common gene mutations detected by recent whole genome sequencing are in tumor suppressor genes [48].

The most frequently mutated gene in lung cancer is the tumor suppressor *p53* which was the initial focus of gene therapy approaches to lung cancer.

The p53 protein monitors cellular stress and DNA damage, either causing growth arrest to facilitate DNA repair or inducing programmed cell death (apoptosis) if DNA damage is extensive [49]. When a cell is stressed by oncogene activation, hypoxia, or DNA damage, an intact p53 pathway may determine whether the cell will receive a signal to arrest at the G1 stage of the cell cycle, whether DNA repair will be attempted, or whether the cell will self-destruct via apoptosis. Previously, it was believed that gene therapy could not replace all the damaged genes in a cancer cell and thus would not have a significant effect. The observation that expression of a wild-type *p53* gene in a cancer cell triggers apoptosis provided the rationale for gene therapy approaches [50]. The fact that restoration of only one of the defective genes is enough to trigger apoptosis suggests that the DNA damage present in a cancer cell may prime it for an apoptotic event that can be provided through a single pathway.

p53 gene replacement

The studies described above suggest that expressing a wild-type *p53* gene in cancer cells defective in p53 function could mediate either apoptosis or cell growth arrest, both of which would be of therapeutic benefit to a cancer patient. Initial studies showed that restoration of functional *p53* using a retroviral vector suppressed the growth of some, but not all, human lung cancer cell lines. The first published study of *p53* gene therapy showed suppression of tumor growth in an orthotopic human lung cancer model using a retroviral expression vector [51]. This was the first study to show that restoring the function of a single tumor suppressor gene could result in the regression of human cancer cells *in vivo*. Because of limitations inherent in the use of retroviruses including genomic integration and unreliable transgene expression, subsequent studies of *p53* gene replacement in lung cancer made use of an adenoviral vector (*Ad-p53*) [52]. The original adenoviral vector was a serotype 5 replication-defective vector with a deleted E1 region. Subsequent studies with *Ad-p53* showed inhibition of tumor growth in a mouse model of human orthotopic lung cancer [53] and induction of apoptosis and suppression of proliferation in various other cancer cell lines and *in vivo* mouse xenograft tumor models [54–56]. Bystander killing (killing of nontransduced cells by transduced cells), which is necessary as the viral vectors do not transduce all cancer cells, appears to involve regulation of angiogenesis [57, 58], immune upregulation [59–61], and secretion of soluble proapoptotic proteins [62].

Clinical trials of *p53* gene replacement

The first clinical trial protocol for *p53* gene-replacement utilized a replication-defective retroviral vector expressing wild-type *p53* driven by a beta-actin promoter [63]. The gene/vector construct was injected into tumors of nine patients with unresectable NSCLC that had progressed after conventional therapy. Three of the nine patients showed evidence of tumor regression with no vector-related toxicity, demonstrating the feasibility and safety of *p53* gene therapy.

Subsequent *p53* clinical trials were conducted with an adenovirus *p53* expression vector. A phase I trial enrolled 28 NSCLC patients whose cancers had not responded to conventional treatments. Successful gene transfer was demonstrated in 80% of evaluable patients [64]. Expression of *p53* was detected in 46% of patients, apoptosis was seen in all but one of the patients expressing the gene, and, importantly, no significant toxicity was observed. More than a 50% reduction in tumor size was observed in two patients, with one patient remaining free of tumor more than a year after concluding therapy and another experiencing nearly complete regression of a chemotherapy- and radiation-resistant upper lobe endobronchial tumor. Additional studies in patients with head and neck cancer helped to establish *Ad-p53* gene transfer as a clinically feasible strategy resulting in successful gene transfer and gene expression, low toxicity, evidence of tumor regression, and the ability of a p53 biomarker to predict response [65–67].

Gene replacement in combination with chemotherapy and radiation

P53 gene therapy combined with cisplatin in cultured NSCLC cells and in human xenografts in nude mice showed that sequential administration of cisplatin and *p53* gene therapy resulted in enhanced expression of the *p53* gene product [68, 69], and studies of *Ad-p53* gene transfer combined with radiation therapy showed that delivery of *Ad-p53* increased the sensitivity of *p53*-deficient tumor cells to external beam radiation [56].

Twenty-four NSCLC patients with tumors previously unresponsive to conventional treatment were treated with *Ad p53* and cisplatin [70]. Seventy-five percent of the patients had tumor progression on cisplatin- or carboplatin-containing regimens. Up to six monthly courses of intravenous cisplatin, followed three days later by intratumoral injection of *Ad-p53*, resulted in 17 patients remaining stable for at least two months and two patients achieving partial responses. Seventy-nine percent of tumor biopsies showed an increase in the number of apoptotic cells.

A phase II clinical trial evaluated two comparable metastatic lesions in each NSCLC patient enrolled in the study [71]. All patients received chemotherapy, either three cycles of carboplatin plus paclitaxel or three cycles of cisplatin plus vinorelbine, and then *Ad-p53* was injected directly into one lesion. Patients receiving carboplatin plus paclitaxel, the combination of drugs that provided the greatest benefit on its own, did not realize additional benefit from *Ad-p53* gene transfer. However, patients treated with the less-successful cisplatin and vinorelbine regimen experienced significantly greater mean local tumor regression, as measured by size, in the *Ad-p53*-injected lesion than in the control lesion.

Preclinical studies suggesting that *p53* gene replacement might confer radiation sensitivity to some tumors [56. 72–75] led to a clinical trial of *p53* gene transfer combined with external beam radiation therapy [76]. Patients with a poor performance status who could not undergo surgery and would be at high risk for combined chemotherapy and radiation received 60 Gy over six weeks with *Ad-p53* injected on days 1, 18, and 32. Nineteen patients with localized NSCLC were treated, resulting in a complete response in one patient (5%), partial response in 11 patients (58%), and stable disease in three patients (16%). Three months after the completion of therapy, biopsies revealed no viable tumor in 12 patients (63%) and viable tumor in three (16%). Tumors of four patients (21%) were not biopsied because of tumor progression, early death, or weakness. The one-year progression-free survival rate was 45.5%. Among 13 evaluable patients after one year, five (39%) had a complete response and three (23%) had a partial response or disease stabilization. Most treatment failures were caused by metastatic disease without local progression.

In that study, biopsies of the tumor were performed before and after treatment so that detailed studies of gene expression were possible. *Ad-p53* vector-specific DNA was detected in biopsy specimens from 9 of 12 patients with paired biopsies. For 11 patients with adequate samples for both vector DNA and mRNA analysis, 8 showed a postinjection increase in mRNA expression associated with detectable vector DNA. Postinjection increases in *p53* mRNA were detected in 11 of 12 paired biopsies obtained 24 hours after *Ad-p53* injection, with 10 of 11 increasing threefold or more. Preinjection biopsy specimens that were shown by immunohistochemistry to be negative for p53 protein expression were stained for p53 protein expression after *Ad-p53* injection. Staining results confirmed that the p53 protein was expressed in the posttreatment samples in the nuclei of cancer cells. For *p21* (*CDKN1A*) mRNA, increases of statistical significance were noted 24 hours after *Ad-p53* injection and during treatment, as compared with the pretreatment biopsy. *MDM2* mRNA levels were higher during treatment than before treatment. Levels of *FAS* mRNA did not change significantly during treatment. BAK mRNA expression increased significantly 24 hours after injection of *Ad-p53* and thus appeared to be the marker most acutely upregulated by *Ad-p53* injection.

The safety profile for intratumoral injection of *Ad-p53* has been excellent. The most frequently reported adverse events related to treatment with *Ad-p53* injection were fever and chills, asthenia, injection site pain, nausea, and vomiting. The vast majority of these events were mild to moderate. To date, no maximum tolerated dose for *Ad-p53* injection has been established. Based on an increased number of complete responses in head and neck cancers treated with *Ad-p53* combined with radiation, *Ad-p53* was approved for human use in China, the first gene therapy agent to be so designated [22].

Systemic gene therapy for metastases

Local control of lung cancer is important, but most patients with lung cancer die from systemic metastases. Cancer vaccines could potentiate a systemic immune response to aberrantly expressed proteins in cancer cells such as mutant p53. Mutant p53 is conformationally altered and has a prolonged half-life in cancer cells suggesting that p53 could function as a tumor antigen and vaccine target [77–80]. A clinical trial for patients with small cell lung cancer (SCLC) with extensive stage disease was initiated using dendritic cells, which are the most effective antigen-presenting cells, transduced with *Ad-p53* [81]. SCLC patients with extensive stage disease have a median survival of two to four months untreated or six to eight months with chemotherapy. Patients were first treated with conventional chemotherapy. Patients' autologous dendritic cells were treated *ex vivo* with *Ad-p53*, which activates the cells and results in the expression of high levels of p53 protein. Those who achieved at least stable disease with chemotherapy received the vaccine biweekly for a total of 3–6 injections. If patients progressed, they were treated with chemotherapy. Of the 29 patients treated, one had a partial response, seven had stable disease, and 21 had progression. Patients having progression then received second-line chemotherapy. Clinical follow-up was completed for 21 patients. Complete or partial responses to the second-line chemotherapy were observed in 61.9% of the 21 patients treated. Eleven of the patients were alive one year after the first vaccine treatment. Clinical responses were correlated with induction of immune responses to the vaccine. Published objective response rates for second-line chemotherapy in extensive-stage SCLC patients range from 5% to 30%.

Whole genome sequencing has identified driver mutations which are the basis for targeted small molecule development. Many small molecule drugs targeting critical cancer survival pathways are now in clinical trials. Three major challenges have emerged. Driver mutations are infrequent, generally being detected in less than 10% of human cancers. Although dramatic responses initially occur, the responses are transient generally lasting six months or less. Finally, the most frequent mutations are found in tumor suppressor genes, with p53 the most common, and to date, small molecules have not been able to restore tumor suppressor gene function. If gene delivery to distant sites of cancer were feasible, successful restoration of tumor suppressor gene function could be accomplished. Recently, the development of nanoscale synthetic vesicles that can encapsulate plasmid DNA and deliver it to cells after intravenous injection has been reported [82, 83]. This has been studied in mouse xenograft models of disseminated human lung cancer. In addition to p53, other tumor suppressor genes have been delivered using this technique. Multiple 3p21.3 genes show different degrees of tumor suppression activities in various human cancers in vitro and in preclinical animal models. One of the tumor suppressor genes at this locus is TUSC2 (also known as FUS1), which is not expressed in most lung cancers. When wild-type TUSC2 is expressed in a lung cancer cell, the apoptotic pathway is activated and cell death occurs. To translate these findings to clinical applications for molecular cancer therapy, a systemic treatment strategy was developed using a novel TUSC2-expressing plasmid vector complexed with *N*-[1-(2,3-dioleoyloxy)propyl]-*N*,*N*,*N*-trimethylammonium chloride (DOTAP):cholesterol (DOTAP:Chol) nanovesicles, termed TUSC2 nanovesicle, for treating lung cancer and lung metastases [82, 83]. Intravenous injections of TUSC2 nanovesicles into mice bearing experimental A549 lung metastasis significantly decreased the number of metastases, and lung tumor-bearing animals treated with TUSC2 nanovesicles survived significantly longer than control animals. These studies provided the rationale for a clinical trial of intravenous TUSC2-mediated molecular therapy in stage IV lung cancer patients [84]. Patients with recurrent or metastatic lung cancer previously treated with platinum-based chemotherapy were treated with escalating doses of intravenous N-[1-(2,3-dioleoyloxy)propyl]-N,N,N-trimethylammonium chloride (DOTAP):cholesterol nanovesicles encapsulating a FUS-1 expression plasmid (DOTAP:chol-FUS-1) every three weeks. Thirty-one patients were treated at six dose levels (range 0.01 to 0.09 milligrams per kilogram). The MTD was determined to be 0.06 mg/kg. Five patients achieved stable disease (2.6–10.8 months, including two minor responses). One patient had a complete metabolic response on positron emission tomography (PET) imaging. RT-PCR analysis detected FUS-1 plasmid expression in seven of eight post-treatment tumor specimens but not in pretreatment specimens and peripheral blood lymphocyte controls. Proximity ligation assay immunostaining, performed on paired biopsies from three patients, demonstrated low background FUS-1 protein staining in pretreatment tissues compared with intense (10–25 fold increase) FUS-1 protein staining in posttreatment tissues. RT-PCR gene expression profiling analysis of apoptotic pathway genes in two patients with high posttreatment levels of FUS-1 mRNA and protein showed significant posttreatment changes in the intrinsic apoptotic pathway. Twenty-nine genes of the 82 tested in the apoptosis array were altered posttreatment in both patients. The study concluded that DOTAP:chol-FUS-1 can be safely administered intravenously in lung cancer patients and results in uptake of the gene by human primary and metastatic tumors, transgene and gene product expression, specific alterations in FUS-1-regulated pathways, and antitumor effects which is the first time this has been reported for systemic DOTAP:cholesterol nanovesicle gene therapy. Future studies are planned combining gene therapy with other targeted therapies.

Future directions for gene therapy

The clinical trials summarized in this chapter clearly demonstrate that, contrary to initial predictions that gene therapy would not be suitable for cancer, gene replacement therapy targeted to a tumor suppressor gene can cause cancer regression by activation of known pathways with minimal toxicity.

As gene therapy for cancer matures several issues will need to be addressed including the development of more efficient vectors for systemic gene delivery, identification of the optimal genes targeted, optimization of combination therapy, more sensitive and predictive techniques for monitoring gene uptake and expression by cancer cells, and strategies for overcoming treatment resistance.

A broad array of targeted gene-based therapies is under active clinical development in NSCLC. At the same time quantitative proteomic and genomic technology is becoming more accessible, thereby enabling personalized attempts to match a particular targeted gene therapy with a unique cancer specific molecular signal.

References

1 Sequist LV, Gettinger S, Senzer NN, *et al.* (2010) Activity of IPI-504, a novel heat-shock protein 90 inhibitor, in patients with molecularly defined non-small-cell lung cancer. *J Clin Oncol*, 28: 4953–60.

2 Wong K, Koczywas M, Goldman J, *et al.* (2011) An open-label phase II study of the Hsp90 inhibitor ganetespib (STA-9090) as monotherapy in patients with advanced NSCLC [abstract 7500]. *J Clin Oncol*, 29: 7500.

3 Engelman JA, Zejnullahu K, Mitsudomi T, *et al.* (2007) MET amplification leads to gefitinib resistance in lung cancer by activating ERBB3 signaling. *Science*, 316: 1039–43.

4 Spigel D, Ervin T, Ramlau R, *et al.* (2011) Final efficacy results from OAM4558g, a randomized phase II study evaluating MetMAb or placebo in combination with erltoinib in advanced NSCLC. [Abstract 7505]. *J Clin Oncol*, 29: 7505.

5 Sequist LV, von Pawel J, Garmey EG, *et al.* (2011) Randomized phase II study of erlotinib plus tivantinib versus erlotinib plus placebo in previously treated non-small-cell lung cancer. *J Clin Oncol*, 29: 3307–15.

6 Mok T, Park K, Jac J, Han M, Payumo FC, Credi M, McKee K, Cotreau MM, Bhargava P, Slichenmyer W (2011) Randomized phase II study of ficlatuzumab (formerly AV-299), an anti-hepatocyte growth factor (HGF) monoclonal antibody (MAb) in combination with gefitinib (G) in Asian patients (pts) with NSCLC. *J Clin Oncol*, 29: TPS213.

7 Davies BR, Logie A, McKay JS, *et al.* (2007) AZD6244 (ARRY-142886), a potent inhibitor of mitogen-activated protein kinase/extracellular signal-regulated kinase kinase 1/2 kinases: mechanism of action in vivo, pharmacokinetic/pharmacodynamic relationship, and potential for combination in preclinical models. *Mol Cancer Ther*, 6: 2209–19.

8 Hainsworth JD, Cebotaru CL, Kanarev V, *et al.* (2010) A phase II, open-label, randomized study to assess the efficacy and safety of AZD6244 (ARRY-142886) versus pemetrexed in patients with non-small cell lung cancer who have failed one or two prior chemotherapeutic regimens. *J Thorac Oncol*, 5: 1630–6.

9 Pasi A, Janne ATS, Pereira JR, Jeannin G, Vansteenkiste J, Barrios CH, Franke FA, Grinsted L, Smith PD, Zazulina V, Smith IC, Crino L (2012) Phase II double-blind, randomized study of selumetinib (SEL) plus docetaxel (DOC) versus DOC plus placebo as second-line treatment for advanced KRAS mutant non-small cell lung cancer (NSCLC). *J Clin Oncol*, 30: 7503.

10 Engelman JA (2009) Targeting PI3K signalling in cancer: opportunities, challenges and limitations. *Nat Rev Cancer*, 9: 550–62.

11 Sansal I, Sellers WR (2004) The biology and clinical relevance of the PTEN tumor suppressor pathway. *J Clin Oncol*, 22: 2954–63.

12 Katso R, Okkenhaug K, Ahmadi K, *et al.* (2001) Cellular function of phosphoinositide 3-kinases: Implications for development, homeostasis, and cancer. *Annu Rev Cell Dev Biol*, 17: 615–75.

13 Maira SM, Pecchi S, Huang A, *et al.* (2012) Identification and characterization of NVP-BKM120, an orally available pan-class I PI3-kinase inhibitor. *Mol Cancer Ther*, 11: 317–28.

14 Bendell JC, Rodon J, Burris HA, *et al.* (2012) Phase I, dose-escalation study of BKM120, an oral pan-Class I PI3K inhibitor, in patients with advanced solid tumors. *J Clin Oncol*, 30: 282–90.

15 Besse B, Gomez-Roca C, Ware JA, Adjei AA, Dy GK, Shankar G, Brachmann RK, Groen HJ (2011) A phase Ib study to evaluate the PI3-kinase inhibitor GDC-0941 with paclitaxel (P) and carboplatin (C), with and without bevacizumab (BEV), in patients with advanced non-small cell lung cancer (NSCLC). *J Clin Oncol*, 29: 3044.

16 Hong DS, Bowles DW, Falchook GS, *et al.* (2012) A multicenter phase I trial of PX-866, an oral irreversible phosphatidylinositol 3-kinase inhibitor, in patients with advanced solid tumors. *Clin Cancer Res*, 18: 4173–82.

17 Yap TA, Yan L, Patnaik A, *et al.* (2011) First-in-man clinical trial of the oral pan-AKT inhibitor MK-2206 in patients with advanced solid tumors. *J Clin Oncol*, 29: 4688–95.

18 Price KA, Azzoli CG, Krug LM, *et al.* (2010) Phase II trial of gefitinib and everolimus in advanced non-small cell lung cancer. *J Thorac Oncol*, 5: 1623–9.

19 Gridelli C, Rossi A, Morgillo F, *et al.* (2007) A randomized phase II study of pemetrexed or RAD001 as second-line treatment of advanced non-small-cell lung cancer in elderly patients: treatment rationale and protocol dynamics. *Clin Lung Cancer*, 8: 568–71.

20 Papadimitrakopoulou VA, Soria JC, Jappe A, *et al.* (2012) Everolimus and erlotinib as second- or third-line therapy in patients with advanced non-small-cell lung cancer. *J Thorac Oncol*, 7: 1594–1601.

21 Soria JC, Shepherd FA, Douillard JY, *et al.* (2009) Efficacy of everolimus (RAD001) in patients with advanced NSCLC previously treated with chemotherapy alone or with chemotherapy and EGFR inhibitors. *Ann Oncol*, 20: 1674–81.

22 Vansteenkiste J, Solomon B, Boyer M, *et al.* (2011) Everolimus in combination with pemetrexed in patients with advanced non-small cell lung cancer previously treated with chemotherapy: a phase I study using a novel, adaptive Bayesian dose-escalation model. *J Thorac Oncol*, 6: 2120–9.

23 Hidalgo M, Buckner JC, Erlichman C, *et al.* (2006) A phase I and pharmacokinetic study of temsirolimus (CCI-779) administered intravenously daily for 5 days every 2 weeks to patients with advanced cancer. *Clin Cancer Res*, 12: 5755–63.

24 Pandya KJ, Dahlberg S, Hidalgo M, *et al.* (2007) A randomized, phase II trial of two dose levels of temsirolimus (CCI-779) in patients with extensive-stage small-cell lung cancer who have responding or stable disease after induction chemotherapy: A trial of the Eastern Cooperative Oncology Group (E1500). *J Thorac Oncol*, 2: 1036–41.

25 Maira SM, Stauffer F, Brueggen J, *et al.* (2008) Identification and characterization of NVP-BEZ235, a new orally available dual phosphatidylinositol 3-kinase/mammalian target of rapamycin inhibitor with potent in vivo antitumor activity. *Mol Cancer Ther*, 7: 1851–63.

26 Burris H, Sharma S, Herbst RS, Tabernero J, Infante JR, Silva A, Demanse D, Hackl W, Baselga J (2010) First-in-human phase I study of the oral PI3K inhibitor BEZ235 in patients (pts) with advanced solid tumors. *J Clin Oncol*, 28: 3005.

27 NCI: http://clinicaltrials.gov/show/NCT01343498.

28 Xu CX, Li Y, Yue P, *et al.* (2011) The combination of RAD001 and NVP-BEZ235 exerts synergistic anti-cancer activity against non-small cell lung cancer in vitro and in vivo. *PLoS One*, 6: e20899.
29 Annunziata CM, O'Shaughnessy J (2010) Poly (ADP-ribose) polymerase as a novel therapeutic target in cancer. *Clin Cancer Res*, 16: 4517–26.
30 Helleday T (2011) The underlying mechanism for the PARP and BRCA synthetic lethality: Clearing up the misunderstandings. *Mol Oncol*, 5: 387–93.
31 Fong PC, Boss DS, Yap TA, *et al.* (2009) Inhibition of poly(ADP-ribose) polymerase in tumors from BRCA mutation carriers. *N Engl J Med*, 361: 123–34.
32 Ledermann J, Harter P, Gourley C, *et al.* (2012) Olaparib maintenance therapy in platinum-sensitive relapsed ovarian cancer. *N Engl J Med*, 366: 1382–92.
33 Alison MR, Lin WR, Lim SM, *et al.* (2012) Cancer stem cells: In the line of fire. *Cancer Treat Rev*, 38: 589–98.
34 Guruharsha KG, Kankel MW, Artavanis-Tsakonas S (2012) The Notch signalling system: recent insights into the complexity of a conserved pathway. *Nat Rev Genet*, 13: 654–66.
35 Kopan R, Ilagan MX (2009) The canonical Notch signaling pathway: unfolding the activation mechanism. *Cell*, 137: 216–33.
36 Artavanis-Tsakonas S, Rand MD, Lake RJ (1999) Notch signaling: Cell fate control and signal integration in development. *Science*, 284: 770–6.
37 Weiss GJ (2012) Doubling down with inhibitors of Notch and Hedgehog signaling pathways. *J Thorac Oncol*, 7: S409–10.
38 Rahnama F, Shimokawa T, Lauth M, *et al.* (2006) Inhibition of GLI1 gene activation by Patched1. *Biochem J*, 394: 19–26.
39 Tang JY, Mackay-Wiggan JM, Aszterbaum M, *et al.* (2012) Inhibiting the hedgehog pathway in patients with the basal-cell nevus syndrome. *N Engl J Med*, 366: 2180–8.
40 Von Hoff DD, LoRusso PM, Rudin CM, *et al.* (2009) Inhibition of the hedgehog pathway in advanced basal-cell carcinoma. *N Engl J Med*, 361: 1164–72.
41 Seve P, Mackey J, Isaac S, *et al.* (2005) Class III beta-tubulin expression in tumor cells predicts response and outcome in patients with non-small cell lung cancer receiving paclitaxel. *Mol Cancer Ther*, 4: 2001–7.
42 Dumontet C, Jordan MA, Lee FF (2009) Ixabepilone: Targeting betaIII-tubulin expression in taxane-resistant malignancies. *Mol Cancer Ther*, 8: 17–25.
43 Socinski MA, Bondarenko I, Karaseva NA, *et al.* (2012) Weekly nab-paclitaxel in combination with carboplatin versus solvent-based paclitaxel plus carboplatin as first-line therapy in patients with advanced non-small-cell lung cancer: final results of a phase III trial. *J Clin Oncol*, 30: 2055–62.
44 Kawata E, Ashihara E, Kimura S, *et al.* (2008) Administration of PLK-1 small interfering RNA with atelocollagen prevents the growth of liver metastases of lung cancer. *Mol Cancer Ther*, 7: 2904–12.
45 Denissenko MF, Pao A, Tang M, *et al.* (1996) Preferential formation of benzo[a]pyrene adducts at lung cancer mutational hotspots in p53. *Science*, 274: 430–2.
46 Thu KL, Vucic EA, Chari R, *et al.* (2012) Lung adenocarcinoma of never smokers and smokers harbor differential regions of genetic alteration and exhibit different levels of genomic instability. *PLoS One*, 7: e33003.
47 Pal SK, Figlin RA, Reckamp K (2010) Targeted therapies for non-small cell lung cancer: An evolving landscape. *Mol Cancer Ther*, 9: 1931–44.
48 Hammerman PS, Hayes DN, Wilkerson MD, *et al.* (2012) Comprehensive genomic characterization of squamous cell lung cancers. *Nature*, 489: 519–25.
49 Burns TF, El-Deiry WS (1999) The p53 pathway and apoptosis. *J Cell Physiol*, 181: 231–9.
50 Fujiwara T, Grimm EA, Mukhopadhyay T, *et al.* (1993) A retroviral wild-type p53 expression vector penetrates human lung cancer spheroids and inhibits growth by inducing apoptosis. *Cancer Res*, 53: 4129–33.
51 Fujiwara T, Cai DW, Georges RN, *et al.* (1994) Therapeutic effect of a retroviral wild-type p53 expression vector in an orthotopic lung cancer model. *J Natl Cancer Inst*, 86: 1458–62.
52 Zhang WW, Fang X, Mazur W, *et al.* (1994) High-efficiency gene transfer and high-level expression of wild-type p53 in human lung cancer cells mediated by recombinant adenovirus. *Cancer Gene Ther*, 1: 5–13.
53 Georges RN, Mukhopadhyay T, Zhang Y, *et al.* (1993) Prevention of orthotopic human lung cancer growth by intratracheal instillation of a retroviral antisense K-ras construct. *Cancer Res*, 53: 1743–6.
54 Bouvet M, Fang B, Ekmekcioglu S, *et al.* (1998) Suppression of the immune response to an adenovirus vector and enhancement of intratumoral transgene expression by low-dose etoposide. *Gene Ther*, 5: 189–95.
55 Nielsen LL, Dell J, Maxwell E, *et al.* (1997) Efficacy of p53 adenovirus-mediated gene therapy against human breast cancer xenografts. *Cancer Gene Ther*, 4: 129–38.
56 Spitz FR, Nguyen D, Skibber JM, *et al.* (1996) Adenoviral-mediated wild-type p53 gene expression

sensitizes colorectal cancer cells to ionizing radiation. *Clin Cancer Res*, 2: 1665–71.

57 Dameron KM, Volpert OV, Tainsky MA, *et al.* (1994) Control of angiogenesis in fibroblasts by p53 regulation of thrombospondin-1. *Science*, 265: 1582–4.

58 Miyashita T, Reed JC (1995) Tumor suppressor p53 is a direct transcriptional activator of the human bax gene. *Cell*, 80: 293–9.

59 Carroll JL, Nielsen LL, Pruett SB, *et al.* (2001) The role of natural killer cells in adenovirus-mediated p53 gene therapy. *Mol Cancer Ther*, 1: 49–60.

60 Molinier-Frenkel V, Le Boulaire C, Le Gal FA, *et al.* (2000) Longitudinal follow-up of cellular and humoral immunity induced by recombinant adenovirus-mediated gene therapy in cancer patients. *Hum Gene Ther*, 11: 1911–20.

61 Yen N, Ioannides CG, Xu K, *et al.* (2000) Cellular and humoral immune responses to adenovirus and p53 protein antigens in patients following intratumoral injection of an adenovirus vector expressing wild-type. P53 (Ad-p53). *Cancer Gene Ther*, 7: 530–6.

62 Owen-Schaub LB, Zhang W, Cusack JC, *et al.* (1995) Wild-type human p53 and a temperature-sensitive mutant induce Fas/APO-1 expression. *Mol Cell Biol*, 15: 3032–40.

63 Roth JA, Nguyen D, Lawrence DD, *et al.* (1996) Retrovirus-mediated wild-type p53 gene transfer to tumors of patients with lung cancer. *Nat Med*, 2: 985–91.

64 Swisher SG, Roth JA, Nemunaitis J, *et al.* (1999) Adenovirus-mediated p53 gene transfer in advanced non-small-cell lung cancer. *J Natl Cancer Inst*, 91: 763–71.

65 Clayman GL, El-Naggar AK, Lippman SM, *et al.* (1998) Adenovirus-mediated p53 gene transfer in patients with advanced recurrent head and neck squamous cell carcinoma. *Journal of Clinical Oncology*, 16: 2221–32.

66 Peng Z (2005) Current status of gendicine in China: Recombinant human Ad-p53 agent for treatment of cancers. *Human Gene Therapy*, 16: 1016–27.

67 Nemunaitis J, Clayman G, Agarwala SS, *et al.* (2009) Biomarkers predict p53 gene therapy efficacy in recurrent squamous cell carcinoma of the head and neck. *Clin Cancer Res*, 15: 7719–25.

68 Fujiwara T, Grimm EA, Mukhopadhyay T, *et al.* (1994) Induction of chemosensitivity in human lung cancer cells in vivo by adenovirus-mediated transfer of the wild-type p53 gene. *Cancer Res*, 54: 2287–91.

69 Nguyen DM, Spitz FR, Yen N, *et al.* (1996) Gene therapy for lung cancer: enhancement of tumor suppression by a combination of sequential systemic cisplatin and adenovirus-mediated p53 gene transfer. *J Thorac Cardiovasc Surg*, 112: 1372–6; discussion 1376–7.

70 Nemunaitis J, Swisher SG, Timmons T, *et al.* (2000) Adenovirus-mediated p53 gene transfer in sequence with cisplatin to tumors of patients with non-small-cell lung cancer. *J Clin Oncol*, 18: 609–22.

71 Schuler M, Herrmann R, De Greve JL, *et al.* (2001) Adenovirus-mediated wild-type p53 gene transfer in patients receiving chemotherapy for advanced non-small-cell lung cancer: results of a multicenter phase II study. *J Clin Oncol*, 19: 1750–8.

72 Broaddus WC, Liu Y, Steele LL, *et al.* (1999) Enhanced radiosensitivity of malignant glioma cells after adenoviral p53 transduction. *J Neurosurg*, 91: 997–1004.

73 Feinmesser M, Halpern M, Fenig E, *et al.* (1999) Expression of the apoptosis-related oncogenes bcl-2, bax, and p53 in Merkel cell carcinoma: can they predict treatment response and clinical outcome? *Hum Pathol*, 30: 1367–72.

74 Jasty R, Lu J, Irwin T, *et al.* (1998) Role of p53 in the regulation of irradiation-induced apoptosis in neuroblastoma cells. *Mol Genet Metab*, 65: 155–64.

75 Sakakura C, Sweeney EA, Shirahama T, *et al.* (1996) Overexpression of bax sensitizes human breast cancer MCF-7 cells to radiation-induced apoptosis. *Int J Cancer*, 67: 101–5.

76 Swisher S, Roth JA, Komaki R, *et al.* (2000) A phase II trial of adenoviral mediated p53 gene transfer (RPR/INGN 201) in conjunction with radiation therapy in patients with localized non-small cell lung cancer (NSCLC). *Amer Soc Clin Oncol*, 19: 461a.

77 Chada S, Mhashilkar A, Roth JA, *et al.* (2003) Development of vaccines against self-antigens: The p53 paradigm. *Curr Opin Drug Discov Devel*, 6: 169–73.

78 Ishida T, Chada S, Stipanov M, *et al.* (1999) Dendritic cells transduced with wild-type p53 gene elicit potent anti-tumour immune responses. *Clin Exp Immunol*, 117: 244–51.

79 Mayordomo JI, Loftus DJ, Sakamoto H, *et al.* (1996) Therapy of murine tumors with p53 wild-type and mutant sequence peptide-based vaccines. *J Exp Med*, 183: 1357–65.

80 Nikitina EY, Clark JI, Van Beynen J, *et al.* (2001) Dendritic cells transduced with full-length wild-type p53 generate antitumor cytotoxic T lymphocytes from peripheral blood of cancer patients. *Clin Cancer Res*, 7: 127–35.

81 Antonia SJ, Mirza N, Fricke I, *et al.* (2006) Combination of p53 cancer vaccine with chemotherapy in patients with extensive stage small cell lung cancer. *Clin Cancer Res*, 12: 878–87.

82 Ito I, Ji L, Tanaka F, *et al.* (2004) Liposomal vector mediated delivery of the 3p FUS1 gene demonstrates potent antitumor activity against human lung cancer in vivo. *Cancer Gene Ther,* 11: 733–9.

83 Uno F, Sasaki J, Nishizaki M, *et al.* (2004) Myristoylation of the fus1 protein is required for tumor suppression in human lung cancer cells. *Cancer Res,* 64: 2969–76.

84 Lu C, Stewart DJ, Lee JJ, *et al.* (2012) Phase I clinical trial of systemically administered TUSC2(FUS1)-nanoparticles mediating functional gene transfer in humans. *PLoS One,* 7: e34833.

CHAPTER 31
Novel Clinical Trial Designs for Metastatic Lung Cancer

Vassiliki A. Papadimitrakopoulou
Department of Thoracic/Head and Neck Medical Oncology, The University of Texas MD Anderson Cancer Center, Houston, TX, USA

Introduction

Lung cancer is a debilitating disease responsible for most cancer deaths yearly among all malignancies [1] since it is usually diagnosed at advanced stages not amenable to curative therapy [2]. Despite the recognized benefits of chemotherapy, no significant improvement of clinical outcomes have been reported with use of alternative chemotherapy agents and combinations over others in unselected patient populations [3].

Recent advances in molecular biology and genomic profiling have resulted in development of many new anticancer agents that specifically target aberrant pathways and/or genes and proteins that are specific to cancer cells. This wide availability of new agents suggests that there is a need for a more efficient system aimed at quickly and accurately identifying promising agents for phase III testing. The US Food and Drug Administration (FDA) has two mechanisms for approval of drugs and biologics – regular and accelerated approval [4]. Regular approval requires demonstration of clinical benefit, i.e., a longer life, better life, or benefit in an established surrogate for clinical benefit. Accelerated approval, introduced exclusively for new drugs or biologics for the treatment of serious or life-threatening illness, requires favorable effect on a surrogate endpoint that is deemed "reasonably likely to predict clinical benefit," and always requires confirmation of clinical benefit in subsequent trials. Although this second type of approval provides earlier access to novel therapies it is also associated with doubt regarding the choice of the surrogate as well as uncertainty about ultimate drug approval. Appropriate endpoints correlating with benefit in targeted patient populations have included overall survival (OS) and progression-free survival (PFS) in metastatic NSCLC, while key new approaches and other potential surrogate endpoints of interest (e.g., response rate [RR], disease control at 8 weeks) are currently in active development and discussion. In addition to identifying good surrogates, which could be imaging biomarkers or biochemical, genetic, or molecular biology biomarkers, novel phase II study designs are needed.

Alternative endpoints in clinical trials

The correlation between RR and OS in advanced NSCLC has been systematically reviewed and found in randomized trials of first-line cancer therapy to correlate with improved OS ($P < 0.0001$) but large differences in RR were required for benefit

Lung Cancer, Fourth Edition. Edited by Jack A. Roth, Waun Ki Hong and Ritsuko U. Komaki.

detection [5]. Systematic review of phase II and III trials of single-agent gefitinib or erlotinib for advanced NSCLC, identified a strong correlation between RR and median OS was identified with a positive but weaker correlation between disease control rate (DCR) and median OS; with RR emerging as a potential surrogate for OS in EGFRTKI monotherapy-treated populations [6], which is thought to reflect both RR and PFS were acting as surrogates for EGFR mutations, with RR being a better surrogate than DCR, as DCR would be anticipated to include both patients with EGFR mutations as well as those with indolent disease, while RR would be expected to include almost exclusively patients with EGFR mutations. Stable disease (SD) appears to contribute to long-term benefit in early clinical trials [7], however it may not be a valid endpoint in the setting of indolent tumors. Randomized discontinuation studies have utilized SD as an endpoint for targeted treatments [8]. In a placebo-controlled randomized phase II discontinuation trial in pretreated metastatic NSCLC, sorafenib monotherapy was associated with significant PFS benefit and a significantly higher SD rate [9]. The use of RR based on conventional imaging endpoints that dichotomize the continuous variable of tumor burden to response or no response fails frequently to capture such patient benefit, because they may miss the fact that residual tumor remaining on imaging after treatment may be largely composed of necrotic tissue. The main advantage of using overall survival as the endpoint in clinical trials is that it is a clinically relevant outcome, however it requires a control cohort it is affected by crossover designs and subsequent therapies and requires longer follow-up. In contrast tumor response rate is easily standardized and is an early outcome, but can be burdened by measurement imprecision, while progression-free survival (PFS) is not confounded by salvage therapy, but is subject to investigator bias and is only partially validated as a surrogate of survival benefit.

As discussed more extensively later in this chapter, the BATTLE trial used 8-week DCR (complete response, partial response, or SD by RECIST) as the primary endpoint, as this endpoint requires shorter time and was found to be predictive of OS, with median OS of 11.3 months in the 104 patients with disease control at 8 weeks versus 7.5 months in patients without disease control at 8 weeks ($P = 0.002$) [10].

Other novel endpoints include molecular and imaging biomarkers. Molecular biomarkers may prove to be predictive and may provide insight into resistance mechanisms when used as surrogate endpoints; however, they are not usually validated during early clinical development of agents. If the drug target is not ubiquitous, patients need to be selected according to the presence or absence of specific tumor-related molecular signatures to enhance clinical benefit [11]. Frequently, however, the true target of the agent in tumors is unknown and even when it is known target inhibition may be necessary but not sufficient for tumor shrinkage or patient benefit [12, 13]. Imaging can be costly and may add little to response assessment, however novel positron emission tomography imaging agents and other novel imaging methodologies are being investigated.

The need for novel trial designs

Pharmaceutical innovation remains inefficient because it is increasingly risky with rising costs of Phase II and III trials that represent key components [14, 15]. Despite the increased investment in research and development by the industry, the number of new molecular entities achieving marketing authorization is not increasing. The traditional approach to drug development separates clinical development into sequential phases, in which progress is measured at discrete milestones. Novel approaches to clinical development and trial design could have a key role in overcoming some of these challenges by improving efficiency and reducing attrition rates. Over the last two decades increasingly randomized phase II study designs have been adopted testing experimental agents or combinations in the phase II setting usually with PFS as the primary endpoint [16, 17]. The randomized discontinuation design [18] has been adopted by many investigators for molecularly targeted agents. In this design all patients are initially treated with the study agent for a defined period and then patients with stable disease are randomized to continuation or a discontinuation for a defined period to assess the effect of the drug in a population of presumably responsive and more homogeneous patients. This type of design referenced above in the case of sorafenib [9], is useful when the agent is anticipated to provide significant additional benefit after an initial response or disease stabilization. The disadvantage of this design is that a large number of patients needs to be treated initially, therefore unnecessarily exposing many to nonefficacious therapy in order to define a smaller subgroup that benefits that may not have been readily identifiable initially. Even so, further testing of these agents may be difficult if the subgroup that derives benefit is not molecularly or otherwise defined.

Central to a new model for drug development are novel tools, including modeling and simulation, Bayesian methodologies, and adaptive designs.

The impact of molecularly targeted agents in trial design

Molecular dissection of the pathogenesis of the disease [19] has facilitated the pairing of targeted therapy with biomarker selected cohorts of patients which in turn has revolutionized the field with clearly defined benefit from epidermal growth factor receptor (EGFR) tyrosine kinase inhibitors (TKI) in *EGFR* mutated tumors and from ALK TKIs in *EML-ALK* translocated tumors [20, 21]. Testing NSCLC patients for these and other biomarkers at the time of diagnosis is becoming an increasingly acceptable approach since it affects treatment decisions and patient outcomes [22]. Crizotinib which among other targets inhibits echinoderm microtubule-associated protein like-4/anaplastic lymphoma kinase(EML4-ALK) fusion protein implicated in up to 7% of patients with advanced NSCLC (mainly adenocarcinomas and nonsmokers) [23] was unique in the speed of clinical development, receiving orphan drug status in the United States in September 2010 and approved by the FDA in August 2011 [24]. Activity in the biomarker-positive setting was seen in the phase I trial, with RR of 61% with median survival not reached [20, 25, 26]. To compensate for the lack of controlled data for crizotinib, an analysis was conducted comparing outcomes of 82 patients relative to historical controls with crizotinib-untreated/ALK-positive disease or ALK-negative/EGFRnegative disease [26], demonstrating a significant OS benefit for crizotinib. The approval of crizotinib differs from current convention for anticancer agents, as it was based on RR rather than PFS or OS benefit.

However, clinical trial designs have not traditionally and in their majority been based on research advances, and have been mostly histology-based, "all-comers" phase I and II trial designs leading to failure in phase III studies or demonstration of a marginal statistical but clinically questionable benefit in these patient populations. Indeed, only two drugs that target signaling pathways have been approved by the FDA for the treatment of unselected NSCLC patients:the EGFR TKI erlotinib and bevacizumab (monoclonal antibody targeting vascular endothelial growth factor (VEGF)).

Exploration of biomarkers in early clinical trials of targeted therapies is also hampered by the fact that most novel targeted therapies studied in NSCLC clinical trials are not administered as initial therapies but rather as second, third, or later lines of treatment, settings that do not traditionally mandate tumor tissue upfront and where molecular analyses are usually done in a subset of cases at the conclusion of the clinical trial [27,28] and are based on the archival diagnostic specimen, therefore possibly missing biologic and mutational evolution of the recurrent and refractory tumor. Another reason is the difficulty of selecting a diagnostic test to identify responsive patient subgroups in early clinical trials, since cancer pathways are not simple or linear and perturbation by therapeutics frequently results in feedback mechanisms and activation of other parallel signaling pathways. Also application of molecular predictive signatures derived from preclinical systems is not usually reliable in the clinic [29, 30], and development of clinical predictive signatures requires large clinical datasets for signature validation not available in early phase clinical trials.

groupings did not allow for confirmation of the pairing of multiple biomarker-treatment matches. This can be avoided by taking a more exploratory approach for biomarkers as is attempted in this new iteration of the BATTLE trial. The study also allows the agility required to adapt biomarker selection in the second half of the study to emerging biomarker-treatment matches and modifications to the trial in case such data emerge. As outlined for the I-SPY 2 study above, apart from the clinically validated biomarkers, a set of candidate and exploratory biomarkers are being studied in an effort to define a set of biomarkers that can best drive adaptive randomization to each of the four arms in the second half of the clinical trial.

The BATTLE study design may provide a more distinct advantage in the study of novel drugs without clearly understood mechanisms of action or in situations when the biologic characteristics of the target are uncertain. In these situations, real-time, complex biomarker analyses may accelerate the identification and further testing of potential biomarker–therapy relationships. Conversely, when hypotheses about the drug target and its biologic features are well understood, the adaptive randomization strategy may be less efficient than either prospective biomarker-directed trials addressing mature hypotheses or conventional targeted therapy studies in less restricted patient populations that incorporate retrospective analyses of well-defined biomarkers. The BATTLE approach may represent an alternative, more efficient approach to co-development of new therapeutics with matching predictive biomarkers. The operational innovation of the BATTLE trial is the pioneering of the goal of incorporating 4 different treatment arms and 5 biomarker classifiers in a single study with assignments based on the pretreatment biopsy, thus allowing for small numbers of screen failures which imposes significant impediments to accrual of biomarker-positive only separate phase II studies and substantially increases the sample size. This type of design also allows for a simple control arm, in this case erlotinib for all other three investigational arms. A similar approach is used in the Investigation of Serial Studies to Predict Your Therapeutic Response with Imaging and Molecular Analysis 2 (I-SPY 2) trial, which involves patients with newly diagnosed breast cancer who are eligible for neoadjuvant treatment with a taxane [34]. I-SPY 2 represents a unique approach toward addressing biomarkers, since apart from the primary endpoint of pathologic complete response, it will also test, analytically validate, and qualify biomarkers as new drugs are tested, use adaptive design to enable learning each drug's biomarker signature; and utilize organizational management principles and sophisticated bioinformatics in order to eliminate the current inefficiencies in clinical trials. The goal is to identify improved treatment regimens for patient subsets on the basis of molecular characteristics (biomarker signatures) of their disease. Regimens that show a high Bayesian predictive probability of being more effective than standard therapy will graduate from the trial with their corresponding biomarker signature(s). Regimens will be dropped if they show a low probability of improved efficacy with any biomarker signature. Biomarkers in I-SPY 2 are categorized in three distinct classes, standard biomarkers that Food and Drug Administration (FDA) approved, qualifying biomarkers not yet FDA approved, but promising in either determining trial eligibility or measuring tumor response and exploratory biomarkers that are of interest on the basis of promising preliminary data suggesting predictive or prognostic value.

Statistical designs different from those of BATTLE and I-SPY 2 have been proposed for randomized trials that include predictive biomarker hypotheses [35, 36]. These designs do not require a prespecified biomarker test used for treatment assignment, which avoids the screen failure problem. Not having to prespecify a set of biomarkers to test before enrollment has the major advantage of accommodating how little we often know at the beginning of a pivotal trial about which subgroups may benefit from a novel treatment regimen.

Moving forward with innovative clinical trial designs

For regulatory approval of anticancer drugs, although OS is the traditional endpoint in oncology trials, demonstrating OS benefit may pose insurmountable challenges in the targeted therapy era, when taking into account the confounding impact of subsequent therapies. At the same time, the magnitude of prolonged PFS must not only be statistically significant but also clinically meaningful. The effectiveness of clinical development can be improved by adopting a more integrated model that increases flexibility and maximizes the use of accumulated knowledge. Central to this model of drug development are novel tools, including modeling and simulation, Bayesian methodologies, and adaptive designs, such as seamless adaptive designs and sample-size re-estimation methods. These new trial designs require significant statistical analyses, simulations and logistical considerations to verify their operating characteristics, and therefore tend to require more time for the planning and protocol development phase. Regulatory agencies and institutional review boards also need to approve the design format for interim analysis, and these discussions can sometimes take considerable time. Applications of these methodologies to drug development described with specific examples in this chapter offer advantages but also pose challenges, and barriers to implementation. The BATTLE trials offer proof that we can successfully raise the bar for lung cancer clinical trials research to include comprehensive pretreatment biopsies and genotyping for all participants. We believe that such efforts have great potential to exponentially increase our understanding of patients who benefit from targeted therapies and are likely to accelerate and improve the drug development process. A new standard has been set for acquiring tissue and performing comprehensive biomarker evaluation in real time that will allow implementation in studies of novel agents with distinct targets currently under investigation and will accelerate progress. Indeed, building on these designs, an alternative to traditional drug development and design is currently being discussed.

This development strategy is a master protocol for a Phase III registration trial in which multiple new therapies are tested simultaneously in a specific disease setting. However, this proposed trial would not be a Phase II adaptive screening trial like I-SPY 2 and BATTLE, but rather would be a multi-arm, multi-marker/drug Phase III trial powered to allow FDA approval of new therapeutics, along with matching companion diagnostics when applicable. Unlike the adaptive screening trials, where unknown associations between marker and drug are analyzed, screening in the Master Protocol Multi-drug Registration trial is specifically for appropriate treatment-arm assignment and validation of clinical utility. Each biomarker included in the Master Protocol Multi-drug Registration trial would have a corresponding treatment; assignment to that treatment would be based on results of a validated diagnostic assay. This type of trial would be a nationwide effort with the ability to screen patients upon enrollment and direct them to an arm of the trial based on the results of screening diagnostic tests.

There are multiple advantages to a multi-armed registration study, compared to the traditional alternative of multiple 2-arm registration studies. First, for drugs that have shown promise in a biomarker-selected patient population, grouping these studies under a single trial, with a common control (standard-of-care) arm reduces the overall screen failure rate. Second, there are process and operational efficiencies gained by having a single master protocol, which could be amended as needed as drugs enter and exit the study. A master protocol will also provide consistency, as every drug for the disease would be tested in the identical manner. Sponsors may be encouraged to include their drug in a master registration trial if there were assurances that if pre-specified efficacy and safety criteria were met, the drug and accompanying companion diagnostic would be approved. Finally, by improving the overall efficiency of drug development in a specific disease setting, this trial offers the advantage of bringing safe and effective drugs to patients sooner than they might otherwise be available.

Overcoming internal resistance and aversion to change represents a major hurdle for incorporating the prospective use of novel trial designs and methodologies into clinical development programs. Greater awareness of the distinct advantages of innovative designs by regulators and sponsors are crucial to increasing the adoption of these modern tools.

References

1 Siegel R, Naishadham D, Jemal A (2012) Cancer statistics, 2012. *CA Cancer J Clin*, 62: 10–29.

2 NCCN (2012) Clinical Practice Guidelines in Oncology, National Comprehensive Cancer Network. Non-small cell lung cancer.

3 Schiller JH, Harrington D, Belani CP, *et al.* (2002) Comparison of four chemotherapy regimens for advanced non-small-cell lung cancer. *N Engl J Med*, 346: 92–8.

4 Johnson JR, Ning YM, Farrell A, *et al.* (2011) Accelerated approval of oncology products: The food and drug administration experience. *J Natl Cancer Inst*, 103: 636–44.

5 Johnson KR, Ringland C, Stokes BJ, *et al.* (2006) Response rate or time to progression as predictors of survival in trials of metastatic colorectal cancer or non-small-cell lung cancer: A meta-analysis. *Lancet Oncol*, 7: 741–6.

6 Tsujino K, Kawaguchi T, Kubo A, *et al.* (2009) Response rate is associated with prolonged survival in patients with advanced non-small cell lung cancer treated with gefitinib or erlotinib. *J Thorac Oncol*, 4: 994–1001.

7 Tolcher AW (2009) Stable disease is a valid end point in clinical trials. *Cancer J*, 15: 374–8.

8 Hales RK, Banchereau J, Ribas A, *et al.* (2010) Assessing oncologic benefit in clinical trials of immunotherapy agents. *Ann Oncol*, 21: 1944–51.

9 Wakelee HA, *et al.* (2012) A double-blind randomized discontinuation phase-II study of sorafenib (BAY 43-9006) in previously treated non-small-cell lung cancer patients: Eastern cooperative oncology group study E2501. *J Thorac Oncol*, 7(10): 1574–82.

10 Kim ES, Herbst RS, Wistuba, II, *et al.* (2011) The BATTLE trial: personalizing therapy for lung cancer. *Cancer Discov*, 1: 44–53.

11 Dy GK, Adjei A (2007) Patient selection for rational development of novel anticancer agents. In: Kaufman H, Wadler S, Antman K (eds), *Cancer Drug Discovery and Development Molecular Targeting in Oncology*. Totowa, NJ, Humana Press, Inc., pp. 639–46.

12 Adjei AA, Cohen RB, Franklin W, *et al.* (2008) Phase I pharmacokinetic and pharmacodynamic study of the oral, small-molecule mitogen-activated protein kinase kinase 1/2 inhibitor AZD6244 (ARRY-142886) in patients with advanced cancers. *J Clin Oncol*, 26: 2139–46.

13 Friday BB, Yu C, Dy GK, *et al.* (2008) BRAF V600E disrupts AZD6244-induced abrogation of negative feedback pathways between extracellular signal-regulated kinase and Raf proteins. *Cancer Res*, 68: 6145–53.

14 Adams CP, Brantner VV (2010) Spending on new drug development. *Health Econ*, 19(2): 130–41.

15 Adams CP, Brantner VV (2006) Estimating the cost of new drug development: Is it really 802 million dollars? *Health Aff (Millwood)*, 25: 420–8.

16 Phase II trials in the EORTC. The Protocol Review Committee, the Data Center, the Research and Treatment Division, and the New Drug Development Office (1997) European Organization for Research and Treatment of Cancer. *Eur J Cancer*, 33: 1361–3.

17 Van Glabbeke M, Steward W, Armand JP (2002) Non-randomised phase II trials of drug combinations: Often meaningless, sometimes misleading. Are there alternative strategies? *Eur J Cancer*, 38: 635–8.

18 Rosner GL, Stadler W, Ratain MJ (2002) Randomized discontinuation design: Application to cytostatic antineoplastic agents. *J Clin Oncol*, 20: 4478–84.

19 Kris MG, Johnson BE, Kwiatkowski DJ, *et al.* (2011) Identification of driver mutations in tumor specimens from 1000 patient with lung adenocarcinoma: The NCI's Lung Cancer Mutation Consortium (LCMC). *J Clin Oncol*, 29 (Suppl.).

20 Kwak EL, Bang YJ, Camidge DR, *et al.* (2010) Anaplastic lymphoma kinase inhibition in non-small-cell lung cancer. *N Engl J Med*, 363: 1693–1703.

21 Mok TS, Wu YL, Thongprasert S, *et al.* (2009) Gefitinib or carboplatin-paclitaxel in pulmonary adenocarcinoma. *N Engl J Med*, 361: 947–57.

22 Azzoli CG, Baker S, Jr., Temin S, *et al.* (2009) American Society of Clinical Oncology Clinical Practice Guideline update on chemotherapy for stage IV non-small-cell lung cancer. *J Clin Oncol*, 27: 6251–66.

23 Horn L, Pao W (2009) EML4-ALK: Honing in on a new target in non-small-cell lung cancer. *J Clin Oncol*, 27: 4232–5.

24 XALKORI (Crizotinib) capsules, oral (package insert) New York, Pfizer Labs.

25 Camidge DR, Bang YJ, Kwak EL, *et al.* (2011) Progression-free survival (PFS) from a phase I study of crizotinib (PF-02341066) in patients with ALK-positive non-small cell lung cancer (NSCLC). *J Clin Oncol*, 29: 15S.

26 Shaw AT, Yeap B, Solomon B, *et al.* (2011) Impact of crizotinb on survival in patients with advanced ALK-positive NSCLC compared with historical controls. *J Clin Oncol*, 29: 15S.

27 Eberhard DA, Johnson BE, Amler LC, *et al.* (2005) Mutations in the epidermal growth factor receptor

and in KRAS are predictive and prognostic indicators in patients with non-small-cell lung cancer treated with chemotherapy alone and in combination with erlotinib. *J Clin Oncol*, 23: 5900–9.

28 Tsao MS, Sakurada A, Cutz JC, *et al.* (2005) Erlotinib in lung cancer – molecular and clinical predictors of outcome. *N Engl J Med*, 353: 133–44.

29 Baggerly K, Coombes K (2009) Deriving chemosensitivity from cell lines: Forensic bioinformatics and reproducible research in highthroughput biology. *Ann Appl Stat*, 3: 1309–34.

30 Potti A, Dressman HK, Bild A, *et al.* (2006) Genomic signatures to guide the use of chemotherapeutics. *Nat Med*, 12: 1294–1300.

31 Lara PN, Jr., Redman MW, Kelly K, *et al.* (2008) Disease control rate at 8 weeks predicts clinical benefit in advanced non-small-cell lung cancer: Results from Southwest Oncology Group randomized trials. *J Clin Oncol*, 26: 463–7.

32 Massarelli E, Varella-Garcia M, Tang X, *et al.* (2007) KRAS mutation is an important predictor of resistance to therapy with epidermal growth factor receptor tyrosine kinase inhibitors in non-small-cell lung cancer. *Clin Cancer Res*, 13: 2890–6.

33 Thall PF, Wathen JK (2007) Practical Bayesian adaptive randomisation in clinical trials. *Eur J Cancer*, 43: 859–66.

34 Barker AD, Sigman CC, Kelloff GJ, *et al.* (2009) I-SPY 2: An adaptive breast cancer trial design in the setting of neoadjuvant chemotherapy. *Clin Pharmacol Ther*, 86: 97–100.

35 Baker SG, Sargent DJ (2010) Designing a randomized clinical trial to evaluate personalized medicine: A new approach based on risk prediction. *J Natl Cancer Inst*, 102: 1756–9.

36 Freidlin B, Jiang W, Simon R (2010) The cross-validated adaptive signature design. *Clin Cancer Res*, 16: 691–8.

CHAPTER 32

Novel Statistical Models for NSCLC Clinical Trials

J. Jack Lee and Caleb T. Chu

Department of Biostatistics, The University of Texas MD Anderson Cancer Center, Houston, TX, USA

Introduction

The rapid advancement in cancer biology over the recent years has not only brought us into a deeper understanding of the molecular and genomic mechanism of lung cancer but has also laid a fertile ground for the development of new and more effective treatments. For example, Figure 32.1a [1] shows the traditional view of lung cancer being classified generally by histology, into adenocarcinoma, squamous cell carcinoma, and large cell carcinoma. In 1987, the KRAS mutation was identified followed by the discovery of activating EGFR mutations in 2004. Then in 2009 and beyond, an increasing number of rare mutations including the EML4-ALK translocation were identified in lung cancer. As individual mutations emerged, some were also found to overlap with each other and formed interesting intersections between molecular profiles (Figure 32.1b) [2]. Despite the prevalent discovery of mutations, the presentation of a specific type of activating mutation in patients was still rare. However, if all of the known mutations were considered collectively, more than 50% of the patients are with known molecular aberrations. This suggested that treatments directed towards molecular targets could be a promising approach for cancer therapy.

Biological discoveries of mutations paved the way for the development of many targeted agents within the past 20 years. The most notable example is that of imatinib. The Philadelphia chromosome in chronic myelogenous leukemia (CML) was first reported in 1960. However, it wasn't until 30 years had passed before the function of the BCR-ABL translocation and its role in carcinogesis was understood. It was this functional understanding that was key to the later synthesis of an inhibitor to the hyperactive BCR-ABL protein known as STI571 (imatinib). After convincing evidence demonstrated that imatinib can effectively inhibit the growth of BCR-ABL expressing cells in vitro and in animal studies, the novel drug began to be tested in human patients in 1998. Promising results from phase I studies led to phase II trials in 1999. Amazingly, 31 out of 31 patients who received at least 300 milligrams of imatinib daily had their blood counts return to normal. In nine of the 20 patients who were treated for five months or longer, no cells with the Philadelphia chromosome could be found. The result led to a phase III trial in 2000 and the drug was approved soon after by the FDA for CML in 2001 and GIST in 2002 [3].

In parallel, EGFR tyrosine kinase inhibitors were first identified in 1994. In 1997, phase I clinical trials of gefitinib tested its tolerability and confirmed its mode of action. In 2000, phase II trials demonstrated that 250 mg/d of gefitinib had clinically meaningful activity in non-small cell lung cancer.

Lung Cancer, Fourth Edition. Edited by Jack A. Roth, Waun Ki Hong and Ritsuko U. Komaki.

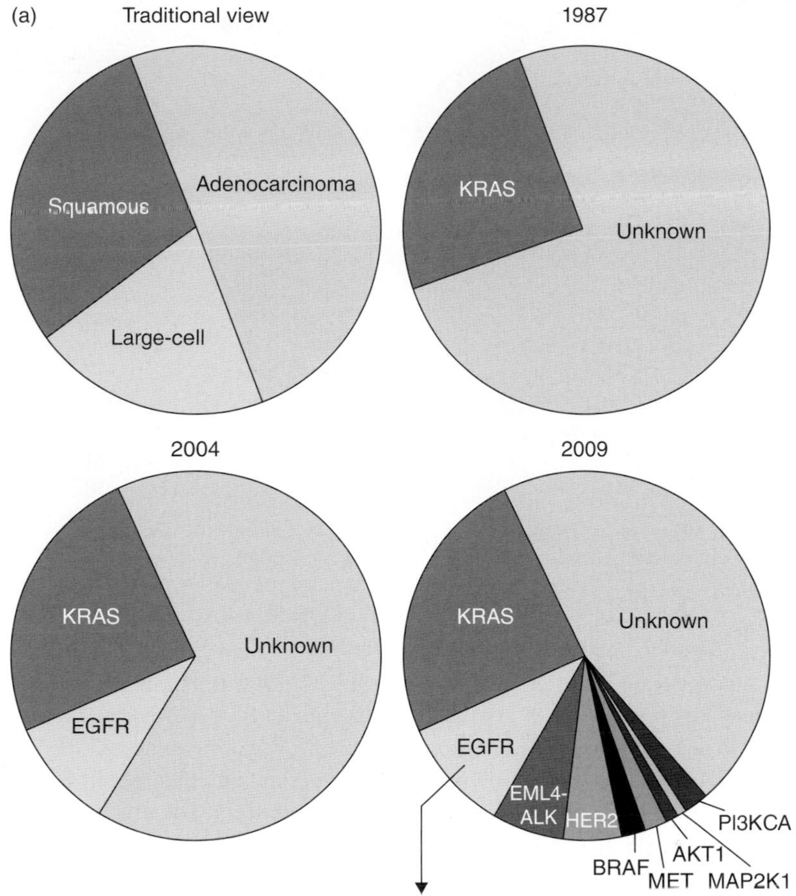

Figure 32.1 Evolution of knowledge in classifying non-small cell lung cancer. a: Traditional view by histology; 1987 with the discovery of KRAS mutation; 2004 with the discovery of EGFR mutation; 2009 with many new mutations identified. b: Common, rare, and overlapping mutations.
Source: (a) Pao W, Girard N (2011) New driver mutations in non-small-cell lung cancer. *Lancet Oncology*, 12(2): 175–80. Reproduced with permission of Elsevier. (b) Sequist LV, Heist RS, Shaw AT, *et al.* (2011) Implementing multiplexed genotyping of non-small-cell lung cancers into routine clinical practice. *Ann Oncol*, Dec; 22(12): 2616–24. Reproduced with permission of Oxford University Press.

In 2003, FDA granted accelerated approval for the third line use of gefitinib in advanced non-small cell lung cancer (NSCLC) patients who had failed standard chemotherapy. However, subsequent phase III trials demonstrated that there was no added benefit of adding gefitinib to standard first-line chemotherapy in NSCLC. In 2005 the FDA withdrew approval for the use of gefitinib in new lung cancer patients

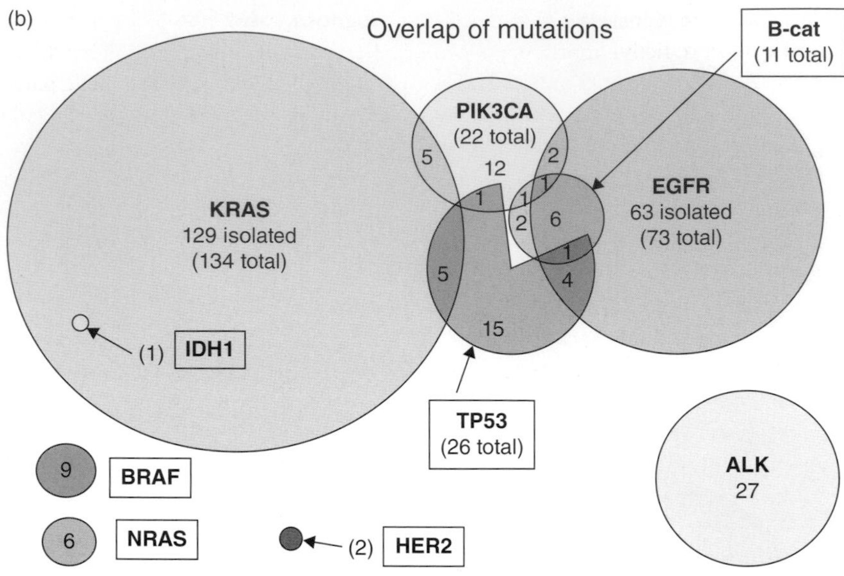

Figure 32.1 (*Continued*)

due to its failure to demonstrate a benefit to overall survival. However, the recent IPASS trial reconfirmed that gefitinib is beneficial specifically for patients with an EGFR mutation [4]. Gefitinib was approved and is now used in more than 60 countries worldwide but not in the US. In contrast, a similar EGFR TKI, erlotinib, received the FDA approval in 2004 for treating patients with locally advanced or metastatic NSCLC after failure of at least one prior chemotherapy regimen. Even with an active agent on the market, this example illustrates the importance of clinical trial designs and strategies for successful drug development [5].

Another fascinating story is the development of crizotinib. The lead compound of its class was identified in 2005. Clinical testing in NSCLC began in 2006 and the discovery of EML4-ALK translocation was reported in 2007. The first clinical responses from crizotinib were observed in tumors with EML4-ALK translocation in 2008. By 2009, a phase 3 trial in lung cancer was initiated, and crizotinib was approved by FDA in 2011 with a companion diagnostic of the EML4-ALK translocation [6].

The development of targeted agents with the companion discovery of the EGFR mutation and EML4-ALK translocation revolutionized both the clinical diagnosis and treatment of lung cancer. Patients with newly diagnosed lung cancer are now subject to routine genomic profiling from diagnostic material (e.g., core needle biopsy) in many major medical centers. The practice is now also extending to smaller clinics. With cheaper and more powerful genomic testing methods arriving at an unprecedented pace, we expect the growing trend to only continue. In the near future, newly diagnosed lung cancer patients will promptly have genetic maps of their tumors by the time they make clinic appointments for medical care. In addition, patients with recurrent lung cancer are likely to have repeat biopsies done to collect fresh tissues for further molecular/genomic analysis and to identify of the most effective second or third-line treatments.

Matching anomalous molecular drivers with targeted treatments present a promising direction in the field of oncology. However it is also apparent that targeted agents do not work for all patients. The overall landscape of lung cancer, the number one killer in cancer, has been persistently dismal as the five-year survival rate for NSCLC continues to hover around 15%. Known actionable mutations are rare and patients who have been treated with targeted therapy for a period of time are likely to develop drug resistance. The identification and validation of prognostic and predictive markers pose a long and challenging task. We need to continue asking ourselves: Do we have sufficient information to make an intelligent choice for treatment? How can we use the information that we have to choose the most effective treatment for each patient? For most cases with matching activated mutations and drugs, effective treatments are available and patients can be treated accordingly. In many other cases, we still do not have enough validated markers to consistently choose effective treatments. However in the past decade, we have seen an explosion in the number of targeted agents and potential biomarkers being discovered. This has far outnumbered the number of trials that can be run at one given time simply because of limited resources. This places great importance upon the need to develop highly efficient and innovative clinical trials for the testing of new agents and gathering of information on the prognostic and predictive ability of biomarkers. In this chapter, we will begin by providing an overview on how standard and innovative clinical trial designs can be applied to seek out effective treatments for non-small cell lung cancer (NSCLC). Statistical issues pertinent to efficient, ethical and novel clinical trial designs will also be discussed.

Clinical trials are bedrocks in the rigorous field of drug development. Such trials are necessary for seeking out safe and effective treatments for diseases while also laying the foundation of evidence-based medicine. Without properly and rigorously conducted clinical trials, progress in clinical medicine would be severely limited. This places great importance on the collaboration of clinical trials with clinical practice in the advancement of knowledge and improvement of disease treatments [7–10].

In the process of drug development, when a molecular aberration is isolated and the corresponding targeted agent is developed, effective treatments for patients may be potentially identified. However, the effectiveness of targeted agents varies from patient to patient and for some drugs, there may be no effectiveness at all. The challenge in developing targeted agents is in requiring the evaluation of treatment efficacy as well as the identification of prognostic and predictive markers. Furthermore, upon the identification of each patient's marker profile, it is desirable to treat patients with comparatively the best treatment available. Therefore a good clinical trial design should be able to (1) test the treatment efficacy, (2) identify prognostic and predictive markers, and (3) provide the most superior treatment for patients who are enrolled in the trial.

Although clinical trials have been around for more than half a century, standard clinical trial designs tend to be rigid and requires a long study duration. Recent efforts have been proposed to apply new methods to improve the efficiency of trials while placing patients in more effective treatment arms. One major emerging statistical innovation that meets such requirements is the application of Bayesian methods in adaptive designs. In the next two sections, we will introduce both Bayesian statistics and adaptive designs. Subsequently, we will illustrate how the Bayesian adaptive design is applied in a seminal trial: the BATTLE trial as an example for advancing lung cancer research. Finally, we will give an overview of other novel designs and conclude with a chapter summary.

Bayesian statistics and its relevance in clinical trials

Statistics is a science of quantitative reasoning. It provides a framework for assessing information contained in the data in the midst of uncertainty. Statistics is used to quantify the probability of an event so that a proper inference can be made. Statistics can also be applied to design more efficient clinical trials such that accurate inference can be attained timely to advance knowledge in clinical research.

There are two main approaches for statistical inference: the predominant frequentist approach and the lesser known Bayesian approach. Although the famous Bayes theorem developed by Reverend Thomas Bayes was published posthumously in 1763, long before frequentist methods became popular, the Bayesian method has historically been underutilized and underappreciated compared to its frequentist counterpart. The Bayesian method treats an unknown parameter (e.g., the response rate of a new agent in untreated stage IV NSCLC) as random and the known data as fixed. The Bayesian approach calculates the probability of the parameters given the data; whereas the frequentist approach computes the probability of the data given the parameters. Hence, these two methods are complementary.

How does the Bayesian method work? Simply put, the Bayesian method follows these three steps: (1) obtain a prior distribution (a pre-defined measure on what is already known or estimated from past data) of the parameter of interest; (2) compute the data likelihood (information gathered during the study); and (3) synthesize these two pieces of information to form a posterior distribution. The posterior distribution then becomes the prior distribution for subsequent evaluations. Some unique strengths of the Bayesian approach are as follows: (i) Compared to the frequentist approach, the Bayesian approach is more intuitive and addresses the problem at hand directly. For example, it can directly calculate the probability that the null hypothesis is true whereas the frequentist approach calculates the probability of the data given that the null hypothesis is true (e.g., the *P* value) – providing an indirect assessment of whether the null hypothesis is true. (ii) The Bayesian approach models the unknown parameter with a distribution and properly addresses various levels of uncertainty. For example, a hierarchical Bayes model can be constructed to evaluate the response rate of a drug in subgroups of patients and/or in multicenter trials. (iii) The Bayesian method accommodates more frequent monitoring and interim decision making during a trial; thus, it provides a platform for sequential learning. Most clinical trials are conducted over an extended period of time. Hence, it is desirable to frequently monitor the interim results so decisions can be made early on when sufficient evidence has accumulated. (iv) The Bayesian method takes the "learn as we go" approach. The built-in "learning" feature makes the Bayesian approach adaptive in nature. The conduct of a clinical trial can be adapted according to the knowledge gained from the currently observed data. For example, a trial design that incorporates outcome-adaptive randomization can assign more patients to better treatments as the trial moves along. In addition, an adaptive sample size estimation procedure can adjust the size of the trial according to the observed outcome. (v) The Bayesian method can incorporate a utility function for informed decision making. Taking the Bayesian decision theoretic approach, clinical trial investigators can specify the "utility" or "loss" of various events. For example, "what is the utility (or importance) to the patient of being cured of cancer, and what is the loss to the patient if a long-term toxicity occurred due to the treatment?" The Bayesian method formulates the subjective preference for outcomes explicitly and quantitatively to aid investigators/patients in making informed decisions. The optimal decision of the trial conduct can be made by maximizing the utility function or minimizing the loss function.

However, Bayesian methods have their limitations as they require the proper specification of the prior distribution. Formally incorporating prior information gathered before, during, and outside of the trial can enhance the trial efficiency but results may be sensitive based upon the chosen prior. Bayesian methods are also more computationally intensive – a challenge that has been alleviated by the development of better computing algorithms and faster computers. Additional infrastructure is often necessary for implementing Bayesian designs in clinical trials. Specialized software programs are required for the study design, simulation, conduct, and analysis of data. Web-based applications are particularly useful for timely data entry, interim analysis, and reporting. Trial success requires not only the development of proper tools, but also timely and accurate execution of outcome evaluation, adaptive randomization, data analysis, and inference making.

Bayesian methods hold great promise for improving the efficiency and flexibility of conducting clinical trials, and are ideal for learning and adaptation. Bayesian methods provide excellent tools for searching for effective treatments and predictive markers in the quest for biomarker-based personalized medicine – all toward the goal of treating more patients with more effective therapies both inside and outside of the trial. Later on, examples such as the BATTLE trial, the BATTLE-2 trial will be illustrated. The relative merit of the Bayesian and frequentist approaches continues to be the subject of debate in statistics. Better statistical methods can lead to more efficient clinical trials designs, lower sample sizes, more accurate conclusions, and better outcomes for patients enrolled in trials and beyond. The Bayesian approach offers an attractive alternative for better trials. Such types of trials should be more commonly designed and conducted so to demonstrate its true benefit [11].

Adaptive designs

Clinical drug development is a long and costly process with a success rate of only 5% in oncology [12, 13]. Adaptive designs allow for adjustments to be made on the trial conduct, based on interim data, making it ideally suited for drug development. In the early phase of drug development, the efficacy and toxicity of new agents and/or their combinations under investigation are often unknown before the study. As the trial progresses, an adaptive design can use the observed information to guide the study conduct. The resulting design is often more efficient in requiring less patients to achieve the study objective and ethically appealing by adaptively moving patients over to safer and more efficacious regimens in a study [12–16]. Many adaptive designs have been proposed in the literature [17–21]. Most relevant features of adaptive designs for early drug development can be classified into the following categories: (1) adaptively determining dose levels, (2) adaptively allocating or randomizing patients into doses or treatments, (3) allowing adding, dropping, or graduating treatments and/or doses based on interim analysis, and (4) adaptively adjusting sample size as the trial progresses. Many, but not all, of the adaptive designs are constructed under the Bayesian framework. Due to the fact that inference is not constrained on the sampling scheme, the Bayesian method by nature is more flexible and adaptive, even when the conduct of a study deviates from the original design [22, 23]. For all adaptive designs, design parameters should be carefully chosen and simulation studies should be performed beforehand to calibrate the design such that desirable operating characteristics can be achieved.

Several adaptive designs are chosen to illustrate how they are used in drug development.

Continual reassessment method (CRM)

CRM [24] is a model-based method used to estimate the dose-toxicity curve and subsequently to identify the maximum tolerated dose (MTD). A one-parameter dose-toxicity curve such as hyperbolic tangent, logistic, or power model, needs to be specified in advance. After specifying a prior distribution of the model parameter, the dose closest to the target toxicity level can be determined for treating the next patient. CRM allows the investigator to treat patients at the dose closest to the estimated MTD level based on the current data. Subsequent modifications proposed for CRM incorporate additional safety measures, such as starting with the lowest dose and not skipping dose levels, etc. [25]. CRM results in a more rapid dose escalation and it uses all available information in determining the MTD. An excellent tutorial of the CRM can be found in a paper by Garrett-Mayer [26]. Several recent papers extend the original CRM in different ways to enhance its applicability and accuracy, which include, the time-to-event CRM (TITE-CRM), the escalation with over-dose control (EWOC) methods, and the Bayesian Model Averaging CRM (BMA-CRM), etc [27–29].

Predictive probability design (PPD)

Two- or three-stage designs are commonly used for initial efficacy assessment of new agents [30]. Although these designs control for false positive and negative error rates and allow early futility stopping based on the interim data, the rigid study design can be difficult to follow because the response has to be evaluated at a pre-specified fixed number of patients. PPD is an efficient and flexible design based on Bayesian predictive probability [31]. Predictive probability is obtained by calculating the probability of a positive conclusion (rejecting the null hypothesis) should the current trend continue and the trial conducted to the maximum planned sample size given the interim observed data. The decision to continue or to stop the trial can be made according to the strength of the predictive probability. The design allows for continuous monitoring of the trial outcome. Consequently, PPD is more efficient in stopping the trial early and results in a smaller than expected sample size when the new treatment is not efficacious. PPD remains robust in controlling the error rates when the trial conduct deviates from the original design. It is more adaptable than traditional multistage designs in evaluating the study outcome, hence, easier to implement.

Biomarker stratified Bayesian adaptive randomization design (BSBARD)

Molecular signature of tumors can be used for identifying predictive markers in searching for the best-fit targeted therapy for individual patients. BSBARD takes an outcome-based adaptive randomization approach to align patient characteristics with targeted agents. All patients have biopsy samples taken for a biomarker assessment prior to randomization. A short-term study endpoint such as the response rate or the disease control rate at a pre-specified time (e.g., 8 weeks) is often used. The Bayesian probit model or the Bayesian logistic model can be applied to characterize the response outcome. Patients are adaptively randomized to treatments with the randomization rate based on the updated response rate from the accumulated data in the trial. For each biomarker profile, high-performing arms have higher randomization rates, and vice versa. An early stopping rule can be added so that low-performing arms can be suspended from randomization. The proposed design can have the desirable operating characteristics to: (1) identify effective agents with a high probability; (2) suspend ineffective agents; and (3) treat more patients with effective agents that correspond to their biomarker profiles. As the trial progresses, the trial design continues to adapt by refining the parameter estimates and assigning patients into better performing arms accordingly.

Comparison of standard and novel designs

Several designs have been proposed in the literature for evaluating targeted agent in this setting [32]. We compare the operating characteristics of five recently proposed designs, namely, the simple randomization design, the marker stratified design, the marker strategy design [33], the efficient targeted design [34, 35] and the Biomarker stratified Bayesian adaptive randomization design (BSBARD). The schematic diagram of these designs is given in Figure 32.2. In the simple randomization design, patients are randomized equally into the standard or the targeted treatment without the knowledge of the marker status. Simple randomization design can be used to test the overall treatment effect in the whole patient population. Based on the post-hoc analysis by patients' marker status, it can also be used to test treatment effect in the M− and M+ patients separately. However, the marker distribution may not be balanced between the two treatment groups for small samples. If markers are measured retrospectively, a higher missing rate could occur. On the other hand, the marker stratified design requires that marker values be obtained at baseline. After stratifying based on marker status, patients are equally randomized into the standard and targeted treatments. The prognostic effect of the marker can be tested by comparing A vs. C. Testing A vs. B or C vs. D can be used to assess the treatment effects in patients within each marker group. The predictive effect can be tested by comparing the odds of treatment response between M− and M+ patients (A/B vs. C/D). In the marker strategy design, patients are first randomized between strategies. Patients randomized into the nonstrategy arm can either receive the standard treatment (not shown in the figure), or be equally randomized to the standard and targeted treatments. For patients randomized into the marker-based strategy arm, the treatment assignment is deterministic. M− patients receive standard treatment while M+ patients receive targeted treatment. The differential effect of the two strategies can be compared by testing A+B vs. C+D. The comparison between A and B can test the treatment effect in the unselected population. Similarly, the treatment effect in the

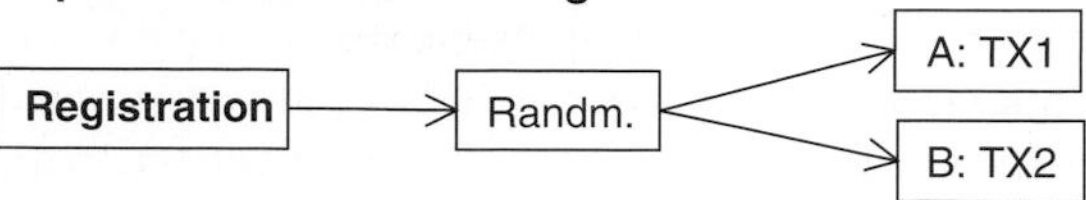

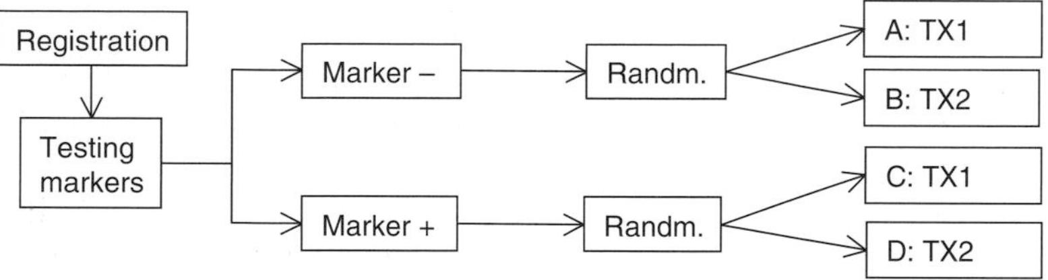

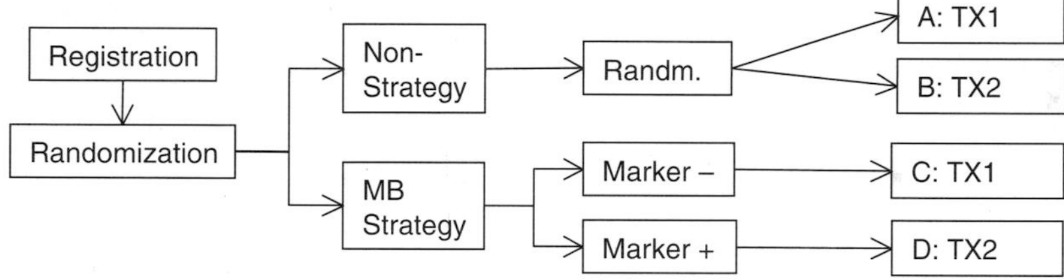

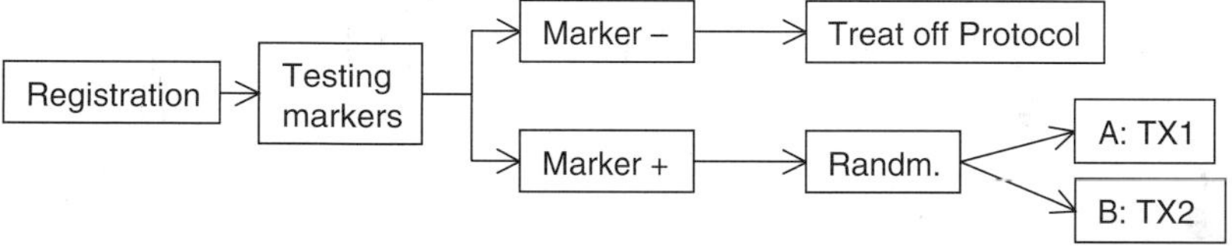

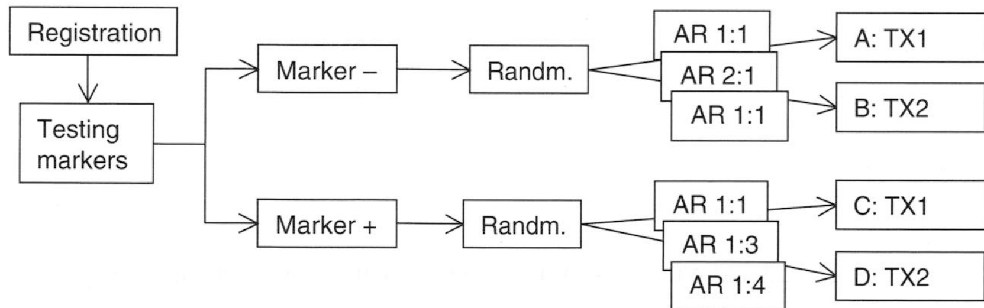

Figure 32.2 Schematic diagram of simple randomization design, marker stratified design, marker strategy design, efficient targeted design, and Biomarker stratified Bayesian adaptive randomization design (BSBARD). Randm: Randomization; AR: Adaptive Randomization; MB: Marker Based; TX1: Standard Therapy; TX2: Targeted Therapy.

selected population can be tested by the comparison between C and D. The marker strategy design is, however, very inefficient and requires a large sample size when comparing various strategies as the overlapping nature of similar patient types could place them in the same treatment arms in different strategies. In the marker-based strategy arm, the marker effect and the treatment effect can not be separated because they are totally confounded per design. Efficient targeted design is an enrichment design which only treats M+ patients in the trial. M− patients are treated off protocol. It can answer the question whether targeted treatment works in the M+ patients, but its effectiveness in M− patients cannot be assessed.

BSBARD is a model-based approach, where the treatment effects are evaluated in marker groups progressively. The design structure is similar to marker stratified design, where randomization is conducted conditionally on marker status. However, instead of using ER, covariate-adjusted AR by marker is applied to allocate more patients to the putatively superior treatment. The design can yield the answers of treatment effect, marker effect, and treatment by marker interaction, as well as treating patients with more effective treatments using the available data collected during the trial.

Challenges for adaptive designs

Adaptive designs provide a sensible and flexible approach to facilitate learning. In order to adapt based on the interim data, study endpoints need to be measured objectively and observed within a reasonably short period of time. Patient accrual cannot be faster than the accumulation of data. Additional infrastructure support is required, which includes a robust mechanism for endpoint evaluation during the trial, timely data entry into a centralized database, and the development of specialized software for allocating patients into treatments. Many useful tools can be downloaded from http://biostatistics.mdanderson.org/SoftwareDownload.

The BATTLE trial: a case study

The Biomarker-integrated Approaches of Targeted Therapy for Lung Cancer Elimination (BATTLE) trial is the first prospective, biopsy-mandated, biomarker-based, adaptively randomized study in patients with heavily pre-treated lung cancer [36, 37]. From 2006 to 2009, 341 patients were enrolled in the BATTLE trial and among them, 255 were randomized. Upon biopsy, tissue samples were analyzed for their biomarker profiles. Patients were assigned to one of the five biomarker groups according to the rank order of the estimated predictive value as follows: (1) EGFR mutation, amplification, or high polysomy; (2) KRAS or BRAF mutation; (3) VEGF or VEGFR-2 overexpression; (4) RXR α, β, or γ overexpression and/or Cyclin D1 overexpression/amplification; or (5) no study biomarkers. Following an initial equal randomization period ($N = 97$), patients were adaptively randomized ($N = 158$) to one of the four study arms: erlotinib, vandetanib, erlotinib plus bexarotene, or sorafenib, based on each patient's relevant molecular biomarkers.

The primary endpoint of the study was the 8-week disease control rate (DCR) which has been shown to be a good surrogate for the overall survival in this patient population [38]. Based on our preliminary data, we considered that the 8-week DCR is 30% under the null hypothesis and 50% under the alternative hypothesis. The statistical design was based on adaptive randomization under a Bayesian hierarchical model that would assign more patients into more effective treatments with the randomization probability proportional to the observed efficacy based on patients' individual biomarker profiles. Prior to the adaptive randomization, patients were equally randomized to the four treatments to train the model for calculating the randomization probability. The trial design also allowed for the suspension of underperforming treatments in marker groups if the probability of a DCR >50% was <0.1. At the end of the trial, a treatment is considered efficacious in a marker group if the posterior probability of the 8-week DCR >30% is >0.80. The study schema is shown in Figure 32.3a.

At the conclusion of the study, the overall 8-week DCR was 46%. The study confirmed several pre-specified hypotheses such as erlotinib working well in patients with EGFR mutation, vandetanib working well for patients with high VEGFR-2 expression, and erlotinib plus bexarotene working

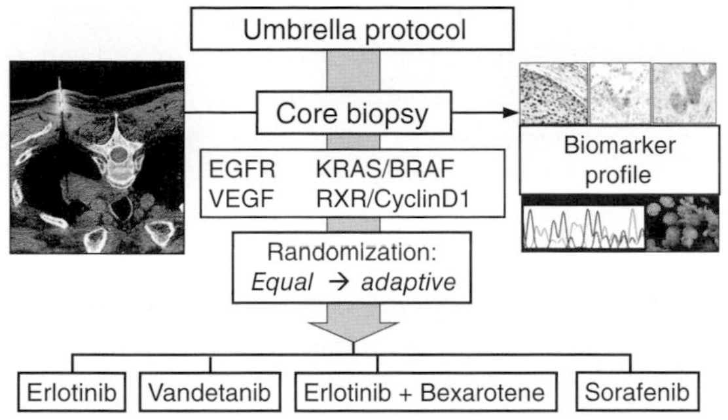

(a)

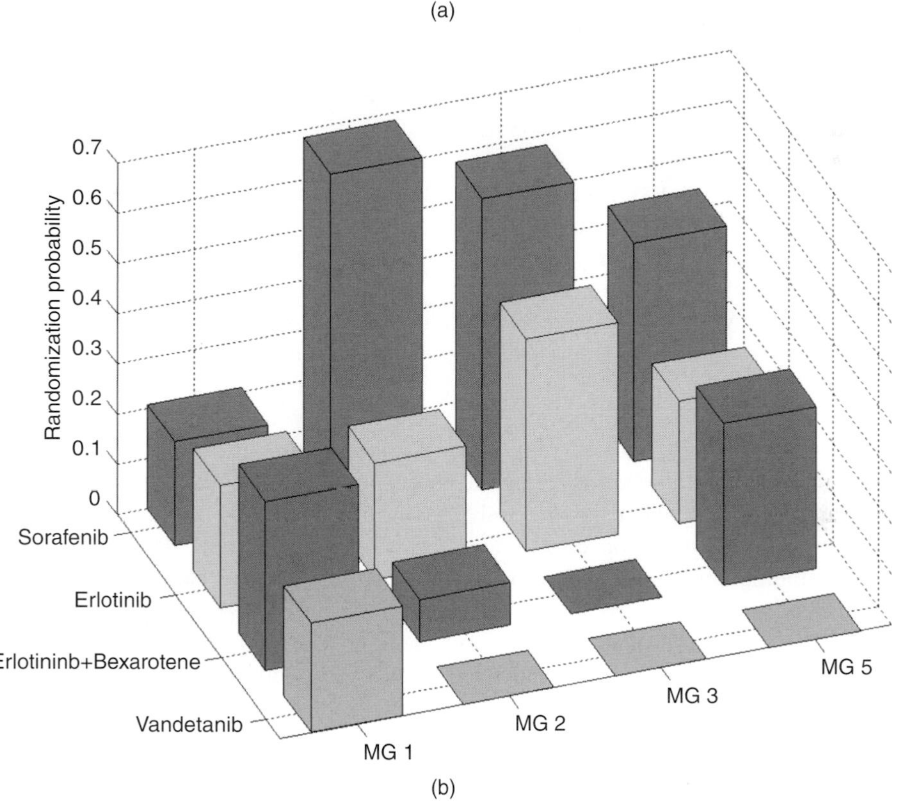

(b)

Figure 32.3 BATTLE trials. a: BATTLE trial design schema. b: Probability of adaptive randomization by treatment and marker group at the end of the BATTLE trial. (For a color version, see the color plate section.)

well for patients with high Cyclin D1 expression. The study also generated some intriguing hypothesis. For example, sorafenib showed efficacy among mutant-KRAS patients, which will be investigated in a greater extent in future trials. The distribution of the final randomization probability into the four treatments for the biomarker groups 1, 2, 3, and 5 is given in Figure 32.4. (Note that only 6 patients were in marker group 4; hence marker group 4 is not shown.)

One adaptive feature in the BATTLE trial is the suspension of randomization in the

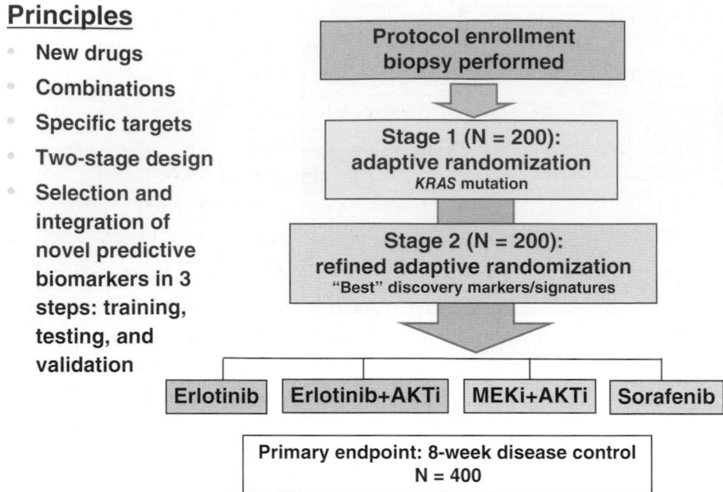

Figure 32.4 BATTLE-2 trial principles and design schema.

underperforming treatment/marker pairs. For example, toward the end of the BATTLE trial, the data suggested that vandetanib did not work for the KRAS/BRAF mutation group and both vandetanib and erlotinib plus bexarotene did not work for the VEGF/VEGFR-2 overexpression group. Hence, the randomization probability was set to 0 (Figure 32.3b). The suspension or early stopping rule can avoid assigning patients to ineffective treatments and redirect them to more effective treatments. Bayesian framework allows the information to be updated continuously in the trial. The updated posterior distribution can be used for guiding the study conduct such as the outcome-adaptive randomization, early stopping due to futility or efficacy, etc.

The BATTLE trial establishes a new paradigm for a personalized approach to treat lung cancer [39, 40]. There are many precious lessons learned from this pioneering trial. It has demonstrated that acquiring a fresh biopsy in recurrent lung cancer patients is not only feasible but also important in determining the marker profiles of tumor at the time of recurrence [41]. This allows the study to search for the most effective treatment for each individual patient. Prospective tissue collection and biomarker analysis provide a wealth of information for future discovery work. The trial had robust accrual with an average of 9.5 patients enrolling each month, proving that the outcome-adaptive randomization design is well received by both the clinical team and patients. Under the Bayesian hierarchical model, the treatment effect and predictive markers are efficiently assessed. This "learn-as-we-go" approach is appealing as it leverages accumulating patient data to improve the treatment outcome as the trial moves along.

Despite its innovation, the BATTLE trial also faced many challenges. To capture the plethora of information including biomarker data, patient eligibility, and efficacy and toxicity outcomes in real time, we had to develop a web-based data management system. The web-based application allows for remote data entry and performs data quality control by the built-in data type, value, and range checking. It also has automatic e-mail/report generation and data download capability for monitoring the study conduct. For example, when the research nurse entered the patients' baseline information, data was used for checking the patient's eligibility. The patient biomarker profile was analyzed and directly entered into the web-based system by members in the molecular pathology laboratory within two weeks of the biopsy. Upon verification of patient eligibility and completion of the biomarker profiling, the research nurse could perform the randomization by hitting the randomization button in the web-based application. This would call an adaptive randomization code written in R via web services. The R code would read the data currently available, perform Bayesian computation, and randomize patients accordingly. The randomization result would then be sent to the pharmacy for the dispensing of appropriate drugs. In addition to meeting the general database security requirements, the system also has a role-based security control feature in which each study collaborator has his/her own read/write privilege to the relevant data. Such a database system was essential for conducting the BATTLE trial and similar adaptive trials following. As a result, high quality data was collected in a more accurate, complete and timely manner.

In our study, 38% of the patients were equally randomized and the remaining 62% were adaptively randomized. In retrospect, we consider that the adaptive randomization could have been triggered earlier. Our trial design called for enrolling at least one patient in each treatment/marker group pair before adaptive randomization. Due to the fact that there were very few patients in biomarker group 4, the adaptive randomization was delayed. The initial equal randomization can be replaced by using a fair prior with the proper effective sample size to control the percentage of patients being equally randomized. More discussion of the use of outcome adaptive randomization can be found in Lee *et al.* [42] Another drawback of the design is that we pre-specified biomarkers and combined markers into marker groups in designing the BATTLE trial. It turned out that some markers (such as the RXR's) were not informative in predicting the treatment outcome at all. Furthermore, grouping markers for dimension reduction is not a good idea because markers in the same group have different predictive strength. For example, to predict DCR using erlotinib, EGFR mutation was the strongest followed by the EGFR gene amplification. The EGFR protein expression had little predictive value. Hence grouping markers ended up diluting the predictive strength of some of the more important markers. Learning from the BATTLE trial, we are currently conducting the BATTLE-2 trial with a two-stage design. Predictive markers will be identified in the first stage and applied in the second stage (Figure 32.4). An important lesson learned is that the outcome-adaptive randomization would benefit patients most if there are effective treatments and associated predictive markers. We are in the quest of finding the best treatments and markers. Adaptive randomization is a sensible way to facilitate this process.

Although many Bayesian methods have been developed in clinical trials over the years, few of them are actually put into practice. However, the use of Bayesian methods in clinical trials has substantially increased recently [11]. Due to the inherent nature of continually updating information, the Bayesian framework is ideal for adaptive clinical trial designs. The design parameters can be calibrated to control the frequentist's type I and type II errors.

In conclusion, the BATTLE study is the first completed, biomarker-based, Bayesian adaptive randomized study in lung cancer. It continually inspires the development of similar adaptive trials [43–49]. The real-time biopsy and biomarker profiling, coupled with adaptive randomization have taken a substantial step toward the realization of personalized lung cancer therapy. More trials such as BATTLE should be conducted to refine the design and conduct of adaptive trials. This will further improve the efficiency of discovering effective treatments against cancer.

Other novel designs

There are many other novel designs proposed in the literature for the development of targeted agents. We list some of them below with a brief discussion on each design.

1 *Adaptive signature design (ASD)* [50]: This is an efficient design to identify effective treatments using genomic signature as predictive markers. The design can sort out whether a treatment is broadly effective or only effective in a subset of patients. It is a two-stage design. Stage 1 is devoted to develop the "classifier." For example, identifying a group of genes that are either highly expressed or lowly expressed and are correlated with drug sensitivity or resistance. Stage 2 is for hypothesis testing that takes place in two steps. First, the treatment effect is tested in all subjects with the type I

error α_1. If the result is significant, one can claim that the treatment is effective in all patients. If results are not significant, the treatment effect is tested among the "sensitive" subgroup (identified in Stage 1) using the type I error α_2. If the result then becomes significant, one can claim that the treatment works only in the sensitive subgroup. The overall level of significance is controlled at α with $\alpha = \alpha_1 + \alpha_2$. For example, we can set $\alpha_1 = 0.04$, $\alpha_2 = 0.01$ and $\alpha = 0.05$.

2 *Adaptive threshold design (ATD)* [51]: After a gene signature is identified, the question of how to select the threshold still remains. The ATD combines a test for overall treatment effect in all patients, with the establishment and validation of a cutpoint for a prespecified biomarker in the sensitive subpopulation. The ATD preserves the power to detect the overall effect when the new treatment is broadly effective. When the proportion of sensitive patients is low, the design provides a substantial improvement in efficiency compared to the design with unselected populations. A recent paper adds cross-validation to enhance the prediction accuracy [52].

3 *Randomized discontinuation design (RDD)* [53, 54]: In a randomized study, certain patients will be randomized into the "standard treatment" or the control group and others will be randomized into the "new treatment" or the experimental group. To alleviate the concern that some patients may not receive the new treatment, the RDD gives the new treatment to all patients up front. For patients who respond to the new treatment, the treatment will continue until progression. For patients with disease progression on the treatment, the treatment will be discontinued and next line therapies will be given. For patients who reach stable disease, they will be equally randomized into the control group and the experimental group. The design does not require the study to have known predictive markers and advantageously allows all patients to receive the new treatment. It can also select a more homogeneous study population to evaluate the effect of discontinuing the new treatment. However, the design may be less efficient than simple randomization studies. There is also an ethical concern in stopping the potentially effective treatment in patients who are randomized into the discontinuation arm [55–57].

4 *Seamless phase II/III designs (SP23D)* [58–60]: The design starts with a randomized Phase II trial with an active control (standard treatment) and several experimental arms with different treatments and/or doses. It uses a short-term endpoint in the phase II trail component (e.g. the objective response rate after 2 cycles of treatment), to inform the long-term endpoint (e.g. overall survival (OS)). At the interim of the trial, inefficacious arms or arms with high toxicities are dropped. If at least one experimental arm is promising, the study will roll into the phase III component with one standard treatment and one or more selected experimental treatments. The phase III trial uses the longer-term endpoint (e.g. OS), as the primary endpoint. Information collected in the phase II component is used in phase III to increase the efficiency. The SP23D also eliminates the "white space" between the phase II and phase III and saves time in trial conduct.

5 *N-of-1 design* [61–64]: As genomic testing becomes more comprehensive in both coverage and depth, it is foreseeable that no two patients will share exactly the same genomic profile. The challenge is how to develop the most effective treatment for each patient when the marker profile of every individual patient is uniquely defined. The N-of-1 design allows for the comparison of the effect of multiple treatments in a multi-period cross-over trial in a single patient. In cancer, a patient condition tends to deteriorate over time. Hence, the time trend needs to be corrected as time passes. For example, when deciding on what therapy to give based upon the time-to progression comparisons of different treatments, the line of therapy should be properly modeled. Furthermore, the Bayesian hierarchical model can be applied to aggregate the information from multiple N-of-1 trials.

6 *Basket Studies*: Basket studies are genotype-focused clinical trial designs. The study takes all comers regardless of disease site or histology and performs comprehensive genomic testing. Depending on the mutation types, molecular aberrations, or pathway abnormalities, patients are classified into "baskets". Matching targeted therapies are then identified and assigned to baskets where patients are treated accordingly. The goal is to enroll at least 10–15 subjects per tumor type per basket [65]. For example, patients who are grouped into EGFR, EML4-ALK, HER-2, BRAF, AKT/MTOR, KRAS, etc. "baskets" are given matched targeted therapies. The effect of therapy by molecular profiles and tumor sites can be determined later. If the drug worked for a certain molecular subgroup in a certain disease site, further studies can be designed to enrich that cohort. If the result is overwhelming positive, only a small number of patients need to be treated to validate the finding before the drug can be approved. The design is efficient for studying rare genomic aberrations.

7 *Dynamic treatment regimen (DTR)* [66, 67]: Unlike most clinical trials with the objective of finding the best treatment in a static setting, DTR seeks for the optimal treatment sequence which yields the best outcome, such as extending the overall survival. For example, treatment A may be the best initial treatment in achieving a highest response rate. Upon disease progression, the best salvage treatment is treatment B, but it is not very effective in extending overall survival. Another option is treatment C, which may be slightly less effective than treatment A as the front-line therapy. But when disease progresses, following with treatment D is highly effective in controlling the disease and extending the overall survival. In this case, DTR indicates that the treatment sequence C-D is better than treatment sequence A-B. For DTR to be effective, it requires a well defined process in a complex setting with the application of complex dynamic programming algorithms. This is an exciting area for both methodology development and clinical application. However, the field is still in its infancy stage.

8 *Platform design*: It is well known that only a very small fraction of cancer patients participate in clinical trials. The estimated participation rates range from 3% to 5% despite much effort to increase the enrollment rate [68, 69]. In contrast to the trial-centric approach for traditional clinical trials, the platform design takes the patient-centric approach. The main themes of the platform design is that there is something for every patient and all the information from all patients are collected consistently and uniformly to form a knowledge database to benefit future patients. Traditional clinical trials have well-defined and often strict eligibility criteria to ensure that a homogeneous group of patients are enrolled to reduce the variability among patients. This is done so that treatments can be compared without the influence of other unduly factors. For trials with very selective eligibility criteria, we may need to screen a vary large number of patients to reach the required sample size, such as identifying patients for enrollment with EML4-ALK translocation. The process is long and inefficient. In the platform design, all patients are subject to genomic profiling. Depending on the results, different patients are channeled to different trial settings and no patients are left behind. For example, for patients with actionable mutations and when tier 1 evidence is available to match the molecular profile with targeted therapy, the patients are treated accordingly. This includes lung cancer patients with EGFR mutations treated with EGFR inhibitors such as gefitinib and erlotinib. Another example is patients with EML4-ALK translocation treated with crizotinib.

Patients who do not have actionable mutations but carry aberrant molecular profiles with putatively effective targeted agents in development, they are considered to have tier 2 evidence. Such patients may be enrolled in corresponding trials and be adaptively randomized into the most effective treatments. For example, there are active developments in AKT inhibitors and MEK inhibitors. Similar to the concept of basket trials, patients with AKT or MEK mutations can be entered into AKT or MEK trials. If no trials are available, patients may be treated with agents of physicians choice. The treatment outcome can be considered as part of the N-of-1 trial and be later combined via the individual patient meta-analysis.

Tier 3 evidence is defined by weakly-associated information or a lack of information on a targeted therapy's effect toward a predictive marker. For patients without any actionable mutations or putative treatments, they can be enrolled into trials with unselected patient populations to screen for drug activities. When an unusual response is found, the information can be aggregated and tested to form new hypothesis in designing future trials. Under the platform design, each clinical trial is considered as a module and can be plugged in or taken out from the platform as needed. All patients are directed to the best treatments and/or trials. All of the information is collected and can be used for current and future drug development, thereby greatly enhancing the efficiency of clinical research.

Summary

In conclusion, the adaptive design is a smart and ethical way for drug development. It can be used to efficiently identify effective agents, eliminate ineffective ones, test and validate prognostic and predictive markers, and match effective treatments with patients' biomarker profile. The adaptive design is suitable for the development of targeted therapy and offers a rational approach toward the goal of personalized medicine. Other novel designs including the N-of-1 design, basket trials, seamless phase II/III design, dynamic treatment regime, platform design, and so forth, offer attractive alternatives to conventional study designs by allowing any patient to be enrolled and treated with treatments based on factors such as the patients' marker profiles, available treatments, physician's choice, or the statistical algorithm. These designs allow for information to be collected in a uniform way, then aggregating them to form a knowledge database for the advance of science and benefit of future patients. More novel trial designs should continue to be developed and implemented to turn promise into progress.

References

1 Pao W, Girard N (2011) New driver mutations in non-small-cell lung cancer. *Lancet Oncology*, 12(2): 175–80.
2 Sequist LV, Heist RS, Shaw AT, *et al.* (2011) Implementing multiplexed genotyping of non-small-cell lung cancers into routine clinical practice. *Ann Oncol*, Dec. 22(12): 2616–24.
3 Capdeville R, Buchdunger E, Zimmermann J, *et al.* (2002) Glivec (STI571, imatinib), a rationally developed, targeted anticancer drug. *Nat Rev Drug Discov*, Jul; 1(7): 493–502.
4 Mok TS, Wu YL, Thongprasert S, *et al.* (2009) Gefitinib or carboplatin-paclitaxel in pulmonary adenocarcinoma. *New England Journal of Medicine*, 361 (10): 947–57.
5 Herbst RS, Fukuoka M, Baselga J (2004) Gefitinib – a novel targeted approach to treating cancer. *Nat Rev Cancer*, Dec; 4(12): 956–65.
6 Shaw AT, Yasothan U, Kirkpatrick P (2011) Crizotinib. *Nat Rev Drug Discov*, Dec; 10(12): 897–8.
7 Rosenberg WM, Sackett DL (1996) On the need for evidence-based medicine. *Therapie*, May–Jun; 51(3): 212–7.
8 Sackett DL, Rosenberg WM, Gray JA, *et al.* (1996) Evidence based medicine: what it is and what it isn't. *BMJ*, Jan 13; 312(7023): 71–2.
9 Guyatt G (2008) *Users' Guides to the Medical Literature: Essentials of Evidence-based Clinical Practice*, 2nd edn. New York: McGraw-Hill Medical, xxii, 359 pp.
10 Montori VM, Guyatt GH (2008) Progress in evidence-based medicine. *JAMA*, Oct 15; 300(15): 1814–16.
11 Lee JJ, Chu CT (2012) Bayesian clinical trials in action. *Stat Med*, Nov 10; 31(25): 2955–72.
12 Chen EX, Siu LL (2005) Development of molecular targeted anticancer agents: Successes, failures and future directions. *Curr Pharm Des*, 11(2): 265–72.
13 Schmidt C (2007) Adaptive design may hasten clinical trials. *J Natl Cancer Inst*, Jan 17; 99(2): 108–9.
14 Bauer P, Brannath W (2004) The advantages and disadvantages of adaptive designs for clinical trials. *Drug Discov Today*, Apr 15; 9(8): 351–7.
15 Booth CM, Calvert AH, Giaccone G, *et al.* (2008) Design and conduct of phase II studies of targeted anticancer therapy: Recommendations from the task force on methodology for the development of innovative cancer therapies (MDICT). *Eur J Cancer*, Jan; 44(1): 25–9.
16 Chang M, Chow SC, Pong A (2006) Adaptive design in clinical research: issues, opportunities, and recommendations. *J Biopharm Stat*, May; 16(3): 299–309; discussion 11–12.
17 Cheung YK, Inoue LY, Wathen JK, *et al.* (2006) Continuous Bayesian adaptive randomization based on event times with covariates. *Stat Med*, Jan 15; 25(1): 55–70.
18 Jones CL, Holmgren E (2007) An adaptive Simon Two-Stage Design for Phase 2 studies of targeted therapies. *Contemp Clin Trials*, Sep; 28(5): 654–61.
19 Smith MK, Jones I, Morris MF, *et al.* (2006) Implementation of a Bayesian adaptive design in a proof of concept study. *Pharm Stat*, Jan–Mar; 5(1): 39–50.

20 Yin G, Li Y, Ji Y (2006) Bayesian dose-finding in phase I/II clinical trials using toxicity and efficacy odds ratios. *Biometrics*, Sep; 62(3): 777–84.

21 Zohar S, Chevret S (2007) Recent developments in adaptive designs for Phase I/II dose-finding studies. *J Biopharm Stat*, 17(6): 1071–83.

22 Berry DA (2005) Introduction to Bayesian methods III: use and interpretation of Bayesian tools in design and analysis. *Clin Trials*, 2(4): 295–300; discussion 1–4, 64–78.

23 Berry DA (2006) Bayesian clinical trials. *Nat Rev Drug Discov*, Jan; 5(1): 27–36.

24 O'Quigley J, Pepe M, Fisher L (1990) Continual reassessment method: a practical design for phase 1 clinical trials in cancer. *Biometrics*, Mar; 46(1): 33–48.

25 Goodman SN, Zahurak ML, Piantadosi S (1995) Some practical improvements in the continual reassessment method for phase I studies. *Stat Med*, Jun 15; 14(11): 1149–61.

26 Garrett-Mayer E (2006) The continual reassessment method for dose-finding studies: A tutorial. *Clin Trials*, 3(1): 57–71.

27 Ying Kuen Cheung, Chappell R (2000) Sequential designs for phase I clinical trials with late-onset toxicities. *Biometrics*, 56(4): 1177–82.

28 Babb J, Rogatko A, Zacks S (1998) Cancer phase I clinical trials: Efficient dose escalation with overdose control. *Statistics in Medicine*, 17(10): 1103–20.

29 Yin G, Yuan Y (2009) Bayesian model averaging continual reassessment method in phase I clinical trials. *Journal of the American Statistical Association*, 104(487): 954–68.

30 Simon R (1989) Optimal two-stage designs for phase II clinical trials. *Control Clin Trials*, Mar; 10(1): 1–10.

31 Lee JJ, Liu DD (2008) A predictive probability design for phase II cancer clinical trials. *Clin Trials*, 5(2): 93–106.

32 Sargent DJ, Conley BA, Allegra C, *et al.* (2005) Clinical trial designs for predictive marker validation in cancer treatment trials. *J Clin Oncol*, Mar 20; 23(9): 2020–7.

33 Lee JJ, Xuemin G, Suyu L (2010) Bayesian adaptive randomization designs for targeted agent development. *Clin Trials*, 7(5): 584–96.

34 Maitournam A, Simon R (2005) On the efficiency of targeted clinical trials. *Stat Med*, Feb 15; 24(3): 329–39.

35 Simon R, Maitournam A (2004) Evaluating the efficiency of targeted designs for randomized clinical trials. *Clin Cancer Res*, Oct 15; 10(20): 6759–63.

36 Zhou X, Liu S, Kim ES, *et al.* (2008) Bayesian adaptive design for targeted therapy development in lung cancer: A step toward personalized medicine. *Clin Trials*, 5(3): 181–93.

37 Kim ES, Herbst RS, Wistuba, II, *et al.* (2011) The BATTLE trial: personalizing therapy for lung cancer. *Cancer Discov*, Jun; 1(1): 44–53.

38 Lara PN, Jr., Redman MW, Kelly K, *et al.* (2008) Disease control rate at 8 weeks predicts clinical benefit in advanced non-small-cell lung cancer: Results from Southwest Oncology Group randomized trials. *J Clin Oncol*, Jan 20; 26(3): 463–7.

39 Rubin EH, Anderson KM, Gause CK (2011) The BATTLE trial: A bold step toward improving the efficiency of biomarker-based drug development. *Cancer Discov*, Jun; 1(1): 17–20.

40 Sequist LV, Muzikansky A, Engelman JA (2011) A new BATTLE in the evolving war on cancer. *Cancer Discov*, Jun; 1(1): 14–16.

41 Tam AL, Kim ES, Lee JJ, *et al.* (2013) Feasibility of image-guided transthoracic core-needle biopsy in the BATTLE lung trial. *J Thorac Oncol*, Apr; 8(4): 436–42.

42 Lee JJ, Chen N, Yin G (2012) Worth adapting? Revisiting the usefulness of outcome-adaptive randomization. *Clin Cancer Res*, Sep 1; 18(17): 4498–4507.

43 Allison M (2012) Reinventing clinical trials. *Nat Biotechnol*, Jan; 30(1): 41–9.

44 Berry DA, Herbst RS, Rubin EH (2012) Reports from the 2010 Clinical and Translational Cancer Research Think Tank meeting: design strategies for personalized therapy trials. *Clin Cancer Res*, Feb 1; 18(3): 638–44.

45 Gold KA, Kim ES, Lee JJ, *et al.* (2011) The BATTLE to personalize lung cancer prevention through reverse migration. *Cancer Prev Res (Phila)*, Jul; 4(7): 962–72.

46 Kelloff GJ, Sigman CC (2012) Cancer biomarkers: Selecting the right drug for the right patient. *Nat Rev Drug Discov*, Mar; 11(3): 201–14.

47 Lai TL, Lavori PW, Shih MC, *et al.* (2012) Clinical trial designs for testing biomarker-based personalized therapies. *Clin Trials*, Apr; 9(2): 141–54.

48 Printz C (2010) BATTLE to personalize lung cancer treatment. Novel clinical trial design and tissue gathering procedures drive biomarker discovery. *Cancer*, Jul 15; 116(14): 3307–8.

49 Rubin EH, Gilliland DG (2012) Drug development and clinical trials: The path to an approved cancer drug. *Nat Rev Clin Oncol*, Apr; 9(4): 215–22.

50 Freidlin B, Simon R (2005) Adaptive signature design: an adaptive clinical trial design for generating and

prospectively testing a gene expression signature for sensitive patients. *Clin Cancer Res*, Nov 1; 11(21): 7872–8.

51 Jiang W, Freidlin B, Simon R (2007) Biomarker-adaptive threshold design: A procedure for evaluating treatment with possible biomarker-defined subset effect. *J Natl Cancer Inst*, Jul 4; 99(13): 1036–43.

52 Freidlin B, Jiang W, Simon R (2010) The cross-validated adaptive signature design. *Clin Cancer Res*, Jan 15; 16(2): 691–8.

53 Ratain MJ, Eisen T, Stadler WM, *et al.* (2006) Phase II placebo-controlled randomized discontinuation trial of sorafenib in patients with metastatic renal cell carcinoma. *J Clin Oncol*, Jun 1; 24(16): 2505–12.

54 Rosner GL, Stadler W, Ratain MJ (2002) Randomized discontinuation design: application to cytostatic antineoplastic agents. *J Clin Oncol*, Nov 15; 20(22): 4478–84.

55 Capra WB (2004) Comparing the power of the discontinuation design to that of the classic randomized design on time-to-event endpoints. *Control Clin Trials*, Apr; 25(2): 168–77.

56 Stadler WM, Rosner G, Small E, *et al.* (2005) Successful implementation of the randomized discontinuation trial design: An application to the study of the putative antiangiogenic agent carboxyaminoimidazole in renal cell carcinoma – CALGB 69901. *J Clin Oncol*, Jun 1; 23(16): 3726–32.

57 Pacey S, Ratain MJ, Flaherty KT, *et al.* (2011) Efficacy and safety of sorafenib in a subset of patients with advanced soft tissue sarcoma from a Phase II randomized discontinuation trial. *Invest New Drugs*, Jun; 29(3): 481–8.

58 Bretz F, Schmidli H, Konig F, *et al.* (2006) Confirmatory seamless phase II/III clinical trials with hypotheses selection at interim: General concepts. *Biom J*, Aug; 48(4): 623–34.

59 Inoue LY, Thall PF, Berry DA (2002) Seamlessly expanding a randomized phase II trial to phase III. *Biometrics*, Dec; 58(4): 823–31.

60 Stallard N (2010) A confirmatory seamless phase II/III clinical trial design incorporating short-term endpoint information. *Stat Med*, Apr 30; 29(9): 959–71.

61 Gabler NB, Duan N, Vohra S, *et al.* (2011) N-of-1 trials in the medical literature: a systematic review. *Med Care*, Aug; 49(8): 761–8.

62 Lillie EO, Patay B, Diamant J, *et al.* (2011) The n-of-1 clinical trial: the ultimate strategy for individualizing medicine? *Per Med*, Mar; 8(2): 161–73.

63 Zucker DR, Ruthazer R, Schmid CH (2010) Individual (N-of-1) trials can be combined to give population comparative treatment effect estimates: methodologic considerations. *J Clin Epidemiol*, Dec; 63(12): 1312–23.

64 Zucker DR, Schmid CH, McIntosh MW, *et al.* (1997) Combining single patient (N-of-1) trials to estimate population treatment effects and to evaluate individual patient responses to treatment. *J Clin Epidemiol*, Apr; 50(4): 401–10.

65 Willyard C (2013) 'Basket studies' will hold intricate data for cancer drug approvals. *Nature medicine*, 19(6): 655.

66 Murphy SA (2003) Optimal dynamic treatment regimes. *Journal of the Royal Statistical Society: Series B (Statistical Methodology)*, 65(2): 331–55.

67 Wang L, Rotnitzky A, Lin X, *et al.* (2012) Evaluation of viable dynamic treatment regimes in a sequentially randomized trial of advanced prostate cancer. *J Am Stat Assoc*, Jun; 107(498): 493–508.

68 Murthy VH, Krumholz HM, Gross CP (2004) Participation in cancer clinical trials: race-, sex-, and age-based disparities. *JAMA*, Jun 9; 291(22): 2720–6.

69 Nass SJ, Balogh E, Mendelsohn J (2011) A National Cancer Clinical Trials Network: Recommendations from the Institute of Medicine. *Am J Ther*, Sep; 18(5): 382–91.

CHAPTER 33

Tumor Microenvironment, Angiogenesis Biology, and Targeted Therapy

John V. Heymach[1] *and Tina Cascone*[2]

[1]Department of Thoracic/Head and Neck Medical Oncology, The University of Texas MD Anderson Cancer Center, Houston, TX, USA

[2]Department of Medicine, Division of Medical Education, Barnes-Jewish Hospital/Washington University School of Medicine in St. Louis, St. Louis, MO, USA

Tumor angiogenesis

The growth and spread of solid tumors depend upon access to functional blood supply [1, 2]. In fact, tumor growth beyond a few millimeters in diameter results in low oxygen tension and depletion of nutrients, which triggers the angiogenic switch and allows progression [3]. Angiogenesis consists of the formation of a new vascular supply from pre-existing blood vessels occurring during development and vascular remodeling to ensure increasing requirements in growing tissues. This process is tightly regulated by a complex balance between pro- and anti-angiogenic factors that ultimately leads to neovascularization in physiologic conditions, such as wound healing, and the reproductive cycle. In pathologic states, such as cancer, the sustained response to uncontrolled stimulation ultimately leads to pathological angiogenesis [4]. The tumor microenvironment becomes enriched in growth factors that bind to their receptors on stromal and tumor cells in a paracrine and autocrine manner, and activated tumor-associated endothelial cells undergo a series of cellular processes (e.g., migration, protease production, cell division) that lead to new vascular networks. However, the tumor vasculature is different from blood vessels found in normal organs in that it is inherently leaky [5], in part because of a lack of coverage by supporting pericytes, which causes the interstitial fluid pressure to increase above that of normal organs [6] and potentially exert a negative impact on treatment efforts by limiting the uptake of anticancer therapies [6]. Moreover, loss of pericyte support of tumor blood vessels has shown to result in an increased frequency of metastasis [7].

Efforts to limit tumor growth and prevent cancer cell metastasis by inhibiting the angiogenic process are an active area of investigation. In the following sections, we discuss the factors that regulate angiogenesis in lung cancer, the molecular mechanisms whereby cancers of the lung may become resistant to antiangiogenic therapies and the clinical development of angiogenesis inhibitors in lung cancer.

Lung Cancer, Fourth Edition. Edited by Jack A. Roth, Waun Ki Hong and Ritsuko U. Komaki.

Regulation of tumor angiogenesis

The onset of angiogenesis is thought to be the result of an imbalance between angiogenesis inhibitors and stimulators [8]. One of the most potent stimulators for the production of proangiogenic proteins is a reduction in the normal level of tissue oxygen tension [9]. Hypoxia stabilizes the transcription factor hypoxia inducible factor-1 α (HIF-1α), which leads to upregulation of genes that regulate angiogenesis and glycolysis [10]. HIF-1α is overexpressed in a number of human tumors and their metastases, including lung cancers [11]. Intraoperative measurements of the pO_2 in lung tumors confirmed the presence of hypoxia in patients with early stage non-small cell lung cancer (NSCLC) [12]. Hypoxia-induced HIF-1α upregulation in NSCLC cells is clinically relevant as it can induce tumor resistance to the effects of chemotherapy [13] and radiation therapy.

Oncogene activation and mutation of tumor suppressor genes can also induce the angiogenic switch in tumors. For example, loss of *p53* [14] or *Ras* activation [15] correlate with increased levels of the proangiogenic protein vascular endothelial growth factor (VEGF). Activation of the EGFR receptor, via mutations or ligand binding, can lead to HIF-1α upregulation and increased secretion of VEGF and other proangiogenic molecules. Loss of the LKB1 tumor suppressor can also result in HIF-1α upregulation and increased aggressiveness [16–18]. Reports suggest that tumor-associated stromal cells may be a major cellular source of proangiogenic proteins in NSCLC [19]. Tumor-associated macrophages express a significant number of angiogenic factors [20] and a high density of macrophages in human lung tumors is associated with angiogenesis and poor outcome [21].

Reports indicate that the extent of angiogenic response varies between different tumor types and that lung cancers possess the fewest number of dividing endothelial cells [22]. Indeed, a study performed on 500 stage I NSCLC tumors reported that 16% of tumors lacked histological evidence of new blood vessel development [23]. The lack of robust angiogenesis in some cancers of the lung may be related to the remarkable number of capillaries present in the normal lung and may have important implications for antiangiogenic therapies in this type of cancer. One way that angiogenesis-independent tumors continue to progress is by proliferating very near to the preexisting blood vessels in a process referred as "vessel co-option" [24]. In the next sections, we discuss several angiogenic proteins and review the evidence for their role in lung cancer.

Vascular endothelial growth factor receptor signaling

One of the key angiogenic regulators is vascular endothelial growth factor (VEGF). This cytokine can stimulate all of the processes required for the formation of new blood vessels [5, 25]. VEGF belongs to a family of growth factors that includes five VEGF ligands (VEGFs A-E) and placental growth factor (PlGF). These ligands mediate their effects by binding to three different VEGF receptors: VEGFR1-VEGFR3 [26]. VEGFA is thought to be the most important VEGF ligand involved in angiogenesis and it mediates its activity by binding to VEGFR2, which is expressed primarily on endothelial cells [27]. Activation of VEGFR2 signaling stimulates receptor autophosphorylation and dimerization that signal for a number of endothelial cells properties, including migration, protease production, cell division, and survival [28]. VEGFC and VEGFD ligands have been shown to signal for lymphangiogenesis when they bind to the VEGFR3 on lymphatic endothelial cells [29].

To a large extent, VEGFA expression is regulated by HIF1-α and the oxygenation status of the tissue. In the normal lung, VEGF is expressed by alveolar type II pneumocytes, bronchiolar Clara cells, smooth muscle cells and alveolar myofibroblasts [30]. A correlation exists between VEGF expression and microvascular density in stage I NSCLC, which is associated with a poor prognosis [31]. Small cell lung cancers (SCLCs) are also highly vascularized, but this feature appears to be independent of VEGF expression [32]. Previous reports showed that VEGF is expressed in both primary NSCLC and matched brain metastases, however the proportion of mature, pericyte-covered blood vessels associated with brain metastases is 60% greater than in primary tumors [33]. Phosphorylated VEGFR2 is expressed on tumor-associated endothelial cells in experimental NSCLC xenografts and its inhibition can lead to improved survival times in some tumor models [19]. The precise role of VEGFR3 signaling and lymphangiogenesis in lung cancer remains unclear.

Fibroblast growth factor receptor signaling

Fibroblast growth factors (FGFs) are a large family of heparin-binding proteins that play a role in neovascularization, wound healing, development and cancer [34]. The most studied FGFs in cancer are acidic FGF (FGF1) and basic FGF (FGF2). FGF2 was among the first cancer cell-derived angiogenic proteins to be isolated and cloned [35]. FGFs exert their effects by binding to one of four high-affinity receptors, known as FGFR1-4 [36]. The FGFs and their receptors are expressed on a number of different cell types including endothelial cells, smooth muscle cells, glial cells, fibroblast cells and macrophages.

The export of FGF was found to trigger the "angiogenic switch" of nonangiogenic fibromas to highly vascular metastatic fibrosarcomas [37]. FGF, FGFR1 and FGFR2 are frequently overexpressed in squamous cell carcinoma of the lung [38] and FGFR1 amplifications have been observed [39]. Elevated levels of FGF2 have been found in the serum and urine of patients with various types of tumors, including lung cancer [40]. In fact, serum FGF2 levels were shown to correlate with tumor volume, higher relapse risk and poorer survival in NSCLC [41]. Recent evidence suggests that tumor cell expression of FGF is an independent negative predictor of loco-regional control, metastasis-free, and overall survival in patients irradiated for stage II-III NSCLC [42]. In experimental models of NSCLC, the acquired resistance of tumors to VEGFR pathway inhibition is associated with the upregulation of members of the FGFR family [19].

Epidermal growth factor receptor signaling

The epidermal growth factor receptor (EGFR) belongs to the ErbB family of receptors that also includes HER2 (ErbB2), Her3 (ErbB3) and Her4 (ErbB-4). Activation of EGFR by EGF or transforming growth factor alpha (TGFα) ligands stimulates formation of homo- and heterodimers and ultimately activation of intracellular effector proteins that activate the intracellular effector proteins mitogen-activated protein (MAP) kinase, phosphatidylinositol 3-kinase/Akt, and signal transducer and activator of transcription (STAT). Activation of EGFR signaling promotes tumor progression by stimulating cancer cell division, invasion, survival and metastasis [43, 44]. EGFR and its ligands are frequently overexpressed during the development and progression of NSCLC [45]. Recent reports suggest that EGFR may play a role in stimulating the formation of new capillaries, and endothelial cells isolated from experimental tumors differ from endothelial cells of normal organs in that they express EGFR and are responsive to EGF ligands [46]. Moreover, the treatment of TGFα-expressing experimental NSCLC tumors with small molecule tyrosine kinase inhibitors (TKIs) of EGFR and VEGFR signaling has shown to exert significant antiangiogenic effects, reduce frequency of metastasis, and improve survival [47].

Platelet derived growth factor receptor signaling

The platelet derived growth factors and receptors (PDGF/Rs) are widely recognized key regulators of vessel maturation through their ability to recruit and retain pericytes to the sites of developing vascular networks [48]. The family of PDGF ligands consists of four structurally related soluble polypeptides that exist as homo- and heterodimers that bind to two tyrosine kinase receptors, PDGFR-α and -β [49]. Most solid tumors express PDGFRs on endothelial or perivascular cells [50], and overexpression has been associated with poor prognosis in a number of cancers [51, 52]. PDGFs have also been shown to stimulate angiogenesis *in vivo* [53, 54], suggesting that some endothelial cells possess high-affinity PDGFRs. The PDGFR signaling contributes to tumor angiogenesis by increasing pericyte recruitment and vessel maturation [55]. In fact, for vessels to function properly, they must be mature and covered by mural cells. To stabilize endothelial cell channels, angiogenic endothelial cells release PDGF-B to attract PDGFR-β^+ pericytes [56, 57]. In support of this concept, experimental studies demonstrated the PDGF-dependent recruitment of pericytes to tumor vessels in a mouse model of glioma [58]. Upregulation of PDGFRs on tumor-associated endothelial cells has been described in a mouse model of prostate cancer bone metastasis in which PDGF β-receptor expression was observed on endothelial cells of tumors growing in the bone, but not on endothelial cells of normal bone or of tumors growing in surrounding muscle [59]. Pericyte deficiency after PDGF-B ablation causes vessel leakage, tortuosity, microaneurysm formation and bleeding, and PDGFR inhibition diminishes tumor growth by causing pericyte detachment leading to immature vessels that are prone to regression [60]. Because the survival of endothelial cells depends on pericyte VEGF production, pericytes protect endothelial cells from VEGF withdrawal and confer resistance to VEGF blockade [61]. Several multi-target receptor tyrosine kinase inhibitors (TKIs) have been developed and initial studies showed that blocking PDGF signaling pathway increases the sensitivity of mature normalized vessel to VEGF inhibition by depleting pericytes [4].

Therapeutic strategies to inhibit angiogenesis in lung cancer

Therapeutic targeting of tumor-associated endothelial cells as a means to control tumor growth is considered attractive for several reasons. For example, endothelial cells are genetically stable and therefore less likely to develop resistance to therapy [62]. In addition, antiangiogenic therapies are targeted therapies and, therefore, less likely to produce systemic toxicities associated with chemotherapy.

Most efforts to inhibit the neovascularization response of tumors have focused on the VEGF/R signaling pathway. Studies examining the effects of anti-VEGF therapies in tumors determined that these agents may "normalize" the tumor vasculature by reducing the size and tortuosity of vessels, increasing vessel maturation by actively recruiting pericytes to the vascular wall, and by normalizing the basement membrane [63]. Collectively, these effects result in a transient reduction in the microvessel density and a decrease tumor interstitial fluid pressure, which lead to improved delivery of oxygen and drugs [64]. Promising results of preclinical studies led to test several classes of agents inhibiting tumor vasculature in clinical trials for the treatment of a variety of cancers.

VEGF targeted therapies: FDA approved agents

The anti-VEGF monoclonal antibody bevacizumab (Avastin®) binds to and inhibits the activity of human VEGF [65]. Bevacizumab was the first antiangiogenic agent to receive approval from the United States Food and Drug Administration for the treatment of human cancers. Specifically, this approval was based on the results of phase III clinical trials revealing significant improvement in progression free survival (PFS) and/or overall survival (OS), as well as objective tumor responses in patients with colon cancer and NSCLC receiving bevacizumab in combination with standard chemotherapy [66, 67]. Bevacizumab monotherapy was determined to be ineffective for NSCLC [68], however, when this agent was combined with standard first line chemotherapy in patients with advanced nonsquamous NSCLC it produced a significant increase in PFS and OS compared with chemotherapy alone [67].

Currently, the use of bevacizumab in combination with chemotherapy in the neoadjuvant or adjuvant settings (stage I-III NSCLC) is being evaluated. The BEACON (Bevacizumab and Chemotherapy for Operable NSCLC) phase II study, a single institution trial for patients with clinical Stage IB-IIIA NSCLC (T1-3N0-2M0) who have resectable disease, has been completed at Memorial Sloan Kettering Cancer Center (NCT00130780). The primary goal of this trial is to show that the addition of bevacizumab to a cisplatin-based chemotherapy in the neoadjuvant setting for non-squamous NSCLC improves the rate of pathologic downstaging, defined as any decrease in the final pathologic stage compared with the clinical stage before induction therapy. The phase III randomized ECOG trial (E1505) of adjuvant chemotherapy with or without bevacizumab for patients with completely resected stage IB (>4 cm) – IIIA NSCLC, including squamous histology, is currently recruiting patients and results are pending (NCT00324805).

The combination of bevacizumab with concurrent chemo-radiation for inoperable stage IIIB NSCLC is not recommended due to a significant risk of developing tracheoesophageal fistulae [70]. The inhibition of VEGF pathway is directed not only against the growth of tumor-associated vasculature, but exerts several effects on blood vessels in normal organs. This may explain why bevacizumab toxicities include thromboembolic events, bleeding, complicated wound healing, hypertension, and proteinuria [71]. Furthermore, squamous cell tumor histology generally represents a contraindication to bevacizumab use, as patients with this histological subtype experience increased rate of hemoptysis.

Combined VEGF/R and EGFR targeted therapies

Targeting multiple key pathways driving cancer growth, progression and metastasis has resulted in improved outcomes across multiple tumor types. This can be achieved with a single compound or a combination of agents. Preclinical experiments performed in xenograft models of NSCLC have identified VEGFR and EGFR pathways as rational therapeutic targets. In fact, a greater tumor growth inhibitory effect was obtained by combining bevacizumab and the anti-EGFR TKI erlotinib (Tarceva®) compared with either agent alone [72]. The anti-EGFR monoclonal antibody cetuximab (Erbitux®) was evaluated in combination with bevacizumab and chemotherapy in a phase II Southwest Oncology Group (SWOG) trial, which revealed a promising antitumor activity and a tolerable toxicity profile [73]. The combination of erlotinib plus bevacizumab was tested in a phase I/II study of patients with pretreated non-squamous, advanced NSCLC, revealing a median OS of 12.6 months and a PFS duration of 6.2 months [74]. In addition, in another phase II trial testing this combination in a similar population of NSCLC patients, bevacizumab plus erlotinib achieved activity comparable with that of bevacizumab plus chemotherapy, with a median OS of 13.7 vs. 12.6 months, respectively [75]. Finally, the phase III BeTa Lung trial investigated this combination therapy in pretreated patients with advanced NSCLC and although its primary endpoint of prolonged OS time compared with erlotinib alone was not met (median OS 9.3 vs. 9.2 months, P=0.75), the PFS was notably increased in patients receiving combination therapy [76]. ATLAS, a phase III trial investigating bevacizumab plus erlotinib versus bevacizumab and placebo as maintenance therapy following first-line treatment was stopped early after an interim analysis showed that the combination led to a significant improvement in the PFS interval than with bevacizumab plus placebo [77].

Tyrosine kinase inhibitors of VEGFR pathway

Several small molecule TKIs of critical signaling pathways involved in tumor angiogenesis, such as VEGFR, PDGFR, FGFR, Raf, and c-KIT, have demonstrated higher anticancer activity over agents with single targets and are currently under clinical development. In addition, these agents are orally available and therefore, more convenient for patients. Conversely, a broader toxic profile results from off-target kinase inhibition, and the additive toxicity may be particularly significant when these compounds are administered in combination with chemotherapy. Multi-targeted, antiangiogenic agents that have received FDA approval for cancer treatment include sunitinib (renal cell carcinoma [RCC], hepatocellular carcinoma [HCC], pancreatic neuroendocrine tumors [PNET]), sorafenib (RCC, HCC), vandetanib (medullary thyroid cancer), pazopanib and axitinib (RCC). However, these compounds failed to induce any significant survival benefit in NSCLC treatment.

Sunitinib (Sutent®, SU11248), an oral small molecule tyrosine kinase inhibitor (TKI) that targets VEGFR-1, VEGFR-2, VEGFR-3, PDGFRs, KIT, FLT3, RET, and CSF-1R, is approved in the USA and Europe for the treatment of advanced RCC and imatinib-resistant or -intolerant gastrointestinal stromal tumor (GIST). Results obtained from preclinical studies revealed the promising antitumor activity of sunitinib in multiple xenograft models, including NSCLC [78]. In fact, in combination with docetaxel, pemetrexed, gemcitabine, or platinum agents, sunitinib provided a greater tumor growth inhibitory effect compared with monotherapy [79, 80]. Phase II trials evaluating single agent sunitinib in a continuous or intermittent dosing schedule demonstrated activity in patients with previously treated NSCLC, with a generally well tolerated toxicity profile [81]. In addition, a phase I study investigating sunitinib in combination with platinum and gemcitabine demonstrated promising tumor responses [82]. Dual EGFR and VEGF/R signaling pathway blockade is being investigated in phase II (SUN 1058) and phase III (SUN 1087) trials evaluating the activity and efficacy of erlotinib alone or in combination with sunitinib in patients with advanced NSCLC (www.clinicaltrial.gov). In a recently reported phase III trial, Scagliotti *et al.* found that the combination sunitinib plus erlotinib did not improve OS compared with erlotinib alone in refractory NSCLC [83]; however, the experimental arm was associated with a significantly prolonged PFS, improved ORR, and greater incidence of grade 3 adverse events (AEs).

Sorafenib (Nexavar®) targets Raf, VEGFR-2 and -3, PDGFR and KIT and is approved for the treatment of advanced RCC and HCC [84]. Preclinical experiments performed in cell lines and xenograft models showed that sorafenib in combination with EGFR inhibitors, vinorelbine, cisplatin, or gefitinib significantly delays tumor growth [85–87]. Data from phase II trials evaluating sorafenib monotherapy in heavily pretreated patients with metastatic NSCLC revealed a significant increase in disease stabilization at 2 months [88], an OS time of 6.8 months and a median PFS time of 2.8 month [89]. The recent phase II BATTLE trial found significant benefit for the use of sorafenib in pretreated lung cancers harboring KRAS mutations, emphasizing the importance of biomarkers to identify those patients most likely to benefit from targeted therapies [90]. Sorafenib has also been studied in combination with pemetrexed versus pemetrexed alone as second-line therapy. The NCCTG N0626 phase II study demonstrated similar median PFS (3.4 vs. 4.1 months; P = 0.22) and OS (9.4 vs. 9.7 months; P = 0.49) in patients with nonsquamous NSCLC [91]. In combination with erlotinib, sorafenib showed no significant improvements in RR, PFS, or OS in 168 patients with previously treated, advanced NSCLC [92]. Similar efficacy was observed in an additional phase II trial evaluating such combination in 50 chemotherapy-naive patients with advanced NSCLC [93]. Gridelli et al. evaluated sorafenib in combination with gemcitabine or erlotinib in elderly patients with previously untreated advanced NSCLC [94]. No significant improvement in RR and median OS were noticed (6.5% vs. 6.5 months with sorafenib plus gemcitabine and 10.3% and 12.6 months with sorafenib plus erlotinib, respectively). The phase III trial ESCAPE comparing the efficacy of carboplatin plus paclitaxel with and without sorafenib, failed to detect any significant improvement in OS with the addition of sorafenib in nonsquamous hystotype and, in a planned subgroup analysis, demonstrated a detrimental effect in patients with squamous cell carcinoma [95]. A similarly designed phase III study, NExUS (NCT00449033), evaluated the doublet cisplatin-gemcitabine with and without sorafenib and was stopped early due to failure in meeting its primary endpoint of OS.

Vandetanib (Zactima®, ZD6474), an oral TKI that targets the rearranged during transfection receptor (RET), VEGFR2-3, and EGFR, is the first systemic therapy approved by the U.S. FDA for the treatment of symptomatic or progressive advanced medullary thyroid cancer [96]. In vitro and preclinical experiments revealed a more portent VEGFR2 than EGFR inhibitory activity at much lower concentrations of vandetanib [97]. In combination with standard platinum-based chemotherapy, vandetanib induced higher response rates and increased PFS when compared with vandetanib alone in chemotherapy-naïve NSCLC patients [98]. In phase II trials, vandetanib plus docetaxel demonstrated superiority to docetaxel alone in patients who had failed prior chemotherapy [99], and significantly prolonged PFS compared with gefitinib in the second-line setting [100]. The phase III ZEAL study revealed no survival benefit in adding vandetanib to pemetrexed; however, the combination therapy improved the ORR, as well as the time to deterioration of symptoms [101]. The phase III ZODIAC trial, comparing vandetanib plus docetaxel versus placebo plus docetaxel in patients with advanced NSCLC following progression to first-line therapy, achieved the primary endpoint of PFS in the vandetanib arm (PFS HR = 0.79, P < 0.001), but this prolonged PFS did not translate in significantly improved OS [102]. The most common serious adverse event was febrile neutropenia (7%) in vandetanib group vs. (6%) in placebo. The antitumor activity and the efficacy of vandetanib compared to standard second line erlotinib has been investigated in the phase III ZEST study in unselected patients with advanced NSCLC who previously failed at least 1 chemotherapy regimen [103]. No significant improvement in PFS was detected for patients treated with vandetanib versus erlotinib (median PFS 2.6 months for vandetanib group and 2.0 months for erlotinib group). In addition, no significant differences were detected for the secondary end points of OS (HR = 1.01; P = 0.83), ORR (both 12%), and time to deterioration of symptoms for pain (HR = 0.92; P = 0.28). Both agents showed equivalent PFS and OS in a noninferiority analysis. Furthermore, the toxicity profile was more severe with vandetanib, as indicated by the overall incidence of grade ≥3 AEs, which was higher with vandetanib than with erlotinib (50% vs. 40%, respectively). ZEPHYR, a placebo-controlled, randomized, double-blind phase III study of vandetanib plus best supportive care versus best supportive care alone in patients with advanced NSCLC after prior treatment with an EGFR TKI and one or two chemotherapy regimens failed to show any significant OS benefit in vandetanib-treated patients (HR = 0.95, P = 0.52; median OS 8.5 months with vandetanib vs. 7.8 months with placebo). However, vandetanib therapy was favored in terms of PFS (HR = 0.63; P < 0.001) and ORR objective response rate (2.6% v 0.7%; P = 0.028) [104].

Cediranib (Recentin®, AZD2171) is an oral TKI that targets VEGFR-1, VEGFR-2, VEGFR-3, PDGFRs, and KIT [105]. It has been primarily evaluated in combination with chemotherapy. Findings of phase I studies indicated promising antitumor activity of this agent in combination with standard chemotherapy [106]. Given these encouraging results, the phase II/III trial BR.24 investigated carboplatin/paclitaxel plus cediranib or placebo as first-line therapy for advanced NSCLC. Although the phase II revealed a higher RR with cediranib vs. placebo (38% vs. 16%; P < 0.0001), and the PFS favored the combination of chemotherapy plus cediranib (HR = 0.77), the study was prematurely closed due to excessive toxicity, despite an initial reduction in cediranib dose reduction to 30 mg [107]. Given the concern regarding the toxicity profile, the NCIC BR29 phase III trial was similarly designed to further investigate cediranib 20 mg with carboplatin and paclitaxel, however, due to an interim analysis revealing insufficient efficacy, the study was recently close [108]. In a similar patient setting, the phase II N0528 study investigated the safety and efficacy of gemcitabine/carboplatin with or without cediranib (45 mg orally daily). No significant differences in terms of RR (20% vs. 18%; P = 1.0) were reported, although median PFS (6.3 vs. 4.5 months; HR, 0.69; P = 0.15), median OS (11.8 vs. 9.9 months; HR, 0.66; P = 0.16), as well as grade 3 and higher toxicities (71% vs. 45%; P = 0.01) were slightly increased in the experimental arm [109].

Pazopanib (GW786034, GlaxoSmithKline) is a small molecule TKI with activity against VEGFR-1, -2, -3, PDGFR-α/β, FGFR-1 and FGFR-3 [110]. In nonmetastatic setting, pazopanib monotherapy induced encouraging responses as neoadjuvant therapy in previously patients with stage I/II NSCLC [111], with common AEs of grade 1–2, including hypertension, diarrhea, and fatigue. The activity and efficacy of this agent is currently under investigation in the adjuvant and advanced setting [112].

Novel agents

Newer antiangiogenic agents directed against the VEGFR, PDGFR, or FGFR signaling pathways have been investigated in the preclinical setting revealing promising antitumor activity and are currently being evaluated in clinical trials at different stages of development.

Axitinib (AG-013736, Pfizer) is an oral TKI that targets VEGFR-1, VEGFR-2, and VEGFR-3, PDGFR-beta, and c-KIT, with a modest antitumor activity in a number of solid tumors [113]. In a phase II study of patients with advanced NSCLC receiving single-agent axitinib, the median OS was 14.6 months, a greater time than expected in this patient population with an acceptable toxicity profile [114]. Additional phase II trials evaluating axitinib in combination with standard chemotherapy in the first line setting are currently ongoing, including AGILE 1030 comparing axitinib plus paclitaxel-carboplatin vs. bevacizumab plus paclitaxel/carboplatin, and AGILE 1039, evaluating the benefit of adding axitinib to cisplatin-pemetrexed vs. doublet chemotherapy only. The phase II AGILE 1038 is currently studying axitinib plus cisplatin-gemcitabin in squamous cell carcinoma.

Motesanib (AMG 706, Amgen) targets all the VEGFRs, PDGFR, c-kit, and RET [115]. Recent results demonstrated equivalence of daily motesanib in combination with carboplatin-paclitaxel versus bevacizumab plus carboplatin-paclitaxel in the first line setting for advanced nonsquamous NSCLC [116]. The MONET1 phase III study of motesanib plus carboplatin-paclitaxel is currently recruiting patients with advanced nonsquamous NSCLC only (NCT00460317), due to higher mortality rates and incidence of hemoptysis observed in squamous lung carcinoma. Preliminary results reported at ASCO 2011 revealed statistically significant improvement in median PFS (5.6 vs. 5.4 months; HR = 0.78; P = 0.0006) and RR (40% vs. 26%; P < 0.0001) in patients receiving chemotherapy plus motesanib, with no differences in median OS (13.0 vs. 11.0 months; HR = 0.89; P = 0.13).

Nintedanib BIBF 1120 (Boehringer Ingelheim; Ingelheim, Germany) is an oral small molecule inhibitor of all VEGFRs, PDGFR-α/β, and FGFR1, -2, -3, Src family members and flt-3 [117]. The single agent activity of BIBF1120 in NSCLC has been shown in a phase II of pretreated NSCLC with 48% of patients achieving disease stabilization [118], a median PFS and OS of 6.9 and 21.9 week, respectively. Currently, phase III trials are assessing the efficacy of BIBF 1120 in combination with chemotherapy (LUME-Lung 2, NCT00806819, and LUME-Lung 1, NCT00805194).

Vascular disrupting agents (VDAs)

While angiogenesis inhibitors prevent the formation of new blood vessels from preexisting vasculature, vascular disrupting agents (VDAs) target the endothelial cells of established tumor vessels, leading to tumor vasculature disruption and oxygen and nutrient deprivation in the tumor [119].

Vadimezan (ASA404), an analog of flavone acetic acid, demonstrated initial encouraging results in combination with chemotherapy as treatment for patients with NSCLC in a phase II trial [120]; however these findings were not validated in the phase III setting. In fact, a phase III trial of vadimezan in combination with the carboplatin/paclitaxel as first line treatment in NSCLC failed to meet its primary endpoint, as no significant differences were detected in OS between vadimezan and placebo arms (median OS 13.4 vs. 12.7 months respectively (HR = 1.01; P = 0.535)) [121]. Given these results and the failure of this agent in demonstrating any advantage in the second line setting, the development of vedimezan in lung cancer has been halted by Novartis.

ABT-751 is another VDA with potent preclinical anticancer activity. This agent has been evaluated in a phase I/II study in combination with docetaxel as second line treatment for NSCLC [122]. The trial unfortunately failed to demonstrate any improvement in PFS (primary endpoint) with a median of

2.3 months for ABT-751 vs. 1.9 months for placebo; P = 0.82). However, a subgroup analysis favored ABT-751 in squamous NSCLC in terms of OS (P = 0.034; median 3.3 months vs. 8.1 months).

Antiangiogenic therapy in SCLC

The clinical application of antiangiogenic agents in small cell lung cancer (SCLC) has been less extensively investigated. The randomized, double-blind, placebo-controlled phase III trial IFTC 00-01 compared combination chemotherapy (cisplatin, etoposide, epidoxorubicin, and cyclophosphamide) with or without thalidomide (400 mg) in patients with untreated extensive stage disease [123], after the first two PCDE cycles, ORR was 81.5%, and 92 patients were randomly assigned to placebo (n = 43) or thalidomide (n = 49). The median survival time in patients who received thalidomide was prolonged compared to placebo, but this result was not statistically significant (HR = 0.74; 11.7 vs. 8.7 months, respectively, P = 0.16) with a minimal follow up time of 3 years. An exploratory analysis revealed that patients with performance status (PS) of 1–2 who received thalidomide had a significantly longer survival (HR = 0.59; P = 0.02) and a slower time to disease progression (HR = 0.54, P = 0.02). The use of thalidomide was associated with higher incidence of neuropathy, constipation and requirements for red cell transfusions, and about one-third of patients discontinued thalidomide due to side effects. Unfortunately, it is debatable whether the results of this trial can be generalized to support the efficacy of antiangiogenic agents in SCLC due to the relative small number of patients enrolled, and the alternative mechanisms of action exerted by thalidomide in addition to its antiangiogenic properties, including immune-modulatory effects.

Several phase II trials investigating anti-VEGFR therapies have been conducted in previously untreated extensive stage SCLC (ES-SCLC). Horn et al. recently published the final results of the phase II E3501 trial that studied efficacy and safety of bevacizumab in combination with first-line cisplatin, and etoposide as first line therapy in ED-SCLC [124]. A total of 63 patients were treated with bevacizumab plus cisplatin and etoposide followed by bevacizumab alone until death or onset of disease progression. The 6-month PFS was 30.2%, the median PFS was 4.7 months, and the OS was 10.9 months, with a RR of 63.5%. In regard with the toxicity profile, the experimental regimen appeared to be well tolerated, with minimal increase in side effects compared with chemotherapy alone. Biomarker analyses revealed that high baseline VCAM levels predicted significantly higher risk of progression or death, but no additional relationships among treatment, biomarkers, and outcome were identified.

A multicenter phase II study investigated the addition of bevacizumab to irinotecan and carboplatin as first-line treatment in patients ECOG PS 0–1 with ED-SCLC, with bevacizumab maintenance in absence of progression at the end of the planned number of administered cycles [125]. Fifty-one patients were enrolled, with a reported ORR of 84%, including 1 complete and 42 partial responses. Median TTP and OS were 9.13 and 12.1 months, respectively. The most common severe AEs were neutropenia, thrombocytopenia, GI symptoms and fatigue (20%), without significant bleeding events. A similar recently published phase II study, the CALGB 30306 trial reported the efficacy of cisplatin, irinotecan, and bevacizumab in 72 patients with untreated ES-SCLC [126]. The median PFS and OS times were higher 7.0 and 11.6 months, respectively, and the ORR was 75%. However, the primary end point of differentiating between 50% and 65% 12-month survival rates was not met. Three patients died while on treatment due to pneumonitis, stroke, and heart failure. Hypertension was associated with improved survival (P = 0.04), and lower baseline VEGF predicted poorer PFS after adjusting for age and PS (P = 0.03).

Given the promising efficacy of anti-VEGF therapy in single-arm studies, the phase II, placebo-controlled, double-blind, randomized SALUTE trial assessed the efficacy and safety of adding bevacizumab versus placebo to first-line therapy with cisplatin or carboplatin plus etoposide, for 4 cycles followed by single-agent bevacizumab or placebo until progression or unacceptable toxicity in 52 patients with ES-SCLC [127]. The median PFS was higher in bevacizumab group than placebo (5.5 vs. 4.4 months), while no OS differences were found (9.4 vs. 10.9 months for bevacizumab and placebo groups, respectively). ORRs were 58% vs. 48%, with a median duration of response of 4.7 s. 3.2 months for bevacizumab and placebo, respectively. Grade 3 or higher AEs occurred more frequently in bevacizumab-treated patients, however no new or unexpected safety signals were observed. The Hellenic Oncology Research Group evaluated the efficacy and the tolerance of paclitaxel combined with bevacizumab in a phase II trial of patients with relapsed, chemo-resistant SCLC [128]. Thirty patients with a PS 0-2 who experienced relapse within 3 months after completion of 1st line chemotherapy for SCLC were enrolled. The overall ORR was 20%, and the disease control rate (DCR) was 36.7%, with reported median PFS and OS of 2.7 and 6.3 months, respectively. Grades ≥ 3 and 4 toxicities were limited in neutropenia, diarrhea and fatigue, with one case of nonfatal pulmonary embolism. The Hoosier Oncology Group LUN06-113 study is an ongoing randomized, double blind phase II trial of cisplatin plus etoposide with or without concurrent vandetanib in patients with previously untreated ED-SCLC. Patients are currently being recruited and preliminary results have not been reported yet (NCT00613626). The National Cancer Center of Korea, in collaboration with Bayer, is currently conducting a randomized phase II study evaluating whether Sorafenib maintenance therapy prolongs PFS and OS in patients with ED-SCLC who achieved CR or PR after platinum-based induction chemotherapy (NCT01159327).

The benefit of incorporating an antiangiogenic agent into the therapeutic regimen administered to patients with limited stage SCLC (LS-SCLS) has also been investigated in clinical trials. The first study in 60 patients with limited stage SCLC evaluated chemotherapy plus radiation (four cycles of irinotecan and carboplatin with concurrent RT) followed by maintenance single-agent bevacizumab (10 mg/kg every 2 weeks for 10 doses) for patients with response or stable disease [129]. The complete and partial response rates were 27% and 53%, respectively, the median PFS was unreached with a median follow-up time of 24 months, and median OS was 17.5 months. One-year and 2-year survival rates were 70 and 29%, respectively. In a second phase II study, patients with limited stage SCLC received chemoradiation with irinotecan and carboplatin regimen given for 4 cycles, with concurrent bevacizumab [70]. Patients with stable disease or response after the 4 cycles of systemic therapy also received single-agent bevacizumab as maintenance therapy until disease progression or a further 6 months. The median patient follow-up for this trial was 14 months; however, due to safety issues, the trial was closed early in March 2007, and the primary endpoint PFS was unreached. Eight patients discontinued chemoradiation early due to trial closure and were not evaluated for treatment efficacy; 21 patients completed all planned induction therapy, and 8 patients completed 25 cycles of bevacizumab maintenance therapy. The ORR was 88%, with 4 CRs, 11 PRs, and 1 SD. Overall survival end points could not be assessed due to trial discontinuation. Grade 3–4 AEs included diarrhea (21%), esophagitis (14%), fatigue (17%), pain (14%), neutropenia (18%), leukopenia (10%), and thrombocytopenia (28%), with one death from treatment-related bowel perforation.

Biomarkers of response to antiangiogenic therapy

The clinical use of antiangiogenic therapies would be greatly facilitated by the identification of biomarkers modulated by treatment. In fact, activity biomarkers could be beneficial to determine the optimal antitumor dose [130]; to select patients whose tumors are likely to benefit from a specific agent, while sparing others from toxicity; to monitor responses to therapy; and to enhance our understanding of the mechanisms underlying angiogenesis inhibitor resistance. Thus, much effort is currently devoted to identify biomarkers that can predict outcomes and help individualize antiangiogenic therapies. To date, several predictive biomarkers of outcomes have been identified, none has yet been validated and routinely used as a reliable tool to identify patients most likely to benefit from angiogenesis inhibitors.

High blood pressure

Hypertension is the most frequent grade 3 or higher toxic effect of antiangiogenic therapy [131, 132]. By decreasing the synthesis of nitric oxide, bevacizumab leads to high blood pressure (HBP), which correlates with an effective VEGF blockade on the vasculature. Dahlberg et al. recently reported the results of a subgroup analysis of the phase III ECOG 4599 trial of bevacizumab in NSCLC, consisting in a positive correlation between the onset of HBP (>150/100 mmHg or at least a 20-mmHg increase in diastolic BP from baseline) and improved clinical outcomes in patients receiving bevacizumab [133]. In fact, a significant OS improvement was observed when hypertensive patients on PCB arm were compared with those on PC (HR = 0.60; P = 0.001), with an adjusted PFS HR of 0.54 (P < 0.0001). When nonhypertensive patients receiving PCB were compared with those on PC alone, the OS HR was 0.86 (P = 0.05), and the PFS HR was 0.72 (P < 0.0001). Overall, these data indicate that onset of HBP while receiving bevacizumab in combination with standard chemotherapy may be associated with improved outcomes. Similarly, final analysis of data obtained from six phase II trials of axitinib in 230 patients with various tumor types, including 30 patients with NSCLC, suggested the potential role of diastolic blood pressure > 90 mmHg as biomarker of longer OS [134]. Prospective studies to validate hypertension as a reliable biomarker of response in clinical practice are warranted.

Circulating cytokines

The expression of VEGF has been one of the most extensively studied predictive biomarkers. Increased circulating VEGF and decreased soluble VEGFR2 concentrations have been repetitively reported in phase I and II studies evaluating the safety and antitumor activity of VEGFR TKIs, indicating that such changes may represent a specific class effect of these agents [135–137]. However, only some studies have found associations between these factor changes and improved outcomes. Recently, Ebos et al. showed that the changes in VEGF and VEGFR-2 levels in tumor-bearing and nontumor-bearing mice receiving sunitinib might represent the result of a systemic, tumor-independent, dose-dependent, host-derived response and correlate with the optimal antitumor dose of sunitinib [135]. Using multiplexed bead arrays and ELISA, Hanrahan et al. performed an exploratory retrospective analysis of the correlation between baseline circulating VEGF levels and PFS in three phase II trials evaluating vandetanib in NSCLC, which suggested that low baseline circulating VEGF may predict for PFS advantage in patients with advanced NSCLC receiving vandetanib versus gefitinib or vandetanib plus docetaxel versus docetaxel alone. Analysis of cytokine and angiogenic factors (CAFs) from 123 patients with NSCLC randomized in the phase II study of vandetanib monotherapy (V) versus carboplatin and paclitaxel (CP), or the combination (VCP) in the first line setting, at baseline and during treatment revealed an increase in VEGF and a sVEGFR2 decrease by day 43 in the V arm only, and increases in VEGF were associated with an increased risk of disease progression in patients receiving treated with V [138]. In the same study, high baseline concentrations of HGF significantly correlated with a poorer PFS in V group, but not in the combination or chemotherapy arms [139]. These findings are in accordance with our recently reported preclinical results showing that in xenograft models of NSCLC treated with V until progression, elevated HGF/c-MET pathway expression and activation is associated with onset of therapeutic resistance [140]. In plasma samples of early NSCLC patients treated with pazopanib, post-treatment changes in plasma sVEGFR2 and IL-4 significantly correlated with tumor shrinkage, and baseline HGF and IL-12 were associated with tumor response to pazopanib, suggesting that CAF profiling may be useful for identifying patients likely to benefit from VEGFR blockade with small molecule TKIs [137]. However, conflicting data have been reported in regard with the effectiveness of using baseline (pretreatment) VEGF levels as a predictive biomarker of clinical outcome. For example, a phase II/III trial evaluating chemotherapy plus bevacizumab in patients with advanced NSCLC failed to demonstrate the role of high baseline circulating plasma VEGF as a predictive marker of survival (PFS and OS), although a significant correlation with improved ORR was reported [141]. Given these findings, it is clear that the use of circulating VEGF as predictive biomarker of survival benefit in NSCLC warrants further investigation.

VEGF single nucleotide polymorphisms (SNPs)

A growing area of research is investigating the role of VEGF genotype and VEGF single nucleotide polymorphisms (SNPs). It has been demonstrated that SNPs may affect the efficiency of drug metabolism and excretion, and influence the responses to drugs through gene-expression alterations or posttranscriptional modifications. The variant C allele of the *VEGF* +405G>C polymorphism has been associated with a significant survival improvement in early stage NSCLC [142]. A study of 133 patients with advanced NSCLC enrolled in the ECOG 4599 trial showed that a SNP signature of VEGFA −634GG, ICAM1 469T/C, and IL8 −251T/A was the best predictor of OS and PFS [143], suggesting a critical association between genetic variants of molecules involved in angiogenic pathways and clinical outcomes. SNP biomarkers for sorafenib have been assessed in a correlative study of the E2501 trial [144], a randomized discontinuation, phase II study of sorafenib versus placebo in patients with metastatic NSCLC that progressed after prior two chemotherapy regimens. Analysis of DNA obtained from 88 plasma samples indicated that VEGFA −1498CC and −634CC genotypes correlated with improved PFS [145].

Other biomarkers

A significant correlation between high microvascular density (MVD), which reflects the amount of vessels supplying a tumor, and poor survival, tumor progression and metastasis has been demonstrated in patients with NSCLC [146]. Given this association, MVD has been hypothesized to correlate with response to and benefit from antiangiogenic therapies. However, while preclinical models proved the role of MVD as a predictive marker of response to therapy, this was not validated in the clinical setting [147].

Circulating endothelial cells (CECs) originate from the wall of blood vessels and express the phenotype of mature ECs. A vast body of evidence demonstrated that CECs are increased in cancer patients [148]. Antiangiogenic therapies may induce the endothelial cells to dissociate from the tumor vasculature, which increases the amount of CECs in the bloodstream of patient whose tumors are responding to treatment [149, 150]. These findings led to the identification of CECs as a novel biomarker of response to angiogenesis inhibition [151], as high levels of CECs may indicate that a patient is responding to therapy. Measurement of CEC levels in clinical trials evaluating antiangiogenic treatments demonstrated a positive correlation between decreased concentration while on therapy and improved PFS [152]. In addition, greater baseline levels of CECs have been correlated with greater response rates; however, at time of progression a significant decrease in CEC levels was detected [153]. Taken together, these data indicate that while much effort is ongoing to identify biomarkers predictive of improved clinical outcomes and resistance to antiangiogenic therapies, to date no marker is validated and approved for the routine use into the clinical setting.

Tumor resistance to antiangiogenic therapies

Unfortunately, despite the initial encouraging results obtained from the clinical use of antiangiogenic agents, it is clear that the magnitude of clinical responses and survival benefit is far less than predicted from preclinical studies. In fact, not all tumors respond to therapy and tumors that showed an initial response eventually relapse and progress. In this section, we review what is known regarding the cellular and molecular mechanisms that enable tumors to become refractory to anti-VEGF therapies.

Recent preclinical studies suggest that one way in which tumors circumvent blockade of the VEGFR signaling pathway is by exploiting alternative angiogenic signaling pathways. In fact, it has been extensively shown that while anti-VEGFR therapy initially blocks neovascularization and tumor growth in preclinical models of cancer, angiogenesis and tumor progression eventually rebound by an increased production of FGF family associated molecules by cancer cells [154]. Commonly occurring genetic alterations in cancer cells have also been also been shown to permit tumors to become less dependent on angiogenesis. Cancer cells that lose activity of the *p53* tumor suppressor gene are able to better withstand hypoxic conditions [155] and *p53*-deficient tumors are much less sensitive to the effects of antiangiogenic therapy [156]. There is also evidence suggesting that some cancer cells may alter their pattern of growth in response to antiangiogenic therapies. In experimental models of brain metastasis, melanoma cells progressed while receiving anti-VEGF therapy by co-opting the preexisting cerebral vasculature [157].

A vast body of evidence also suggests that in addition to cancer cells themselves, stromal cells residing within the tumor microenvironment play a critical role in mediating tumor resistance to antiangiogenic therapy. In some experimental tumor models, VEGF/R inhibitor resistance was dependent on the ability of tumors to recruit $CD11b^+Gr\text{-}1^+$ granulocytic myeloid cells [158]. $CD11b^+Gr\text{-}1^+$ myeloid cells comprise several subpopulations of cells including neutrophils, macrophages, and dendritic cells and localize to tumors in response to cytokines produced by cancer cells (e.g., granulocyte macrophage colony stimulating factor). $CD11b^+Gr\text{-}1^+$ cells are a significant source of proangiogenic proteins and also produce several immunosuppressive molecules [159], both of which favor tumor progression. Other investigations suggest a role for tumor-associated fibroblasts in mediating tumor resistance to anti-VEGF agents. Antibody-mediated neutralization of VEGF in murine lymphoma models resulted in upregulation of platelet-derived growth factor (PDGF-C) from tumor-associated fibroblasts, which was sufficient to sustain angiogenesis and ensure tumor progression [160].

The relative contribution of cancer and stromal cells to resistance to antiangiogenic therapies varies in each cancer subtype [161, 162]. Our group recently reported a previously unknown stromal adaptation in VEGFR-inhibitor resistance murine models of human NSCLC, that include upregulation of stromal EGFR and FGFR family members, as well EGFR-driven pericyte recruitment and vascular remodeling promoting resistance to VEGF inhibition. Furthermore, our results demonstrated that, dual VEGFR and EGFR pathway targeting significantly prolonged survival and delayed the onset of resistance, which is partially in line with the findings of clinical trials investigating this therapeutic strategy in patients with advanced NSCLC [19, 163].

Conclusion

Despite the extensive research performed over the past few decades to advance the field of antiangiogenic therapy as an anticancer strategy, at this time, bevacizumab is the only angiogenesis inhibitor approved for clinical use in the treatment of patients with advanced/metastatic NSCLC in combination with standard platinum-based chemotherapy. This success has resulted in a rapid escalation in the number of antiangiogenic agents, including monoclonal antibodies and receptor TKIs and VDAs, which are currently at various stages of preclinical and clinical development. Results of antiangiogenic therapy use in early stage NSCLC are pending. Much effort is currently directed toward a better understanding of the molecular abnormalities associated with NSCLC cell growth and proliferation and their impact on therapeutic response and clinical outcomes. This will guide the discovery and validation of activity biomarkers modulated by therapy that can identify those patients most likely to benefit from therapies targeting the tumor vasculature.

The incremental benefit of bevacizumab in NSCLC is modest and emergence of resistance occurs in all patients. Therefore, future investigations also include a better understanding of the cellular and molecular mechanisms mediating intrinsic or acquired resistance to these agents to improve clinical outcomes for patients with lung cancer.

References

1 Folkman J (2002) Role of angiogenesis in tumor growth and metastasis. *Semin Oncol*, 29: 15–18.

2 Folkman J (1990) What is the evidence that tumors are angiogenesis dependent? *J Natl Cancer Inst*, 82: 4–6.

3 Weis SM, Cheresh DA (2011) Tumor angiogenesis: molecular pathways and therapeutic targets. *Nat Med*, 17: 1359–70.

4 Carmeliet P, Jain RK (2011) Molecular mechanisms and clinical applications of angiogenesis. *Nature*, 473: 298–307.

5 Dvorak HF, Brown LF, Detmar M, Dvorak AM (1995) Vascular permeability factor/vascular endothelial growth factor, microvascular hyperpermeability, and angiogenesis. *Am J Pathol*, 146: 1029–39.

6 Jain RK (1990) Vascular and interstitial barriers to delivery of therapeutic agents in tumors. *Cancer Metastasis Rev*, 9: 253–66.

7 Xian X, Hakansson J, Stahlberg A, Lindblom P, Betsholtz C, Gerhardt H, Semb H (2006) Pericytes limit tumor cell metastasis. *J Clin Invest*, 116: 642–51.

8 Carmeliet P, Jain RK (2000) Angiogenesis in cancer and other diseases. *Nature*, 407: 249–57.

9 Harris AL (2002) Hypoxia – a key regulatory factor in tumour growth. *Nat Rev Cancer*, 2: 38–47.

10 Semenza GL (1999) Regulation of mammalian O2 homeostasis by hypoxia-inducible factor 1. *Annu Rev Cell Dev Biol*, 15: 551–78.

11 Zhong H, De Marzo AM, Laughner E, Lim M, Hilton DA, Zagzag D, Buechler P, Isaacs WB, Semenza GL, Simons JW (1999) Overexpression of hypoxia-inducible factor 1alpha in common human cancers and their metastases. *Cancer Res*, 59: 5830–5.

12 Le QT, Chen E, Salim A, Cao H, Kong CS, Whyte R, Donington J, Cannon W, Wakelee H, Tibshirani R, *et al.* (2006) An evaluation of tumor oxygenation and gene expression in patients with early stage non-small cell lung cancers. *Clin Cancer Res*, 12: 1507–14.

13 Song X, Liu X, Chi W, Liu Y, Wei L, Wang X, Yu J (2006) Hypoxia-induced resistance to cisplatin and doxorubicin in non-small cell lung cancer is inhibited by silencing of HIF-1alpha gene. *Cancer Chemother Pharmacol*, 58: 776–84.

14 Niklinska W, Burzykowski T, Chyczewski L, Niklinski J (2001) Expression of vascular endothelial growth factor (VEGF) in non-small cell lung cancer (NSCLC): Association with p53 gene mutation and prognosis. *Lung Cancer*, 34(Suppl 2): S59–64.

15 Rak J, Mitsuhashi Y, Bayko L, Filmus J, Shirasawa S, Sasazuki T, Kerbel RS (1995) Mutant ras oncogenes upregulate VEGF/VPF expression: implications for induction and inhibition of tumor angiogenesis. *Cancer Res*, 55: 4575–80.

16 Ji H, Ramsey MR, Hayes DN, Fan C, McNamara K, Kozlowski P, Torrice C, Wu MC, Shimamura T, Perera SA, *et al.* (2007) LKB1 modulates lung cancer differentiation and metastasis. *Nature*, 448: 807–10.

17 Gao Y, Xiao Q, Ma H, Li L, Liu J, Feng Y, Fang Z, Wu J, Han X, Zhang J, *et al.* (2010) LKB1 inhibits lung cancer progression through lysyl oxidase and extracellular matrix remodeling. *Proceedings of the National Academy of Sciences of the United States of America*, 107: 18892–7.

18 Marcus AI, Zhou W (2010) LKB1 regulated pathways in lung cancer invasion and metastasis. *Journal of Thoracic Oncology*, 5: 1883–6.

19 Cascone T, Herynk MH, Xu L, Du Z, Kadara H, Nilsson MB, Oborn CJ, Park YY, Erez B, Jacoby JJ, *et al.* (2011) Upregulated stromal EGFR and vascular remodeling in mouse xenograft models of angiogenesis inhibitor-resistant human lung adenocarcinoma. *J Clin Invest*, 121: 1313–28.

20 Sica A, Allavena P, Mantovani A (2008) Cancer related inflammation: the macrophage connection. *Cancer Lett*, 267: 204–15.

21 Takanami I, Takeuchi K, Kodaira S (1999) Tumor-associated macrophage infiltration in pulmonary adenocarcinoma: Association with angiogenesis and poor prognosis. *Oncology*, 57: 138–42.

22 Eberhard A, Kahlert S, Goede V, Hemmerlein B, Plate KH, Augustin HG (2000) Heterogeneity of angiogenesis and blood vessel maturation in human tumors: Implications for antiangiogenic tumor therapies. *Cancer Res*, 60: 1388–93.

23 Pezzella F, Pastorino U, Tagliabue E, Andreola S, Sozzi G, Gasparini G, Menard S, Gatter KC, Harris AL, Fox S, *et al.* (1997) Non-small-cell lung carcinoma tumor growth without morphological evidence of neo-angiogenesis. *Am J Pathol*, 151: 1417–23.

24 Ribatti D, Vacca A, Dammacco F (2003) New non-angiogenesis dependent pathways for tumour growth. *Eur J Cancer*, 39: 1835–41.

25 Ferrara N (2004) Vascular endothelial growth factor: basic science and clinical progress. *Endocr Rev*, 25: 581–611.

26 Nilsson M, Heymach JV (2006) Vascular endothelial growth factor (VEGF) pathway. *J Thorac Oncol*, 1: 768–70.

27 Ferrara N, Davis-Smyth T (1997) The biology of vascular endothelial growth factor. *Endocr Rev*, 18: 4–25.

28 Hicklin DJ, Ellis LM (2005) Role of the vascular endothelial growth factor pathway in tumor growth and angiogenesis. *J Clin Oncol*, 23: 1011–27.

29 He Y, Karpanen T, Alitalo K (2004) Role of lymphangiogenic factors in tumor metastasis. *Biochim Biophys Acta*, 1654: 3–12.

30 Fehrenbach H, Kasper M, Haase M, Schuh D, Muller M (1999) Differential immunolocalization of VEGF in rat and human adult lung, and in experimental rat lung fibrosis: light, fluorescence, and electron microscopy. *Anat Rec*, 254: 61–73.

31 Han H, Silverman JF, Santucci TS, Macherey RS, d'Amato TA, Tung MY, Weyant RJ, Landreneau RJ (2001) Vascular endothelial growth factor expression in stage I non-small cell lung cancer correlates with neoangiogenesis and a poor prognosis. *Ann Surg Oncol*, 8: 72–9.

32 Stefanou D, Batistatou A, Arkoumani E, Ntzani E, Agnantis NJ (2004) Expression of vascular endothelial growth factor (VEGF) and association with microvessel density in small-cell and non-small-cell lung carcinomas. *Histol Histopathol*, 19: 37–42.

33 Jubb AM, Cesario A, Ferguson M, Congedo MT, Gatter KC, Lococo F, Mule A, Pezzella F (2011) Vascular phenotypes in primary non-small cell lung carcinomas and matched brain metastases. *Br J Cancer*, 104: 1877–81.

34 Beenken A, Mohammadi M (2009) The FGF family: Biology, pathophysiology and therapy. *Nat Rev Drug Discov*, 8: 235–53.

35 Shing Y, Folkman J, Sullivan R, Butterfield C, Murray J, Klagsbrun M (1984) Heparin affinity: purification of a tumor-derived capillary endothelial cell growth factor. *Science*, 223: 1296–9.

36 Eswarakumar VP, Lax I, Schlessinger J (2005) Cellular signaling by fibroblast growth factor receptors. *Cytokine Growth Factor Rev*, 16: 139–49.

37 Kandel J, Bossy-Wetzel E, Radvanyi F, Klagsbrun M, Folkman J, Hanahan D (1991) Neovascularization is associated with a switch to the export of bFGF in the multistep development of fibrosarcoma. *Cell*, 66: 1095–1104.

38 Behrens C, Lin HY, Lee JJ, Raso MG, Hong WK, Wistuba II, Lotan R (2008) Immunohistochemical expression of basic fibroblast growth factor and fibroblast growth factor receptors 1 and 2 in the pathogenesis of lung cancer. *Clin Cancer Res*, 14: 6014–22.

39 Weiss J, Sos ML, Seidel D, Peifer M, Zander T, Heuckmann JM, Ullrich RT, Menon R, Maier S, Soltermann A, *et al.* (2010) Frequent and focal FGFR1 amplification associates with therapeutically tractable FGFR1 dependency in squamous cell lung cancer. *Sci Transl Med* 2: 62ra93.

40 Nguyen M, Watanabe H, Budson AE, Richie JP, Hayes DF, Folkman J (1994) Elevated levels of an angiogenic peptide, basic fibroblast growth factor, in the urine of patients with a wide spectrum of cancers. *J Natl Cancer Inst*, 86: 356–61.

41 Brattstrom D, Bergqvist M, Hesselius P, Larsson A, Lamberg K, Wernlund J, Brodin O, Wagenius G (2002) Elevated preoperative serum levels of angiogenic cytokines correlate to larger primary tumours and poorer survival in non-small cell lung cancer patients. *Lung Cancer*, 37 57–63.

42 Rades D, Setter C, Dahl O, Schild SE, Noack F (2012) Fibroblast growth factor 2 – a predictor of outcome for patients irradiated for stage II-III non-small-cell lung cancer. *Int J Radiat Oncol Biol Phys*, 82: 442–7.

43 Hynes NE, Lane HA (2005) ERBB receptors and cancer: The complexity of targeted inhibitors. *Nat Rev Cancer*, 5: 341–54.

44 Ciardiello F, Tortora G (2008) EGFR antagonists in cancer treatment. *New England Journal of Medicine*, 358: 1160–74.

45 Herbst RS, Heymach JV, Lippman SM (2008) Lung cancer. *N Engl J Med*, 359: 1367–80.

46 Amin DN, Hida K, Bielenberg DR, Klagsbrun M (2006) Tumor endothelial cells express epidermal growth factor receptor (EGFR) but not ErbB3 and are responsive to EGF and to EGFR kinase inhibitors. *Cancer Res*, 66: 2173–80.

47 Wu W, Onn A, Isobe T, Itasaka S, Langley RR, Shitani T, Shibuya K, Komaki R, Ryan AJ, Fidler IJ, *et al.* (2007) Targeted therapy of orthotopic human lung cancer by combined vascular endothelial growth factor and epidermal growth factor receptor signaling blockade. *Mol Cancer Ther*, 6: 471–83.

48 Lindahl P, Johansson BR, Leveen P, Betsholtz C (1997) Pericyte loss and microaneurysm formation in PDGF-B-deficient mice. *Science*, 277: 242–5.

49 Cao Y, Cao R, Hedlund EM (2008) Regulation of tumor angiogenesis and metastasis by FGF and

PDGF signaling pathways. *J Mol Med (Berl)*, 86: 785–9.

50 Pietras K, Sjoblom T, Rubin K, Heldin CH, Ostman A (2003) PDGF receptors as cancer drug targets. *Cancer Cell*, 3: 439–43.

51 Hermanson M, Funa K, Hartman M, Claesson-Welsh L, Heldin CH, Westermark B, Nister M (1992) Platelet-derived growth factor and its receptors in human glioma tissue: expression of messenger RNA and protein suggests the presence of autocrine and paracrine loops. *Cancer Res*, 52: 3213–19.

52 Nister M, Libermann TA, Betsholtz C, Pettersson M, Claesson-Welsh L, Heldin CH, Schlessinger J, Westermark B (1988) Expression of messenger RNAs for platelet-derived growth factor and transforming growth factor-alpha and their receptors in human malignant glioma cell lines. *Cancer Res*, 48: 3910–18.

53 Oikawa T, Onozawa C, Sakaguchi M, Morita I, Murota S (1994) Three isoforms of platelet-derived growth factors all have the capability to induce angiogenesis in vivo. *Biol Pharm Bull*, 17: 1686–8.

54 Risau W, Drexler H, Mironov V, Smits A, Siegbahn A, Funa K, Heldin CH (1992) Platelet-derived growth factor is angiogenic in vivo. *Growth Factors*, 7: 261–6.

55 Hellstrom M, Kalen M, Lindahl P, Abramsson A, Betsholtz C (1999) Role of PDGF-B and PDGFR-beta in recruitment of vascular smooth muscle cells and pericytes during embryonic blood vessel formation in the mouse. *Development*, 126: 3047–55.

56 Hellberg C, Ostman A, Heldin CH (2010) PDGF and vessel maturation. *Recent Results Cancer Res*, 180: 103–14.

57 Gaengel K, Genove G, Armulik A, Betsholtz C (2009) Endothelial-mural cell signaling in vascular development and angiogenesis. *Arterioscler Thromb Vasc Biol*, 29: 630–8.

58 Guo P, Hu B, Gu W, Xu L, Wang D, Huang HJ, Cavenee WK, Cheng SY (2003) Platelet-derived growth factor-B enhances glioma angiogenesis by stimulating vascular endothelial growth factor expression in tumor endothelia and by promoting pericyte recruitment. *Am J Pathol*, 162: 1083–93.

59 Uehara H, Kim SJ, Karashima T, Shepherd DL, Fan D, Tsan R, Killion JJ, Logothetis C, Mathew P, Fidler IJ (2003) Effects of blocking platelet-derived growth factor-receptor signaling in a mouse model of experimental prostate cancer bone metastases. *J Natl Cancer Inst*, 95: 458–70.

60 Bergers G, Song S, Meyer-Morse N, Bergsland E, Hanahan D (2003) Benefits of targeting both pericytes and endothelial cells in the tumor vasculature with kinase inhibitors. *J Clin Invest*, 111: 1287–95.

61 Bergers G, Hanahan D (2008) Modes of resistance to anti-angiogenic therapy. *Nat Rev Cancer*, 8: 592–603.

62 Kerbel RS (1991) Inhibition of tumor angiogenesis as a strategy to circumvent acquired resistance to anti-cancer therapeutic agents. *Bioessays*, 13: 31–6.

63 Jain RK (2003) Molecular regulation of vessel maturation. *Nat Med*, 9: 685–93.

64 Jain RK, Duda DG, Clark JW, Loeffler JS (2006) Lessons from phase III clinical trials on anti-VEGF therapy for cancer. *Nat Clin Pract Oncol*, 3: 24–40.

65 Ferrara N, Hillan KJ, Gerber HP, Novotny W (2004) Discovery and development of bevacizumab, an anti-VEGF antibody for treating cancer. *Nat Rev Drug Discov*, 3: 391–400.

66 Hurwitz H, Fehrenbacher L, Novotny W, Cartwright T, Hainsworth J, Heim W, Berlin J, Baron A, Griffing S, Holmgren E, *et al.* (2004) Bevacizumab plus irinotecan, fluorouracil, and leucovorin for metastatic colorectal cancer. *N Engl J Med*, 350: 2335–42.

67 Sandler A, Gray R, Perry MC, Brahmer J, Schiller JH, Dowlati A, Lilenbaum R, Johnson DH (2006) Paclitaxel-carboplatin alone or with bevacizumab for non-small-cell lung cancer. *N Engl J Med*, 355: 2542–50.

68 Johnson DH, Fehrenbacher L, Novotny WF, Herbst RS, Nemunaitis JJ, Jablons DM, Langer CJ, DeVore RF, 3rd, Gaudreault J, Damico LA, *et al.* (2004) Randomized phase II trial comparing bevacizumab plus carboplatin and paclitaxel with carboplatin and paclitaxel alone in previously untreated locally advanced or metastatic non-small-cell lung cancer. *J Clin Oncol*, 22: 2184–91.

69 Reck M, von Pawel J, Zatloukal P, Ramlau R, Gorbounova V, Hirsh V, Leighl N, Mezger J, Archer V, Moore N, *et al.* (2009) Phase III trial of cisplatin plus gemcitabine with either placebo or bevacizumab as first-line therapy for nonsquamous non-small-cell lung cancer: AVAil. *Journal of Clinical Oncology*, 27: 1227–34.

70 Spigel DR, Hainsworth JD, Yardley DA, Raefsky E, Patton J, Peacock N, Farley C, Burris HA, 3rd, Greco FA (2010) Tracheoesophageal fistula formation in patients with lung cancer treated with chemoradiation and bevacizumab. *Journal of Clinical Oncology*, 28: 43–8.

71 Kamba T, McDonald DM (2007) Mechanisms of adverse effects of anti-VEGF therapy for cancer. *British Journal of Cancer*, 96: 1788–95.

72 Sandler A, Herbst R (2006) Combining targeted agents: Blocking the epidermal growth factor and vascular endothelial growth factor pathways. *Clinical Cancer Research*, 12: 4421s–5s.

73 Gandara D, Kim ES, Herbst RS, Moon J, Redman, M, Dakhil SR, Hirsch F, Mack PC, Franklin W (2009) S0536: Carboplatin, paclitaxel, cetuximab and bevacizumab followed by cetuximab and bevacizumab maintenance in advanced NSCLC: A SWOG phase II study. *J Clin Oncol*, 27: 15s (suppl; abstr 8015).

74 Herbst RS, Johnson DH, Mininberg E, Carbone DP, Henderson T, Kim ES, Blumenschein G, Jr, Lee JJ, Liu DD, Truong MT, *et al.* (2005) Phase I/II trial evaluating the anti-vascular endothelial growth factor monoclonal antibody bevacizumab in combination with the HER-1/epidermal growth factor receptor tyrosine kinase inhibitor erlotinib for patients with recurrent non-small-cell lung cancer. *J Clin Oncol*, 23(11): 2544–55.

75 Herbst RS, O'Neill VJ, Fehrenbacher L, Belani CP, Bonomi PD, Hart L, Melnyk O, Ramies D, Lin M, Sandler A (2007) Phase II study of efficacy and safety of bevacizumab in combination with chemotherapy or erlotinib compared with chemotherapy alone for treatment of recurrent or refractory non small-cell lung cancer. *J Clin Oncol*, 25: 4743–50.

76 Herbst RS, Ansari R, Bustin F, Flynn P, Hart L, Otterson GA, Vlahovic G, Soh CH, O'Connor P, Hainsworth J (2011) Efficacy of bevacizumab plus erlotinib versus erlotinib alone in advanced non-small-cell lung cancer after failure of standard first-line chemotherapy (BeTa): A double-blind, placebo-controlled, phase 3 trial. *Lancet*, 377: 1846–54.

77 Miller VA, O'Connor P, Soh C, Kabbinavar F (2009) A randomized, double-blind, placebo-controlled, phase IIIb trial (ATLAS) comparing bevacizumab (B) therapy with or without erlotinib (E) after completion of chemotherapy with B for first-line treatment of locally advanced, recurrent, or metastatic non-small cell lung cancer (NSCLC). *J Clin Oncol, 2009 ASCO Annual Meeting Proceedings* 27:abstr LBA8002.

78 Christensen JG (2007) A preclinical review of sunitinib, a multitargeted receptor tyrosine kinase inhibitor with anti-angiogenic and antitumour activities. *Annals of Oncology*, 18(Suppl 10): x3–10.

79 Wang D, Jiang Z, Zhang L (2012) Concurrent and sequential administration of sunitinib malate and docetaxel in human non-small cell lung cancer cells and xenografts. *Medical Oncology*, 29: 600–6.

80 Christensen J, Hall C, Hollister B (2008) Antitumor efficacy of sunitinib malate in concurrent and sequential combinations with standard chemotherapeutic agents in non-small cell lung cancer (NSCLC) nonclinical models. In: *99th Annual Meeting of the American Association for Cancer Research*. San Diego, California.

81 Socinski MA, Novello S, Brahmer JR, Rosell R, Sanchez JM, Belani CP, Govindan R, Atkins JN, Gillenwater HH, Pallares C, *et al.* (2008) Multicenter, phase II trial of sunitinib in previously treated, advanced non-small-cell lung cancer. *J Clin Oncol*, 26: 650–6.

82 Reck M, Frickhofen N, Cedres S, Gatzemeier U, Heigener D, Fuhr HG, Thall A, Lanzalone S, Stephenson P, Ruiz-Garcia A, *et al.* (2010) Sunitinib in combination with gemcitabine plus cisplatin for advanced non-small cell lung cancer: a phase I dose-escalation study. *Lung Cancer*, 70: 180–7.

83 Scagliotti GV, Krzakowski M, Szczesna A, Strausz J, Makhson A, Reck M, Wierzbicki RF, Albert I, Thomas M, Miziara JE, *et al.* (2012) Sunitinib plus erlotinib versus placebo plus erlotinib in patients with previously treated advanced non-small-cell lung cancer: a phase III trial. *Journal of Clinical Oncology*, 30: 2070–8.

84 Escudier B, Eisen T, Stadler WM, Szczylik C, Oudard S, Siebels M, Negrier S, Chevreau C, Solska E, Desai AA, *et al.* (2007) Sorafenib in advanced clear-cell renal-cell carcinoma. *N Engl J Med*, 356: 125–34.

85 Morgillo F, Martinelli E, Troiani T, Orditura M, De Vita F, Ciardiello F (2011) Antitumor activity of sorafenib in human cancer cell lines with acquired resistance to EGFR and VEGFR tyrosine kinase inhibitors. *PloS One*, 6: e28841.

86 Martinelli E, Troiani T, Morgillo F, Rodolico G, Vitagliano D, Morelli MP, Tuccillo C, Vecchione L, Capasso A, Orditura M, *et al.* (2010) Synergistic antitumor activity of sorafenib in combination with epidermal growth factor receptor inhibitors in colorectal and lung cancer cells. *Clinical Cancer Research*, 16: 4990–5001.

87 Carter CA, Chen C, Brink C, Vincent P, Maxuitenko YY, Gilbert KS, Waud WR, Zhang X (2007) Sorafenib is efficacious and tolerated in combination with cytotoxic or cytostatic agents in preclinical models of human non-small cell lung carcinoma. *Cancer Chemotherapy and Pharmacology*, 59: 183–95.

88 Schiller J, Lee J, Hanna N, Traynor A, Carbone D (2008) A randomized discontinuation phase II study

of sorafenib versus placebo in patients with non-small cell lung cancer who have failed at least two prior chemotherapy regimens: E2501. *J Clin Oncol*, 26: abstr 8014.

89 Blumenschein GR, Jr, Gatzemeier U, Fossella F, Stewart DJ, Cupit L, Cihon F, O'Leary J, Reck M (2009) Phase II, multicenter, uncontrolled trial of single-agent sorafenib in patients with relapsed or refractory, advanced non-small-cell lung cancer. *J Clin Oncol*, 27: 4274–80.

90 Kim E, Herbst R, Wistuba I, Lee J, Blumenschein G, Tsao A, Stewart D, Hicks M, Erasmus J, Gupta S, *et al.* (2011) The BATTLE trial (Biomarker-integrated Approaches of Targeted Therapy for Lung Cancer Elimination): Personalizing therapy for lung cancer. *Cancer Discovery*, 1: 43–51.

91 Molina J, Dy G, Foster N, Allen Ziegler K, Adjei A, Rowland K, Aubry M, Flynn P, Mandrekar S, Schild S, *et al.* (2011) A randomized phase II study of pemetrexed (PEM) with or without sorafenib (S) as second-line therapy in advanced non-small cell lung cancer (NSCLC) of nonsquamous histology: NCCTG N0626 study. *J Clin Oncol*, 29: (suppl; abstr 7513).

92 Spigel DR, Burris HA, 3rd, Greco FA, Shipley DL, Friedman EK, Waterhouse DM, Whorf RC, Mitchell RB, Daniel DB, Zangmeister J, *et al.* (2011) Randomized, double-blind, placebo-controlled, phase II trial of sorafenib and erlotinib or erlotinib alone in previously treated advanced non-small-cell lung cancer. *Journal of Clinical Oncology*, 29: 2582–9.

93 Lind JS, Dingemans AM, Groen HJ, Thunnissen FB, Bekers O, Heideman DA, Honeywell RJ, Giovannetti E, Peters GJ, Postmus PE, *et al.* (2010) A multicenter phase II study of erlotinib and sorafenib in chemotherapy-naive patients with advanced non-small cell lung cancer. *Clinical Cancer Research*, 16: 3078–87.

94 Gridelli C, Morgillo F, Favaretto A, de Marinis F, Chella A, Cerea G, Mattioli R, Tortora G, Rossi A, Fasano M, *et al.* (2011) Sorafenib in combination with erlotinib or with gemcitabine in elderly patients with advanced non-small-cell lung cancer: a randomized phase II study. *Annals of Oncology*, 22: 1528–34.

95 Scagliotti GV, Parikh P, von Pawel J, Biesma B, Vansteenkiste J, Manegold C, Serwatowski P, Gatzemeier U, Digumarti R, Zukin M, *et al.* (2008) Phase III study comparing cisplatin plus gemcitabine with cisplatin plus pemetrexed in chemotherapy-naive patients with advanced-stage non-small-cell lung cancer. *J Clin Oncol*, 26: 3543–51.

96 Wells SA, Jr, Gosnell JE, Gagel RF, Moley J, Pfister D, Sosa JA, Skinner M, Krebs A, Vasselli J, Schlumberger M (2010) Vandetanib for the treatment of patients with locally advanced or metastatic hereditary medullary thyroid cancer. *Journal of Clinical Oncology*, 28: 767–72.

97 Wedge SR, Ogilvie DJ, Dukes M, Kendrew J, Chester R, Jackson JA, Boffey SJ, Valentine PJ, Curwen JO, Musgrove HL, *et al.* (2002) ZD6474 inhibits vascular endothelial growth factor signaling, angiogenesis, and tumor growth following oral administration. *Cancer Research*, 62: 4645–55.

98 Heymach JV, Paz-Ares L, De Braud F, Sebastian M, Stewart DJ, Eberhardt WE, Ranade AA, Cohen G, Trigo JM, Sandler AB, *et al.* (2008) Randomized phase II study of vandetanib alone or with paclitaxel and carboplatin as first-line treatment for advanced non-small-cell lung cancer. *J Clin Oncol*, 26: 5407–15.

99 Heymach JV, Johnson BE, Prager D, Csada E, Roubec J, Pesek M, Spasova I, Belani CP, Bodrogi I, Gadgeel S, *et al.* (2007) Randomized, placebo-controlled phase II study of vandetanib plus docetaxel in previously treated non small-cell lung cancer. *J Clin Oncol*, 25: 4270–7.

100 Natale RB, Bodkin D, Govindan R, Sleckman BG, Rizvi NA, Capo A, Germonpre P, Eberhardt WE, Stockman PK, Kennedy SJ, *et al.* (2009) Vandetanib versus gefitinib in patients with advanced non-small-cell lung cancer: Results from a two-part, double-blind, randomized phase II Study. *J Clin Oncol*, 27: 2523–9.

101 de Boer RH, Arrieta O, Yang CH, Gottfried M, Chan V, Raats J, de Marinis F, Abratt RP, Wolf J, Blackhall FH, *et al.* (2011) Vandetanib plus pemetrexed for the second-line treatment of advanced non-small-cell lung cancer: A randomized, double-blind phase III trial. *Journal of Clinical Oncology*, 29: 1067–74.

102 Herbst RS, Sun Y, Eberhardt WE, Germonpre P, Saijo N, Zhou C, Wang J, Li L, Kabbinavar F, Ichinose Y, *et al.* (2010) Vandetanib plus docetaxel versus docetaxel as second-line treatment for patients with advanced non-small-cell lung cancer (ZODIAC): A double-blind, randomised, phase 3 trial. *Lancet Oncol*, 11: 619–26.

103 Natale RB, Thongprasert S, Greco FA, Thomas M, Tsai CM, Sunpaweravong P, Ferry D, Mulatero C, Whorf R, Thompson J, *et al.* (2011) Phase III trial of vandetanib compared with erlotinib in patients with previously treated advanced non-small-cell lung cancer. *J Clin Oncol*, 29: 1059–66.

104 Lee JS, Hirsh V, Park K, Qin S, Blajman CR, Perng RP, Chen YM, Emerson L, Langmuir P, Manegold C (2012) Vandetanib versus placebo in patients with advanced non-small-cell lung cancer after prior therapy with an epidermal growth factor receptor tyrosine kinase inhibitor: a randomized, double-blind phase III trial (ZEPHYR). *Journal of Clinical Oncology*, 30: 1114–21.

105 Wedge SR, Kendrew J, Hennequin LF, Valentine PJ, Barry ST, Brave SR, Smith NR, James NH, Dukes M, Curwen JO, *et al.* (2005) AZD2171: A highly potent, orally bioavailable, vascular endothelial growth factor receptor-2 tyrosine kinase inhibitor for the treatment of cancer. *Cancer Res*, 65: 4389–4400.

106 Laurie SA, Gauthier I, Arnold A, Shepherd FA, Ellis PM, Chen E, Goss G, Powers J, Walsh W, Tu D, *et al.* (2008) Phase I and pharmacokinetic study of daily oral AZD2171, an inhibitor of vascular endothelial growth factor tyrosine kinases, in combination with carboplatin and paclitaxel in patients with advanced non-small-cell lung cancer: the National Cancer Institute of Canada clinical trials group. *Journal of Clinical Oncology*, 26: 1871–8.

107 Goss GD, Arnold A, Shepherd FA, Dediu M, Ciuleanu TE, Fenton D, Zukin M, Walde D, Laberge F, Vincent MD, *et al.* (2010) Randomized, double-blind trial of carboplatin and paclitaxel with either daily oral cediranib or placebo in advanced non-small-cell lung cancer: NCIC clinical trials group BR24 study. *J Clin Oncol*, 28: 49–55.

108 Laurie S, Solomon B, Seymour L, Ellis P, Goss G, Shepherd F, Boyer M, Arnold A, Clingan P, Laberge F, *et al.* (2012) A randomized double-blind trial of carboplatin plus paclitaxel (CP) with daily oral cediranib (CED), an inhibitor of vascular endothelial growth factor receptors, or placebo (PLA) in patients (pts) with previously untreated advanced non-small cell lung cancer (NSCLC): NCIC Clinical Trials Group study BR29. *Journal of Clinical Oncology; 2012 ASCO Annual Meeting Proceedings*.

109 Dy GK, Mandrekar SJ, Nelson GD, Meyers JP, Adjei AA, Ross HJ, Ansari RH, Lyss AP, Stella PJ, Schild SE, *et al.* (2013) A randomized phase II Study of gemcitabine and carboplatin with or without cediranib as first-line therapy in advanced non-small-cell lung cancer: North Central Cancer Treatment Group Study N0528. *Journal of Thoracic Oncology*, 8: 79–88.

110 Kumar R, Knick VB, Rudolph SK, Johnson JH, Crosby RM, Crouthamel MC, Hopper TM, Miller CG, Harrington LE, Onori JA, *et al.* (2007) Pharmacokinetic-pharmacodynamic correlation from mouse to human with pazopanib, a multikinase angiogenesis inhibitor with potent antitumor and antiangiogenic activity. *Molecular Cancer Therapeutics*, 6: 2012–21.

111 Altorki N, Lane ME, Bauer T, Lee PC, Guarino MJ, Pass H, Felip E, Peylan-Ramu N, Gurpide A, Grannis FW, *et al.* (2010) Phase II proof-of-concept study of pazopanib monotherapy in treatment-naive patients with stage I/II resectable non-small-cell lung cancer. *Journal of Clinical Oncology*, 28: 3131–7.

112 Ellis PM, Al-Saleh K (2012) Multitargeted anti-angiogenic agents and NSCLC: Clinical update and future directions. *Critical Reviews in Oncology/Hematology*, 84: 47–58.

113 Choueiri TK (2008) Axitinib, a novel anti-angiogenic drug with promising activity in various solid tumors. *Current Opinion in Investigational Drugs*, 9: 658–71.

114 Schiller JH, Larson T, Ou SH, Limentani S, Sandler A, Vokes E, Kim S, Liau K, Bycott P, Olszanski AJ, *et al.* (2009) Efficacy and safety of axitinib in patients with advanced non-small-cell lung cancer: Results from a phase II study. *Journal of Clinical Oncology*, 27: 3836–41.

115 Polverino A, Coxon A, Starnes C, Diaz Z, DeMelfi T, Wang L, Bready J, Estrada J, Cattley R, Kaufman S, *et al.* (2006) AMG 706, an oral, multikinase inhibitor that selectively targets vascular endothelial growth factor, platelet-derived growth factor, and kit receptors, potently inhibits angiogenesis and induces regression in tumor xenografts. *Cancer Research*, 66: 8715–21.

116 Blumenschein GR, Jr, Reckamp K, Stephenson GJ, O'Rourke T, Gladish G, McGreivy J, Sun YN, Ye Y, Parson M, Sandler A (2010) Phase 1b study of motesanib, an oral angiogenesis inhibitor, in combination with carboplatin/paclitaxel and/or panitumumab for the treatment of advanced non-small cell lung cancer. *Clinical Cancer Research*, 16: 279–90.

117 Hilberg F, Roth GJ, Krssak M, Kautschitsch S, Sommergruber W, Tontsch-Grunt U, Garin-Chesa P, Bader G, Zoephel A, Quant J, *et al.* (2008) BIBF 1120: Triple angiokinase inhibitor with sustained receptor blockade and good antitumor efficacy. *Cancer Research*, 68: 4774–82.

118 Reck M, Kaiser R, Eschbach C, Stefanic M, Love J, Gatzemeier U, Stopfer P, von Pawel J (2011) A phase II double-blind study to investigate efficacy and safety of two doses of the triple angiokinase inhibitor BIBF 1120 in patients with relapsed advanced non-small-cell lung cancer. *Annals of Oncology*, 22: 1374–81.

119 Thorpe PE (2004) Vascular targeting agents as cancer therapeutics. *Clinical Cancer Research*, 10: 415–27.

120 McKeage MJ, Von Pawel J, Reck M, Jameson MB, Rosenthal MA, Sullivan R, Gibbs D, Mainwaring PN, Serke M, Lafitte JJ, *et al.* (2008) Randomised phase II study of ASA404 combined with carboplatin and paclitaxel in previously untreated advanced non-small cell lung cancer. *British Journal of Cancer*, 99: 2006–12.

121 Lara PN, Jr, Douillard JY, Nakagawa K, von Pawel J, McKeage MJ, Albert I, Losonczy G, Reck M, Heo DS, Fan X, *et al.* (2011) Randomized phase III placebo-controlled trial of carboplatin and paclitaxel with or without the vascular disrupting agent vadimezan (ASA404) in advanced non-small-cell lung cancer. *Journal of Clinical Oncology*, 29: 2965–71.

122 Rudin CM, Mauer A, Smakal M, Juergens R, Spelda S, Wertheim M, Coates A, McKeegan E, Ansell P, Zhou X, *et al.* (2011) Phase I/II study of pemetrexed with or without ABT-751 in advanced or metastatic non-small-cell lung cancer. *Journal of Clinical Oncology*, 29: 1075–82.

123 Pujol JL, Breton JL, Gervais R, Tanguy ML, Quoix E, David P, Janicot H, Westeel V, Gameroff S, Geneve J, *et al.* (2007) Phase III double-blind, placebo-controlled study of thalidomide in extensive-disease small-cell lung cancer after response to chemotherapy: An intergroup study FNCLCC cleo04 IFCT 00–01. *Journal of Clinical Oncology*, 25: 3945–51.

124 Horn L, Dahlberg SE, Sandler AB, Dowlati A, Moore DF, Murren JR, Schiller JH (2009) Phase II study of cisplatin plus etoposide and bevacizumab for previously untreated, extensive-stage small-cell lung cancer: Eastern Cooperative Oncology Group Study E3501. *Journal of Clinical Oncology*, 27: 6006–11.

125 Spigel DR, Hainsworth JD, Simons L, Meng C, Burris HA, 3rd, Yardley DA, Grapski R, Schreeder M, Mallidi PV, Greco FA (2007) Irinotecan, carboplatin, and imatinib in untreated extensive-stage small-cell lung cancer: A phase II trial of the Minnie Pearl Cancer Research Network. *J Thorac Oncol*, 2: 854–61.

126 Ready NE, Dudek AZ, Pang HH, Hodgson LD, Graziano SL, Green MR, Vokes EE (2011) Cisplatin, irinotecan, and bevacizumab for untreated extensive-stage small-cell lung cancer: CALGB 30306, a phase II study. *Journal of Clinical Oncology*, 29: 4436–41.

127 Spigel DR, Townley PM, Waterhouse DM, Fang L, Adiguzel I, Huang JE, Karlin DA, Faoro L, Scappaticci FA, Socinski MA (2011) Randomized phase II study of bevacizumab in combination with chemotherapy in previously untreated extensive-stage small-cell lung cancer: results from the SALUTE trial. *Journal of Clinical Oncology*, 29: 2215–22.

128 Mountzios G, Emmanouilidis C, Vardakis N, Kontopodis E, Hatzidaki D, Popis E, Karachaliou N, Kotsakis A, Agelidou M, Georgoulias V (2012) Paclitaxel plus bevacizumab in patients with chemoresistant relapsed small cell lung cancer as salvage treatment: a phase II multicenter study of the Hellenic Oncology Research Group. *Lung Cancer*, 77: 146–50.

129 Patton J, Spigel D, Greco F, Liggett W, Zubkus J, Baskette M, Schreeder M, Woytowitz D, Nelson E, Hainsworth J (2006) Irinotecan (I), carboplatin (C), and radiotherapy (RT) followed by maintenance bevacizumab (B) in the treatment (tx) of limited-stage small cell lung cancer (LS-SCLC): Update of a phase II trial of the Minnie Pearl Cancer Research Network. *J Clin Oncol, 2006 ASCO Annual Meeting Proceedings*, 24: 7085.

130 Norden-Zfoni A, Desai J, Manola J, Beaudry P, Force J, Maki R, Folkman J, Bello C, Baum C, DePrimo SE, *et al.* (2007) Blood-based biomarkers of SU11248 activity and clinical outcome in patients with metastatic imatinib-resistant gastrointestinal stromal tumor. *Clin Cancer Res*, 13: 2643–50.

131 Launay-Vacher V, Deray G (2009) Hypertension and proteinuria: a class-effect of antiangiogenic therapies. *Anti-Cancer Drugs*, 20: 81–2.

132 Izzedine H, Ederhy S, Goldwasser F, Soria JC, Milano G, Cohen A, Khayat D, Spano JP (2009) Management of hypertension in angiogenesis inhibitor-treated patients. *Annals of Oncology*, 20: 807–15.

133 Dahlberg SE, Sandler AB, Brahmer JR, Schiller JH, Johnson DH (2010) Clinical course of advanced non-small-cell lung cancer patients experiencing hypertension during treatment with bevacizumab in combination with carboplatin and paclitaxel on ECOG 4599. *Journal of Clinical Oncology*, 28: 949–54.

134 Rini BI, Schiller JH, Fruehauf JP, Cohen EE, Tarazi JC, Rosbrook B, Bair AH, Ricart AD, Olszanski AJ, Letrent KJ, *et al.* (2011) Diastolic blood pressure as a biomarker of axitinib efficacy in solid tumors. *Clinical Cancer Research*, 17: 3841–9.

135 Ebos JM, Lee CR, Christensen JG, Mutsaers AJ, Kerbel RS (2007) Multiple circulating proangiogenic factors induced by sunitinib malate are tumor-independent and correlate with antitumor efficacy. *Proc Natl Acad Sci USA*, 104: 17069–74.

136 Batchelor TT, Sorensen AG, di Tomaso E, Zhang WT, Duda DG, Cohen KS, Kozak KR, Cahill DP, Chen PJ,

Zhu M, *et al.* (2007) AZD2171, a pan-VEGF receptor tyrosine kinase inhibitor, normalizes tumor vasculature and alleviates edema in glioblastoma patients. *Cancer Cell*, 11: 83–95.

137 Nikolinakos PG, Altorki N, Yankelevitz D, Tran HT, Yan S, Rajagopalan D, Bordogna W, Ottesen LH, Heymach JV (2010) Plasma cytokine and angiogenic factor profiling identifies markers associated with tumor shrinkage in early-stage non-small cell lung cancer patients treated with pazopanib. *Cancer Res*, 70: 2171–9.

138 Hanrahan EO, Lin HY, Kim ES, Yan S, Du DZ, McKee KS, Tran HT, Lee JJ, Ryan AJ, Langmuir P, *et al.* (2010) Distinct patterns of cytokine and angiogenic factor modulation and markers of benefit for vandetanib and/or chemotherapy in patients with non-small-cell lung cancer. *Journal of Clinical Oncology*, 28: 193–201.

139 Hanrahan E, Lin H, Du D, Yan S, Kim E, Lee J, Ryan A, Tran H, Johnson B, Heymach J (2007) Correlative analyses of plasma cytokine / angiogenic factor (C/AF) profile, gender and outcome in a randomized, three-arm, phase II trial of 1st-line vandetanib (VAN) and/or carboplatin plus paclitaxel (CP) for advanced non small cell lung cancer (NSCLC). *J Clin Oncol, 2007 ASCO Annual Meeting Proocedings*, 25: 7593.

140 Cascone T, Herynk MH, Xu L, Kadara H, Hanrahan EO, Saigal B, Lee JJ, Langley RR, *et al.* (2010) Increased HGF is associated with resistance to VEGFR tyrosine kinase inhibitors (TKIs) in non-small cell lung cancer (NSCLC). *AACR Annual Meeting* #376.

141 Dowlati A, Gray R, Sandler AB, Schiller JH, Johnson DH (2008) Cell adhesion molecules, vascular endothelial growth factor, and basic fibroblast growth factor in patients with non-small cell lung cancer treated with chemotherapy with or without bevacizumab – an Eastern Cooperative Oncology Group Study. *Clin Cancer Res*, 14: 1407–12.

142 Heist RS, Zhai R, Liu G, Zhou W, Lin X, Su L, Asomaning K, Lynch TJ, Wain JC, Christiani DC (2008) VEGF polymorphisms and survival in early-stage non-small-cell lung cancer. *Journal of Clinical Oncology*, 26: 856–62.

143 Zhang W, Dahlberg S, Yang D, Sandler A, Brahmer J, Schiller J, Carbone D, Johnson D, Lenz H (2009) Genetic variants in angiogenesis pathway associated with clinical outcome in NSCLC patients (pts) treated with bevacizumab in combination with carboplatin and paclitaxel: Subset pharmacogenetic analysis of ECOG 4599. *J Clin Oncol*, 27: abstr 8032.

144 Wakelee HA, Lee JW, Hanna NH, Traynor AM, Carbone DP, Schiller JH (2012) A double-blind randomized discontinuation phase-II study of sorafenib (BAY 43–9006) in previously treated non-small-cell lung cancer patients: Eastern cooperative oncology group study E2501. *Journal of Thoracic Oncology*, 7: 1574–82.

145 Zhang W, Lee J, Schiller J, Carbone D, Chung C, Lenz H (2010) Use of germline polymorphisms in VEGF to predict tumor response and progression-free survival in non-small cell lung cancer (NSCLC) patients treated with sorafenib: subset pharmacogenetic analysis of Eastern Cooperative Oncology Group (ECOG) trial E2501. In: *Proc Am Soc Clin Oncol*, 28 (suppl): abstr 7607.

146 Trivella M, Pezzella F, Pastorino U, Harris AL, Altman DG (2007) Microvessel density as a prognostic factor in non-small-cell lung carcinoma: a meta-analysis of individual patient data. *Lancet Oncol*, 8: 488–99.

147 Sessa C, Guibal A, Del Conte G, Ruegg C (2008) Biomarkers of angiogenesis for the development of antiangiogenic therapies in oncology: tools or decorations? *Nat Clin Pract Oncol*, 5: 378–91.

148 Mancuso P, Burlini A, Pruneri G, Goldhirsch A, Martinelli G, Bertolini F (2001) Resting and activated endothelial cells are increased in the peripheral blood of cancer patients. *Blood*, 97: 3658–61.

149 Goon PK, Lip GY, Stonelake PS, Blann AD (2009) Circulating endothelial cells and circulating progenitor cells in breast cancer: relationship to endothelial damage/dysfunction/apoptosis, clinicopathologic factors, and the Nottingham Prognostic Index. *Neoplasia*, 11: 771–9.

150 Bertolini F, Shaked Y, Mancuso P, Kerbel RS (2006) The multifaceted circulating endothelial cell in cancer: towards marker and target identification. *Nat Rev Cancer*, 6: 835–45.

151 Mancuso P, Calleri A, Cassi C, Gobbi A, Capillo M, Pruneri G, Martinelli G, Bertolini F (2003) Circulating endothelial cells as a novel marker of angiogenesis. *Adv Exp Med Biol*, 522: 83–97.

152 Ronzoni M, Manzoni M, Mariucci S, Loupakis F, Brugnatelli S, Bencardino K, Rovati B, Tinelli C, Falcone A, Villa E, *et al.* (2010). Circulating endothelial cells and endothelial progenitors as predictive markers of clinical response to bevacizumab-based first-line treatment in advanced colorectal cancer patients. *Annals of Oncology*, 21: 2382–9.

153 Dellapasqua S, Bertolini F, Bagnardi V, Campagnoli E, Scarano E, Torrisi R, Shaked Y, Mancuso P, Goldhirsch A, Rocca A, *et al.* (2008) Metronomic

cyclophosphamide and capecitabine combined with bevacizumab in advanced breast cancer. *Journal of Clinical Oncology*, 26: 4899–4905.

154 Casanovas O, Hicklin DJ, Bergers G, Hanahan D (2005) Drug resistance by evasion of antiangiogenic targeting of VEGF signaling in late-stage pancreatic islet tumors. *Cancer Cell*, 8: 299–309.

155 Graeber TG, Osmanian C, Jacks T, Housman DE, Koch CJ, Lowe SW, Giaccia AJ (1996) Hypoxia-mediated selection of cells with diminished apoptotic potential in solid tumours. *Nature*, 379: 88–91.

156 Yu JL, Rak JW, Coomber BL, Hicklin DJ, Kerbel RS (2002) Effect of p53 status on tumor response to antiangiogenic therapy. *Science*, 295: 1526–8.

157 Leenders WP, Kusters B, Verrijp K, Maass C, Wesseling P, Heerschap A, Ruiter D, Ryan A, de Waal R (2004) Antiangiogenic therapy of cerebral melanoma metastases results in sustained tumor progression via vessel co-option. *Clin Cancer Res*, 10: 6222–30.

158 Shojaei F, Wu X, Malik AK, Zhong C, Baldwin ME, Schanz S, Fuh G, Gerber HP, Ferrara N (2007) Tumor refractoriness to anti-VEGF treatment is mediated by CD11b+Gr1+ myeloid cells. *Nat Biotechnol*, 25: 911–20.

159 Ferrara N (2010) Role of myeloid cells in vascular endothelial growth factor-independent tumor angiogenesis. *Curr Opin Hematol*, 17: 219–24.

160 Crawford Y, Kasman I, Yu L, Zhong C, Wu X, Modrusan Z, Kaminker J, Ferrara N (2009) PDGF-C mediates the angiogenic and tumorigenic properties of fibroblasts associated with tumors refractory to anti-VEGF treatment. *Cancer Cell*, 15: 21–34.

161 Ebos JM, Kerbel RS (2011) Antiangiogenic therapy: impact on invasion, disease progression, and metastasis. *Nat Rev Clin Oncol*, 8: 210–21.

162 Weis SM, Cheresh DA (2011) Tumor angiogenesis: Molecular pathways and therapeutic targets. *Nature Medicine*, 17: 1359–70.

163 Casanovas O (2011) The adaptive stroma joining the antiangiogenic resistance front. *J Clin Invest*, 121: 1244–7.

CHAPTER 34

Anti-angiogenic Agents in Metastatic NSCLC

Millie Das[1,2] *and Heather Wakelee*[2]
[1]VA Palo Alto Heath Care System, Palo Alto, CA, USA
[2]Division of Oncology, Stanford University/Stanford Cancer Institute, Stanford, CA, USA

Introduction

Since the discovery that angiogenesis plays a critical role in tumor growth and progression, there has been considerable interest in developing anti-angiogenic agents for the treatment of various malignancies, including non-small cell lung cancer (NSCLC) [1]. Vascular endothelial growth factor (VEGF) is one of the key mediators of angiogenesis and has emerged as an important therapeutic target in NSCLC. The VEGF family consists of 5 glycoproteins (VEGF-A, VEGF-B, VEGF-C, VEGF-D, and placental growth factor) that bind to three tyrosine kinase receptors: VEGF receptor 1 (VEGFR-1)/fms-like tyrosine kinase I (flt1), VEGFR-2/kinase insert domain receptor (KDR), and VEGFR-3/flt4. Ligand receptor binding results in downstream signaling that leads to endothelial cell proliferation and migration, as well as increased permeability of existing blood vessels [2]. Anti-angiogenic agents being studied in NSCLC include monoclonal antibodies against VEGF, tyrosine kinase inhibitors (TKIs) directed at VEGF receptors, as well as vascular disrupting agents (VDAs) which do not involve inhibition of VEGF (Table 34.1). This chapter reviews the data for a number of these different anti-angiogenic therapies in NSCLC.

Monoclonal antibodies to VEGF/VEGFR

Bevacizumab

Bevacizumab, a humanized monoclonal antibody to VEGF-A, remains the only anti-angiogenic agent that has been approved by the United States Federal Drug Administration (FDA) for the treatment of NSCLC. Approval was granted based upon the results of a number of key studies. In the initial phase II study, 99 patients were randomized into 3 treatment arms: chemotherapy (carboplatin/paclitaxel) alone, chemotherapy plus bevacizumab 7.5 mg/kg, and chemotherapy plus bevacizumab 15 mg/kg. Patients receiving bevacizumab plus chemotherapy arm were allowed to continue bevacizumab monotherapy for up to 18 cycles after completion of the chemotherapy. Importantly, patients in the chemotherapy alone arm who progressed were allowed to crossover and receive bevacizumab at the time of progression. Results indicated that both overall response rate (ORR) (31.5% vs. 18.8%) and progression-free survival (PFS) (7.4 months vs. 4.2 months, $p = 0.023$) were superior in the high-dose bevacizumab arm compared to the chemotherapy alone arm, although overall survival (OS) was not statistically different between the

Lung Cancer, Fourth Edition. Edited by Jack A. Roth, Waun Ki Hong and Ritsuko U. Komaki.

Table 34.1 Specific targets of investigational antiangiogenic agents

Tumor cells	VEGF ligand	Vasculature/ endothelial cell
TKIs	Bevacizumab	VDAs
Ramucirumab	Aflibercept	TKIs

TKI, tyrosine kinase inhibitor; VDA, vascular disrupting agent; VEGF, vascular endothelial growth factor.

two arms (17.7 vs. 14.9 months, p = 0.63). Additionally, low-dose bevacizumab did not appear to confer any advantages over chemotherapy alone. The lack of OS benefit may be explained by the relatively small number of patients in this trial and the ability to crossover to maintenance bevacizumab. In this study, pulmonary hemorrhage was observed in 9.0% of patients, including 4 fatalities, which occurred mainly in patients with squamous histology [3], who coincidentally tended to be in the low dose bevacizumab arm. Given the association of bleeding with squamous histology seen in this trial, subsequent phase III trials investigating bevacizumab excluded patients with squamous histology. Based upon the encouraging phase II data, frontline bevacizumab-based therapy has been evaluated in a number of different phase III studies (Table 34.2).

Eastern Cooperative Group (ECOG) 4599 was a landmark phase III study that randomized 878 patients with recurrent or advanced NSCLC to receive first-line chemotherapy consisting of carboplatin/paclitaxel with or without bevacizumab 15 mg/kg given every 3 weeks. No crossover was allowed, and patients with squamous histology, brain metastases, and significant hemoptysis were excluded from this trial. Both ORR (35% vs. 15%, p < 0.001) and PFS (6.2 months vs. 4.5 months, HR: 0.66; 95% CI: 0.57–0.77; p < 0.001) were improved in those patients receiving bevacizumab compared to chemotherapy alone. Additionally, the primary endpoint of OS was also significantly improved in patients receiving bevacizumab (12.3 months vs. 10.3 months; HR: 0.79; 95% CI: 0.67–0.92; p = 0.003). However, bevacizumab was also associated with increased toxicities, including higher rates of hemorrhage and febrile neutropenia, as well as a higher incidence of death (15 deaths compared to 2 deaths in the chemotherapy alone arm) [4].

Table 34.2 Results of frontline bevacizumab-based therapy in phase III studies of NSCLC

Trial	Regimen	Progression-free survival (PFS)	Overall survival (OS)
ECOG 4599 (4)	Carboplatin/paclitaxel	4.5 mos	10.3 mos
	Carboplatin/paclitaxel/bevacizumab	6.2 mos	12.3 mos
		HR: 0.66, p < 0.001	HR: 0.79, p = 0.003
AVAiL (6) (7)	Cisplatin/gemcitabine	6.1 mos	13.1 mos
	Cisplatin/gemcitabine/bevacizumab	6.5 mos	13.4 mos
		HR: 0.82, p = 0.03	HR: 1.03, p = 0.761
POINTBREAK (12)	Carboplatin/paclitaxel/bevacizumab→	5.6 mos	13.4 mos
	Bevacizumab maintenance	6.0 mos	12.6 mos
	Carboplatin/pemetrexed/bevacizumab→	HR: 0.83, p = 0.012	HR: 1.00, p = 0.949
	Pemetrexed/bevacizumab maintenance		
AVAPERL (13)	Cisplatin/pemetrexed/bevacizumab→	6.6 mos	15.7 mos
	Bevacizumab maintenance	10.2 mos	Not reached
	Cisplatin/pemetrexed/bevacizumab→	HR: 0.50, p < 0.001	HR: 0.75, p = 0.23
	Bevacizumab/pemetrexed maintenance		
ATLAS (14) (15)	Platinum-based chemotherapy→	3.7 mos	14.4 mos
	Bevacizumab maintenance	4.8 mos	13.3 mos
	Platinum-based chemotherapy→	HR: 0.72, p = 0.0012	HR: 0.92, p = 0.56
	Bevacizumab/erlotinib maintenance		

In particular, those patients over the age of 70 who received bevacizumab had significantly greater grade 3–5 toxicities compared to those receiving chemotherapy alone (87% vs. 61%, $p < 0.001$), though the ORR and PFS benefit was still seen, arguing for caution with bevacizumab in this subgroup of patients [5]. Despite these limitations, ECOG 4599 was the first trial to demonstrate a survival benefit in patients with advanced NSCLC receiving an anti-angiogenic agent and was important in leading to approval of bevacizumab in the treatment of NSCLC.

The AVAiL phase III trial randomized 1043 patients with recurrent or advanced NSCLC to receive cisplatin/gemcitabine with or without bevacizumab (7.5 or 15 mg/kg). All three drugs were given on day 1 of each 3-week cycle, with additional day 8 gemcitabine. Although the primary endpoint of PFS was significantly improved in patients receiving bevacizumab at both the low dose (6.7 months; HR: 0.75; $p = 0.003$) and the high dose (6.5 months; HR: 0.82, $p = 0.03$) compared to those patients receiving chemotherapy alone (6.1 months), OS was not significantly prolonged in either bevacizumab arm (low-dose: 13.6 months; HR: 0.93; $p = 0.420$ and high-dose: 13.4 months; HR: 1.03; $p = 0.761$) compared to the chemotherapy alone arm (13.1 months) [6, 7]. The relatively high percentage (61–65%) of patients who went on to receive additional post-study treatment may explain the lack of OS benefit seen in this trial [8]. Importantly, this study also indicated that bevacizumab can be safely administered in patients on full-dose anticoagulation as 9% of the patients in this study received therapeutic anticoagulation with either warfarin or low molecular weight heparin after initiation of the trial, and none of these patients developed pulmonary hemorrhage.

In order to further evaluate the safety and efficacy of bevacizumab in NSCLC, there have been a number of other completed and ongoing studies. The PASSPORT study showed that bevacizumab can be administered safely in patients with treated brain metastases [9]. The Phase IV Safety of Avastin in Lung (SAiL) trial evaluated bevacizumab in combination with a number of different chemotherapeutic agents. In this study, patients receiving cisplatin doublets plus bevacizumab had improved OS (14.7 months) compared to patients receiving carboplatin doublets plus bevacizumab (14.3 months), non-platinum doublets plus bevacizumab (8.1 months), or single-agent chemotherapy plus bevacizumab (9.4 months). Grade ≥ 3 pulmonary hemorrhage was noted in 1% of patients, and grade 3–5 bleeding (excluding pulmonary hemorrhage) was noted in 3% of patients [10]. Another study found that bevacizumab is efficacious in combination with other commonly used platinum doublets, including carboplatin/pemetrexed [11]. The recently completed phase III POINTBREAK trial compared 2 arms: carboplatin/pemetrexed/bevacizumab induction followed by pemetrexed/bevacizumab maintenance (arm A) and carboplatin/paclitaxel/bevacizumab induction followed by bevacizumab maintenance (arm B) in patients with advanced non-squamous NSCLC. Results indicated that the primary endpoint of OS was not different between the two arms of treatment (12.6 months on arm A, 13.4 months on arm B, HR: 1.00, $p = 0.949$), and that the secondary endpoints of ORR (34.1% versus 33.0%, arms A and B respectively) and disease control rate (DCR) (65.9% versus 69.8%, arms A and B respectively) were also not significantly different [12]. The AVAPERL trial is another recently completed study that compared bevacizumab maintenance and bevacizumab/pemetrexed maintenance in patients who completed four cycles of cisplatin/pemetrexed/bevacizumab. PFS was significantly improved in those patients receiving bevacizumab/pemetrexed maintenance compared to bevacizumab alone maintenance (10.2 months versus 6.6 months, $p < 0.001$), and preliminary OS data at 11 months of follow-up shows a non-statistically significant trend toward improvement in OS for the bevacizumab/pemetrexed arm ($HR = 0.75$, $p = 0.23$) [13]. The ongoing ECOG 5508 trial is looking at bevacizumab maintenance questions in advanced stage NSCLC patients. Patients on the trial receive the E4599 regimen for 4 cycles and those with stable disease are then randomized to continue on bevacizumab alone, receive pemetrexed (500 mg/m2 q 3 weeks) or both agents until documented progression or intolerable toxicity. Bevacizumab is now also being evaluated in the early stage setting in the ongoing phase III ECOG 1505 study, randomizing patients with stages I-III resected NSCLC to receive 4 cycles of adjuvant cisplatin-based chemotherapy with or without bevacizumab. The study has now completed accrual and, an interim safety analysis revealed no unexpected toxicity concerns [14].

There has been enthusiasm in investigating bevacizumab in combination with other targeted therapies, including erlotinib, an oral epidermal growth factor receptor (EGFR) inhibitor, in both the maintenance and second-line setting. In the phase III ATLAS study, patients with advanced NSCLC who had completed 4 cycles of platinum-based chemotherapy were randomized to receive maintenance bevacizumab (15 mg/kg) plus erlotinib (150 mg daily) versus maintenance bevacizumab plus placebo. Although the primary endpoint of PFS was improved in those patients receiving maintenance bevacizumab/erlotinib compared to those receiving maintenance bevacizumab/placebo (4.8 months vs. 3.7 months; HR: 0.72; $p = 0.0012$) [15], the secondary endpoint of OS was not improved in the bevacizumab/erlotinib arm (14.4 months vs. 13.3 months; 95% CI: 0.70–1.21; $p = 0.56$) [16]. A phase II second-line trial randomized patients to one of 3 arms: erlotinib plus bevacizumab, chemotherapy (docetaxel or pemetrexed) plus bevacizumab, and chemotherapy alone. Median PFS was improved with the addition of bevacizumab to either chemotherapy (4.8 months) or erlotinib (4.4 months) in comparison with chemotherapy alone (3 months) [17]. The phase III BETA trial randomized 636 patients with progressive disease after frontline chemotherapy to receive erlotinib with or without bevacizumab. Despite PFS prolongation seen with the combination therapy (3.4 months vs. 1.7 months; HR: 0.62; $p < 0.0001$), the primary endpoint of OS was not different between the two arms (9.3 months vs. 9.2 months; HR: 0.97; $p = 0.75$) [18]. Finally, results from a phase I/II trial of bevacizumab and erlotinib in the combined-modality treatment of stage III NSCLC were reported with the finding that 29% of the 45 patients enrolled developed grade 3 or 4 esophagitis, including tracheoesophageal fistula, without significant improvement in efficacy [19].

Ramucirumab

Ramucirumab (IMC-1121B) is a monoclonal antibody against VEGFR-2 that has been studied in early clinical trials in several types of malignancies, including NSCLC. A single-arm phase II study involving patients with advanced NSCLC evaluated ramucirumab in combination with carboplatin/paclitaxel as frontline treatment and found that ramucirumab was associated with an ORR of 59% and DCR of 97% [20]. These exciting results have led to additional studies of ramucirumab in metastatic NSCLC, including a phase II trial in which patients are randomized to treatment based upon histology; patients with nonsquamous histology receive platinum/pemetrexed +/− ramucirumab × 4–6 cycles, followed by maintenance pemetrexed in both arms while patients with squamous histology receive platinum/gemcitabine +/− ramucirumab × 4–6 cycles, followed by maintenance ramucirumab in the ramucirumab arm. The nonsquamous enrollment has completed and the squamous enrollment in ongoing (ClinicalTrials.gov identifier: NCT 01160744). The phase III REVEL study is also underway, enrolling patients with metastatic NSCLC who have progressed after receiving frontline platinum-based therapy and randomizing them to receive docetaxel +/− ramucirumab (ClinicalTrials.gov identifier: NCT 01168973).

Small molecule tyrosine kinase inhibitors

There are several anti-angiogenic small molecule tyrosine kinase inhibitors (TKIs) in current clinical development in NSCLC. Advantages of TKIs include the fact that they inhibit multiple receptors simultaneously, thereby potentially providing a higher likelihood of single-agent activity, and that they are often available orally, an added patient convenience. Despite these advantages, toxicity remains

Table 34.3 Antiangiogenesis small molecule tyrosine kinase inhibitors and their targets

Target	Sorafenib	Sunitinib	Pazopanib	Vandetanib	Cediranib	Motesanib	Axitinib	BIBF 1120	Cabozantinib
VEGFR-1	x	x	x		x	x	x		
VEGFR-2	x	x	x	X	x	x	x		
VEGFR-3	x	x	x	X	x	x	x		
PDGFR	x	x	x		x	x	x	x	
c-kit	x	x	x		x	x	x		x
EGFR				X					
Other	Raf, Flt 3	Ret, Flt 3				Ret		FGFR	MET, Ret, Flt 3

a concern given the multi-targeted kinase inhibition and the potential additive adverse events when these agents are combined with chemotherapy. Below we review selected small molecule TKIs that include VEGF as a target for the treatment of NSCLC (Table 34.3).

Sorafenib

Sorafenib is an oral multi-kinase inhibitor of VEGFR-2 and -3, platelet-derived growth factor receptor (PDGFR) beta, RAF-kinase, c-Kit, Ret, and fms-like tyrosine kinase receptor 3 (Flt3) that has been FDA-approved for treatment of patients with metastatic renal cell carcinoma (RCC) and advanced hepatocellular carcinoma (HCC) based upon prolongation in PFS seen in phase III studies [21, 22]. In NSCLC, sorafenib was evaluated in the phase II ECOG 2501 trial, in which 342 patients with advanced NSCLC who had failed at least two prior chemotherapy regimens received sorafenib 400 mg twice daily for two cycles. Patients who had stable disease after two cycles (n = 97) were randomized to receive additional sorafenib or placebo. PFS was prolonged in those patients receiving sorafenib compared to placebo (3.6 months versus 1.9 months, p = 0.01) [23]. Another phase II trial involving 52 patients found that sorafenib, when given continuously at a dose of 400 mg twice daily as a single agent to patients with relapsed or refractory advanced NSCLC, resulted in stable disease (SD) in 59% of evaluable patients and a median PFS of 5.5 months. Treatment-related toxicities were manageable and similar to the toxicities seen in previous trials with sorafenib, including hand-foot reaction seen in 10% of patients [24].

The promising phase II results led to two large phase III trials evaluating sorafenib in combination with chemotherapy. The double-blind, placebo-controlled phase III ESCAPE trial randomized patients with advanced NSCLC to receive front-line treatment with carboplatin/paclitaxel with or without sorafenib. An interim analysis revealed increased toxicity in patients with squamous histology and also indicated that the primary endpoint of OS was unlikely to be reached, leading to early termination of the study [25]. The phase III NEXUS trial investigated sorafenib in combination with cisplatin/gemcitabine and demonstrated a PFS benefit, although the primary endpoint of OS was not improved [26]. Sorafenib has also been studied in the phase II setting in combination with erlotinib with encouraging results, warranting further evaluation [27] [28]. Recently, the BATTLE study was the first completed prospective, biomarker-based adaptively randomized study in which previously treated patients with advanced lung cancer were randomized into one of 4 arms: erlotinib, vandetanib, erlotinib plus bexarotene, or sorafenib, based upon results of biomarker analyses obtained from individual patients. In comparing patients in the adaptive randomization arm against the equal randomization arm, *K-ras* mutant patients treated with sorafenib were found to have a nonstatistically significant trend toward improved DCR (61% versus 32%, p = 0.11), suggesting that *K-ras* mutant patients may derive preferential benefit with sorafenib, although this correlation will need to further tested in additional clinical trials [29].

Sunitinib

Sunitinib is an oral TKI that inhibits VEGFR-1, -2, -3, PDGFR alpha/beta, c-kit, Flt-3, and RET and is FDA-approved for the treatment of advanced RCC and imatinib-resistant gastrointestinal stromal tumor. In NSCLC, sunitinib was evaluated in two separate phase II trials with encouraging results [30, 31]. The subsequent phase III study comparing sunitinib/erlotinib and placebo/erlotinib in patients with previously treated advanced NSCLC noted an improvement in ORR (10.6% versus 6.9%, $p = 0.0471$) and PFS (3.6 months versus 2.0 months, $p = 0.0023$), though no improvement in OS was seen (9.0 months versus 8.5 months, $p = 0.1388$) [32]. There are ongoing studies investigating sunitinib in patients with NSCLC, including the phase II CALGB 30704 trial evaluating sunitinib as second-line therapy (ClinicalTrials.gov identifier: NCT00698815) and the phase III CALGB 30607 study of sunitinib as maintenance therapy (ClinicalTrials.gov identifier: NCT00693992).

Pazopanib

Pazopanib is an oral inhibitor of VEGFR-1, -2, and -3, PDGFR-beta, and c-kit, and was FDA approved in 2009 for the treatment of advanced RCC. In NSCLC, pazopanib demonstrated efficacy in a small phase II trial in which patients with stage I/II NSCLC received neoadjuvant treatment with pazopanib 800 mg/daily for 2–6 weeks (median duration: 16 days) prior to resection. Tumor volume reduction was noted in 30 patients (86%) and the most frequent adverse events were grade 2 hypertension, fatigue, and diarrhea [33]. These promising initial results led to additional studies of pazopanib in NSCLC, including a recently completed phase II open-label multi-center randomized study comparing pazopanib/pemetrexed with cisplatin/pemetrexed as frontline treatment in patients with metastatic NSCLC (ClinicalTrials.gov identifier: NCT00871403). Other studies have completed accrual with results awaited include the phase II randomized, placebo-controlled study of pazopanib in combination with erlotinib in previously treated patients with NSCLC (ClinicalTrials.gov identifier: NCT01027598) and the phase II study comparing pazopanib/paclitaxel with carboplatin/paclitaxel as first-line treatment in advanced NSCLC (ClinicalTrials.gov identifier: NCT00866528).

Vandetanib

Vandetanib is an orally administered inhibitor of VEGFR (VEGFR-2, VEGFR-3), RET, and EGFR. A phase II study of vandetanib in combination with chemotherapy in NSCLC yielded encouraging results, leading to further evaluation of vandetanib in four separate phase III studies in metastatic NSCLC [34]. The phase III ZODIAC trial randomized patients with advanced NSCLC to receive either docetaxel/vandetanib or docetaxel/placebo as second-line treatment. Although the addition of vandetanib improved ORR (17% versus 10%, $p = 0.0001$) and PFS (HR: 0.79, $p < 0.0001$), the primary endpoint of OS was not met (HR: 0.91, $p = 0.196$) [35]. In the phase III ZEAL trial, patients were randomized to receive vandetanib/pemetrexed or placebo/pemetrexed in the second-line setting. Results indicated that ORR (19% for pemetrexed/vandetanib versus 8% for pemetrexed/placebo, $p < 0.001$) and delay in time to worsening of lung cancer symptoms (18.1 weeks for pemetrexed/vandetanib versus 12.1 weeks for pemetrexed/placebo, $p = 0.0052$) favored those patients receiving vandetanib, though this study did not meet its primary endpoint of PFS (HR: 0.86, $p = 0.108$) [36]. The phase III ZEST trial randomized previously treated patients to receive vandetanib or erlotinib and found no significant improvement in PFS seen for patients treated with vandetanib versus erlotinib (HR: 0.98, 95% CI: 0.87–1.10, $p = 0.721$) [37]. Finally, in the phase III ZEPHYR study, patients with advanced NSCLC who had progressed after chemotherapy and erlotinib were randomized to receive vandetanib as a single agent versus placebo. Here, PFS was improved in those patients receiving vandetanib (HR: 0.63, $p < 0.0001$), but the primary endpoint of OS was not met (HR: 0.95, $p = 0.527$) [38]. Altogether, the disappointing results from these studies have led to suspension of any further studies of vandetanib in NSCLC.

Cediranib

Cediranib (AZD2171) inhibits VEGFR-1 and -2, PDGFR-beta, and c-kit and has been studied in combination with chemotherapy in advanced NSCLC in a few separate trials. In the phase II/III BR24 trial, 296 patients with advanced NSCLC were randomized to receive carboplatin/paclitaxel with or without cediranib as frontline treatment. Although interim results indicated a higher ORR and PFS with cediranib, the study was discontinued early due to excessive toxicities associated with cediranib given at the 30 mg dose, including severe hypertension, gastrointestinal toxicity, and febrile neutropenia [39]. The subsequent BR29 phase II/III trial utilized cediranib at a reduced dose of 20 mg daily combined with carboplatin/paclitaxel, but this was also halted due to an interim analysis revealing that cediranib did not meet pre-specified PFS efficacy criteria (ClinicalTrials.gov identifier: NCT00795340). A phase II study of cediranib in combination with pemetrexed in patients with recurrent NSCLC has completed accrual and results are awaited (ClinicalTrials.gov identifier: NCT00410904).

Motesanib

Motesanib (AMG 706) is a selective oral inhibitor of VEGFR-1, -2, and -3, PDGFR-beta, c-kit, and RET that has been studied both as monotherapy and in combination with chemotherapy in various malignancies [40, 41]. In NSCLC, a phase II study of patients with advanced nonsquamous NSCLC evaluated motesanib or bevacizumab in combination with carboplatin/paclitaxel as frontline treatment. Motesanib administered at a dose of 125 mg/day resulted in similar efficacy compared to the bevacizumab arm, with a median PFS of 7.7 months (compared to 8.3 months with bevacizumab) and a median OS of 14.0 months (compared to 14.0 months with bevacizumab) [8]. However, the phase III double-blind, placebo-controlled MONET1 study of motesanib plus carboplatin/paclitaxel in patients with nonsquamous advanced NSCLC did not meet its primary endpoint of improved OS (HR: 0.89, $p = 0.137$), leading to less enthusiasm for further development of this agent in NSCLC [42].

Axitinib

Axitinib (AG-013736) is an oral TKI that targets VEGFR-1, -2, and -3, PDGFR-beta, and c-kit. A phase II trial involving 32 patients with advanced NSCLC evaluated axitinib administered as a single-agent. In this trial, 28% of the patients had received no prior chemotherapy. The ORR was 9%, median PFS was 4.9 months (95% CI: 3.6–7.0 months), and median OS was 14.8 months (95% CI: 10.7-not estimable). Axitinib was also generally well tolerated, with grade 3 toxicities of fatigue (22%), hypertension (9%), and hyponatremia (9%) [43]. Overall, given the favorable single agent activity of axitinib in patients with NSCLC, there are ongoing phase II trials of axitinib in patients with both squamous and nonsquamous histology. In nonsquamous NSCLC, there are two studies: AGILE 1030 comparing axitinib/carboplatin/paclitaxel to bevacizumab/carboplatin/paclitaxel (ClinicalTrials.gov identifier: NCT00600821) and AGILE 1039 comparing axitinib/cisplatin/pemetrexed to cisplatin/pemetrexed (ClinicalTrials.gov identifier: NCT 007687855). In squamous NSCLC, the AGILE 1038 trial randomizes patients to axitinib/cisplatin/gemcitabine versus cisplatin/gemcitabine (Clinical Trials.gov identifier: NCT00735904).

BIBF 1120

BIBF 1120 is an oral inhibitor of VEGFR-1, -2, and -3, PDGFR alpha/beta, and fibroblast growth factor receptors (FGFR) 1–3, which has been studied as a single agent and in combination with chemotherapy in NSCLC. A phase II study of 73 patients with relapsed advanced NSCLC who received BIBF 1120 as a single agent was well tolerated and resulted in a median PFS of 11.6 weeks, median OS of 37.7 weeks, and disease control rate (complete response, partial response, or stable disease) of 46%. The most common grade 3/4 toxicities were nausea, vomiting, diarrhea, and elevation of liver function tests [44]. BIBF 1120 was also studied in combination with carboplatin/paclitaxel as frontline treatment in patients with advanced NSCLC in a phase I dose-escalation study. Results from this study indicated that the MTD of BIBF 1120 was 200 mg administered twice daily when given with carboplatin/paclitaxel and that the combination demonstrated an acceptable safety profile [45]. There are two phase III studies of BIBF 1120 in combination with chemotherapy in the second-line NSCLC setting that have completed accrual and results are awaited: LUME-Lung 1 (in combination with docetaxel) and LUME-Lung 2 (in combination with pemetrexed) (ClinicalTrials.gov identifier: NCT00805194 and NCT00806819, respectively).

Cabozantinib

Cabozantinib (XL-184) is a TKI of VEGFR-2, MET, RET, Kit, and Flt3 that has demonstrated decreased tumor and endothelial cell proliferation in preclinical lung tumor models [46]. In a phase Ib/II study of cabozantinib with or without erlotinib in previously treated patients with advanced NSCLC, the combination of cabozantinib and erlotinib was well tolerated with evidence of clinical activity in a largely erlotinib pretreated patient cohort, including patients with EGFR T790M and MET amplification, and additional results are anticipated [47]. Multiple trials of the drug in NSCLC either alone or in combination with erlotinib and other targeted agents are in development.

Vascular disrupting agents

Vascular disrupting agents (VDAs) directly target established tumor blood vessels, leading to arrest of blood flow and central tumor necrosis. VDAs that have been studied in NSCLC include ASA-404, fosbretabulin, bavituxumab, and omrabulin. In the phase III ATTRACT-1 study of carboplatin/paclitaxel +/- ASA-404, the addition of ASA-404 did not result in an improvement in OS [48], and the subsequent phase III ATTRACT-2 second-line study of docetaxel +/- ASA-404 was stopped early after interim results revealed that the primary endpoint of OS was unlikely to be reached, leading to discontinuation of further development of this agent. The phase II FALCON trial randomized chemotherapy-naïve patients with non-squamous metastatic disease to receive carboplatin/paclitaxel/bevacizumab +/− fosbretabulin. Encouragingly, initial results indicate that the addition of fosbretabulin resulted in an ORR of 56% (compared to 36% in those patients receiving carboplatin/paclitaxel/bevacizumab alone), and that OS was improved in patients receiving fosbretabulin with an aggregate tumor burden of > 10 cm (14. 2 months vs. 11.0 months, HR: 0.67, 95% CI: 0.26–0.7) [49]. Bavituximab is a VDA monoclonal antibody that targets the phosphatidylserine/beta-2 glycoprotein 1 complex and was studied in a single-arm phase II study in NSCLC in combination with carboplatin/paclitaxel [50]. Two phase II randomized studies of bavituximab in the first (in combination with carboplatin/paclitaxel) and second line (in combination with docetaxel) setting in NSCLC (ClinicalTrials.gov identifier: NCT01160601 and NCT01138163, respectively) were presented in 2012. However, preliminary data from the trial have been subsequently retracted due to discrepancies related to the coding and distribution of the investigational drug and the future of the drug remains unknown. Finally, ombrabulin is a novel VDA that is an analog of combretastatin A4 and a tubulin-binding agent that is being studied in the multinational, placebo-controlled, phase II DISRUPT trial, in which patients with metastatic NSCLC are randomized to receive front-line treatment with taxane and platinum with or without ombrabulin (ClinicalTrials.gov identifier: NCT01293630). While the study has completed accrual, results are pending.

Other anti-angiogenic therapies

Aflibercept

Aflibercept (VEGF-Trap, ZALTRAP) is a recombinant fusion protein that binds VEGFR-1, VEGFR-2, and placental growth factor (PlGF) that is FDA-approved for the treatment of macular degeneration. Most recently, aflibercept also gained FDA approval for previously treated patients with metastatic colorectal cancer based upon the improvement in PFS (HR = 0.758, p = 0.00007) and OS (HR = 0.817, p = 0.0032) seen with the addition of aflibercept to FOLFIRI in these patients in the phase III VELOUR study [51]. In NSCLC, a phase II study in which heavily pretreated patients with advanced disease received aflibercept as a single-agent, at a dose of 4.0 mg/kg intravenously every two weeks, demonstrated an ORR of 2% (95% CI: 0.2–7.2%), PFS of 2.7 months, and OS of 6.2 months [52]. The subsequent phase III VITAL trial compared aflibercept/docetaxel and placebo/docetaxel in patients with locally advanced or metastatic NSCLC who had failed platinum-based chemotherapy. Despite an improvement in ORR (23.3% versus 8.9%) and PFS (HR = 0.82, 95% CI: 0.716–0.937) with the addition of aflibercept, the primary endpoint of OS (HR = 1.01, 95% CI: 0.868–1.174) was not statistically significant between the two arms, leading to less certainty in further development of this agent in NSCLC [53]. In addition, a single-arm phase II study of aflibercept in combination with cisplatin/pemetrexed in previously untreated patients with advanced/metastatic NSCLC reported an ORR of 26.3% (95% CI: 12.3–40.3%) and PFS of 5 months (95% CI: 4.3-7.1), though this trial was stopped early after enrollment of 42 patients due to a higher than anticipated rate of reversible posterior leukoencephalopathy syndrome (RPLS) (confirmed in three patients). Interestingly, no RPLS was reported in a meta-analysis of safety involving three large placebo-controlled trials of aflibercept plus chemotherapy [54].

Biomarkers for anti-angiogenic therapies

The identification of predictive biomarkers for anti-angiogenesis agents remains an important goal that has yet to be achieved. The lack of reliable biomarkers has hindered the development of bevacizumab and other anti-angiogenic therapies and the true potential of these agents will not be realized until better biomarkers have been discovered.

Hypertension is a clinically useful biomarker for response to VEGF targeted agents, initially noted in trials involving sunitinib in the treatment of renal cell carcinoma [55]. In NSCLC, an association with development of hypertension and clinical benefit with bevacizumab was noted in an analysis of patients treated on ECOG 4599 [56]. Importantly, this response can only be assessed after initiation of therapy, which has led to efforts to establish surrogate markers that have not yet been identified.

Serum and plasma candidate biomarkers of angiogenesis have been studied extensively. One of the first biomarkers to be evaluated was the plasma concentration of VEGF. In ECOG 4599, high baseline plasma VEGF levels correlated with higher response to bevacizumab, but did not predict for a survival benefit [57]. More recently, the role of baseline circulating VEGF appears to be more promising as a predictive marker for bevacizumab in other types of malignancies, including gastric cancer. In the phase III AVAGAST trial of patients with gastric cancer, patients with high baseline plasma VEGF-A levels were found to have an overall poorer prognosis, although they had a trend toward higher response and survival when treated with bevacizumab [58]. In both renal and pancreatic cancer patients, a similar differential survival benefit from bevacizumab was seen [59].

Aside from VEGF, various other biomarkers have been explored in trials of patients treated with anti-angiogenic therapies. Patients on ECOG 4599 also had measurement of plasma levels of basic fibroblast growth factor (bFGF), soluble intercellular adhesion molecule (ICAM), and E-selectin both at baseline and during therapy. Baseline ICAM levels were shown to be prognostic but not predictive, as patients on both arms with low baseline ICAM had a higher response rate and better overall survival ($p = 0.00005$) compared to those with high ICAM [57]. Genetic variants related to angiogenesis, such as single nucleotide polymorphisms (SNPs), have also been investigated as potentially predictive biomarkers. In E4599, SNPs in VEGF, VEGFR1, ICAM-1, and epidermal growth factor were analyzed without a conclusive result, though one VEGF polymorphism did appear to correlate with survival [60]. A SNP analysis of patients with pancreatic or renal cell carcinoma enrolled on two separate phase III clinical trials of bevacizumab therapy revealed that a single SNP in VEGFR-1 was significantly associated with PFS for patients receiving bevacizumab in both trials, and additionally with OS in the pancreatic cancer study [59]. Additional research on VEGF SNPs continues.

There is also interest in profiling multiple plasma markers in order to identify marker signatures associated with response to VEGFR TKIs. Changes in cytokines and angiogenic factors (CAFs) have been correlated with clinical outcome in lung cancer patients treated with VEGFR TKIs, though the cytokines of interest have been variable between the studies [61, 62]. Investigators are also evaluating other methods in patients receiving VEGF inhibitors, such as detection of circulating endothelial cells (CECs), but there are significant methodological problems that need to be overcome before incorporating these biomarkers into large trials. Finally, using recent advances in gene expression profiling and proteomics, researchers have been able to correlate high levels of proangiogenic cytokines, such as interleukin-6 (IL-6), to poorer prognosis in patients with various malignancies [63, 64] and have also found the high IL-6 levels may predict therapeutic response to sunitinib in ovarian clear cell carcinoma [65]. As the pursuit of clinically useful biomarkers for anti-angiogenic therapies continues, it is imperative that future trials involving these agents incorporate exploratory and confirmatory biomarker analysis to help us reach better understanding.

Conclusion

Anti-angiogenic agents have demonstrated promising results in the treatment of NSCLC, including the monoclonal antibody bevacizumab, which is FDA-approved in patients with advanced nonsquamous NSCLC. In the landmark ECOG 4599 study, bevacizumab improved both PFS and OS when given in combination with carboplatin/paclitaxel as frontline treatment in patients with advanced NSCLC, and additional studies of bevacizumab have expanded its use in combination with other chemotherapy regimens and in patients with treated brain metastases. Other anti-angiogenic therapies, such as small molecule TKIs that include VEGFR as a target and VDAs, remain in various stages of clinical development and the results from ongoing studies are eagerly anticipated. The discovery of reliable predictive biomarkers for anti-angiogenic treatments is a critical goal in order to establish the exact role of these agents in the treatment of lung cancer. Ultimately, to improve patient outcomes, it will be crucial to determine the optimal treatment combinations and dosing schedules from clinical trials, and perhaps more importantly, to identify upfront through the use of biomarkers, which patients are most likely to derive benefit from the anti-angiogenic therapies available.

References

1 Folkman J (1971) Tumor angiogenesis: therapeutic implications. *N Engl J Med*, Nov 18; 285(21): 1182–6. PubMed PMID: 4938153. Epub 1971/11/18. eng.

2 Ferrara N, Gerber HP, LeCouter J (2003) The biology of VEGF and its receptors. *Nat Med*, Jun; 9(6): 669–76. PubMed PMID: 12778165. Epub 2003/06/05. eng.

3 Johnson DH, Fehrenbacher L, Novotny WF, Herbst RS, Nemunaitis JJ, Jablons DM, *et al.* (2004) Randomized phase II trial comparing bevacizumab plus carboplatin and paclitaxel with carboplatin and paclitaxel alone in previously untreated locally advanced or metastatic non-small-cell lung cancer. *J Clin Oncol*, Jun 1; 22(11): 2184–91. PubMed PMID: 15169807. Epub 2004/06/01. eng.

4 Sandler A, Gray R, Perry MC, Brahmer J, Schiller JH, Dowlati A, *et al.* (2006) Paclitaxel-carboplatin alone or with bevacizumab for non-small-cell lung cancer. *N Engl J Med*, Dec 14; 355(24): 2542–50. PubMed PMID: 17167137.

5 Hanna N, Shepherd FA, Fossella FV, Pereira JR, De Marinis F, von Pawel J, *et al.* (2004) Randomized phase III trial of pemetrexed versus docetaxel in patients with non-small-cell lung cancer previously treated with chemotherapy. *J Clin Oncol*, May 1; 22(9): 1589–97. PubMed PMID: 15117980. Epub 2004/05/01. eng.

6 Reck M, von Pawel J, Zatlouka P, Ramlau R, Gorbounova V, Hirsh V, *et al.* (2009) Phase III trial of cisplatin plus gemcitabine with either placebo or bevacizumab as first-line therapy for nonsquamous non-small-cell lung cancer: AVAil. *J Clin Oncol*, Mar 10; 27(8): 1227–34. PubMed PMID: 19188680.

7 Reck M, von Pawel J, Zatloukal P, Ramlau R, Gorbounova V, Hirsh V, *et al.* (2010) Overall survival with cisplatin-gemcitabine and bevacizumab or placebo as first-line therapy for nonsquamous non-small-cell lung cancer: results from a randomised phase III trial (AVAiL). *Ann Oncol*, Sep; 21(9): 1804–9. PubMed

PMID: 20150572. Pubmed Central PMCID: 2924992. Epub 2010/02/13. eng.

8 Blumenschein GR, Jr., Kabbinavar F, Menon H, Mok TS, Stephenson J, Beck JT, *et al.* (2011) A phase II, multicenter, open-label randomized study of motesanib or bevacizumab in combination with paclitaxel and carboplatin for advanced nonsquamous non-small-cell lung cancer. *Ann Oncol*, Sep; 22(9): 2057–67. PubMed PMID: 21321086. Epub 2011/02/16. eng.

9 Socinski MA, Langer CJ, Huang JE, Kolb MM, Compton P, Wang L, *et al.* (2009) Safety of bevacizumab in patients with non-small-cell lung cancer and brain metastases. *J Clin Oncol*, Nov 1; 27(31): 5255–61. PubMed PMID: 19738122. Epub 2009/09/10. eng.

10 Crino L, Dansin E, Garrido P, Griesinger F, Laskin J, Pavlakis N, *et al.* (2010) Safety and efficacy of first-line bevacizumab-based therapy in advanced non-squamous non-small-cell lung cancer (SAiL, MO19390): a phase 4 study. *Lancet Oncol*, Aug; 11(8): 733–40. PubMed PMID: 20650686. Epub 2010/07/24. eng.

11 Patel JD, Hensing TA, Rademaker A, Hart EM, Blum MG, Milton DT, *et al.* (2009) Phase II study of pemetrexed and carboplatin plus bevacizumab with maintenance pemetrexed and bevacizumab as first-line therapy for nonsquamous non-small-cell lung cancer. *J Clin Oncol*, Jul 10; 27(20): 3284–9. PubMed PMID: 19433684. Epub 2009/05/13. eng.

12 Patel J, Socinski M, Garon EB, Reynolds CH, Spigel D, Hermann RC, *et al.* (2012) A randomized, open-label, phase 3, superiority study of Pemetrexed (Pem) + Carboplatin (Cb) +Bevacizumab (B) followed by maintenance Pem + B versus Paclitaxel (Pac) + Cb +B followed by maintenance B in patients (pts) with stage IIIB or IV non-squamous non-small cell lung cancer (NS-NSCLC). *2012 Chicago Multidisciplinary Symposium in Thoracic Oncology*; Sept 7, Chicago, IL.

13 Barlesi F, de Castro J, Dvornichenko V, Kim JH, Pazzola A, Rittmeyer A, *et al.* (2011) Final efficacy outcomes for patients (pts) with advanced non-squamous non-small cell lung cancer (NSCLC) randomised to continuation maintenance (mtc) with Bevacizumab (bev) or Bev + Pemetrexed (pem) after first-line (1L) Bev-cisplatin (cis)-pem treatment (Tx). *Eur J Cancer*, 47(Suppl 2): 16.

14 Wakelee HA, Dahlberg SE, Keller SM, Gandara DR, Graziano SL, Leighl NB, *et al.* (2011) Interim report of on-study demographics and toxicity from E1505, a phase III randomized trial of adjuvant (adj) chemotherapy (chemo) with or without bevacizumab (B) for completely resected early-stage non-small cell lung cancer (NSCLC). *J Clin Oncol*, 29(Suppl.): Abstract 7013.

15 Miller MJ, Lindsay H, Valverde-Ventura R, O'Conner MJ (2009) Evaluation of the BioVigilant IMD-A, a novel optical spectroscopy technology for the continuous and real-time environmental monitoring of viable and nonviable particles. Part I. Review of the technology and comparative studies with conventional methods. *PDA J Pharm Sci Technol*. May–Jun; 63(3): 245–58. PubMed PMID: 20069798. Epub 2010/01/15. eng.

16 Kabbinavar FF, Miller VA, Johnson BE, O'Conner PG, Soh C (2010) Overall survival (OS) in ATLAS, a Phase IIIb trial comparing bevacizumab (B) therapy with or without erlotnib (E) after completion of chemotherapy (chemo) with B for first-line treatment of locally advanced, recurrent, or metastatic non-small-cell lung cancer (NSCLC). *J Clin Oncol*, 28(15S): Abstract 7526.

17 Herbst RS, Prager D, Hermann R, Fehrenbacher L, Johnson BE, Sandler A, *et al.* (2005) TRIBUTE: a phase III trial of erlotinib hydrochloride (OSI-774) combined with carboplatin and paclitaxel chemotherapy in advanced non-small-cell lung cancer. *J Clin Oncol*, Sep 1; 23(25): 5892–9. PubMed PMID: 16043829.

18 Herbst RS, Ansari R, Bustin F, Flynn P, Hart L, Otterson GA, *et al.* (2011) Efficacy of bevacizumab plus erlotinib versus erlotinib alone in advanced non-small-cell lung cancer after failure of standard first-line chemotherapy (BeTa): a double-blind, placebo-controlled, phase 3 trial. *Lancet*, May 28; 377(9780): 1846–54. PubMed PMID: 21621716. Epub 2011/05/31. eng.

19 Socinski MA, Stinchcombe TE, Moore DT, Gettinger SN, Decker RH, Petty WJ, *et al.* (2012) Incorporating bevacizumab and erlotinib in the combined-modality treatment of stage III non-small-cell lung cancer: Results of a phase I/II trial. *J Clin Oncol*, Nov 10; 30(32): 3953–9. PubMed PMID: 23045594.

20 Camidge DR, Ballas MS, Dubey S, Haigentz M, Rosen PJ, Spicer JF, *et al.* (2010) A phase II, open-label study of ramucirumab (IMC-1121B), an IgG1 fully human monoclonal antibody (MAb) targeting VEGFR-2, in combination with paclitaxel and carboplatin as first-line therapy in patients (pts) with stage IIIb/IV non-small cell lung cancer (NSCLC). *J Clin Oncol*, 28(15s): Abstract 7588.

21 Escudier B, Eisen T, Stadler WM, Szczylik C, Oudard S, Siebels M, *et al.* (2007) Sorafenib in advanced clear-cell renal-cell carcinoma. *N Engl J Med*, Jan 11; 356(2): 125–34. PubMed PMID: 17215530. Epub 2007/01/12. eng.

22 Llovet JM, Ricci S, Mazzaferro V, Hilgard P, Gane E, Blanc JF, *et al.* (2008) Sorafenib in advanced

hepatocellular carcinoma. *N Engl J Med*, Jul 24; 359(4): 378–90. PubMed PMID: 18650514. Epub 2008/07/25. eng.

23 Schiller J, Lee JW, Hanna H, Traynor AM, Carbone DP (2008) A randomized discontinuation phase II study of sorafenib versus placebo in patients with non-small cell lung cancer who have failed at least two prior chemotherapy regimens: E2501. *J Clin Oncol*, 26(May 20 suppl): Abstract 8014.

24 Blumenschein GR, Jr., Gatzemeier U, Fossella F, Stewart DJ, Cupit L, Cihon F, *et al.* (2009) Phase II, multicenter, uncontrolled trial of single-agent sorafenib in patients with relapsed or refractory, advanced non-small-cell lung cancer. *J Clin Oncol*, Sep 10; 27(26): 4274–80. PubMed PMID: 19652055. Epub 2009/08/05. eng.

25 Scagliotti G, von Pawel J, Reck M, Cupit L, Cihon F, DiMatteo S, *et al.* (2008) Sorafenib plus carboplatin/paclitaxel in chemonaiive patients with stage IIIB-IV non-small cell lung cancer: interim analysis results from the phase III, randomized, double-blind, placebo-controlled, ESCAPE (Evaluation of Sorafenib, Carboplaitn and Paclitaxel Efficacy in NSCLC) trial. *J Thorac Oncol*, 4(S97).

26 Paz-Ares LG, Biesma B, Heigener D, von Pawel J, Eisen T, Bennouna J, *et al.* (2012) Phase III, randomized, double-blind, placebo-controlled trial of Gemcitabine/Cisplatin alone or with Sorafenib for the first-line treatment of advanced, nonsquamous non-small-cell lung cancer. *J Clin Oncol*, Sep 1; 30(25): 3084–92. PubMed PMID: 22851564. Epub 2012/08/02. eng.

27 Spigel DR, Burris HA, 3rd, Greco FA, Shipley DL, Friedman EK, Waterhouse DM, *et al.* (2011) Randomized, double-blind, placebo-controlled, phase II trial of sorafenib and erlotinib or erlotinib alone in previously treated advanced non-small-cell lung cancer. *J Clin Oncol*, Jun 20; 29(18): 2582–9. PubMed PMID: 21576636. Epub 2011/05/18. eng.

28 Gridelli C, Morgillo F, Favaretto A, de Marinis F, Chella A, Cerea G, *et al.* (2011) Sorafenib in combination with erlotinib or with gemcitabine in elderly patients with advanced non-small-cell lung cancer: A randomized phase II study. *Ann Oncol*, Jul; 22(7): 1528–34. PubMed PMID: 21212155. Epub 2011/01/08. eng.

29 Kim ES, Herbst RS, Wistuba II, Lee JJ, Blumenschein GR, Jr., Tsao A, *et al.* (2011) The BATTLE Trial: Personalizing therapy for lung cancer. *Cancer Discov*, 1(1): 44–53.

30 Socinski MA, Novello S, Brahmer JR, Rosell R, Sanchez JM, Belani CP, *et al.* (2008) Multicenter, phase II trial of sunitinib in previously treated, advanced non-small-cell lung cancer. *J Clin Oncol*, Feb 1; 26(4): 650–6. PubMed PMID: 18235126. Epub 2008/02/01. eng.

31 Novello S, Scagliotti GV, Rosell R, Socinski MA, Brahmer J, Atkins J, *et al.* (2009) Phase II study of continuous daily sunitinib dosing in patients with previously treated advanced non-small cell lung cancer. *Br J Cancer*, Nov 3; 101(9): 1543–8. PubMed PMID: 19826424. Pubmed Central PMCID: 2778527. Epub 2009/10/15. eng.

32 Scagliotti GV, Krzakowski M, Szczesna A, Strausz J, Makhson A, Reck M, *et al.* (2012) Sunitinib plus erlotinib versus placebo plus erlotinib in patients with previously treated advanced non-small-cell lung cancer: a phase III trial. *J Clin Oncol*. Jun 10;30(17):2070-8. PubMed PMID: 22564989. Epub 2012/05/09. eng.

33 Altorki N, Lane ME, Bauer T, Lee PC, Guarino MJ, Pass H, *et al.* Phase II proof-of-concept study of pazopanib monotherapy in treatment-naive patients with stage I/II resectable non-small-cell lung cancer. *J Clin Oncol*, Jul 1; 28(19): 3131–7. PubMed PMID: 20516450. Epub 2010/06/03. eng.

34 Heymach JV, Paz-Ares L, De Braud F, Sebastian M, Stewart DJ, Eberhardt WE, *et al.* (2008) Randomized phase II study of vandetanib alone or with paclitaxel and carboplatin as first-line treatment for advanced non-small-cell lung cancer. *J Clin Oncol*, Nov 20; 26(33): 5407–15. PubMed PMID: 18936474. Epub 2008/10/22. eng.

35 Herbst RS, Sun Y, Eberhardt WE, Germonpre P, Saijo N, Zhou C, *et al.* (2010) Vandetanib plus docetaxel versus docetaxel as second-line treatment for patients with advanced non-small-cell lung cancer (ZODIAC): A double-blind, randomised, phase 3 trial. *Lancet Oncol*, Jul; 11(7): 619–26. PubMed PMID: 20570559. Pubmed Central PMCID: 3225192. Epub 2010/06/24. eng.

36 de Boer RH, Arrieta O, Yang CH, Gottfried M, Chan V, Raats J, *et al.* (2011) Vandetanib plus pemetrexed for the second-line treatment of advanced non-small-cell lung cancer: a randomized, double-blind phase III trial. *J Clin Oncol*, Mar 10; 29(8): 1067–74. PubMed PMID: 21282537. Epub 2011/02/02. eng.

37 Natale RB, Thongprasert S, Greco FA, Thomas M, Tsai CM, Sunpaweravong P, *et al.* (2011) Phase III trial of vandetanib compared with erlotinib in patients with previously treated advanced non-small-cell lung cancer. *J Clin Oncol*, Mar 10; 29(8): 1059–66. PubMed PMID: 21282542. Epub 2011/02/02. eng.

38 Lee JS, Hirsh V, Park K, Qin S, Blajman CR, Perng RP, *et al.* (2012) Vandetanib Versus placebo in patients

with advanced non-small-cell lung cancer after prior therapy with an epidermal growth factor receptor tyrosine kinase inhibitor: a randomized, double-blind phase III trial (ZEPHYR). *J Clin Oncol*, Apr 1; 30(10): 1114–21. PubMed PMID: 22370318. Epub 2012/03/01. eng.

39 Goss GD, Arnold A, Shepherd FA, Dediu M, Ciuleanu TE, Fenton D, *et al.* (2009) Randomized, double-blind trial of carboplatin and paclitaxel with either daily oral cediranib or placebo in advanced non-small-cell lung cancer: NCIC clinical trials group BR24 study. *J Clin Oncol*, Jan 1; 28(1): 49–55. PubMed PMID: 19917841. Epub 2009/11/18. eng.

40 Sherman SI, Wirth LJ, Droz JP, Hofmann M, Bastholt L, Martins RG, *et al.* (2008) Motesanib diphosphate in progressive differentiated thyroid cancer. *N Engl J Med*, Jul 3; 359(1): 31–42. PubMed PMID: 18596272. Epub 2008/07/04. eng.

41 Rosen LS, Kurzrock R, Mulay M, Van Vugt A, Purdom M, Ng C, *et al.* (2007) Safety, pharmacokinetics, and efficacy of AMG 706, an oral multikinase inhibitor, in patients with advanced solid tumors. *J Clin Oncol*, Jun 10; 25(17): 2369–76. PubMed PMID: 17557949. Epub 2007/06/15. eng.

42 Scagliotti GV, Vynnychenko I, Park K, Ichinose Y, Kubota K, Blackhall F, *et al.* (2012) International, randomized, placebo-controlled, double-blind phase III study of motesanib plus carboplatin/paclitaxel in patients with advanced nonsquamous non-small-cell lung cancer: MONET1. *J Clin Oncol*, Aug 10; 30(23): 2829–36. PubMed PMID: 22753922. Epub 2012/07/04. eng.

43 Schiller JH, Larson T, Ou SH, Limentani S, Sandler A, Vokes E, *et al.* (2009) Efficacy and safety of axitinib in patients with advanced non-small-cell lung cancer: results from a phase II study. *J Clin Oncol*, Aug 10; 27(23): 3836–41. PubMed PMID: 19597027. Epub 2009/07/15. eng.

44 Reck M, Kaiser R, Eschbach C, Stefanic M, Love J, Gatzemeier U, *et al.* (2011) A phase II double-blind study to investigate efficacy and safety of two doses of the triple angiokinase inhibitor BIBF 1120 in patients with relapsed advanced non-small-cell lung cancer. *Ann Oncol*, Jun; 22(6): 1374–81. PubMed PMID: 21212157. Epub 2011/01/08. eng.

45 Doebele RC, Conkling P, Traynor AM, Otterson GA, Zhao Y, Wind S, *et al.* (2012) A phase I, open-label dose-escalation study of continuous treatment with BIBF 1120 in combination with paclitaxel and carboplatin as first-line treatment in patients with advanced non-small-cell lung cancer. *Ann Oncol*, Aug; 23(8): 2094–2102. PubMed PMID: 22345119. Epub 2012/02/22. eng.

46 Yakes FM, Chen J, Tan J, Yamaguchi K, Shi Y, Yu P, *et al.* (2011) Cabozantinib (XL 184), a novel MET and VEGFR2 inhibitor, simultanously suppresses metastasis, angiogenesis, and tumor growth. *Mol Cancer Ther*, 10(12): 2298–2308.

47 Wakelee HA, Gettinger SN, Engelman JA, Janne PA, West HJ, Subramanian DS, *et al.* (2010) A phase Ib/II study of XL184 (BMS 907351) with and without erlotinib (E) in ptatients (pts) with non-small cell lung cancer (NSCLC). *J Clin Oncol*, 28(15s): Abstract 3017.

48 Lara PN, Jr., Douillard JY, Nakagawa K, von Pawel J, McKeage MJ, Albert I, *et al.* (2011) Randomized phase III placebo-controlled trial of carboplatin and paclitaxel with or without the vascular disrupting agent vadimezan (ASA404) in advanced non-small-cell lung cancer. *J Clin Oncol*, Aug 1; 29(22): 2965–71. PubMed PMID: 21709202. Epub 2011/06/29. eng.

49 Garon EB, Kabbinavar FF, Neidhart JA, Neidhart JD, Gabrail NY, Oliveira MR, *et al.* (2011) A randomized phase II trial of a vascular disrupting agent (VDA) fosbretabulin tromethamine (CA4P) with carboplatin (C), paclitaxel (P), and bevacizumab (B) in stage 3B/4 nonsquamous non-small cell lung cancer (NSCLC): Analysis of safety and activity of the FALCON trial. *J Clin Oncol*, 29(Suppl.): Abstract 7559.

50 Digumarti R, Suresh AV, Bhattacharyya GS, Dasappa L, Shan J (2010) Phase II study of bavituximab plus paclitaxel and carboplatin in untreated locally advanced or metastatic non-small cell lung cancer: Interim results. *J Clin Oncol*, 28(15 suppl): Abstract 7589.

51 Van Cutsem E, Tabernero J, Lakomy R, Prasouva J, Ruff P, Van Hazel G, *et al.* (eds) (2011) Intravenous (IV) aflibercept versus placebo in combination with irinotecan/5-FU (FOLFIRI) for second-line treatment of metastatic colorectal cancer (MCRC): Results of a multinational phase 3 trial (EFC10262-VELOUR). *13th ESMO World Congress on Gastrointestinal Cancer; 2011 June 22–25; Barcelona, Spain*: Abstract 0-0024.

52 Leighl NB, Raez LE, Besse B, Rosen PJ, Barlesi F, Massarelli E, *et al.* (2010) A multicenter, phase 2 study of vascular endothelial growth factor trap (Aflibercept) in platinum- and erlotinib-resistant adenocarcinoma of the lung. *J Thorac Oncol*, 5(7): 1054–9.

53 Novello S, Ramlau R, Gorbunova VA, Ciuleanu TE, Ozguroglu M, Goskel T, *et al.* (eds) (2011) Aflibercept in combination with docetaxel for second-line treatment of locally advanced or metastatic non-small-cell lung cancer (NSCLC): Final results of a multinational

placebo-controlled phase III trial (EFC10261-VITAL). *14th Biennial World Conference on Lung Cancer; July 3–7; Amsterdam, Netherlands*: Abstract O43.06.

54 Chen H, Modiano MR, Neal JW, Brahmer J, Rigas JR, Jotte RM, *et al.* (2012) A phase II multicenter study of aflibercept (AFL) in combination with cisplatin (C) and pemetrexed (P) in patients with previously untreated advanced/metastatic nonsquamous non-small cell lung cancer (NSCLC). *J Clin Oncol*, 30(Suppl): Abstr 7541.

55 Rini BI, Cohen DP, Lu DR, Chen I, Hariharan S, Gore ME, *et al.* (2011) Hypertension as a biomarker of efficacy in patients with metastatic renal cell carcinoma treated with sunitinib. *J Natl Cancer Inst*, May 4; 103(9): 763–73. PubMed PMID: 21527770. Pubmed Central PMCID: 3086879. Epub 2011/04/30. eng.

56 Dahlberg SE, Sandler AB, Brahmer JR, Schiller JH, Johnson DH (2010) Clinical course of advanced non-small-cell lung cancer patients experiencing hypertension during treatment with bevacizumab in combination with carboplatin and paclitaxel on ECOG 4599. *J Clin Oncol*, Feb 20; 28(6): 949–54. PubMed PMID: 20085937. Pubmed Central PMCID: 2834434. Epub 2010/01/21. eng.

57 Dowlati A, Gray R, Sandler AB, Schiller JH, Johnson DH (2008) Cell adhesion molecules, vascular endothelial growth factor, and basic fibroblast growth factor in patients with non-small cell lung cancer treated with chemotherapy with or without bevacizumab – an Eastern Cooperative Oncology Group Study. *Clin Cancer Res*, Mar 1; 14(5): 1407–12. PubMed PMID: 18316562. Epub 2008/03/05. eng.

58 Van Cutsem E, de Haas S, Kang YK, Ohtsu A, Tebbutt NC, Ming Xu J, *et al.* (2012) Bevacizumab in combination with chemotherapy as first-line therapy in advanced gastric cancer: a biomarker evaluation from the AVAGAST randomized phase III trial. *J Clin Oncol*, Jun 10; 30(17): 2119–27. PubMed PMID: 22565005. Epub 2012/05/09. eng.

59 Lambrechts D, Claes B, Delmar P, Reumers J, Mazzone M, Yesilyurt BT, *et al.* (2012) VEGF pathway genetic variants as biomarkers of treatment outcome with bevacizumab: an analysis of data from the AViTA and AVOREN randomised trials. *Lancet Oncol*, Jul; 13(7): 724–33. PubMed PMID: 22608783. Epub 2012/05/23. eng.

60 Zhang W, Dahlberg SE, Yang D, Sandler AB, Brahmer JR, Schiller JH, *et al.* (2009) Genetic variants in angiogenesis pathway associated with clinical outcome in NSCLC patients (pts) treated with bevacizumab in combination with carboplatin and paclitaxel: Subset pharmacogenetic analysis of ECOG 4599. *J Clin Oncol*, 27(15S): Abstract 8032.

61 Hanrahan EO, Lin HY, Kim ES, Yan S, Du DZ, McKee KS, *et al.* (2009) Distinct patterns of cytokine and angiogenic factor modulation and markers of benefit for vandetanib and/or chemotherapy in patients with non-small-cell lung cancer. *J Clin Oncol*, Jan 10; 28(2): 193–201. PubMed PMID: 19949019. Pubmed Central PMCID: 3040010. Epub 2009/12/02. eng.

62 Nikolinakos PG, Altorki N, Yankelevitz D, Tran HT, Yan S, Rajagopalan D, *et al.* (2010) Plasma cytokine and angiogenic factor profiling identifies markers associated with tumor shrinkage in early-stage non-small cell lung cancer patients treated with pazopanib. *Cancer Res*, Mar 15; 70(6): 2171–9. PubMed PMID: 20215520. Epub 2010/03/11. eng.

63 Zhu AX, Sahani DV, Duda DG, di Tomaso E, Ancukiewicz M, Catalano OA, *et al.* (2009) Efficacy, safety, and potential biomarkers of sunitinib monotherapy in advanced hepatocellular carcinoma: a phase II study. *J Clin Oncol*, Jun 20; 27(18): 3027–35. PubMed PMID: 19470923. Pubmed Central PMCID: 2702235. Epub 2009/05/28. eng.

64 Nilsson MB, Langley RR, Fidler IJ (2005) Interleukin-6, secreted by human ovarian carcinoma cells, is a potent proangiogenic cytokine. *Cancer Res*, Dec 1; 65(23): 10794-800. PubMed PMID: 16322225. Pubmed Central PMCID: 1534114. Epub 2005/12/03. eng.

65 Anglesio MS, George J, Kulbe H, Friedlander M, Rischin D, Lemech C, *et al.* (2011) IL6-STAT3-HIF signaling and therapeutic response to the angiogenesis inhibitor sunitinib in ovarian clear cell cancer. *Clin Cancer Res*, Apr 15; 17(8): 2538-48. PubMed PMID: 21343371. Epub 2011/02/24. eng.

CHAPTER 35
Targeting *ALK* Rearrangements

Justin F. Gainor and Alice T. Shaw
Department of Medicine, Harvard Medical School, Massachusetts General Hospital, Boston, MA, USA

Introduction

Systemic chemotherapy has long been the mainstay of treatment for patients with advanced non-small cell lung cancer (NSCLC); however, the discovery of activating mutations in the epidermal growth factor receptor (*EGFR*) in 2004 marked a major turning point in the management of the disease [1–3]. This discovery established a new paradigm of lung cancer treatment that stratified patients based upon the molecular characteristics of their tumors. The success of this approach in patients with *EGFR* mutations has prompted additional research efforts to find new genetic alterations, or "driver" mutations, which might also serve as drug targets. Such efforts ultimately led to the identification of chromosomal rearrangements involving the anaplastic lymphoma kinase (*ALK*) gene in 2007. Like *EGFR* mutations, *ALK* rearrangements define a unique genetic subset of NSCLC. In this chapter, we will: (1) review the molecular pathogenesis of *ALK* rearrangements; (2) summarize the common clinicopathologic features of ALK-positive patients; (3) outline currently available techniques for detection of *ALK* rearrangements; and (4) review clinical trial data providing support for ALK-directed therapies.

The molecular biology of native ALK

The *ALK* gene is located on chromosome 2 and encodes a 1620 amino acid receptor tyrosine kinase [4, 5]. Native ALK consists of an extracellular domain, short transmembrane region, and an intracellular tyrosine kinase domain (Figure 35.1). A member of the insulin receptor superfamily, *ALK* shares sequence homology with leukocyte tyrosine kinase (*LTK*), c-ros oncogene 1 (*ROS1*), insulin-like growth factor-1 receptor (*IGF-1R*), and the insulin receptor. Native ALK expression is limited to the central nervous system, testes and the small intestine in human adults [6, 7]. In mice, ALK is transiently expressed in the developing embryonic and neonatal nervous systems [8]. This pattern of expression suggests that ALK may be important in neural development. Experiments in *ALK* knockout mice, however, demonstrate that these mice are viable and do not exhibit any apparent developmental or morphologic changes [9]. Additional analysis of ALK knockout mice has revealed age-related increases in hippocampal progenitor cells and changes in behavioral testing.

The function of native ALK is incompletely understood. Activation is believed to occur through

Lung Cancer, Fourth Edition. Edited by Jack A. Roth, Waun Ki Hong and Ritsuko U. Komaki.

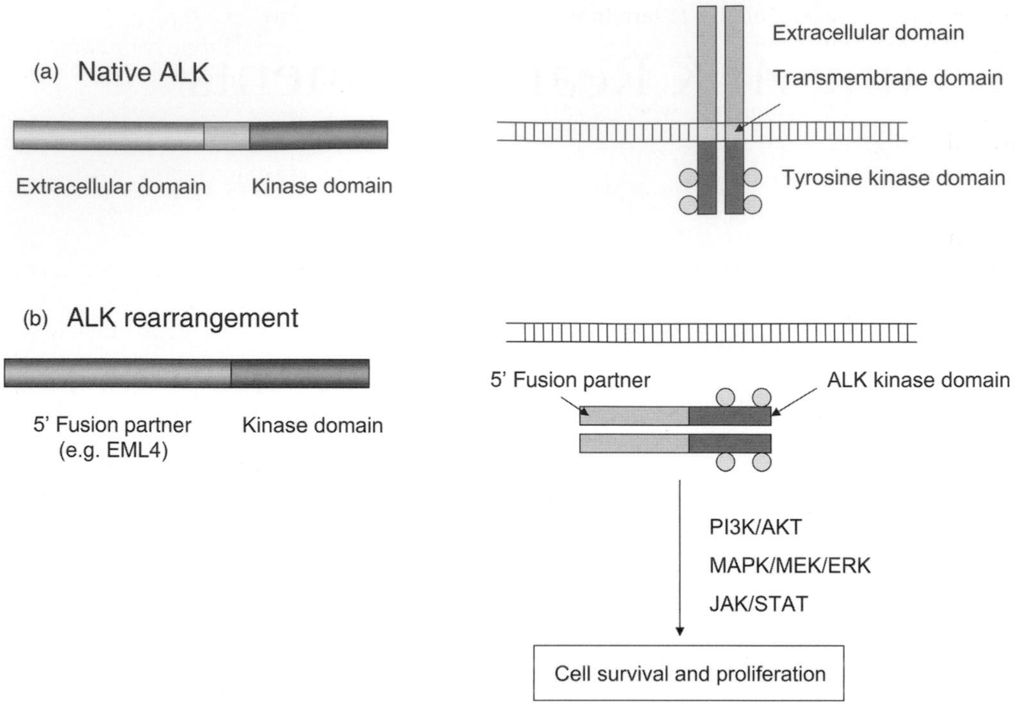

Figure 35.1 a: Schematic of native ALK structure and cellular localization. b: Schematic of an *ALK* fusion oncogene. *ALK* rearrangements, which consist of a 5′ fusion partner and the *ALK* tyrosine kinase domain, most commonly arise through chromosomal inversions involving chromosome 2. The resulting fusion protein is ectopically expressed and redistributed to the cytoplasm, where it is constitutively active.

ligand-induced dimerization [10]. In *Drosophila*, Jelly belly (Jeb) has been identified as the ligand for ALK activation and downstream signaling, though no human homologue of this protein has been recognized to date [11]. In humans, the growth factors pleiotrophin and midkine have been proposed as ALK ligands [12, 13].

EML4-ALK: role in molecular pathogenesis

Oncogenic activation of ALK has been identified in a number of malignancies [14]. In most cases, activation occurs through chromosomal translocations. *ALK* gene rearrangements were first reported in anaplastic large cell lymphoma (ALCL), where a recurring t(2;5)(p23;q35) translocation was identified in 1994 [7]. This rearrangement generates a chimeric fusion protein involving the amino-terminus of nucleophosmin (NPM1) and the carboxy-terminus of ALK. Since this initial description, *ALK* rearrangements have been found in a number of other malignancies, including inflammatory myofibroblastic tumors, NSCLC, and renal cell carcinomas, among others [15–18]. In addition, activating point mutations in the *ALK* tyrosine kinase domain have been reported in neuroblastoma and anaplastic thyroid cancer [19–23].

ALK gene rearrangements in NSCLC were first identified in 2007 [17, 24]. Using retroviral cDNA expression libraries prepared from a human lung adenocarcinoma, Soda and colleagues detected a small inversion on chromosome 2 that produces a fusion gene consisting of exons 1–13 of echinoderm microtubule-associated protein-like 4 (*EML4*) and exons 20–29 of *ALK* [17]. The resulting *EML4-ALK* fusion transcript encodes a chimeric protein composed of the N-terminus of EML4 and the intracellular tyrosine kinase domain of ALK. As a result, ALK is relocated from the cell membrane to the cytoplasm, where EML4 mediates ligand-independent dimerization and autophosphorylation of ALK [17, 25]. This in turn leads to constitutive activation of ALK with downstream signaling through the MAPK/MEK/ERK, PI3K/AKT and JAK/STAT pathways [26, 27]. Accordingly, *EML4-ALK* is transforming *in vitro* and *in vivo* [17, 28]. Indeed, transgenic mice expressing *EML4-ALK* in alveolar type II cells developed multiple adenocarcinoma nodules throughout the lungs [28]. Upon treatment with an ALK inhibitor, however, these animals experienced tumor regression. Together, these results suggest that *EML4-ALK* is a novel oncogenic driver in NSCLC.

Several different *ALK* fusion partners have since been identified in NSCLC, including kinesin family member 5B (*KIF5B*), kinesin light chain 1 (*KCL1*), and transforming growth factor (*TFG*) [24, 29, 30]. These rearrangements appear to possess similar biological properties [31]. In NSCLC, *EML4* is the most common *ALK* fusion partner [32]. Furthermore, multiple *EML4-ALK* variants exist, all of which contain an identical *ALK* tyrosine kinase domain but possess different truncations of *EML4* [17, 26, 33, 34]. *EML4-ALK* variant 1 appears to be the most common (49.6%), followed by variant 3a/b (25.6%) and variant 2 (10%) [35]. Other *EML4-ALK* variants comprise less than 15% of the remaining cases reported to date.

Clinicopathologic features of patients with *ALK* rearrangements

In the initial report of *EML4-ALK* in NSCLC, fusion transcripts were found in 6.7% of 75 specimens [17]. Subsequent screening studies estimated the prevalence of *ALK* rearrangements to be approximately 3–5% in unselected patients [26, 29, 33, 36–41]. *ALK* rearrangements are associated with unique clinical and pathologic features, including younger age, adenocarcinoma histology and lack of smoking history. Patients with *ALK* translocations and *EGFR* mutations share similar clinical characteristics. However, *ALK* rearrangements are essentially mutually exclusive with *EGFR* and *KRAS* mutations [36, 42]; only rare cases of overlapping mutations have been reported [41, 43–51]. Knowledge of the clinico-pathologic features associated with *ALK* rearrangements may guide molecular testing and facilitate identification of this rare population of patients [36].

ALK rearrangements are associated with a relatively younger age at the time of diagnosis [36, 37, 52–54]. The median age is approximately 50 years, which is nearly 10–15 years younger than ALK-negative patients. *ALK* rearrangements are also strongly associated with light or never-smoking history [36, 52, 53]. In recent databases established from clinical trials of crizotinib, approximately 70% of ALK-positive patients were never-smokers [55, 56]. In contrast to *EGFR* mutations, *ALK* rearrangements have no apparent association with gender or ethnicity.

ALK-positive lung cancers are also associated with distinctive morphologic features. The overwhelming majority of ALK-positive patients (approximately 97%) exhibit adenocarcinoma histology [55]. Squamous cell differentiation has also been reported in a rare subset of patients [36, 37, 55, 57, 58]. In studies analyzing resection specimens from a predominantly Asian patient population, *ALK* rearrangements were also associated with the presence of signet-ring cells, a mucinous cribiform pattern, and features of acinar growth [57]. In a more recent analysis of 104 ALK-positive and 215 ALK-negative lung cancer specimens, ALK-positive primary tumors were also associated with signet-ring cells [59]. However, these same specimens did not show higher rates of acinar or mucinous cribiform growth patterns. Collectively, abundant signet-ring cells and a solid-predominant growth pattern have emerged as the most specific morphologic features of *ALK* rearrangements in both primary and metastatic lesions. Over 70% of ALK-positive tumors demonstrate the presence of signet ring cells while nearly half exhibit a solid growth pattern. Nevertheless, these features should not be used as a substitute for tumor genotyping; rather, they may inform prioritization of testing strategies, particularly in cases with limited tissue.

Prognostic implications of *ALK* rearrangements

In early descriptions, *ALK* rearrangements were associated with advanced stage at the time of presentation [36, 52]. Moreover, ALK-positive patients were noted to have distinct patterns of disease spread. In one report of patients with advanced-stage disease, *ALK* rearrangements were significantly associated with pericardial, pleural and liver metastases compared to ALK-negative patients [60]. The prevalence of brain metastases was not different across numerous genotypes, including patients with alterations in *ALK*, *EGFR*, or *KRAS*. In a separate study using FDG PET/CT, Choi *et al.* suggest that *ALK* rearrangements may also be associated with a more aggressive phenotype [61]. In their analysis, ALK-positive tumors demonstrated significantly higher maximum standardized uptake values and more frequent nodal and distant metastases compared to ALK-negative comparators.

As will be discussed more fully below, *ALK* rearrangements are predictive biomarkers of response to the ALK TKI crizotinib. However, the prognostic significance of these genetic alterations is less certain [62]. In early-stage disease, a number of conflicting studies have been reported [47, 63, 64]. Zhang *et al.* identified a nonsignificant trend towards improved overall survival among ALK-positive patients following surgical resection [47]. In contrast, Yang et al. demonstrated that the five-year risk of progression or recurrence was two-fold higher in patients with ALK-positive tumors compared to ALK-negative controls [63]. In a separate report, Kim and colleagues evaluated 119 patients who underwent surgical resection and compared recurrence-free survival (RFS) based upon genotype [64]. There was no significant difference in RFS based upon genotype (*EGFR* mutations – 39.7 months, *ALK* rearrangements – 20.0 months, *KRAS* mutations – 21.4 months, and "triple-negative" – 26.8 months; $p = 0.344$).

In the setting of advanced-stage disease, the prognostic significance of *ALK* rearrangements is similarly unclear. Early studies suggested that *ALK* rearrangements confer no difference in overall survival [36, 65, 66]. In one such study, Shaw *et al.* evaluated overall survival in 36 crizotinib-naïve, ALK-positive patients compared to 253 wild-type (WT) controls, finding no difference in median overall survival between the groups (20 versus 15 months, $p = 0.244$) [66]. More recently, Lee and colleagues reported that *ALK* rearrangements were associated with numerically shorter, though nonsignificant, median overall survival (*ALK* rearrangements – 12.2 months, *EGFR* mutations – 29.6 months, and WT/WT – 19.3 months; *ALK* versus WT/WT, $p = 0.127$) [67]. Similarly, Kim *et al.* compared median overall survival across various genotypes in 229 patients with NSCLC, finding a statistically significant shorter median overall survival for those with *ALK* rearrangements compared to EGFR-positive or WT/WT patients (14.3 versus 37.2 versus 33.3 months, respectively) [64]. In contrast, Wu and colleagues recently reported improved overall survival in 39 patients with *ALK* rearrangements compared to 77 WT controls (14.7 versus 10.3 months, $p = 0.009$) [68]. Collectively, these studies were limited by retrospective assessments, small sample sizes, and variability in testing techniques. On the whole, however, these studies suggest that *ALK* rearrangements are unlikely to be strong positive prognostic biomarkers.

Diagnostic testing for *ALK* rearrangements

A number of different techniques exist for the detection of *ALK* rearrangements. The three most commonly reported methods include: ALK fluorescence *in situ* hybridization (FISH), reverse transcription polymerase chain reaction (RT-PCR), and ALK immunohistochemistry (IHC) [69]. Unfortunately, no one test is perfectly suited to clinical testing of all specimens.

ALK FISH

ALK FISH is the current gold-standard technique for diagnosing *ALK* rearrangements. In clinical trials of crizotinib, *ALK* rearrangements have been primarily confirmed using the Vysis ALK Break-Apart FISH assay (Abbott Molecular) [55, 56, 70]. The test uses red and green fluorescent probes that flank

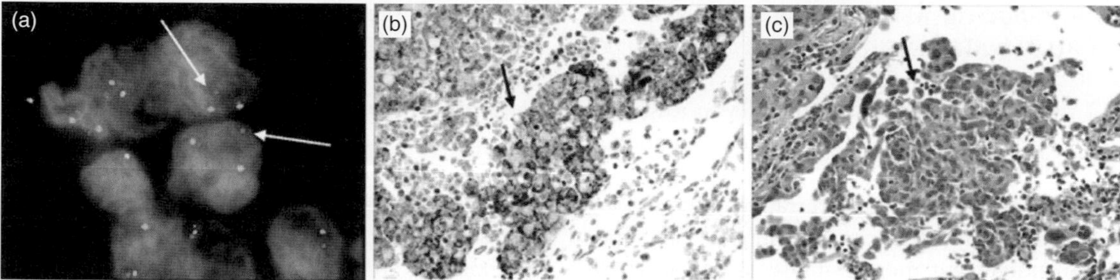

Figure 35.2 a: ALK FISH reveals split red and green probes (arrows), indicative of an *ALK* rearrangement. b: ALK immunohistochemistry demonstrates positive ALK staining. c: Hematoxylin and eosin stain shows signet ring cells, a common morphologic feature of ALK-positive NSCLC. From Shaw AT, Yeap BY, Mino-Kenudson M, *et al.* (2009) Clinical features and outcomes of patients with non-small-cell lung cancer who harbor *EML4-ALK*, 27(26): 4247–53. Reprinted with permission.

the highly conserved breakpoint region within *ALK*. In the absence of an *ALK* rearrangement, the two overlapping probes produce a yellow or fused signal. When an *ALK* rearrangement is present, however, the 5′ green probe and 3′ red probe become separated, resulting in a classic "split" signal (Figure 35.2). A positive signal is defined by the separation of 5′ and 3′ signals by more than two signal diameters. The presence of a single isolated red 3′ probe, which presumably occurs through loss of the 5′ binding site, is also considered to be a positive signal [71]. A given specimen is considered diagnostic for an *ALK* rearrangement if ≥15% of scored nuclei possess split or isolated red signals.

The major advantage of ALK FISH is that it is the only assay that has been validated in clinical trials of crizotinib. ALK FISH can also be performed on formalin-fixed, paraffin-embedded (FFPE) specimens [72]. Even a single unstained slide is usually sufficient for testing. Furthermore, ALK FISH can detect rearrangements without prior knowledge of the *ALK* 5′ fusion partner or *EML4-ALK* variant. Thus, it may permit identification of novel *ALK* rearrangements. On the other hand, ALK FISH also poses a number of challenges for routine clinical testing. In particular, the assay requires technical expertise and experience in interpretation. It may therefore not be widely available in routine pathology labs. On a related note, ALK FISH testing is relatively more expensive than other techniques.

RT-PCR

An alternative technique for detection of *ALK* rearrangements is RT-PCR. This method uses multiplexed primers to amplify in-frame *ALK* fusion transcripts [26, 33]. While this technique is able to capture known *ALK* fusion variants, one major limitation of RT-PCR is that it is unable to detect *ALK* rearrangements involving novel 5′ fusion partners. Additionally, RT-PCR results are dependent on the availability and quality of RNA in tested specimens. Since RNA is often degraded in FFPE tissues, early RT-PCR screening efforts for *ALK* rearrangements required fresh frozen specimens [17, 26, 33, 37]. More recently, commercially available RT-PCR techniques have been developed that allow testing of FFPE specimens [73–75]. Nonetheless, prospective comparisons between RT-PCR and ALK FISH as predictors of response to crizotinib are lacking.

Immunohistochemistry

Given the widespread use of IHC in routine pathology practice and the lack of ALK expression in normal adult tissue, IHC has been proposed as an alternative detection method for *ALK* rearrangements. Indeed, ALK IHC is now used as a screening tool in non-Hodgkin lymphoma. Unfortunately, adoption of ALK IHC has been more problematic in NSCLC since *EML4-ALK* rearrangements result in lower levels of ALK fusion protein expression compared to those observed in ALCL [76].

Three different ALK IHC antibodies have been investigated: ALK1 (DAKO, Carpinteria, CA), D5F3 (Cell Signaling Technologies, Beverly, MA), and 5A4 (Novacastra, Newcastle Upon Tyne, UK) [52, 59, 76–79]. Initial studies used the ALK1 antibody [52]. While specific, this antibody was less sensitive for detection of *ALK* rearrangements among ALK FISH-positive specimens. Subsequent series demonstrated that the sensitivity of this antibody could be improved through various signal amplification strategies [29, 52, 80]. More recently, data has emerged regarding two additional antibodies, D5F3 and 5A4, both of which appear to be highly sensitive and specific for detection of *ALK* rearrangements in NSCLC specimens [59, 76–79].

ALK IHC is promising as a potential low-cost and rapid screening tool for *ALK* rearrangements. Recently, fully automated and standardized ALK IHC systems have been developed for clinical implementation. Once these systems are validated and undergo regulatory approval, screening approaches may consist of ALK IHC alone or in combination with ALK FISH.

ALK Inhibitors: Crizotinib

The discovery of *ALK* rearrangements in NSCLC sparked immediate interest in identifying small molecule inhibitors of this target. In preclinical testing, ALK TKIs demonstrated marked activity against ALK-positive cell lines and murine models, providing a strong rationale for pursuing similar strategies in the clinic [17, 26–28, 81]. The first ALK inhibitor tested in ALK-positive patients was crizotinib, an orally-available small molecule tyrosine kinase inhibitor. Although this agent was initially developed as an inhibitor of mesenchymal epithelial transition growth factor (c-MET), it was soon recognized that crizotinib potently inhibits ALK with half maximum inhibitory concentration values of 25–50 nmol/L in cell-based assays [81, 82].

Clinical efficacy

The phase I, first-in-man study of crizotinib (PROFILE 1001) was activated in 2006, prior to the discovery of *EML4-ALK* in NSCLC (Table 35.1) [17, 70]. This international, multi-center trial included a standard dose escalation cohort as well as a dose expansion cohort at the maximum tolerated dose (MTD). Soon after the report of *EML4-ALK* in NSCLC [17], two ALK-positive patients with NSCLC experienced dramatic symptomatic improvement after receiving crizotinib during the dose escalation phase of the trial [70]. Based upon these early results, study sites began prospectively screening patients for *ALK* rearrangements. The trial was also amended to allow ALK-positive

Table 35.1 Select trials of crizotinib in ALK-positive non-small cell lung cancer (NSCLC)

Name	Phase	Description	ORR	mPFS
PROFILE 1001 (NCT00585195)	I	Safety, pharmacokinetic and pharmacodynamic study of crizotinib in patients with advanced cancer.	60%	9.7 months
PROFILE 1005 (NCT00932451)	II	Safety and efficacy of crizotinib in patients with ALK-positive NSCLC who have received $\geq$1 prior chemotherapy.	60%	8.1 months
PROFILE 1007 (NCT00932893)	III	Randomized trial comparing crizotinib versus second-line docetaxel or pemetrexed in patients with ALK-positive NSCLC.*	NR	NR
PROFILE 1014	III	Randomized trial comparing crizotinib versus first-line platinum/pemetrexed in patients with ALK-positive NSCLC and no prior therapy.	NR	NR

*Preliminary results reported at the 2012 European Society of Medical Oncology.
ALK, anaplastic lymphoma kinase; mPFS, median progression-free survival; NCT, National Clinical Trial; NR, not reported; ORR, objective response rate.

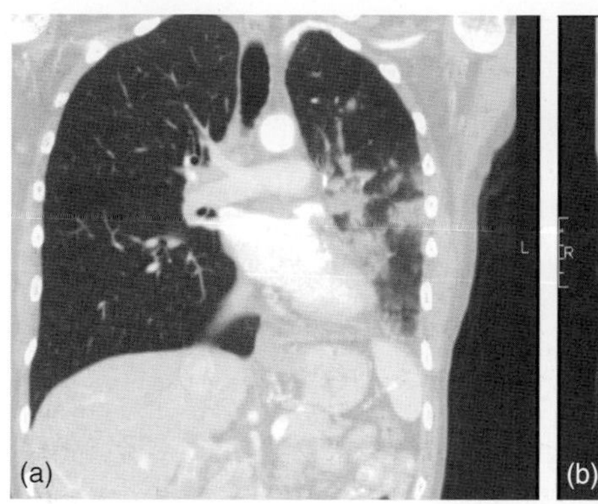

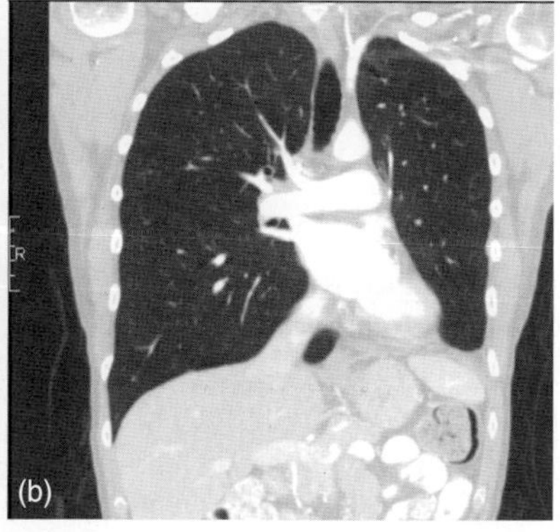

Figure 35.3 Marked radiographic response to crizotinib in an ALK-positive patient with advanced NSCLC. (a) demonstrates a pre-crizotinib radiograph; b represents a radiograph obtained 8 weeks after starting crizotinib.

patients with NSCLC to enter an expanded molecular cohort at the MTD of 250 mg twice daily [70].

In the most recent update from this trial, a total of 149 patients with NSCLC have been enrolled [55]. All participants were positive for *ALK* rearrangement based upon ALK FISH testing. Among 143 evaluable patients, the objective response rate (ORR) was 60.8%, which included 3 complete responses and 84 partial responses. The disease control rate (i.e., complete response, partial response, or stable disease) was 82.5% at week 8 and 70.6% at week 16. In total, over 90% of ALK-positive patients experienced some degree of tumor shrinkage (Figure 35.3). Importantly, these responses appeared to be independent of line of therapy. Moreover, responses appeared durable. The median progression-free survival (PFS) in patients receiving crizotinib was approximately 10 months. Median overall survival had not been reached at the time of data cutoff [55].

A similar ongoing phase II study of crizotinib opened to enrollment in 2009 (PROFILE 1005, ClinicalTrials.gov identifier NCT00932451). This single-arm study includes patients with advanced, ALK-positive NSCLC who have progressed after one or more prior lines of therapy. In a preliminary report of this trial, crizotinib demonstrated a high ORR (60%) and a median PFS of approximately 8 months [56]. Statistically significant improvements in quality of life and patient-reported symptoms (e.g., cough, dsypnea, insomnia, fatigue) were also reported.

In August 2011, crizotinib received accelerated approval by the US Food and Drug Administration based upon response rates from the first 136 patients enrolled on PROFILE 1001 together with 119 patients enrolled on PROFILE 1005 [83]. This approval was conditional upon results from ongoing randomized trials (PROFILE 1007, ClinicalTrials.gov identifier NCT00932893; PROFILE 1014, ClinicalTrials.gov identifier NCT01154140) comparing crizotinib to standard cytotoxic chemotherapy. Preliminary results from one of these trials, PROFILE 1007, were recently presented [84]. In this phase III randomized trial, patients with advanced, ALK-positive NSCLC previously treated with one prior platinum-based regimen were randomized to receive crizotinib or either pemetrexed or docetaxel as second-line therapy. In preliminary reporting, treatment with crizotinib was superior to chemotherapy in prolonging PFS, the primary endpoint of the trial.

Prospective clinical trials comparing crizotinib to conventional chemotherapy may not detect differences in overall survival because crossover between treatment groups is likely to be common. Given the current lack of randomized data, the impact of crizotinib on overall survival was assessed in a retrospective analysis of patients enrolled in the phase I study of crizotinib [66]. Overall survival rates at one-year and two-year were significantly higher in ALK-positive patients treated with crizotinib in the second- or third-line compared to a crizotinib-naïve, ALK-positive control cohort given any second-line therapy (70% versus 44% and 55% versus 12%, respectively; $p = 0.004$). This provides indirect evidence that crizotinib may be associated with improved overall survival.

Safety profile

In general, treatment with crizotinib has been well tolerated. Common treatment-related adverse events (TRAE) include gastrointestinal effects, such as nausea, vomiting, constipation and diarrhea [55, 56, 70]. A majority of patients (50–64%) also experience visual disturbances, which typically occur within days of starting the drug. These visual disturbances, commonly described as light trails, flashes or image-persistence, are almost always associated with transitions from dark to light environments. The majority of visual disturbances reported to date have been grade 1 in severity. Detailed ophthalmological examinations performed in a subset of patients enrolled on PROFILE 1005 showed no ophthalmological changes associated with these visual disturbances [85].

Peripheral edema may also be observed in a subset of patients treated with crizotinib [55, 70]. In these patients, peripheral edema typically occurs after 2–3 months of treatment with crizotinib. It is believed that this edema may be associated with crizotinib's ability to inhibit MET [86]. Additional key toxicities associated with crizotinib include elevations in liver function tests. Specifically, elevations in alanine aminotransferase (ALT) and aspartate aminotransferase (AST) have been identified in 13% and 9% of patients, respectively [55, 83]. These elevations typically occur within eight weeks of initiating therapy and are usually reversible. However, grade 3/4 ALT or AST elevations have been reported in 7% and 3% of patients, respectively. Additionally, five cases (<1%) of severe, potentially drug-related hepatotoxicity have been reported, two of which were fatal [87]. Treatment interruption followed by dose reduction may permit continued treatment with crizotinib, though some patients require permanent discontinuation.

One rare adverse event related to crizotinib is severe or life-threatening pneumonitis, which has been reported in 1.6% of patients [70, 83]. This toxicity should result in permanent discontinuation of crizotinib. Other adverse events associated with crizotinib include renal cysts, QTc prolongation and asymptomatic sinus bradycardia [70, 83, 88]. Lastly, one small series has reported rapid reductions in total testosterone levels in men receiving crizotinib [89]. The clinical impact of this abnormality and the importance of testosterone replacement are presently unclear.

Acquired resistance to crizotinib

The long-term effectiveness of crizotinib has been uniformly limited by the development of acquired resistance. Mechanisms of acquired crizotinib resistance can be broadly characterized as involving either: (1) genetic alterations in the target (i.e., ALK) or 2) activation of alternative, or bypass, signaling pathways. The earliest report of acquired resistance to crizotinib involved a 28-year-old, ALK-positive patient who experienced a partial response to crizotinib but progressed 5 months later [90]. Deep sequencing of a pleural fluid specimen from this patient revealed 2 nonoverlapping secondary mutations, L1196M and C1156Y, in the *ALK* tyrosine kinase domain. Each mutation independently conferred resistance to crizotinib *in vitro*. Of note, the L1196M mutation occurs at the conserved "gatekeeper" residue of *ALK*, which is analogous to T790M in *EGFR* and T315I in *ABL*. In subsequent reports of acquired crizotinib resistance, secondary mutations in *ALK* have been identified in approximately 30% of cases [91–93]. These mutations are distributed throughout the kinase and include both missense mutations (L1152R, G1202R, S1206Y, G1269Y) and insertions (1151Tins). In vitro, these secondary mutations demonstrate differential sensitivities to crizotinib and next generation ALK TKIs [91].

Bypass signaling is another potential mechanism of crizotinib resistance. In particular, up-regulation of EGFR signaling has been observed in ALK-positive cell lines that have grown resistant to crizotinib [48, 91, 94]. Consistent with these preclinical findings, Katayama and colleagues found that nearly half of ALK-positive patients demonstrated immunohistochemical evidence of EGFR activation at the time of crizotinib resistance [91]. In this same study, *KIT* gene amplification was also identified in crizotinib-resistant patients, suggesting that aberrant KIT activation may mediate resistance as well. Other potential mechanisms of crizotinib resistance that have been reported to date include the emergence of mutations in *EGFR* and *KRAS* [92]. A subset of patients may also exhibit amplification of the ALK fusion gene at the time of crizotinib resistance [91, 92]. Lastly, multiple different mechanisms of resistance have been identified within the same patient [91, 92], suggesting that combination therapies may be necessary to overcome resistance.

Other systemic therapies

The efficacy of other systemic therapies in patients with *ALK* rearrangements has been predominantly examined through small retrospective studies [36, 67]. In one such series, patients with *ALK* rearrangements, *EGFR* mutations or wild-type status were found to have similar ORRs and time to progression (TTP) following platinum-based chemotherapy [36]. Median overall survival was similar in all three groups. Additionally, EGFR TKIs have also been examined in ALK-positive patients in a number of retrospective studies [36, 64, 67]. Together, these reports demonstrated ORRs of 0% and median PFS of 1.4–1.6 months in ALK-positive patients receiving EGFR TKIs.

Recently, several retrospective studies have suggested that the cytotoxic agent pemetrexed may be associated with enhanced responses in patients with *ALK* rearrangements [95, 96]. In one report, ALK-positive patients receiving second-line pemetrexed had higher response rates and longer TTP compared to *EGFR* mutant or WT patients [96]. In a separate study, Camidge *et al.* reported a median PFS of 9 months among 19 ALK-positive patients receiving pemetrexed-containing chemotherapy regimens, whereas median PFS was only 4 months in patients who were negative for *ALK, EGFR* and *KRAS* [95]. More recently, Shaw *et al.* reported findings from a multicenter, retrospective study of pemetrexed in 121 ALK-positive and 266 ALK-negative, EGFR-wild-type patients [97]. This study demonstrated no difference in PFS between ALK-positive and ALK-negative patients treated with pemetrexed, except when pemetrexed was used with first-line platinum. In the latter setting, the median PFS was 8.5 months in ALK-positive patients and 5.4 months in patients negative for *ALK, EGFR* and *KRAS* ($p = 0.018$). Interestingly, among never or light-smoking patients, PFS was similar between ALK-positive and ALK-negative patients, suggesting that smoking status may confound associations between pemetrexed sensitivity and ALK rearrangement status. We expect that the results of ongoing randomized trials in ALK-positive patients may help delineate these relationships.

Future directions

Next generation ALK inhibitors

One strategy to combat acquired resistance to crizotinib is to intensify ALK inhibition using more potent, next-generation ALK TKIs. A number of second-generation agents are currently being evaluated in the crizotinib-naïve and crizotinib-resistant settings. Although multiple compounds are in preclinical testing, we will briefly review only those agents being examined in clinical trials.

LDK378

LDK378 is a novel, highly-potent and selective inhibitor of ALK. In preclinical models, this agent has demonstrated potent activity against ALK *in vitro* and *in vivo* [98]. In addition, preliminary reports from the first-in-human phase I study of LDK378 (ClinicalTrials.gov identifier NCT01283516) suggest promising antitumor activity [99]. Based in part on this data, LDK378 was granted breakthrough-therapy designation status by the FDA in March 2013.

AP26113

AP26113 is a structurally distinct, novel ALK inhibitor that possesses approximately five- to tenfold greater potency against ALK compared to crizotinib [100]. In vitro, AP26113 has demonstrated activity in crizotinib-naïve, EML4-ALK-containing cell lines as well as crizotinib-resistant cells harboring the L1196M gatekeeper mutation [100]. AP26113 also exhibits antitumor activity in *ALK* xenograft models. Based upon these preclinical findings, AP26113 is now being investigated in a phase I/II clinical trial (ClinicalTrials.gov identifier NCT01449461). In a preliminary report from this study, the most common adverse events were fatigue and nausea [101]. Partial responses were observed in four of four ALK-positive patients. Like LDK378, activity in the CNS has been observed following treatment with AP26113. The dose finding phase of this study is ongoing as of the last report.

CH5424802

CH5424802 is a potent, orally-available ALK inhibitor with a unique chemical scaffold [102, 103]. In an initial preclinical study, CH5424802 demonstrated selective anti-tumor activity in cell lines and murine xenograft models expressing *EML4-ALK* [102]. Furthermore, CH5424802 induced tumor regression in xenograft models harboring *EML4-ALK* and concomitant L1196M mutations. Given this preclinical activity, a phase I/II trial of CH5424802 is currently underway in the United States for ALK-positive patients in the crizotinib-naïve and crizotinib-resistant settings (ClinicalTrials.gov identifier NCT 01588028). Additionally, results from a separate ongoing phase I/II trial of CH5424802 in crizotinib-naïve, ALK-rearranged NSCLC conducted in Japan were recently reported [104–106]. In the phase I portion of this study, 24 patients were treated with CH5424802 at doses of 20–300 mg twice daily [106]. No dose-limiting toxicities were observed, and 300 mg twice daily was considered the recommended phase II dose. Among 46 crizotinib-naïve, ALK-positive patients treated at this dose in the phase II portion of the study, objective responses were observed in 43 (93.5%) patients. The median treatment duration for this cohort was 7.1 months with a median follow-up period of 7.6 months at the time of reporting. The most common treatment-related adverse events included dysgeusia, increased ALT, increased blood bilirubin, rash and increased blood creatinine. Like LDK378, CH5424802 has been granted breakthrough-therapy status by the FDA.

ASP3026

ASP3026 is a novel, selective ALK inhibitor that has demonstrated activity in EML4-ALK-containing cell lines and xenograft models [107]. In preclinical models, ASP3026 also appears active against the gatekeeper L1196M mutation. A phase I trial of ASP3026 is currently ongoing (ClinicalTrials.gov identifier NCT01401504).

Heat shock protein 90 inhibitors

An alternative approach to acquired crizotinib resistance is to target heat shock protein 90 (HSP90). HSP90 is a molecular chaperone that promotes structural folding and stabilization of a broad range of proteins, including EML4-ALK [108,109]. HSP90 inhibitors have demonstrated activity in ALK-positive cell lines and murine models [109, 110]. Furthermore, cell line data suggests that HSP90 inhibitors retain their effectiveness despite acquired resistance to crizotinib [100, 110]. Clinical data of HSP90 inhibitors in ALK-positive NSCLC is more limited. In a phase II trial of the HSP90 inhibitor, IPI-504, the overall response rate was 7% among 76 patients with advanced NSCLC [111]. However, among the three patients with confirmed *ALK* rearrangements, two patients experienced partial responses and the third had prolonged stable disease. Notably, all three patients were crizotinib-naïve. In a preliminary report of a phase II study using the HSP90 inhibitor AUY922, 6 of 21 (29%) ALK-positive patients experienced partial responses, including two patients with crizotinib resistance [112]. Additional studies of HSP90 inhibitors in the crizotinib-resistant setting are ongoing.

Conclusion

In summary, *ALK* rearrangements now represent an important molecular subtype of NSCLC. Like *EGFR* mutations, *ALK* rearrangements confer an oncogene-addicted state associated with sensitivity to ALK inhibition. The early success of crizotinib has reaffirmed current treatment paradigms based upon tumor genotyping. Crizotinib is already a standard systemic therapy for ALK-positive NSCLC. Nonetheless, a number of important challenges remain. Most ALK-positive patients treated with crizotinib develop disease progression within one year. Understanding the mechanisms of crizotinib resistance and identifying new therapies based upon these findings will be necessary to improve the long-term effectiveness of ALK-directed therapies.

References

1 Lynch TJ, Bell DW, Sordella R, Gurubhagavatula S, Okimoto RA, Brannigan BW, *et al.* (2004) Activating mutations in the epidermal growth factor receptor underlying responsiveness of non-small-cell lung cancer to gefitinib. *N Engl J Med.* 350(21): 2129–39.

2 Paez JG, Jänne PA, Lee JC, Tracy S, Greulich H, Gabriel S, *et al.* (2004) EGFR mutations in lung cancer: correlation with clinical response to gefitinib therapy. *Science,* 304(5676): 1497–1500.

3 Pao W, Miller V, Zakowski M, Doherty J, Politi K, Sarkaria I, *et al.* (2004) EGF receptor gene mutations are common in lung cancers from "never smokers" and are associated with sensitivity of tumors to gefitinib and erlotinib. *Proc Natl Acad Sci USA,* 101(36): 13306–11.

4 Iwahara T, Fujimoto J, Wen D, Cupples R, Bucay N, Arakawa T, *et al.* (1997) Molecular characterization of ALK, a receptor tyrosine kinase expressed specifically in the nervous system. *Oncogene,* 14(4): 439–49.

5 Morris SW, Naeve C, Mathew P, James PL, Kirstein MN, Cui X, *et al.* (1997) ALK, the chromosome 2 gene locus altered by the t(2;5) in non-Hodgkin's lymphoma, encodes a novel neural receptor tyrosine kinase that is highly related to leukocyte tyrosine kinase (LTK). *Oncogene,* 14(18): 2175–88.

6 Pulford K, Lamant L, Morris SW, Butler LH, Wood KM, Stroud D, *et al.* (1997) Detection of anaplastic lymphoma kinase (ALK) and nucleolar protein nucleophosmin (NPM)-ALK proteins in normal and neoplastic cells with the monoclonal antibody ALK1. *Blood,* 89(4): 1394–1404.

7 Morris SW, Kirstein MN, Valentine MB, Dittmer KG, Shapiro DN, Saltman DL, *et al.* (1994) Fusion of a kinase gene, ALK, to a nucleolar protein gene, NPM, in non-Hodgkin's lymphoma. *Science,* 263(5151): 1281–4.

8 Vernersson E, Khoo NK, Henriksson ML, Roos G, Palmer RH, Hallberg B (2006) Characterization of the expression of the ALK receptor tyrosine kinase in mice. *Gene Expr Patterns,* 6(5): 448–61.

9 Bilsland JG, Wheeldon A, Mead A, Znamenskiy P, Almond S, Waters KA, *et al.* (2008) Behavioral and neurochemical alterations in mice deficient in anaplastic lymphoma kinase suggest therapeutic potential for psychiatric indications. *Neuropsychopharmacology,* 33(3): 685–700.

10 Chiarle R, Voena C, Ambrogio C, Piva R, Inghirami G (2008) The anaplastic lymphoma kinase in the pathogenesis of cancer. *Nat Rev Cancer,* 8(1): 11–23.

11 Lee HH, Norris A, Weiss JB, Frasch M (2003) Jelly belly protein activates the receptor tyrosine kinase Alk to specify visceral muscle pioneers. *Nature,* 425(6957): 507–12.

12 Stoica GE, Kuo A, Aigner A, Sunitha I, Souttou B, Malerczyk C, *et al.* (2001) Identification of anaplastic lymphoma kinase as a receptor for the growth factor pleiotrophin. *J Biol Chem,* 276(20): 16772–9.

13 Stoica GE, Kuo A, Powers C, Bowden ET, Sale EB, Riegel AT, *et al.* (2002) Midkine binds to anaplastic lymphoma kinase (ALK) and acts as a growth factor for different cell types. *J Biol Chem,* 277(39): 35990–8.

14 Mano H (2012) ALKoma: a cancer subtype with a shared target. *Cancer Discov,* 2(6): 495–502.

15 Griffin CA, Hawkins AL, Dvorak C, Henkle C, Ellingham T, Perlman EJ (1999) Recurrent involvement of 2p23 in inflammatory myofibroblastic tumors. *Cancer Res,* 59(12): 2776–80.

16 Coffin CM, Patel A, Perkins S, Elenitoba-Johnson KS, Perlman E, Griffin CA (2001) ALK1 and p80 expression and chromosomal rearrangements involving 2p23 in inflammatory myofibroblastic tumor. *Mod Pathol,* 14(6): 569–76.

17 Soda M, Choi YL, Enomoto M, Takada S, Yamashita Y, Ishikawa S, *et al.* (2007) Identification of the transforming EML4-ALK fusion gene in non-small-cell lung cancer. *Nature,* 448(7153): 561–6.

18 Sugawara E, Togashi Y, Kuroda N, Sakata S, Hatano S, Asaka R, *et al.* (2012) Identification of anaplastic lymphoma kinase fusions in renal cancer: large-scale immunohistochemical screening by the intercalated antibody-enhanced polymer method. *Cancer,* 118(18): 4427–36.

19 Murugan AK, Xing M (2011) Anaplastic thyroid cancers harbor novel oncogenic mutations of the ALK gene. *Cancer Res,* 71(13): 4403–11.

20 Mossé YP, Laudenslager M, Longo L, Cole KA, Wood A, Attiyeh EF, *et al.* (2008) Identification of ALK as

a major familial neuroblastoma predisposition gene. *Nature*, 455(7215): 930–5.

21 Janoueix-Lerosey I, Lequin D, Brugières L, Ribeiro A, de Pontual L, Combaret V, *et al.* (2008) Somatic and germline activating mutations of the ALK kinase receptor in neuroblastoma. *Nature*, 455(7215): 967–70.

22 Chen Y, Takita J, Choi YL, Kato M, Ohira M, Sanada M, *et al.* (2008) Oncogenic mutations of ALK kinase in neuroblastoma. *Nature*, 455(7215): 971–4.

23 George RE, Sanda T, Hanna M, Fröhling S, Luther W, Zhang J, *et al.* (2008) Activating mutations in ALK provide a therapeutic target in neuroblastoma. *Nature*, 455(7215): 975–8.

24 Rikova K, Guo A, Zeng Q, Possemato A, Yu J, Haack H, *et al.* (2007) Global survey of phosphotyrosine signaling identifies oncogenic kinases in lung cancer. *Cell*, 131(6): 1190–1203.

25 Webb TR, Slavish J, George RE, Look AT, Xue L, Jiang Q, *et al.* (2009) Anaplastic lymphoma kinase: Role in cancer pathogenesis and small-molecule inhibitor development for therapy. *Expert Rev Anticancer Ther*, 9(3): 331–56.

26 Koivunen JP, Mermel C, Zejnullahu K, Murphy C, Lifshits E, Holmes AJ, *et al.* (2008) EML4-ALK fusion gene and efficacy of an ALK kinase inhibitor in lung cancer. *Clin Cancer Res*, 14(13): 4275–83.

27 McDermott U, Iafrate AJ, Gray NS, Shioda T, Classon M, Maheswaran S, *et al.* (2008) Genomic alterations of anaplastic lymphoma kinase may sensitize tumors to anaplastic lymphoma kinase inhibitors. *Cancer Res*, 68(9): 3389–95.

28 Soda M, Takada S, Takeuchi K, Choi YL, Enomoto M, Ueno T, *et al.* (2008) A mouse model for EML4-ALK-positive lung cancer. *Proc Natl Acad Sci USA*, 105(50): 19893–7.

29 Takeuchi K, Choi YL, Togashi Y, Soda M, Hatano S, Inamura K, *et al.* (2009) KIF5B-ALK, a novel fusion oncokinase identified by an immunohistochemistry-based diagnostic system for ALK-positive lung cancer. *Clin Cancer Res*, 15(9): 3143–9.

30 Togashi Y, Soda M, Sakata S, Sugawara E, Hatano S, Asaka R, *et al.* (2012) KLC1-ALK: A novel fusion in lung cancer identified using a formalin-fixed paraffin-embedded tissue only. *PLoS One*, 7(2): e31323.

31 Pulford K, Lamant L, Espinos E, Jiang Q, Xue L, Turturro F, *et al.* (2004) The emerging normal and disease-related roles of anaplastic lymphoma kinase. *Cell Mol Life Sci*, 61(23): 2939–53.

32 Sasaki T, Rodig SJ, Chirieac LR, Jänne PA (2010) The biology and treatment of EML4-ALK non-small cell lung cancer. *Eur J Cancer*, 46(10): 1773–80.

33 Takeuchi K, Choi YL, Soda M, Inamura K, Togashi Y, Hatano S, *et al.* (2008) Multiplex reverse transcription-PCR screening for EML4-ALK fusion transcripts. *Clin Cancer Res*, 14(20): 6618–24.

34 Choi YL, Takeuchi K, Soda M, Inamura K, Togashi Y, Hatano S, *et al.* (2008) Identification of novel isoforms of the EML4-ALK transforming gene in non-small cell lung cancer. *Cancer Res*, 68(13): 4971–6.

35 Ou SH, Bartlett CH, Mino-Kenudson M, Cui J, Iafrate AJ (2012) Crizotinib for the treatment of ALK-rearranged non-small cell lung cancer: A success story to usher in the second decade of molecular targeted therapy in oncology. *Oncologist*, 17(11): 1351–75.

36 Shaw AT, Yeap BY, Mino-Kenudson M, Digumarthy SR, Costa DB, Heist RS, *et al.* (2009) Clinical features and outcome of patients with non-small-cell lung cancer who harbor EML4-ALK. *J Clin Oncol*, 27(26): 4247–53.

37 Wong DW, Leung EL, So KK, Tam IY, Sihoe AD, Cheng LC, *et al.* (2009) The EML4-ALK fusion gene is involved in various histologic types of lung cancers from nonsmokers with wild-type EGFR and KRAS. *Cancer*, 115(8): 1723–33.

38 Boland JM, Erdogan S, Vasmatzis G, Yang P, Tillmans LS, Johnson MR, *et al.* (2009) Anaplastic lymphoma kinase immunoreactivity correlates with ALK gene rearrangement and transcriptional up-regulation in non-small cell lung carcinomas. *Hum Pathol*, 40(8): 1152–8.

39 Inamura K, Takeuchi K, Togashi Y, Nomura K, Ninomiya H, Okui M, *et al.* (2008) EML4-ALK fusion is linked to histological characteristics in a subset of lung cancers. *J Thorac Oncol*, 3(1): 13–17.

40 Shinmura K, Kageyama S, Tao H, Bunai T, Suzuki M, Kamo T, *et al.* (2008) EML4-ALK fusion transcripts, but no NPM-, TPM3-, CLTC-, ATIC-, or TFG-ALK fusion transcripts, in non-small cell lung carcinomas. *Lung Cancer*, 61(2): 163–9.

41 Martelli MP, Sozzi G, Hernandez L, Pettirossi V, Navarro A, Conte D, *et al.* (2009) EML4-ALK rearrangement in non-small cell lung cancer and non-tumor lung tissues. *Am J Pathol*, 174(2): 661–70.

42 Takahashi T, Sonobe M, Kobayashi M, Yoshizawa A, Menju T, Nakayama E, *et al.* (2010) Clinicopathologic features of non-small-cell lung cancer with EML4-ALK fusion gene. *Ann Surg Oncol*, 17(3): 889–97.

43 Kris M, Johnson B, Kwiatkowski D, *et al.* (2011) Identification of driver mutations in tumor specimens from 1000 patients with lung adenocarcinoma: The NCI's Lung Cancer Mutation Consortium (LCMC). *J Clin Oncol.* 29 (suppl; abstr CRA7506).

44 Popat S, Vieira de Araújo A, Min T, Swansbury J, Dainton M, Wotherspoon A, *et al.* (2011) Lung adenocarcinoma with concurrent exon 19 EGFR mutation and ALK rearrangement responding to erlotinib. *J Thorac Oncol,* 6(11): 1962–3.

45 Kuo YW, Wu SG, Ho CC, Shih JY (2010) Good response to gefitinib in lung adenocarcinoma harboring coexisting EML4-ALK fusion gene and EGFR mutation. *J Thorac Oncol,* 5(12): 2039–40.

46 Tiseo M, Gelsomino F, Boggiani D, Bortesi B, Bartolotti M, Bozzetti C, *et al.* (2011) EGFR and EML4-ALK gene mutations in NSCLC: a case report of erlotinib-resistant patient with both concomitant mutations. *Lung Cancer,* 71(2): 241–3.

47 Zhang X, Zhang S, Yang X, Yang J, Zhou Q, Yin L, *et al.* (2010) Fusion of EML4 and ALK is associated with development of lung adenocarcinomas lacking EGFR and KRAS mutations and is correlated with ALK expression. *Mol Cancer,* 9: 188.

48 Sasaki T, Koivunen J, Ogino A, Yanagita M, Nikiforow S, Zheng W, *et al.* (2011) A novel ALK secondary mutation and EGFR signaling cause resistance to ALK kinase inhibitors. *Cancer Res,* 71(18): 6051–60.

49 Rimkunas VM, Crosby K, Kelly M, Gu TL, Mack J, Silver M, *et al.* (2012) Analysis of receptor tyrosine kinase ROS1 positive tumors in non-small cell lung cancer: Identification of a FIG-ROS1 fusion. *Clin Cancer Res,* 18(16): 4449–57.

50 Lee JK, Kim TM, Koh Y, Lee SH, Kim DW, Jeon YK, *et al.* (2012) Differential sensitivities to tyrosine kinase inhibitors in NSCLC harboring EGFR mutation and ALK translocation. *Lung Cancer,* 77(2): 460–3.

51 Yang J, Zhang X, Su J, *et al.* (2011) Concomitant EGFR mutation and EML4-ALK gene fusion in non-small cell lung cancer. *J Clin Oncol,* 29 (suppl; abstr 10517).

52 Rodig SJ, Mino-Kenudson M, Dacic S, Yeap BY, Shaw A, Barletta JA, *et al.* (2009) Unique clinicopathologic features characterize ALK-rearranged lung adenocarcinoma in the western population. *Clin Cancer Res,* 15(16): 5216–23.

53 Shaw AT, Solomon B (2011) Targeting anaplastic lymphoma kinase in lung cancer. *Clin Cancer Res,* 17(8): 2081–6.

54 Inamura K, Takeuchi K, Togashi Y, Hatano S, Ninomiya H, Motoi N, *et al.* (2009) EML4-ALK lung cancers are characterized by rare other mutations, a TTF-1 cell lineage, an acinar histology, and young onset. *Mod Pathol,* 22(4): 508–15.

55 Camidge DR, Bang YJ, Kwak EL, Iafrate AJ, Varella-Garcia M, Fox SB, *et al.* (2012) Activity and safety of crizotinib in patients with ALK-positive non-small-cell lung cancer: updated results from a phase 1 study. *Lancet Oncol,* 13(10): 1011–19.

56 Kim D, Ahn M, Shi Y, *et al.* (2012) Results of a global phase II study with crizotinib in advanced ALK-positive non-small cell lung cancer (NSCLC). *J Clin Oncol,* 30 (suppl; abstr 7533).

57 Yoshida A, Tsuta K, Nakamura H, Kohno T, Takahashi F, Asamura H, *et al.* (2011) Comprehensive histologic analysis of ALK-rearranged lung carcinomas. *Am J Surg Pathol,* 35(8): 1226–34.

58 Yoshida A, Tsuta K, Watanabe S, Sekine I, Fukayama M, Tsuda H, *et al.* (2011) Frequent ALK rearrangement and TTF-1/p63 co-expression in lung adenocarcinoma with signet-ring cell component. *Lung Cancer,* 72(3): 309–15.

59 Nishino M, Klepeis VE, Yeap BY, Bergethon K, Morales-Oyarvide V, Dias-Santagata D, *et al.* (2012) Histologic and cytomorphologic features of ALK-rearranged lung adenocarcinomas. *Mod Pathol,* 25(11): 1462–72.

60 Doebele RC, Lu X, Sumey C, Maxson DA, Weickhardt AJ, Oton AB, *et al.* (2012) Oncogene status predicts patterns of metastatic spread in treatment-naive non-small cell lung cancer. *Cancer,* 118(18): 4502–11.

61 Choi H, Paeng JC, Kim DW, Lee JK, Park CM, Kang KW, *et al.* (2013) Metabolic and metastatic characteristics of ALK-rearranged lung adenocarcinoma on FDG PET/CT. *Lung Cancer,* 79(3): 242–7.

62 Solomon B, Shaw AT (2012) Are anaplastic lymphoma kinase gene rearrangements in non-small cell lung cancer prognostic, predictive, or both? *J Thorac Oncol,* 7(1): 5–7.

63 Yang P, Kulig K, Boland JM, Erickson-Johnson MR, Oliveira AM, Wampfler J, *et al.* (2012) Worse disease-free survival in never-smokers with ALK+ lung adenocarcinoma. *J Thorac Oncol,* 7(1): 90–7.

64 Kim HR, Shim HS, Chung JH, Lee YJ, Hong YK, Rha SY, *et al.* (2012) Distinct clinical features and outcomes in never-smokers with nonsmall cell lung cancer who harbor EGFR or KRAS mutations or ALK rearrangement. *Cancer,* 118(3): 729–39.

65 Varella-Garcia M, Cho Y, Lu X, *et al.* (2010) ALK gene rearrangements in unselected caucasians with non-small cell lung carcinoma (NSCLC). *J Clin Oncol,* 28(15s): (suppl; abstr 10533).

66 Shaw AT, Yeap BY, Solomon BJ, Riely GJ, Gainor J, Engelman JA, *et al.* (2011) Effect of crizotinib on overall survival in patients with advanced non-small-cell lung cancer harbouring ALK gene rearrangement: A retrospective analysis. *Lancet Oncol,* 12(11): 1004–12.

67 Lee JK, Park HS, Kim DW, Kulig K, Kim TM, Lee SH, *et al.* (2012) Comparative analyses of overall survival in patients with anaplastic lymphoma kinase-positive and matched wild-type advanced nonsmall cell lung cancer. *Cancer,* 118(14): 3579–86.

68 Wu SG, Kuo YW, Chang YL, Shih JY, Chen YH, Tsai MF, *et al.* (2012) EML4-ALK translocation predicts better outcome in lung adenocarcinoma patients with wild-type EGFR. *J Thorac Oncol,* 7(1): 98–104.

69 Shaw AT, Solomon B, Kenudson MM (2011) Crizotinib and testing for ALK. *J Natl Compr Canc Netw,* 9(12): 1335–41.

70 Kwak EL, Bang YJ, Camidge DR, Shaw AT, Solomon B, Maki RG, *et al.* (2010) Anaplastic lymphoma kinase inhibition in non-small-cell lung cancer. *N Engl J Med,* 363(18): 1693–1703.

71 Camidge DR, Kono SA, Flacco A, Tan AC, Doebele RC, Zhou Q, *et al.* (2010) Optimizing the detection of lung cancer patients harboring anaplastic lymphoma kinase (ALK) gene rearrangements potentially suitable for ALK inhibitor treatment. *Clin Cancer Res,* 16(22): 5581–90.

72 Weickhardt AJ, Aisner DL, Franklin WA, Varella-Garcia M, Doebele RC, Camidge DR (2012) Diagnostic assays for identification of anaplastic lymphoma kinase-positive non-small cell lung cancer. *Cancer,* 119(8): 1467–77.

73 Sanders HR, Li HR, Bruey JM, Scheerle JA, Meloni-Ehrig AM, Kelly JC, *et al.* (2011) Exon scanning by reverse transcriptase-polymerase chain reaction for detection of known and novel EML4-ALK fusion variants in non-small cell lung cancer. *Cancer Genet,* 204(1): 45–52.

74 Danenberg P, Stephens C, Cooc J, *et al.* (2010) A novel RT-PCR approach to detecting EML4-ALK fusion genes in archival NSCLC tissue. *J Clin Oncol,* 28(15s): (suppl; abstr 10535).

75 Li T, Mack P, Desai S, *et al.* (2011) Large-scale screening of ALK fusion oncogene transcripts in archival NSCLC tumor specimens using multiplexed RT-PCR assays. *J Clin Oncol,* 29: (suppl; abstr 10520).

76 Mino-Kenudson M, Chirieac LR, Law K, Hornick JL, Lindeman N, Mark EJ, *et al.* (2010) A novel, highly sensitive antibody allows for the routine detection of ALK-rearranged lung adenocarcinomas by standard immunohistochemistry. *Clin Cancer Res,* 16(5): 1561–71.

77 McLeer-Florin A, Moro-Sibilot D, Melis A, Salameire D, Lefebvre C, Ceccaldi F, *et al.* (2012) Dual IHC and FISH testing for ALK gene rearrangement in lung adenocarcinomas in a routine practice: A French study. *J Thorac Oncol,* 7(2): 348–54.

78 Paik JH, Choe G, Kim H, Choe JY, Lee HJ, Lee CT, *et al.* (2011) Screening of anaplastic lymphoma kinase rearrangement by immunohistochemistry in non-small cell lung cancer: correlation with fluorescence in situ hybridization. *J Thorac Oncol,* 6(3): 466–72.

79 Park HS, Lee JK, Kim DW, Kulig K, Kim TM, Lee SH, *et al.* (2012) Immunohistochemical screening for anaplastic lymphoma kinase (ALK) rearrangement in advanced non-small cell lung cancer patients. *Lung Cancer,* 77(2): 288–92.

80 Yi ES, Boland JM, Maleszewski JJ, Roden AC, Oliveira AM, Aubry MC, *et al.* (2011) Correlation of IHC and FISH for ALK gene rearrangement in non-small cell lung carcinoma: IHC score algorithm for FISH. *J Thorac Oncol,* 6(3): 459–65.

81 Christensen JG, Zou HY, Arango ME, Li Q, Lee JH, McDonnell SR, *et al.* (2007) Cytoreductive antitumor activity of PF-2341066, a novel inhibitor of anaplastic lymphoma kinase and c-Met, in experimental models of anaplastic large-cell lymphoma. *Mol Cancer Ther,* 6(12 Pt 1): 3314–22.

82 Cui JJ, Tran-Dubé M, Shen H, Nambu M, Kung PP, Pairish M, *et al.* (2011) Structure based drug design of crizotinib (PF-02341066), a potent and selective dual inhibitor of mesenchymal-epithelial transition factor (c-MET) kinase and anaplastic lymphoma kinase (ALK). *J Med Chem,* 54(18): 6342–63.

83 Food and Drug Administration [1/8/2013]. Available from: http://www.accessdata.fda.gov/drugsatfda_docs/label/2012/202570s003lbl.pdf.

84 Shaw A, Kim D, Nakagawa K, *et al.* (eds) (2012) Phase III study of crizotinib versus pemetrexed or docetaxel chemotherapy in patients with advanced ALK-positive non-small cell lung cancer. *European Society Medical Oncology,* abstr LBA1_PR.

85 Besse B, Salgia R, Solomon B, *et al.* (2012) Visual disturbances in patients (PTs) with anaplastic lymphoma kinase (ALK)-positive advanced non-small cell lung cancer (NSCLC) treated with crizotinib. *Ann Oncol,* 23(9s): (abstr 1268P).

86 Spigel D, Ervin T, Ramlau R, *et al.* (2011) Final efficacy results from OAM4558g, a randomized phase II study evaluating MetMab or placebo in combination

with erlotinib in advanced NSCLC. *J Clin Oncol*, 29: suppl; abstr 7505.

87 Schnell P, Safferman A, Barlett C, *et al*. (2012) Clinical presentation of hepatotoxicity-associated crizotinib in ALK-positive (ALK+) advanced non-small cell lung cancer (NSCLC). *J Clin Oncol*, 30: suppl; abstr 7598.

88 Ou SH, Azada M, Dy J, Stiber JA (2011) Asymptomatic profound sinus bradycardia (heart rate ≤45) in non-small cell lung cancer patients treated with crizotinib. *J Thorac Oncol*, 6(12): 2135–7.

89 Weickhardt AJ, Rothman MS, Salian-Mehta S, Kiseljak-Vassiliades K, Oton AB, Doebele RC, *et al*. (2012) Rapid-onset hypogonadism secondary to crizotinib use in men with metastatic nonsmall cell lung cancer. *Cancer*, 118(21): 5302–9.

90 Choi YL, Soda M, Yamashita Y, Ueno T, Takashima J, Nakajima T, *et al*. (2010) EML4-ALK mutations in lung cancer that confer resistance to ALK inhibitors. *N Engl J Med*, 363(18): 1734–9.

91 Katayama R, Shaw AT, Khan TM, Mino-Kenudson M, Solomon BJ, Halmos B, *et al*. (2012) Mechanisms of acquired crizotinib resistance in ALK-rearranged lung Cancers. *Sci Transl Med*, 4(120): 120ra17.

92 Doebele RC, Pilling AB, Aisner DL, Kutateladze TG, Le AT, Weickhardt AJ, *et al*. (2012) Mechanisms of resistance to crizotinib in patients with ALK gene rearranged non-small cell lung cancer. *Clin Cancer Res*, 18(5): 1472–82.

93 Lovly CM, Pao W (2012) Escaping ALK inhibition: mechanisms of and strategies to overcome resistance. *Sci Transl Med*, 4(120): 120ps2.

94 Tanizaki J, Okamoto I, Okabe T, Sakai K, Tanaka K, Hayashi H, *et al*. (2012) Activation of HER family signaling as a mechanism of acquired resistance to ALK inhibitors in EML4-ALK-positive non-small cell lung cancer. *Clin Cancer Res*, 18(22): 6219–26.

95 Camidge DR, Kono SA, Lu X, Okuyama S, Barón AE, Oton AB, *et al*. (2011) Anaplastic lymphoma kinase gene rearrangements in non-small cell lung cancer are associated with prolonged progression-free survival on pemetrexed. *J Thorac Oncol*, 6(4): 774–80.

96 Lee JO, Kim TM, Lee SH, Kim DW, Kim S, Jeon YK, *et al*. (2011) Anaplastic lymphoma kinase translocation: A predictive biomarker of pemetrexed in patients with non-small cell lung cancer. *J Thorac Oncol*, 6(9): 1474–80.

97 Shaw AT, Varghese AM, Solomon BJ, Costa DB, Novello S, Mino-Kenudson M, *et al*. (2013) Pemetrexed-based chemotherapy in patients with advanced, ALK-positive non-small cell lung cancer. *Ann Oncol*, 24(1): 59–66.

98 Marsilje TH, Pei W, Chen B, Lu W, Uno T, Jin Y, *et al*. (2013) Synthesis, structure-activity relationship and in vivo efficacy of the novel potent and selective anaplastic lymphoma kinase (ALK) inhibitor 5-Chloro-*N*2-(2-isopropoxy-5-methyl-4-(piperidin-4-yl)phenyl)-*N*4-(2-(isopropylsulfonyl) phenyl)pyrimidine-2,4-diamine (LDK378) currently in phase I and II clinical trials. *J Med Chem*, June 26 [Epub ahead of print].

99 Shaw A, Camidge R, Felip E, *et al*. (2012) Results of a first-in-human phase I study of the ALK inhibitor LDK378 in advanced solid tumors. *Ann Oncol*, 23(9s): abstr 4400.

100 Katayama R, Khan TM, Benes C, Lifshits E, Ebi H, Rivera VM, *et al*. (2011) Therapeutic strategies to overcome crizotinib resistance in non-small cell lung cancers harboring the fusion oncogene EML4-ALK. *Proc Natl Acad Sci USA*, 108(18): 7535–40.

101 Gettinger S, Weiss G, Salgia R, *et al*. (2012) A first-in-human dose-finding study of the ALK/EGFR inhibitor AP26113 in patients with advanced malignancies. *Ann Oncol*, 23(9s): abstr 4390.

102 Sakamoto H, Tsukaguchi T, Hiroshima S, Kodama T, Kobayashi T, Fukami TA, *et al*. (2011) CH5424802, a selective ALK inhibitor capable of blocking the resistant gatekeeper mutant. *Cancer Cell*, 19(5): 679–90.

103 Kinoshita K, Asoh K, Furuichi N, Ito T, Kawada H, Hara S, *et al*. (2012) Design and synthesis of a highly selective, orally active and potent anaplastic lymphoma kinase inhibitor (CH5424802). *Bioorg Med Chem*, 20(3): 1271–80.

104 Kiura K, Seto T, Yamamoto N, *et al*. (2012) A first-in-human phase I/II study of ALK inhibitor CH5424802 in patients with ALK-positive NSCLC. *J Clin Oncol*, 30: suppl; abstr 7602.

105 Nishio M, Kiura K, Nakagawa K, *et al*. (2012) A phase I/II study of ALK inhibitor CH5424802 in patients with ALK-positive NSCLC; safety and efficacy interim results of the phase II portion. *Ann Oncol*, 23(9s): abstr 4410.

106 Seto T, Kiura K, Nishio M, *et al*. (2013) CH5424802 (R0542802) for patients with ALK-rearranged advanced non-small-cell lung cancer (AF-001JP study): A single-arm, open-label, phase 1–2 study. *Lancet Oncol*, April 29 [E-pub ahead of print].

107 Kuromitsu S, Mori M, Shimada I, *et al*. (eds) (2011) Antitumor activities of ASP3026 against EML4-ALK-dependent tumor models. Presented at the *International Conference of the American Association for*

Cancer Research-National Cancer Institute-European Organization for Research and Treatment of Cancer, San Francisco, CA, November 12–16.

108 Whitesell L, Lindquist SL (2005) HSP90 and the chaperoning of cancer. *Nat Rev Cancer,* 5(10): 761–72.

109 Chen Z, Sasaki T, Tan X, Carretero J, Shimamura T, Li D, *et al.* (2010) Inhibition of ALK, PI3K/MEK, and HSP90 in murine lung adenocarcinoma induced by EML4-ALK fusion oncogene. *Cancer Res,* 70(23): 9827–36.

110 Normant E, Paez G, West KA, Lim AR, Slocum KL, Tunkey C, *et al.* (2011) The Hsp90 inhibitor IPI-504 rapidly lowers EML4-ALK levels and induces tumor regression in ALK-driven NSCLC models. *Oncogene,* 30(22): 2581–6.

111 Sequist LV, Gettinger S, Senzer NN, Martins RG, Jänne PA, Lilenbaum R, *et al.* (2010) Activity of IPI-504, a novel heat-shock protein 90 inhibitor, in patients with molecularly defined non-small-cell lung cancer. *J Clin Oncol,* 28(33): 4953–60.

112 Felip E, Carcereny E, Barlesi F, *et al.* (2012) Phase II activity of the HSP90 inhibitor AUY922 in patients with ALK-rearranged (ALK+) or EGFR-mutated advanced non-small cell lung cancer (NSCLC). *Ann Oncol,* 23(9s): abstr 4380.

CHAPTER 36

Non-small Cell Lung Cancers (NSCLC) with Mutations in *BRAF*

Renata Ferrarotto and George R. Simon

Department of Thoracic/Head and Neck Medical Oncology, The University of Texas MD Anderson Cancer, Center, Houston, TX, USA

Introduction

Non-small cell lung cancers (NSCLC) are now divided into several distinct molecular entities, each with its own divergent natural histories and targeted therapies. BRAF, a protein kinase, is a member of the RAF family and is encoded by the *BRAF* gene. The RAF family of proteins includes 3 isoforms: ARAF, BRAF, and CRAF. BRAF, however, is the principal activator of key downstream signaling molecules MEK and ERK. Constitutive activation of the RAS-RAF signaling cascade through mutations in BRAF leads to uncontrolled proliferation, growth and metastases of tumor cells. Preclinical studies also demonstrate that mutations in the *BRAF* gene allow for BRAF to signal independently of upstream cues [1,2]. Identification of these mutations has allowed us to specifically treat tumors with targeted therapies. Outlined below are the molecular pathogenesis of BRAF deregulated tumors, its clinical characteristics and the targeted approaches used to treat these tumors.

Biology of *BRAF* mutant malignancies

RAF is a family of serine/threonine kinases in the mitogen-activated protein kinase (MAPK) signaling cascade that regulates cell growth, proliferation and differentiation. The pathway mediates the signal transduction from the cell surface to nuclear and cytosolic targets. It is also able to 'cross-talk' with other pathways, most importantly the phosphoinositide 3-kinase (PI3K/AKT/mTOR) cascade [3, 4].

As noted above, there are three RAF protein homologues identified in humans: ARAF, BRAF and CRAF. They all share sequence homology and contain a RAS binding domain necessary for membrane recruitment, a serine-threonine domain essential for activation and binding to regulatory proteins, and a protein-kinase domain at the C-terminus [5]. BRAF, however, has a significantly higher basal kinase activity than the other two RAFs and mutations in BRAF constitutively activate key downstream molecules, MEK and ERK [1, 6, 7].

RAS-GTP association with the RAS binding domain in the N-terminal regulatory region initiates BRAF activation through conformational changes that promote BRAF phosphorylation. The phosphorylation of BRAF stimulates its serine-threonine kinase activity that leads to phosphorylation and activation of MEK1/2 and ERK1/2 that will ultimately induce the activation of this pathway leading to its oncogenic transformation [7].

Lung Cancer, Fourth Edition. Edited by Jack A. Roth, Waun Ki Hong and Ritsuko U. Komaki.

Constitutive activation of BRAF can occur through multiple single-site missense mutations. These mutations cluster within the kinase domain at exons 11 and 15. The most common mutation, accounting for up to 90% of the cases in solid human malignancies, correspond to the hotspot transversion mutation T1799A at exon 15, that causes a valine (V) to glutamine (E) substitution at residue 600. The kinase activity of this mutation is 500-fold more potent than wild-type BRAF [1].

The vast majority of *BRAF* mutations are activating, however 'dominant-negative' mutations that lead to decreased kinase activity have also been described. These inactivating mutations can transactivate wild type *CRAF* and still phosphorylate and thus activate ERK [8]. Therefore, BRAF mutations in solid tumors can be characterized as high, intermediate or impaired kinase activity [7].

Molecular pathogenesis and frequency of *BRAF* mutations in human malignancies

Somatic mutation in *BRAF* occurs in approximately 60% of melanomas, 36% of papillary thyroid carcinoma and 10% of colorectal cancer [1,9–11].

The high incidence of *BRAF* mutation in melanomas and thyroid cancer lead to screening studies that sequenced exons 11 and 15 of *BRAF* in lung cancer. Missense mutations were identified in 1.6 to 3% of lung adenocarcinomas [2, 11]. Recent studies including larger patient populations and better screening techniques have identified mutations in 3 to 4.9% of patients screened [12–14].

Importantly, about 50% of *BRAF* mutations in NSCLC are V600E. They tend to occur in females and never-smokers. The other 50% of *BRAF* mutations, commonly referred to as non-V600E mutations, are distributed in narrow areas between codons 594 and 606 (exon 15) and 446 and 449 (exon 11), the most common being G469A in exon 11 (39%). The non-V600E mutations are almost exclusively found in current or former smokers, are very rare in melanoma and may reflect a tobacco-related carcinogenic effect [12, 13].

All *BRAF* mutations in NSCLC tend to be mutually exclusive of *EGFR* and *KRAS* mutations and *EML4–ALK* translocations, with anecdotal reports of mutations co-occurring with *EGFR*. It is also almost exclusive found in adenocarcinomas, with an incidence of non-V600E mutations in 0.2% of lung squamous cell carcinomas [13].

BRAF V600E mutant melanomas and colorectal cancers

To contextually understand *BRAF* mutant NSCLC, the results of major clinical trials in BRAF mutants melanoma and colorectal cancer are described in this section. Seventy to ninety percent of *BRAF* mutations in melanoma are of the V600E type; while 10 to 30% are due to the substitution of lysine to glutamic acid in codon 600 (V600K) [15].

The high frequency of V600E mutations in melanoma led to the development of drugs that target this genetic abnormality. Vemurafenib (Zelboraf, Genentech Inc. San Francisco, CA) is the first-in-class inhibitor of the kinase domain of V600E mutant *BRAF*. In a pivotal phase III trial comparing vemurafenib with dacarbazine in the first-line treatment of 675 patients with metastatic melanoma harboring the *BRAF* V600E mutation, vemurafenib demonstrated a response rate of 48% vs. 5%, and a median progression-free survival (PFS) of 5.3 months vs. 1.6 months ($P < 0.001$). At 6 months, overall survival (OS) was 84% (95% confidence interval [CI], 78 to 89) in the vemurafenib group and 64% (95% CI, 56 to 73) in the dacarbazine group [16]. A second phase III trial comparing dabrafenib (Tafinlar, GlaxoSmithKline Inc. Philadelphia, PA), a newer-generation kinase inhibitor of mutant V600E BRAF, to dacarbazine as first-line treatment for BRAF V600E positive metastatic melanoma, showed a response rate of 50% versus 6%, and a median PFS of 5.1 months for dabrafenib and 2.7 months for dacarbazine, with a hazard ratio (HR) of 0.30 (95% CI 0.18–0.51; $p < 0.0001$). Notably, shrinkage of brain metastases was seen in patients treated with dabrafenib [17].

The experience with BRAF inhibitors in colorectal cancer has not been as exciting. In a phase IB study evaluating vemurafenib in V600E *BRAF* mutant metastatic colorectal cancer, partial response was seen only in 1 out of 21 patients, with a median PFS of 3.7 months [18]. One of the postulated reasons for the low activity of BRAF inhibitors in colorectal cancer is the activation of epidermal growth factor receptor (EGFR), through a feedback loop, which triggers sustained MAPK signaling, and/or activation of the anti-apoptotic PI3K/AKT pathway, that results in the de novo or acquired resistance to BRAF inhibitors [19–21].

Vemurafenib and dabrafenib are now US FDA approved drugs for use in patients with metastatic melanoma harboring BRAF V600E mutations. In colorectal cancer, studies evaluating the combination of BRAF inhibitors with EGFR or PI3K inhibitors are currently underway [21].

BRAF mutant NSCLC

Diagnosis of BRAF mutations

BRAF mutations are most commonly diagnosed when reverse transcriptase – polymerase chain reaction (RT-PCR) is carried out in the multiplexed setting. An advantage of RT-PCR is that it can identify all the BRAF mutant transcripts, with high sensitivity. In practice, the institution of routine PCR testing technique faces several challenges [22]. Firstly, the complexity of the technique itself may confine this form of testing to larger cancer centers or to specialized commercialized CLIA (clinical laboratory improvement amendments) certified laboratories. Secondly, any PCR based strategy must incorporate validated primer pairs for all of the known BRAF mutant transcripts. Thirdly, RNA extraction of sufficient quality could be difficult from formalin fixed and paraffin embedded (FFPE) tissues. Given these caveats, it may be difficult to implement the routine testing for *BRAF* mutations in a clinical diagnostic laboratory and thus may entail sending the tissue to a specialized center or laboratory for testing [23, 24].

Clinical characteristics of BRAF mutated NSCLC

The clinical features of this distinct molecular entity await further accumulation of experience before firm conclusions regarding demographic characteristics can be discerned. From the limited published information available, the median age of a cohort of NSCLC patients (n = 18) with *BRAF* mutations was 64 years, 61% were female and all patients were Caucasian. Rare as this mutation is in Caucasians, it appears to be even rarer in Asians. It is also mutually exclusive of other more common molecular aberrations like *EGFR* and *KRAS* mutations and *ALK* translocations. Unlike *EGFR* mutations and *ALK* translocations, *BRAF* mutations are more commonly seen in former or current smokers. Indeed, 100% of the 18 patients in the Memorial Sloan Kettering case series were either former or current smokers. Other than these details, further clinical characteristics namely, the natural history of the disease, responses to chemotherapy, predilection for brain metastases and other clinical features will become evident once experience accumulates [12].

The treatment of V600E BRAF mutant NSCLC

The clinical data with BRAF inhibitors in lung cancer is currently limited. Gautschi *et al.* reported the first case of a patient with a V600E metastatic lung adenocarcinoma who responded to vemurafenib. Unfortunately, the patient did not have significant clinical benefit from the drug as he died shortly after treatment started, owing to poor performance status and complications of comorbidities [25].

More recently, Peters et al. reported the case of a 66-year-old male, never-smoker, diagnosed with an adenocarcinoma of the lung metastatic to the pleura, lymph nodes and liver, who progressed after cisplatin and pemetrexed first-line followed by pemetrexed maintenance. Tumor analysis revealed a V600E BRAF mutation and the patient started vemurafenib in September 2012, achieving a complete metabolic response after 6 weeks. The patient was still under treatment at the time of the report, in July 2013, and remains asymptomatic from his tumor [26].

The most robust clinical data in lung adenocarcinomas comes from a preliminary analysis of a phase II study evaluating dabrafenib in 40 patients with metastatic disease harboring BRAF V600E mutations. Eligibility criteria included progression after at least one line of platinum based chemotherapy. The population included 32% never-smokers, 48% with less than or equal to 40-pack year exposure and 20% with more than 40 pack-year smoking history. Only one patient out of 25 patients available for safety analysis was a current smoker. The primary objective of the trial was response rate (RR) and secondary objectives were progression free survival (PFS), overall survival (OS), safety, tolerability, pharmacokinetics and duration of response. Out of the 20 patients available for efficacy analysis, eight (40%) had a partial response (PR) and three (15%) had stable disease (SD). The patients who were heavy smokers did not seem to benefit from treatment. The duration of treatment response was between 6 and 12 months for 16% of the patients and over 12 months for two patients (8%). Data from 25 patients were available for safety analyses. Grade 3 adverse events were observed in 44% of the patients, leading to treatment discontinuation in 8%. Two patients (8%) developed squamous cell carcinoma of the skin, a known side effect of V600E BRAF inhibitors. Most common adverse events included fatigue, decreased appetite, asthenia, rash and nausea. The most common grade 3 toxicity was hypophosphatemia in two patients (8%)[27].

These preliminary results are encouraging and suggest that *BRAF* V600E can be used as a biomarker to predict sensitivity to BRAF V600E inhibitors. However, firm conclusions will have to await the emergence of mature data from this and other future studies.

The non-V600E *BRAF* mutants

BRAF V600E accounts for approximately 50% of BRAF mutations in NSCLC. The remainder, categorized as non-V600E BRAF mutations, comprises in the majority of the cases other activating mutations, but also includes BRAF inactivating mutations.

The type I BRAF inhibitors such as vemurafenib and dabrafenib specifically target the V600E mutant kinase. The activity against other BRAF activating mutations is unknown. Preclinical data suggest that non-V600E mutations are resistant to vemurafenib, however, they are sensitive to MEK inhibitors [28, 29]. Clinical studies evaluating MEK inhibitors in BRAF mutant NSCLC are ongoing [NCT00888134].

BRAF inactivating mutations

In a phase II study including 32 patients with stage IV NSCLC treated with dasatinib (Sprycel, Bristol Myers Squibb, Inc. Princeton, NJ), one patient achieved a complete response and was disease free without any further cancer treatments for 4 years, when the last follow-up was reported [30]. Sen *et al.*, studying the sample of the responding patient, identified a kinase inactivating *BRAF* mutation in exon 11, Y472C, that was able to activate MEK and ERK via transactivation of CRAF [8]. Further studies demonstrated that cell lines with G466V *BRAF* mutation, another kinase inactivating mutation found in approximately 0.87% of lung adenocarcinomas, were also sensitive to dasatinib in vitro, undergoing irreversible senescence after 72 hours of treatment. These observations could not be replicated in cell lines with BRAF wild type or activating mutations. Dasatinib indirectly inhibits CRAF and induces BRAF dimerization in NSCLC cell lines with impaired BRAF kinase activity, leading to oncogene induced senescence through ERK activation [8]. This mechanism explains the remarkable response the patient had to dasatinib and suggests that *BRAF* inactivating mutation predicts sensitivity to this drug [31]. Prospective clinical trials evaluating dasatinib in patients with lung cancer harboring BRAF inactivating mutations is needed to confirm these retrospective clinical and laboratory findings.

Mechanisms of resistance to BRAF inhibitors

Mechanisms of resistance to BRAF inhibitors in NSCLC are yet to be elucidated. However, attempts have been made to model resistance in BRAF V600E positive melanomas. Development of secondary mutations in the target gene has not been identified in BRAF V600E mutant melanoma cell lines with acquired resistance to BRAF inhibitors. Through preclinical modeling, three potential pathways of resistance have been identified and these include:

1 *Reactivation of the MAPK pathway in a BRAF-independent manner.* The BRAF inhibitor sensitive parental cell lines rely on BRAF for MAPK activation. The BRAF-inhibitor resistant cells had elevated expression of CRAF and ARAF, and thus were able to use these two RAF isoforms to activate MAPK signaling downstream. This would suggest that these resistant cell lines would be sensitive to inhibitors of molecules downstream of Ras. However, treatment of BRAF-inhibitor resistant cells with various structurally different MEK inhibitors had only cytostatic effects, suggesting that additional bypass mechanisms could be coexistent [32, 33].

2 *Differential activation of alternative receptor tyrosine kinase (RTK) signaling.* Other signaling pathways could be activated and, in particular, up regulation of IGF-1R has been noted in BRAF inhibitor resistant BRAF V600E mutant cell lines. Although the parental melanoma cells express the IGF-1R receptor, some of the BRAF-resistant melanomas expressed higher surface levels of IGF-1R. Interestingly, it was also reported that the enhanced IGF-1 mediated signaling was not due to amplification or mutations of the IGF-1R gene. Thus, the mechanism of enhanced IGF-1R expression and signaling in the context of chronic BRAF inhibition remains to be elucidated. Possible crosstalk between BRAF and RTKs, particularly IGF-1R-dependent networks, could be postulated [33–35].

3 *Activation of PI3K and phosphorylation of AKT.* Activation of the PI3K/Akt anti-apoptotic pathway, either through the increased phosphorylation of Akt or through the homozygous loss of PTEN, has also been described. This increased PI3K signaling could be induced by the up regulation of the IGF/IGF-1R axis. However, even though exogenous IGF-1 increases PI3K signalling in vitro, it is not sufficient to induce resistance. Thus it appears that the MAPK and IGF-1R/PI3K/AKT signaling pathways jointly cooperate to promote survival and expansion of the BRAF-inhibitor resistant cells [36].

Therefore the combined inhibition of the RAF/MEK pathway and the PI3K/AKT pathway may be an approach to treat BRAF inhibitor resistant BRAF V600E mutants. This has been observed pre-clinically where the combination of MEK and PI3K inhibitors has led to dramatic cytotoxic effects in BRAF-inhibitor resistant melanoma cell lines. Currently, there are several clinical trials underway testing the combination of MEK and PI3K inhibitors in this setting.

Summary

BRAF mutations are seen in about 3% of lung adenocarcinomas. Approximately 50% of *BRAF* mutations are V600E. The remainder, classified as non-V600E, are most commonly identified in exons 11 and 15. Inactivating mutations of *BRAF* have also been reported but are very rare. The *BRAF* V600E mutant lung adenocarcinomas may be treated with vemurafenib or dabrafenib and durable responses lasting at least 6 months have been reported in 50% of the patients [27]. The non-V600E *BRAF* mutants are under clinical investigation and combination targeted therapy such as MEK and PI3K/AKT inhibitors may be beneficial. It has also been reported in a rare inactivating BRAF mutated patient that dasatinib has clinical activity [30]. In the future, as experience accumulates, we will inevitably learn more about this relatively rare subset of BRAF mutated NSCLC.

References

1 Davies H, Bignell GR, Cox C, Stephens P, Edkins S, Clegg S, *et al.* (2012) Mutations of the BRAF gene in human cancer. *Nature*, 417(6892): 949–54. Epub 2002/06/18.

2 Brose MS, Volpe P, Feldman M, Kumar M, Rishi I, Gerrero R, *et al.* (2002) BRAF and RAS mutations in human lung cancer and melanoma. *Cancer Res*, 62(23): 6997–7000. Epub 2002/12/04.

3 Dhillon AS, von Kriegsheim A, Grindlay J, Kolch W (2007) Phosphatase and feedback regulation of Raf-1 signaling. *Cell Cycle*, 6(1): 3–7. Epub 2007/01/16.

4 Ramjaun AR, Downward J (2007) Ras and phosphoinositide 3-kinase: partners in development and tumorigenesis. *Cell Cycle*, 6(23): 2902–5. Epub 2007/11/13.

5 Moelling K, Heimann B, Beimling P, Rapp UR, Sander T (1984) Serine- and threonine-specific protein kinase activities of purified gag-mil and gag-raf proteins. *Nature*, 312(5994): 558–61. Epub 1984/12/06.

6 Rajagopalan H, Bardelli A, Lengauer C, Kinzler KW, Vogelstein B, Velculescu VE (2002) Tumorigenesis: RAF/RAS oncogenes and mismatch-repair status. *Nature*, 418(6901): 934. Epub 2002/08/29.

7 Wan PT, Garnett MJ, Roe SM, Lee S, Niculescu-Duvaz D, Good VM, *et al.* (2004) Mechanism of activation of the RAF-ERK signaling pathway by oncogenic mutations of B-RAF. *Cell*, 116(6): 855–67. Epub 2004/03/24.

8 Sen B, Peng S, Tang X, Erickson HS, Galindo H, Mazumdar T, *et al.* (2012) Kinase-impaired BRAF mutations in lung cancer confer sensitivity to dasatinib. *Sci Transl Med*, 4(136): 136ra70. Epub 2012/06/01.

9 Kimura ET, Nikiforova MN, Zhu Z, Knauf JA, Nikiforov YE, Fagin JA (2003) High prevalence of BRAF mutations in thyroid cancer: genetic evidence for constitutive activation of the RET/PTC-RAS-BRAF signaling pathway in papillary thyroid carcinoma. *Cancer Res*, 63(7): 1454–7. Epub 2003/04/03.

10 Samowitz WS, Sweeney C, Herrick J, Albertsen H, Levin TR, Murtaugh MA, *et al.* (2005) Poor survival associated with the BRAF V600E mutation in microsatellite-stable colon cancers. *Cancer Res*, 65(14): 6063–9. Epub 2005/07/19.

11 Naoki K, Chen TH, Richards WG, Sugarbaker DJ, Meyerson M (2002) Missense mutations of the BRAF gene in human lung adenocarcinoma. *Cancer Res*, 62(23): 7001–3.

12 Paik PK, Arcila ME, Fara M, Sima CS, Miller VA, Kris MG, *et al.* (2011) Clinical characteristics of patients with lung adenocarcinomas harboring BRAF mutations. *J Clin Oncol*, 29(15): 2046–51. Epub 2011/04/13.

13 Marchetti A, Felicioni L, Malatesta S, Grazia Sciarrotta M, Guetti L, Chella A, *et al.* (2011) Clinical features and outcome of patients with non-small-cell lung cancer harboring BRAF mutations. *J Clin Oncol*, 29(26): 3574–9. Epub 2011/08/10.

14 Cardarella S, Ogino A, Nishino M, Butaney M, Shen J, Lydon C, *et al.* (2013) Clinical, pathological and biological features associated with BRAF mutations in non-small cell lung cancer. *Clin Cancer Res*, Epub 2013/07/09.

15 Menzies AM, Haydu LE, Visintin L, Carlino MS, Howle JR, Thompson JF, *et al.* (2012) Distinguishing clinicopathologic features of patients with V600E and V600K BRAF-mutant metastatic melanoma. *Clin Cancer Res*, 18(12): 3242–9. Epub 2012/04/27.

16 Chapman PB, Hauschild A, Robert C, Haanen JB, Ascierto P, Larkin J, *et al.* (2011) Improved survival with vemurafenib in melanoma with BRAF V600E mutation. *N Engl J Med*, 364(26): 2507–16. Epub 2011/06/07.

17 Hauschild A, Grob JJ, Demidov LV, Jouary T, Gutzmer R, Millward M, *et al.* (2012) Dabrafenib in BRAF-mutated metastatic melanoma: a multicentre, open-label, phase 3 randomised controlled trial. *Lancet*, 380(9839): 358–65. Epub 2012/06/28.

18 Kopetz S, Hoff PM, Morris JS, Wolff RA, Eng C, Glover KY, *et al.* (2010) Phase II trial of infusional fluorouracil, irinotecan, and bevacizumab for metastatic colorectal cancer: efficacy and circulating angiogenic biomarkers associated with therapeutic resistance. *J Clin Oncol*, 28(3): 453–9. Epub 2009/12/17.

19 Corcoran RB, Ebi H, Turke AB, Coffee EM, Nishino M, Cogdill AP, *et al.* (2012) EGFR-mediated re-activation of MAPK signaling contributes to insensitivity of BRAF mutant colorectal cancers to RAF inhibition with vemurafenib. *Cancer Discov*, 2(3): 227–35. Epub 2012/03/27.

20 Prahallad A, Sun C, Huang S, Di Nicolantonio F, Salazar R, Zecchin D, *et al.* (2012) Unresponsiveness of colon cancer to BRAF(V600E) inhibition through feedback activation of EGFR. *Nature*, 483(7387): 100–3. Epub 2012/01/28.

21 Mao M, Tian F, Mariadason JM, Tsao CC, Lemos R, Jr., Dayyani F, *et al.* (2012) Resistance to BRAF inhibition in BRAF-mutant colon cancer can be overcome with PI3K inhibition or demethylating agents. *Clin Cancer Res*, 19(3): 657–67. Epub 2012/12/20.

22 Szankasi P, Reading NS, Vaughn CP, Prchal JT, Bahler DW, Kelley TW (2013) A quantitative allele-specific PCR test for the BRAF V600E mutation using a single heterozygous control plasmid for quantitation: A model for qPCR testing without standard curves. *Journal of Molecular Diagnostics*, 15(2): 248–54. Epub 2013/01/15.

23 Gonzalez D, Fearfield L, Nathan P, Taniere P, Wallace A, Brown E, *et al.* (2013) BRAF mutation testing algorithm for vemurafenib treatment in melanoma: recommendations from an expert panel. *British Journal of Dermatology*, 168(4): 700–7. Epub 2013/01/31.

24 Lade-Keller J, Romer KM, Guldberg P, Riber-Hansen R, Hansen LL, Steiniche T, *et al.* (2013) Evaluation of

BRAF mutation testing methodologies in formalin-fixed, paraffin-embedded cutaneous melanomas. *Journal of Molecular Diagnostics*, 15(1): 70–80. Epub 2012/11/20.

25 Gautschi O, Pauli C, Strobel K, Hirschmann A, Printzen G, Aebi S, *et al.* (2012) A patient with BRAF V600E lung adenocarcinoma responding to vemurafenib. *J Thorac Oncol*, 7(10): e23–4. Epub 2012/06/30.

26 Peters S, Michielin O, Zimmermann S (2013) Dramatic response induced by vemurafenib in a BRAF V600E-mutated lung adenocarcinoma. *J Clin Oncol*, 31(20): e341–4. Epub 2013/06/05.

27 Planchard D, Mazieres J, Riely GJ, Rudin CM, Barlesi F, Quoix E, *et al.* (2013) Interim results of phase II study BRF113928 of dabrafenib in BRAF V600E mutation-positive non-small cell lung cancer (NSCLC) patients. *J Clin Oncol*, 31(Suppl).

28 Yang H, Higgins B, Kolinsky K, Packman K, Go Z, Iyer R, *et al.* (2010) RG7204 (PLX4032), a selective BRAFV600E inhibitor, displays potent antitumor activity in preclinical melanoma models. *Cancer Res*, 70(13): 5518–27. Epub 2010/06/17.

29 Trejo CL, Juan J, Vicent S, Sweet-Cordero A, McMahon M. (2012) MEK1/2 inhibition elicits regression of autochthonous lung tumors induced by KRASG12D or BRAFV600E. *Cancer Res*, 72(12): 3048–59. Epub 2012/04/19.

30 Johnson FM, Bekele BN, Feng L, Wistuba I, Tang XM, Tran HT, *et al.* (2010) Phase II study of dasatinib in patients with advanced non-small-cell lung cancer. *J Clin Oncol*, 28(30): 4609–15. Epub 2010/09/22.

31 Collado M, Serrano M (2010) Senescence in tumours: Evidence from mice and humans. *Nat Rev Cancer*, 10(1): 51–7. Epub 2009/12/24.

32 Alcala AM, Flaherty KT (2012) BRAF inhibitors for the treatment of metastatic melanoma: Clinical trials and mechanisms of resistance. *Clin Cancer Res*, 18(1): 33–9. Epub 2012/01/05.

33 Villanueva J, Vultur A, Lee JT, Somasundaram R, Fukunaga-Kalabis M, Cipolla AK, *et al.* (2010) Acquired resistance to BRAF inhibitors mediated by a RAF kinase switch in melanoma can be overcome by cotargeting MEK and IGF-1R/PI3K. *Cancer Cell*, 18(6): 683–95. Epub 2010/12/16.

34 Villanueva J, Vultur A, Herlyn M (2011) Resistance to BRAF inhibitors: Unraveling mechanisms and future treatment options. *Cancer Res*, 71(23): 7137–40. Epub 2011/12/02.

35 Girotti MR, Marais R (2013) Deja vu: EGF receptors drive resistance to BRAF inhibitors. *Cancer Discov*, 3(5): 487–90. Epub 2013/05/10.

36 Atefi M, von Euw E, Attar N, Ng C, Chu C, Guo D, *et al.* (2011) Reversing melanoma cross-resistance to BRAF and MEK inhibitors by co-targeting the AKT/mTOR pathway. *PLoS One*, 6(12): e28973. Epub 2011/12/24.

CHAPTER 37
Prognostic and Predictive Biomarker Signatures

Johannes R. Kratz[1] *and David M. Jablons*[2]
[1]Department of Surgery, Massachusetts General Hospital, Boston, MA, USA
[2]Department of Surgery, University of California, San Francisco, CA, USA

Introduction

Five-year survival rates after the diagnosis of non-small cell lung cancer (NSCLC) range from 73% for pathologically diagnosed stage IA lung cancer to 17% for metastatic stage IV lung cancers [1]. Surgical resection represents the mainstay of treatment for patients with stage I and stage II lung NSCLC and remains the only hope for cure in patients with localized disease [2,3]. The poor 5-year survival rate of localized NSCLC (53%) [4] after complete surgical resection compared to that of breast (98%) [4] and colorectal cancer (91%), however, indicates that TNM staging alone does not adequately risk stratify patients and predict outcome [5,6].

Although differences in the demographics of these patient cohorts may explain some of the discrepancies in outcome for early stage lung cancer vs. other solid tumors, it is widely accepted that lung cancers are particularly aggressive relative to other solid tumors and much more likely to harbor a component of micrometastatic disease at the time of diagnosis [7]. This is supported by the clinical observation that patients undergoing lobectomy have less locoregional recurrence in the only randomized prospective trial to-date of patients with stage I lung cancer undergoing lobectomy vs. limited (segment or wedge) resection [8]. For this reason, lobectomy is widely considered the standard of care in patients with adequate lung reserve as it more completely excises occult micrometastases at the time of resection. One of the biggest challenges that remains is being able to more accurately predict which patients with early stage disease are likely to have subclinical metastases undetectable by our current imaging and pathological modalities.

The ability to predict which patients have subclinical metastases putting them at risk for early mortality could change treatment regimens in a variety of ways. Despite relatively poor overall outcomes in localized disease, multiple randomized control trials do not support a significant benefit of adjuvant therapy in most patients with stage I disease [9]. Identifying which patients may harbor highly aggressive tumors may select a subset of patients with local disease that may, in fact, benefit from adjuvant therapy and/or more radical operations. Select patients with regional and even distant spread may similarly benefit from aggressive treatment regimens if shown to have less aggressive tumors. At the same, patients with less aggressive forms of the disease may be spared from both toxic chemotherapy

Lung Cancer, Fourth Edition. Edited by Jack A. Roth, Waun Ki Hong and Ritsuko U. Komaki.

regimens as well as more substantial pulmonary resections. The potential to both change our treatment regimens as well as improve patient outcomes by providing targeted therapy has been the driving force behind recent efforts to improve patient prognostic classification to the level of breast and colorectal cancers in recent years.

The TNM lung cancer staging system was revised in 2009 upon recommendations of the International Association for the Study of Lung Cancer International Staging Committee in an attempt to modernize the current staging system to reflect updated technological and treatment advances as well as globalize the staging system by including multiple international cohorts [10]. Despite the truly outstanding effort that was poured into the project, only relatively minor changes to the established TNM staging system were made [11]. The improvement in prognostic discrimination was similarly modest in nature [12], leading more than one author to speculate that the next major advance in the lung cancer staging system would come in the form of biomarker classifiers that conveyed important prognostic information about tumor biology [10, 12, 13].

Prognostic biomarker signatures

Several studies have demonstrated the potential power of molecular biomarker signatures in refining lung cancer prognosis. As early as 2001, multiple independent groups reported substantial differences in gene expression in lung tumors compared to normal lung tissues. Several of these groups noted strong correlations between gene expression patterns and patient outcomes, leading to the first reported prognostic biomarker signatures in lung cancer. Bhattacharjee *et al.* reported that a subclass of lung adenocarcinomas with high expression levels of several neuroendocrine markers had significantly worse outcomes (median survival of 21 months compared to 41 months for lung adenocarcinomas not belonging to this subclass) [14]. Conversely a subclass of lung adenocarcinomas with high expression levels of type II alveolar markers was associated with significantly better outcomes (median survival of 50 months compared to 33 months for lung adenocarcinomas not belonging to this subclass) [14]. In 2002, Beer *et al.* reported a 50-gene prognostic signature that conferred increased risk of mortality at 3 years in a validation cohort of stage I patients (HR of 2.78) [15].

Since these early reports, a multitude of other groups have reported biomarker signatures prognostic of survival in NSCLC [16–30]. In fact, the multiple prognostic biomarker signatures that have been published have led us to the point where clinicians are no longer asking whether prognostic biomarker signatures may someday be helpful in improving risk discrimination in patients with NSCLC. Instead, clinicians are beginning to ask which of these signatures is not only ready for practical clinical application now, but has evidence supporting its everyday use in the clinic [31].

The translation of these prognostic biomarker signatures from bench to bedside has proven difficult. The majority of the proposed prognostic biomarker signatures are microarray-based [30, 31]. Microarrays have been a notoriously difficult platform to translate into the clinical setting. Traditionally, they have required high-quality RNA extracted from snap frozen tissue samples not typically available in a community setting [30]. In addition, microarray data is difficult to manage, interpret and standardize [32], leading to significant barriers to widespread and rapid adoption by commercial laboratories. Results from microarray-based gene expression studies performed at multiple institutions have not always been consistent [33, 34], leading to the standard practice of many academic laboratories to confirm their microarray results by real-time PCR. Cognizant of these recognized difficulties with microarray-based signatures, quantitative PCR-based prognostic signatures have recently been reported [17, 19, 21, 22, 25, 35]. In contrast to the technical and logistical difficulties of translating microarray-based signatures into the clinical setting, quantitative PCR is widely available, inexpensive, easy to understand and replicate, and highly reliable. No special substrate is required; in fact, the use of formalin-fixed paraffin embedded tissues specimens as the test substrate has been reported in lung [35] and other solid tumors [36, 37].

The second barrier to bedside translation has been the lack of rigorous clinical evidence supporting the use of the majority of these prognostic biomarker signatures. Like any clinical model, prognostic biomarker signatures must be both developed as well as validated before they can be adopted into clinical practice [38]. With the multitude of biomarker signatures already proposed, the development of additional prognostic signatures is unlikely to yield anything but a relatively modest improvement in performance. This is especially true in cases where publically available microarray datasets [20] are used and reused to generate additional prognostic biomarker signatures. The real challenge, therefore, lies in validating prognostic biomarker signatures in a clinically-relevant and rigorous manner. In statistics, model overfitting is a frequent outcome of studies in which a large number of predictors and small number of outcomes are used to develop a model [38]. Because such a large number of predictors are used, there is a high chance that many of the final predictors included in the model may be more related to statistical noise rather than truly relevant biological properties associated with patient outcomes. Unfortunately, the widespread approach of using microarrays containing tens of thousands of predictors in the context of relatively small developmental cohorts makes many of the proposed prognostic biomarker signatures in NSCLC especially vulnerable to this statistical phenomenon. In fact, it has been reported that a random microarray-based biomarker signature results in a statistically significant improvement in prognosis approximately 10% and up to 40% of the time, depending on the cohort tested [39]. Although various ways to reduce statistical overfitting in clinical models have been described [38], the litmus test of model overfitting is blinded validation of the proposed biomarker signature on an independent cohort of patients. Although validation on previously published publicly available microarray datasets is frequently employed, this technique is not equivalent to an independent blinded validation, as the proposed biomarker signature may be modified or rejected in favor of another once its performance in the validation cohort has been explored, but before it has been reported.

To date, only two groups have reported the results of blinded, independent validation of prognostic biomarker signatures. In 2008, Shedden reported the results from the National Cancer Institute Directors Challenge, a large multi-institutional study that subjected multiple proposed prognostic biomarker signatures to blinded validation using independent cohorts [20]. 442 stage I-III resected adenocarcinomas were divided into two training cohorts of 177 and 79 patients as well as two validation cohorts of 82 and 104 patients. Microarray data was acquired by four participating institutions that independently developed eight prognostic biomarker signatures using the training cohort datasets. These eight signatures were submitted to a fifth institution acting as a referee that redistributed the biomarker signatures amongst all institutions for blinded independent validation. Unfortunately, of the 8 signatures developed, none was able to reliably separate stage I patients without the addition of clinical covariates. In addition, the signature that was able to reliably separate stage I patients with clinical covariates in their model performed worse than a model using clinical covariates alone [20]. The results from this study should not discourage further attempts to develop a robust, independently validated prognostic biomarker signature. Rather, the study serves as an ideal model of prognostic assay development and validation and underscores the importance of blinded, independent validation before a prognostic biomarker signature can be considered appropriate for clinical use.

Recently, our group reported the development and blinded large-scale validation of a quantitative PCR based prognostic biomarker signature for non-squamous NSCLC [35]. This signature was unique in a number of respects:

1 The use of formalin-fixed, paraffin-embedded (FFPE) tissues as a substrate and quantitative PCR to measure gene expression, resulting in a highly practical and robust prognostic signature ready for immediate clinical use.

2 The use of only 11 predictors, a variety of statistical techniques, and a large training cohort of 361 patients to minimize overfitting.

3 Blinded international validation using multiple large-scale independent cohorts including 433 patients who underwent resection of stage I disease at community hospitals belonging to the Kaiser Permanente Northern California system as well as over 1000 patients who underwent resection in hospitals belonging to the China Clinical Trials Consortium (CCTC).

The prognostic biomarker signature was derived by measuring expression of 11 genes intimately related to known lung cancer pathways to assign patients to low-, intermediate-, and high-risk categories using an algorithm and cut-off points developed on a training cohort of 361 patients who underwent surgical resection of nonsquamous NSCLC at the University of California, San Francisco. Kaplan-Meier analysis of low-, intermediate- and high-risk tumors demonstrated highly significant differences in outcomes of patients with stage I disease in the Kaiser Permanente validation cohort as well as within all stages of the CCTC validation cohort [35]. Multivariable analysis demonstrated that risk category was the strongest predictor of outcome after adjustment for age, sex, smoking history, histology, and stage, and improved risk discrimination in stage I patients beyond both the National Comprehensive Cancer Network (NCCN) criteria [40] used to identify high-risk stage I patients (Kaiser cohort) as well as stage (CCTC cohort). The assay was also able to successfully risk-stratify patients with T1a node-negative tumors, identifying patients with almost 50% 5-year mortality despite surgical resection of these small node-negative tumors [41]. The performance of prognostic biomarker signatures in this patient population is increasingly relevant as the number of surgical resections performed for T1a node-negative tumors is expected to increase dramatically with the adoption of new lung cancer screening guidelines [42].

Predictive biomarker signatures

As opposed to prognostic biomarker signatures which attempt to improve risk stratification of patients with respect to overall outcome, predictive biomarker signatures attempt to risk stratify patients with respect to specific types of treatment they receive; i.e., responders vs. nonresponders. The potential clinical utility of predictive signatures is immediately apparent. By directing therapies only at patients likely to respond, the prognosis of these patients is expected to improve dramatically while the toxic effects of these therapies are avoided entirely in the nonresponders. In an ideal world in which multiple predictive biomarker signatures exist, each individual patient would receive therapies to which their tumors are most likely to respond.

The literature describing the predictive ability of molecular biomarker signatures is not as robust as the evidence supporting single-gene predictive biomarkers such as those associated with the eGFR pathway (see Chapter 29). However, a few notable studies add to the growing body of evidence that suggests prognostic biomarker signatures are also predictive of response to chemotherapy. In 2010, Zhu *et al.* described a prognostic biomarker signature developed on patients randomized to receive either observation or cisplatin/vinorelbine as part of the JBR.10 trial [43]. The signature was found to be prognostic of survival in four independent previously published microarray datasets. In addition, this prognostic biomarker signature was predictive of improved disease-specific survival in high-risk patients randomized to receive adjuvant chemotherapy, but not in low-risk patients (HR 0.33 [95% CI 0.17–0.63] and 3.67 [95% CI 1.22–11.06] respectively) [43]. A separate group recently described both the development of a separate signature predictive of response to chemotherapy using the Director's Challenge dataset and independent validation of this predictive signature on 69 patients from the JBR.10 trial dataset [44]. A signature that correlates with premetrexed response and resistance in squamous cell lung carcinoma has also been proposed [45].

Although definitive proof of the predictive ability of molecular biomarker signatures will come in the form of future prospective randomized trials, it is important to note that current clinical practice guidelines such as those proposed by the National Comprehensive Cancer Network (NCCN) recommend adjuvant chemotherapy in patients with "high-risk" stage IB tumors. Many of the criteria qualifying tumors as "high-risk" (poor differentiation, vascular invasion, wedge resection, visceral pleural involvement, lack of adequate lymph node sampling) have never undergone prospective validation demonstrating a survival benefit for adjuvant chemotherapy in patients with such criteria. Nonetheless, in light of the extremely poor outcomes patients with "localized" NSCLC experience compared to other solid tumors, consensus groups such as the NCCN recommend adjuvant chemotherapy in patients with these high-risk criteria. It is easy to envision, therefore, how validated tools that improve risk stratification above and beyond these criteria proposed by the NCCN may therefore provide clinicians with much stronger reasons to consider additional therapy for patients with biomarker proven high-risk disease.

Future directions

Lung oncology continues to trend towards increasing personalized prognosis and individualized treatment regimens. The next major revision of the lung cancer staging system will almost certainly include the use of molecular biomarkers [10,12,13]. Several promising novel developments are on the horizon, including the development of prognostic biomarker signatures from sputum [46], serum [47], and pleural fluid samples [48], prognostic biomarker signatures derived from lung cancer stem cell populations [49, 50], and new techniques that enable microarray-based gene expression analysis from formalin-fixed paraffin-embedded tissue specimens [51, 52]. The adoption of clinically validated prognostic and predictive biomarker signatures in lung oncology is underway and is expected to soon mirror the widespread use of such signatures in the field of breast oncology [53].

References

1 Mountain CF (1997) Revisions in the international system for staging lung cancer. *Chest*, Jun; 111(6): 1710–17. PubMed PMID: 9187198. Epub 1997/06/01. eng.

2 Spira A, Ettinger DS (2004) Multidisciplinary management of lung cancer. *N Engl J Med*, Jan 22; 350(4): 379–92. PubMed PMID: 14736930. eng.

3 Spiro SG, Silvestri GA (2005) One hundred years of lung cancer. *Am J Respir Crit Care Med*, Sep 1; 172(5): 523–9. PubMed PMID: 15961694. eng.

4 Jemal A, Siegel R, Xu J, Ward E (2010) Cancer statistics, 2010. *CA Cancer J Clin*, Sep–Oct; 60(5): 277–300. PubMed PMID: 20610543. Epub 2010/07/09. eng.

5 Pfannschmidt J, Muley T, Bulzebruck H, Hoffmann H, Dienemann H (2007) Prognostic assessment after surgical resection for non-small cell lung cancer: Experiences in 2083 patients. *Lung Cancer*, Mar; 55(3): 371–7. PubMed PMID: 17123661.eng.

6 Fang D, Zhang D, Huang G, Zhang R, Wang L (2001) Results of surgical resection of patients with primary lung cancer: A retrospective analysis of 1,905 cases. *Ann Thorac Surg*, Oct; 72(4): 1155–9. PubMed PMID: 11603429. eng.

7 Coello MC, Luketich JD, Litle VR, Godfrey TE (2004) Prognostic significance of micrometastasis in non-small-cell lung cancer. *Clin Lung Cancer*, Jan; 5(4): 214–25. PubMed PMID: 14967073.

8 Ginsberg RJ, Rubinstein LV (1995) Randomized trial of lobectomy versus limited resection for T1 N0 non-small cell lung cancer. Lung Cancer Study Group. *Ann Thorac Surg*, Sep; 60(3): 615–22; discussion 22–3. PubMed PMID: 7677489. eng.

9 Pignon JP, Tribodet H, Scagliotti GV, Douillard JY, Shepherd FA, Stephens RJ, *et al.* (2008) Lung adjuvant cisplatin evaluation: A pooled analysis by the LACE Collaborative Group. *Journal of Clinical Oncology*, Jul 20; 26(21): 3552–9. PubMed PMID: 18506026. Epub 2008/05/29. eng.

10 Goldstraw P, Shepherd FA, Pass HI (2009) The International Staging System for Lung Cancer. *Am Soc Clin Oncol*, 29: 462–8.

11 Rami-Porta R, Crowley JJ, Goldstraw P (2009) The revised TNM staging system for lung cancer. *Ann Thorac Cardiovasc Surg*, Feb; 15(1): 4–9. PubMed PMID: 19262443.

12 Detterbeck FC, Boffa DJ, Tanoue LT (2009) The new lung cancer staging system. *Chest*, Jul; 136(1): 260–71. PubMed PMID: 19584208. eng N1 – Journal Article N1 – Review.

13 D'Amico TA (2008) Molecular biologic staging of lung cancer. *Ann Thorac Surg*, Feb; 85(2): S737–42. PubMed PMID: 18222207.

14 Bhattacharjee A, Richards WG, Staunton J, Li C, Monti S, Vasa P, *et al.* (2001) Classification of human lung carcinomas by mRNA expression profiling reveals

distinct adenocarcinoma subclasses. *Proc Natl Acad Sci USA*, Nov 20; 98(24): 13790–5. PubMed PMID: 11707567. eng.

15 Beer DG, Kardia SL, Huang CC, Giordano TJ, Levin AM, Misek DE, *et al.* (2002) Gene-expression profiles predict survival of patients with lung adenocarcinoma. *Nat Med*, Aug; 8(8): 816–24. PubMed PMID: 12118244. Epub 2002/07/16. eng.

16 Roepman P, Jassem J, Smit EF, Muley T, Niklinski J, van de Velde T, *et al.* (2009) An immune response enriched 72-gene prognostic profile for early-stage non-small-cell lung cancer. *Clin Cancer Res*, Jan 1; 15(1): 284–90. PubMed PMID: 19118056. Epub 2009/01/02.eng.

17 Boutros PC, Lau SK, Pintilie M, Liu N, Shepherd FA, Der SD, *et al.* (2009) Prognostic gene signatures for non-small-cell lung cancer. *Proc Natl Acad Sci USA*, Feb 24; 106(8): 2824–8. PubMed PMID: 19196983. Pubmed Central PMCID: 2636731. Epub 2009/02/07. eng.

18 Sun Z, Wigle DA, Yang P (2008) Non-overlapping and non-cell-type-specific gene expression signatures predict lung cancer survival. *J Clin Oncol*, Feb 20; 26(6): 877–83. PubMed PMID: 18281660. Epub 2008/02/19. eng.

19 Skrzypski M, Jassem E, Taron M, Sanchez JJ, Mendez P, Rzyman W, *et al.* (2008) Three-gene expression signature predicts survival in early-stage squamous cell carcinoma of the lung. *Clin Cancer Res*, Aug 1; 14(15): 4794–9. PubMed PMID: 18676750. Epub 2008/08/05. eng.

20 Shedden K, Taylor JM, Enkemann SA, Tsao MS, Yeatman TJ, Gerald WL, *et al.* (2008) Gene expression-based survival prediction in lung adenocarcinoma: A multi-site, blinded validation study. *Nat Med*, Aug; 14(8): 822–7. PubMed PMID: 18641660. Pubmed Central PMCID: 2667337. Epub 2008/07/22. eng.

21 Raz DJ, Ray MR, Kim JY, He B, Taron M, Skrzypski M, *et al.* (2008) A multigene assay is prognostic of survival in patients with early-stage lung adenocarcinoma. *Clin Cancer Res*, Sep 1; 14(17): 5565–70. PubMed PMID: 18765549. Epub 2008/09/04. eng.

22 Lau SK, Boutros PC, Pintilie M, Blackhall FH, Zhu CQ, Strumpf D, *et al.* (2007) Three-gene prognostic classifier for early-stage non small-cell lung cancer. *J Clin Oncol*, Dec 10; 25(35): 5562–9. PubMed PMID: 18065728. Epub 2007/12/11. eng.

23 Larsen JE, Pavey SJ, Passmore LH, Bowman RV, Hayward NK, Fong KM (2007) Gene expression signature predicts recurrence in lung adenocarcinoma. *Clin Cancer Res*, May 15; 13(10): 2946–54. PubMed PMID: 17504995. Epub 2007/05/17. eng.

24 Larsen JE, Pavey SJ, Passmore LH, Bowman R, Clarke BE, Hayward NK, *et al.* (2007) Expression profiling defines a recurrence signature in lung squamous cell carcinoma. *Carcinogenesis*, Mar; 28(3): 760–6. PubMed PMID: 17082175. Epub 2006/11/04. eng.

25 Chen HY, Yu SL, Chen CH, Chang GC, Chen CY, Yuan A, *et al.* (2007) A five-gene signature and clinical outcome in non-small-cell lung cancer. *N Engl J Med*, Jan 4; 356(1): 11–20. PubMed PMID: 17202451. Epub 2007/01/05. eng.

26 Raponi M, Zhang Y, Yu J, Chen G, Lee G, Taylor JM, *et al.* (2006) Gene expression signatures for predicting prognosis of squamous cell and adenocarcinomas of the lung. *Cancer Res*, Aug 1; 66(15): 7466–72. PubMed PMID: 16885343. Epub 2006/08/04. eng.

27 Lu Y, Lemon W, Liu PY, Yi Y, Morrison C, Yang P, *et al.* (2006) A gene expression signature predicts survival of patients with stage I non-small cell lung cancer. *PLoS Med*, Dec; 3(12): e467. PubMed PMID: 17194181. Pubmed Central PMCID: 1716187. Epub 2006/12/30. eng.

28 Guo L, Ma Y, Ward R, Castranova V, Shi X, Qian Y (2006) Constructing molecular classifiers for the accurate prognosis of lung adenocarcinoma. *Clin Cancer Res*, Jun 1; 12(11 Pt 1): 3344–54. PubMed PMID: 16740756. Epub 2006/06/03.eng.

29 Tomida S, Koshikawa K, Yatabe Y, Harano T, Ogura N, Mitsudomi T, *et al.* (2004) Gene expression-based, individualized outcome prediction for surgically treated lung cancer patients. *Oncogene*, Jul 8; 23(31): 5360–70. PubMed PMID: 15064725. Epub 2004/04/06.eng.

30 Kratz JR, Jablons DM (2009) Genomic prognostic models in early-stage lung cancer. *Clin Lung Cancer*, May; 10(3): 151–7. PubMed PMID: 19443334. Epub 2009/05/16. eng.

31 Subramanian J, Simon R (2010) Gene expression-based prognostic signatures in lung cancer: Ready for clinical use? *J Natl Cancer Inst*, Apr 7; 102(7): 464–74. PubMed PMID: 20233996. Pubmed Central PMCID: PMC2902824. Epub 2010/03/18. eng.

32 Michiels S, Koscielny S, Hill C (2007) Interpretation of microarray data in cancer. *Br J Cancer*, Apr 23; 96(8): 1155–8. PubMed PMID: 17342085.eng.

33 Parmigiani G, Garrett-Mayer ES, Anbazhagan R, Gabrielson E (2004) A cross-study comparison of gene expression studies for the molecular classification of lung cancer. *Clin Cancer Res*, May 1; 10(9): 2922–7. PubMed PMID: 15131026. eng.

34 Xu JZ, Wong CW (2010) Hunting for robust gene signature from cancer profiling data: sources of variability, different interpretations, and recent methodological developments. *Cancer Lett*, Oct 1; 296(1): 9–16. PubMed PMID: 20579805. Epub 2010/06/29. eng.

35 Kratz JR, He J, Van Den Eeden SK, Zhu ZH, Gao W, Pham PT, *et al.* (2012) A practical molecular assay to predict survival in resected non-squamous, non-small-cell lung cancer: Development and international validation studies. *Lancet*, Mar 3; 379(9818): 823–32. PubMed PMID: 22285053. Pubmed Central PMCID: 3294002. Epub 2012/01/31. eng.

36 Gray RG, Quirke P, Handley K, Lopatin M, Magill L, Baehner FL, *et al.* Validation study of a quantitative multigene reverse transcriptase-polymerase chain reaction assay for assessment of recurrence risk in patients with stage II colon cancer. *Journal of Clinical Oncology*, Dec 10; 29(35): 4611–19. PubMed PMID: 22067390. Epub 2011/11/10. eng.

37 Paik S, Shak S, Tang G, Kim C, Baker J, Cronin M, *et al.* (2004) A multigene assay to predict recurrence of tamoxifen-treated, node-negative breast cancer. *N Engl J Med*, Dec 30; 351(27): 2817–26. PubMed PMID: 15591335. eng N1 – Clinical Trial N1 – Journal Article N1 – Randomized Controlled Trial N1 – Research Support, Non-US Gov't.

38 Steyerberg EW (2009) *Clinical Prediction Models: A Practical Approach to Development, Validation, and Updating*. New York, NY: Springer, xxviii, 497 pp.

39 Starmans MH, Fung G, Steck H, Wouters BG, Lambin P (2011) A simple but highly effective approach to evaluate the prognostic performance of gene expression signatures. *PLoS One*, 6(12): e28320. PubMed PMID: 22163293. Pubmed Central PMCID: PMC3233554. Epub 2011/12/14. eng.

40 NCCN Clinical Practice Guidelines in Oncology Non-Small Cell Lung Cancer: National Comprehensive Cancer Network; 2012. Available from: http://www.nccn.org/professionals/physician_gls/PDF/nscl.pdf.

41 Kratz JR, Van den Eeden SK, He J, Jablons DM, Mann MJ (2012) A prognostic assay to identify patients at high risk of mortality despite small, node-negative lung tumors. *JAMA*, Oct 24; 308(16): 1629–31. PubMed PMID: 23093159. Epub 2012/10/25. eng.

42 Bach PB, Mirkin JN, Oliver TK, Azzoli CG, Berry DA, Brawley OW, *et al.* (2012) Benefits and harms of CT screening for lung cancer: A systematic review of benefits and harms of CT screening for lung cancer. *JAMA*, May 20: 1–12. PubMed PMID: 22610500. Epub 2012/05/23. Eng.

43 Zhu CQ, Ding K, Strumpf D, Weir BA, Meyerson M, Pennell N, *et al.* (2010) Prognostic and predictive gene signature for adjuvant chemotherapy in resected non-small-cell lung cancer. *J Clin Oncol*, Oct 10; 28(29): 4417–24. PubMed PMID: 20823422. Pubmed Central PMCID: 2988634. Epub 2010/09/09. eng.

44 Van Laar RK (2012) Genomic signatures for predicting survival and adjuvant chemotherapy benefit in patients with non-small-cell lung cancer. *BMC Med Genomics*, 5: 30. PubMed PMID: 22748043. Pubmed Central PMCID: PMC3407714. Epub 2012/07/04. eng.

45 Hou J, Lambers M, den Hamer B, den Bakker MA, Hoogsteden HC, Grosveld F, *et al.* (2012) Expression profiling-based subtyping identifies novel non-small cell lung cancer subgroups and implicates putative resistance to pemetrexed therapy. *J Thorac Oncol*, Jan; 7(1): 105–14. PubMed PMID: 22134068. Epub 2011/12/03. eng.

46 Leng S, Do K, Yingling CM, Picchi MA, Wolf HJ, Kennedy TC, *et al.* (2012) Defining a gene promoter methylation signature in sputum for lung cancer risk assessment. *Clin Cancer Res*, Jun 15; 18(12): 3387–95. PubMed PMID: 22510351. Pubmed Central PMCID: PMC3483793. Epub 2012/04/19. eng.

47 Bianchi F, Nicassio F, Marzi M, Belloni E, Dall'olio V, Bernard L, *et al.* (2011) A serum circulating miRNA diagnostic test to identify asymptomatic high-risk individuals with early stage lung cancer. *EMBO Molecular Medicine*, Aug; 3(8): 495–503. PubMed PMID: 21744498. Pubmed Central PMCID: PMC3377091. Epub 2011/07/12. eng.

48 Wang T, Lv M, Shen S, Zhou S, Wang P, Chen Y, *et al.* (2012) Cell-free microRNA expression profiles in malignant effusion associated with patient survival in non-small cell lung cancer. *PLoS One*, 7(8): e43268. PubMed PMID: 22937028. Pubmed Central PMCID: PMC3427341. Epub 2012/09/01. eng.

49 Perumal D, Singh S, Yoder SJ, Bloom GC, Chellappan SP (2012) A novel five gene signature derived from stem-like side population cells predicts overall and recurrence-free survival in NSCLC. *PLoS One*, 7(8): e43589. PubMed PMID: 22952714. Pubmed Central PMCID: PMC3430700. Epub 2012/09/07.eng.

50 Onaitis M, D'Amico TA, Clark CP, Guinney J, Harpole DH, Rawlins EL (2011) A 10-gene progenitor cell signature predicts poor prognosis in lung adenocarcinoma. *Ann Thorac Surg*, Apr; 91(4): 1046–50; discussion 50. PubMed PMID: 21353202. Pubmed Central PMCID: PMC3376444. Epub 2011/03/01.eng.

51 Xie Y, Xiao G, Coombes KR, Behrens C, Solis LM, Raso G, *et al.* (2011) Robust gene expression signature

from formalin-fixed paraffin-embedded samples predicts prognosis of non-small-cell lung cancer patients. *Clin Cancer Res*, Sep 1; 17(17): 5705–14. PubMed PMID: 21742808. Pubmed Central PMCID: PMC3166982. Epub 2011/07/12. eng.

52 Jacobson TA, Lundahl J, Mellstedt H, Moshfegh A (2011) Gene expression analysis using long-term preserved formalin-fixed and paraffin-embedded tissue of non-small cell lung cancer. *Int J Oncol*, Apr; 38(4): 1075–81. PubMed PMID: 21305253. Epub 2011/02/10. eng.

53 Paik S (2007) Development and clinical utility of a 21-gene recurrence score prognostic assay in patients with early breast cancer treated with tamoxifen. *Oncologist*, Jun; 12(6): 631–5. PubMed PMID: 17602054. eng N1 – Journal Article N1 – Research Support, N.I.H., Extramural.

CHAPTER 38
Brain Metastasis from Lung Cancer

Ritsuko U. Komaki and Amol J. Ghia
Department of Radiation Oncology, The University of Texas MD Anderson Cancer Center, Houston, TX, USA

Introduction

Brain metastases from lung cancer represent a significant portion of all brain metastases. Between 10% and 25% of patients with lung cancer present with brain metastases, and about 40% to 50% of all patients with lung cancer will develop brain metastasis during the course of the disease [1]. Some evidence exists to suggest that improved control of locally advanced disease may be associated with increased incidence of brain metastases [2, 3]. The prognosis for patients with brain metastasis is poor with median survival times usually less than 1 year.

The manifestations of brain metastases vary and depend on the location and number of lesions and the amount of associated edema, hemorrhage, or both. Presenting symptoms can include headache, nausea and emesis, focal weakness, seizures, confusion, ataxia, visual disturbances, or occasionally cranial nerve palsies. Magnetic resonance imaging (MRI) is currently the gold standard for identifying brain metastases and is more sensitive than CT scanning for this purpose [4].

Initial management of brain metastases usually involves oral or intravenous corticosteroids [5]. Patients with seizures should be treated with antiseizure medications. However, prophylactic use of antiseizure medication is controversial because of the high risk of adverse effects [6]. Subsequent management of brain metastases depends on size, number, location of the lesions as well as the presence of extracranial disease and the general condition of the patient. Whole-brain radiation therapy (WBRT) may be used as primary therapy for brain metastases, as adjuvant treatment after surgery or stereotactic radiosurgery (SRS) or as salvage therapy following local treatment. SRS confers local control rates comparable to those for surgery with minimal toxicity and may be used as primary therapy or salvage therapy. Its versatility makes it useful for multiple or deep-seated lesions and for patients who are medically unfit for surgery. Surgery provides rapid relief of mass effect and may be the best choice for a large single metastasis.

This chapter comprises a brief review of the pathophysiology of brain metastases followed by the roles of various forms of therapy for treatment of brain metastases from lung cancer, including surgical resection, SRS, WBRT, and prophylactic cranial irradiation (PCI). Other topics covered include the toxicity of radiation to the brain and the current state of knowledge on biomarkers in non-small cell lung cancer and brain metastases.

Pathophysiology of brain metastasis

The numerous mechanisms underlying the metastatic spread of cancer are enormously complex, and their discussion is beyond the scope of this chapter. In simple terms, the formation of

Lung Cancer, Fourth Edition. Edited by Jack A. Roth, Waun Ki Hong and Ritsuko U. Komaki.

metastases requires that cells separate from the primary tumor and reach distant tissues specific to the type of primary tumor, where they must adapt to the local microenvironment [7, 8]. The epithelial-to-mesenchymal transition has been implicated in this process, the molecular mechanisms of which continue to be investigated [8]. Other steps involved in the development of metastases include angiogenesis, cellular invasion of basement membranes, and cellular transportation [9]. Cells destined to become brain metastases most likely access the brain via the arterial circulation. Tumor cells within primary tumors of the lung have direct access to the arterial circulation, which contributes to the relatively high rate of brain metastases from primary lung cancers [9]. Within the brain parenchyma, metastases tend to localize at the grey–white matter junction, where the capillary beds are located. The distribution of brain metastases also roughly follows the cerebral blood flow, consistent with the so-called "mechanical hypothesis" proposed by Ewing [10]. Another hypothesis to explain metastatic dissemination and distribution is that of the "seed and soil." Originally developed by Paget, the modern version of the seed and soil hypothesis suggests that genetic changes in cancer cells define the predilection of those cells for particular microenvironments within host tissues [11], such as the preferential metastasis of prostate cancer cells to bone and cells from breast cancer or melanoma to the brain. The molecular basis for these relationships continues to be investigated [9].

Treatment options

Surgical resection

The surgical resection of brain metastases has traditionally been reserved for the palliation of symptomatic lesions or in situations in which pathologic confirmation is necessary. However, subgroups of patients with favorable prognosis have undergone surgical resection to improve survival. In a pivotal study, Patchell *et al.* performed a randomized trial in the 1980s to evaluate the role of surgery in 48 patients with a single brain metastasis receiving WBRT [12]. Specifically, patients with a suspected brain metastasis were randomly assigned to undergo either biopsy followed by WBRT or surgical resection followed by WBRT. WBRT was to be delivered to a dose of 36 Gy in 12 fractions. Patients with a suspected brain metastasis were randomized to undergo either a biopsy followed by WBRT or a surgical resection followed by WBRT. WBRT was delivered to a dose of 36 Gy in 12 fractions. Local recurrence was improved (52% vs. 20%) and quality of life (2 months vs. 9 months of functional independence) was improved in those receiving a resection. Moreover, survival was improved (3 months vs. 9 months) and neurologic death improved (6 months vs. 14 months) in the surgery arm. The operative mortality (4%) and morbidity (8%) were deemed acceptable.

Another phase III trial conducted in the Netherlands involved patients with a single brain metastasis receiving WBRT (40 Gy in 2-Gy fractions twice a day), alone or with surgical resection [13]. Surgical resection was again associated with extended median survival time (10 months vs. 6 months), with particular benefits seen among those with stable extracranial disease. Indeed, local therapy is generally advocated for those with favorable performance status, a single brain metastasis, and stable extracranial disease. The need for adjuvant radiotherapy after surgical resection to maintain intracranial disease control is discussed further later in this chapter.

Stereotactic radiosurgery

The neurosurgeon Lars Leksell formulated the principles of radiosurgery in 1951, about 17 years before the launch of the first Gamma Knife prototype at the Karolinska Institute. SRS is commonly defined as a single high dose of radiation directed by stereotaxis conformally to the target minimizing dose to the normal surrounding tissue [14]. The first Gamma Knife unit was installed in the United States at the University of Pittsburgh Medical Center in 1987 [15]. Today, brain metastases represent the most common indication for SRS [16]. The goals of SRS can be achieved with several types of technologies, including Gamma Knife, linear accelerator, or Cyberknife.

The Radiation Therapy Oncology Group (RTOG) has conducted several trials investigating SRS for brain metastases. The prospective RTOG 90-05 trial sought to determine the optimal dose for radiosurgery of brain metastases by evaluating the maximum tolerated radiosurgical dose in 168 patients who had previously undergone irradiation for primary or metastatic brain lesions [17]. The maximum tolerated doses depended on the size of the lesion, being 24 Gy for tumors ≤20 mm in diameter, 18 Gy for those 21–30 mm, and 15 Gy for tumors 31–40 mm. However, the actual maximum tolerated dose for lesions ≤20 mm was not met because the investigators were reluctant to exceed 24 Gy. Notably, the rate of radionecrosis at 2 years was 11%. Subsequent research suggested that treating tumors ≤20 mm with 20 Gy rather than 24 Gy produced equivalent control with lower complication rates [18, 19].

RTOG 95–08 was a randomized controlled trial comparing WBRT alone versus WBRT with SRS for 333 patients with 1–3 brain metastases [20]. The WBRT dose was 37.5 Gy delivered in 15 fractions, and the SRS dose was delivered according to the guidelines established by RTOG 90-05. Although no difference was found in overall survival between the two groups, subgroup analyses revealed that SRS improved overall survival for patients with a single brain metastasis. The addition of SRS to WBRT also led to higher response rates and better local control rates at 1 year (82% vs. 71%); receipt of SRS was the only factor predictive of local control in a Cox proportional hazards analysis. The risk of developing a local recurrence was 43% higher in the WBRT alone arm than in the WBRT with SRS arm. Moreover, patients receiving SRS were more likely to have had stable or improved Karnofsky Performance Status scores at 6 months after treatment.

To date, no randomized controlled trials have been undertaken to compare surgery with SRS for single brain metastases. Findings from retrospective analyses are mixed and fraught with selection bias [21–23]. The indications for SRS remain controversial, with factors contributing to the choice of treatment including the number of metastases, performance status, status of extracranial disease, and tumor histology. Further clinical trials are necessary to define an SRS treatment algorithm for patients with brain metastases.

Whole-brain radiation therapy

WBRT has been used to treat brain metastases since the early 20th century. The first report of its efficacy in a large series came from Memorial Hospital, where Chao *et al.* described 38 patients with brain metastases treated from 1949 to 1953 with fractionated WBRT [24]. Palliation was successful for 63% of patients so treated, and the recommended dose was 30–40 Gy given over 3–5 weeks. A subsequent report of an additional 218 patients at Memorial Hospital given WBRT to a goal dose of 30 Gy in 3 weeks revealed a survival benefit among those who responded to this therapy [25], further establishing the role of WBRT in the treatment of intracranial metastatic disease. WBRT is still used for effective palliation of gross brain metastases and as prophylaxis against the development of new brain metastases. These topics are described further in the following sections.

WBRT as primary therapy for gross disease

Prospective trials led by the RTOG have been used to help ascertain the optimal dose and fractionation for WBRT. In general, WBRT to a dose of 20–40 Gy given over 1–4 weeks has resulted in median survival times of 4–6 months for patients with brain metastases (Table 38.1) [26]. Although the treatment schedules varied somewhat, they were comparable with regard to the incidence and the duration of improvement, time to progression, survival, and palliative index. In RTOG 7361, approximately 900 patients were randomly assigned to receive 20 Gy in 5 fractions over 1 week, 30 Gy in 10 fractions over 2 weeks, or 40 Gy in 15 fractions over 3 weeks. The median survival times were similar among the three treatment groups at 15 weeks for

Table 38.1 Studies of postoperative whole-brain radiation therapy for brain metastases by the Radiation Therapy Oncology Group

Protocol and reference	Period of study	No. of patients	Treatment scheme	Median survival time
RTOG 6901	1971–1973	233	30 Gy in 10 Fx over 2 wks	21 wks
Borgelt *et al.*, 1980 [27]		217	30 Gy in 15 Fx over 3 wks	18 wks
		233	40 Gy in 15 Fx over 3 wks	18 wks
		227	40 Gy in 20 Fx over 4 wks	16 wks
RTOG 7361	1973–1976	447	20 Gy in 5 Fx over 1 wk	15 wks
Borgelt *et al.*, 1981 [28]		228	30 Gy in 10 Fx over 2 wks	15 wks
		227	40 Gy in 15 Fx over 3 wks	18 wks
RTOG 6901 ultra-rapid	1971–1973	26	10 Gy in 1 Fx over 1 day	15 wks
Borgelt *et al.*, 1981 [27]				
RTOG 7361 ultra-rapid	1973–1976	33	12 Gy in 2 Fx over 2 days	13 wks
Borgelt *et al.*, 1981 [28]				
RTOG 7606 favorable pts	1976–1979	130	30 Gy in 10 Fx over 2 wks	18 wks
Kurtz *et al.*, 1981 [123]		125	50 Gy in 20 Fx over 4 wks	17 wks
RTOG 8528	1986–1989	30	48 Gy in 1.6-Gy bid	4.8 months
Accelerated		53	54.5 Gy in 1.6-Gy bid	5.4 months
HFX		44	64 Gy in 1.6-Gy bid	7.2 months
Sause *et al.*, 1993 [29]		36	70.4 Gy in 1.6-Gy bid	8.2 months
RTOG 9104	1991–1995	213	30 Gy in 10 Fx	4.5 months
Murray *et al.*, 1997 [30]		216	54.4 Gy in 1.6-Gy fx bid	4.5 months
RTOG 7916	1979–1983	193	30 Gy in 10Fx over 2 wks	4.5 months
Misonidazole		200	5 Gy in 6 Fx over 3 wks	4.1 months
Phillips *et al.*, 1995 [32]		196	30 Gy in 10 Fx+Miso	3.1 months
		190	5 Gy in 6 Fx+Miso	3.9 months
RTOG 8905	1989–1993	36	37.5 Gy in 15 Fx over 3 wks	6.1 months
BrdU		34	37.5 Gy in 15 Fx+BrdUrd	4.3 months
Komarnicky *et al.*, 1991 [31]				

BrdU, bromodeoxyuridine; Fx, fraction; HFX, hyperfractionated.
Source: Modified from Sneed PK, Larson DA, Wara WM (1996) *Neurosurg Clin N Am*, 7: 505–15[26]. Reproduced with permission of Elsevier.

the 20-Gy and 30-Gy groups and 18 weeks for the 40-Gy group. WBRT was shown to improve neurological function for about half of the patients in this study, without much improvement in survival, depending on dose or fractionation [27]. Another randomized study of an ultra-rapid high-dose radiation schedule (10 Gy in 1 fraction or 12 Gy in 2 fractions) [28] revealed median survival times that were not much different than those in RTOG 7361; however, patients who received the ultra-rapid high-dose WBRT had more treatment-related neurological toxicity. The rapidity of the response to therapy was also similar between the two treatment groups in this study, but the duration of improvement, time to worsening of neurological status, and rate of complete disappearance of neurological symptoms were generally less for patients receiving 10–12 Gy in one or two fractions than for those receiving more prolonged treatment such as 30 Gy in 10 fractions.

The RTOG 8528 trial investigated accelerated hyperfractionated WBRT, with patients receiving 1.6-Gy twice-daily fractionation to a total dose of 48 Gy, 54.4 Gy, 64 Gy, or 70.4 Gy [29].

Although median survival times seemed to increase with increasing dose (4.8 months, 5.4 months, 7.2 months and 8.2 months), this apparent difference was not statistically significant. A follow-up randomized RTOG phase III study included 445 patients with Karnofsky Performance Status scores of ≥60 who were given either hyperfractionated RT at 1.2-Gy twice-daily fractionation to a total tumor dose of 54.4 Gy or 30 Gy in 10 fractions [30]. The median survival time was 4.5 months in both treatment groups. Given the lack of superiority of the hyperfractionated regimens and the toxicity of ultra-rapid high-dose fractionations, modern clinical trials involving WBRT for gross disease typically use either 30 Gy in 10 fractions or 37.5 Gy in 15 fractions.

Various radiosensitizers have also been investigated in prospective randomized clinical trials. The RTOG 7916 trial evaluated one such radiosensitizer, misonidazole, in patients with brain metastases [31]. This study involved 779 patients who received 30 Gy in 10 fractions over 2 weeks with or without 1 g/m^2 of misonidazole or 30 Gy in 6 fractions over 3 weeks with or without 2 g/m^2 misonidazole. The median survival times ranged from 3.1 months to 4.5 months and were not affected by the use of misonidazole. Other sensitizers tested have included the halogenated pyrimidine bromodeoxyuridine (BrdU) and gadolinium texaphyrins. In investigating the role of BrdU as a radiosensitizer for brain metastases, RTOG 89–05 [32] enrolled 72 patients and treated them with WBRT to 37.5 Gy in 15 fractions over 3 weeks, with BrdU at 0.8 g/m^2 per day for 4 days given each week for 3 weeks. Five patients who received BrdU manisfested significant grade 4 and 5 hematologic or skin toxicities. There was no significant survival benefit for patients receiving BrdU.

Another randomized controlled trial, RTOG 9801, evaluated the role of motaxefin gadolinium (MGd) as a radiosensitizer for patients with brain metastases treated with WBRT [33]. In that study, 401 patients received either WBRT alone (30 Gy in 10 fractions) or WBRT with MGd, injected intravenously at a dose of 5 mg/kg/d at 2–5 hours before each fraction. Receipt of MGd did not affect median survival time, which was 5.2 months for those given MGd and WBRT and 4.9 months for those given WBRT alone. Regression after WBRT correlated with survival and preservation of neurocognitive function [34]. Time to neurological progression was improved in the subset of patients with metastatic lung cancer receiving MGd. In a subsequent phase III study, 554 patients with brain metastases from non-small cell lung cancer (NSCLC) were randomly assigned to the same treatments as were given for 9801 [35]. The median interval to neurological progression seemed to be better in the MGd group (15.4 months vs. 10.0 months), although this apparent difference was not statistically significant at $p = 0.11$.

Thalidomide was investigated as a radiosensitizer in patients with brain metastases in RTOG 0118 [36]. Patients were randomly assigned to receive WBRT alone (37.5 Gy in 15 fractions) or WBRT with thalidomide. Nearly half of the patients had to discontinue thalidomide because of side effects, and no survival benefit was noted. In the latest published study of radiosensitizers with WBRT, temozolomide or erlotinib was given concurrently with SBRT and SRS for patients with NSCLC and 1–3 brain metastases in RTOG 0320 [37]. In that phase III trial, the addition of radiosensitizer increased the rates of grade 3–5 toxicity (11% control vs. 41% temozolomide vs. 49% erlotinib, $p < 0.001$) and seemed to reduce the median survival time (13.4 months control vs. 6.3 months temozolomide vs. 6.1 months erlotinib). Other radiosensitizers continue to be investigated for their potential efficacy in combination with WBRT.

WBRT as an adjuvant after local therapy

WBRT after surgery

WBRT has an established role in preventing local recurrence after surgical resection of brain metastases. In one prospective, randomized trial reported by Patchell *et al.* [38], 95 patients with a single brain metastasis underwent complete resection followed by either observation or postoperative WBRT to a dose of 50.4 Gy. Receipt of WBRT led to a significant reduction in recurrence anywhere in the brain

Table 38.2 Trials of whole-brain radiation therapy after surgery for brain metastases

Study reference	Primary tumor type	No. of patients		% with brain recurrence			Median survival time (mo)		
		RT	No RT	RT	No RT	*P* value	RT	No RT	*P* value
Doseretz *et al.*, 1980 [40]	any	12	21	50	52	NS	8	10	NS
Smalley *et al.*, 1987 [43]	any	34	51	21	85	NA	21	12	0.02
DeAngelis *et al.*, 1989 [44]	any	79	19	45	65	0.03	21	4	NS
Hagen *et al.*, 1990 [41]	melanoma	12	21	50	52	NS	8	10	NS
Armstrong *et al.*, 1994 [39]	lung	32	32	47	38	NS	10	14	NS
Skibber *et al.*, 1996 [42]	melanoma	22	12	32	72	NA	18	6	0.002
Patchell *et al.*, 1998 [38]	any	49	46	18	70	0.001	11	10	NS

NA, not available; NS, not significant; RT, postoperative whole-brain radiation therapy.
Source: Modified from Komaki R, Chang E (2004) Whole-brain radiation therapy. In: Sawaya R (ed.), *Intracranial Metastases: Current Management Strategies*. Malden, MA: Blackwell Publishing, pp. 126–38 [124]. Reproduced with permission of John Wiley and Sons.

compared with the observation group (18% vs. 70%; $p < 0.001$). Local recurrence in the tumor bed was reduced from 46% to 10%, whereas regional recurrence within the brain and outside the tumor bed was reduced from 37% to 14%. WBRT also reduced the number of deaths from neurological causes from 44% to 14% but did not affect median survival.

A series of retrospective studies evaluating the role of WBRT after surgical resection is listed in Table 38.2 [38–44]. Most of these studies found no significant reduction in brain recurrence after postoperative WBRT except for that of DeAngelis *et al.* ($p = 0.03$) [44]. Only two retrospective studies have shown an increase in median survival from postoperative WBRT ($p = 0.02$) [42,43].

In general, more patients who received WBRT at recurrence died from neurological causes than did those given WBRT immediately after surgery, findings that support the immediate postoperative delivery of WBRT. Although the routine use of postoperative WBRT seems to prevent deaths from neurological causes, this practice has become controversial because of growing concerns about the long-term toxicity of WBRT, including neurocognitive decline and dementia. Withholding postoperative WBRT carries the risk of increased neurological morbidity from tumor recurrence within the brain; thus if postoperative WBRT is to be given, it should be given in a timely manner, usually within a few weeks of resection, depending on the aggressiveness of the surgical procedure and the patient's rate of postoperative recovery.

WBRT after stereotactic radiosurgery

WBRT after SRS has also been evaluated in prospective clinical trials. In a study reported by Aoyama *et al.*, 132 patients with 1–4 brain metastases smaller than 3 cm in diameter were randomly assigned to undergo SRS or SRS followed by WBRT to a total dose of 30 Gy in 10 fractions [45]. The SRS dose was reduced by 30% for the patients who were to be given WBRT. The addition of WBRT to SRS improved the 1-year local control rate (89% vs. 73%) and decreased the incidence of new brain metastases at 1 year (42% vs. 63.7% for SRS alone). Because no differences were found in median survival times, percentages with neurological death, or neurocognitive outcomes, the authors concluded that SRS alone could be considered a reasonable strategy, with WBRT reserved for salvage therapy as needed.

In a similar study, Chang *et al.* enrolled 58 patients with 1–3 brain metastases and RTOG recursive partitioning analysis class 1 or 2 status to receive either SRS alone or SRS followed by WBRT to a dose of 30 Gy in 12 fractions [46]. Notably, the primary end point in this study was neurocognitive function as defined by the Hopkins Verbal Learning Test-Revised (HVLT-R) of total recall at 4 months. The study was stopped early when it became clear that SRS followed by WBRT led to declines in learning and memory function. Indeed, the addition of WBRT led to a significant decline in HVLT-R 4-month recall (52% vs. 24%); however, use of WBRT led to improved rates of local control at 1 year (100% vs. 67%) and distant brain control at 1 year (73% vs. 45%). Conversely, median overall survival time was longer in the SRS-only group (15 months vs. 6 months SRS+WBRT).

The European Organization for Research and Treatment of Cancer (EORTC) also performed a randomized trial of 359 patients undergoing either SRS (n = 199) or surgery (n = 160) for 1–3 brain metastases who were then randomly assigned to receive WBRT (30 Gy in 10 fractions) or observation [47]. Those who went on to receive WBRT had reduced rates of relapse at initial sites at 2 years (surgery: 59% vs. 27%; SRS: 31% vs. 19%) and relapse at new sites (surgery: 42% vs. 23%; SRS: 48% vs. 33%). The rates of neurological death were also lower among those who received WBRT (28% vs. 44%). No differences were found in time to worsening performance status or overall survival.

The need for WBRT after SRS for the initial treatment of brain metastases continues to be debated. Although distant intracranial control is undoubtedly improved by the addition of WBRT, the lack of survival benefit and increase in toxicity argue against the routine use of WBRT after SRS. Clinical trials are ongoing to evaluate survival, quality of life, and functional independence for such patients.

Prophylactic cranial irradiation

PCI has been noted to improve survival among pediatric patients with acute lymphocytic leukemia by preventing the disease from involving the central nervous system (CNS) [48]. As systemic chemotherapy has become more effective, isolation of the malignancy in the CNS has been more common among patients with acute lymphocytic leukemia, this phenomenon has also been noted in patients with small cell lung cancer (SCLC) [49].

PCI has been proposed for patients with SCLC since the 1970s because of the high incidence of brain metastases from SCLC [50]. Approximately half of patients with SCLC who do not receive PCI will develop clinically significant brain metastases [51]. However, the incidence of microscopic brain metastases and extracranial CNS metastases had been underestimated given the relatively short survival duration for such patients [52], and PCI became more important when improvements in systemic treatment and earlier use of thoracic RT were shown to improve survival rates for patients with limited SCLC [30]. Because PCI can be neurotoxic and because it had not improved overall survival time, it was not considered for routine use despite its ability to reduce the number of brain metastases (Table 38.3) until neuropsychological testing of patients before and after PCI revealed no significant mental deterioration [53].

In one early trial of PCI, Cox *et al.* with the Veterans Affairs Lung Study Group found that giving 20 Gy in 5 fractions did not reduce brain metastasis [54]. At the time, this was thought to have resulted from the low total dose of RT (20 Gy), although the fraction size was considerably larger than the 2- to 3-Gy fractions in subsequent trials of PCI. In one such study, Bieler *et al.* delivered 24 Gy in 3-Gy fractions and found that no patient given PCI developed a brain tumor relapse, compared with 16% of 54 patients who did not receive PCI ($p < 0.05$) [55].

Another trial involving PCI given in 3-Gy fractions was reported by Maurer *et al.*, who randomly assigned 163 patients to receive or not receive PCI at a total dose of 30 Gy in 10 fractions [56]. Considerably fewer patients in the PCI group developed brain metastasis compared with patients who did not receive PCI (4% vs. 18%; $p < 0.009$). Other groups also found that PCI produced statistically significant reductions in brain metastasis, but PCI did not affect overall survival [57–61]. As Table 38.3 illustrates, use of radiation doses in excees of 30 Gy seemed to reduce brain tumor recurrence in the later studies, although this may also have been related to the advent of more sensitive means of detecting brain metastases, improvements in

Table 38.3 Early trials of prophylactic cranial irradiation for small cell lung cancer

Study reference	No. of patients	Radiation dose	% with brain relapse	
			PCI	No PCI
Cox *et al.*, 1978 [54]	45	20 Gy in 5 Fx	17	20
Bieler *et al.*, 1979 [55]	54	24 Gy in 8 Fx	0	16
Maurer *et al.*, 1980 [56]	163	30 Gy in 10 Fx	4	18
Hansen *et al.*, 1980 [49]	110	40 Gy in 20 Fx	9	12
Eagan *et al.*, 1981 [57]	30	36 Gy in 10 Fx	13	73
Katensis *et al.*, 1982 [59]	38	40 Gy in 10 Fx	12	44
Jackson *et al.*, 1983 [58]	29	30 Gy in 10 Fx	0	27
Seydel *et al.*, 1985 [61]	217	30 Gy in 10 Fx	5	22
Niiranen *et al.*, 1989 [60]	51	40 Gy in 20 Fx	0	27

Fx, fractions; PCI, prophyactic cranial irradiation.
Source: Modified from Gregor A, Cull A (1999) Role of prophylactic cranial irradiation: Benefits and late effects. In: *Progress and Perspectives in the Treatment of Lung Cancer*, Van Houtte P, Klastersk J, Rocmans P (eds), Springer-Verlag, Berlin, pp. 139–49 [62]. Reproduced with permission of Springer Science and Business Media.

systemic chemotherapy, and the use of thoracic RT [62]. Hirsch *et al.* reported a series of 111 patients randomly assigned to receive or not receive PCI to 40 Gy, which did not improve the incidence of brain metastasis (9% with PCI vs. 13% without PCI) [63]. This finding was thought to be related to the late use of the PCI, which was begun 12 weeks after completion of the prolonged systemic treatment.

Twenty years after publication of the previous report, a meta-analysis by Auperin *et al.* showed a survival benefit from PCI for patients with SCLC in complete remission [64]. That analysis involved individualized data from 987 patients who had participated in seven clinical trials comparing PCI with no PCI from 1977 to 1994 (Table 38.4) [65–70]. A minority of patients (12–17%) had extensive disease. An absolute increase of 5.4% in survival at 3 years was noted for patients undergoing PCI (20.7% vs. 15.3% no PCI), and the relative risk of death for the treatment group compared with the control group was 0.84 (95% confidence interval 0.73–0.97, $p = 0.01$). PCI also led to significant increases in rates of brain metastasis–free survival at 3 years (22.3% vs. 13.5% in control patients, $p < 0.001$), and the cumulative incidence of brain metastasis was reduced from 58.6% to 33.3% at 3 years ($p < 0.001$). Analysis of four total radiation doses (8 Gy, 24–25 Gy, 30 Gy, and 36–40 Gy) revealed that the larger doses led to greater decreases in the risk of brain metastasis ($p = 0.02$), but the effect on survival was not proportional to the dose administered. Also recognized in this meta-analysis was a trend toward decrease risk of brain metastasis when PCI was given soon after the initiation of the induction chemotherapy (p = 0.01 for <4 months vs. 4–6 months vs. >6 months). No significant neuropsychological deterioration was noted after the PCI, although systematic evaluations with neuropsychological testing were not done before and after PCI in most of these randomized studies.

In addition to limited-stage SCLC, PCI seems to have a role in extensive-stage SCLC. The EORTC conducted a prospective randomized trial in which 286 patients with extensive-stage SCLC who had had any response to 4–6 cycles of chemotherapy were assigned to receive PCI (20 Gy in 5 fractions or 30 Gy in 12 fractions) or no PCI [71]. Those who received PCI had lower rates of symptomatic brain metastases (15% vs. 40%) and improved overall survival (27% vs. 13%) at 1 year. Notably, no brain imaging was required before randomization in this study, and a follow-up report suggested that those who received PCI had worse health-related quality of life [72].

Ongoing debate regarding the optimal dose for PCI led to an Intergroup trial that enrolled

Table 38.4 Characteristics of seven trials included in a meta-analysis of the effects of prophylactic cranial irradiation for small-cell lung cancer

Trial name or site and reference	Enrollment period	Median follow-up time, yr	Induction therapy	Total dose/No. of fractions (dose/fraction)	Median time between start of induction therapy and enrollment, months	No. of patients	No. of patients surviving
U Maryland Cancer Ctr [65]	1977–1980	18.5	CT	30 Gy/10 (3 Gy)	3.6	29	2
Okayama University [69]	1981–1986	11.7	CT or CT+RT	40 Gy/20 (2 Gy)	2.5	46	4
PCI-85 [66]	1985–1993	8.4	CT or CT+RT	24 Gy/8 (3 Gy)	5.3	300	32
Danish-National Cancer Institute (unpublished)	1985–1991	8.8	CT	24 Gy/8 (3 Gy)	4.4	55	7
UKCCR-EORTC [67]	1987–1995	3.5	CT or CT+RT	8–36 Gy/1–18*	NA	314	54
PCI-88 [68]	1988–1994	5.1	CT or CT+RT	24 Gy/8 (3 Gy)	5.1	211	37
ECOG-RTOG [70]	1991–1994	3.9	CT or CT+RT	25 Gy/10 (2.5 Gy)	NA	32	5

CT, chemotherapy; ECOG-RTOG, Eastern Cooperative Oncology Group-Radiation Therapy Oncology Group; PCI, prophylactic cranial irradiation; RT, thoracic radiation therapy; UKCCR-EORTC, United Kingdom Clinical Cancer Research-European Organisation for Research and Treatment of Cancer.

*The first part of the trial included three treatment groups: no PCI, PCI to 24 Gy in 12 fractions, and PCI to 36 Gy in 18 fractions; the second part of the trial involved only two treatment groups: no PCI and PCI at various doses.

Source: Modified from Auperin A, Arriagada R, Pignon JP, *et al.* (1999) Prophylactic cranial irradiation for patients with small-cell lung cancer in complete remission. Prophylactic Cranial Irradiation Overview Collaborative Group. *N Engl J Med*, 341: 476–84 [64]. Reproduced with permission of the Massachusetts Medical Society.

720 patients with limited-stage SCLC in complete response after chemotherapy and thoracic RT to receive PCI at either a standard dose (25 Gy in 10 fractions) or one of two higher doses (36 Gy in 18 fractions daily or 36 Gy in 24 fractions twice daily) [73]. Brain imaging was used in all cases. No difference was found in the 2-year incidence of brain metastases, but the standard dose produced a better overall survival rate (42% vs. 37%; $p = 0.05$). A subsequent analysis revealed no significant difference between the low-dose versus high-dose groups in quality of life, neurological function and cognitive function over the 3-year period studied [74]. Thus at this time, the standard fractionation regimen for PCI remains a dose of 25 Gy given in 10 fractions.

Randomized studies have also been done to evaluate PCI for patients with NSCLC. One such study was RTOG 84–03, in which patients whose primary tumors were of adenocarcinomatous or large-cell histology and had been controlled were randomly assigned to receive or not receive PCI to a dose of 30 Gy in 10 fractions [75]. The results, reported in 1991, indicated that patients given PCI had fewer brain metastases but no significant improvement in overall survival, an outcome that could reflect either the ineffectiveness of the systemic chemotherapy or the timing of the PCI. A subsequent multicenter study from Germany on the role of neoadjuvant therapy for operable stage IIIA NSCLC offered additional information regarding the role of PCI in NSCLC [76]. In that study, 112 patients were randomly assigned to undergo either primary thoracic resection followed by adjuvant thoracic RT or preoperative chemotherapy followed by concurrent chemoradiotherapy to the primary site and definitive surgery at the primary site. The latter group also received postoperative PCI (30 Gy in 15 fractions). Receipt of PCI reduced the probability of brain metastases as the first site of failure at 5 years (8% vs. 35%) without a discernible difference in neurocognitive toxicity. The RTOG then attempted a phase III trial (RTOG 0214) comparing PCI versus observation for patients with locally advanced NSCLC [77]. In that study, 340 eligible patients who had been treated for stage III NSCLC and had no disease progression after primary therapy were randomly assigned to PCI (30 Gy in 15 fractions) or observation. Overall survival and disease-free survival were the same in the two groups, but the 1-year rate of brain metastases was lower in the PCI group (8% vs. 18%). In subsequent analyses of neurocognition and quality of life, no differences were found at 1 year in global cognitive function or quality of life, although memory (measured by the HVLT) had declined significantly [78]. Based on these prospective findings, the routine use of PCI for NSCLC is not warranted at this time.

In summary, PCI can effectively reduce the incidence of brain metastases without evidence of serious PCI-related complications if it is given appropriately. The use of PCI extends survival times among patients with limited-stage SCLC who achieve a complete response to primary therapy as well as those with extensive-stage SCLC who achieve any response to primary therapy [64, 71]. Dose escalation beyond 25 Gy in 10 fractions offers no additional benefit [73]. The use of PCI does not seem to confer a survival advantage for patients with NSCLC.

Toxicity of radiation to the brain

Complications of RT are generally divided into acute effects (those occurring during the course of radiation), early-delayed effects (at 2–4 months after radiation) and late effects (at months or years after radiation). Common acute effects include reversible alopecia, mild radiation dermatitis, and mild fatigue. Acute encephalopathy is exceedingly rare with modern-day fractionation schedules, although it was noted in one 1970 report to have been fatal in 7% of patients who received 10 Gy in a single fraction [79]. Somnolence syndrome, described as persistent fatigue, anorexia, and irritability (especially in children), can occur 3–10 weeks after WBRT but usually resolves within 6 months [80, 81].

Among long-term survivors after WBRT, some of whom received multiple chemotherapeutic drugs, a syndrome consisting of progressive dementia, ataxia, and urinary incontinence was reported to cause severe disability and the deaths of 7 of 12 patients in one report [44]. CT scans of the brains of those patients showed cortical atrophy and hypodense white matter. All 12 patients had received daily fractions of at least 3 Gy, and 9 patients received some daily fractionation of 5 Gy or more during treatment. On the basis of these findings, the authors of this report advocated use of smaller fractions, 1.8 to 2 Gy per day, for a total dose of 40–45 Gy to reduce long-term sequelae among patients with more favorable prognostic factors. More recently, recursive partitioning analyses have identified subgroups of patients who are likely to experience extended survival. In a recent report of a graded prognostic assessment approach, clinical characteristics such as age, Karnofsky Performance Status, number of CNS metastases, and the presence of extracranial metastases are scored to characterize the prognosis of patients with brain metastases [82]. The subgroup with the most favorable prognosis was noted to have a median survival time of 11 months compared with 2.6 months for the subgroup with the least favorable prognosis. For patients with favorable clinical factors, we advocate a dose per fraction of ≤3 Gy.

The relationship between WBRT, intracranial disease control, and neurocognitive function is complicated. Briefly, intracranial disease progression and WBRT may be competing risk factors in the development of neurocognitive dysfunction [46, 83–85]. Further studies are necessary to adequately characterize the relative risks of these competing factors to help guide therapeutic recommendations for patients with favorable prognosis.

Within the PCI literature, concerns have also been expressed regarding neuropsychological toxicity not only from WBRT but also from systemic treatment. Sheline *et al.*, Leibel *et al.*, and Gregor *et al.* have all documented the effect of ionizing radiation on CNS function [86–88]. Johnson *et al.* described the frequency of neuropsychological deficits in orientation, memory, and language function as occurring in 86% of patients with SCLC who survived for 6–13 years after treatment [89]. Factors or conditions contributing to these impairments include immunologic dysfunction, opportunistic infection, microscopic brain metastasis, toxicity from large irradiated field volumes, use of a neurotrophic chemotherapeutic agent in combination with PCI, and the total dose of RT. Particular concern has been expressed for children with acute lymphocytic leukemia who undergo PCI while receiving methotrexate, and also for patients with SCLC who undergo PCI combined with lomustine [90, 91]. However, at least one group has found a lack of clinical findings corresponding to CT abnormalities among patients who received prophylactic CNS radiation and experienced unexplained late neurologic sequelae [92]. In our own investigation of the lowest effective biological dose for PCI, we found 25 Gy in 10 fractions to be as effective and possibly less toxic than 30 Gy in 10 fractions [93]. In a subsequent prospective study, 30 patients with limited SCLC and no evidence of brain metastasis were evaluated with neuropsychological testing before any treatment and after PCI. The findings revealed 29 of the 30 patients had minor cognitive dysfunction before the PCI. The most common impairment was in verbal memory, followed by frontal lobe dysfunction and fine-motor incoordination. No significant deterioration attributable to the PCI was found after the PCI [53]. Similar results were found in two subsequent randomized trials of PCI for SCLC with prospectively evaluated neurocognitive endpoints [66, 67], that is, neurocognitive impairments were noted before the PCI, but PCI had no detected effects on neurocognitive function.

As systemic therapies continue to improve and patients survive longer, the late effects of WBRT will become increasingly relevant. A recently closed phase III trial by the RTOG randomly assigned patients to receive memantine, an N-methyl-D-aspartate receptor agonist approved for use in patients with Alzheimer's disease, with WBRT. Results of this study are pending. Conformal RT techniques are also being investigated as a way of sparing critical structures involved in neurocognition, as dose to the hippocampus has been implicated in neurocognitive dysfunction [94–96]. The RTOG is currently conducting a phase II trial to assess whether hippocampal-sparing WBRT can help to preserve neurocognitive function.

Biomarkers in non-small cell lung cancer and brain metastases

Previous research has established that the risk of brain metastasis is highest among patients with SCLC, adenocarcinoma, or large cell histology [51, 97–99]. In the modern era of molecular tailored therapy, biomarkers are eagerly sought to help guide therapeutic recommendations for patients with NSCLC. Numerous attempts have been made to correlate gene expression with the development of brain metastases in NSCLC [100–102], but thus far no consistent or independent correlations have been found between expression of Ki-67, p53, bcl-2, the epidermal growth factor receptor (EGFR), cyclooxygenase-2, or BAX and the development of brain metastases [101, 102]. Expression patterns involving multiple markers, however, may hold promise for predicting who is more likely to develop brain metastases [103]. In one retrospective analysis, an 8-marker molecular panel was able to sort patients with stage I NSCLC and identified a subset of patients who had a 37% likelihood of developing isolated cerebral metastases [104]. Serum markers such as carcinoembryonic antigen may also be useful as a risk factor for predicting the development of brain metastases [105–107]. However, any potential biomarker or biomarker panel must be validated in prospective clinical trials before the findings can be used to guide therapeutic recommendations.

EGFR has been investigated in relation to the development and treatment of brain metastases. It is unclear whether the presence of EGFR mutation or amplification can predict the development of brain metastases [101, 108–111]. However, use of the EGFR tyrosine kinase inhibitors gefitinib and erlotinib has been associated with objective intracranial response in patients with NSCLC and brain metastases [112–116]. This response has been shown to correlate with the presence of EGFR mutations in the tyrosine kinase domain [114–116]. Those patients with EGFR mutations have been shown to be more likely to respond to WBRT than those without EGFR mutations, with improved survival independent of age, functional status, extracranial disease status and number of brain metastases [117, 118]. Notably, however, EGFR status may be discordant between primary NSCLC and the corresponding metastases, and metastatic lesions as well as primary tumors should be analyzed for EGFR status if targeted therapies are being considered [109, 119–121].

Although the risk of CNS metastases is relatively high for patients with NSCLC that is treated with conventional chemotherapy [99], those with EGFR mutations treated with targeted therapy have a lower incidence of brain metastases. In one report, for patients with stage IIIB/IV or relapsed NSCLC and somatic EGFR mutations who had been treated with gefitinib or erlotinib as part of the initial therapy, the actuarial risk of CNS progression was 6% at 1 year and 13% at 2 years [110]. The authors of that report proposed that targeted therapy may have a prophylactic effect in preventing the development of brain metastases. In a subsequent analysis, outcomes were compared between patients with NSCLC and EGFR mutations who had been treated with upfront targeted therapy and those treated with conventional chemotherapy [122]. Those given the targeted therapy had a 44% relative risk reduction in the development of CNS progression, suggesting that gefitinib or erlotinib may have a role in chemoprevention of CNS metastases.

These findings, although tantalizing, need to be validated in prospective clinical trials. As mentioned earlier, RTOG 0320, which evaluated temozolomide or erlotinib given concurrently with WBRT and SRS for patients with NSCLC and 1–3 brain metastases [37], showed that the addition of erlotinib increased the rate of grade 3–5 toxicity from 11% for those given SRS and WBRT to 49% ($p < 0.001$) and may have shortened their median survival time (6.1 months vs. 13.4 months for the control; p = NS). Molecular features currently guide the upfront management of NSCLC; however, the role of biomarkers in the management of brain metastases has yet to be established and continues to be investigated.

Conclusions

In summary, WBRT is a valuable tool for treating gross brain metastases, for preventing the recurrence of brain metastases after local therapy, and for preventing the development of brain metastases in patients with SCLC. Many prospective clinical trials have been conducted to identify the ideal dose and fractionation schedules, to clarify the potential role of concurrent systemic agents, and to assess the risk of toxicity. Further advances in neuroimaging, neuropsychological testing, SRS delivery, and predictive biomarker assays will direct the optimal implementation of WBRT in the future.

References

1 Yamanaka R (2009) Medical management of brain metastases from lung cancer (Review). *Oncol Rep*, 22(6): 1269–76.

2 Ceresoli GL, Reni M, Chiesa G, *et al.* (2002) Brain metastases in locally advanced nonsmall cell lung carcinoma after multimodality treatment: risk factors analysis. *Cancer*, 95(3): 605–12.

3 Gandara DR, Chansky K, Albain KS, *et al.* (2003) Consolidation docetaxel after concurrent chemoradiotherapy in stage IIIB non-small-cell lung cancer: Phase II Southwest Oncology Group Study S9504. *J Clin Oncol*, 21(10): 2004–10.

4 Sze G, Milano E, Johnson C, Heier L (1990) Detection of brain metastases: comparison of contrast-enhanced MR with unenhanced MR and enhanced CT. *AJNR Am J Neuroradiol*, 11(4): 785–91.

5 Coia LR, Aaronson N, Linggood R, Loeffler J, Priestman TJ (1992) A report of the consensus workshop panel on the treatment of brain metastases. *Int J Radiat Oncol Biol Phys*, 23(1): 223–7.

6 Cohen N, Strauss G, Lew R, Silver D, Recht L (1988) Should prophylactic anticonvulsants be administered

to patients with newly-diagnosed cerebral metastases? A retrospective analysis. *J Clin Oncol*, 6(10): 1621–4.

7 Hanahan D, Weinberg RA (2000) The hallmarks of cancer. *Cell*, 100(1): 57–70.

8 Hanahan D, Weinberg RA (2011) Hallmarks of cancer: The next generation. *Cell*, 144(5): 646–74.

9 Gavrilovic IT, Posner JB (2005) Brain metastases: Epidemiology and pathophysiology. *J Neurooncol*, 75(1): 5–14.

10 Ewing J (1940) Metastasis. In: Ewing J (ed.), *Neoplastic Diseases: A Treatise on Tumours*. Philadelphia: W.B. Saunders, pp. 62–74.

11 Paget S (1989) The distribution of secondary growths in cancer of the breast. *Cancer Metastasis Rev*, 8(2): 98–101.

12 Patchell RA, Tibbs PA, Walsh JW, *et al.* (1990) A randomized trial of surgery in the treatment of single metastases to the brain. *N Engl J Med*, 322(8): 494–500.

13 Noordijk EM, Vecht CJ, Haaxma-Reiche H, *et al.* (1994) The choice of treatment of single brain metastasis should be based on extracranial tumor activity and age. *Int J Radiat Oncol Biol Phys*, 29(4): 711–17.

14 Leksell L (1951) The stereotaxic method and radiosurgery of the brain. *Acta Chir Scand*, 102(4): 316–19.

15 Lunsford LD, Maitz A, Lindner G (1987) First United States 201 source cobalt-60 gamma unit for radiosurgery. *Appl Neurophysiol*, 50(1–6): 253–6.

16 Jayarao M, Chin LS, Regine WF (2009) Stereotactic radiosurgery for brain metastases. In: Lundsford LD, Sheehan J (eds), *Intracranial Stereotactic Radiosurgery*. New York: Thieme Medical Publishers, pp. 151–62.

17 Shaw E, Scott C, Souhami L, *et al.* (2000) Single dose radiosurgical treatment of recurrent previously irradiated primary brain tumors and brain metastases: Final report of RTOG protocol 90–05. *Int J Radiat Oncol Biol Phys*, 47(2): 291–8.

18 Shehata MK, Young B, Reid B, *et al.* (2004) Stereotatic radiosurgery of 468 brain metastases < or = 2 cm: implications for SRS dose and whole brain radiation therapy. *Int J Radiat Oncol Biol Phys*, 59(1): 87–93.

19 Elliott RE, Rush SC, Morsi A, *et al.* (2011) Local control of newly diagnosed and distally recurrent, low-volume brain metastases using fixed dose (20 Gy) gamma knife radiosurgery. *Neurosurgery*, 68(4): 921–31.

20 Andrews DW, Scott CB, Sperduto PW, *et al.* (2004) Whole brain radiation therapy with or without stereotactic radiosurgery boost for patients with one to three brain metastases: Phase III results of the RTOG 9508 randomised trial. *Lancet*, 363(9422): 1665–72.

21 O'Neill BP, Iturria NJ, Link MJ, Pollock BE, Ballman KV, O'Fallon JR (2003) A comparison of surgical resection and stereotactic radiosurgery in the treatment of solitary brain metastases. *Int J Radiat Oncol Biol Phys*, 55(5): 1169–76.

22 Auchter RM, Lamond JP, Alexander E, *et al.* (1996) A multiinstitutional outcome and prognostic factor analysis of radiosurgery for resectable single brain metastasis. *Int J Radiat Oncol Biol Phys*, 35(1): 27–35.

23 Bindal AK, Bindal RK, Hess KR, *et al.* (1996) Surgery versus radiosurgery in the treatment of brain metastasis. *J Neurosurg*, 84(5): 748–54.

24 Chao JH, Phillips R, Nickson JJ (1954) Roentgen-ray therapy of cerebral metastases. *Cancer*, 7(4): 682–9.

25 Chu FC, Hilaris BB (1961) Value of radiation therapy in the management of intracranial metastases. *Cancer*, 14: 577–81.

26 Sneed PK, Larson DA, Wara WM (1996) Radiotherapy for cerebral metastasis. *Neurosurg Clin N Am*, 7: 505–15.

27 Borgelt B, Gelber R, Kramer S, *et al.* (1980) The palliation of brain metastases: Final results of the first two studies by the Radiation Therapy Oncology Group. *Int J Radiat Oncol Biol Phys*, 6(1): 1–9.

28 Borgelt B, Gelber R, Larson M, Hendrickson F, Griffin T, Roth R (1981) Ultra-rapid high dose irradiation schedules for the palliation of brain metastases: final results of the first two studies by the Radiation Therapy Oncology Group. *Int J Radiat Oncol Biol Phys*, 7(12): 1633–8.

29 Sause WT, Scott C, Krisch R, *et al.* (1993) Phase I/II trial of accelerated fractionation in brain metastases RTOG 85–28. *Int J Radiat Oncol Biol Phys*, 26(4): 653–7.

30 Murray KJ, Scott C, Greenberg HM, *et al.* (1997) A randomized phase III study of accelerated hyperfractionation versus standard in patients with unresected brain metastases: A report of the Radiation Therapy Oncology Group (RTOG) 9104. *Int J Radiat Oncol Biol Phys*, 39(3): 571–4.

31 Komarnicky LT, Phillips TL, Martz K, Asbell S, Isaacson S, Urtasun R (1991) A randomized phase III protocol for the evaluation of misonidazole combined with radiation in the treatment of patients with brain metastases (RTOG-7916). *Int J Radiat Oncol Biol Phys*, 20(1): 53–8.

32 Phillips TL, Scott CB, Leibel SA, Rotman M, Weigensberg IJ (1995) Results of a randomized comparison

of radiotherapy and bromodeoxyuridine with radiotherapy alone for brain metastases: report of RTOG trial 89–05. *Int J Radiat Oncol Biol Phys*, 33(2): 339–48.

33 Mehta MP, Rodrigus P, Terhaard CH, *et al.* (2003) Survival and neurologic outcomes in a randomized trial of motexafin gadolinium and whole-brain radiation therapy in brain metastases. *J Clin Oncol*, 21(13): 2529–36.

34 Li J, Bentzen SM, Renschler M, Mehta MP (2007) Regression after whole-brain radiation therapy for brain metastases correlates with survival and improved neurocognitive function. *J Clin Oncol*, 25(10): 1260–6.

35 Mehta MP, Shapiro WR, Phan SC, *et al.* (2009) Motexafin gadolinium combined with prompt whole brain radiotherapy prolongs time to neurologic progression in non-small-cell lung cancer patients with brain metastases: Results of a phase III trial. *Int J Radiat Oncol Biol Phys*, 73(4): 1069–76.

36 Knisely JP, Berkey B, Chakravarti A, *et al.* (2008) A phase III study of conventional radiation therapy plus thalidomide versus conventional radiation therapy for multiple brain metastases (RTOG 0118). *Int J Radiat Oncol Biol Phys*, 71(1): 79–86.

37 Sperduto PW, Wang M, Robins HI, *et al.* (2012) RTOG 0320: A phase III trial comparing whole brain radiation therapy (WBRT) and stereotactic radiosurgery (SRS) alone versus WBRT with temozolomide (TMZ) or erlotinib for non-small cell lung cancer (NSCLC) and 1–3 brain metastases. *Cancer Res*, 72(8 Supplement).

38 Patchell RA, Tibbs PA, Regine WF, *et al.* (1998) Postoperative radiotherapy in the treatment of single metastases to the brain: A randomized trial. *JAMA*, 280(17): 1485–9.

39 Armstrong JG, Wronski M, Galicich J, Arbit E, Leibel SA, Burt M (1994) Postoperative radiation for lung cancer metastatic to the brain. *J Clin Oncol*, 12(11): 2340–4.

40 Doseretz DE, Blitzer PH, Russel AH (1980) Management of solitary metastasis to the brain: The role of elective brain irradiation following complete surgical resection. *Int J Radiat Oncol Biol Phys*, 6: 1727–30.

41 Hagen NA, Cirrincione C, Thaler HT, DeAngelis LM (1990) The role of radiation therapy following resection of single brain metastasis from melanoma. *Neurology*, 40(1): 158–60.

42 Skibber JM, Soong SJ, Austin L, Balch CM, Sawaya RE (1996) Cranial irradiation after surgical excision of brain metastases in melanoma patients. *Ann Surg Oncol*, 3(2): 118–23.

43 Smalley SR, Schray MF, Laws ER, O'Fallon JR (1987) Adjuvant radiation therapy after surgical resection of solitary brain metastasis: association with pattern of failure and survival. *Int J Radiat Oncol Biol Phys*, 13(11): 1611–16.

44 DeAngelis LM, Delattre JY, Posner JB (1989) Radiation-induced dementia in patients cured of brain metastases. *Neurology*, 39(6): 789–96.

45 Aoyama H, Shirato H, Tago M, *et al.* (2006) Stereotactic radiosurgery plus whole-brain radiation therapy vs stereotactic radiosurgery alone for treatment of brain metastases: A randomized controlled trial. *JAMA*, 295(21): 2483–91.

46 Chang EL, Wefel JS, Hess KR, *et al.* (2009) Neurocognition in patients with brain metastases treated with radiosurgery or radiosurgery plus whole-brain irradiation: A randomised controlled trial. *Lancet Oncol* 10(11): 1037–44.

47 Kocher M, Soffietti R, Abacioglu U, *et al.* (2011) Adjuvant whole-brain radiotherapy versus observation after radiosurgery or surgical resection of one to three cerebral metastases: Results of the EORTC 22952–26001 study. *J Clin Oncol*, 29(2): 134–41.

48 Bleyer WA, Poplack DG (1985) Prophylaxis and treatment of leukemia in the central nervous system and other sanctuaries. *Semin Oncol*, 12(2): 131–48.

49 Hansen HH, Dombernowsky P, Hirsch FR, Hansen M, Rygård J (1980) Prophylactic irradiation in bronchogenic small cell anaplastic carcinoma. A comparative trial of localized versus extensive radiotherapy including prophylactic brain irradiation in patients receiving combination chemotherapy. *Cancer*, 46(2): 279–84.

50 Hansen HH (1973) Should initial treatment of small cell carcinoma include systemic chemotherapy and brain irradiation? *Cancer Chemother Rep*, 3; 4(2): 239–41.

51 Komaki R (1985) Prophylactic cranial irradiation for small cell carcinoma of the lung. *Cancer Treat Symp*, 2: 35–9.

52 Nugent JL, Bunn PA, Matthews MJ, *et al.* (1979) CNS metastases in small cell bronchogenic carcinoma: Increasing frequency and changing pattern with lengthening survival. *Cancer*, 44(5): 1885–93.

53 Komaki R, Meyers CA, Shin DM, *et al.* (1995) Evaluation of cognitive function in patients with limited small cell lung cancer prior to and shortly following prophylactic cranial irradiation. *Int J Radiat Oncol Biol Phys*, 33(1): 179–82.

54 Cox JD, Petrovich Z, Paig C, Stanley K (1978) Prophylactic cranial irradiation in patients with

inoperable carcinoma of the lung: preliminary report of a cooperative trial. *Cancer*, 42(3): 1135–40.

55 Beiler DD, Kane RC, Bernath AM, Cashdollar MR (1979) Low dose elective brain irradiation in small cell carcinoma of the lung. *Int J Radiat Oncol Biol Phys*, 5(7): 941–5.

56 Maurer LH, Tulloh M, Weiss RB, *et al.* (1980) A randomized combined modality trial in small cell carcinoma of the lung: Comparison of combination chemotherapy-radiation therapy versus cyclophosphamide-radiation therapy effects of maintenance chemotherapy and prophylactiv whole brain irradiation. *Cancer*, 45(1): 30–9.

57 Eagan RT, Frytak S, Lee RE, Creagan ET, Ingle JN, Nichols WC (1981) A case for preplanned thoracic and prophylactic whole brain radiation therapy in limited small-cell lung cancer. *Cancer Clin Trials*, 4(3): 261–6.

58 Jackson DV, Richards F, Cooper MR (1983) II, Prophylactic cranial irradiation in small cell lung cancer 237: 2730–33.

59 Katensis AT, Karpastis N, Giannakakis D (1982) Elective brain irradiation in patients with small cell carcinoma of the lung: A preliminary report. *Excerpta Medica*, Amsterdam, Lung Cancer International Congress series no 558: 277–84.

60 Niiranen A, Holsti P, Salmo M (1989) Treatment of small cell lung cancer. Two-drug versus four-drug chemotherapy and loco-regional irradiation with or without prophylactic cranial irradiation. *Acta Oncol*, 28(4): 501–5.

61 Seydel HG, Creech R, Pagano M, *et al.* (1985) Prophylactic versus no brain irradiation in regional small cell lung carcinoma. *Am J Clin Oncol*, 8(3): 218–23.

62 Gregor A, Cull A, Lung P, Klastersk J, Van C, Rocmans P (1999) Role of prophylactic cranial irradiation: Benefits and late effects. In P Van Houtte, J Kalstersk, P Rocmans (eds), *Progress and Perspectives in the Treatment of Lung Cancer*. Berlin, Springer-Verlag, pp. 139–49.

63 Hirsch FR, Hansen HH, Paulson OB, *et al.* (1979) Development of brain metastasis in small cell anaplastic carcinoma of the lung. In: Kayjn, Whitehouse J (eds), *CNS Complications of Malignant Disease*. Berlin: Springer-Verlag, pp. 175–84.

64 Auperin A, Arriagada R, Pignon JP, *et al.* (1999) Prophylactic cranial irradiation for patients with small-cell lung cancer in complete remission. Prophylactic Cranial Irradiation Overview Collaborative Group. *N Engl J Med*, 341(7): 476–84.

65 Aroney RS, Aisner J, Wesley MN, *et al.* (1983) Value of prophylactic cranial irradiation given at complete remission in small cell lung carcinoma. *Cancer Treat Rep*, 67(7–8): 675–82.

66 Arriagada R, Le Chevalier T, Borie F, *et al.* (1995) Prophylactic cranial irradiation for patients with small-cell lung cancer in complete remission. *J Natl Cancer Inst*, 87(3): 183–90.

67 Gregor A, Cull A, Stephens RJ, *et al.* (1990) Prophylactic cranial irradiation is indicated following complete response to induction therapy in small cell lung cancer: results of a multicentre randomised trial. United Kingdom Coordinating Committee for Cancer Research (UKCCCR) and the European Organization for Research and Treatment of Cancer (EORTC). *Eur J Cancer*, 33(11): 1752–8.

68 Laplanche A, Monnet I, Santos-Miranda JA, *et al.* (1998) Controlled clinical trial of prophylactic cranial irradiation for patients with small-cell lung cancer in complete remission. *Lung Cancer* (Amsterdam, Netherlands), 21(3): 193–201.

69 Ohonoshi T, Ueoka H, Kawahara S, *et al.* (1993) Comparative study of prophylactic cranial irradiation in patients with small cell lung cancer achieving a complete response: A long-term follow-up result. *Lung Cancer* (Amsterdam, Netherlands), 10(1–2): 47–54.

70 Wagner H, Kim K, Turrisi A (1996) A randomized phase III study of prophylactic cranial irradiation versus observation in patients with small cell lung cancer achieving a complete response: Final report of an incomplete trial by the Eastern Cooperative Oncology Group and Radiation Therapy Oncology Group (E3589/). *Proc Am Soc Clin Oncol*, 376, abstract 1996; 15: R92–01.

71 Slotman B, Faivre-Finn C, Kramer G, *et al.* (2007) Prophylactic cranial irradiation in extensive small-cell lung cancer. *N Engl J Med*, 357(7): 664–72.

72 Slotman BJ, Mauer ME, Bottomley A, *et al.* (2009) Prophylactic cranial irradiation in extensive disease small-cell lung cancer: short-term health-related quality of life and patient reported symptoms: Results of an international Phase III randomized controlled trial by the EORTC Radiation Oncology and Lung Cancer Groups. *J Clin Oncol*, 27(1): 78–84.

73 Le Pechoux C, Dunant A, Senan S, *et al.* (2009) Standard-dose versus higher-dose prophylactic cranial irradiation (PCI) in patients with limited-stage small-cell lung cancer in complete remission after chemotherapy and thoracic radiotherapy (PCI 99–01,

EORTC 22003–08004, RTOG 0212, and IFCT 99–01): A randomised clinical trial. *Lancet Oncol*, 10(5): 467–74.

74 Le Pechoux C, Laplanche A, Faivre-Finn C, *et al.* (2011) Clinical neurological outcome and quality of life among patients with limited small-cell cancer treated with two different doses of prophylactic cranial irradiation in the intergroup phase III trial (PCI99–01, EORTC 22003–08004, RTOG 0212 and IFCT 99–01). *Ann Oncol*, 22(5): 1154–63.

75 Russell AH, Pajak TE, Selim HM, *et al.* (1991) Prophylactic cranial irradiation for lung cancer patients at high risk for development of cerebral metastasis: Results of a prospective randomized trial conducted by the Radiation Therapy Oncology Group. *Int J Radiat Oncol Biol Phys*, 21(3): 637–43.

76 Pottgen C, Eberhardt W, Grannass A, *et al.* (2007) Prophylactic cranial irradiation in operable stage IIIA non small-cell lung cancer treated with neoadjuvant chemoradiotherapy: Results from a German multicenter randomized trial. *J Clin Oncol*, 25(31): 4987–92.

77 Gore EM, Bae K, Wong SJ, *et al.* (2011) Phase III comparison of prophylactic cranial irradiation versus observation in patients with locally advanced non-small-cell lung cancer: primary analysis of radiation therapy oncology group study RTOG 0214. *J Clin Oncol*, 29(3): 272–8.

78 Sun A, Bae K, Gore EM, *et al.* (2011) Phase III trial of prophylactic cranial irradiation compared with observation in patients with locally advanced non-small-cell lung cancer: Neurocognitive and quality-of-life analysis. *J Clin Oncol*, 29(3): 279–86.

79 Hindo WA, DeTrana FA, 3rd, Lee MS, Hendrickson FR (1970) Large dose increment irradiation in treatment of cerebral metastases. *Cancer*, 26(1): 138–41.

80 Boldrey ES, Heline GE (1996) Delayed transitory clinical manifestations after radiation treatment of intracranial tumors. *Acta Radiol*, 5 SRC – GoogleScholar.

81 Littman P, Rosenstock J, Gale G, *et al.* (1984) The somnolence syndrome in leukemic children following reduced daily dose fractions of cranial radiation. *Int J Radiat Oncol Biol Phys*, 10(10): 1851–3.

82 Sperduto PW, Berkey B, Gaspar LE, Mehta M, Curran W (2008) A new prognostic index and comparison to three other indices for patients with brain metastases: an analysis of 1,960 patients in the RTOG database. *Int J Radiat Oncol Biol Phys*, 70(2): 510–14.

83 Li J, Bentzen SM, Renschler M, Mehta MP (2008) Relationship between neurocognitive function and quality of life after whole-brain radiotherapy in patients with brain metastasis. *Int J Radiat Oncol Biol Phys*, 71(1): 64–70.

84 Meyers CA, Smith JA, Bezjak A, *et al.* (2004) Neurocognitive function and progression in patients with brain metastases treated with whole-brain radiation and motexafin gadolinium: results of a randomized phase III trial. *J Clin Oncol*, 22(1): 157–65.

85 Corn BW, Moughan J, Knisely JP, *et al.* (2008) Prospective evaluation of quality of life and neurocognitive effects in patients with multiple brain metastases receiving whole-brain radiotherapy with or without thalidomide on Radiation Therapy Oncology Group (RTOG) trial 0118. *Int J Radiat Oncol Biol Phys*, 71(1): 71–8.

86 Gregor A, Cull A, Traynor E, Stewart M, Lander F, Love S. (1996) Neuropsychometric evaluation of long-term survivors of adult brain tumours: relationship with tumour and treatment parameters. *Radiother Oncol*, 41(1): 55–9.

87 Leibel SA, Sheline GE, Lett JT, Altman KI, New A (1987) Tolerance of the central and peripheral nervous system to therapeutic irradiation. In: *Advances in Radiation Biology*, pp. 257–88.

88 Sheline GE, Wara WM, Smith V (1980) Therapeutic irradiation and brain injury. *Int J Radiat Oncol Biol Phys*, 6(9): 1215–28.

89 Johnson BE, Patronas N, Hayes W, *et al.* (1990) Neurologic, computed cranial tomographic, and magnetic resonance imaging abnormalities in patients with small-cell lung cancer: Further follow-up of 6- to 13-year survivors. *J Clin Oncol*, 8(1): 48–56.

90 Blyer WA (1981) Neurogenic sequellae of methotrexate and ionizing radiation: A new classification. *Cancer Treat Rep*, 65: 89–98.

91 Ellison N, Bernath A, Kane R (1982) Disturbing problems of success: Clinical status of long term survivors of small cell lung cancer (SCLC). *Proc Am Soc Clin Oncol*, 1:149.

92 Catane R, Schwade JG, Yarr I, *et al.* (1981) Follow-up neurological evaluation in patients with small cell lung carcinoma treated with prophylactic cranial irradiation and chemotherapy. *Int J Radiat Oncol Biol Phys*, 7(1): 105–9.

93 Komaki R, Cox JD, Hartz AJ, *et al.* (1985) Characteristics of long-term survivors after treatment for inoperable carcinoma of the lung. *Am J Clin Oncol*, 8(5): 362–70.

94 Cheung MC, Chan AS (2003) Memory impairment in humans after bilateral damage to lateral temporal neocortex. *Neuroreport*, 14(3): 371–4.

95 Gondi V, Tome WA, Mehta MP (2010) Why avoid the hippocampus? A comprehensive review. *Radiother Oncol*, 97(3): 370–6.

96 Gondi V, Hermann BP, Mehta MP, Tome WA (2012) Hippocampal dosimetry predicts neurocognitive function impairment after fractionated stereotactic radiotherapy for benign or low-grade adult brain tumors. *Int J Radiat Oncol Biol Phys*, 83(4): e487–93.

97 Curran WJ, Jr., Paulus R, Langer CJ, *et al.* (2011) Sequential vs. concurrent chemoradiation for stage III non-small cell lung cancer: randomized phase III trial RTOG 9410. *J Natl Cancer Inst*, 103(19): 1452–60.

98 Komaki R, Derus SB, Perez-Tamayo C, Byhardt RW, Hartz A, Cox JD (1987) Brain metastasis in patients with superior sulcus tumors. *Cancer*, 59(9): 1649–53.

99 Chen AM, Jahan TM, Jablons DM, Garcia J, Larson DA (2007) Risk of cerebral metastases and neurological death after pathological complete response to neoadjuvant therapy for locally advanced nonsmall-cell lung cancer: Clinical implications for the subsequent management of the brain. *Cancer*, 109(8): 1668–75.

100 Grinberg-Rashi H, Ofek E, Perelman M, *et al.* (2009) The expression of three genes in primary non-small cell lung cancer is associated with metastatic spread to the brain. *Clin Cancer Res*, 15(5): 1755–61.

101 Milas I, Komaki R, Hachiya T, *et al.* (2003) Epidermal growth factor receptor, cyclooxygenase-2, and BAX expression in the primary non-small cell lung cancer and brain metastases. *Clin Cancer Res*, 9(3): 1070–6.

102 Bubb RS, Komaki R, Hachiya T, *et al.* (2002) Association of Ki-67, p53, and bcl-2 expression of the primary non-small-cell lung cancer lesion with brain metastatic lesion. *Int J Radiat Oncol Biol Phys*, 53(5): 1216–24.

103 Saad AG, Yeap BY, Thunnissen FB, *et al.* (2008) Immunohistochemical markers associated with brain metastases in patients with nonsmall cell lung carcinoma. *Cancer*, 113(8): 2129–38.

104 D'Amico TA, Aloia TA, Moore MB, *et al.* (2001) Predicting the sites of metastases from lung cancer using molecular biologic markers. *Ann Thorac Surg*, 72(4): 1144–8.

105 Arrieta O, Saavedra-Perez D, Kuri R, *et al.* (2009) Brain metastasis development and poor survival associated with carcinoembryonic antigen (CEA) level in advanced non-small cell lung cancer: A prospective analysis. *BMC Cancer*, 9: 119.

106 Horinouchi H, Sekine I, Sumi M, *et al.* (2012) Brain metastases after definitive concurrent chemoradiotherapy in patients with stage III lung adenocarcinoma: Carcinoembryonic antigen as a potential predictive factor. *Cancer Sci*, 103(4): 756–9.

107 Lee DS, Kim YS, Jung SL, *et al.* (2012) The relevance of serum carcinoembryonic antigen as an indicator of brain metastasis detection in advanced non-small cell lung cancer. *Tumour Biol*, 33(4): 1065–73.

108 Matsumoto S, Takahashi K, Iwakawa R, *et al.* (2006) Frequent EGFR mutations in brain metastases of lung adenocarcinoma. *Int J Cancer*, 119(6): 1491–4.

109 Sun M, Behrens C, Feng L, *et al.* (2009) HER family receptor abnormalities in lung cancer brain metastases and corresponding primary tumors. *Clin Cancer Res*, 15(15): 4829–37.

110 Heon S, Yeap BY, Britt GJ, *et al.* (2010) Development of central nervous system metastases in patients with advanced non-small cell lung cancer and somatic EGFR mutations treated with gefitinib or erlotinib. *Clin Cancer Res*, 16(23): 5873–82.

111 Lee YJ, Park IK, Park MS, *et al.* (2009) Activating mutations within the EGFR kinase domain: A molecular predictor of disease-free survival in resected pulmonary adenocarcinoma. *J Cancer Res Clin Oncol*, 135(12): 1647–54.

112 Hotta K, Kiura K, Ueoka H, *et al.* (2004) Effect of gefitinib ('Iressa', ZD1839) on brain metastases in patients with advanced non-small-cell lung cancer. *Lung Cancer*, 46(2): 255–61.

113 Namba Y, Kijima T, Yokota S, *et al.* (2004) Gefitinib in patients with brain metastases from non-small-cell lung cancer: Review of 15 clinical cases. *Clin Lung Cancer*, 6(2): 123–8.

114 Shimato S, Mitsudomi T, Kosaka T, *et al.* (2006) EGFR mutations in patients with brain metastases from lung cancer: association with the efficacy of gefitinib. *Neuro Oncol*, 8(2): 137–44.

115 Porta R, Sanchez-Torres JM, Paz-Ares L, *et al.* (2011) Brain metastases from lung cancer responding to erlotinib: The importance of EGFR mutation. *Eur Respir J*, 37(3): 624–31.

116 Bai H, Han B (2012) The effectiveness of erlotinib against brain metastases in non-small-cell lung cancer patients. *Am J Clin Oncol*, 36(2): 110–15.

117 Gow CH, Chien CR, Chang YL, *et al.* (2008) Radiotherapy in lung adenocarcinoma with brain metastases: effects of activating epidermal growth factor receptor mutations on clinical response. *Clin Cancer Res*, 14(1): 162–8.

118 Eichler AF, Kahle KT, Wang DL, *et al.* (2010) EGFR mutation status and survival after diagnosis of brain metastasis in nonsmall cell lung cancer. *Neuro Oncol*, 12(11): 1193–9.

119 Daniele L, Cassoni P, Bacillo E, *et al.* (2009) Epidermal growth factor receptor gene in primary tumor and metastatic sites from non-small cell lung cancer. *J Thorac Oncol*, 4(6): 684–8.

120 Gomez-Roca C, Raynaud CM, Penault-Llorca F, *et al.* (2009) Differential expression of biomarkers in primary non-small cell lung cancer and metastatic sites. *J Thorac Oncol*, 4(10): 1212–20.

121 Han HS, Eom DW, Kim JH, *et al.* (2011) EGFR mutation status in primary lung adenocarcinomas and corresponding metastatic lesions: discordance in pleural metastases. *Clin Lung Cancer*, 12(6): 380–6.

122 Heon S, Yeap BY, Lindeman NI, *et al.* (2012) The impact of initial gefitinib or erlotinib versus chemotherapy on central nervous system progression in advanced non-small cell lung cancer with EGFR mutations. *Clin Cancer Res*, 18(16): 4406–14.

123 Kurtz JM, Gelber R, Brady LW, Carella RJ, Cooper JS (1981) The palliation of brain metastases in a favorable patient population: A randomized clinical trial by the Radiation Therapy Oncology Group. *Int J Radiat Oncol Biol Phys*, 7(7): 891–5.

124 Komaki R, Chang E (2004) Whole-brain radiation therapy. In: Sawaya R (ed.), *Intracranial Metastases: Current Management Strategies*. Malden, MA: Blackwell Publishing, pp. 126–38.

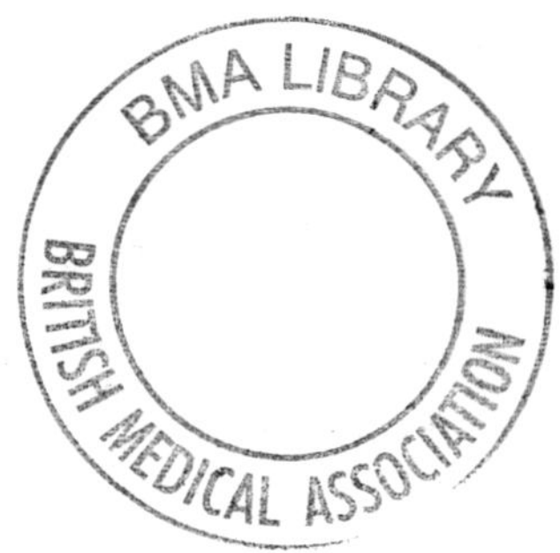